The Natural Pharmacy

The Natural Pharmacy

2nd Edition

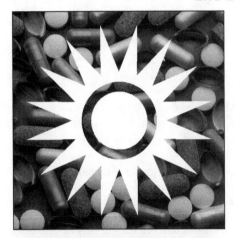
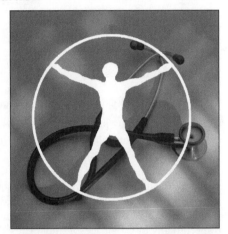
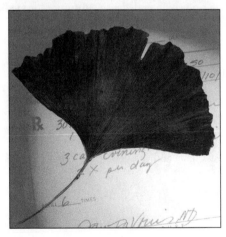
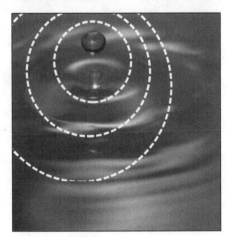

Schuyler W. Lininger, Jr. DC, Editor-in-Chief

Alan R. Gaby MD

Steve Austin ND

Donald J. Brown ND

Jonathan V. Wright MD

Alice Duncan DC, CCH

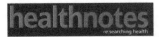

Prima Health *A Division of Prima Publishing*

For Jane, Cory, and Ciel

Disclaimer: Prima Publishing has designed this book to provide information in regard to the subject matter covered. It is sold with the understanding that the publisher and the author are not liable for the misconception or misuse of information provided. Every effort has been made to make this book as complete and as accurate as possible. The purpose of this book is to educate. The author and Prima Publishing shall have neither liability nor responsibility to any person or entity with respect to any loss, damage, or injury caused or alleged to be caused directly or indirectly by the information contained in this book. The information presented herein is in no way intended as a substitute for medical counseling.

All products mentioned in this book are trademarks of their respective companies.

Published in association with Healthnotes Online, Inc.

PRIMA HEALTH and colophon are trademarks of Prima Communications, Inc.
HEALTHNOTES is a registered trademark of Healthnotes, Inc.

Cover photos © Superstock (front cover, top row, right) and © Eyewire (all other photos).

Library of Congress Cataloging-in-Publication Data on file.

ISBN 0-7615-1967-X

00 01 02 DD 10 9 8 7 6 5 4 3 2

Printed in the United States of America

How to Order
Single copies may be ordered from Prima Publishing, P.O. Box 1260BK, Rocklin, CA 95677; telephone (916) 632-4400. Quantity discounts are also available. On your letterhead, include information concerning the intended use of the books and the number of books you wish to purchase.

Visit us online at www.primahealth.com and www.healthnotes.com

Contents

Part One

Health Concerns **1**

Part Two

Nutritional Supplements

Part Three

Herbs 385

Part Four

Homeopathic Remedies .505

Foreword

I first met and really enjoyed the company of Dr. Skye Lininger on a trip to Costa Rica in 1998 sponsored by the American Botanical Council. As we rode buses through the mountains, Skye ran a red pencil across the printouts for what would later become the *Healthnotes Online* computer program—and now the second edition of the book you are holding in your hands. We enjoyed stimulating and animated conversations from the hot coasts of Tortuguero on the Atlantic to the cloud forests of Monte Verde.

At that time, I had the pleasure of reading over some of the pages in the herbal section that had been mostly written by Dr. Don Brown, a noted naturopath and teacher, whom I also respect. I was impressed with how easy the information was to access.

Most of the important information about the herb's use and elusive dosage data, cross-referenced to the condition, including potential side effects and interactions, all make this book especially useful. I'm even more impressed with the information about the more than 130 herbs, complete with backup citations from the scientific literature (including many articles from German journals).

The fact that Dr. Lininger used some of the foremost experts on herbs and nutrition makes this reference an excellent source book for help with 115 common health conditions. This second edition has called on the expertise of even more natural medicine experts to cover the latest information. I think you'll find yourself turning to this book often!

Enjoy it in good health. Think green, the green of natural medicines, with which you co-evolved.

Dr. Jim Duke
Economic Botanist, USDA (Retired)

Preface

An evolution is taking place in healthcare. It is quite obvious as more nutritional supplements and herbal medicines gain acceptance that they are becoming part of the mainstream. What has driven this growing acceptance is that the public is gaining access to reliable, sound information on the value of these natural medicines, as well as increased scientific investigation. Unfortunately, the public has also been duped and misled by marketing hype on natural products. The public and physicians want unbiased, factual information on natural products—not hyperbole or hype. *The Natural Pharmacy* delivers scientifically sound information from leading experts. In fact, the greatest accomplishment of *The Natural Pharmacy* is that it provides a clear, concise interpretation of the science behind natural medicine.

The primary authors of *The Natural Pharmacy* are respected for their expertise and knowledge in an emerging form of medicine that relies on nature rather than drugs or surgery. Their contributions to this field go beyond their expertise as they are true visionaries and pioneers who have dedicated their lives to make a difference in the lives of others by educating physicians, their patients, and the public at large on the value of natural products. This book, *The Natural Pharmacy*, is their gift to all of us. From it you will learn what works and what does not. Although written primarily for the public, this book also serves as a valuable resource for physicians as well.

One of the great myths about nutritional supplements and herbal products has been the belief that there is no firm scientific evidence to support them. However, this argument is quickly becoming outdated. There is more than enough reasonable certainty to employ nutritional supplements and/or herbal products for virtually every common health condition.

Unfortunately, for some reason there has always been resistance to natural products and nutrition within the medical community. The bias today against nutritional supplementation is nothing new; it has a very long history. For example, the medical community and the British Navy did not adopt the use of lime juice rations for its crews until 1804, 62 years after the discovery and proof offered by the British physician James Lind in 1742. The timeline seems to run a little faster now, but it is still too long between the period when a vitamin or mineral is proven to be effective for preventing or treating a certain health condition and the time it becomes widely accepted and is recommended by physicians. A case in point is the time lag between the demonstration and the acceptance of the role folic acid plays in the prevention of neural tube defects such as spina bifida, a defect in which the vertebrae do not form a complete ring to protect the spinal cord.

The discovery that folic acid supplementation (400 mg per day) in early pregnancy can reduce the incidence of neural tube defects by as much as 80% has been referred to as one of the greatest discoveries of the last part of the 20th century. The evidence became so overwhelming that the Food and Drug Administration reversed a previous position and now acknowledge the association, allowing folic acid supplements and foods high in folic acid to claim that "daily consumption of folic acid by women of childbearing age may reduce the risk of neural tube defects."

The interesting thing concerning the discovery of the link between folic acid deficiency and neural tube defects is how long it took for obstetricians and other medical doctors to begin making the recommendation of folic acid supplementation to pregnant women, even though folic acid deficiency has been linked to neural tube defects for more than 30 years.

There are countless examples of how supplementing one's diet with an inexpensive vitamin, mineral, or herb can provide significant preventive or therapeutic effects. The growing popularity of nutritional supplements and herbal products is a sign that the public is bridging the gap between information and utilization faster than most healthcare practitioners. Providing sound scientifically based information about natural medicine is what *The Natural Pharmacy* is all about.

Michael T. Murray, ND
Author of *The Encyclopedia of Natural Medicine*
and *The Healing Power of Herbs*

Acknowledgments

No book of this size and scope comes into existence without the inspiration and help of many people—most of whom labor behind the scenes.

Gratitude for a job well done to all the contributors to this book—especially Drs. Alan Gaby, Steve Austin (our Chief Science Officer), Don Brown, Eric Yarnell, and Alice Duncan who wrote with energy and whose integrity and attention to detail has ensured the second edition of this book will surely set a new standard for excellence, and to Drs. Jonathan Wright and Alan Gaby (again), who have served as mentors to us.

Special thanks to Victoria Dolby Toews MPH for her diligent and professional job in serving as managing editor to all editions of *Healthnotes Online* software and both editions of this book.

Thanks to my family for their love and putting up with long hours, a demanding travel schedule, and an exciting yet stressful period in our lives; to all the team at Healthnotes, Inc., who are the best at what they do of any I have ever worked with; to our Chief Technical Officer, Rick Wilkes (and his team) and the person who brought us together, Thom Hartmann (an expert author of books on ADD and someone who also belongs in the mentor category); to those talented people who helped make the original *Healthnotes Online* software a reality from a graphics and programmatic perspective, Marcia Barrentine and Loren Jenkins; to those who were there at the beginning (and helped inspire, motivate, and create), Michael Peet and his sister, Margaret, Stan Amy, Cheryl Bottger, and Eileen Brady; to our friends from Catalyst II, Jill Higgins and David Cole, for their support, encouragement, and mentoring.

To our publishing partners at Prima; to Dr. Joe Pizzorno, the President of Bastyr University; to all the retailers in health and natural food stores, grocery stores, and pharmacies and departments who offer high-quality supplements; and to the pioneers and innovators in natural medicine who have kept as their credo the care of their patients . . . naturally.

Introduction

In 1975, when I first became interested in "alternative" medicine, it was hard to sort out the fact from the folklore. While millions of people took supplements to either protect their health or help with a problem their doctors were unable to cure, most were relying on anecdotes and hearsay.

Two decades ago, many scientific articles had been written about most of the vitamins and a few of the herbs, but getting hold of that information was challenging. It is only in recent years that medicine has become interested in the use of nutritional supplements as a complement to conventional medicine. In most cases, the subject is just now being added to the curriculum in some medical schools.

In the 1970s, books about supplements were of mixed quality. Despite being poorly referenced and filled with errors, the books provided enough information (much of which later proved true) to help millions of people with their health problems.

Beginning in the early 1980s, a steady stream of articles about antioxidants and other dietary supplements began appearing in the medical literature. By the late 1980s, the stream had become a flood and some 15,000 articles began forming a solid foundation for nutritional therapies. Books appearing in those years began to take advantage of the scientific underpinnings and gradually became more reliable and useful. However, they were still aimed squarely at those who accepted the premise that only natural was good.

By the time we began working on our electronic database "Healthnotes Online," which is the basis for this book, the number of useful scientific articles on the role of vitamins and herbs in human health exceeded 25,000. Our team of researchers combed the libraries of medical schools on a weekly basis to keep up-to-date on breaking research. I can say without reservation that those who contributed to this book are among the most knowledgeable physicians in the world on the subject of natural medicine.

Our expert scientific and evidence-based medical team consists of MDs (Drs. Gaby and Wright), NDs—naturopaths—(Drs. Austin, Brown, Yarnell, Reichert, Aesoph, Seligman, Meletis, and Hudson), and DCs (myself and Drs. Gerber and Duncan). Our goal was to create a book that stressed an integrated approach to self-care, to create a tool that would let readers assess the pluses and minuses of the use of vitamins, minerals, herbs, homeopathic remedies, and other nutrients for the most common and troublesome health conditions.

The first edition of this book was a bestseller. Its first printing sold out immediately, making it the fastest-selling book on natural medicine ever published. This second edition has almost three times the information and all the topics are either new or have been completely revised. Without a doubt, this is the most reliable and complete book on natural medicine ever published.

This book has numerous unique characteristics.

- All statements that might be controversial have been documented with a reference from the scientific literature (from some of those 25,000 articles I mentioned). Thousands of citations are included so the serious reader can retrieve the article and review the material we relied on. In addition, we have used primarily human studies; very little of our information depended on either animal or test-tube trials.

- Contraindications and side effects include information on possible areas of concern when taking a certain supplement or herb. Millions of people who have never before taken vitamins or herbs are now doing so. This mainstream consumer is legitimately concerned about the safety (and efficacy) of these products. The information we provide gives you a way to make sensible choices for yourself and your family. For a complete look at drug-nutrient depletions and interactions, see our book, *A to Z Guide to Drug-Herb-Vitamin Interactions* (Prima Health and Healthnotes, Inc., 1999).

- All of our key contributors have actually been in practice with real patients. They are not biochemists or researchers writing theoretically or from an ivory tower—but from real-life experience in their clinics.

In short, we have created the most useful, comprehensive, and balanced book that has ever been made available on this topic and believe that it will be the first place many people will turn for information about complementary or alternative medicine. Because some people have asked for this book to be available on their computer, we have also created a special CD-ROM version of the program. Please look at the back of this book for information about how you can obtain your own personal copy.

All the authors join me in wishing you good health.

Schuyler W. Lininger, Jr., DC
Editor-in-Chief

How to Use This Book

The Natural Pharmacy, 2nd Edition is divided into four sections. Each section is easily found by looking for the tabs on the side of the book. Once found, you can flip through the pages to find the specific topic you are looking for, alphabetized within each section. You can also use the table of contents or the index to locate topics. The synonym tables found at the beginning of each section can help you locate an entry by synonym or closely related term.

Once you have located the information you want in one of the four sections, you can easily navigate throughout the rest of the book with our unique cross-referencing approach. Next to key words (such as Vitamin C or High Cholesterol) are page number "links" that direct you to more detailed information. By flipping back and forth in the book using the page number links, you can mimic the ease of use you'd find in a computer hypertext document. We think this feature makes *The Natural Pharmacy, 2nd Edition* the easiest-to-use reference book we've ever seen.

It is very important to realize this book is provided for information or educational purposes only and should only be used in consultation with a nutritionally oriented physician.

Following is a list of the four sections of the book and information about what you'll find in each one.

Part One: Health Concerns Look here for information about specific health concerns ranging from acne to yeast infections. Each entry includes a section that describes the concern, makes dietary and lifestyle recommendations when appropriate, and suggests which nutrients and herbs might be of help.

At the end of each condition is a summary checklist of the nutritional supplements and herbs discussed in the text. When applicable, a page number is also given to find out information about homeopathic remedies. These items are ranked as either "primary," "secondary," or "other" according to the strength of the scientific documentation.

If you can try only a few nutrients or herbs, try the ones that are listed as "primary."

Part Two: Nutritional Supplements Look here for information about specific vitamins, minerals, amino acids, and other nutrients (such as CoQ_{10}). Each nutrient entry includes information about where it is found, health concerns in which the nutrient might be supportive, suggested dosage ranges, and possible side effects or interactions.

Part Three: Herbs Look here for information about specific herbs. Each herb includes information about where it is found, what part is used, in which concerns the herb might be supportive, information about historical and traditional use (which may or may not be supported by scientific studies), data on the active compounds (if known), suggested dosage ranges, and possible side effects or interactions.

Part Four: Homeopathic Remedies Look here if you are interested in homeopathy. Information in this section is found by looking up a specific health condition and then matching symptoms to find the specific homeopathic remedy. Refer to p. 509 for complete information about homeopathy dosage directions.

Important Features

This book has many unique features that help make it useful. Take a moment to read over this list to learn how to get the most out of *The Natural Pharmacy, 2nd Edition*.

- In **Part One: Health Concerns,** nutritional supplements and herbs are clearly ranked in the checklist as to which have the most scientific evidence and work the best. In our practices, the items ranked as "primary" are the ones we'd usually have patients use initially.
- The checklist in **Part One: Health Concerns** is also a very useful reminder of what nutrients and herbs might be supportive.

- Information about potential side effects or interactions for nutrients and herbs is located in the individual nutritional supplement or herb. You should refer to each supplement or herb for safety information.
- In **Part Two: Nutritional Supplements** and **Part Three: Herbs,** general information is given. To find out how a particular compound is used for a specific condition, refer to the **Part One: Health Concerns** section that is cross-referenced.
- In **Part Three: Herbs,** the active ingredient(s) of an herb is described if it is known. Many herbs are available in multiple forms: dried (usually in capsules, tablets, poultice, or tea), liquid (as tinctures or extracts), or standardized (where a particular compound is measured and quantified). We have tried to give you dosages for all the various forms when that information was available.
- In all the sections (except **Part Four: Homeopathic Remedies**), we have tried not to make any statements without providing scientific documentation in the form of a footnote. If you or your doctor need to find out more on a particular subject, we hope we have made it easier for you by providing a full citation from the scientific literature. We have used, almost exclusively, human studies from the major medical and scientific journals. We have rarely fallen back on a book or a secondary source.
- In all the sections we have tried to be balanced in our approach to giving you the information. We have tried to avoid overstating the case and have attempted to present information about any negative or equivocal studies. We feel by taking this path, you have a book in which you can have confidence.

About Doses and When to Take Supplements

Each health condition covered in this book includes specific, useful information about nutritional, herbal, and homeopathic support for the condition. Keep in mind that, unless the text specifies differently, the suggested amounts of vitamins, minerals, amino acids, herbs, or homeopathic ingredients apply only to an average-size male or female adult. Children's doses should be determined in consultation with a nutritionally oriented physician.

Unless otherwise specified in the text, nutritional supplements and herbs should be taken with meals.

Continue the Healthnotes Experience

Register online at www.healthnotes.com/tnp and you can receive at no charge, via e-mail, the "Healthnotes Newsletter." This newsletter (an $18 per year value) is published monthly and focuses on specific health concerns and related natural remedies. (For more details, see Also Available from Healthnotes p. 617.)

About the Tables

Information about the effects of a particular supplement or herb on a particular condition has been qualified in terms of the methodology or source of supporting data (for example: clinical, double-blind, meta-analysis, or traditional use). For the convenience of the reader, the information in the table listing the supplements for particular conditions is also categorized. The criteria for the categorizations are:

Primary	Indicates there are reliable and relatively consistent scientific data showing a health benefit.
Secondary	Indicates there are conflicting, insufficient, or only preliminary studies suggesting a health benefit or that the health benefit is minimal.
Other	Indicates that an herb is primarily supported by traditional use or that the herb or supplement has little scientific support and/or minimal proven health benefit.

Health Concerns

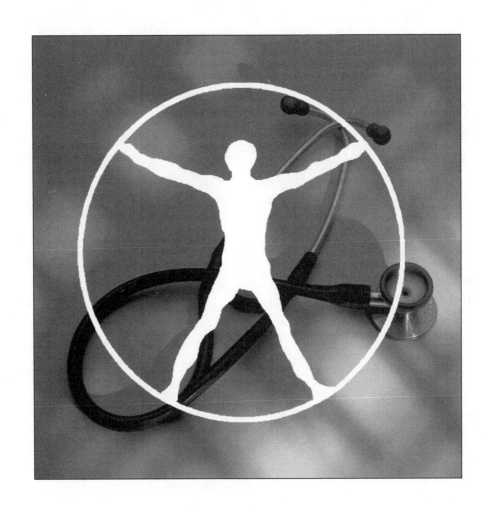

Acne

Acne (also called acne vulgaris) is a skin condition characterized by reddened, inflamed lesions (sometimes called pustules or "whiteheads") on the face, neck, shoulders, and elsewhere. Acne occurs most commonly in teenagers and to a lesser extent in young adults. The condition results in part from excessive stimulation of the skin by androgens (male hormones). Bacterial infection of the skin also appears to play a role.

Dietary Changes That May Be Helpful

Many people assume certain aspects of diet are linked to acne, but there isn't much evidence. Preliminary research found chocolate was not implicated, for example.[1] Similarly, though a diet high in **iodine** (p. 303) can create an acne-like rash in a few people, this is rarely the cause of acne. In a preliminary study, people who thought that certain foods triggered their acne turned out to be consistently wrong.[2] Despite the lack of evidence, some doctors of natural medicine continue to believe that **food allergy** (p. 8) can play a role, at least in adult acne.[3]

Nutritional Supplements That May Be Helpful

Several studies indicate that **zinc** (p. 346) supplements reduce the severity of acne.[4] In one study, zinc was found to be as effective as oral antibiotic therapy.[5] Nutritionally oriented doctors sometimes suggest that people with acne take 30 mg of zinc 2 or 3 times per day for a few months, then 30 mg per day thereafter. It often takes 12 weeks before any improvement is seen.

Large quantities of **vitamin A** (p. 336)—such as 300,000 IU per day for females and 400–500,000 IU per day for males—have been used successfully to treat severe acne.[6] However, those quantities of vitamin A are quite toxic. Moreover, unlike the permanent actions of synthetic prescription versions of vitamin A (such as Accutane), the acne will return several months after real vitamin A is discontinued. Therefore, vitamin A is generally a poor treatment for acne and should be taken only under the supervision of a health professional if at all.

An isolated trial using **pantothenic acid** (p. 340) reported good results.[7] In that trial, people with acne were given 2.5 grams of pantothenic acid 4 times per day (for a total of 10 grams per day)—a remarkably high amount. A cream containing 20% pantothenic acid was also applied topically 4 to 6 times per day. With moderate acne, near-complete relief was seen within 2 months, but severe conditions took at least 6 months to respond. Eventually, the level of pantothenic acid was reduced to 1–5 grams per day—still a very high level.

Niacinamide (p. 339) was found to substantially help people with acne in a double-blind trial lasting 2 months and using topical gel containing 4% niacinamide applied twice per day.[8] There is little reason to believe that the vitamin would have similar actions if taken orally, however.

Vitamin B$_6$ (p. 340) at 50 mg per day may alleviate premenstrual flare-ups of acne experienced by some women.[9]

Are There Any Side Effects or Interactions? Refer to the individual supplement for information about any side effects or interactions.

Checklist for Acne

Ranking	Nutritional Supplements	Herbs
Primary		Tea tree oil (p. 463)
Other	Niacinamide (topical) (p. 339) Pantothenic acid (p. 340) Vitamin A (p. 336) Vitamin B$_6$ (p. 340) Zinc (p. 346)	Burdock (p. 405) Vitex (p. 467)

See also: Homeopathic Remedies for **Acne** (p. 509)

Herbs That May Be Helpful

A large study compared the topical use of 5% **tea tree oil** (p. 463) to 5% benzoyl peroxide for common acne. Although the tea tree oil was slower and less potent in its action, it had far fewer side effects and was thus considered more effective overall.[10] For topical treatment of acne, the oil may be used at a dilution of 5–15%.

Historically, tonic or alterative herbs, such as **burdock** (p. 405), have been used in the treatment of skin conditions. These herbs are believed to have a cleansing action when taken internally.[11] Burdock root tincture may be taken in 2–4 ml amounts per day. Dried root preparations in a capsule or tablet can be used at 1–2 grams 3 times per day. Many herbal preparations combine burdock root with other alterative herbs, such as **yellow dock** (p. 472), **red clover** (p. 453), or **cleavers** (p. 412).

Some older German literature suggests that **vitex** (p. 467) might contribute to clearing of premenstrual acne.[12] Women in these studies used 40 drops of a concentrated liquid product once daily.[13]

Are There Any Side Effects or Interactions? Refer to the individual herb for information about any side effects or interactions.

Alcohol Withdrawal

A majority of people who have been drinking alcohol and decide to stop (often for health-related reasons) are able to do so without much trouble. Alcohol withdrawal typically becomes difficult only when problem drinkers—alcoholics—attempt to quit. Almost inevitably, alcoholics need help in achieving this goal. Sometimes, this help requires medical intervention in detoxification centers.

Although treatments in "detox" centers may involve natural substances, such as B vitamins and vitamin C, these substances are often administered intravenously and therefore require a doctor's intervention. Oral vitamins are not believed to be very helpful in the initial stages of detoxification, because excessive drinking damages the gastrointestinal tract, leading to malabsorption. Intravenous (IV) administration of vitamins bypasses the gastrointestinal tract and therefore supplies vitamins even in the absence of a healthy gut.

> **Warning:** All mention of oral supplement use in this section assumes either that a person does not need intravenous vitamins or that intravenous vitamins have already been administered and oral absorption is now possible.

Deciding whether someone needs intravenous vitamins or when the person can switch from IV to oral supplementation requires a doctor's help. Finding doctors who work with alcohol detoxification is often as easy as calling the local chapter of Alcoholics Anonymous (AA) and asking for referral information. Most programs successful in getting alcoholics to quit drinking are either part of the AA network or employ AA techniques. Natural approaches to alcohol withdrawal should not substitute for detox centers or for AA or AA-related programs.

Lifestyle Changes That May Be Helpful

Most doctors of all kinds agree that alcoholics must stop drinking completely in order to overcome the addiction. Moreover, before nutritional supplements can be used, effective treatment of the malabsorption problems requires a complete avoidance of alcohol.

Dietary Changes That May Be Helpful

Some of the nutritional deficiencies associated with alcoholism can be caused by a poor diet—a factor that needs correction on an individual basis. Improving the overall diet should be done in conjunction with a nutritionally oriented doctor. Sometimes liver or pancreatic disease associated with alcoholism also contributes to nutritional deficiencies. These problems require medical assessment and intervention.

In one trial, a hospital diet was compared with a special diet including fruit and wheat germ and excluding caffeinated coffee, junk food, dairy products, and peanut butter.[1] After 6 months, fewer than 38% of those on the hospital diet remained sober, compared with over 81% of those eating the special diet. A review of the research shows that diets loaded with junk food increase alcohol intake in animals.[2] In a human trial, restricting sugar, increasing complex carbohydrates, and eliminating caffeine also led to a reduction in alcohol craving.[3] While the support for dietary intervention remains somewhat unclear, many doctors of natural medicine suggest that alcoholics reduce sugar and junk food intake and avoid caffeine.

Nutritional Supplements That May Be Helpful

One of the early goals of alcohol detoxification is to allow the body to heal from alcohol-induced damage to the gastrointestinal tract. This damage causes malabsorption, which may initially require IV vitamin supplementation. If alcohol-induced malabsorption is present, supplements should not be taken by mouth until after there has been sufficient healing of the gastrointestinal tract. However, not all alcoholics giving up alcohol require intravenous nutrition. Each case should be assessed by a doctor used to working with alcohol detoxification.

Vitamin B$_3$ (p. 339) is needed to metabolize alcohol—a process that is abnormal in chronic alcoholics. As a result, John Cleary, M.D., has hypothesized that vitamin B$_3$ might help alcoholics.[4] Preliminary research by Cleary found that 500 mg of niacin per day was helpful for a group of twelve alcoholics.[5] Using several grams per day, other preliminary research has also found niacin therapeutic.[6] Activated vitamin B$_3$ used intravenously has helped alcoholics quit drinking.[7] Niacinamide—a safer form of the same vitamin—might have similar actions and has been reported to improve alcohol metabolism in animals.[8]

Deficiencies of the **B-complex** (p. 341) vitamins are well established with chronic alcohol use.[9] The situation is exacerbated by the fact that alcoholics have an increased need for B vitamins.[10] Doctors eventually switch to oral B vitamins after malabsorption is successfully treated by a combination of abstinence from alcohol and IV vitamins (if intravenous vitamins are required). Many doctors of natural medicine use at least 100 mg of B-complex vitamins when oral supplementation is called for. It is possible that successful treatment of the B-complex vitamin deficiencies may actually reduce alcohol cravings because animals crave alcohol when fed a B-complex-deficient diet.[11]

The daily combination of 3 grams of **vitamin C** (p. 341), 3 grams of **niacin** (p. 339), 600 mg of **vitamin B**$_6$ (p. 340), and 600 IU of **vitamin E** (p. 344) has been used by researchers from the University of Mississippi Medical Center in an attempt to reduce anxiety and depression in alcoholics.[12] Although the effect of vitamin supplementation was no better than placebo in treating alcohol-associated depression, the vitamins did result in a significant drop in anxiety within 3 weeks of use. Because of possible side effects, anyone taking such high amounts of niacin and vitamin B$_6$ must do so only under the care of a nutritionally oriented doctor.

Although the incidence of B-complex deficiencies is known to be high in alcoholics, the incidence of other vitamin deficiencies remains less clear.[13] Nonetheless, deficiencies of **vitamin A** (p. 336), **vitamin D** (p. 343), **vitamin E** (p. 344), and **vitamin C** (p. 341) are seen in many alcoholics. It may be safer for some alcoholics to supplement **beta-carotene** (p. 268) instead of vitamin A[14]—a decision that requires a doctor's assessment of liver function. Supplementing with vitamin C appears to help the body rid itself of alcohol.[15] Many nutritionally oriented doctors recommend several grams per day of vitamin C.

Kenneth Blum and researchers at the University of Texas have examined neurotransmitter deficiencies in alcoholics. Neurotransmitters are the chemicals the body makes to allow nerve cells to pass messages (of pain, touch, thought, etc.) from cell to cell. **Amino acids** (p. 265) are the precursors of these neurotransmitters. In preliminary double-blind research, Blum et al. gave alcoholics 1.5 grams of **D,L-phenylalanine** (p. 320), 900 mg of **tyrosine** (p. 335), 300 mg of **glutamine** (p. 300), and 400 mg of **tryptophan** (p. 295) (now available only by prescription) per day, plus a **multivitamin-mineral** (p. 314) supplement.[16] This nutritional supplement regimen led to a reduction in withdrawal symptoms and decreased stress in alcoholics.

The amino acid **glutamine** (p. 300) has also been used as an isolated supplement. Animal research finds that glutamine supplementation reduces alcohol intake, a finding that has been confirmed in double-blind human research.[17] In that trial, 1 gram of glutamine per day given in divided portions with meals decreased both the desire to drink and anxiety levels.

Alcoholics can be deficient in **magnesium** (p. 320). Initially, medical doctors can add magnesium to intravenous vitamin preparations used in detoxification centers.[18] The effect of following short-term IV magnesium with oral supplements has not been well researched.

Alcoholics may be deficient in a substance called prostaglandin E1 (PGE1) and in gamma linolenic acid, a precursor to PGE1.[19] Double-blind though preliminary evidence suggests that supplementation with **evening primrose oil** (p. 292) (which contains gamma linolenic acid) may facilitate withdrawal from alcohol.[20]

Because of the multiple nutrient deficiencies associated with alcoholism, it makes sense for all heavy drinkers who quit alcohol to supplement with a high-potency **multivitamin** (p. 314) for at least several months after the detoxification period.

Are There Any Side Effects or Interactions? Refer to the individual supplement for information about any side effects or interactions.

Herbs That May Be Helpful

Kudzu (p. 438) is most famous as a quick-growing weed in the southern United States. It has a long tradition of use in Chinese herbal medicine. Alcoholic hamsters (one of the few animals to become so besides humans) were found to have decreased interest in drinking when fed kudzu extract.[21] These results have not been confirmed in humans, although traditional Chinese medicine practitioners generally recommend 3–5 grams of root 3 times each day. Tincture in the amount of 3–4 ml 3 times each day can also be helpful to reduce alcohol cravings.

Milk thistle (p. 445) extract is commonly recommended to counteract the harmful effects of alcohol on the liver.[22] Milk thistle extract may protect the cells of the liver by both blocking the entrance of harmful toxins and helping remove these toxins from the liver cells.[23,24] As with other bioflavonoids, silymarin is a powerful antioxidant.[25] Milk thistle also regenerates injured liver cells.[26]

Allergies and Sensitivities

Dandelion (p. 415) can be helpful to those recovering from liver damage caused by alcohol abuse.

Are There Any Side Effects or Interactions? Refer to the individual herb for information about any side effects or interactions.

Checklist for Alcohol Withdrawal

Ranking	Nutritional Supplements	Herbs
Primary	Vitamin B$_3$ (p. 339) Vitamin B-complex (p. 341)	Milk Thistle (p. 445)
Secondary	Evening Primrose Oil (p. 292)	
Other	Beta-carotene (p. 268) D, L-phenylalanine (p. 320) Glutamine (p. 300) Magnesium (p. 310) Multiple vitamin/mineral (p. 314) Tyrosine (p. 335) Vitamin B$_6$ (p. 340) Vitamin C (p. 341) Vitamin D (nutrient depletion) (p. 343) Vitamin E (nutrient depletion) (p. 344)	Dandelion (p. 415) Kudzu (p. 438)

See also: Homeopathic Remedies for **Alcohol Withdrawal** (p. 510)

Allergies and Sensitivities
(Food and Chemical)

What Is an Allergy or Sensitivity?

Allergies are responses mounted by the immune system to a particular food, inhalant, or chemical. The term "sensitivity" is general and may include true allergies, reactions that do not affect the immune system (and therefore are not technically allergies), and reactions for which the cause has yet to be determined. In popular terminology, the terms "allergies" and "sensitivities" are often used to mean the same thing and will be used interchangeably in this section, although from a conventional medical point of view, many sensitivities would not be considered allergies.

What Conditions Are Related to Allergies?

According to J. C. Breneman, M.D., author of the book *Basics of Food Allergy,*[1] many health conditions are related to allergies and have been the subject of independent studies. Even so, any relationship between the condition and the allergy needs to be considered with the aid of a nutritionally oriented doctor. For information on testing and treatment, see **Information About Allergy Testing** (p. 10).

Acne (p. 5) Although supported primarily by anecdotes, some doctors of natural medicine believe that food allergy may play a role in at least adult acne.[2]

Arthritis, Rheumatoid (p. 151) Rheumatoid arthritis (RA) may be linked to food allergies and sensitivities. In many people, RA is made worse when they eat foods to which they are allergic or sensitive and is made better by avoiding these foods.[3,4,5,6] English researchers have suggested that one-third of people with RA can control the disease completely through allergy elimination.[7]

Asthma (p. 15) Unrecognized food allergy is a contributing factor in a significant number of asthmatics,[8] a link that has been confirmed by double-blind research, particularly for nuts, peanuts, dairy, eggs, and soy,[9] though other substances have been implicated elsewhere.[10] Some allergic reactions in asthmatics can be life-threatening.[11]

Attention Deficit (p. 26)—**Hyperactivity Disorder** (p. 26) **ADD** (or **ADHD**), learning disability, and/or childhood hyperactivity has been linked in some studies to certain foods, inhalant allergens, and food colors.[12,13,14] In a study of twenty children, their poor ability to concentrate and behavior problems vanished when allergic foods were removed from their diets.[15] The Feingold diet and a hypoallergenic diet have been used with ADD. In some studies the Feingold diet helped,[16,17,18] though in another study it did not.[19] Studies have shown that eliminating individual allergenic foods and additives from the diet can help children with attention problems.[20,21]

Bed-Wetting (Nocturnal Enuresis) If there is no medical cause for bed-wetting, allergies should be investigated. Several researchers have found allergies to be an important cause of bed-wetting.[22,23]

Urinary Tract Infection (p. 160) People who have recurrent or chronic urinary tract infections should discuss the possible role of allergies with a nutritionally oriented doctor. Chronic infections have been linked to allergies in many reports.[24,25,26,27]

Yeast infection (p. 169) Allergies have been reported to cause recurrent yeast vaginitis. When the allergens are avoided and the allergies treated, the chronic recurring yeast infections sometimes are resolved.[28]

Canker Sores (p. 30) Some studies show food sensitivities or allergies may make mouth ulcers worse.[29,30,31] However, a double-blind study found allergies to play only a minor role.[32]

Colic (p. 40) Thirty-eight bottle-fed and seventy-seven breast-fed babies who had colic were studied in a double-blind, randomized, placebo-controlled trial. Distress was reduced by 25–39% on a diet free of milk, wheat, and nuts.[33] Other foods are also likely to exacerbate colic in some infants.

Constipation (p. 44) A double-blind trial found that chronic constipation and problems associated with it can be triggered by intolerance to cow's milk in two-thirds of constipated infants studied.[34] Symptoms went away in most of those infants kept away from cow's milk. Foods other than dairy might also trigger chronic constipation in some individuals (adults).

Crohn's Disease (p. 48) One study reported that people with Crohn's disease were most likely to react to cereals, dairy, and yeast.[35] Other reports confirm that Crohn's can be exacerbated by food sensitivities.[36]

Depression (p. 50) Although some of the research has produced mixed results,[37] several double-blind studies have shown that food allergies may trigger mental symptoms, including depression.[38,39]

Diarrhea (p. 58) Sensitivity to a food is a common cause of noninfectious diarrhea.[40] People with chronic diarrhea problems not attributable to other causes should discuss the possibility of food sensitivity with a nutritionally oriented doctor.

Ear Infections (recurrent) (p. 63) The incidence of allergy among children with recurrent ear infections is much higher than among the general public.[41] In one study, more than half of all children with recurrent ear infections were found to be allergic to foods. Removing those foods led to significant improvement in 86% of the allergic children tested.[42] Other reports show similar results.[43,44]

Eczema (p. 64) Eczema may be triggered by allergies.[45,46] A nutritionally oriented doctor should be consulted to determine if allergies are a factor. Once the trigger for the allergy has been identified, avoidance of the allergen can lead to significant improvement.[47]

Gallstones (p. 69) Some doctors report that food sensitivities may exacerbate gallbladder attacks in people who have gallstones. Preliminary research has found that foods most commonly reported to be triggers include eggs, pork, and onion, though specific offending foods may vary considerably from person to person.[48]

Gastrointestinal Symptoms Vague gastrointestinal (GI) symptoms (such as abdominal pain, bloating, gas, and diarrhea) that are not caused by serious disease, can sometimes be triggered by food sensitivities. In one double-blind trial, people with vague GI problems believed to be caused by dairy were given dairy to see how their bodies would react.[49] These people were not lactose intolerant. Various indicators of immunity changed as a result of the dairy challenge, showing that their bodies were reacting to the dairy in an abnormal way. However, the indicator of a true dairy allergy—what doctors call milk-specific immunoglubulin E—was normal in most of these people. This study suggests that vague GI symptoms unrelated to serious disease can be caused by food sensitivities that are neither lactose intolerance nor true allergies.

Glaucoma (p. 74) At least two older reports claim that allergy may exacerbate, though not cause, glaucoma.[50,51]

Hay Fever (p. 76) Hay fever may be related to food allergies.[52]

High Blood Pressure (p. 89) Limited research has reported that food allergy may contribute to high blood pressure in some people.[53]

Hives Double-blind research has shown that most chronic hives (urticaria) is caused by food sensitivities and that avoiding these offending food leads to long-term improvement.[54] In this report evidence showed that many of these reactions may not be true allergies, which makes proper diagnosis more difficult though not impossible for nutritionally oriented doctors.

Hypoglycemia (p. 92) Some symptoms of low blood sugar may be related to or made worse by food allergies.[55]

Irritable Bowel Syndrome (IBS) (p. 109) Some,[56] and perhaps most,[57] people with IBS are sensitive to certain foods. People who have IBS often experience improvement when food sensitivities are discovered and the particular foods are avoided.

Migraine Headaches (p. 121) Migraines can be triggered by allergies and may be relieved by identifying and avoiding the "problem" foods.[58,59,60,61] In fact, the preponderance of this research shows that most migraines appear to be triggered by allergies. Uncovering these foods, with the help of a nutritionally oriented doctor, is often a useful way to treat migraines. In children suffering migraines who also have epilepsy, there is evidence that eliminating offending foods may also reduce seizures.[62]

Musculoskeletal Pain (Including Back Pain) Ingestion of allergenic foods has been reported to

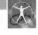

produce a variety of musculoskeletal syndromes in susceptible individuals.[63]

Nephrotic Syndrome Several studies have found a link between nephrotic syndrome (a kidney disease) and allergies. In one study people with nephrotic syndrome responded when the allergens were removed from their diet;[64] in another study, those with nephrotic syndrome did not respond.[65]

Obesity (p. 165) Although the relationship between food sensitivities and body weight remains uncertain, according to one researcher, chronic food allergy may lead to overeating, resulting in obesity.[66]

Psoriasis (p. 147) Anecdotal evidence suggests that people with psoriasis may improve on a hypoallergenic diet.[67] One study reported that eliminating gluten (found in wheat, oats, rye, and barley) improved psoriasis in some people.[68]

Rhinitis Chronic or recurrent infection in the nose or sinuses (p. 156) may be related to food and/or inhalant allergies.[69,70] Similarly, **hay fever** (p. 76) may also be related to food allergies.[71]

Ulcer (duodenal) (p. 158), Eating foods that a person is allergic to can aggravate peptic ulcers,[72] and exposure to allergic foods may actually cause stomach bleeding.[73]

Upper Respiratory Infection (Chronic/Recurring) People who have recurrent or chronic infections should discuss the possible role of allergies with a nutritionally oriented doctor. Chronic infections have been linked to allergies in many reports.[74,75,76,77]

Information About Allergy Testing

There are several tests or procedures that are used by physicians to detect allergies. Most of these tests remain controversial.[78] Some clinicians (cited below), however, believe some of these tests can be effective.

Scratch Testing This form of testing is one of the most widely used. A patient's skin is scratched with a needle that contains a portion of the food, inhalant, or chemical that is being tested. After a period of time, the skin is examined for reactions. If there is a reaction, it is determined that an allergy exists. Although this test is accepted by most allergists, scratch testing is subject to a relatively high incidence of inaccurate results, some tests showing positive when the person is not truly allergic to the substance (false positive) and some tests showing negative when an allergy really exists (false negative).

RAST/MAST/PRIST/ELISA (and Other Tests That Measure Immunoglobulins) The radioallergosorbent test (RAST) indirectly measures antibodies in the blood that react to specific foods. It is used by many nutritionally oriented physicians and has been shown to be a somewhat reliable indicator of allergies.[79,80] It does not, however, pick up nonallergic food sensitivities and is therefore associated with a high risk of false negative readings. In an attempt to avoid this problem, a variety of modifications have been made to tests related to RAST (such as MAST, PRIST, and ELISA). Some of these changes may have reduced the risk of false negative readings somewhat but are likely to have increased the risk of false positive readings. A number of conditions associated with food sensitivities, such as migraine headaches and irritable bowel syndrome, have shown remarkably poor correlation between RAST results and proven sensitivities.

Cytotoxic Testing The cytotoxic test views a patient's serum under a microscope to see whether it is reacting to certain substances. The test is subject to numerous errors and is not generally considered to be reliable.[81]

Clinical Ecology (Also Called "Provocative Neutralization" or "End-Point Titration") This branch of medicine is considered very controversial. Testing is done using intradermal injections of minute dilutions of foods, inhalants, or (in some cases) chemicals. Based on reactions, additional dilutions are used. This test not only determines whether an allergy exists but also operates on the theory that one dilution can trigger a reaction while another can neutralize a reaction. Preliminary research suggests that this approach may have beneficial effects,[82,83] though negative research exist.[84]

Elimination and Reintroduction It is universally acknowledged that the most reliable way to determine a food allergy is to have the patient eliminate a suspected food from the diet for a period of time and then reintroduce it at a later date. The theory behind doing this is that once a food is eliminated, the symptoms that food is causing stop. The body then becomes more sensitive to the food, so when it is reintroduced, the symptom is more likely to recur. This tool lets the patient know with a high degree of certainty which foods are problem foods. This sort of testing requires a great deal of patience and, as with all other forms of allergy testing, is best undertaken with the help of a nutritionally oriented physician who can monitor the diet.[85] Reintroduction of an allergic food has been reported to lead to occasionally dangerous reactions in some patients with certain conditions—another reason this approach should not be attempted without supervision.

Environmental Allergies Some people react to chemicals in the environment. There are chemicals indoors and outdoors, as well as in food, water, medications, cosmetics, perfumes, textiles, and plastics that can trigger allergies. Detecting which chemicals are problems and then eliminating or reducing exposure to them is a time-consuming and challenging task that is difficult to undertake without the assistance of an expert in this area.[86,87]

Alzheimer's Disease

Alzheimer's disease is a brain disorder that occurs in the later years of life. Individuals with Alzheimer's disease develop progressive loss of memory and gradually lose the ability to function and to take care of themselves. The cause of this disorder is not known. Some studies suggest that it may be related to an accumulation of aluminum in the brain.[1] Despite this, aluminum toxicity has been studied in humans, and it is quite distinct from Alzheimer's disease.[2] Therefore, the importance of aluminum in causing Alzheimer's disease remains an unresolved issue.

Dietary Changes That May Be Helpful

Whether aluminum in the diet can cause Alzheimer's disease remains controversial.[3,4] Until this issue is resolved, it seems prudent for healthy people to take steps to minimize exposure to this unnecessary and potentially toxic metal. This can be done by reducing intake of foods cooked in aluminum pots, foods that come into direct contact with aluminum foil, and beverages stored in aluminum cans. Some water authorities add aluminum to the water supply to prevent the accumulation of particulate matter in the water. In such areas, bottled water may be preferable. It appears most unlikely, however, that avoidance of aluminum exposure after the diagnosis of Alzheimer's disease could significantly affect the course of the disease.

Preliminary evidence has linked populations at high risk for Alzheimer's disease with higher levels of dietary fat and calories; similarly, fish intake has been linked with low-risk populations.[5,6,7] Whether these foods can actually increase or reduce the risk of Alzheimer's disease, however, remains unknown.

Nutritional Supplements That May Be Helpful

Phosphatidylserine (p. 321), which is related to **lecithin** (p. 307), is a naturally occurring compound present in the brain. Though it is clearly not a cure, phosphatidylserine (100 mg 3 times per day) has been shown to improve mental function (such as ability to remember names and ability to recall the location of frequently misplaced objects) in individuals with Alzheimer's disease.[8] However, the phosphatidylserine used in these studies was obtained from the brain of cows, which at least in England has been found to sometimes be infected with a virus that could cause Creutzfeldt-Jakob syndrome, a rare and fatal disease in humans. A totally safe plant source of phosphatidylserine is also available; however, this is a different form of phosphatidylserine, and its effectiveness has not yet been documented.[9]

Large amounts of **vitamin E** (p. 344) may slow the progression of Alzheimer's disease, according to researchers from the Alzheimer's Disease Cooperative Study. A 2-year double-blind study of 341 individuals with Alzheimer's disease of moderate severity found that 2,000 IU per day of vitamin E extended the time people with Alzheimer's disease were able to care for themselves (such as bathing, dressing, and other necessary daily functions), compared with those taking placebo.[10] Preliminary evidence has linked people who use antioxidant supplements (vitamins E or C [p. 267]) to a lower risk of Alzheimer's disease compared with people not taking supplements.[11] Other preliminary research shows that higher blood levels of vitamin E correlate with better brain functioning in middle-aged and older adults.[12] The link between antioxidants and protection might make sense because in conditions related to Alzheimer's disease, oxidative damage appears to be part of the disease process.[13]

DMAE (2-dimethylaminoethanol) (p. 290), like choline, may increase levels of the brain neurotransmitter acetylcholine. One uncontrolled 4-week trial of fourteen senile people given DMAE supplements of 600 mg 3 times per day did not show any changes in memory (based on ability to recall faces, numbers, or names) but did produce positive behavior changes in some of the subjects.[14] However, subsequent research of a double-blind, placebo-controlled design did not find a significant benefit from the use of DMAE in people with Alzheimer's disease.[15]

The acetyl group that is part of **acetyl-L-carnitine** (p. 263) contributes to the production of the neurotransmitter acetylcholine. Several clinical trials suggest that acetyl-L-carnitine delays the progression of Alzheimer's disease,[16] improves memory,[17] and enhances overall performance in some individuals with Alzheimer's disease.[18] One double-blind study found that acetyl-L-carnitine slowed progression of the disease in people under the age of 65 but paradoxically appeared to have the opposite effect in older people with Alzheimer's disease.[19] Overall, however, most research indicates improvement in short-term studies and reduction in the rate of deterioration in longer studies (lasting 1 year).[20] A typical supplemental amount is 1 gram taken 3 times per day (total amount equaling 3 grams per day). Alzheimer's research has been done with the acetyl-L-carnitine, rather than the L-carnitine form of this nutrient.

Huperzine A (p. 302) is a substance first found in *Huperzia serrata,* a Chinese medicinal herb. In a well-designed, placebo-controlled trial, 58% of people with Alzheimer's disease had significant improvement in memory and cognitive and behavioral functions after taking 200 mcg of huperzine A twice per day for 8 weeks—a statistically significant improvement over the 36% who responded to placebo.[21] Another double-blind report using injected huperzine A confirmed a positive effect in people with dementia, including, but not limited to, Alzheimer's disease.[22]

Mitochondrial function appears to be impaired in people with Alzheimer's disease. Due to its effects on mitochondrial functioning, one group of researchers has given **coenzyme Q₁₀** (p. 283) (along with **iron** [p. 304] and **vitamin B₆** [p. 340]) to several people with Alzheimer's disease and reported that the progression of the disease was prevented for 1½ to 2 years.[23]

Preliminary research had suggested that people with Alzheimer's disease should avoid zinc supplements.[24] More recently, preliminary evidence in four people with Alzheimer's disease actually showed improved mental function with zinc supplementation.[25] In a convincing review of the zinc/Alzheimer's disease research, perhaps the most respected zinc researcher in the world concluded that zinc does not cause or exacerbate Alzheimer's disease symptoms.[26]

A small uncontrolled study showed that oral **NADH** (p. 317) improved mental function in people with Alzheimer's disease.[27]

Some researchers have found links between Alzheimer's disease and evidence of vitamin B₁₂ and folic acid deficiencies,[28] while others consider the problem to be of only minor significance.[29] Little is known about whether supplementation with either vitamin would significantly help people with this disease. Nonetheless, it makes sense for people with Alzheimer's disease to be medically tested for vitamin B₁₂ and folate deficiencies and to be treated if they are deficient.

Are There Any Side Effects or Interactions? Refer to the individual supplement for information about any side effects or interactions.

Herbs That May Be Helpful

An extract made from the leaves of the *Ginkgo biloba* tree is a leading treatment for early-stage Alzheimer's disease in Europe. While not a cure for this serious condition, **Ginkgo biloba** (p. 427) extract (GBE) may improve memory and quality of life and slow progression in the early stages of the disease. In addition, three double-blind studies have shown that GBE is helpful for people in early stages of Alzheimer's disease, as well as the closely related multi-infarct dementia.[30,31,32] People with other types of dementia, including problems due to poor blood flow to the brain, also respond to GBE.

The tonic, or adaptogenic, class of herb is often used traditionally for elderly persons experiencing mental decline, although this use does not have scientific studies to support it. Examples include **Asian ginseng** (p. 394) (100 to 200 mg per day of the standardized herbal extract), **eleuthero (Siberian ginseng)** (p. 419) (2–3 grams per day of the dried root or 300–400 mg per day of the concentrated solid extract standardized on eleutherosides B and E), **astragalus** (p. 395) (two to three 500 mg capsules 3 times per day), and ashwagandha.

Ashwagandha (p. 393) has been shown to improve memory, although it has not been studied in people who have Alzheimer's disease.[33]

Asian ginseng (p. 394) has the longest history of use in traditional Chinese medicine and is commonly used for older individuals showing signs of memory loss. Asian ginseng improves and sharpens mental concentration and performance, including attention and memory.[34,35] While not as thoroughly researched as GBE for this condition, studies show that ginseng is effective at improving memory and also countering depression in the elderly. Some herbal supplements combine GBE with Asian ginseng.

Are There Any Side Effects or Interactions? Refer to the individual herb for information about any side effects or interactions.

Checklist for Alzheimer's Disease

Ranking	Nutritional Supplements	Herbs
Primary	Acetyl-L-carnitine (p. 263) Phosphatidylserine (p. 321)	*Ginkgo biloba* (p. 427)
Secondary	Huperzine A (p. 302) Vitamin E (p. 344)	
Other	Coenzyme Q₁₀ (p. 283) DMAE (2-dimethylam inoethanol) (p. 290) Folic acid (p. 297) NADH (p. 317) Vitamin B₁₂ (p. 337)	Ashwagandha (p. 393) Asian ginseng (p. 394) Astragalus (p. 395) Eleuthero (p. 419)

Angina

Chest pain due to reduced blood flow to the heart is known as angina or angina pectoris. Hardening of the coronary arteries (**atherosclerosis** [p. 17]) that feed the heart is usually the underlying problem. Therefore it is very important that anyone with angina read the chapter on atherosclerosis; the information there is important for treatment and prevention of angina. The only items covered here are those that specifically relate to angina. Coronary artery spasms may also cause angina.

There are three main types of angina. The first is called stable angina. This type of chest pain comes on during exercise and is both common and predictable. Stable angina is most associated with atherosclerosis. A second type, called variant angina, can occur at rest or during exercise. This type is primarily due to sudden coronary artery spasm, though atherosclerosis may also be a component. The third, most severe type is called unstable angina. It occurs with no predictability and can quickly lead to a heart attack. Anyone with significant, new chest pain or a worsening of previously mild angina must seek medical care immediately.

Lifestyle Changes That May Be Helpful

Cigarette smoking causes damage to the coronary arteries and, in this way, can contribute to angina. Stopping smoking is critical for anyone with angina who smokes. Smoking has also been shown to reduce the effectiveness of treatment of angina.[1] Secondhand smoke should be avoided as well.[2]

Increasing physical exercise has been clearly demonstrated to reduce symptoms of angina as well as to relieve the underlying causes. One study found that intense exercise daily for 10 minutes was as effective as beta-blocker drugs in one group of people with angina.[3] Anyone with a heart condition including angina or anyone over the age of 40 should consult a doctor before beginning an exercise plan.

Dietary Changes That May Be Helpful

Coffee should probably be avoided. Drinking five cups or more a day has been shown to increase the risk of angina, although specifics about the relationship between different forms of coffee and angina remain unclear.[4] (See also the chapter on **atherosclerosis** [p. 17].)

Nutritional Supplements That May Be Helpful

Carnitine (p. 279) is an amino acid important for transporting fats that can be turned into energy in the heart. Several studies using 1 gram of carnitine 2 to 3 times per day show improvement in heart function and reduced symptoms people with angina.[5,6,7] **Coenzyme Q$_{10}$** (p. 283) also contributes to the energy-making mechanisms of the heart. People with angina given 150 mg of coenzyme Q$_{10}$ each day have experienced greater ability to exercise without problems.[8] This has been confirmed in independent investigations.[9]

Low levels of antioxidant vitamins in the blood, particularly **vitamin E** (p. 344), are associated with greater rates of angina.[10] This is true even when smoking and other risk factors for angina are taken into account. Early, short-term studies using 300 IU per day of vitamin E could not find a beneficial action on angina.[11] A later study supplementing small doses of vitamin E (50 IU per day) for longer periods of time showed a minor benefit in people suffering angina.[12] Those affected by variant angina have been found to have the greatest deficiency of vitamin E compared with other people who have angina.[13]

Fish oil (p. 294), which contains the beneficial fatty acids known as EPA and **DHA** (p. 287), has been studied in the treatment of angina. In some studies, 3 grams or more of fish oil 3 times per day (providing a total of about 3 grams of EPA and 2 grams of DHA) have reduced chest pain as well as the need for nitroglycerin, a common medication used to treat angina;[14] other investigators could not confirm these findings.[15] If fish oil is supplemented, **vitamin E** (p. 344) should be taken with it, as vitamin E may protect the fragile oil against free radical damage.[16]

Magnesium (p. 310) deficiency may be responsible for spasms that occur in coronary arteries, particularly in variant angina.[17,18] While studies have used injected magnesium to stop such attacks effectively,[19,20] it is unclear if oral magnesium would be effective.

Nitroglycerin and similar drugs cause dilation of arteries by interacting with nitric oxide, a potent stimulus for dilation. Nitric oxide is made from **arginine** (p. 268), a common amino acid. Blood cells in people with angina are known to make insufficient nitric oxide,[21] which may in part be due to abnormalities of arginine metabolism. Taking 2 grams of arginine 3 times per day for as little as 3 days has improved the ability of angina sufferers to exercise.[22] Detailed studies have investigated the mechanism of arginine and have proven that it operates by stimulating blood vessel dilation.[23]

Bromelain (p. 276) is a natural blood thinner because it prevents excessive blood platelet stickiness.[24] This may explain, in part, the positive reports in a few clinical trials of bromelain to decrease

Angina

thrombophlebitis (inflammation of veins) and pain from angina and thrombophlebitis.[25][26]

Are There Any Side Effects or Interactions? Refer to the individual supplement for information about any side effects or interactions.

Herbs That May Be Helpful

The fruits, leaves, and flowers of the **hawthorn** (p. 433) tree contain anthocyanidins, which protect blood vessels from damage. A 60-mg hawthorn extract containing 18.75% proanthocyanidins taken 3 times per day improved heart function and exercise tolerance in people with angina.[27]

Kudzu (p. 438) is used in modern Chinese medicine as a treatment for angina.

Are There Any Side Effects or Interactions? Refer to the individual herb for information about any side effects or interactions.

Checklist for Angina

Ranking	Nutritional Supplements	Herbs
Primary	Carnitine (p. 279) Coenzyme Q₁₀ (p. 283)	Hawthorn (p. 433)
Secondary	Arginine (p. 268) Vitamin E (p. 344)	
Other	Bromelain (p. 276) Fish oil (p. 294) (EPA/DHA [p. 287])	Kudzu (p. 438)
See also: Atherosclerosis (p. 17)		

Anxiety

Anxiety describes any feeling of worry or dread, usually about potential events that might happen. Some anxiety about stressful events is normal. However, in some people, anxiety interferes with the ability to function. Severe anxiety usually lasts more than 6 months, though it may not be a problem every day. Physical symptoms can sometimes result, including fatigue, insomnia, and irritability. Some people who think they are anxious may actually be depressed. Because of all these factors, it is important for people who are anxious to seek expert medical care. Natural therapies can be one part of the approach to helping relieve mild to moderate anxiety.

Lifestyle Changes That May Be Helpful

Reducing exposure to stressful situations can help decrease anxiety. In some cases, meditation, counsel-ing, or group therapy can greatly facilitate this process.[1]

Dietary Changes That May Be Helpful

All sources of caffeine should be avoided, including coffee, tea, chocolate, caffeinated sodas, and caffeine-containing medications. People with high levels of anxiety appear to be more susceptible to the actions of caffeine.[2]

Nutritional Supplements That May Be Helpful

For mild anxiety, **magnesium** (p. 310) may be relaxing.[3] Typically, 200–300 mg of magnesium are taken 2 to 3 times per day. Some doctors of natural medicine recommend soaking in a hot tub containing 1–2 cups of magnesium sulfate crystals (such as Epsom salts) for 15 to 20 minutes, though support for this approach remains anecdotal.

Inositol (p. 303) has been used to help people with anxiety who have panic attacks. Up to 4 grams 3 times per day has been reported to control such attacks in one double-blind trial.[4]

Vitamin B₃ (p. 339) as niacinamide may be beneficial. It has been shown in animals to work in the brain in ways similar to drugs, such as Valium, which are used to treat anxiety.[5] One study found that niacinamide could help people get through withdrawal from Valium-type drugs—a common problem.[6] A reasonable amount of niacinamide (not niacin) to take for anxiety, according to some doctors of natural medicine, is up to 500 mg 4 times per day.

Are There Any Side Effects or Interactions? Refer to the individual supplement for information about any side effects or interactions.

Herbs That May Be Helpful

The preeminent botanical remedy for anxiety is **kava** (p. 438), an herb from the South Pacific. It has been extensively studied for this purpose.[7] One 100-mg capsule standardized to 70% kava-lactone is given 3 times per day in many studies. Double-blind studies have validated the effectiveness of kava for people with anxiety,[8,9] including menopausal women.[10] Although kava is safer and rarely causes side effects at the given amount, it may cause problems if combined for more than a few days with benzodiazepines in some people.[11] A previous study found kava to be just as effective as benzodiazepines over the course of 6 weeks.[12] The latest research shows that use of kava for up to 6 months is safe and effective compared with placebo.[13]

St. John's wort (p. 461) is very popular for the treatment of mild depression. It has also been reported in at least one double-blind study to reduce anxiety.[14] Like kava, a flavonoid compound from St. John's wort known as amentoflavone has been found to act in the central nervous system in a way similar to benzodiazepine drugs.[15]

An old folk remedy for anxiety, particularly when it causes insomnia, is **chamomile** (p. 409) tea. There is evidence from test tube studies that chamomile contains compounds with a calming action.[16] There are also animal studies that suggest a benefit of chamomile for anxiety.[17] Often one cup of tea is taken 3 or more times per day.

A number of other botanicals known as "nerve tonics" are also used in traditional herbal medicine with anxious people. These have not been rigorously investigated by scientific means to confirm their efficacy, although they have a long track record of safety. These include **oats (oat straw)** (p. 448), **hops** (p. 434), **passion flower** (p. 449), **scullcap** (p. 459), and **valerian** (p. 467). A German study has found the combination of valerian and passion flower to be useful for anxiety.[18]

Are There Any Side Effects or Interactions? Refer to the individual herb for information about any side effects or interactions.

Checklist for Anxiety

Ranking	Nutritional Supplements	Herbs
Primary		Kava (p. 438) Passion flower (p. 449)
Secondary		St. John's wort (p. 461) Valerian (p. 467)
Other	Inositol (p. 303) Magnesium (p. 310) Vitamin B$_3$ (niacinamide) (p. 339)	Chamomile (p. 409) Hops (p. 434) Oats (oat straw) (p. 448) Scullcap (p. 459)
See also: Homeopathic Remedies for Anxiety (p. 512)		

Asthma

Asthma is a lung disorder in which spasms of the bronchial passages restrict the flow of air in and out of the lungs. The number of people with asthma and the death rate from this condition have been increasing since the late 1980s. Environmental pollution may be one of the causes of this growing epidemic.

Dietary and Other Natural Therapies That May Be Helpful

A vegan (pure vegetarian) diet given for 1 year in conjunction with many specific dietary changes (such as

avoidance of caffeine, sugar, salt, and chlorinated tap water) and combined with a variety of herbs and supplements led to significant improvement in a group of asthmatics.[1] Although sixteen out of twenty-four people who continued the intervention for the full year were much better and one person was actually cured, it remains unclear how much of the action was purely a result of the dietary changes compared with the many other therapies employed.

Although most people with asthma do not suffer from food allergies,[2] unrecognized **food allergy** (p. 8) can be an exacerbating factor.[3] A medically supervised "allergy elimination diet" followed by reintroduction of the eliminated foods often helps identify problematic foods. A health-care professional must supervise this allergy test, because there is a chance of triggering a severe asthma attack during the reintroduction.[4]

Some asthmatics react to food additives, such as sulfites, tartrazine (yellow dye #5), aspirin, and aspirin-like substances found in foods called natural salicylates.[5][6] A nutritionally oriented doctor or an allergist can help determine whether chemical sensitivities are present.

Ionized air may also play a role in allergies. Research suggests that some allergy-provoking substances, such as dust and pollen, have a positive electrical charge. Meanwhile, negative ions appear to counteract the allergenic actions of these positively charged ions on respiratory tissues. Negative ions generally lead to favorable actions, and many individuals experience relief from their respiratory allergies.[7] Other allergy sufferers report considerable relief, with a few allergy reactions resolving completely, after negative ion therapy. The majority of allergy sufferers appear to be able to reduce reliance on other treatments (nutritional, biochemical, or prescription) during negative ion therapy.

A set of breathing exercises called Buteyko breathing techniques has been reported to significantly reduce the need for prescription drugs for people with asthma.[8] Although the people in this blinded randomized trial had improved quality of life while doing these exercises, objective measures of breathing capacity did not improve despite the decreased need for drugs.

Nutritional Supplements That May Be Helpful

Vitamin B$_6$ (p. 340) deficiency is common in asthmatics.[9] This deficiency may relate to the asthma itself or to certain asthma drugs (such as theophylline and aminophylline) that deplete vitamin B$_6$.[10] In a double-blind study of asthmatic children, 200 mg per day of vitamin B$_6$ for 2 months reduced the severity of their

Asthma

illness and reduced the amount of asthma medication needed.[11] In another study, asthmatic adults experienced a dramatic decrease in the frequency and severity of asthma attacks while taking 50 mg of vitamin B_6 twice a day.[12] Nonetheless, the research remains somewhat inconsistent, and at least one double-blind study did not find high levels of B_6 to help asthmatics who require the use of steroid drugs.[13]

Magnesium (p. 310) levels are frequently low in asthmatics.[14] Magnesium supplements might help prevent asthma attacks because magnesium can prevent spasms of the bronchial passages. Intravenous injection of magnesium has been reported to stop acute asthma attacks within minutes in double-blind research.[15] Although the effect of oral magnesium has not been appropriately studied, many doctors recommend magnesium supplements for people who have asthma. The usual amount of magnesium taken by an adult is 200–400 mg per day (children take proportionately less based on their body weight).

Supplementation with 1 gram of **vitamin C** (p. 341) per day reduces the tendency of the bronchial passages to go into spasm,[16] an action that has been confirmed in double-blind research.[17] Some individuals with asthma have shown improvement after taking 1–2 grams of vitamin C per day. A buffered form of vitamin C (such as sodium ascorbate or calcium ascorbate) may work better for some asthmatics than regular vitamin C (ascorbic acid).[18]

Very high amounts of **vitamin B_{12}** (p. 337) supplements (1,500 mcg per day) have been found to reduce the tendency for asthmatics to react to sulfites.[19] The trace mineral **molybdenum** (p. 314) also helps the body detoxify sulfite,[20] though the ability of supplemental molybdenum to help people with asthma remains mostly unexplored. A nutritionally oriented physician should be involved in any evaluation and treatment of sulfite sensitivity.

People with low levels of **selenium** (p. 331) have a high risk of asthma.[21][22] Asthma involves free radical damage[23] that selenium might protect against. A double-blind trial gave 45 mcg of selenium to twelve people with asthma.[24] Half showed clear clinical improvement even though lung function tests did not change. Most doctors of natural medicine recommend 200 mcg per day for adults (and proportionately less for children)—a much higher, though still safe level.

Double-blind research shows that **fish oil** (p. 294) partially reduces reactions to allergens that can trigger attacks in some asthmatics.[25] Although a few researchers report small but significant improvements when asthmatics supplement fish oil,[26][27] a review of the research shows that most fish oil studies with asth-

matics come up empty-handed.[28] Nonetheless, there is evidence that children who eat oily fish may have a much lower risk of getting asthma.[29] Therefore, even though evidence supporting the use of fish oils remains weak, eating more fish may still be worth considering.

Stomach levels of hydrochloric acid were reported to be low in asthmatic children many years ago. Supplementation with **betaine HCl** (p. 269) in combination with avoidance of known food allergens led to clinical improvement.[30]

Quercetin (p. 328), a flavonoid found in most plants, has an inhibiting action on lipoxygenase, an enzyme that contributes to problems with asthma.[31] No human studies have confirmed whether quercetin decreases asthma symptoms. Some nutritionally oriented doctors are currently experimenting with 400–1,000 mg of quercetin 3 times per day.

Bromelain (p. 276) reduces the thickness of mucus, which may be beneficial for those with asthma,[32] though clinical actions in asthmatics remain unproven.

Are There Any Side Effects or Interactions? Refer to the individual supplement for information about any side effects or interactions.

Herbs That May Be Helpful

Ephedrine, an alkaloid extracted from **ephedra** (p. 420), is an approved over-the-counter treatment for bronchial tightness associated with asthma.[33] Over-the-counter drugs containing ephedrine can be safely used by adults in the amount of 12.5–25 mg every 4 hours. Adults should take a total dose of no more than 150 mg every 24 hours. They should refer to labels for children's dosages. Ephedrine has largely been replaced by other bronchodilating drugs, such as alupent and albuterol. *Ephedra sinica*, also known as ma huang, continues to be a component of traditional herbal preparations for asthma, often in amounts of 1–2 grams of the herb per day.

Traditionally, herbs that have a soothing action on bronchioles are also used for asthma. These would include **marshmallow** (p. 444), **mullein** (p. 446), and **licorice** (p. 440).

Ginkgo (p. 427) extracts have been considered a potential therapy for asthma for some time. This is because the extracts block the action of platelet-activating factor (PAF), a compound the body produces that in part causes asthma symptoms. A study using isolated ginkgolides from ginkgo (not the whole extract) found they reduced asthma symptoms.[34] A controlled study used a highly concentrated tincture of ginkgo leaf and found this helped decrease asthma symptoms.[35] For asthma, 120–240 mg of standardized extract or 3–4 ml of regular tincture 3 times daily can be used.

Eclectic physicians—doctors at the turn of the century in North America who used herbs as their main medicine—considered **lobelia** (p. 442) to be one of the most important plant medicines.[36] Traditionally, it was used by Eclectics to treat **coughs** (p. 47) and spasms in the lungs from all sorts of causes.[37]

Are There Any Side Effects or Interactions? Refer to the individual herb for information about any side effects or interactions.

Checklist for Asthma

Ranking	Nutritional Supplements	Herbs
Secondary	Selenium (p. 331) Vitamin B$_6$ (p. 340)	Ephedra (p. 420)
Other	Betaine HCl (p. 269) Bromelain (p. 276) Fish Oil (EPA) (p. 294) Magnesium (p. 310) Molybdenum Quercetin (p. 328) Vitamin B$_{12}$ (p. 337) Vitamin C (p. 341)	Elecampane (p. 418) *Ginkgo Biloba* (p. 427) Licorice (p. 440) Lobelia (p. 442) Marshmallow (p. 444) Mullein (p. 446)
See also: Homeopathic Remedies for **Asthma** (p. 514)		

Atherosclerosis
(Hardening of the Arteries)

Atherosclerosis, or hardening of the arteries, is a very common disease of the major blood vessels. It is characterized by fatty streaks along the vessel walls and deposits of cholesterol and calcium. Atherosclerosis of arteries supplying the heart is called coronary artery disease. It can restrict the flow of blood to the heart, which often triggers heart attacks—the leading cause of death in Americans and Europeans. Atherosclerosis of the arteries supplying the legs causes a condition called **intermittent claudication** (p. 106).

People with elevated cholesterol levels are much more likely to have atherosclerosis than people with low cholesterol levels. Many important nutritional approaches to protecting against atherosclerosis are aimed at lowering serum cholesterol levels. People concerned about atherosclerosis should also read the chapter on **cholesterol** (p. 79), *particularly regarding specific dietary information.*

People with diabetes are also at very high risk for atherosclerosis. Those with diabetes who are concerned about atherosclerosis should also read the chapter on **diabetes** (p. 53).

People with elevated triglycerides may be at high risk for atherosclerosis. For a discussion about natural substances that lower triglycerides and may also reduce the risk of atherosclerosis, see the chapter on **high triglycerides** (p. 85).

Lifestyle Changes That May Be Helpful

Virtually all doctors acknowledge that smoking is directly linked to atherosclerosis and heart disease. Quitting smoking protects many people from atherosclerosis and heart disease and is a critical step in the process of disease prevention.

Obesity (p. 165) and type A behavior (time-conscious, impatient, and aggressive) are both associated with an increased risk of atherosclerosis, while exercise is linked to protection from this condition. These are discussed in more detail in the chapter on **cholesterol** (p. 79).

Dietary Changes That May Be Helpful

The most important dietary changes in protecting arteries from atherosclerosis include avoiding meat and dairy fat, increasing fiber, and avoiding foods that contain trans fatty acids (margarine, some vegetable oils, and many processed foods containing vegetable oils). Increasingly, the importance of avoiding trans fatty acids is being accepted by the scientific community.[1] The fibers most linked to the reduction of cholesterol levels are found in oats, psyllium seeds, fruit (pectin), and beans (guar gum).[2] The importance of making these changes is widely accepted by many researchers. Leading researchers have recently begun to view the evidence linking trans fatty acids to markers for heart disease as "unequivocal."[3]

Independent of their action on serum cholesterol, foods that contain high amounts of cholesterol—mostly egg yolks—can induce atherosclerosis.[4] It makes sense to reduce the intake of egg yolks. However, eating eggs does not increase serum cholesterol as much as eating saturated fat, and eggs may not increase serum cholesterol at all if the overall diet is low in fat. A decrease in atherosclerosis resulting from a pure vegetarian diet—meaning no meat, poultry, dairy, or eggs—combined with exercise and stress reduction has been proven by medical research.[5] These and other dietary issues for people with atherosclerosis are discussed in more detail in the chapter on **cholesterol** (p. 79).

Nutritional Supplements That May Be Helpful

Many cardiologists agree that LDL—low-density lipoproteins, or "bad" cholesterol—triggers atherosclerosis only when it has been damaged by reactive molecules called free radicals. Several **antioxidant** (p. 267) supplements protect LDL cholesterol.

Vitamin E (p. 344) is an antioxidant that serves to protect LDL from oxidative damage[6] and has been linked to prevention of heart disease in double-blind research.[7] Virtually all nutritionally oriented doctors recommend 400–800 IU of vitamin E per day to lower the risk of atherosclerosis and heart attacks. However, some leading researchers suggest taking only 100–200 IU per day as studies that have explored the long-term effects of different supplemental levels suggest no further benefit beyond that amount, and research reporting positive effects with 400–800 IU per day have not investigated the effects of lower intakes.[8]

In some studies, people who consume more **selenium** (p. 331) from their diet have a lower risk of heart disease.[9][10] In one double-blind report, individuals who already had one heart attack were given 100 mcg of selenium per day or placebo for 6 months.[11] At the end of the trial, there were four deaths from heart disease in the placebo group but none in the selenium group (although the numbers were too small for this difference to be statistically significant). Some nutritionally oriented doctors recommend that people with atherosclerosis supplement with 100–200 mcg of selenium per day.

Quercetin (p. 328), a **bioflavonoid** (p. 271), also protects LDL cholesterol from damage.[12] Several studies have found eating foods high in quercetin lowers the risk of heart disease,[13,14,15] but the research on this subject is not always consistent,[16] and some research finds no protective link.[17] Quercetin is found in apples, onions, black tea, and as a supplement. In some studies, dietary amounts linked to protection from heart disease are as low as 35 mg per day.

Blood levels of an amino acid called homocysteine have been linked to atherosclerosis and heart disease in most research,[18] though uncertainty remains about whether elevated homocysteine actually causes heart disease.[19,20] Although some reports have found associations between homocysteine levels and dietary factors such as coffee and protein intakes,[21] evidence linking specific foods to homocysteine remains preliminary. Higher blood levels of vitamins B_6 (p. 340), B_{12} (p. 337), and **folic acid** (p. 297) are associated with low levels of homocysteine,[22] and supplementing with these vitamins lowers homocysteine levels.[23][24] For the few cases in which B_6, B_{12}, and folic acid

fail to normalize homocysteine, adding 6 grams per day of betaine may be effective.[25] The form of betaine used to lower homocysteine levels is different from the betaine HCl supplement used to acidify the stomach. Of these four supplements, folic acid appears to be the most important.[26] Attempts to lower homocysteine by simply changing the diet rather than using vitamin supplements have not been successful.[27]

While several trials have consistently shown that B_6, B_{12}, and folic acid lower homocysteine, the amounts used vary from study to study. Many nutritionally oriented doctors recommend 50 mg of vitamin B_6, 100–300 mcg of vitamin B_{12}, and 500–800 mcg of folic acid. Even researchers finding only inconsistent links between homocysteine and heart disease have acknowledged that a B vitamin might offer protection against heart disease independent of the homocysteine-lowering effect.[28]

Experimentally increasing homocysteine levels in humans has led to temporary dysfunction of the cells lining blood vessels. Researchers are concerned that this dysfunction may be linked to atherosclerosis and heart disease. **Vitamin C** (p. 341) has been reported to reverse the dysfunction caused by increases in homocysteine.[29] Vitamin C also protects LDL.[30]

Despite these protective mechanisms attributed to vitamin C, some research has been unable to link vitamin C intake to protection against heart disease. These negative trials have mostly been conducted using people who consume 90 mg of vitamin C per day or more—a level beyond which further protection of LDL may not occur. Trials studying people who eat foods containing lower amounts of vitamin C *have* been able to show a link between dietary vitamin C and protection from heart disease. Therefore, leading vitamin C researchers have begun to suggest that vitamin C may be important in preventing heart disease, but only up to 100 to 200 mg of intake per day.[31] Many nutritionally oriented doctors suggest that people take vitamin C—often 1 gram per day—despite the fact that research does not yet support levels higher than 200 mg per day. See the chapter on **cholesterol** (p. 79) for more details.

Though low levels (2 grams per day) of **evening primrose oil** (p. 292) appear to be without action,[32] 3–4 grams per day have lowered cholesterol in double-blind research.[33] Lowering cholesterol levels should in turn reduce the risk of atherosclerosis.

Preliminary research shows that **chondroitin sulfate** (p. 281) may prevent atherosclerosis in animals and humans and may also prevent heart attacks in people who already have atherosclerosis.[34][35] However, further research is needed to determine the value of chondroitin sulfate supplements for preventing or treating atherosclerosis.

Resveratrol (p. 329), found primarily in red wine, is a naturally occurring antioxidant that decreases the "stickiness" of blood platelets and may help blood vessels remain open and flexible.[36][37][38] Resveratrol research remains very preliminary, however, and as yet there is no clear evidence that the levels found in supplements will help in any significant way.

Preliminary evidence suggests that **octacosanol** (p. 318) may reduce atherosclerosis,[39] but the significance of this research remains unknown.

In 1992, a Finnish study found a strong link between unnecessary exposure to **iron** (p. 304) and increased risk for heart disease.[40] Since then many studies have not found that link,[41,42,43] though several others have.[44,45] A 1999 analysis of twelve studies looking at iron status and heart disease found no overall relationship.[46] While unnecessary exposure to iron, including iron supplements, might not increase the risk of heart disease, there is no benefit in supplementing iron in the absence of a diagnosed deficiency. **Are There Any Side Effects or Interactions?** Refer to the individual supplement for information about any side effects or interactions.

Herbs That May Be Helpful

Several herbs have been shown in research to lower lipid levels. Of these, **psyllium** (p. 452) has the most consistent backing from multiple double-blind studies showing lower cholesterol and triglyceride levels.[47]

Garlic (p. 425) has also lowered cholesterol levels in double-blind research,[48] though more recently, some double-blind studies have not found garlic to be effective.[49,50,51] Some of the negative studies have flaws in their design.[52] Nonetheless, the relationship between garlic and cholesterol lowering is somewhat unclear.[53]

Garlic has also been shown to prevent excessive platelet adhesion in humans.[54] Allicin, often considered the main active component of garlic, is not alone in this action. The constituent known as ajoene has also shown beneficial effects on platelets.[55]

Ginkgo (p. 427) may reduce the risk of atherosclerosis by interfering with a chemical the body sometimes makes in excess called platelet activating factor (PAF).[56] PAF stimulates platelets to stick together too much; ginkgo stops this from happening. Refer to the chapter on **intermittent claudication** (p. 106) for an example of how garlic and ginkgo can directly affect an atherosclerosis-induced disorder. Ginkgo also increases blood circulation, both to the brain and to the arms and legs.[57]

Checklist for Atherosclerosis

Ranking	Nutritional Supplements	Herbs
Primary	Vitamin E (p. 344)	Fenugreek (p. 424) Guggul (p. 432) Psyllium (p. 452)
Secondary	Folic acid (p. 297) Octacosanol (p. 318) Selenium (p. 331) Vitamin B$_6$ (p. 340) Vitamin B$_{12}$ (p. 337)	Garlic (p. 425) *Ginkgo biloba* (p. 427)
Other	Betaine (not HCl) Chondroitin sulfate (p. 281) Evening primrose oil (p. 292) Quercetin (p. 328) Resveratrol (p. 329) Vitamin C (p. 341)	Bilberry (p. 396) Butcher's broom (p. 405) Fo-ti (p. 425) Ginger (p. 427) Hawthorn (p. 433) Rosemary (p. 455) Turmeric (p. 465)

Garlic (p. 425) and **ginkgo** (p. 427) also decrease excessive blood coagulation. Both have been shown in double-blind[58] or single blind[59] studies to decrease the overactive coagulation of blood that may contribute to atherosclerosis.

Guggul (p. 432) has been less extensively studied but double-blind evidence suggests it can significantly improve cholesterol and triglyceride levels in people.[60] Numerous medicinal plants and plant compounds have demonstrated an ability to protect LDL cholesterol from being damaged by free radicals. Garlic,[61] ginkgo,[62] and guggul[63] are of particular note in this regard. Garlic and ginkgo have been most convincingly shown to protect LDL cholesterol in humans.

The evidence supporting the ability of **fenugreek** (p. 424) to lower lipid levels is not as complete, coming from smaller, less complete studies.[64] Preliminary Chinese research found that **fo-ti** (p. 425) may lower cholesterol levels.[65]

The research on **ginger's** (p. 427) ability to reduce platelet stickiness indicates that 10 grams (approximately 1 heaping teaspoon) per day is the minimum necessary amount to be effective.[66] Lower amounts of dry ginger,[67] as well as various levels of fresh ginger,[68] have not been shown to affect platelets.

Turmeric's (p. 465) active compound curcumin has shown potent antiplatelet activity in animal studies.[69] It has also demonstrated this effect in preliminary human studies.[70] In a similar vein, **bilberry** (p. 396) has been shown to prevent platelet aggregation.[71]

Hawthorn (p. 433) also increases circulation, but mostly to the heart.[72] Refer to the **angina** (p. 13)

Athlete's Foot

chapter on how hawthorn can affect people with this atherosclerosis-related disease.

Butcher's broom (p. 405) and **rosemary** (p. 455) are not well studied as being circulatory stimulants but are traditionally reputed to have such actions. While butcher's broom is useful for various diseases of veins, it can protect arteries, too.[73]

Are There Any Side Effects or Interactions? Refer to the individual herb for information about any side effects or interactions.

Athlete's Foot

A number of different fungi can infect the skin and nails of the toes. This results in the condition known as athlete's foot. Generally this does not cause any problem more serious than flaking or itching skin. However, it can be a source of significant infections in people with impaired blood flow to the feet, such as **diabetics** (p. 53), or in people with impaired **immune systems** (p. 94). Infections of the nails are more difficult to treat than those affecting only the skin.

Lifestyle Changes That May Be Helpful

Keeping the feet dry is very important for preventing and fighting athlete's foot. After showering or bathing, drying or careful use of a hair dryer is recommended. Light is also an anathema to fungi. People with athlete's foot should change socks daily to decrease contact with the fungus or wear sandals occasionally to get sunlight exposure.

Herbs That May Be Helpful

Tea tree (p. 463) oil has been shown to help athlete's foot. One report found that application of a 10% tea tree cream reduced symptoms of athlete's foot just as effectively as drugs and better than placebo, although it did not eliminate the fungus.[1]

The compound known as ajoene, found in **garlic** (p. 425), is a powerful antifungal agent. Of a group of thirty-four people using a 0.4% ajoene cream (applying once per day), 79% saw complete clearing of athlete's foot over 7 days; the rest saw complete clearing within 14 days.[2] All participants remained cured 3 months later. Ajoene cream is not yet available, but topical application of crushed, raw garlic is a potential alternative application.

Myrrh (p. 446) can be applied in the tincture form topically to athlete's foot.

Many doctors of natural medicine have used highly diluted grapefruit seed extract in a footbath for ath-

lete's foot. Four to five drops at most need to be added to sufficient water to cover the affected areas on the feet, including toenails; soak for 5 to 10 minutes 1 to 4 times per day.

Are There Any Side Effects or Interactions? Refer to the individual herb for information about any side effects or interactions.

Checklist for Athlete's Foot

Ranking	Nutritional Supplements	Herbs
Primary		Tea tree oil (p. 463)
Secondary		Garlic (p. 425)
Other		Grapefruit seed extract Myrrh (p. 446)

Athletic Performance

Aside from training, nutrition may be the most important influence on athletic performance.[1] However, in seeking a competitive edge, athletes are often susceptible to fad diets or supplements that have not been scientifically validated. Nevertheless, there is much useful research to guide the exerciser toward optimum health and performance.

Lifestyle Changes That May Be Helpful

Many athletes use exercise and weight-modifying diets as tools to change their body composition, assuming that a lower percent body fat and/or higher lean body mass is desirable in any sport. There is no single standard for body weight and body composition that applies to all types of athletic activities. Different sports, even different roles in the same sport (e.g., running vs. blocking in football), require different body types. These body types are largely determined by genetics. However, within each athlete's genetic predisposition, variations occur due to diet and exercise that may impact performance. In general, excess weight is a disadvantage in activities that require quickness and speed. However, brief, intense bursts of power depend partly on muscle size, so this type of activity may favor athletes with higher body weights due to increased lean body mass. On the other hand, participants in endurance sports, which require larger energy reserves, should not attempt to lower their body fat so much as to compromise long-term performance.[2]

Athletic Performance

Dietary Changes That May Be Helpful

Calorie requirements for athletes depend on the intensity of their training and performance. The athlete who trains to exhaustion on a daily basis needs more fuel than one who performs a milder regimen 2 or 3 times per week. Calorie requirements can be as much as 23 to 39 kcal per pound of body weight per day for the training athlete who exercises vigorously for many hours per day.[3,4] Many athletes compete in sports having weight categories (such as wrestling and boxing), sports that favor small body size (such as gymnastics and horse racing), or sports that may require a specific socially accepted body shape (such as figure skating). These athletes may feel pressured to restrict calories to extreme degrees to gain a competitive edge.[5] Excessive calorie restriction can result in chronic fatigue, sleep disturbances, reduced performance, impaired ability for intensive training, and increased vulnerability to injury.[6]

Carbohydrate is the most efficient fuel for energy production and can also be stored as glycogen in muscle and liver, functioning as a readily available energy source for prolonged, strenuous exercise. For these reasons, carbohydrate may be the most important nutrient for sports performance.[7] Depending on training intensity and duration, athletes require up to 4.5 grams per day of carbohydrate per pound of body weight or 60–70% of total dietary calories from carbohydrate, whichever is greater.[8,9] Emphasizing grains, starchy vegetables, fruits, low-fat dairy products, and carbohydrate-replacement beverages and reducing intake of fatty foods results in a relatively high carbohydrate diet.

Carbohydrate beverages should be consumed during endurance training or competition (30–70 grams of carbohydrate per hour) to help prevent carbohydrate depletion that might otherwise occur near the end of the exercise period. At the end of endurance exercise, body carbohydrate stores must be replaced to prepare for the next session. This replacement can be achieved most rapidly if 40–60 grams of carbohydrate are consumed right after exercise, repeating this intake every hour for at least 5 hours after the event.[10] Standard sport drinks containing 6–8% carbohydrate can be used during exercise, while high-density carbohydrate beverages containing 20–25% carbohydrate are useful for immediate post-exercise repletion. Addition of protein or a blend of essential amino acids to these products may increase their effectiveness for carbohydrate repletion,[11] may help athletes recover from anaerobic (short-term and intense) exercise,[12]

and, according to preliminary research,[13,14] may facilitate muscle growth during weight-training.

Carbohydrate-loading, or "supercompensation," is a pre-event strategy that improves performance for some endurance athletes.[15,16] Carbohydrate-loading can be achieved by consuming a 70% carbohydrate diet (or 4.5 grams per pound of body weight) for 3 to 5 days before competition, while gradually reducing training time, and ending with a day of no training while continuing the diet just before the event date.

Protein requirements are often higher for both strength and endurance athletes than for people who are not exercising vigorously; however, the increased food intake needed to supply necessary calories and carbohydrate also supplies extra protein. As long as the diet contains at least the typical 12–15% of calories as protein, or up to 0.75 grams per day per pound of body weight, protein supplements are neither necessary nor likely to be of benefit.[17,18]

Some athletes have speculated that consuming a high-fat diet for 2 or more weeks prior to endurance competition might cause the body to shift its fuel utilization toward more abundant fat stores ("fat adaptation"). In general, high-fat diets have not been found to consistently improve performance, and may even be detrimental;[19,20,21] however, one study did report that a high-fat diet supported endurance training and performance as effectively as a high carbohydrate diet after 2 to 4 weeks of adaptation to the diets.[22]

Water is the most abundant substance in the human body and is essential for normal physiological function. Water loss due to sweating during exercise can result in decreased performance and other problems. The athlete should not wait until thirst occurs before drinking water but should instead drink before the need is felt. Fluids should be ingested prior to, during, and after exercise, especially when extreme conditions of climate, exercise intensity, and exercise duration exist.[23] Approximately two glasses of fluid should be consumed 2 hours before exercise and at regular intervals during exercise; fluid should be cool, not cold, (59–72 degrees F). Flavored sports drinks containing electrolytes are not necessary for fluid replacement during brief periods of exercise, but they may be more effective in encouraging the athlete to drink frequently in larger amounts.[24]

Nutritional Supplements That May Be Helpful

Many athletes do not eat an optimal diet, especially when they are trying to control their weight while training strenuously.[25] These athletes may experience micronutrient deficiencies that, even if marginal, could affect performance or cause health problems.[26,27,28,29] However, athletes who receive recommended daily allowances of vitamins and minerals from their diet do not appear to benefit from additional **multivitamin/mineral supplements** (p. 314) with increased performance.[30,31,32] The importance of individual vitamins and minerals is discussed below.

Electrolyte replacement is not as important as water intake in most athletic endeavors. It usually takes several hours of exercise in warm climates before sodium depletion becomes significant, and even longer for **potassium** (p. 323), chloride, and **magnesium** (p. 310).[33] However, the presence of sodium in fluids will often make it easier to drink as well as retain more fluid.[34]

Most research has demonstrated that strenuous exercise increases production of harmful substances called **free radicals** (p. 267), which can damage muscle tissue and result in inflammation and muscle soreness. Exercising in cities or smoggy areas also increases exposure to free radicals. **Antioxidants** (p. 267), including **vitamin C** (p. 341) and **vitamin E** (p. 344), neutralize free radicals before they can damage the body, so antioxidants may aid in exercise recovery. Regular exercise increases the efficiency of the antioxidant defense system, potentially reducing the increased intake otherwise needed for protection. However, supplements of antioxidant vitamins may be at least theoretically beneficial in older or untrained individuals or athletes who are undertaking an especially vigorous training protocol or athletic event, although research focusing on recovery from exercise is lacking.[35,36] Placebo-controlled research, some of it double-blind, has shown that taking 400–3,000 mg of vitamin C per day may reduce pain and speed up muscle strength recovery after intense exercise.[37,38] Reductions in blood indicators of muscle damage and free radical activity have also been reported for supplementation with 400–1,200 IU per day of vitamin E in most studies,[39,40,41] but no measurable benefits in exercise recovery have been reported.[42] A combination of 90 mg per day of **coenzyme Q$_{10}$** (p. 283) and a very small amount of **vitamin E** (p. 344) did not produce any protective effects in one double-blind study,[43] while in another double-blind study, a combination of 50 mg per day of **zinc** (p. 346) and 3 mg per day of **copper** (p. 285) significantly reduced evidence of post-exercise free radical activity.[44]

In most well-controlled studies, *exercise performance* has not been shown to benefit from supplementation of **vitamin C** (p. 341), unless a deficiency exists.[45,46] Similarly, **vitamin E** (p. 344) has not benefit-

ed exercise performance,[47] except possibly at high altitudes.[48,49]

The **B-complex vitamins** (p. 341) are important for athletes, because they are needed to produce energy from carbohydrates. Exercisers may have slightly increased requirements for some of the B vitamins, including **vitamin B$_2$** (p. 337), **vitamin B$_6$** (p. 340), and **pantothenic acid** (p. 340);[50] athletic performance can suffer if these slightly increased needs are not met.[51] However, most athletes obtain enough B vitamins from their diet without supplementation,[52] and supplementation studies have found no effect on performance measures for vitamin B$_2$,[53,54] **niacin** (p. 339),[55] or vitamin B$_6$.[56]

Chromium (p. 282), primarily in a form called chromium picolinate, has been studied for its potential role in altering body composition. Preliminary research in animals[57] and humans[58 59] suggested that chromium picolinate increases fat loss and lean muscle tissue gain when used with a weight-training program. However, several recent studies have found little to no effect of chromium on body composition or strength,[60,61,62] though one group of researchers has reported significant reductions in body fat measured with precise techniques in double-blind trials using 200–400 mcg per day of chromium for 6 to 12 weeks in middle-aged adults.[63,64]

Iron (p. 304) is important for the athlete because it transports oxygen to and within muscle cells. Some athletes, especially women, do not get enough of this mineral, and endurance athletes, such as marathon runners, frequently have low body iron levels for reasons that are unclear.[65,66,67] A severe deficiency of iron can impair performance, but mild deficiency appears harmless; as a result, supplementing non-anemic athletes does not usually improve performance.[68] Anemia in athletes is often not due to iron deficiency and may be a normal adaptation to the stress of exercise.[69] Therefore, it is unwise to supplement with iron unless a significant deficiency has been diagnosed. Athletes who experience undue fatigue (an early warning sign of iron deficiency) should have their iron status evaluated by a nutritionally oriented physician.

Magnesium (p. 310) deficiency can reduce exercise performance and contribute to muscle cramps, but it is not clear whether the occasional suboptimal intake found in some athletes is particularly important.[70] One recent study found no effect of supplementation with 500 mg per day of magnesium on performance or muscle symptoms in athletes with blood levels of magnesium in the low end of the normal range.[71] However, two double-blind studies have reported intriguing results. One suggested that magnesium at

3.6 mg per pound body weight per day (including both diet and supplements) may benefit strength training,[72] and the other trial used 390 mg per day of magnesium in triathletes and demonstrated reduced swimming, cycling, and running times.[73]

Very little research has been done to evaluate the ergogenic effects of other vitamins or minerals. Supplementation with **selenium** (p. 331) had no effect on the results of endurance training in one double-blind study.[74] Vanadyl sulfate, a form of **vanadium** (p. 335) that may have an insulin-like action, was given to weight-training athletes in a double-blind study using 225 mcg per pound of body weight per day, but no effect on body composition was seen after 12 weeks, and effects on strength were inconsistent.[75]

Certain **amino acids** (p. 265), the building blocks for protein, might be ergogenic aids as discussed below. However, while athletes have an increased need for protein compared with non-exercising adults, the maximum amount of protein suggested by many researchers—0.75 grams per pound of body weight—is already in the diet of most athletes as long as they are not restricting calories. Supplements of amino acids are therefore not needed to fulfill protein requirements for either strength or endurance exercise.[76]

Some research has shown that supplemental **branched-chain amino acids (BCAA)** (p. 274) (typically 10–20 grams per day) do not result in meaningful changes in body composition,[77] nor do they improve exercise performance[78,79,80,81] or enhance the effects of physical training.[82,83] However, BCAA supplementation may be useful in special situations, such as the prevention of muscle loss at high altitudes[84] and prolonging endurance performance in the heat.[85] Studies by one group of researchers suggest that BCAA supplementation may also improve exercise-induced declines in some aspects of mental functioning.[86,87,88]

L-carnitine (p. 279), which is normally manufactured by the human body, has been popular as a potential ergogenic aid because of its role in the conversion of fat to energy.[89] However, while some studies have found that L-carnitine improves certain measures of muscle physiology, research on the effects of 2–4 grams of carnitine per day on performance have produced inconsistent results.[90] L-carnitine may be effective in certain intense exercise activities leading to exhaustion,[91] but recent studies have reported that L-carnitine supplementation does not benefit non-exhaustive or even marathon-level endurance exercise,[92,93] anaerobic performance,[94] or lean body mass in weight-lifters.[95]

At very high intakes (approximately 250 mg per 2.2 pounds of body weight) the amino acid **arginine** (p. 268) has increased growth hormone levels,[96] an effect that has interested body builders. Large quantities (170 mg per 2.2 pounds of body weight per day) of a related amino acid, **ornithine** (p. 318), has also raised growth hormone levels in some athletes.[97] High amounts of arginine[98] or ornithine[99] do not appear to raise levels of insulin, another anabolic hormone. More reasonable amounts of a combination of these amino acids have not had measurable effects on any anabolic hormone levels during exercise.[100,101] Nonetheless, double-blind trials combining weight training with either arginine/ornithine (500 mg of each, twice per day, five times per week) or placebo, found that the amino acid combination produced decreases in body fat,[102] higher total strength and lean body mass, and reduced evidence of tissue breakdown after only 5 weeks.[103] These remarkable results need independent confirmation before gaining acceptance among health-care professionals who work with athletes.

The amino acid **glutamine** (p. 300) appears to play a role in muscle function and and in the immune system.[104] Intense exercise lowers blood levels of glutamine, which can remain indefinitely low with over-training.[105] Glutamine supplementation raises levels of growth hormone at an intake of 2 grams per day,[106] and intravenous glutamine is better than other amino acids at helping replenish muscle glycogen after exercise.[107] However, glutamine supplementation (30 mg per 2.2 pounds body weight) has not improved performance of short-term, high-intensity exercise by trained athletes,[108] and no studies on endurance performance have been done. Although the effects of glutamine supplementation on immune function after exercise have been inconsistent,[109,110] a double-blind study giving athletes glutamine (2.5 grams after exercise and again 2 hours later) reported 81% without subsequent infection compared with 49% in the placebo group.[111]

Strenuous physical activity lowers blood levels of **coenzyme Q$_{10}$ (CoQ$_{10}$)** (p. 283).[112] However, the effects of CoQ$_{10}$ on how the healthy body responds to exercise have been inconsistent, with several studies finding no improvement.[113,114] A few studies using at least 4 weeks of CoQ$_{10}$ supplementation at 60–100 mg per day, have reported improvements in measures of work capacity ranging from 3 to 29% in sedentary people and from 4 to 32% in trained athletes.[115] However, recent double-blind and/or placebo-controlled trials in trained athletes, using performance measures such as time to exhaustion and total performance, have found either no significant improvement[116] or significantly *poorer* results in those taking CoQ$_{10}$.[117,118]

One group of researchers has reported on two small placebo-controlled trials showing that 100 grams of a combination of dihydroxyacetone and **pyruvate** (p. 328) enhanced the endurance of certain muscles.[119,120] No follow-up research has appeared in the last decade to confirm these preliminary results.

Aspartic acid is a non-essential amino acid that participates in many biochemical reactions relating to energy and protein. Preliminary, though conflicting, animal and human research suggested a role for aspartic acid (in the form of potassium and magnesium aspartate) in reducing fatigue during exercise.[121] However, most studies have found aspartic acid useless in improving either athletic performance or the body's response to exercise.[122,123,124,125,126]

Whey protein (p. 346) is a dairy-based source of amino acids. While whey is a high-quality source of protein, there is no evidence that currently supports its use for strength-training or body-building.

Ornithine alpha-ketoglutarate (OKG) (p. 319) is formed from the amino acids ornithine and glutamine and is believed to facilitate muscle growth by enhancing the body's release of anabolic hormones. While this effect has been found in studies on hospitalized patients[127] and elderly people,[128] no studies on muscle growth in athletes using OKG have been published.

Creatine (p. 285) (creatine monohydrate) is used in muscle tissue for the production of phosphocreatine, a factor in the formation of ATP, the source of energy for muscle contraction and many other functions in the body.[129,130] Creatine supplementation increases phosphocreatine levels in muscle, especially when accompanied by exercise or carbohydrate intake.[131,132] It may also increase exercise-related gains in lean body mass, though it is unclear whether this represents more muscle or simply water retention.[133] Most controlled studies have shown that 20 grams per day of creatine monohydrate taken for 5 or 6 days in sedentary or moderately active people have improved performance and delayed muscle fatigue during short-duration, high-intensity exercise such as sprinting and weight lifting.[134,135]

However, performance does not appear to be improved for *trained athletes* supplementing with **creatine** (p. 285) in competitive situations, according to most,[136] though not all,[137,138] studies. Creatine supplementation does not appear to increase endurance performance and may impair it by contributing to weight gain.[139] Only one controlled study lasting over 1 month has been done to evaluate the effects of creatine mono-

hydrate supplementation.[140] More long-term research is needed to evaluate creatine's positive effects on athletic performance, particularly in trained athletes.

Gamma oryzanol (p. 298) is a mixture of sterols and ferulic acid esters. Despite claims that gamma oryzanol or its components increase testosterone levels, the release of endorphins, and the growth of lean muscle tissue, research has provided little support and has also shown gamma-oryzanol to be poorly absorbed.[141] A recent 9-week double-blind trial of 500 mg per day of gamma-oryzanol in weightlifters found no benefit compared with placebo in strength performance gains or circulating anabolic hormones;[142] however, a small, double-blind study using 30 mg per day of ferulic acid for 8 weeks in trained weightlifters did find significantly more weight gain (though lean body mass was not measured) and increased strength in one of three measures compared with placebo.[143]

Medium chain triglycerides (MCT) (p. 312) contain a class of fatty acids found only in very small amounts in the diet, which are more rapidly absorbed and burned as energy than are other fats.[144] For this reason, athletes have been interested in their use, especially during prolonged endurance exercise. However, no effect on carbohydrate sparing or endurance exercise performance has been shown with moderate amounts of MCT (30 to 45 grams over 2 to 3 hours).[145,146] Trials using very large amounts (approximately 85 grams over 2 hours) have resulted in both increased[147] and decreased performance.[148]

Wheat germ oil, which contains a waxy substance known as **octacosanol** (p. 318), was investigated long ago as an ergogenic agent. These preliminary studies suggested that octacosanol had promising effects on endurance, reaction time, and other measures of exercise capacity.[149] In a more recent controlled trial, 1 mg per day of octacosanol for 8 weeks was found to improve grip strength and visual reaction time, but it had no effect on chest strength, auditory reaction time, or endurance.[150]

HMB (beta hydroxy-beta-methylbutyrate) (p. 301) is a metabolite of **leucine** (p. 274), one of the essential **branched-chain amino acids** (p. 274). As with other amino acid-related substances, HMB appears to play a role in the synthesis of protein, including the protein that builds new muscle tissue. Animal research suggests that HMB may improve the growth of lean muscle tissue,[151] but only preliminary and limited research in humans supports the potential link between HMB and enhanced muscle building in athletes.[152] One study of twenty-eight individuals involved in a weight-lifting program reported that supplements of 3 grams of HMB, compared with no supplementation, contributed to greater gains of muscle in 7 weeks.[153]

The use of alkalinizing agents, such as bicarbonate, citrate, and phosphate, to enhance athletic performance is designed to neutralize the acids produced during exercise that may interfere with energy production or muscle contraction.[154] Placebo-controlled studies have found that sodium bicarbonate typically improves exercise performance for events lasting 1 to 7 minutes when at least 135 mg per pound of body weight is used.[155] This amount is taken either as a single ingestion at least 1 hour before exercise or divided into smaller amounts taken over several hours before exercise. Similar results have been reported for sodium citrate ingestion at 225 mg per pound of body weight in placebo-controlled studies demonstrating improved performance of exercise of short to intermediate duration.[156,157,158,159] However, performance during periods less than 1 minute[160,161,162] or greater than 7 minutes is not improved by taking alkalinizing agents.[163,164] Sodium citrate may be preferable to sodium bicarbonate because it causes less gastrointestinal upset.[165] Another alkalinizing agent, phosphate, has been investigated primarily as an endurance performance enhancer, with very inconsistent results.[166,167]

Inosine is a purine-like substance that appears in exercising muscle tissue. Its role in various cellular reactions has led to suggestions that it may have ergogenic effects.[168] However, two placebo-controlled studies demonstrated no beneficial effects on performance and suggested that inosine may impair some aspects of exercise performance.[169,170] Therefore, use of inosine is discouraged.

Caffeine is present in many popular beverages and appears to have an effect on fat utilization.[171] Caffeine does not benefit short-term, high-intensity exercise, according to most,[172,173] but not all, studies.[174,175] However, placebo-controlled research, much of it double blind, has shown that *endurance* performance does appear to be enhanced by caffeine in many athletes.[176,177,178,179] Inconsistency in reported effectiveness of caffeine in some trials can been explained by differences in caffeine sensitivity among athletes, variable effect of caffeine on different forms of exercise and under different environmental conditions, and effects of other dietary components on the response to caffeine.[180,181] Effective amounts of caffeine appear to be about 2.5 mg per pound of body weight, which would require 2–3 cups brewed coffee or the equivalent taken 1 hour before exercise. However, most research has used caffeine supplements in capsules, and a recent study found caffeine was not effective when taken as coffee.[182] Caffeine consumption is banned by the International Olympic Committee at levels that produce urinary concentrations of 12 mg/ml or more. These levels would require ingestion of considerably more than 2.5 mg per pound of body weight, or several cups of coffee over a short period of time.[183]

Androstenedione (p. 266) is an androgen hormone. It is produced in the adrenal glands and gonads from dehyroepiandrosterone (**DHEA** [p. 288]) or 17 alpha-hydroxyprogesterone and is converted to testosterone by several tissues, including muscle. One study reported that 100 mg of androstenedione raised testosterone levels in women to six times the normal range and was significantly more effective in this than a similar amount of DHEA.[184] A German patent claims that oral androstenedione briefly raises blood levels of testosterone in men,[185] but no published data are available to corroborate this. Despite interest by some athletes, no studies have investigated the effects of androstenedione on body composition or athletic performance.

Are There Any Side Effects or Interactions? Refer to the individual supplement for information about any side effects or interactions.

Herbs That May Be Helpful

Extensive but often poorly executed studies have been conducted on the use of **Asian ginseng** (p. 394) *(Panax ginseng)* to improve athletic performance.[186] Some of these studies have reported that Asian ginseng is beneficial[187] while others have not.[188] One study also found that an extract of the related plant, **American ginseng** *(Panax quinquefolium)* (p. 392), was not effective at improving exercise performance in untrained people after 1 week's supplementation.[189] Despite a lack of consistent evidence, some doctors of natural medicine recommend taking extracts containing 5% ginsenosides at a level of 150–200 mg 3 times per day for at least several weeks.

Siberian ginseng or **eleuthero** (p. 419) *(Eleutherococcus senticosus)* has also been investigated as an herb that may improve athletic performance. Research from Russia indicates it may be effective for this purpose.[190] Other studies have been inconclusive[191] or have shown no beneficial effect.[192] Although many doctors of natural medicine suggest taking 1–4 ml (¼–½ teaspoon) of fluid extract of eleuthero 3 times per day, supportive evidence remains weak.

Some athletes take **guaraná** (p. 431) during their training; however, there is no scientific research to support this use. Guaraná contains caffeine, which is discussed above.

Are There Any Side Effects or Interactions? Refer to the individual herb for information about any side effects or interactions.

ADHD

Checklist for Athletic Performance

Ranking	Nutritional Supplements	Herbs
Primary	Citrate (for high-intensity, short-intermediate duration exercise) Iron (p. 304) (for iron-deficiency anemia [p. 107] only) Sodium bicarbonate (for high-intensity, short-intermediate duration exercise) Vitamin C (p. 341) (for deficiency only)	
Secondary	Creatine monohydrate (p. 285) Electrolyte replacement (for ultra-endurance competition only) Glutamine (p. 300) (for reducing risk of post-exercise infection) Multiple vitamin-mineral (p. 314) (for deficiency prevention in weight-conscious athletes only) Vitamin C (p. 341) (for exercise recovery) Vitamin E (p. 344) (for exercise recovery and high-altitude exercise performance only)	American ginseng (p. 392) Asian ginseng (p. 394) Eleuthero (p. 419) (Siberian ginseng)
Other	Arginine (p. 268)/ Ornithine (p. 318) (for body composition and strength) B-complex (p. 341) (B_2 [p. 338] B_6 [p. 340] pantothenic acid [p. 340]) Branched-chain amino acids (BCAAs) (p. 274) (for high altitude and extreme temperature only) Chromium (p. 282) Carnitine (p. 279) (for ultra-endurance only) Coenzyme Q_{10} (p. 283) Ferulic acid, HMB (p. 301) (for strength and body composition)	Guaraná (p. 431)

(continued)

Ranking	Nutritional Supplements	Herbs
Other	Magnesium (p. 310) Octacosanol (p. 318) Pyruvate (p. 328) Zinc (p. 346)	

See also: Homeopathic Remedies for **Athletic Performance** (p. 515)

Attention Deficit–Hyperactivity Disorder

Attention deficit–hyperactivity disorder (ADD or ADHD) is defined as age-inappropriate impulsiveness, lack of concentration, and sometimes excessive physical activity. ADD has been associated with learning difficulties and lack of social skills. Obviously what constitutes "normal" in these areas covers a wide spectrum, and thus it is unclear which child suffers true ADD and which child is just more rambunctious or rebellious than another. No objective criteria exists to accurately confirm the presence of ADD.

The main drug treatment for ADD, Ritalin (methylphenidate), is similar to amphetamine drugs. Paradoxically, these drugs are stimulants in adults but most often have a calming effect in those with ADD. Nevertheless, some parents have expressed growing concern about treating their children with an amphetamine-like drug. A variety of natural approaches to this condition have been investigated as alternatives to drug therapy.

Lifestyle Changes That May Be Helpful

Smoking during pregnancy should be avoided, as it appears to increase the risk of giving birth to a child who develops ADD.[1]

Lead[2] and other heavy-metal exposures[3] have been linked to ADD. If other therapies do not seem to be helping a child with ADD, the possibility of heavy-metal exposure can be explored with a nutritionally oriented health practitioner.

Dietary Changes That May Be Helpful

The two most studied dietary approaches to ADD are the Feingold diet and a hypoallergenic diet (See also the **Allergies and Sensitivities** [p. 8] chapter). The Feingold diet was developed by Benjamin Feingold,

M.D., on the premise that salicylates (chemicals similar to aspirin that are found in a wide variety of foods) are an underlying cause of hyperactivity. In some studies, this hypothesis did not appear to hold up.[4] But in studies where markedly different levels of salicylates were investigated, a causative role for salicylates could be detected in some hyperactive children.[5] As many as 10–25% of children may be sensitive to salicylates.[6] Parents of ADD children can contact local Feingold Associations for more information about which foods and medicines contain salicylates.

The Feingold diet also eliminates synthetic additives, dyes, and chemicals, which are commonly added to processed foods. The yellow dye, tartrazine, has been specifically shown to provoke symptoms in controlled studies of ADD-affected children.[7] Again, not every child reacts, but enough do so that a trial avoidance may be worthwhile. The Feingold diet in any form is complex and requires help from an experienced healthcare professional.

In another study, twenty-six children diagnosed with ADD were put on a hypoallergenic diet, and the nine children who improved were then challenged with food additives. All nine showed an exacerbation of symptoms when given these additives.[8] Other studies have shown that eliminating individual allergenic foods and additives from the diet can help children with attention problems.[9,10]

Some parents believe that sugar may exacerbate ADD. One study found that avoiding sugar reduced aggressiveness and restlessness in hyperactive children.[11] Girls who restrict sugar have been reported to improve more than boys.[12] However, a study using large amounts of sugar and aspartame (Nutrasweet) found that negative actions were limited to a few children,[13] and most studies have not found sugar to stimulate hyperactivity except in rare cases.[14]

Nutritional Supplements That May Be Helpful

A deficiency of several essential fatty acids has been observed in some children with ADD compared with unaffected children.[15,16] One study gave children with ADD **evening primrose oil** (p. 292) in an attempt to correct the problem.[17] Although a degree of benefit was seen, results were not promising.

B vitamins (p. 340), particularly **vitamin B**$_6$ (p. 340), have also been used for ADD. Low levels of vitamin B$_6$ have been detected in some children with ADD.[18] A study of six children with low vitamin B$_6$ levels found that vitamin B6 and Ritalin were both effective at reducing symptoms, while only vitamin B$_6$ corrected the vitamin deficiency.[19] High doses of other B vitamins have shown mixed results in relieving

ADD symptoms.[20,21] A practitioner knowledgeable in nutrition must be consulted when using high doses of vitamin B$_6$.

Some children with ADD have lowered levels of **magnesium** (p. 310). In a preliminary but controlled trial, fifty ADD children with low magnesium (as determined by red blood cell, hair, and serum levels of magnesium) were given 200 mg of magnesium per day for 6 months.[22] Compared with twenty-five other magnesium-deficient ADD children, those given magnesium supplementation had a significant decrease in hyperactive behavior.

Are There Any Side Effects or Interactions? Refer to the individual supplement for information about any side effects or interactions.

Checklist for Attention Deficit–Hyperactivity Disorder

Ranking	Nutritional Supplements	Herbs
Secondary	Magnesium (p. 310)	
Other	B vitamins (p. 341) (vitamin B$_6$ [p. 340]) Evening primrose oil (p. 292)	

Autism

Autism is a severe psychiatric disorder that begins in childhood. Autistic individuals generally have only weak contact with reality.

Dietary Changes That May Be Helpful

Preliminary research suggests that some autistic children may be **allergic** (p. 8) or sensitive to certain foods, and that removal of these foods from the diet has appeared to improve some behaviors.[1] As a result, one prominent nutritionally oriented doctor has recommended a trial hypoallergenic diet.[2] Such a trial requires supervision by a nutritionally oriented doctor.

Nutritional Supplements That May Be Helpful

Vitamin B$_6$ (p. 340) has helped normalize the function of nerve cells in autistic children.[3] Uncontrolled and double-blind research shows that vitamin B$_6$ can be helpful for autistic children.[4,5] In these trials, children typically took between 3.5 mg and almost 100 mg of B$_6$ for every 2.2 pounds of body weight, with some researchers recommending 30 mg per 2.2 pounds of body weight. Although toxicity was not reported, such amounts are widely considered to have potential toxicity that can damage the nervous system, and should only be administered by a nutritionally oriented doctor. One prominent researcher has suggested that vitamin B$_6$ is better supported by research than is drug treatment in dealing with autism.[6]

Some researchers have added **magnesium** (p. 310) to vitamin B6, reporting that taking both nutrients may have better effects than taking B$_6$ alone.[7] The amount of magnesium—10–15 mg per 2.2 pounds of body weight—is high enough to cause diarrhea in some people and should be administered by a nutritionally oriented doctor. Doctors of natural medicine will often try vitamin B$_6$ or the combination of B$_6$ and magnesium for at least 3 months to see if these nutrients help autistic children.

In one double-blind trial lasting 10 weeks, autistic children given 1 gram **vitamin C** (p. 341) for each 20 pounds of body weight showed a reduction in symptom severity compared with placebo.[8] The authors speculate that vitamin C may play a positive role because of it known effects on a hormone pathway typically disturbed in children with autism.

Are There Any Side Effects or Interactions? Refer to the individual supplement for information about any side effects or interactions.

Checklist for Autism

Ranking	Nutritional Supplements	Herbs
Primary	Vitamin B$_6$ (p. 340)	
Secondary	Vitamin C (p. 341)	
Other	Magnesium (p. 310)	

Brittle Nails

The common condition of brittle nails is often not definitively linked with any known cause. Nonetheless, natural medicine may be able to help strengthen brittle nails.

Most conditions that affect nails are unrelated to nutrition; instead they are caused by a lack of oxygen associated with lung conditions, hemorrhage due to infection, or inflammation around the nail due to infection. If there is any question about what the problem is, it is important to get a diagnosis from a health-care practitioner.

Nutritional Supplements That May Be Helpful

Nutrition can affect the health of nails in a variety of ways. **Iron** (p. 304) deficiency can cause spoon-shaped nails.[1] For years, some doctors of natural medicine have believed that **zinc** (p. 346) deficiency can cause white spots to appear on nails.[2] In China, excessive **selenium** (p. 331) has been linked to nails actually falling out.[3]

Biotin (p. 272), a B vitamin, is known to strengthen hooves in animals. As a result, Swiss researchers investigated the use of biotin in strengthening brittle fingernails in humans, despite the fact that it remains unclear exactly how biotin affects nail structure.[4] Using 2.5 mg of biotin per day, women with brittle nails who had nail thickness measured before and after 6 to 15 months, found their nail thickness increased by 25%. As a result, splitting of nails was reduced. In a follow-up study of people who had been taking biotin for brittle nails in America, 63% showed improvement from taking biotin.[5] Although the amount of research on the subject is quite limited and positive effects do not appear in all people, people with brittle nails may want to consider a trial period of at least several months using 2.5 mg per day of biotin.

Are There Any Side Effects or Interactions? Refer to the individual supplement for information about any side effects or interactions.

Herbs That May Be Helpful

Anecdotal reports suggest that **horsetail** (p. 436) may be of some use in the treatment of brittle nails.

Are There Any Side Effects or Interactions? Refer to the individual herb for information about any side effects or interactions.

Checklist for Brittle Nails

Ranking	Nutritional Supplements	Herbs
Secondary	Biotin (p. 272)	
Other		Horsetail (p. 436)

Bruising

With sufficient trauma, anyone will suffer a bruise; this is both natural and often unavoidable. It is only when bruising occurs often and from very minor (often unnoticed) trauma that a problem may exist.

Refer to the **capillary fragility** (p. 32) chapter for more information. One cause of easy bruising—leukemia—can usually be ruled out by any doctor with a simple blood test. More often, no clear cause for easy bruising is found.

Dietary Changes That May Be Helpful

Many Americans eat insufficient amounts of foods containing **vitamin C** (p. 341); the disease caused by vitamin C deficiency, scurvy, causes easy bruising. While very few people actually have scurvy, even minor deficiencies of vitamin C can increase bruising. People who experience easy bruising may want to try eating more fruits and vegetables—common dietary sources of vitamin C. The diet can be assessed by nutritionally oriented doctors by using a diet diary, sometimes accompanied by computerized diet analysis. A diet diary is a written record of what and how much a person is eating, usually divided into sections by meal and/or by day. As used by nutritionally oriented doctors, diet diaries lasting one week are most common. If such an analysis reveals a lack of dietary vitamin C and **bioflavonoids** (p. 271) (related compounds), the diet requires more fruits and vegetables to correct the problem.

Nutritional Supplements That May Be Helpful

Doctors of natural medicine will often suggest that people who experience easy bruising supplement with 1–3 grams of **vitamin C** (p. 341) per day for several months. This is usually accompanied by at least several hundred milligrams of **bioflavonoids** (p. 271)—vitamin-like substances that are needed to strengthen capillaries and therefore might also help with bruising.[1] If the vitamin C/bioflavonoid combination is helpful, it strongly suggests that the person's diet was inadequate.

Are There Any Side Effects or Interactions? Refer to the individual supplement for information about any side effects or interactions.

Herbs That May Be Helpful

Aescin, a compound found in **horse chestnut** (p. 435), has been used effectively as a gel applied at least twice daily to treat bruises.[2] Although aescin gel is not readily available, oral preparations of horse chestnut seed extract have recently appeared in health-food stores and some pharmacies. An appropriate amount of horse chestnut seed extract standardized for aescin

content (16–21%) taken orally is likely to provide 50–75 mg of aescin twice per day.

In traditional herbal medicine, a compress or ointment of sweet clover (*Melilotus officinalis*) is applied to bruises.[3,4] Enough should be applied to cover the bruise, and several applications per day may be necessary to improve healing.

Comfrey (p. 413) has a long, consistent history of use as a topical agent for improving healing of wounds, skin ulcers, thrombophlebitis, strains, and sprains.[5,6]

Are There Any Side Effects or Interactions? Refer to the individual herb for information about any side effects or interactions.

Checklist for Bruising

Ranking	Nutritional Supplements	Herbs
Primary	Vitamin C (p. 341) (only if deficiency)	
Secondary	Bioflavonoids (p. 271)	Horse chestnut (p. 435)
Other		Comfrey (p. 413) Sweet clover
See also: Homeopathic Remedies for **Bruising** (p. 520)		

Burns, Minor

Extensive burns or burns causing more than minor discomfort should be treated by a health-care professional. For superficial burns caused by temperature (picking up a hot object, for example), natural medicine may be helpful after the burn is cleaned with soap and cold water and gently dried.

Nutritional Supplements That May Be Helpful

Despite a lack of research on the subject, many doctors of natural medicine recommend using **vitamin E** (p. 344) topically on minor burns. This makes sense, because some of the damage done to the skin is oxidative, and vitamin E is an **antioxidant** (p. 267).

Vitamin E can be found in both the tocopherol and tocopheryl forms. In the tocopheryl forms (such as alpha tocopheryl acetate), the vitamin E is attached to another molecule (like acetate) to keep the vitamin E protected. While the body has no problem separating vitamin E from the other molecule when swallowed, it remains unknown whether the skin can free vitamin E in the same way. Therefore, people using vitamin E topically on minor burns should use the tocopherol form, which is immediately usable by the skin.

Are There Any Side Effects or Interactions? Refer to the individual supplement for information about any side effects or interactions.

Herbs That May Be Helpful

Aloe (p. 391) has been historically used for many of the same conditions it is used for today, particularly minor burns. Topically for minor burns, the stabilized aloe gel is applied to the affected area of skin 3 to 5 times per day. Treatment of more serious burns should only be done after first consulting a health-care professional.

Calendula (p. 406) cream can be applied to minor burns to soothe pain and help promote tissue repair. It has been shown in animal studies to be anti-inflammatory[1] and to aid repair of damaged tissues.[2] The cream is applied 3 times per day.

Gotu kola (p. 430) has been used in the medicinal systems of central Asia for centuries to treat numerous skin diseases. Saponins in gotu kola beneficially affect collagen (the material that makes up connective tissue) to inhibit its production in hyperactive scar tissue. Dried gotu kola leaf can be made into a tea by adding 1–2 teaspoons to 150 ml boiling water and allowing it to steep for 10 to 15 minutes. Three cups are usually drunk per day. Tincture can also be used at a dose of 10–20 ml 3 times per day. Standardized extracts containing up to 100% total triterpenoids are generally taken in the amount of 60 mg once or twice per day.

Are There Any Side Effects or Interactions? Refer to the individual herb for information about any side effects or interactions.

Checklist for Minor Burns

Ranking	Nutritional Supplements	Herbs
Secondary		Aloe (p. 391)
Other	Vitamin E (p. 344)	Calendula (p. 406) Gotu kola (p. 430)
See also: Homeopathic Remedies for **Minor Burns** (p. 521)		

Bursitis

Bursitis is an inflammation of fluid-filled sacs (bursa) that the body situates in places where movement would otherwise cause friction. The most common

bursa to become inflamed is in the shoulder. The cause of bursitis is mostly unknown, but trauma or arthritis may be involved.

Nutritional Supplements That May Be Helpful

Intramuscular or deep subcutaneous injections of **vitamin B_{12}** (p. 337)[1] or the combination of B_{12} and B_3 (p. 339) in niacin form[2] have not only relieved symptoms but have also decreased calcifications in chronically inflamed bursae. The mechanism is not understood. Oral B vitamins are unlikely to have the same effect because absorption of vitamin B_{12} is quite limited. A nutritionally oriented doctor should be consulted regarding B_{12} or B_{12}/niacin injections.

Are There Any Side Effects or Interactions? Refer to the individual supplement for information about any side effects or interactions.

Herbs That May Be Helpful

While there have been few studies on herbal therapy for bursitis, most practitioners of natural medicine would consider using anti-inflammatory herbs that have proven useful in conditions such as rheumatoid arthritis. These would include **boswellia** (p. 403), **turmeric** (p. 465), **white willow** (p. 468), and topical **cayenne** (p. 408) ointment. Refer to **rheumatoid arthritis** (p. 571) for specific recommendations for these herbs.

Are There Any Side Effects or Interactions? Refer to the individual herb for information about any side effects or interactions.

Checklist for Bursitis

Ranking	Nutritional Supplements	Herbs
Secondary	Vitamin B_{12} (p. 337)	
Other	Vitamin B_3 (p. 339)	Boswellia (p. 403) Cayenne (p. 408) Turmeric (p. 465) White willow (p. 468)
See also: Homeopathic Remedies for **Bursitis** (p. 522)		

Canker Sores (Mouth Ulcers)

Mouth ulcers, or canker sores, are small ulcerations within the mouth. Doctors call this common condition aphthous stomatitis.

Lifestyle Changes That May Be Helpful

Minor trauma from poor-fitting dentures, rough fillings, or braces can aggravate mouth ulcers and should be remedied by a dentist.

Several reports have incriminated sodium lauryl sulfate (SLS), a component of some toothpastes, as a potential cause of canker sores.[1] In one trial, *most* recurrent canker sores were eliminated just by avoiding SLS-containing toothpaste for 3 months.[2] Positive effects of eliminating SLS have been confirmed in double-blind research.[3] SLS is thought to increase the risk of canker sores by removing a protective coating (mucin) in the mouth. People with recurrent canker sores should use an SLS-free toothpaste for several months to see if such a change helps.

Dietary Changes That May Be Helpful

Food sensitivities (p. 8) or allergies (p. 8) can make mouth ulcers worse.[4,5,6] While a double-blind study found that allergies play only a minor role,[7] people with recurrent mouth ulcers should discuss the diagnosis and treatment of food sensitivities with a nutritionally oriented doctor. For some people, treating allergies may be a key component to restoring health.

Nutritional Supplements That May Be Helpful

Several reports have found a surprisingly high incidence of iron (p. 304) and B vitamin (p. 341) deficiency among people with recurrent mouth ulcers.[8,9,10] Supplementing with B vitamins—300 mg vitamin B_1 (p. 337), 20 mg vitamin B_2 (p. 338), and 150 mg vitamin B_6 (p.340)—has been reported to provide some people with relief.[11] Thiamine (B_1) deficiency specifically has been linked to an increased risk.[12] The right supplemental level of iron requires diagnosis of an iron deficiency by a health-care professional using lab tests.

Some people with recurrent mouth ulcers have been reported to respond to lactobacillus acidophilus (p. 325)[13] and lactobacillus bulgaricus.[14] Chewing four lactobacillus tablets 3 times per day may reduce soreness in some people with recurrent mouth ulcers.[15]

Are There Any Side Effects or Interactions? Refer to the individual supplement for information about any side effects or interactions.

Herbs That May Be Helpful

Licorice (p. 440) that has had the glycyrrhizic acid removed is called deglycyrrhizinated licorice (DGL). Glycyrrhizic acid is the portion of licorice root that can increase blood pressure and cause water retention in some people. The wound-healing and soothing components of the root remain in DGL.

A mixture of DGL and warm water applied to the inside of the mouth may shorten the healing time for mouth ulcers.[16] This DGL mixture is made by combining 200 mg of powdered DGL and 200 ml of warm water. It can then be swished in the mouth for 2 to 3 minutes and then spit out. This can be continued each morning and evening for 1 week.

The antiviral, immune-enhancing, and wound-healing properties of echinacea (p. 417) make this herb a reasonable choice for mouth ulcers. Liquid echinacea in the amount of 4 ml can be swished in the mouth for 2 to 3 minutes, then swallowed. This can be repeated 3 times per day. Tablets and capsules containing echinacea may also be helpful.

Because of its soothing effect on mucous membranes (including the lining of the mouth) and healing properties, chamomile (p. 409) can be tried for mouth ulcers and other mouth irritations.[17] A strong tea made from chamomile tincture can be swished in the mouth 3 to 4 times per day.

An extract from aloe vera (p. 391) has been shown to be beneficial in one preliminary study.[18] Some doctors of natural medicine recommend 1 to 3 tablespoons of aloe vera juice be used as a mouthwash then swallowed 3 times daily.

Myrrh (p. 446), another traditional remedy with good wound-healing properties, has a long history of use for mouth and gum irritations. Some herbalists suggest mixing 200 to 300 mg of herbal extract or 4 ml of myrrh tincture with warm water and swishing it in the mouth 2 to 3 times per day.

Are There Any Side Effects or Interactions? Refer to the individual herb for information about any side effects or interactions.

Checklist for Canker Sores (Mouth Ulcers)

Ranking	Nutritional Supplements	Herbs
Secondary	B-complex (p. 341) (B_1 [p. 337] B_2 [p. 338] B_6 [p. 340]) Acidophilus (p. 325)	Aloe vera (p. 391) Licorice (DGL) (p. 440)
Other	Iron (p. 304)	Chamomile (p. 409) Echinacea (p. 417) Myrrh (p. 446)

See also: Homeopathic Remedies for **Canker Sores** (p. 523)

Capillary Fragility

When the smallest blood vessels, capillaries, become weak, a person is said to have capillary fragility. This leads to small spots of bleeding in the skin and easy bruising. Refer to the **bruising** (p. 28) chapter for more information. There are no serious complications from having capillary fragility, but it may signify that a more serious, underlying problem exists. Therefore, individuals should consult a physician if there is bleeding in the skin.

Dietary Changes That May Be Helpful

Eating plenty of fruits and vegetables will provide more of the nutrients mentioned in the following chapter that support the structure of capillaries.

Nutritional Supplements That May Be Helpful

People undergoing dialysis may develop low levels of **vitamin C** (p. 341), which leads to capillary fragility.[1] As little as 100 mg per day may help people with artificially induced fragility. For others, higher amounts may be necessary (1 gram or more).[2] Vitamin C has been used to treat capillary weakness accompanying **diabetes** (p. 53).[3]

Widespread plant compounds called **bioflavonoids** (p. 271) help strengthen weakened capillaries. In test tube and animal studies, they have been shown to protect collagen, one of the most important components of capillary walls.[4,5] Use of bioflavonoids, particularly **quercetin** (p. 328), rutin, and hesperidin, with vitamin C is sometimes recommended for capillary fragility.[6] Doctors of natural medicine often recommend 400 mg of rutin or quercetin 3 times per day or 1 gram of citrus flavonoids 3 times per day.

Are There Any Side Effects or Interactions? Refer to the individual supplement for information about any side effects or interactions.

Checklist for Capillary Fragility

Ranking	Nutritional Supplements	Herbs
Primary	Bioflavonoids (p. 271) (quercetin [p. 328], rutin, hesperidin) Vitamin C (p. 341)	

Cardiovascular Disease Overview

Cardiovascular disease is the number one cause of death in the United States. This introductory chapter briefly discusses several diseases that have a role in the development of cardiovascular disease. Refer to these chapters for further information: **angina** (p. 13), **atherosclerosis** (p. 17), **high cholesterol** (p. 79), **high homocysteine** (p. 84), **high triglycerides** (p. 85), and **hypertension** (p. 89).

Many risk factors are associated with cardiovascular disease; most can be managed, but some cannot. The aging process and hereditary predisposition are risk factors that cannot be altered. Until age 50, men are at greater risk than women of developing heart disease, though once a woman enters menopause, her risk triples.[1]

Many people with cardiovascular disease have elevated cholesterol levels.[2] Low-HDL cholesterol (known as the "good" cholesterol) and high-LDL cholesterol (known as the "bad" cholesterol) are more specifically linked to cardiovascular disease than is total cholesterol.[3] A blood test, administered by most health-care professionals, is used to determine cholesterol levels. Read the **high cholesterol** (p. 79) chapter for information about how to lower cholesterol levels using dietary modification, nutritional supplements, and herbs.

Atherosclerosis (p. 17) (hardening of the arteries) of the vessels that supply the heart with blood is the most common cause of heart attacks. Atherosclerosis and high cholesterol usually occur together, though cholesterol levels can change quickly and atherosclerosis generally takes decades to develop. Read the **atherosclerosis** (p. 17) chapter for information about preventing atherosclerosis with dietary, lifestyle, and other changes.

The link between **high triglyceride** (p. 85) levels and heart disease is less well established than the link between high cholesterol and heart disease. According to some studies, a high triglyceride level is an independent risk factor for heart disease in some people.[4] See **high triglycerides** (p. 85) for information about how to lower triglyceride levels with dietary and other means.

High homocysteine (p. 84) levels have been identified as an independent risk factor for coronary heart disease.[5] Homocysteine can be measured by a blood test that must be ordered by a health-care professional. Read the **homocysteine** (p. 84) chapter for information about lowering homocysteine levels with nutritional supplements.

Hypertension (p. 89) (high blood pressure) is a major risk factor for cardiovascular disease, and the risk increases as blood pressure rises.[6] Glucose intolerance and **diabetes** (p. 53) constitute a separate risk factor for heart disease. Smoking potentiates the risk of heart disease caused by hypertension.

Abdominal fat or a "beer belly," versus fat that accumulates on the hips, is associated with increased risk of cardiovascular disease and heart attack.[7] Overweight individuals are more likely to have additional risk factors related to heart disease, specifically **hypertension** (p. 89), high blood sugar levels, **high cholesterol** (p. 79), **high triglycerides** (p. 85), and **diabetes** (p. 53).

Both smoking[8] and exposure to second-hand smoke[9] increase cardiovascular disease risk. Moderate alcohol consumption appears protective for coronary heart disease,[10] and moderate exercise protects both lean and obese individuals from cardiovascular disease.[11] A diet high in fruits and vegetables,[12] fiber,[13] and possibly fish[14] appears protective against heart disease, while high intake of saturated fat (found in meat and dairy fat) and trans fatty acids (in margarine and processed foods containing hydrogenated vegetable oils)[15] may contribute to heart disease. For more information on these topics, see the diet and lifestyle chapters in the **atherosclerosis** (p. 17) chapter.

Carpal Tunnel Syndrome

In many cases, carpal tunnel syndrome (CTS) is thought to result from long-term repetitive motions of the hands and wrists, such as from computer use. Although repetitive motion is often a culprit, it does not explain the frequent occurrence of CTS with non-motion-related conditions, such as pregnancy. Conventional treatment includes splinting, rest, anti-inflammatory drugs, or surgery.

Nutritional Supplements That May Be Helpful

Vitamin B_6 (p. 340) is needed for normal function of nerve cells and is the most frequently used and well-known nutritional treatment for CTS. It has been reported that people with CTS are frequently deficient in vitamin B_6.[1] Direct links between lower levels of vitamin B_6 and increased symptoms have been reported in men not taking B_6 supplements.[2] However, some trials have not found a link between CTS and vitamin B_6 deficiency.[3,4]

Several studies report that people with CTS are helped when given 100 mg of vitamin B6 three times per day.[5,6] Although some researchers have found benefits with lesser amounts,[7,8,9,10] using *less* than 100 mg taken 3 times per day for several months has often failed.[11,12,13] Most nutritionally oriented doctors assume that people with CTS who respond to vitamin B_6 supplementation do so because of an underlying deficiency, as discussed in the previous paragraph. However, at least one group of researchers has found vitamin B_6 to "dramatically" reduce pain in people with CTS who did not appear to be B_6 deficient.[14] Moreover, some nutritionally oriented doctors believe that B_6 is therapeutic because it reduces swelling around the carpal tunnel in the wrist; this theory remains completely undocumented. Thus, although vitamin B_6 appears useful for people with CTS when the full 100 mg is given 3 times per day for several months, details of how it helps remain unclear.

Checklist for Carpal Tunnel Syndrome

Ranking	Nutritional Supplements	Herbs
Secondary	Vitamin B_6 (p. 340)	
See also: Homeopathic Remedies for **Carpal Tunnel Syndrome** (p. 524)		

At very high levels vitamin B_6 can damage sensory nerves, leading to numbness in the hands and feet as well as difficulty walking; supplementation should be stopped if these symptoms develop. Vitamin B_6 is usually safe in amounts of 200–500 mg per day,[15] although occasional problems have been reported in this range.[16] Higher amounts are clearly toxic.[17] Any adult taking more than 100–200 mg of vitamin B_6 per day for more than a few months should consult a doctor.

In order to be effective, vitamin B_6 must be transformed in the body to pyridoxal-5¹-phosphate (PLP). Some doctors of natural medicine have suggested that people who do not respond well to vitamin B_6 supplements should try 50 mg of PLP 3 times per day. As yet there is no clear evidence that using PLP provides any advantage in reducing symptoms of CTS.

Cataracts

Are There Any Side Effects or Interactions? Refer to the individual supplement for information about any side effects or interactions.

Cataracts

Cataracts develop when damage to the protein of the lens of the eye clouds the lens and impairs vision.

Most people who live long enough will develop cataracts.[1] Cataracts are more likely to occur in those who smoke, have **diabetes** (p. 53), or are exposed to excessive sunlight. All of these factors lead to *oxidative* damage. Oxidative damage to the lens of the eye appears to cause cataracts in animals[2] and people.[3]

It is unlikely that any nutritional supplements of herbs can reverse existing cataracts, although no research has explored this possibility.

Nutritional Supplements That May Be Helpful

People with low blood levels of **antioxidants** (p. 267) and those who eat few antioxidant-rich fruits and vegetables have been reported to be at high risk for cataracts.[4,5]

The major antioxidants in the lens of the eye are **vitamin C** (p. 341)[6] and glutathione (an antioxidant enzyme).[7] Vitamin C is needed to activate **vitamin E** (p. 344),[8] which in turn activates glutathione. Both nutrients are important for healthy vision.

Vitamin C (p. 341) levels in the eye decrease with age;[9] however, supplementing with vitamin C prevents this decrease[10] and has been linked to a lower risk of developing cataracts.[11,12] Healthy people have been reported to be more likely to take vitamin C and vitamin E supplements than those with cataracts in some[13] but not all studies.[14] Nonetheless, because people who supplement with vitamin C have developed far fewer cataracts in some research,[15,16] nutritionally oriented doctors often recommend 500–1,000 mg of vitamin C supplementation as part of a cataract prevention program. The difference between successful and unsuccessful trials may be tied to the length of time people actually supplement vitamin C. In one trial, people taking vitamin C for at least 10 years showed a dramatic reduction in cataract risk, but those taking vitamin C for less than 10 years showed no evidence of protection at all.[17]

Low blood levels of **vitamin E** (p. 344) have been linked to 3.7 times the risk of forming cataracts compared with people in the highest 20% of blood vitamin E levels.[18] Vitamin E supplements have been reported to protect against cataracts in animals[19] and people,[20] though the evidence remains inconsistent.[21] In one trial, people who took vitamin E supplements had less than half the risk of developing cataracts compared with others in the 5-year study.[22] Nutritionally oriented doctors typically recommend 400 IU of vitamin E per day as prevention. Smaller amounts (approximately 50 IU per day) have been proven in double-blind research to provide no protection.[23]

Some studies have reported that eating more foods rich in **beta-carotene** (p. 268) or supplementing with **vitamin A** (p. 336) lowers the risk of cataracts.[24] Synthetic beta-carotene supplementation has not been found to reduce the risk of cataract formation.[25] It remains unclear whether natural beta-carotene from food or supplements would protect the eye or whether beta-carotene in food is merely a marker for other protective factors in fruit and vegetables high in beta-carotene.

People who eat a lot of spinach, which is high in **lutein** (p. 308), a nutrient similar to beta-carotene, have been reported to be at low risk for cataracts.[26] Both lutein and beta-carotene offer the promise of protection because they are antioxidants. It is quite possible, however, that lutein is more important than beta-carotene because lutein is found in the lens of the eye while beta-carotene is not.[27]

Vitamin B$_2$ (p. 338) and **vitamin B$_3$** (p. 339) are needed to protect glutathione, an important antioxidant in the eye. Vitamin B$_2$ deficiency has been linked to cataracts.[28,29] Older people taking 3 mg of vitamin B$_2$ and 40 mg of vitamin B$_3$ per day were partly protected against cataracts in a Chinese trial.[30] Most researchers in the field do not believe that higher amounts would be helpful, and it remains unclear whether these vitamins would help protect people in societies that eat higher levels of B vitamins than do the Chinese, whose intake appears to be low.

The flavonoid **quercetin** (p. 328) may also help by blocking sorbitol accumulation in the eye.[31] This may be especially helpful for people with **diabetes** (p. 53), though no clinical trials have yet explored whether quercetin actually prevents diabetic cataracts.

Are There Any Side Effects or Interactions? Refer to the individual supplement for information about any side effects or interactions.

Herbs That May Be Helpful

Bilberry (p. 396), a close relative of blueberry, is high in the **bioflavonoid** (p. 271) complex anthocyanosides.[32] Anthocyanosides protect both the lens and the retina from oxidative damage. This bioflavonoid also helps with adaptation to bright light and improves night vision. The potent antioxidant activity of anthocyanosides appears to make bilberry useful for reducing the risk of cataracts.[33][34]

Doctors well versed in the use of herbs sometimes recommend 240–480 mg per day of bilberry extract, capsules, or tablets standardized to contain 25% anthocyanosides.

Are There Any Side Effects or Interactions? Refer to the individual herb for information about any side effects or interactions.

Checklist for Cataracts

Ranking	Nutritional Supplements	Herbs
Secondary	B-Complex (p. 341) (B_2 [p. 338], B_3 [p. 339]) Vitamin C (p. 341)	
Other	Beta-Carotene (p. 268) Lutein (p. 308) Quercetin (p. 328) Vitamin A (p. 336) Vitamin E (p. 344)	Bilberry (p. 396)
See also: Homeopathic Remedies for **Cataracts** (p. 524)		

Celiac Disease

Celiac disease (also called gluten-induced enteropathy) is an intestinal disorder that results from intolerance to gluten, a protein found in wheat, oats, barley, and rye. Individuals with celiac disease typically have cramping, abdominal pain, diarrhea, and bloating. Microscopic examination of the small-intestinal lining reveals severe damage, especially in the jejunum. Individuals with untreated celiac disease may eventually experience malaise and weight loss and have an increased risk of developing **anemia** (p. 107), **osteoporosis** (p. 133), osteomalacia, and certain types of cancer. Neurological disorders and emotional problems may also complicate celiac disease in some cases.

Lifestyle Changes That May Be Helpful

In one study, children who were breast-fed for less than 30 days were 4 times more likely to develop celiac disease, compared with children who were breast-fed for more than 30 days.[1] Although this study does not prove that breast-feeding prevents the development of celiac disease, it is consistent with other research showing that breast-feeding promotes a healthier gastrointestinal tract than does formula-feeding.[2]

Dietary Changes That May Be Helpful

It is generally accepted that ingestion of gluten-containing grains (wheat, barley, and rye) is the primary cause of celiac disease. While **oats** (p. 448) contain a substance similar to gluten, modern research has found that eating moderate amounts of oats does not appear to cause problems for people with celiac disease.[3,4] In one of these reports, approximately 95% of people with celiac disease tolerated 50 grams of oats per day for up to 12 months.[5] Strict avoidance of wheat, barley, and rye usually results in an improvement in gastrointestinal symptoms within a few weeks, although in some cases the improvement may take many months. Tests of absorptive function usually improve after a few months on a gluten-free diet.[6]

Avoiding gluten may also influence cancer risk. In one trial, 210 individuals with celiac disease were observed for 11 years. Those who followed a gluten-free diet had an incidence of cancer similar to that in the general population. However, those who only reduced their gluten intake or consumed a normal diet had an increased risk of developing cancer (mainly lymphomas and cancers of the mouth, pharynx, and esophagus).[7]

Children with untreated celiac disease were found to have abnormally low bone mineral density. However, after approximately 1 year on a gluten-free diet, bone mineral density increased rapidly and approximated the level seen in healthy children.[8] Adults with celiac disease also had significantly lower bone mineral density than did healthy individuals. After consumption of a gluten-free diet for 1 year, bone mineral density of the hip and lumbar spine increased by an average of more than 15%.[9]

Infertility, which is common in individuals with celiac disease, has been reportedly reversed in both men and women after commencement of a gluten-free diet.[10]

Some individuals with celiac disease may be intolerant to other foods, in addition to gluten. Foods that have been reported to trigger symptoms include cow's milk[11] and soy.[12,13,14]

Nutritional Supplements That May Be Helpful

The malabsorption that occurs in celiac disease can lead to multiple nutritional deficiencies, some of which may be severe enough to cause illnesses such as anemia or bone disease. The most common nutritional deficiencies in people with celiac disease include essential fatty acids, **iron** (p. 304), **vitamin D** (p. 343), **vitamin K** (p. 345), **calcium** (p. 277), **magnesium** (p. 310), and **folic acid** (p. 297).[15] **Zinc** (p. 346) malabsorption also occurs frequently in celiac disease,[16] and may result in zinc deficiency, even in people who are otherwise in remission.[17] Individuals with newly diagnosed celiac disease should be treated for nutritional deficiencies by a nutritionally oriented doctor.

After commencement of a gluten-free diet, overall nutritional status gradually improves. However, deficiencies of some nutrients may persist, even in people who are strictly avoiding gluten. For example, magnesium deficiency was found in eight of twenty-three adults with celiac disease who had been following a gluten-free diet and were symptom-free. When these individuals were supplemented with magnesium for 2 years, their bone mineral density increased significantly.[18]

Checklist for Celiac Disease

Ranking	Nutritional Supplements	Herbs
Primary	Calcium (p. 277) (if deficient) Folic acid (p. 297) (if deficient) Iron (p. 304) (if deficient) Magnesium (p. 310) (if deficient) Multiple vitamin/ mineral (p. 314) Vitamin A (p. 336) (if deficient) Vitamin B₆ (p. 340) (if deficient) Vitamin D (p. 343) (if deficient) Vitamin K (p. 345) (if deficient) Zinc (p. 346) (if deficient)	
Secondary	Magnesium (p. 310) Vitamin A (p. 336) Vitamin B₆ (p. 340)	
Other	Lipase (p. 307)	

In another study, six people with diet-treated celiac disease had abnormal dark-adaptation tests (indicative of "night blindness"), even though some were taking a multivitamin that contained **vitamin A** (p. 336). Some of these people showed an improvement in dark adaptation after receiving larger amounts of vitamin A, either orally or by injection.[19]

In another trial, eleven people with celiac disease suffered from persistent **depression** (p. 50) despite being on a gluten-free diet for more than 2 years. However, after supplementation with **vitamin B₆** (p. 340) (80 mg per day) for 6 months, the depression disappeared.[20]

It is possible that subtle deficiencies of other nutrients may exist in people with celiac disease who are in remission on a gluten-free diet. Individuals who are not strictly avoiding gluten are likely to have more severe deficiencies. Because of the complexity of this condition and the multiple nutritional factors involved, people with celiac disease should be under the care of a nutritionally oriented doctor.

Are There Any Side Effects or Interactions? Refer to the individual supplement for information about any side effects or interactions.

Chronic Fatigue Syndrome

No single cause for chronic fatigue syndrome (CFS) has been identified; therefore, it is defined by symptoms and by eliminating other known causes of fatigue, which needs to be done by a health-care practitioner. Suggested causes include chronic viral infections, **food allergy** (p. 8), adrenal gland dysfunction, and many others. None of these have been convincingly documented in more than a minority of sufferers. The current definition is disabling fatigue lasting more than 6 months, reducing activity by more than half. In some people there is also difficulty sleeping, swollen lymph nodes, and/or mild fever. When there is muscle soreness, **fibromyalgia** (p. 68) may be the actual problem. Although CFS is considered a modern diagnosis, it may have existed for centuries under other names, such as "the vapors," neurasthenia, "effort syndrome" (diagnosed in World War I veterans), **hypoglycemia** (p. 92), and chronic mononucleosis.

Lifestyle Changes That May Be Helpful

Exercise is important to prevent the worsening of fatigue. Many people report feeling better after undertaking a moderate exercise plan.[12] If exercise seems to lead to consistently worsening fatigue, individuals should consult a physician before continuing. Highly stressful situations should be avoided; coping mechanisms for dealing with stress can sometimes be maximized by behavioral therapy.[3]

Dietary Changes That May Be Helpful

Some nutritionally oriented doctors believe that for people with CFS who have low blood pressure, salt should not be restricted. In CFS sufferers who have a form of low blood pressure triggered by changes in position (orthostatic hypotension), some have been reported to be helped by additional salt intake.[4] People with CFS considering increasing salt intake should consult a nutritionally oriented doctor before making such a change. See the section on herbs for more information on blood pressure and CFS.

Nutritional Supplements That May Be Helpful

The combination of potassium aspartate and magnesium aspartate has shown benefits for chronically fatigued people in several studies.[5,6] Usually 1 gram is taken twice per day. Results have been reported within 1 to 2 weeks.

Magnesium (p. 310) levels have been reported to be low in CFS sufferers.[7] In that double-blind trial, injections with magnesium improved symptoms for most people. Oral magnesium supplementation has also improved symptoms in those people with CFS who had low magnesium levels in another report, although magnesium injections were sometimes necessary.[8] These researchers report that magnesium deficiency appears to be very common in people with CFS. Nonetheless, several other researchers report no evidence of magnesium deficiency in people with CFS.[9,10,11] The reason for this discrepancy remains unclear. If people with CFS do consider magnesium supplementation, it makes sense to have magnesium status checked beforehand by a nutritionally oriented doctor. It appears that only people with magnesium deficiency benefit from this therapy.

Vitamin B$_{12}$ (p. 337) deficiency can cause fatigue. Occasionally, however, reports,[12] even double-blind,[13] have shown that people who are not deficient in B$_{12}$ nonetheless have increased energy following a series of vitamin B$_{12}$ injections. Some sources in conventional medicine have discouraged such people from getting B$_{12}$ shots despite evidence to the contrary.[14] However, some nutritionally oriented doctors have continued to take the limited scientific support for B$_{12}$ seriously.[15] In one unblind trial, 2,500–5,000 mcg of vitamin B$_{12}$ given by injection every two to three days, led to improvement in 50–80% of a group of people with CFS; most improvement appeared after several weeks of B$_{12}$ shots.[16] While the research in this area remains preliminary, people with CFS considering a trial of vitamin B$_{12}$ injections should consult a nutritionally oriented doctor. Oral or sublingual B$_{12}$ supplements are unlikely to obtain the same results as injectable B$_{12}$ because the body's ability to absorb large amounts is relatively poor.

Carnitine (p. 279) is required for energy production in the powerhouses of the cells (the mitochondria). There may be a problem in the mitochondria in people with CFS. Deficiency of carnitine has been seen in some CFS sufferers.[17] One gram of carnitine taken 3 times daily led to improvement in CFS symptoms in a recent preliminary investigation.[18]

NADH (p. 317) (nicotinamide adenine dinucleotide) helps make ATP, the energy source the body runs on. One study suggested that NADH may help people with chronic fatigue syndrome.[19] In the double-blind portion of that report, almost one-third of people with CFS showed evidence of significant improvement. Some nutritionally oriented doctors suggest amounts of at least 2.5 mg per day. However, research in this area remains preliminary.

Are There Any Side Effects or Interactions? Refer to the individual supplement for information about any side effects or interactions.

Checklist for Chronic Fatigue Syndrome

Ranking	Nutritional Supplements	Herbs
Secondary	Carnitine (p. 279) Potassium-magnesium asparate Vitamin B$_{12}$ (p. 337)	
Other	Magnesium (p. 310) NADH (p. 317)	Eleuthero (p. 419) Licorice (p. 440)

Herbs That May Be Helpful

Newer research suggests that CFS may be partially due to low adrenal function resulting from different stressors (for example, mental stress, physical stress, and even viral illness) impacting the normal communication between the hypothalamus, pituitary gland, and the adrenal glands.[20] **Licorice** (p. 440) root is known to stimulate the adrenal glands and to block the breakdown of active cortisol in the body. One case report found that taking 2.5 grams of licorice root daily led to a significant improvement in a man with CFS.[21] While there have been no large clinical trials to test licorice in people with CFS, it may be worth a trial of 6 to 8 weeks using 2–3 grams of licorice root daily.

Adaptogenic herbs such as **Asian ginseng** (p. 394) and **Eleuthero** (p. 419) may also be useful for people with CFS—they not only have an immunomodulating effect but also help support the normal function of the hypothalamic-pituitary-adrenal axis, the hormonal stress system of the body.[22] These herbs are useful follow-ups to the 6 to 8 weeks of licorice root and may be used for long-term support of adrenal function in persons with CFS.

Are There Any Side Effects or Interactions? Refer to the individual herb for information about any side effects or interactions.

Chronic Venous Insufficiency

Chronic venous insufficiency (CVI) can occur after excessive clotting and inflammation of the leg veins, a disease known as deep vein thrombosis. CVI also results from a simple failure of the valves in leg veins to hold blood against gravity, leading to sluggish movement of blood out of the veins. It can cause feet and calves to become swollen, often accompanied by a dull ache made worse with prolonged standing. If CVI is allowed to progress, the skin tends to darken and ulcers can occur. CVI often causes **varicose veins** (p. 163).

Lifestyle Changes That May Be Helpful

People affected by chronic venous insufficiency should not sit or stand for long periods of time and when sitting should elevate their legs. Walking helps move blood out of the veins. Wearing tight-fitting compression stockings available from pharmacies further supports the veins.

Nutritional Supplements That May Be Helpful

Bioflavonoids (p. 271) promote venous strength and integrity. Most studies of bioflavonoids in people with CVI have used a type of bioflavonoid called hydroxyethylrutosides (HR), which are derived from rutin. These studies have consistently shown a beneficial effect of HR in clearing leg edema and other signs of CVI.[12] Positive results from double-blind research have occurred using 500 mg taken twice per day for 12 weeks.[3] HR have also been used to treat ulcers due to CVI,[4] although this use of HR should not be attempted without medical supervision. It is not clear if other bioflavonoids are as effective as HR for chronic venous insufficiency. However, nutritionally oriented doctors will sometimes suggest 300–500 mg 3 to 4 times per day of readily available citrus bioflavonoids.

Are There Any Side Effects or Interactions? Refer to the individual supplement for information about any side effects or interactions.

Checklist for Chronic Venous Insufficiency

Ranking	Nutritional Supplements	Herbs
Primary	Bioflavonoids (p. 271) (rutin) Proanthocyanidins (p. 324)	Grape seed extract Horse chestnut (p. 435)
Secondary	Bioflavonoids (p. 324) (hesperidin)	
Other		Butcher's broom (p. 405) Gotu kola (p. 430)

Herbs That May Be Helpful

Horse chestnut (p. 435) contains the compound aescin, which has shown to be effective in both partially blind[5] and double-blind[6] research, supporting the traditional use of horse chestnut for venous problems. In the medical studies, capsules of horse chestnut extract containing 50 mg of aescin were given twice daily for CVI. The positive effect results in part from horse chestnut's ability to strengthen capillaries, which leads to less swelling.[7]

Grape seed extracts (p. 324) containing oligomeric proanthocyanidins (OPCs), a group of bioflavonoids, have also been shown to strengthen capillaries in double-blind research using as little as two 50 mg tablets per day.[8] Using a total of 150 mg per day, French researchers reported that women with CVI were helped in a double-blind trial.[9] Using a total of 300 mg per day (100 mg taken 3 times), yet another French double-blind trial has reported good effects in just 4 weeks.[10]

Very few doctors working with herbal medicine are aware of these and other double-blind studies supporting the use of OPCs for people with CVI because virtually all publications of these data are in French; and the studies appear in obscure French medical journals not readily available to health-care professionals. Nonetheless, the research has been consistent, and OPC-containing grape seed extract products are available.

Another traditional remedy for vein problems is **butcher's broom** (p. 405). One study used a combination of butcher's broom, the **bioflavonoid** (p. 271) hesperidin, and **vitamin C** (p. 341) and found it better than placebo for treating CVI.[11] Studies have used one capsule—containing standardized extracts providing 15–30 mg ruscogenins—3 times each day.

Gotu kola (p. 430) is another herb recommended by some herbalists for chronic venous insufficiency.

Are There Any Side Effects or Interactions? Refer to the individual herb for information about any side effects or interactions.

Cold Sores

Cold sores (sometimes called fever blisters) are caused by a herpes virus, most often the herpes simplex 1 virus. Cold sores should not be confused with **canker sores** (p. 30), which are small ulcerations in the mouth. Rather, cold sores are fluid-filled blisters that form on the gums and the outside of the mouth and lips. The blisters, which are contagious, later break, ooze, and crust over before healing. Recurrences are common and can be triggered by stress, sun exposure, illness, and menstruation. If the infection is transmitted to the eyes, it can lead to blindness. Genital herpes infection (usually caused by herpes simplex 2) is a related condition and potentially can be treated in much the same way as herpes simplex 1.

Dietary Changes That May Be Helpful

It has been reported that people with cold sores on average eat about the same amount of the amino acids **arginine** (p. 268) and **lysine** (p. 309) compared with people without cold sores.[1] Nonetheless, the herpes simplex virus has a high requirement for arginine. Conversely, lysine inhibits viral replication.[2] For this reason, a diet that is low in arginine and high in lysine is unfavorable to the replication of the herpes simplex virus.[3] A review of research that has studied the effects of lysine in people with cold sores shows that most reports find some significant efficacy.[4] Many nutritionally oriented doctors therefore tell people to avoid foods with high lysine-to-arginine ratios, including nuts, peanuts, and chocolate. Nonfat yogurt and other nonfat dairy can be a healthful way to increase lysine intake.

Nutritional supplements and other natural approaches that may be helpful: The amino acid **lysine** (p. 309), in the amount of 1–3 grams per day, is effective in inhibiting the recurrence of herpes simplex infections in some individuals,[5,6] although occasional positive reports have used lower amounts.[7] Reduction in symptoms and number of infections from lysine supplementation (using 3 grams per day) has been confirmed with double-blind research.[8] At 1 gram per day given for 12 weeks, other double-blind research found that some people appeared to be helped.[9] Not every double-blind study finds lysine effective,[10] and when lysine is supplemented for only a few days after each outbreak, it appears to fail.[11]

Zinc (p. 346), applied topically in a cream, has been reported to prevent the replication of the herpes simplex virus.[12] According to one trial of thirty people with herpes simplex infection, zinc sulfate solution

was applied daily to the skin at the site of a flare-up, and then twice a month to prevent recurrence; results were successful in all of the herpes sufferers.[13] The sooner the zinc is applied to blisters and the more frequently it is applied, the quicker the recovery. Zinc in the form of zinc monoglycerate has been reported to be more effective than zinc oxide.[14] Oral zinc supplements have not shown effectiveness.

Vitamin E (p. 344) oil applied topically and allowed to remain on the lesion for 15 minutes has been reported to reduce pain in an uncontrolled trial;[15] this outcome has been independently confirmed in other uncontrolled research.[16]

Boric acid (p. 272) has antiviral activity. Topical diluted boric acid ointment in the form of sodium borate has been used to shorten the outbreak of cold sores in a double-blind trial.[17] Duration of cold sores was approximately 4 days with boric acid and 6 days with placebo. Concerns about potential toxicity, however, have led some doctors to avoid the use of boric acid.

Are There Any Side Effects or Interactions? Refer to the individual supplement for information about any side effects or interactions.

Checklist for Herpes Simplex/Cold Sores

Ranking	Nutritional Supplements	Herbs
Secondary	Lysine (p. 309) Vitamin E (p. 344) Zinc (p. 346) (topical)	Lemon balm (p. 440) (topical)
Other	Boric acid (p. 272)	Chaparral (p. 410) Echinacea (p. 417) Elderberry (p. 418) Goldenseal (p. 429) Licorice (p. 440) (topical) Myrrh (p. 446) Soapwort St. John's wort (p. 461) (topical/oral)

See also: Homeopathic Remedies for **Cold Sores** (p. 543)

Herbs That May Be Helpful

Lemon balm (p. 440) has antiviral properties. A cream containing an extract of has been shown in double-blind German research to speed the healing of cold sores.[18] Application of concentrated lemon balm creams or ointments several times per day is most likely to be effective.

Licorice (p. 440) in a cream or gel form is applied directly to herpes sores 3 to 4 times per day. Licorice extracts containing glycyrrhizin should be used. Studies have not proven this works, but it is common practice among some doctors of natural medicine.

Colic

According to test tube research, an extract from **elderberry** (p. 418) leaves, combined with **St. John's wort** (p. 461) and soapwort, inhibits the herpes simplex virus.[19]

In traditional herbal medicine, tinctures of a variety of herbs have been applied topically to herpes outbreaks to speed healing. The alcohol in tinctures will dry out the cold sores and thereby reduce some symptoms, and the herbs may have additional benefits. Some of the herbs used include **chaparral** (p. 410), St. John's wort, **goldenseal** (p. 429), **myrrh** (p. 446), and **echinacea** (p. 417).

Are There Any Side Effects or Interactions? Refer to the individual herb for information about any side effects or interactions.

Colic

Colic is a common problem in infants. A colicky baby is healthy but has periods of inconsolable crying. During the crying spell, the infant may experience abdominal distention and excessive gas, drawing up his or her legs. Colic usually develops within a few weeks of birth and disappears by the baby's fourth month.

Lifestyle Changes That May Be Helpful

All infants, particularly those with colic, need to be fed on demand and not by a specific clock schedule. Often the cry is triggered by discomfort caused by low blood sugar; unlike adults, infants do not have a carefully regulated ability to maintain healthy blood sugar levels in the absence of food. This physiological shortcoming found just in infants can only be solved by feeding on demand.

In one trial, parents were taught to not let babies cry unnecessarily but rather to attempt feeding first in response to the infant's cry.[1] If that failed, parents were taught to try to respond to the cry in other ways (such as holding the infant or providing the opportunity to sleep). These parents were also given the solid medical advice that overfeeding is never caused by feeding on demand, nor will the baby be "spoiled" by such an approach. As a result of this intervention, colic was dramatically (and statistically significantly) reduced compared with a group of mothers given different instructions.

Dietary Changes That May Be Helpful

Allergies (p. 8) play a role in some colicky infants.[2] If the child is fed with formula, the problem may be an intolerance to milk proteins from a cow's milk-based formula.[3] Switching to a soy formula may ease colic in such cases.[4] Infants who are sensitive to both milk and soy can be given a nonallergenic formula.

If the child is breast-fed, certain foods in the mother's diet may provoke an allergic reaction in the child. Cow's milk consumed by a breast-feeding mother has been shown in some,[5] but not all,[6] studies to trigger colic. Cow's milk proteins (a trigger of allergy reactions) have been found at higher levels in milk from breast-feeding mothers with colicky infants than mothers with noncolicky infants.[7] A double-blind study of colicky infants (either bottle-fed or breast-fed) showed that changing to a low-allergenic formula or restricting the mother's diet to exclude certain allergy-triggering foods significantly reduced colic symptoms in the infants.[8] A nutritionally oriented physician can help determine which foods in the breast-feeding mothers may be contributing to colic.

Checklist for Colic

Ranking	Nutritional Supplements	Herbs
Secondary		Cardamom, Chamomile (p. 409) Garden angelica Peppermint (p. 451) Vervain, Licorice (p. 440) Fennel (p. 423) Lemon balm (p. 440) (in combination) Yarrow (p. 471)

See also: Homeopathic Remedies for **Colic** (p. 526)

Herbs That May Be Helpful

Chamomile (p. 409) has a long history of use as a calming herb and can be used to ease intestinal cramping in colicky infants. A soothing tea made from chamomile, vervain, **licorice** (p. 440), **fennel** (p. 423), and **lemon balm** (p. 440) has been shown to relieve colic more effectively than placebo.[9] In this study, approximately ½ cup (150 ml) of tea was given during each colic episode for a maximum of 3 times per day.

A tea of **peppermint** (p. 451) is a traditional therapy for colic in infants, and a double-blind study has confirmed its effectiveness.[10] The tea used in this study contained mint, licorice, vervain, fennel, and lemon balm. However, peppermint should be used cautiously in infants.

Several other herbs have been used in traditional medicine for colic, and are approved by the German government's Commission E.[11] These include **yarrow** (p. 471), garden angelica *(Angelica archangelica),* and cardamom *(Carum carvi)*. These are generally administered by doctors of natural medicine as teas or decoctions to the infant or to the mother if she is breastfeeding.

Are There Any Side Effects or Interactions? Refer to the individual herb for information about any side effects or interactions.

Common Cold/Sore Throat

The common cold is an acute (short-term) viral infection of the upper respiratory tract that often causes runny nose, sore throat, and malaise. Sore throat is sometimes a symptom of a more serious condition distinct from the common cold (such as strep throat) that may require medical diagnosis and treatment with appropriate antibiotics.

Lifestyle Changes That May Be Helpful

Colds can be spread through the air, such as when a person sneezes, or by contact with contaminated objects.

Dietary Changes That May Be Helpful

Sugar, dietary fat, and alcohol have been reported to affect the immune system negatively, though no specific information is yet available on how much these foods may actually affect the course of the common cold. For more information, see **immune function** (p. 94).

Nutritional Supplements That May Be Helpful

A review of twenty-one placebo-controlled studies using 1–8 grams of **vitamin C** (p. 341) found that "in each of the twenty-one studies, vitamin C reduced the duration of episodes and the severity of the symptoms of the common cold by an average of 23%."[1] The optimum amount of vitamin C to take for cold treatment remains in debate, but 1–3 grams per day is commonly used and is generally supported by much of the scientific literature.

Zinc (p. 346) interferes with viral replication in test tubes; may interfere with the ability of viruses to enter cells of the body; may help immune cells to fight a cold; and may relieve cold symptoms by affecting prostaglandin metabolism.[2] Certain zinc lozenges have been helpful to adult cold sufferers,[3,4] though this effect has not been reported in children.[5] Most successful studies have used zinc gluconate or zinc gluconate-glycine lozenges containing 15–25 mg of zinc per lozenge.

An analysis of the major zinc trials has claimed that evidence for efficacy is "still lacking."[6] However, despite a lack of *statistical* significance, this compilation of data from six double-blind trials found that people assigned to zinc had a 50% decreased risk of still having symptoms after 1 week compared with those given placebo. Some trials included in this analysis used formulations containing substances that may inactivate zinc salts. Other reasons for failure to show statistical significance could be small sample size (not enough people) or too low an amount of zinc, according to a recent analysis of these studies.[7] Thus, there are plausible reasons why the authors were unable to show statistical significance, even though positive effects are well supported in most trials using either gluconate or gluconate-glycine forms.

Cold sufferers should avoid lozenges that contain citric acid[8] or tartaric acid, substances that may interfere with efficacy and have been used in most trials that fail to get good results.[9] With one exception,[10] trials using forms other than zinc gluconate or zinc gluconate-glycine have failed, as do trials that use insufficient amounts of zinc.[11] Therefore, until more is known, it makes sense to only use zinc gluconate or gluconate-glycine, and in proper amounts (see above). Zinc lozenges are not to be taken long term, but rather only at the onset of a cold and stopped when symptoms have disappeared. The best effect is obtained when lozenges are used at the first sign of a cold; up to 10 lozenges per day can be taken for several days during the cold.

Are There Any Side Effects or Interactions? Refer to the individual supplement for information about any side effects or interactions.

Herbs That May Be Helpful

Fresh pressed juice of the flowers of echinacea *(E. purpurea)* preserved with alcohol and tinctures of root of **echinacea** (p. 417) *(E. pallida)* have been shown to reduce symptoms of the common cold in double-blind studies.[12] In addition, several double-blind studies have found that echinacea *(E. angustifolia)* root tinctures in combination with **wild indigo** (p. 469), **boneset** (p. 402), and homeopathic arnica have been shown to reduce symptoms of the common cold.[13] The minimum effective amount of echinacea tincture or juice that it is necessary to take according to these studies is 3 ml 3 times per day. More (3–5 ml every 2 hours) is generally better and is safe, even for children.[14] Encapsulated products may also be effective, according to a double-blind study involving *E. pallida;*[15] generally 300–600 mg capsules 3 times per day are used.

Common Cold/Sore Throat

Recent studies indicate that regular use of echinacea to prevent colds does not work.[16,17] Therefore, it is currently recommended to limit use of echinacea to the onset of a cold and to use it for only 10 to 14 days consecutively.

In traditional herbal medicine, **goldenseal** (p. 429) root is often taken with echinacea. Two alkaloids in the root (berberine and canadine) have an antimicrobial and mild immune-stimulating effect.[18] However, due to small amounts in the root, it is unlikely that these effects would occur. Goldenseal soothes irritated mucous membranes in the throat,[19] making it useful for those experiencing a sore throat with their cold.

Goldenseal root should only be used for short periods of time. Goldenseal root extract, capsules, or tablets are typically taken in amounts of 4–6 grams 3 times per day. Using goldenseal powder as a tea or tincture may soothe a sore throat.

Herbal supplements can play a role in long-term attempts to strengthen the immune system and fight infections. Adaptogens, which include **eleuthero** (p. 419) (Siberian ginseng), **Asian ginseng** (p. 394), **astragalus** (p. 395), and **schisandra** (p. 458), are thought to help keep various body systems—including the immune system—functioning optimally. Another immune stimulant, **boneset** (p. 402), helps fight off minor viral infections, such as the common cold.

Elderberry (p. 418) has shown antiviral activity in laboratory tests, and thus may be useful for some people with common colds. **Horseradish** (p. 436) has antibiotic properties, which may account for its easing of throat and upper respiratory tract infections.

Herbs high in mucilage, such as **slippery elm** (p. 460) and **marshmallow** (p. 444), are often helpful for symptomatic relief of coughs and irritated throats. **Mullein** (p. 446) has expectorant and demulcent properties, which accounts for this herb's historical use as a remedy for the respiratory tract, particularly in cases of irritating coughs with bronchial congestion.

The resin of the herb **myrrh** (p. 446) has been shown to kill various microbes and to stimulate macrophages (a type of white blood cell). **Usnea** (p. 465) has a traditional reputation as an antiseptic and was sometimes used for people with common colds.

Red raspberry (p. 454), **blackberry** (p. 398), and **blueberry** (p. 401) leaves contain astringent tannins that are helpful for soothing sore throats.[20] **Sage** (p. 456) tea can be gargled to soothe a sore throat. **Yarrow** (p. 471) has been used for sore throats. All of these remedies are not supported by modern research at this time, but are traditionally used.

Wild indigo (p. 469) also stimulates the immune system, according to test-tube experiments,[21] which might account for its role against the common cold and flu. In combination with echinacea, boneset, and homeopathic arnica, as mentioned above, it has been shown in double-blind research to prevent and reduce symptoms of the common cold.

Eucalyptus (p. 421) oil is often used in a steam inhalation to help clear nasal and **sinus congestion** (p. 156). It is said to function in a fashion similar to that of menthol by acting on receptors in the nasal mucosa, leading to a reduction in the symptoms of, for example, nasal stuffiness.[22]

Meadowsweet (p. 444) was used historically for a wide variety of conditions, including treating rheumatic complaints of the joints and muscles and even arthritis.[23] Culpeper, a seventeenth century pharmacist, mentions its use to help break fevers and promote sweating during a cold or **flu** (p. 104). Meadowsweet contains salicylates, which give the herb a possible aspirin-like effect.

Are There Any Side Effects or Interactions? Refer to the individual herb for information about any side effects or interactions.

Checklist for Common Cold/Sore Throat

Ranking	Nutritional Supplements	Herbs
Primary	Vitamin C (p. 341) Zinc (p. 346)	Echinacea (p. 417) (for symptoms)
Secondary		Echinacea (p. 417) (for prevention) Elderberry (p. 418)
Other		Asian Ginseng (p. 394) Astragalus (p. 395) Blackberry (p. 398) Blueberry (p. 401) Boneset (p. 402) Coltsfoot (p. 412) Eleuthero (p. 419) Eucalyptus (p. 421) Goldenseal (p. 429) Horseradish (p. 436) Marshmallow (p. 444) Meadowsweet (p. 444) Mullein (p. 446) Myrrh (p. 446) Red Raspberry (p. 454) Sage (p. 456) Schisandra (p. 458) Slippery Elm (p. 460) Usnea (p. 465) Wild indigo (p. 469) Yarrow (p. 471)

See also: Homeopathic Remedies for **Common Cold/Sore Throat** (p. 527)

Congestive Heart Failure (CHF)

Congestive heart failure (CHF) is a chronic condition that results when the heart muscle is unable to pump blood as quickly as is needed. It leads to breathlessness, fatigue, and accumulation of fluid in the lungs or the veins (primarily in the legs), or both. **High blood pressure** (p. 89) can cause congestive heart failure. Failure of the heart pump can also result from many other causes such as severe anemia, hyperthyroidism, heart attacks, and arrhythmias of the heart.

Cautions: Congestive heart failure is a serious medical condition that requires expert management, rather than self-treatment.

Lifestyle Changes That May Be Helpful

Even with severe disease, appropriate exercise can benefit those with CHF.[1] In a controlled trial, long-term (1 year) exercise training led to improvements in quality of life and functional capacity in people with CHF.[2] Nonetheless, too much exercise can be life-threatening for those with CHF. How much is "too much" varies from person to person; therefore, any exercise program undertaken by someone with CHF requires professional supervision.

Nutritional Supplements That May Be Helpful

As is true for several other heart conditions, **coenzyme Q$_{10}$** (p. 283) has been reported to help people with CHF,[3] an effect confirmed in double-blind research.[4] Much of the research uses 90–150 mg per day. Coenzyme Q$_{10}$ may take several months to show beneficial results. People with CHF taking coenzyme Q$_{10}$ should not stop taking it suddenly, since sudden withdrawal has resulted in severe relapse.[5]

People with CHF have insufficient oxygenation of the heart, which can damage the heart muscle. Such damage may be reduced by taking **carnitine** (p. 279) supplements.[6] Carnitine is a natural substance made from the amino acids **lysine** (p. 309) and **methionine** (p. 313). Levels of carnitine are low in people with CHF;[7] therefore, many nutritionally oriented doctors recommend that those with CHF take 500 mg of carnitine 2 to 3 times per day.

Most carnitine/CHF research has used a modified form of the supplement called propionyl-L-carnitine (PC). In one double-blind trial, using 500 mg PC per day led to a 26% increase in exercise capacity after 6 months.[8] Other indices of heart function have also been reported to improve in double-blind research using 1 gram PC taken twice per day.[9] It remains unclear whether the propionyl-L-carnitine has unique advantages, as limited research in both animals and humans with the more common L-carnitine has also shown very promising effects.[10]

Magnesium (p. 310) deficiency frequently occurs with CHF, which can lead to heart arrhythmias. Magnesium supplements have reduced the risk of these arrhythmias.[11] Those with CHF are often given drugs that deplete both magnesium and **potassium** (p. 323). It is important to protect against the arrhythmias, which could result from a lack of either mineral.[12] Many nutritionally oriented doctors suggest magnesium supplements of 300 mg per day.

Whole fruit and fruit and vegetable juice, all of which are high in potassium, are also recommended by some doctors; however, this dietary change should be discussed with a health-care provider, because several drugs given to people with CHF can actually cause *retention* of potassium, making dietary potassium, even from fruit, dangerous.

Taurine (p. 334), an amino acid, helps the heart pump. Research (some double blind) has repeatedly shown that taurine helps those with CHF.[13,14,15,16] Most nutritionally oriented doctors suggest taking 2 grams 3 times per day.

The body needs **arginine** (p. 268), another amino acid, to make nitric oxide, which increases blood flow. This process is impaired in those with CHF. Arginine has been used successfully in double-blind research in amounts of 5.6 to 12.6 grams per day in people with CHF.[17]

Are There Any Side Effects or Interactions? Refer to the individual supplement for information about any side effects or interactions.

Herbs That May Be Helpful

Studies have shown that standardized extracts made from the leaves and flowers of **hawthorn** (p. 433) *(Crataegus oxyacantha)* are effective in the support of early-stage congestive heart failure.[18,19] Hawthorn extracts appear to help people with early-stage CHF by increasing blood flow to the heart, increasing the strength of heart contractions, reducing resistance to blood flow in the extremities, and acting as an **antioxidant** (p. 267).[20,21,22]

Hawthorn extracts exist in capsules or tablets standardized to either total flavonoid content (usually 2.2%) or oligomeric procyanidins (usually 18.75%). Doctors who work with herbal medicine often suggest 80–300 mg 2 to 3 times per day. Hawthorn berry products that are not standardized may be weaker, and the recommended amount is typically 4 to 6 grams per day for the whole herb or 4–5 ml of the tincture 3 times per day.

Are There Any Side Effects or Interactions? Refer to the individual herb for information about any side effects or interactions.

Checklist for Congestive Heart Failure

Ranking	Nutritional Supplements	Herbs
Primary	Coenzyme Q$_{10}$ (p. 283) Magnesium (p. 310) Propionyl-L-carnitine (p. 279) Taurine (p. 334)	Hawthorn (p. 433)
Secondary	Arginine (p. 268) Potassium (p. 323)	
Other	Creatine monohydrate (p. 285)	

Conjunctivitis (Pinkeye) and Blepharitis

Conjunctivitis is inflammation of the clear membrane that lines the eye. It is caused most commonly by infection with viruses or bacteria or an allergic reaction, though other causes exist, such as over exposure to sun, wind, smog, chorine, or contact lens solution. Pinkeye is a common name for conjunctivitis. Blepharitis is inflammation of the eyelid; most commonly, it is caused by a bacterial infection.

Nutritional Supplements That May Be Helpful

Vitamin A (p. 336) deficiency has been reported in people with chronic conjunctivitis.[1] It is unknown whether vitamin A supplementation can prevent conjunctivitis or help people who already have the condition.

Are There Any Side Effects or Interactions? Refer to the individual supplement for information about any side effects or interactions.

Herbs That May Be Helpful

A number of herbs are traditionally used to treat eye inflammations. To avoid infection, all preparations must be boiled and kept sterile before applying to the eyes. **Calendula** (p. 406), **eyebright** (p. 422), and **chamomile** (p. 409) are used to help reduce the swelling and redness when applied topically. Comfrey

is a soothing herb used for conjunctivitis. **Goldenseal** (p. 429) or **Oregon grape** (p. 449) are antimicrobial and should be applied only if the cause is an infection.[2] None of these herbs has been studied for use in conjunctivitis or blepharitis, although they have a long history of use. When using herbal medicines in the eyes, it is important to work with a doctor of natural medicine.

Are There Any Side Effects or Interactions? Refer to the individual herb for information about any side effects or interactions.

Checklist for Conjunctivitis and Blepharitis

Ranking	Nutritional Supplements	Herbs
Other	Vitamin A (p. 336)	Calendula (p. 406) Chamomile (p. 409) Comfrey (p. 413) Eyebright (p. 422) Goldenseal (p. 429) Oregon grape (p. 449)

See also: Homeopathic Remedies for **Conjunctivitis and Blepharitis** (p. 529)

Constipation

Constipation results when food moves too slowly through the gastrointestinal (GI) tract. No exact frequency of bowel movements or amount of symptoms associated with constipation (such as hard stools and excessive straining) precisely defines constipation. The most common cause is probably dietary (discussed below). However, constipation can be a component of **irritable bowel syndrome** (p. 109) or can result from a wide range of causes, such as a drug side effect or physical immobility. Serious diseases, including colon cancer, can sometimes first appear as bowel blockage leading to acute constipation. Therefore, particularly constipation of recent onset should be diagnosed by a physician. Dietary and other natural approaches discussed below should be used by people with constipation only when there is reason to believe no serious underlying condition exists.

Dietary Changes That May Be Helpful

Insoluble **fiber** (p. 293) from food acts like a sponge. Adding water to the "sponge" makes it soft and easy to push through the GI tract. Insoluble fiber comes mostly from vegetables, beans, brown rice, whole wheat, rye, and other whole grains. Switching from white bread and white rice to whole wheat bread and brown rice often helps relieve constipation. It is important to drink lots of fluid along with the fiber—at least 16 ounces of water per serving of fiber. Otherwise, a "dry sponge" is now in the system, which can worsen the constipation.

In addition, wheat bran can be added to the diet. Nutritionally oriented doctors frequently suggest a quarter cup or more per day of wheat bran along with fluid. An easy way to add wheat bran to the diet is to add it to breakfast cereal or to switch to high-bran cereals. Wheat bran often helps reduce constipation, although not all research shows it to be successful.[1] Higher amounts of wheat bran are sometimes more successful.[2] Some doctors of natural medicine also recommend 15 ml per day of **flaxseed oil** (p. 296) to help relieve constipation, though there is little evidence to support this approach.

A double-blind trial found that chronic constipation and problems associated with it can be triggered by intolerance to cow's milk in two-thirds of constipated infants studied.[3] Symptoms went away in most infants kept away from cow's milk. The possibility exists that constipation occurring in adults and/or constipation triggered by other food allergies might also sometimes be responsible for chronic constipation in some individuals. If other approaches do not help, these possibilities can be discussed with a nutritionally oriented physician.

Lifestyle Changes That May Be Helpful

Exercise may increase the muscular contractions of the intestine, which sometimes helps move the contents through the body.[4] Nonetheless, the effect of exercise on constipation remains unclear.[5]

Nutritional Supplements That May Be Helpful

Chlorophyll (p. 281), the substance responsible for the green color in plants, may be useful for a number of gastrointestinal problems. Evidence supporting its use in people with constipation, however, remains preliminary.[6]

Are There Any Side Effects or Interactions? Refer to the individual supplement for information about any side effects or interactions.

Herbs That May Be Helpful

The most frequently used laxatives worldwide come from plants. Herbal laxatives are either bulk-forming or stimulating.

Bulk-forming laxatives come from plants with a high fiber and mucilage content that expand when they come into contact with water; examples include **psyllium** (p. 452), flaxseed, and **fenugreek** (p. 424). As the volume in the bowel increases, a reflex contraction is stimulated. These mild laxatives are best suited for long-term use in people with constipation.

Many nutritional doctors recommend taking 7.5 grams of psyllium seeds or 5 grams of psyllium husks, mixed with water or juice, 1 to 2 times per day. Some doctors use a combination of senna (18%) and psyllium (82%) for the treatment of chronic constipation. This has been shown to work for people in nursing homes.[7]

Stimulant laxatives are high in anthraquinone glycosides, which stimulate bowel muscle contraction. The most frequently used stimulant laxatives are senna leaves, cascara bark, and aloe latex. While senna is the most popular, cascara has a somewhat milder action. Aloe is very potent and should be used with caution.

The unprocessed roots of **fo-ti** (p. 425) possess a mild laxative effect. The bitter compounds in **dandelion** (p. 415) leaves and root are also mild laxatives.

Are There Any Side Effects or Interactions? Refer to the individual herb for information about any side effects or interactions.

Checklist for Constipation

Ranking	Nutritional Supplements	Herbs
Primary	Fiber (p. 293)	Aloe (p. 391) Cascara (p. 407) Flaxseed Psyllium (p. 452) Senna (p. 459)
Other	Chlorophyll (p. 281) Flaxseed oil (p. 296)	Dandelion (root) (p. 415) Fenugreek (p. 424) Fo-ti (p. 425)

See also: Homeopathic Remedies for **Constipation** (p. 529)

COPD (Chronic Obstructive Pulmonary Disease)

Chronic obstructive pulmonary disease (COPD) (also called chronic obstructive lung disease or COLD) refers to the combination of chronic bronchitis and emphysema resulting in obstruction of airways.

COPD

Although chronic bronchitis and emphysema are distinct conditions, smokers and former smokers often have aspects of both. In chronic bronchitis, the linings of the bronchial tubes are inflamed and thickened, leading to a chronic, mucus-producing **cough** (p. 47) and shortness of breath. In emphysema, the alveoli (tiny air sacs in the lungs) are damaged, also leading to shortness of breath. COPD is generally irreversible and can be fatal.

Lifestyle Changes That May Be Helpful

Smoking is the underlying cause of the majority of cases of emphysema and chronic bronchitis. Anyone who smokes should stop, and although quitting smoking will not reverse the symptoms of COPD, it can help preserve the remaining lung function. Exposure to other respiratory irritants, such as air pollution, dust, toxic gases, or fumes, can aggravate COPD and should be avoided when possible.

The **common cold** (p. 41) or other respiratory infections can aggravate COPD. Avoiding exposure to infections or bolstering resistance with immune-enhancing nutrients and herbs can be valuable.

Dietary and Other Natural Therapies That May Be Helpful

Although clues about the relationship between COPD and diet have surfaced, as yet they have not formed a coherent picture. Malnutrition is common in individuals with COPD and can further compromise lung function and overall health of people with this disease.[1] However, evidence of malnutrition may occur despite adequate dietary intake.[2] Researchers have found that increasing dietary carbohydrate increases carbon dioxide production, which leads to reduced exercise tolerance and increased breathlessness in people with COPD.[3] Despite this evidence, a study comparing the diets of men over a 25-year period found that those with a higher intake of fruit (high in carbohydrate) were at lower risk of developing lung diseases.[4] People with COPD should talk with a nutritionally oriented doctor before making significant dietary changes.

Chronic bronchitis has been linked to **allergies** (p. 8) in many reports.[5,6,7] In a preliminary trial, long-term reduction of some COPD symptoms occurred when people with COPD avoided allergenic foods and (in some cases) were also desensitized to pollen.[8] People with COPD interested in testing the effects of a food allergy elimination program should talk with a nutritionally oriented doctor.

Negative ions may counteract the allergenic effects of positively charged ions on respiratory tissues and potentially ease symptoms of allergic bronchitis, according to preliminary research.[9,10]

Nutritional Supplements That May Be Helpful

N-acetyl cysteine (NAC) (p. 317) helps break down mucus. For that reason, inhaled NAC is used in hospitals to treat bronchitis. NAC may also protect lung tissue through its antioxidant activity.[11] Oral NAC (200 mg taken twice per day) is also effective, improving symptoms in people with bronchitis in double-blind research.[12,13] Results may take 6 months.

Vitamin C (p. 310) has mucus-thinning properties and may be helpful to respiratory conditions. A review of nutrition and lung health reported that people with a higher dietary intake of vitamin C were less likely to be diagnosed with bronchitis.[14] Vitamin C was also shown to be related to greater volume of air expired from the lungs—a sign of healthy lung function. As yet, the effects of supplementing with vitamin C in people with COPD have not been studied.

Antioxidants (p. 267) in general are hypothesized to be important for neutralizing the large amounts of free radicals associated with COPD. However, use of antioxidant supplements (synthetic **beta-carotene** [p. 268] and **vitamin E** [p. 344]) did help people with COPD in a double-blind trial despite the fact that people who ate higher amounts of these nutrients in their diets appeared to have lower risk.[15]

A greater intake of the omega-3 fatty acids found in **fish oils** (p. 294) has been linked to reduced risk of COPD,[16] though research has yet to investigate whether fish oil supplements would help people with COPD.

Many prescription drugs commonly taken by people with COPD have been linked to **magnesium** (p. 310) deficiency, a potential problem because magnesium is needed for normal lung functioning.[17] One group of researchers reported that a magnesium deficiency was found in 47% of people with COPD (as determined by muscle biopsy) but was not reflected in blood levels of magnesium.[18] In this study, magnesium deficiency was also linked with increased hospital stays. Thus it appears that many people with COPD may be magnesium deficient, a problem that could worsen their condition; moreover, the deficiency is not easily diagnosed.

Intravenous magnesium has improved breathing capacity in people experiencing an acute exacerbation of COPD.[19] In this double-blind study, the need for hospitalization was also reduced in the magnesium group (28% versus 42% with placebo), but this difference was not statistically significant. Intravenous magnesium is known to be a powerful bronchodilator.[20] The effect of oral magnesium supplementation in people with COPD has yet to be investigated.

Carnitine (p. 279) has been given to people with chronic lung disease in trials investigating how the body responds to exercise.[21,22] In these double-blind reports, 2 grams of carnitine taken twice per day for 2 to 4 weeks led to positive changes in breathing response to exercise.

Researchers have also given **coenzyme Q$_{10}$ (CoQ$_{10}$)** (p. 283) to people with COPD after discovering their blood levels of CoQ$_{10}$ are lower than those found in healthy people.[23] In that trial, 90 mg of CoQ$_{10}$ given for 8 weeks led to no change in lung function, though oxygenation of blood improved, as did exercise performance and heart rate. Until more research is done, the importance of supplementing with CoQ$_{10}$ for people with COPD remains unclear.

Are There Any Side Effects or Interactions? Refer to the individual supplement for information about any side effects or interactions.

Checklist for Chronic Obstructive Pulmonary Disease

Ranking	Nutritional Supplements	Herbs
Primary	N-acetyl cysteine (p. 317) (for bronchitis)	
Secondary	Carnitine (p. 279)	
Other	Coenzyme Q$_{10}$ (p. 283) Fish oil (p. 294) (EPA/DHA [p. 287]) Magnesium (p. 310) Vitamin C (p. 341)	Anise Elecampane (p. 418) Ephedra (p. 420) Eucalyptus (p. 421) Gumweed Horehound (p. 434) Lobelia (p. 442) Mullein (p. 446) Wild cherry bark (p. 468) Yerba santa

Herbs That May Be Helpful

Mullein (p. 446) is classified in the herbal literature as an expectorant (to promote the discharge of mucus) and demulcent (to soothe and protect mucous membranes) herb. Historically, mullein has been used as a remedy for the respiratory tract, particularly in cases of irritating coughs with bronchial congestion.[24] Other herbs commonly used as expectorants in traditional medicine include **elecampane** (p. 418), **lobelia** (p. 442), yerba santa *(Eriodicyton californica),* **wild cherry** (p. 468) bark, **horehound** (p. 434) *(Marrubium vulgare),* gumweed, anise, and **eucalyptus** (p. 421). Animal studies have suggested that some

of these increase discharge of mucus.[25] However, none of these herbs have been studied for efficacy in humans.

Ephedra sinica (Ma huang) (p. 420) has been used by the Chinese for medicinal purposes for over 5,000 years, including for lung and bronchial constriction, coughing, and shortness of breath. However, this herb has the potential for serious side effects and is best used only with the guidance of a nutritionally oriented physician.

Are There Any Side Effects or Interactions? Refer to the individual herb for information about any side effects or interactions.

Cough

Cough is a symptom of many diseases. Most coughs come from simple viral infections, such as the **common cold** (p. 41). Sometimes but not always mucus is produced with the cough. If the color is green or yellow, it may be a hint of a more serious bacterial infection, although this is not a reliable indicator. If the color is red, there may be bleeding in the lungs. Any cough that produces blood or blood-stained mucus, as well as any cough that lasts more than 2 weeks, requires a visit to a medical professional for diagnosis.

Herbs That May Be Helpful

A number of herbs have a rich history of use for treating coughs due to colds, bronchitis, or other mild conditions. Only a few studies have examined the effectiveness of these herbs. Among those herbs that have been shown to have some degree of cough-relieving activity are **marshmallow** (p. 444),[1] **sundew** (p. 462),[2] and **coltsfoot** (p. 412).[3] Coltsfoot has also been shown to increase the activity of the ciliary hairs lining the bronchial passages, thereby helping expel mucus and the viruses and debris it traps.[4]

Two other herbs traditionally used for cough are **elecampane** (p. 418) and **mullein** (p. 446); however, these have not yet been shown to help a cough in scientific investigations. Both may be helpful in dealing with the underlying cause of the cough if it is infectious. Both have documented effects at killing bacteria and viruses.[5,6]

The mucilage of **slippery elm** (p. 460) gives it a soothing effect for coughs. **Usnea** (p. 465) also contains mucilage, which can be helpful in easing irritating coughs. There is a long tradition of using **wild cherry** (p. 468) syrups to treat coughs. Other traditional remedies to relieve coughs include **bloodroot**

(p. 399), **catnip** (p. 407), **comfrey** (p. 413), **horehound** (p. 434), **lobelia** (p. 442), **ephedra** (p. 420), and **red clover** (p. 453).

The early nineteenth-century Eclectic physicians in the United States (who used herbs as their main medicine) not only employed **eucalyptus** (p. 421) oil to sterilize instruments and wounds but recommended a steam inhalation of the vapor of the oil to help treat **asthma** (p. 15), bronchitis, whooping cough, and emphysema.[7]

Thyme (p. 464) has a long history of use in Europe for the treatment of dry, spasmodic coughs as well as bronchitis.[8] Its antispasmodic actions have made it a common traditional recommendation for whooping cough. Many constituents in thyme team up to provide its antitussive (preventing and treating a cough), antispasmodic, and expectorant actions. The primary constituents are the volatile oils, which include the phenols thymol and carvacol.[9] These are complemented by the actions of flavonoids as well as saponins. Thyme, either alone or in combination with herbs such as **sundew** (p. 462), continues to be one of the most commonly recommended herbs in Europe for the treatment of dry, spasmodic coughs as well as whooping cough.[10] Due to the low toxicity of the herb, it has become a favorite for treating coughs in small children.

Are There Any Side Effects or Interactions? Refer to the individual herb for information about any side effects or interactions.

Checklist for Cough

Ranking	Nutritional Supplements	Herbs
Primary		Sundew (p. 462)
Secondary		Ephedra (p. 420) Thyme (p. 464) Wild cherry (p. 468)
Other		Bloodroot (p. 399) Catnip (p. 407) Coltsfoot (p. 412) Comfrey (p. 413) Elecampane (p. 418) Eucalyptus (p. 421) Horehound (p. 434) Lobelia (p. 442) Marshmallow (p. 444) Mullein (p. 446) Red clover (p. 453) Slippery elm (p. 460) Usnea (p. 465)
See also: Homeopathic Remedies for **Cough** (p. 530)		

Crohn's Disease

Crohn's disease is a poorly understood inflammatory disease that affects the final part of the small intestine and the beginning section of the colon. It often causes bloody stools and malabsorption problems.

Dietary Changes That May Be Helpful

A person with Crohn's disease might consume more sugar than does the average healthy person.[1] A high-fiber, low-sugar diet led to a 79% reduction in hospitalizations compared with no dietary change in one group of people with Crohn's disease.[2] Another trial compared the effects of high- and low-sugar diets in people with Crohn's disease.[3] In that report, those with more active disease fared better on the low-sugar diet compared with those eating more sugar. Several people on the high-sugar diet had to stop eating sugar because their disease grew worse. While details of how sugar injures the intestine are still being uncovered, nutritionally oriented doctors often suggest eliminating all sugar (including soft drinks and processed foods with added sugar) from the diets of those with Crohn's disease.

A high animal protein and high-fat diet (other than fish) has been linked to Crohn's disease in preliminary research.[4] As with many other health conditions, it may be beneficial to eat less meat and dairy fat and more fruits and vegetables.

Some people with Crohn's disease have **food allergies** (p. 8) and have been reported to do better when they avoid foods to which they are allergic. One study found that people with Crohn's are most likely to react to cereals, dairy, and yeast.[5] Yeast and some dairy (cheese) are high in histamine, which is secreted during an allergenic response. People with Crohn's disease lack the ability to break down histamine at a normal rate[6] so it is possible that the link reported to yeast and dairy may not be coincidental.

In one trial, people with Crohn's disease (rather than doctors) were asked which foods exacerbated their symptoms.[7] Those without ileostomies found nuts, raw fruit, and tomatoes to be most problematic, though responses varied from person to person, and other reports have come up with different lists.[8] People with Crohn's wishing to identify and avoid potential allergens should consult a nutritionally oriented doctor.

Lifestyle Changes That May Be Helpful

People with Crohn's disease are more likely to smoke, and there is evidence that continuing to smoke aggravates disease progression.[9]

Nutritional Supplements That May Be Helpful

Crohn's disease often leads to malabsorption. As a result, inadequate levels of many nutrients are common. For this reason, it makes sense for people with Crohn's disease to take a high potency **multiple-vitamin/mineral supplement** (p. 314). In particular, deficiencies in **zinc** (p. 346), **folic acid** (p. 297), **vitamin B$_{12}$** (p. 337), and **iron** (p. 304) have been reported.[10,11] Zinc, folic acid, and vitamin B$_{12}$ are needed to repair intestinal cells damaged by Crohn's disease. Some doctors recommend 25 to 50 mg of zinc (balanced with 2 to 4 mg of copper), 800 mcg of folic acid, and 800 mcg of vitamin B$_{12}$. Iron status should be evaluated by a nutritionally oriented doctor before considering supplementation.

Vitamin A (p. 336) is needed for the growth and repair of cells that line both the small and large intestine.[12] Reports of people with Crohn's responding to vitamin A have appeared.[13,14] However, in one trial of eighty-six people with Crohn's who were in remission, vitamin A supplementation for 14 months led to no benefit.[15] Therefore, although some nutritionally oriented doctors recommend 50,000 IU per day for adults with Crohn's disease, this approach remains unproven. A dose this high should never be taken without qualified guidance, nor should it be given to a woman who is or could become pregnant.

Vitamin D (p. 343) malabsorption is common in Crohn's[16] and can lead to a deficiency.[17] Successful treatment with vitamin D for **osteomalacia** (p. 154) (bone brittleness caused by vitamin D deficiency) triggered by Crohn's disease has been reported.[18] A nutritionally oriented doctor can evaluate vitamin D status and suggest the right level of vitamin D supplements.

Inflammation within the gut occurs in people suffering from Crohn's. EPA and **DHA** (p. 287), the omega-3 fatty acids found in **fish oil** (p. 294), have anti-inflammatory activity. A 2-year trial compared the effects of having people with Crohn's eat 3.5 to 7 ounces of fish high in EPA and DHA per day or a diet low in fish.[19] In that trial, the fish-eating group had a 20% relapse rate compared with 58% in those not eating fish. Salmon, herring, mackerel, albacore tuna, and sardines are all high in EPA and DHA.

Supplementing 2.7 grams per day of a combination of EPA and DHA reduced the recurrence rate of Crohn's disease at 1 year from 59% with placebo to 26% with fish oil in a double-blind trial.[20] This highly statistically significant improvement resulted from the use of a special enteric-coated, "free fatty acid" form of EPA/DHA taken from fish oil. However, other blinded trials using other fish oil supplements that are not enteric coated nor in the free fatty acid form have reported no clinical improvement.[21,22] These disparate outcomes suggest that the enteric-coated free fatty acid form may have important advantages. The enteric-coated free fatty acid form has also been reported to not cause gastrointestinal symptoms often resulting from taking regular fish oil supplements, again suggesting unique benefit.[23]

Diarrhea caused by Crohn's disease has partially responded to *Saccharomyces boulardii* supplementation in double-blind research.[24] Although the amount used in this trial—250 mg taken 3 times per day—was helpful, research successfully using Saccharomyces boulardii supplements with people suffering from other forms of diarrhea has used as much as 500 mg taken 4 times per day.[25]

Individuals with Crohn's disease may be deficient in pancreatic enzymes, including **lipase** (p. 307).[26] In theory, supplemental enzymes might improve malabsorption associated with Crohn's. People with Crohn's disease considering supplementation with enzymes should consult a nutritionally oriented doctor.

Are There Any Side Effects or Interactions? Refer to the individual supplement for information about any side effects or interactions.

Herbs That May Be Helpful

Doctors who use herbal medicine sometimes use a combination of herbs to soothe inflammation throughout the digestive tract. The formula contains **marshmallow** (p. 444), **slippery elm** (p. 460), **wild indigo** (p. 469), **goldenseal** (p. 429), **echinacea** (p. 417), and **cranesbill** (p. 414). Marshmallow and slippery elm are mucilaginous plants that help soothe inflamed tissues. Wild indigo and goldenseal help inhibit growth of abnormal gut bacteria and also have astringent effects. Cranesbill is another astringent. Echinacea promotes normal immune function. Goldenseal is traditionally viewed as a tonic for the intestines as well as an antimicrobial agent. Clinical trials using this combination have not been conducted.

A variety of anti-inflammatory herbs have historically been recommended by doctors using botanical

Crohn's Disease

medicine for people with Crohn's disease. These include **yarrow** (p. 471), **chamomile** (p. 409), **licorice** (p. 440), and **aloe** (p. 391) juice. Cathartic preparations of aloe should be avoided. No research has been conducted to validate the use of these herbs for Crohn's disease.

Tannin-containing herbs may be helpful to decrease diarrhea during acute flare-ups and have been used for this purpose in traditional medicine. An uncontrolled study using isolated tannins in the course of usual drug therapy found them more effective for reducing diarrhea than no additional treatment.[27] Tannin-containing herbs of potential benefit include agrimony, **green tea** (p. 430) (also anti-inflammatory), **oak** (p. 448), **witch hazel** (p. 470), and **cranesbill** (p. 414). Use of such herbs should be discontinued before the diarrhea is completely resolved, otherwise the disease could be exacerbated.

Are There Any Side Effects or Interactions? Refer to the individual herb for information about any side effects or interactions.

Checklist for Crohn's Disease

Ranking	Nutritional Supplements	Herbs
Primary	Fish oil (p. 294) (enteric-coated free fatty acid form) Multiple Vitamin/Mineral (p. 314) (Folic acid [p. 297], Iron [p. 304]). Vitamin B$_{12}$ [p. 337] Vitamin D (p. 343) (Crohn's associated osteomalacia [p. 154])	
Secondary	*Saccharomyces boulardii*, Zinc (p. 346)	
Other	Lipase (p. 307) Vitamin A (p. 336)	Aloe (p. 391) Agrimony Chamomile (p. 409) Cranesbill (p. 414) Echinacea (p. 417) Goldenseal (p. 429) Green tea (p. 430) (also anti-inflammatory) Licorice (p. 440) Marshmallow (p. 444) Oak (p. 448) Slippery Elm (p. 460) Wild Indigo (p. 469) Witch hazel (p. 470) Yarrow (p. 471)

Depression

Depression, characterized by unhappy feelings of hopelessness, can be a response to stressful events, hormonal imbalances, biochemical abnormalities, or other causes. Mild depression that passes quickly may not require any diagnosis or treatment. However, when depression becomes recurrent, constant, or severe, it should be diagnosed by a licensed counselor, psychologist, or psychiatrist. Diagnosis may be crucial to determining appropriate treatment. For example, depression caused by **low thyroid** (p. 93) function can be successfully treated with prescription thyroid medication. Suicidal depression often requires prescription antidepressants. Persistent mild-to-moderate depression triggered by stressful events is often best treated with counseling and not necessarily with medications.

When depression is not a function of external events, it is called endogenous. Endogenous depression can be due to biochemical abnormalities. Lifestyle changes and herbs may be used with people whose depression results from a variety of causes, but dietary and nutrient interventions are usually best geared to endogenous depression.

Dietary Changes That May Be Helpful

Although some research has produced mixed results,[1] several double-blind studies have shown that **food allergies** (p. 8) can trigger mental symptoms, including depression.[2,3] Individuals with depression who do not respond to other natural or conventional approaches should consult a nutritionally oriented doctor to diagnose possible food sensitivities and avoid offending foods.

Restricting sugar and caffeine in people with depression has been reported to elevate mood in preliminary research.[4] How much of this effect resulted from sugar and how much from caffeine remains unknown. Researchers have reported that psychiatric patients who are heavy coffee drinkers are more likely to be depressed than other such patients.[5] However, it remains unclear whether caffeine caused depression or whether depressed people were more likely to want the "lift" associated with drinking a cup of coffee. In fact, "improvement in mood" is considered an effect of long-term coffee consumption by some researchers, a concept supported by the fact that people who drink coffee have been reported to have a 58 to

66% decreased risk of committing suicide compared with non-coffee drinkers.[6] Nonetheless, a symptom of caffeine addiction can be depression.[7] Thus, consumption of caffeine (mostly from coffee) has paradoxically been linked with both improvement in mood and depression, by different researchers. People with depression may want to avoid caffeine as well as sugar for 1 week to see how it affects their mood.

Lifestyle Changes That May Be Helpful

Exercise increases the body's production of endorphins—chemical substances that can relieve depression. Scientific research shows that routine exercise can positively affect mood and help with depression.[8] As little as 3 hours per week of aerobic exercises can profoundly reduce the level of depression.[9]

Nutritional Supplements and Other Natural Therapies That May Be Helpful

Oral contraceptives can deplete the body of **vitamin B₆** (p. 340), a nutrient needed for maintenance of normal mental functioning. Double-blind research shows that women who are depressed and who have become depleted of vitamin B_6 while taking oral contraceptives typically respond to vitamin B_6 supplementation.[10] In one trial, 20 mg of vitamin B_6 were taken twice per day. Some evidence suggests that people who are depressed—even when not taking the oral contraceptive—are still more likely to be B_6 deficient than people who are not depressed.[11]

Several studies also indicate that vitamin B_6 supplementation helps alleviate depression associated with **premenstrual syndrome** (p. 141)[12] (PMS), although the research remains inconsistent.[13] Many nutritionally oriented doctors suggest that women who have depression associated with PMS take 100 to 300 mg of vitamin B_6 per day—a level of intake that requires supervision by a nutritionally oriented doctor.

Iron (p. 304) deficiency is known to affect mood and can exacerbate depression, but it can be diagnosed and treated by any nutritionally oriented doctor. While iron deficiency is easy to fix with iron supplements, people who have not been diagnosed with iron deficiency should not supplement iron.

Deficiency of **vitamin B₁₂** (p. 337) can create disturbances in mood that respond to B_{12} supplementation.[14] Depression caused by vitamin B_{12} deficiency can occur in the absence of anemia.[15] Diagnosis of deficiency

requires a doctor knowledgeable in the field of nutrition.

Mood has been reported to sometimes improve with high amounts of vitamin B_{12} (given by injection) even in the absence of a B_{12} deficiency.[16] Supplying the body with high amounts of vitamin B_{12} can only be done by injection. However, in the case of overcoming a diagnosed B_{12} deficiency, following an initial injection by oral maintenance supplementation (1,000 micrograms per day) is possible even when the cause of the deficiency is pernicious anemia. (See the Vitamin B_{12} information above for more information.)

A deficiency of the B vitamin **folic acid** (p. 297) can also disturb mood. A large percentage of depressed people have low folic acid levels.[17] Folic acid supplements appear to improve the effects of lithium in treating manic-depressives.[18] Depressed alcoholics report feeling better with large amounts of a modified form of folic acid.[19] Anyone suffering from chronic depression should be evaluated for possible folic acid deficiency by a nutritionally oriented doctor. Those with abnormally low levels of folic acid are sometimes given short-term, high amounts of folic acid (10,000 mcg per day).

A deficiency of other B vitamins not discussed above (including **B₁** [p. 337], **B₂** [p. 338], **B₃** [p. 339], **pantothenic acid** [p. 340], and **biotin** [p. 272]) can also lead to depression. However, the level of deficiency of these nutrients needed to induce depression is rarely found in Western societies.

Omega-3 oils (p. 287) found in fish, particularly **DHA** (p. 287), are needed for normal functioning of the nervous system. Depressed people have been reported to have lower DHA levels than people who are not depressed.[20] Low levels of the other omega-3 oil from fish, EPA, have correlated with increased severity of depression.[21] However, researchers have yet to investigate whether omega-3 fish oil supplements help people with depression.

The amino acid **tyrosine** (p. 335) can convert into norepinephrine—a neurotransmitter that affects mood. Women taking oral contraceptives have lower levels of tyrosine, and some researchers think this might be related to depression caused by the Pill.[22] Tyrosine metabolism may be abnormal in other depressed people as well,[23] and preliminary research suggests supplementation might help.[24,25] Several nutritionally oriented doctors recommend a 12-week trial of tyrosine supplementation for people who are depressed. Published research has used a very high amount—100 mg per 2.2 pounds of body weight (or about 7 grams per day for an average adult). It remains unclear whether such high levels are necessary for optimal effect.

L-Phenylalanine (p. 320) is another amino acid that converts to mood-affecting substances (including phenylethylamine). Preliminary research reported that L-phenylalanine improved mood in most depressed people studied.[26] **DLPA** (p. 320) is a mixture of the essential amino acid L-phenylalanine and its synthetic mirror image, D-phenylalanine. DLPA (or the D- or L-form alone) reduced depression in thirty-one of forty people in an uncontrolled study.[27] Some doctors of natural medicine suggest a 1-month trial with 3 to 4 grams per day of phenylalanine for people with depression, although some researchers have found that even very low amounts—75 to 200 mg per day— were helpful in preliminary studies.[28] In one double-blind trial, depressed people given 150 to 200 mg of DLPA experienced results comparable to that of an antidepressant drug.[29]

Phosphatidylserine (PS) (p. 321), a natural substance derived from the amino acid serine, affects neurotransmitter levels in the brain that affect mood. In a controlled trial, older women given 300 mg of PS had significantly less depression compared with placebo.[30] After 45 days, the level of depression in the PS group was more than 60% lower than the level achieved with placebo.

Levels of the hormone dehydroepiandrosterone (**DHEA** [p. 288]) may be lower in depressed people. Supplementation with DHEA improved depression in an uncontrolled study with only six subjects.[31] A double-blind trial reported a significant reduction in major depression in 6 weeks using a maximum of 90 mg per day of DHEA.[32] In that trial, no people had significant improvement with placebo, but five of eleven people given DHEA had a 50% or greater decrease in symptoms. Depressed people considering taking DHEA should consult a nutritionally oriented doctor. In addition, experts have concerns about the safe use of DHEA, particularly because long-term safety data do not exist. See the DHEA chapter for more information about the safety concerns.

Preliminary evidence indicates that individuals with depression may have lower levels of **inositol** (p. 303); however, the clinical application of this remains to be determined.[33]

An isolated preliminary trial suggests that the supplement **NADH** (p. 317) may help people with depression.[34] Controlled trials are needed before any conclusions can be drawn.

S-adenosyl methionine (**SAMe** [p. 330]) is a substance synthesized in the body that has recently been made available as a supplement. SAMe appears to raise levels of dopamine, an important neurotransmitter in mood regulation, and higher SAMe levels in the brain are associated with successful drug treatment of depression. Oral SAMe has been demonstrated to be an effective treatment for depression in most,[35,36,37] but not all,[38] controlled studies. While it does not seem to be as powerful as full doses of antidepressant medications[39] or **St. John's wort** (p. 461), SAMe's effects are felt more rapidly, often within 1 week.[40]

Disruptions in emotional well-being, including depression, have been linked to serotonin imbalances in the brain.[41] Supplementation with **5-HTP** (p. 295) may increase serotonin synthesis, and thus researchers are studying the possibility that 5-HTP might help people with depression. Some[42,43] trials using 5-HTP with people suffering from depression have shown sign of efficacy.[44,45,46] Depressed people interested in considering this hormone precursor should consult a nutritionally oriented doctor.

Are There Any Side Effects or Interactions? Refer to the individual supplement for information about any side effects or interactions.

Herbs That May Be Helpful

St. John's wort (p. 461) extracts are among the leading medicines used in Germany by medical doctors for the treatment of mild to moderate depression. Using St. John's wort extract can significantly relieve the symptoms of depression. People taking St. John's wort show an improvement in mood and ability to carry out their daily routine. Symptoms such as sadness, hopelessness, worthlessness, exhaustion, and poor sleep also decrease.[47,48]

The St. John's wort extract LI 160 has been compared to the prescription antidepressants imipramine,[49] amitriptyline,[50] and maprotiline.[51] The improvement in symptoms of mild to moderate depression was similar with notably fewer side effects in people taking St. John's wort. It is important to note, however, that the above studies compared 900 mg per day of St. John's wort extract with only 75 mg per day of the prescription antidepressants. Health-care professionals consider this a very low amount.

A more recent study compared a higher dose of the St. John's wort extract LI 160 (1,800 mg per day) with a higher dose of imipramine (150 mg per day) in more severely depressed persons.[52] Again, the improvement was virtually the same for both groups with far fewer side effects for the St. John's wort group. While this may point to St. John's wort as a possible treatment for more severe cases of depression, this treatment should only be pursued under the guidance of a health-care professional.

In the German Commission E monograph, the amount of St. John's wort taken is typically based on hypericin concentration in the extract, which should be approximately 1 mg per day.[53] For example, an extract standardized to contain 0.2% hypericin would require a daily intake of 500 mg (usually given in two divided dosages). Many European studies use higher intakes of 900 mg daily and this has become the accepted daily dosage in modern herbal medicine. Recent research suggests, however, that hypericin is not the antidepressant compound in St. John's wort, and attention is starting to shift to the compound known as hyperforin.[54] As an antidepressant, St. John's wort should be monitored for 4 to 6 weeks to check effectiveness. If possible, St. John's wort should be taken near mealtime.

Checklist for Depression

Ranking	Nutritional Supplements	Herbs
Primary	Folic acid (p. 297) (for folate deficiency) Iron (p. 304) (for iron deficiency) Vitamin B$_6$ (p. 340) (with oral contraceptives) Vitamin B$_{12}$ (p. 337) (for B$_{12}$ deficiency)	St. John's wort (p. 461)
Secondary	5-HTP (p. 295) Phenylalanine/DLPA (p. 320) SAMe (p. 330) Tyrosine (p. 335) Vitamin B$_6$ (p. 340) (for premenstrual syndrome [p. 141])	*Ginkgo biloba* (p. 427) (for elderly people)
Other	Fish oil (p. 294) (EPA/DHA [p. 287]) Inositol (p. 303) NADH (p. 317) Phosphatidylserine (p. 321)	*Ginkgo biloba* (p. 427) Damiana (p. 415) Yohimbe (p. 472)
See also: Homeopathic Remedies for **Depression** (p. 532)		

Ginkgo (p. 427) is supportive in the alleviation of depression and has been shown in one double-blind study to be helpful for depressed elderly people not responding to antidepressant drugs.[55] **Damiana**

(p. 415) also has a tradition of being used to stimulate people with depression. Yohimbine (the active component of the herb **yohimbe** [p. 472]) inhibits monoamine oxidase (MAO) and therefore may be beneficial in depressive disorders. However, clinical research has not been conducted for its use in treating depression.

Are There Any Side Effects or Interactions? Refer to the individual herb for information about any side effects or interactions.

Diabetes
Section 1: Introduction

Diabetes here refers to diabetes mellitus. Other uncommon forms of diabetes are not covered in this discussion.

People with diabetes cannot properly process glucose, a sugar the body uses for energy. As a result, glucose stays in the blood, causing blood glucose to rise. At the same time, however, the cells of the body can be starved for glucose. Diabetes can lead to poor **wound healing** (p. 167), higher risk of infections, and many other problems involving the eyes, kidneys, nerves, and heart.

There are two types of diabetes mellitus. Adult-onset diabetes is also called type 2 or non-insulin-dependent diabetes (NIDDM). With NIDDM, the pancreas often makes enough insulin, but the body has trouble using the insulin. NIDDM responds so well to natural medicine that even conventional practitioners recommend starting treatment with dietary and lifestyle changes.

Childhood-onset diabetes is the other form of diabetes mellitus. It is also called type 1 or insulin-dependent diabetes (IDDM). In IDDM, the pancreas cannot make the insulin needed to process glucose. Natural medicine cannot cure IDDM, but by making the body more receptive to insulin supplied by injection, it may help. It is particularly critical for people with IDDM to work carefully with the doctor prescribing insulin before contemplating the use of any herbs, supplements, or dietary changes mentioned in this section. Any change that makes the body more receptive to insulin could require critical changes in insulin dosage that must be determined by the treating physician.

People with diabetes have a high risk for heart disease. As a result, information in the chapter on **atherosclerosis** (p. 17) is also important to read.

Continue reading Section 2: **Dietary and Lifestyle Changes**.

Diabetes

Section 2: Dietary and Lifestyle Changes

Dietary Changes That May Be Helpful

People with diabetes cannot properly process sugar. Although short-term high-sugar diets do not cause blood sugar problems for diabetics,[1][2][3] sugar is not necessarily innocent. Research shows that sugar causes diabetes in animals.[4]

The **fiber** (p. 293) in carbohydrates may help protect against diabetes. Most sugar comes from low-fiber foods, while high-fiber foods are often low in sugar. Therefore, eating more sugar usually means decreasing fiber—probably a mistake for diabetics. When whole foods (such as beans, whole raw fruit, and pasta) are compared with processed sugary foods, the high-sugar foods increase blood sugar more than the whole foods.[5]

Most doctors of natural medicine recommend that diabetics cut intake of sugar from snacks and processed foods. The best replacements for low-fiber, high-sugar foods (such as fruit juice) or starch (such as white bread) are high-fiber, whole foods.

High-fiber supplements, such as **psyllium** (p. 452),[6][7] guar gum (found in beans),[8] pectin (from fruit),[9] oat bran,[10] and glucomannan,[11] have improved glucose tolerance in some studies. Good results have also been reported with the consumption of 1 to 3 ounces of powdered **fenugreek seeds** (p. 424) per day.[12][13] A review of the research revealed that the extent to which moderate amounts of fiber help people with diabetes in the long term is still unknown, and the lack of many long-term studies has led some researchers to question the importance of fiber in improving diabetes.[14] Nonetheless most doctors advise people with diabetes to eat a diet high in fiber. Focus should be placed on fruits, vegetables, seeds, oats, and whole-grain products, although psyllium and glucomannan supplements also help in some studies.

Eating fish also may afford some protection from diabetes.[15] See **Part 3** (p. 55) of the Diabetes chapter for information about fish oil supplements and diabetes.

Vegetarians have been reported to have a low risk of NIDDM.[16] When people with diabetic nerve damage switch to a vegan diet (no meat, dairy, or eggs), improvements have been reported after only several days.[17] In one study, pain completely disappeared in seventeen of twenty-one people.[18] Fats from meat and dairy also cause **heart disease** (p. 32), the leading killer of people with diabetes.

Vegetarians eat less protein than meat eaters. Reducing protein intake has lowered kidney damage caused by diabetes[19][20] and may also improve glucose tolerance.[21] Switching to a low-protein diet should be discussed with a nutritionally oriented doctor.

Monounsaturated oils may be good for diabetics.[22] The easiest way to incorporate monounsaturates into the diet is to use olive oil. However, those who are overweight need to be careful—olive oil is high in calories.

Should children avoid milk to avoid IDDM? Countries with high milk consumption have a high risk of IDDM.[23] Animal research indicates that avoiding milk affords protection from IDDM.[24] Milk contains a protein that is related to a protein in the pancreas, the organ where insulin is made. Some researchers believe that children who are allergic to milk may develop antibodies that attack the pancreas, causing IDDM. Most, but not all, studies indicate that children with IDDM drink cow's milk at an earlier age than other children.[25] Children with IDDM may have high levels of antibodies that attack milk protein.[26]

Immune problems in people with IDDM have been tied to other allergies as well,[27] and the importance of focusing only on the avoidance of dairy products remains unclear.[28] Nonetheless, until more is known, most doctors of natural medicine recommend abstaining from dairy products in infancy and early childhood, particularly for children with a family history of IDDM. Recent research also suggests a possible link between milk consumption in infancy and an increased risk of NIDDM.[29]

Lifestyle Changes That May Be Helpful

Most people with NIDDM are obese.[30] Excess abdominal weight does not stop insulin formation,[31] but it does make the body insensitive to insulin.[32] Excess weight even makes healthy people pre-diabetic.[33] Weight loss reverses this problem.[34] NIDDM improves with weight loss in most studies.[35][36][37]

Being overweight does not cause IDDM, but it does increase the need for more insulin. Therefore, people with IDDM should achieve and maintain appropriate body weight.

Exercise helps decrease body fat[38] and improves insulin sensitivity.[39] Exercisers are less likely to develop NIDDM.[40] People with IDDM who exercise require less insulin.[41] However, exercise can induce low blood sugar or even occasionally *increased* blood sugar.[42] Therefore, diabetics should never begin an exercise program without consulting a health-care professional.

Moderate drinking in *healthy* people improves glucose tolerance.[43,44,45,46] However, alcohol worsens glucose tolerance in the elderly[47] and in diabetics.[48] Diabetics who drink have a high risk for eye[49] and nerve damage.[50] Until more is known, people with diabetes should avoid alcohol. For healthy people, light drinking will not increase the risk of diabetes, but heavy drinking will, and should therefore be avoided.

Diabetics who smoke are at higher risk for kidney damage,[51] heart disease,[52] and other diabetes-linked problems. Smokers are more likely to become diabetic.[53] It is important to quit smoking.

Continue reading Section 3: **Dietary Supplements and Herbs.**

Diabetes
Section 3: Dietary Supplements and Herbs

Nutritional Supplements That May Be Helpful

People with low blood levels of **vitamin E** (p. 344) are more likely to develop NIDDM.[1] Double-blind studies show that vitamin E improves glucose tolerance in people with NIDDM in most,[2 3 4] but not all studies.[5] Vitamin E has also improved glucose tolerance in elderly non-diabetics.[6,7] Three months or more of supplementation may be required for benefits to become apparent. The most common amount used is 900 IU of vitamin E per day. In one of the few trials to not find vitamin E helpful with glucose intolerance in people with NIDDM, damage to nerves caused by the diabetes was nonetheless partially reversed by supplementing with vitamin E for 6 months.[8]

Vitamin E prevents blood from clotting too fast[9] and has other actions that protect diabetics' blood vessels from damage.[10] Vitamin E has protected animals from diabetic cataracts.[11]

Higher blood levels of vitamin E—a reflection of dietary intake—have been associated with a dramatically reduced risk of being diagnosed with IDDM.[12] The possibility that vitamin E supplementation might be protective has not yet been directly explored by researchers. The way vitamin E is thought to protect against IDDM (by reducing oxidative damage in the pancreas) appears unrelated to the possible protective roles vitamin E appears to play in NIDDM.

Glycosylation is an important index of diabetes. It refers to how much sugar attaches abnormally to proteins. Vitamin E reduces this problem in some,[13,14] although not all studies.[15]

People with IDDM appear to have low **vitamin C** (p. 341) levels.[16] As with vitamin E, vitamin C may reduce glycosylation.[17] Vitamin C also lowers sorbitol in diabetics;[18] sorbitol is a sugar that can accumulate and damage the eyes, nerves, and kidneys of diabetics. Vitamin C may improve glucose tolerance in NIDDM,[19,20] although not every study confirms this benefit.[21] Many doctors of natural medicine suggest that diabetics supplement with 1 to 3 grams per day of vitamin C.

One study compared antioxidant supplement intake, including both vitamins E and C, with diabetic retinopathy (damage to the eyes caused by diabetes).[22] Surprisingly, several correlations were found between extensive retinopathy and *greater* likelihood of taking vitamin C and vitamin E supplements. The outcome of this trail, however, does not fit with most other published data and might simply reflect the fact that sicker people are more likely to take supplements in hopes of getting better. For the present, most nutritionally oriented doctors remain relatively unconcerned about the unexpected outcome of this isolated report.

Many diabetics have low blood levels of **vitamin B$_6$** (p. 340).[23,24] Levels are even lower in diabetics with nerve damage.[25] Vitamin B$_6$ supplements improve glucose tolerance in women with diabetes caused by pregnancy.[26,27] Vitamin B$_6$ is also effective for glucose intolerance induced by the birth control pill.[28] For other people with diabetes, 1,800 mg per day of a special form of vitamin B$_6$—pyridoxine alpha-ketoglutarate—has improved glucose tolerance dramatically in some research.[29] Standard vitamin B$_6$ has helped in some,[30] but not all studies.[31]

Vitamin B$_{12}$ (p. 337) is needed for normal functioning of nerve cells. Vitamin B$_{12}$ taken orally, intravenously, or by injection has reduced nerve damage caused by diabetes in most people studied.[32] Oral vitamin B$_{12}$ up to 500 mcg 3 times per day has been used.

Biotin (p. 272) is a B vitamin needed to process glucose. When people with IDDM were given 16 mg of biotin per day for 1 week, their fasting glucose levels dropped by 50%.[33] Similar results have been reported using 9 mg per day for 2 months in people with NIDDM.[34] Biotin may also reduce pain from diabetic nerve damage.[35] Some doctors of natural medicine try 16 mg of biotin for a few weeks to see if blood sugar levels will fall.

High levels—several grams per day—of niacin, a form of **vitamin B$_3$** (p. 339), impair glucose tolerance and should not be taken by people with diabetes.[36,37] Smaller amounts (500 to 750 mg per day for 1 month followed by 250 mg per day) may help some people with NIDDM,[38] though this research remains preliminary.

Preliminary studies have suggested that **niacinamide** (p. 339), the other form of vitamin B$_3$, might be useful in the very early stages of IDDM,[39] though most research does not support this claim.[40,41,42] Some,[43] but not all,[44] research suggests that healthy children at high risk for IDDM may be protected by supplementing niacinamide. Parents of children with IDDM may discuss the possibility of protecting their other children through niacinamide supplementation with a nutritionally oriented doctor.

Years ago, blood levels of vitamin B$_1$ were reported to be low in people with IDDM.[45] Long before that, a trial using 10 mg of vitamin B$_1$ per day for 4 weeks reported reduced blood sugar levels in six of eleven diabetics.[46] Recently, supplementation with both vitamins B$_1$ (25 mg per day) and B$_6$ (50 mg per day) to a group of people with diabetic neuropathy led to significant improvement in only 4 weeks.[47] However, this was a study conducted in a vitamin B$_1$-deficient third-world country. Therefore, these improvements might not occur in other diabetics. A recent German study also found that combining vitamin B$_1$ (in a special fat-soluble form) and vitamin B$_6$ plus vitamin B$_{12}$ in high but variable amounts led to improvement in some aspects of diabetic neuropathy in 12 weeks.[48] As a result, some doctors of natural medicine recommend that people with diabetic neuropathies supplement vitamin B$_1$, though the optimal level of intake remains unknown.

Vitamin D is needed for adequate blood levels of insulin.[49] Vitamin D receptors have been found in the pancreas where insulin is made and preliminary evidence suggests that supplementation can increase insulin secretion for some people with NIDDM; prolonged supplementation might also help reduce blood sugar levels.[50] Not enough is known about optimal amounts of vitamin D for diabetics, and high levels of vitamin D can be toxic. Therefore, people with diabetes considering vitamin D supplementation should talk with and have vitamin D status assessed by a nutritionally oriented doctor.

Animal studies show that **chromium** (p. 282) improves glucose tolerance.[51] Medical reports dating back to 1853 as well as modern research indicate that chromium-containing **brewer's yeast** (p. 275) can be useful in treating diabetes.[52,53] Double-blind research shows that chromium supplements improve glucose tolerance in people with both NIDDM[54] and IDDM, apparently by increasing sensitivity to insulin.[55] Chromium improves the processing of glucose in people with prediabetic glucose intolerance[56] and in women with diabetes associated with pregnancy.[57] Chromium even helps healthy people,[58] although one such report found chromium useful only when accompanied by 100 mg of niacin.[59] Chromium may also lower **triglycerides** (p. 85) (a risk factor in **heart disease** [p. 32]) in diabetics.[60] The typical amount of chromium used in research trials is 200 mcg per day. Some doctors of natural medicine recommend up to 1,000 mcg per day for diabetics.[61]

People who have diabetes tend to have low **magnesium** (p. 310) levels.[62] Double-blind research indicates that supplementing with magnesium overcomes this problem.[63] Magnesium has led to improved insulin production in elderly people with NIDDM.[64] Elders without diabetes can also produce more insulin as a result of magnesium supplements, according to some,[65] but not all, studies.[66] Insulin requirements are lower in people with IDDM who supplement with magnesium in some trials.[67] However, in people with adult-onset diabetes who nonetheless do require insulin, Dutch researchers have reported no improvement in blood sugar levels.[68]

Diabetes-induced damage to the eyes is more likely to occur to magnesium-deficient people with IDDM.[69] In magnesium-deficient pregnant women with IDDM, the lack of magnesium may even account for the high rate of spontaneous abortion and birth defects associated with IDDM.[70]

The American Diabetes Association admits "strong associations . . . between magnesium deficiency and insulin resistance" but will not say magnesium deficiency is a risk factor.[71] Many doctors of natural medicine, however, recommend that diabetics with normal kidney function supplement with 300 to 400 mg of magnesium per day.

People with IDDM tend to be **zinc** (p. 346) deficient,[72] which may impair immune function.[73] Zinc supplements have lowered blood sugar levels in people with IDDM,[74] though some evidence indicates that zinc supplementation in people with NIDDM does not improve their ability to process sugar.[75] Nonetheless, people with NIDDM also have low zinc levels, caused by excess loss of zinc in their urine.[76]

Many doctors of natural medicine recommend that people with NIDDM supplement with moderate amounts of zinc (15 to 25 mg per day) as a way to correct for the deficit.

Some doctors are concerned about having people with IDDM supplement with zinc because of a report that zinc supplementation increased glycosylation,[77] generally a sign of deterioration of the condition. This study is hard to evaluate because zinc increases the life of blood cells and such an effect artificially increases the lab test results for glycosylation. Until this issue is resolved, those with IDDM should consult a nutritionally oriented doctor before considering supplementation with zinc.

People with diabetes cannot adequately process carbohydrates. **Coenzyme Q$_{10}$ (CoQ$_{10}$)** (p. 283) is needed for normal carbohydrate metabolism. Animals with diabetes have been reported to be CoQ$_{10}$ deficient. In one trial, blood sugar levels fell substantially in 31% of people with diabetes after they supplemented with 120 mg of coenzyme Q$_{10}$ per day.[78] In people with IDDM, however, supplementation with 100 mg of coenzyme Q$_{10}$ per day for 3 months did not improve glucose control nor reduce the need for insulin.[79] Currently, suggesting that diabetics supplement with CoQ$_{10}$ appears premature.

Inositol (p. 303) is needed for normal nerve function. Diabetes can cause nerve damage, or diabetic neuropathy. Some of these abnormalities have been reversed by inositol supplementation in preliminary research (500 mg taken twice per day).[80]

Alpha-lipoic acid (p. 264) is a powerful natural antioxidant. It has been used to improve diabetic neuropathies (at an intake of 600 mg per day) and has reduced pain in several studies.[81]

Carnitine (p. 279) is a substance needed for the body to properly use fat for energy. When diabetics were given carnitine (1 mg per 2.2 pounds of body weight), high blood levels of fats—both cholesterol and triglycerides—dropped 25 to 39% in just 10 days in one trial.[82] In higher amounts (1 gram per day by injection), carnitine has been reported to reduce pain from diabetic nerve damage as well.[83]

Taurine (p. 334) is an amino acid found in protein-rich food. People with IDDM have been reported to have low taurine levels, which leads to "thickened" blood—a condition that increases the risk of heart disease. Supplementing taurine (1.5 grams per day) has restored taurine levels to normal and corrected the problem of blood viscosity within 3 months.[84]

Glucose tolerance improves in *healthy* people taking **omega-3 fish oil** (p. 294) supplements.[85] Some studies find that omega-3 fish oil improves glucose

tolerance,[86,87] **high triglycerides** (p. 85),[88] and **cholesterol** (p. 79) levels in diabetics.[89] However, others report that cholesterol increases[90] and diabetes worsens with fish oil supplements.[91,92,93]

Until this issue is resolved, diabetics should feel free to increase their fish intake, but they should consult a nutritionally oriented doctor before taking omega-3 fish oil supplements. Sometimes, such supplementation may be considered. In one trial, people with diabetic neuropathy and diabetic nephropathy (kidney damage) experienced significant improvement when given 600 mg 3 times per day of purified EPA—one of the two major omega-3 fatty acids found in fish oil supplements—for 48 weeks.[94]

Supplementing with 4 grams of **evening primrose oil** (p. 292) per day for 6 months has been found to reverse the cause of diabetic nerve damage and improve this painful condition. In double-blind research, 6 grams per day helped reduce nerve damage in people with both IDDM and NIDDM.[95]

Nutritionally oriented doctors have suggested that **quercetin** (p. 328) might help people with diabetes because of its ability to reduce levels of sorbitol—a sugar that accumulates in nerve cells, kidney cells, and cells within the eyes of diabetics and has been linked to damage to those organs.[96] Human trials have yet to explore whether quercetin actually protects people with diabetes from neuropathy, nephropathy, or retinopathy.

Vanadyl sulfate, a form of **vanadium** (p. 335), may improve glucose control in individuals with NIDDM,[97,98] though it may not help people with IDDM.[99] The long-term safety of the large amounts of vanadium needed to help people with NIDDM (typically 100 mg per day) remains unknown. Many doctors of natural medicine expect that amounts this high may prove to be unsafe.

Are There Any Side Effects or Interactions? Refer to the individual supplement for information about any side effects or interactions.

Herbs That May Be Helpful

Gymnema (p. 432) may assist the pancreas in the production of insulin in people with NIDDM. Gymnema also improves the ability of insulin to lower blood sugar in people with both IDDM and NIDDM. So far no double-blind studies have confirmed the benefit of gymnema for people with any type of diabetes. One uncontrolled study found that 400 mg daily of a gymnema extract could reduce or eliminate the need for oral blood sugar-lowering drugs in some people with NIDDM.[100] Another uncontrolled study suggested the same amount of the extract could allow

Diabetes

for use of less insulin in people with IDDM.[101] Gymnema is not a substitute for insulin.

Asian ginseng (p. 394) is commonly used in traditional Chinese medicine to treat diabetes. It has been shown to enhance the release of insulin from the pancreas and to increase the number of insulin receptors.[102,103] It also has a direct blood sugar-lowering effect.[104] A recent double-blind study found that 200 mg of ginseng extract per day improved blood sugar control, as well as energy levels in NIDDM.[105]

Checklist for Diabetes

Ranking	Nutritional Supplements	Herbs
Primary	Alpha-lipoic acid (p. 264) Brewer's yeast (p. 275) Chromium (p. 282) Evening primrose oil (p. 292) Fiber (p. 293) Magnesium (p. 310) Vitamin E (p. 344)	Asian ginseng (p. 394) Cayenne (p. 408) (topical for neuropathy) Fenugreek (p. 424) (seeds) Psyllium (p. 452)
Secondary	Biotin (p. 272) Carnitine (p. 279) Coenzyme Q$_{10}$ (p. 283) Thiamine (p. 337) Vitamin B$_6$ (p. 340) (gestational diabetes only) Vitamin C (p. 341)	Aloe vera (p. 391) Bilberry (p. 396) Bitter melon (p. 397) Gymnema (p. 432)
Other	Fish oil (p. 294) (EPA/DHA [p. 287]) Inositol (p. 303) Quercetin (p. 328) Taurine (p. 334) Vanadium (p. 335) (for NIDDM) Vitamin B$_3$ (niacinamide) (p. 339) Vitamin B$_{12}$ (p. 337) Vitamin D (p. 343)	Eleuthero (p. 419) *Ginkgo biloba* (p. 427)

Bilberry (p. 396) may lower the risk of some diabetic complications, such as diabetic cataracts and retinopathy. One uncontrolled study found that a standardized extract of bilberry could improve signs of retinal damage in some people with diabetic retinopathy.[106] *Ginkgo biloba* (p. 427) extract may prove useful for prevention and treatment of early-stage diabetic neuropathy though research is at best very preliminary in this area. Other herbs that may help are **fenugreek** (p. 424) seeds (discussed as a source of fiber in **Part 2: Dietary and Lifestyle Changes** [p. 54]) and **eleuthero** (p. 419) (Siberian ginseng).

Two single-blind studies have found that **aloe vera** (p. 391) juice helps lower blood sugar levels in people with NIDDM. One study found that 1 tablespoon twice daily notably improved the efficacy of the oral blood sugar-lowering drug glibdenclamide.[107] The other study found that the juice by itself was effective.[108]

Preliminary studies have found that the whole, fried slices,[109] water extracts,[110] and juice[111] of **bitter melon** (p. 397) may improve blood sugar control in people with NIDDM. Double-blind studies are needed to confirm this potential benefit.

Topical application of creams containing capsaicin (the main active compound in cayenne) can help relieve symptoms of diabetic neuropathy according to double-blind studies.[112,113] Four or more applications per day may be required to relieve severe pain.

Are There Any Side Effects or Interactions? Refer to the individual herb for information about any side effects or interactions.

Diarrhea

Any attack of frequent watery stools is called diarrhea. Many different conditions can trigger it.

Acute diarrhea is often caused by an infection and may require medical management. The primary role of nutrition in acute diarrhea is to prevent depletion of fluid, sodium, potassium, and calories. Replenishment of all four has been achieved with "rehydration solutions" and with a variety of foods, from salted carrot soup to peeled scraped apple to rice gruel. However, the need for rehydration requires direct medical supervision. Therefore nutritional approaches to overcoming depletion of fluid, sodium, potassium, and calories are not discussed here, but rather should be discussed with a doctor. Diarrhea-induced low blood sugar, dehydration, or electrolyte imbalance can be serious or even life-threatening, particularly if prolonged in children.

A health-care provider should be consulted if diarrhea continues for more than a few days, as it may indicate a more serious health condition. Many people who have diarrhea with intermittent constipation have **irritable bowel syndrome (IBS)** (p. 109). People who have been diagnosed with IBS should read the IBS chapter; the Diarrhea chapter does not apply to people with IBS.

Dietary Changes That May Be Helpful

Some foods contain sugars that absorb slowly, such as fructose in fruit juice or sorbitol in dietetic confectionery. Through a process called osmosis, these unabsorbed sugars hold onto water in the intestines, sometimes leading to diarrhea.[1] By reading labels, people with chronic non-infectious diarrhea can easily avoid fruit juice, fructose, and sorbitol to see if this eliminates the problem.

People who are **lactose intolerant** (p. 114)—meaning they lack the enzyme needed to digest milk sugar—often develop diarrhea after consuming milk or ice cream. People whose lactose intolerance is the cause of diarrhea will rid themselves of the problem by avoiding milk and ice cream or in many cases by taking lactase, the enzyme needed to digest lactose. Lactase is available in a variety of forms in pharmacies (and in grocery stores in the form of lactase-treated milk).

Large amounts of **vitamin C** (p. 341) or **magnesium** (p. 310) found in supplements can also cause diarrhea, although the amount varies considerably from person to person. Unlike infectious diarrhea, diarrhea caused by high amounts of vitamin C or magnesium is not generally accompanied by other signs of illness; the same is true when the problem comes from sorbitol or fructose.[2] In these cases, avoiding the offending supplement or food brings rapid relief.

Drinking lots of coffee causes diarrhea in some people.[3] People with chronic diarrhea who drink coffee should avoid all coffee for a few days to evaluate whether coffee is the culprit.

Allergies and food sensitivities (p. 8) are common triggers for diarrhea.[4] For example, some infants suffer diarrhea when fed cow's milk–based formula but improve when switched to soy-based formula.[5] People with chronic diarrhea not attributable to other causes should discuss the possibility of food sensitivity with a nutritionally oriented doctor.

Nutritional Supplements That May Be Helpful

Acute diarrhea can damage the lining of the intestine. **Folic acid** (p. 297) can help repair this damage. In one preliminary trial, supplementing with very large amounts of folic acid (5,000 mcg 3 times per day for several days) shortened the duration of acute infectious diarrhea by 42% in a preliminary study.[6] However, a double-blind trial failed to show any positive effect with the same level of folic acid.[7] Therefore, evidence that high levels of folic acid supplementation will help people with infectious diarrhea remains weak.

Brewer's yeast (p. 275) has been shown to alter the immune system or the flora living in the intestine and may relieve infectious diarrhea. Three capsules or tablets of brewer's yeast 3 times per day for 2 weeks

was reported to be helpful in three cases of infectious diarrhea caused by *Clostridium difficile*.[8] Animal research has confirmed that brewer's yeast helps fight this unfriendly bacterium.[9] (Note that real brewer's yeast is not identical to nutritional or torula yeast, and that when asking for "brewer's yeast" in health-food stores, people are often directed toward these other products. Real brewer's yeast is bitter whereas other health-food-store yeasts have a relatively more pleasant taste.)

An organism related to brewer's yeast, *Saccharomyces boulardii* (Sb), is sometimes available as a supplement and is widely used in Europe to prevent antibiotic-induced diarrhea. Animal research with Sb shows interference with *Clostridium difficile*, a common cause of diarrhea.[10] In double-blind human trials, Sb has prevented antibiotic-induced[11] and other forms of infectious diarrhea.[12] An intake of 500 mg 4 times per day has been used in some of this research. Sb has also helped tourists prevent traveler's diarrhea in double-blind research.[13] In one trial studying persistent traveler's diarrhea, positive results were obtained at amounts as low as 150 to 450 mg per day.[14] Even diarrhea caused by **Crohn's disease** (p. 48) has partially responded to Sb supplementation in double-blind research.[15] While not every trial shows efficacy,[16] the preponderance of evidence clearly supports the use of Sb in people with diarrhea caused by antibiotics or infection.

Beneficial bacteria, such as lactobacilli and bifidobacteria, normally live in a healthy colon, where they inhibit the overgrowth of disease-causing bacteria.[17] Diarrhea flushes intestinal microorganisms out of the digestive tract, leaving the body vulnerable to opportunistic infections. Replenishing with **acidophilus** (p. 325) and other beneficial bacteria can help prevent new infections.

The combination of bifidobacteria and *Strep thermophilus* (found in certain yogurts) dramatically reduces the incidence of acute diarrhea in hospitalized children.[18] Active-culture yogurt may prevent antibiotic-induced diarrhea.[19]

As mentioned in the dietary changes section above, if **lactose intolerance** (p. 114) is the cause of diarrhea, supplemental use of **lactase** (p. 306) prior to consuming milk or milk-containing products can be helpful.[20] Cheese rarely has enough lactase to cause symptoms in lactose-intolerant people. Lactase products are available that can be chewed while drinking milk or added to milk directly.

The malabsorption problems that develop during diarrhea can lead to deficiencies of many vitamins and minerals.[21] For this reason, it makes sense for people with diarrhea to take a **multiple-vitamin/mineral**

Diarrhea

supplement (p. 314). Two of the nutrients that may not absorb as a result of diarrhea are **zinc** (p. 346) and **vitamin A** (p. 336), both needed to fight infections. In third-world countries, supplementation with zinc and vitamin A has led to a reduction in or prevention of infectious diarrhea.[22] Whether such supplementation would help people in less deficient populations remains unclear.

Are There Any Side Effects or Interactions? Refer to the individual supplement for information about any side effects or interactions.

Checklist for Diarrhea

Ranking	Nutritional Supplements	Herbs
Primary	Acidophilus (p. 325) (for infectious diarrhea) Lactase (p. 306) (for lactose-intolerant people [p. 114]) Multiple-vitamin/mineral (p. 314) (to protect against deficiencies) *S boulardii* (for infectious diarrhea)	
Secondary	Brewer's Yeast (p. 275) (for infectious diarrhea) Fiber (p. 293)	Barberry (p. 395) (berberine) Carob (p. 406) Goldenseal (p. 429) (berberine) Psyllium (p. 452) Oregon grape (p. 449) (berberine)
Other	Folic Acid (p. 297) Vitamin A (p. 336) Zinc (p. 346)	Bilberry (p. 396) Blackberry (p. 398) Blueberry (p. 401) Chamomile (p. 409) Cranesbill (p. 414) Goldenseal (p. 429) Marshmallow (p. 444) Oak (p. 448) Red Raspberry (p. 454) Sweet Annie (p. 463)

See also: Homeopathic Remedies for **Diarrhea** (p. 533)

Herbs That May Be Helpful

The following recommendations are for milder forms of diarrhea. For more serious cases of diarrhea, proper medical evaluation and monitoring should occur before taking any herbal supplements.

While **fiber** (p. 293) from dietary or herbal sources is often useful for constipation, it may also play a role in alleviating diarrhea. For example, 9 to 30 grams per day of **psyllium seed** (p. 452) (an excellent source

of fiber) makes stool more solid and can help resolve symptoms of non-infectious diarrhea.[23]

Carob (p. 406) is rich in tannins that have an astringent or binding effect on the mucous membranes of the intestinal tract. It is often used for young children and infants with diarrhea, and a double-blind study suggests it is effective.[24] Commonly, 15 grams of carob powder is mixed with applesauce (for flavor) when given to children. Carob can also be used for adult diarrhea.

Chamomile (p. 409) reduces intestinal cramping and eases the irritation and inflammation associated with diarrhea, according to test tube studies.[25] Chamomile is typically drunk as a tea. Many doctors of natural medicine recommend dissolving 2 to 3 grams of powdered chamomile or adding 3 to 5 ml of a chamomile liquid extract to hot water and drinking it 3 or more times per day, between meals. Two to three teaspoons of the dried flowers can be steeped in a cup of hot water, covered, for 10 to 15 minutes as well.

Herbs high in mucilage, such as **marshmallow** (p. 444) or **slippery elm** (p. 460), can help reduce the irritation to the walls of the intestinal tract that can occur with diarrhea. A usual amount taken is 1,000 mg of marshmallow extract, capsules, or tablets 3 times per day. Marshmallow may also be taken as a tincture in the amount of 5 to 15 ml 3 times daily.

Other astringent herbs traditionally used for diarrhea include **blackberry** (p. 398) leaves, blackberry root bark, **blueberry** (p. 401) leaves, and **red raspberry** (p. 454) leaves.[26] Raspberry leaves are high in tannins and like its relative, blackberry, may relieve acute diarrhea. A close cousin of the blueberry, **bilberry** (p. 396), has been used in Germany for adults and children with diarrhea.[27] Only dried berries or juice should be used—fresh berries may worsen diarrhea.

Cranesbill (p. 414) has been used by a number of the indigenous tribes of North America to treat diarrhea, and the tannins in cranesbill likely account for the antidiarrheal activity[28]—although there has been little scientific research to clarify cranesbill's constituents and actions.

A tannin in **oak** (p. 448) known as ellagitannin, inhibits intestinal secretion in laboratory experiments,[29] which may help resolve diarrhea. The non-irritating nature of oak is well regarded in Germany, where it is recommended even to treat mild, acute diarrhea in children (along with plenty of electrolyte-containing fluids).[30]

Because of its antimicrobial activity, **goldenseal** (p. 429) has a long history of use for infectious diarrhea. Its major alkaloid, berberine (also found in **barberry** [p. 395] and **Oregon grape** [p. 449]), has been shown to be beneficial for people with infectious diarrhea in some double-blind studies.[31] Negative studies have generally focused on people with cholera, while positive studies have looked at viral diarrhea or diarrhea due to strains of *E. coli*. These studies generally used 400 to 500 mg berberine 1 to 3 times per day. Goldenseal extracts with standardized berberine content can be substituted, or 3 to 5 ml of tincture 3 times per day can be used.

Are There Any Side Effects or Interactions? Refer to the individual herb for information about any side effects or interactions.

Dupuytren's Contracture

In Dupuytren's contracture, a poorly understood formation of fibrous tissue occurs in the palm of the hand that can cause the last two fingers to curl up. Conventional treatments involve injection of steroids into the hand or removal of some of the diseased tissue with surgery. Even with surgery, however, recurrences are not uncommon.

Nutritional Supplements That May Be Helpful

Many decades ago, researchers investigated the effects of taking **vitamin E** (p. 344) to treat Dupuytren's contracture. Several studies reported that taking 200 to 2,000 IU of vitamin E per day for several months was helpful;[1] other studies did not find it useful.[2] Overall, there are more positive trials than negative ones,[3] although none of the published research is recent. Nonetheless, many doctors of natural medicine believe that a 3-month trial using very high amounts of vitamin E (2,000 IU per day) is worth a try.

Checklist for Dupuytren's Contracture

Ranking	Nutritional Supplements	Herbs
Other	DMSO (p. 291) Vitamin E (p. 344)	

DMSO (p. 291) may reduce pain by inhibiting transmission of pain messages, and may also soften the abnormal connective tissue associated with disorders such as Dupuytren's contracture, keloids, Peyronie's disease, and scleroderma. Research with Dupuytren's contracture remains preliminary and unproven.[4]

Are There Any Side Effects or Interactions? Refer to the individual supplement for information about any side effects or interactions.

Dysmenorrhea (Painful Menstruation)

Dysmenorrhea, or painful menstruation, is classified as either primary or secondary. Primary dysmenorrhea generally occurs within a couple of years of the first menstrual period. The pain tends to decrease with age and very often resolves after childbirth. Secondary dysmenorrhea is commonly a result of endometriosis, starts later in life, and tends to increase in intensity over time.

As many as half of menstruating women are affected by dysmenorrhea, and of these, about 10% have severe dysmenorrhea, which greatly limits activities for 1 to 3 days each month.[1]

Lifestyle Changes That May Be Helpful

Many women feel the need to lie still while experiencing menstrual cramps, while others find that exercise helps relieve the pain of dysmenorrhea. This variation from woman to woman may explain why some researchers report that exercise makes symptoms worse,[2] though most studies report that exercise appears helpful.[3]

Relaxation techniques have been used with some success to alleviate dysmenorrhea in some young women. According to one study, the symptoms of menstrual cramps, nausea, irritability, and poor concentration greatly improved after 20-minute relaxation sessions twice per week.[4]

Dietary Changes That May Be Helpful

Some nutritionally oriented physicians advise that alcohol should be avoided by women experiencing menstrual pain, because it depletes stores of certain nutrients and alters the metabolism of carbohydrates—which in turn might worsen muscle spasms. Alcohol can also interfere with the liver's ability to metabolize hormones. In theory, this might result in elevated estrogen levels, increased fluid and salt retention, and heavier menstrual flow. Despite these theoretical arguments, however, most[5,6] studies find no link between drinking alcohol and dysmenorrhea.[7]

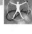

Dysmenorrhea

Nutritional Supplements That May Be Helpful

Niacin (p. 339) has been reported to be effective in relieving menstrual cramps in 87% of a group of forty women taking 200 mg of niacin per day throughout the menstrual cycle; they then took 100 mg every 2 or 3 hours while experiencing menstrual cramps.[8] In a follow-up study of 220 women, this protocol was combined with 300 mg of **vitamin C** (p. 341) and 60 mg of the **bioflavonoid** (p. 271) rutin per day, which resulted in a 90% effectiveness for relieving menstrual cramps.[9] Since these two preliminary studies were published many years ago, no further research has explored the relationship between niacin and dysmenorrhea. The effect of niacin may not be effective unless taken for 7 to 10 days before the onset of menstrual flow.

In theory, **calcium** (p. 277) may help prevent menstrual cramps by maintaining normal muscle tone. Muscles that are calcium-deficient tend to be hyperactive and therefore might be more likely to cramp. Calcium was reported to reduce pain during menses in one double-blind trial,[10] though another such study found that calcium relieved only *pre*menstrual cramping and not pain during menses.[11] Some nutritionally oriented doctors recommend calcium, suggesting 1,000 mg per day throughout the month and 250 to 500 mg every 4 hours for pain relief during acute cramping (up to a total of 2,000 mg per day).

In one double-blind trial, **fish oil** (p. 294) led to a statistically significant 37% drop in menstrual symptoms. In that report, adolescent girls with dysmenorrhea were given 1,080 mg of EPA and 720 mg of **DHA** (p. 294) per day for 2 months to achieve this result.[12] Other trials have yet to study the relationship between fish oil and dysmenorrhea. To achieve the approximate level of EPA and DHA used in this trial often takes 6,000 mg fish oil per day.

Are There Any Side Effects or Interactions? Refer to the individual supplement for information about any side effects or interactions.

Herbs That May Be Helpful

Cramp bark *(Viburnum opulus)* has been a favorite traditional herb for menstrual cramps, thus its signature name. Cramp bark may help ease severe cramps that are associated with nausea, vomiting, and sweaty chills. It has been shown to block smooth muscle spasms in experiments.[13] To use this herb, place 2 teaspoonfuls of the dried bark into a cup of water and bring to a boil; simmer gently for 10 to 15 minutes. This may be drunk 3 times per day.[14] Alternatively, 4 to 8 ml of tincture can be used 3 times per day.

Black cohosh (p. 397) has a history as a folk medicine for relieving menstrual cramps. Black cohosh can be taken in several forms, including crude, dried root, or rhizome (300 to 2,000 mg per day) or as a solid, dry powdered extract (250 mg 3 times per day). Standardized extracts of the herb are available although they have primarily been researched for use with **menopausal** (p. 118) women suffering from hot flashes. The recommended amount is 20 to 40 mg twice per day.[15] The best researched form provides 1 mg of deoxyactein per 20 mg of extract. Tinctures can be taken at 2 to 4 ml 3 times per day.[16] Black cohosh can be taken for up to 6 months, and then it should be discontinued.[17]

Blue cohosh (p. 400), although unrelated to black cohosh, also has been used traditionally for easing painful menstrual periods. Blue cohosh, which is generally taken as a tincture, should be limited to no more than 1 to 2 ml taken 3 times per day. The average single dose of the whole herb is 300 to 1,000 mg. Blue cohosh is generally used in combination with other herbs. Women of child-bearing age using this herb should cease using it as soon as they become pregnant—the herb was shown to cause heart problems in an infant born following maternal use of blue cohosh.[18]

False unicorn (p. 423) was used in the Native American tradition for a large number of women's health conditions, including painful menstruation. Generally, false unicorn root is taken as a tincture in the amount of 2 to 5 ml 3 times per day. The dried root may be used at a dose of 1 to 2 grams 3 times daily. It is almost always taken in combination with other herbs supportive of the female reproductive organs, particularly **vitex** (p. 467).

Yarrow (p. 471) was used traditionally to treat inflammation in a number of conditions, especially in female reproductive system. The German Commission E monograph suggests 4.5 grams of yarrow daily or 3 teaspoons of the fresh pressed juice.[19] A tea can be prepared by steeping 1 to 2 U.S. teaspoons (5 to 10 grams) of yarrow in 250 ml (1 cup) boiling water for 10 to 15 minutes. Three cups a day can be drunk. If tincture is preferred, 3 to 4 ml can be taken 3 times per day. The tea, or cloths dipped in the tea, can be used topically as needed.

Dong quai (p. 417) is a traditional Chinese herb that may also ease dysmenorrhea. The powdered root can be used in capsules, tablets, tinctures, or as a tea. Many women take 3 to 4 grams per day.

Chaparral (p. 410) is another herb that has been used historically for dysmenorrhea, although it should only be used topically in this regard.

Are There Any Side Effects or Interactions? Refer to the individual herb for information about any side effects or interactions.

Checklist for Dysmenorrhea (Painful Menstruation)

Ranking	Nutritional Supplements	Herbs
Secondary	Vitamin B₃ (niacin) (p. 339)	
Other	Calcium (p. 277) Fish oil (p. 294) (EPA/DHA [p. 287])	Black cohosh (p. 397) Blue cohosh (p. 400) Chaparral (p. 410) Cramp bark Dong quai (p. 417) False unicorn (p. 423) Yarrow (p. 471)
	See also: Homeopathic Remedies for **Dysmenorrhea** (p. 556)	

Ear Infections, Recurrent

Many children suffer recurrent infections of the middle ear. Antibiotics are frequently used, but the benefit is very small and side effects can result.[1,2] Likewise, inserting tubes surgically in the ear—another common conventional treatment—has not consistently provided any long-term benefit.[3]

Dietary Changes That May Be Helpful

The incidence of **allergy** (p. 8) among children with recurrent ear infections is much higher than among the general public.[4] In one study, more than half of all children with recurrent ear infections were found to be allergic to foods. Removing those foods led to significant improvement in 86% of the allergic children tested.[5] Other reports show similar results.[6,7] People with recurrent ear infections should discuss allergy diagnosis and elimination with a nutritionally oriented doctor.

Although sugar intake has not been studied in relation to recurrent ear infections, eating sugar is known to impair immune function.[8,9] Therefore, some nutritionally oriented doctors recommend that children with recurrent ear infections reduce or eliminate sugar from their diets.

Xylitol, a natural sugar found in some fruits, interferes with the growth of some bacteria that may cause ear infections. In double-blind research, children who chew gum sweetened with xylitol have a reduced risk of ear infections.[10,11]

Lifestyle Changes and Other Natural Therapies That May Be Helpful

When parents smoke, their children are more likely to have recurrent ear infections.[12] It is important that children are not exposed to passive smoke.

Humidifiers are sometimes used to help children with recurrent ear infections, and animal research has supported this approach.[13] Nonetheless, human research studying the effect of humidity on recurrent ear infections has yet to conclusively show that use of humidifiers is of significant benefit.

Nutritional Supplements That May Be Helpful

Vitamin C (p. 341) has stimulated **immune function** (p. 94) in most studies.[14,15] Vitamin C has not been studied by itself in regard to ear infections; nonetheless, some nutritionally oriented doctors recommend between 500 mg and 1,000 mg of vitamin C per day for people with ear infections.

Zinc (p. 346) supplements increase immune function,[16,17] although research showing this has not studied people with ear infections. Some nutritionally oriented doctors nonetheless recommend zinc supplements for people with recurrent ear infections, suggesting 25 mg per day for adults and lower amounts for children. For example, a 30-pound child could be given 5 mg of zinc.

Are There Any Side Effects or Interactions? Refer to the individual supplement for information about any side effects or interactions.

Herbs That May Be Helpful

It has been suggested that some children with recurrent ear infections may benefit from **echinacea** (p. 417), which helps support healthy short-term **immune response** (p. 341).[18] Echinacea should be started as soon as symptoms start to appear and continued until a few days after they are gone. It has been recommended that children take 1 to 2 ml (depending on age) of tincture 3 times per day or more.[19] Research has not been done to determine if taking echinacea regularly will reduce symptoms or prevent recurrences of ear infections.

Ear drops with **mullein** (p. 446), **St. John's wort** (p. 461), and **garlic** (p. 425) in an oil or glycerin base are traditional remedies used to alleviate symptoms, particularly pain, during acute ear infections. Oil preparations may obscure a physician's view of the eardrum.

Eczema

Are There Any Side Effects or Interactions? Refer to the individual herb for information about any side effects or interactions.

Checklist for Recurrent Ear Infections

Ranking	Nutritional Supplements	Herbs
Other	Vitamin C (p. 341) Zinc (p. 346)	Echinacea (p. 417) Garlic (p. 425) Mullein (p. 446) St. John's wort (p. 461)
See also: Homeopathic Remedies for **Ear Infections** (p. 534)		

Eczema

Eczema is a common skin condition characterized by an itchy, red rash. Many skin diseases cause somewhat similar rashes, so it is important to have the disease properly diagnosed before it can be treated.

Dietary Changes That May Be Helpful

Eczema can be triggered by **allergies** (p. 8).[1,2] Most children with eczema have food allergies, according to data from double-blind research.[3] A nutritionally oriented doctor should be consulted to determine if allergies are a factor. Once the trigger for the allergy has been identified, avoidance of the allergen can lead to significant improvement.[4]

It has been reported that when heavy coffee drinkers with eczema avoided coffee, eczema symptoms improved.[5] In this study, the reaction was to coffee—not caffeine, indicating that some people with eczema may be allergic to coffee. People with eczema who are using a hypoallergenic diet (with the guidance of a nutritionally oriented doctor) to investigate food allergies should avoid coffee as part of this trial.

Nutritional Supplements That May Be Helpful

Researchers have reported that people with eczema do not have the normal ability to process fatty acids, which can result in a deficiency of gamma-linolenic acid (GLA).[6] GLA is found in **evening primrose oil (EPO)** (p. 292), **borage** (p. 402) oil, and black currant seed oil. Most double-blind research has shown that EPO overcomes this block and is useful in the treatment of eczema.[7,8,9] An analysis of nine placebo-controlled trials reported that effects for reduced itching were most striking.[10] Much of the research uses 12 pills per day; each pill contains 500 mg of EPO, of which 45 mg is GLA. Smaller amounts have been shown to lack efficacy.[11] One study questioned the effectiveness of evening primrose oil for treating eczema;[12] however, this negative study has been criticized.[13]

Borage oil has also been employed for eczema in open clinical trials, which showed reductions in skin inflammation, dryness, scaliness, and itch.[14] However, a controlled study using 360 mg of GLA daily from borage in people with eczema was unable to reproduce these results.[15]

Older reports using large amounts of vegetable oil (containing precursors to GLA) claimed some success,[16,17] but these studies were not controlled and do not meet modern standards of research. As a result, it makes more sense to use GLA-containing oils (particularly EPO), rather than vegetable oil.

Ten grams of **fish oil** (p. 294) providing 1.8 grams of EPA (eicosapentaenoic acid) per day were given to a group of eczema sufferers in a double-blind trial. After 12 weeks, those using the fish oil experienced significant improvement.[18,19] According to the researchers, fish oil may be effective because it reduces levels of leukotriene B$_4$, a substance that has been linked to eczema.[20] The eczema-relieving effects of fish oil may require taking 10 pills per day of fish oil taken for at least 12 weeks. Smaller amounts of fish oil have been shown to lack efficacy.[21]

One trial reporting that fish oil was barely more effective than placebo (30% versus 24% improvement) used vegetable oil as the placebo.[22] As vegetable oil has previously been reported to have therapeutic activity, the apparent negative outcome of this trial should not dissuade people with eczema from considering fish oil.

Although **vitamin E** (p. 344) at 400 IU per day has been reported in anecdotal accounts to alleviate eczema,[23] research has not supported this effect.[24] Moreover, rare cases of topical vitamin E potentially causing *eczema have appeared.[25] People with eczema should not expect vitamin E to be helpful with their condition.*

In 1989, *Medical World News* reported that researchers from the University of Texas found that **vitamin C** (p. 341), at 50 to 75 mg per 2.2 pounds of body weight, reduced symptoms of eczema in a double-blind trial.[26] In theory, vitamin C might be beneficial in treating eczema by affecting the immune system, but further research has yet to investigate any role for this vitamin in people with eczema.

Are There Any Side Effects or Interactions? Refer to the individual supplement for information about any side effects or interactions.

Herbs That May Be Helpful

Licorice root (p. 440), used either internally or topically, may help alleviate symptoms of eczema. A traditional Chinese herbal preparation, which includes licorice, has been successful in treating childhood and adult eczema in double-blind studies.[27,28] The product, known as Zemaphyte, is currently under investigation in England. One or two packets of the combination is mixed in hot water and taken once per day. Topically, glycyrrhetinic acid, a constituent of licorice root, reduces the inflammation and itching associated with eczema.[29] Some doctors who use herbal medicine suggest applying creams or ointments containing glycyrrhetinic acid 3 or 4 times per day. Licorice root may also be taken as a tincture in the amount of 2 to 5 ml 3 times daily.

Numerous other herbal preparations are used topically to relieve the redness and itching of eczema. A cream prepared with **witch hazel** (p. 470) and **phosphatidyl choline** (p. 307) has been reported to be as effective as 1% hydrocortisone in the topical management of eczema, according to one double-blind study.[30]

Other topical herbal preparations to consider based on traditional herbal medicine are **chamomile** (p. 409), **calendula** (p. 406), and **chickweed** (p. 411) creams. Chamomile and calendula have anti-inflammatory properties, while chickweed is historically used to reduce itching. Research studies have not documented the efficacy of creams of any of these three herbs for people with eczema.

Although **burdock** (p. 405) root is listed in traditional herbal books for the treatment of eczema, there is little evidence to support its use for this condition. It was used historically on the theory that supporting healthy liver function could help the body to remove potentially skin-damaging compounds from circulation.

Sarsaparilla (p. 457) may be beneficial as an anti-inflammatory based on historical accounts. Capsules or tablets should provide at least 9 grams of the dried root per day, usually taken in divided doses. Tincture is used in the amount of 3 ml 3 times per day.

In traditional herbal medicine, **red clover** (p. 453) is considered beneficial for all manner of chronic conditions, particularly those afflicting the skin. However, the mechanism of action and responsible constituents for red clover's purported benefit in skin conditions is unknown. **Wild oats** (p. 448) has historically been used to treat a variety of skin conditions, including eczema, but it, too, is without scientific investigation.

Tannins, the main therapeutic component of **oak** (p. 448) bark, bind liquids, absorb toxins, and soothe inflamed tissues. For eczema characterized by oozing or weeping, oak is applied topically by first boiling 1 to 2 U.S. tablespoons (15 to 30 grams) of the bark for 15 minutes in 500 ml (2 cups) of water. After cooling, a cloth is dipped into the liquid and applied directly to the rash several times a day. The liquid prepared this way in the morning can be used throughout the day; unused portions should be discarded after that. This approach has been helpful in clinical practice[31] but has yet to be scrutinized scientifically.

Are There Any Side Effects or Interactions? Refer to the individual herb for information about any side effects or interactions.

Checklist for Eczema

Ranking	Nutritional Supplements	Herbs
Primary	Evening primrose oil (p. 292)	
Secondary	Fish oil (p. 294) (EPA/DHA [p. 287])	Borage (p. 402) Licorice (p. 440) Oak (p. 448) Witch hazel (p. 470)
Other	Vitamin C (p. 341)	Calendula (p. 406) Chamomile (p. 409) Chickweed (p. 411) Oak (p. 448) Oats (p. 448) Red clover (p. 453) Sarsaparilla (p. 457)

See also: Homeopathic Remedies for **Eczema** (p. 535)

Edema (Water Retention)

Abnormal accumulation of fluid beneath the skin is known as edema. This leads to a puffy appearance often to a limb, most commonly a leg. There are many causes of edema. In some cases, the underlying problem (for example **congestive heart failure** [p. 43] or preeclampsia of pregnancy) must be medically treated in order for the edema to resolve. In other cases (such as **chronic venous insufficiency** [p. 38] or edema following **minor trauma** [p. 122]) it is possible with both conventional and natural approaches to focus specifically on the edema. Unless it is clearly due to minor trauma, edema should never be treated until the underlying cause has been properly diagnosed by a health-care professional. The discussion below deals only with situations in which it is safe to focus on the edema itself and not the underlying cause.

Lifestyle Changes That May Helpful

The affected limb should be kept elevated whenever possible. This uses gravity to pull fluid out of the congested area. To decrease fluid buildup in the legs, individuals should avoid sitting or standing for long periods of time without moving.

Dietary Changes That May Be Helpful

High salt intake should be avoided, as it tends to lead to water retention and in some people may worsen edema.

Nutritional Supplements That May Be Helpful

Coumarin is a bioflavonoid-like compound, found in a variety of herbs, that has been used for edema. Because coumarin is not widely available in the U.S., other **bioflavonoids** (p. 271) such as **quercetin** (p. 328) and rutin can be substituted in an attempt to get similar benefits. Both animal[1] and human[2] studies have found that coumarin can be beneficial in treating edema. Even edema after surgery (when lymph drainage is damaged) has been helped by coumarin. However, a large double-blind study detected no benefit using 200 mg coumarin twice daily for 6 months in women who had arm edema after mastectomy.[3] (Coumarin should not be confused with the anticlotting drug Coumadin.)

Other bioflavonoid-type compounds from medicinal plants, known as hydroxyethylrutosides, are also beneficial for edema.[4] The ideal amount of the bioflavonoids quercetin and rutin is unknown, but 1,000 mg of mixed bioflavonoids taken 3 times each day is a standard recommendation by many doctors of natural medicine.

Are There Any Side Effects or Interactions? Refer to the individual supplement for information about any side effects or interactions.

Herbs That May Be Helpful

Herbs that stimulate the kidneys were traditionally used to reduce edema. Herbal diuretics do not work the same way that drugs do; thus it is unclear if such herbs would be effective for this purpose. Goldenrod is considered one of the strongest herbal diuretics.[5] Although human trials have not yet been conducted, animal research shows another commonly used diuretic herb, **dandelion** (p. 415) leaves, to be as powerful as the drug Lasix.[6] Corn silk *(Zea mays)* has also long been used as a diuretic, though a human study did not find that it increased urine output.[7] Thus,

diuretic herbs are not yet well supported for use in reducing edema.

Aescin isolated from **horse chestnut** (p. 435) seed has been shown to effectively reduce postsurgical edema.[8,9] Generally, extracts standardized to provide 90 to 120 mg aescin per day are used. If these are not available, horse chestnut tincture can be substituted at a dose of 2 to 3 ml (½ teaspoon) 3 times each day by mouth, usually in combination with other approaches. Creams applied topically 3 or more times per day are also sometimes recommended by doctors of natural medicine.

Horsetail (p. 436) contains several types of bioflavonoids that are believed to be responsible for this herb's diuretic action and that help account for its traditional use in reducing mild edema. The volatile oils in **juniper** (p. 437) cause an increase in urine volume and in this way can theoretically lessen edema.[10] In either case, there is no clinical research that yet supports their use for people with edema.

Cleavers (p. 412) is one of numerous plants considered diuretic in ancient times.[11] It was therefore used to relieve edema and to promote urine formation during bladder infections. **Meadowsweet** (p. 444) was also used historically as a diuretic for persons with poor urinary flow.

Are There Any Side Effects or Interactions? Refer to the individual herb for information about any side effects or interactions.

Checklist for Edema (Water Retention)

Ranking	Nutritional Supplements	Herbs
Secondary	Coumarin, Hydroxyethylrutosides	
Other	Bioflavonoids (p. 271) (quercetin [p. 328], rutin)	Cleavers (p. 412) Corn silk Dandelion (leaves) (p. 415) Goldenrod Horse chestnut (p. 435) Horsetail (p. 436) Juniper (p. 437) Meadowsweet (p. 444)

See also: Homeopathic Remedies for **Edema** (p. 536)

Fibrocystic Breast Disease

Fibrocystic breast disease is a term colloquially given to a group of benign conditions affecting the breast.

This group of conditions is very common in younger women. Both breasts become tender or painful and lumpy, and the symptoms vary at different times in the menstrual cycle. Despite the fact that signs and symptoms of fibrocystic disease appear to be quite distinct from textbook signs and symptoms of breast cancer, any lump in the breast should be diagnosed by a health-care professional to rule out the possibility of cancer.

Dietary Changes That May Be Helpful

Long-term and complete avoidance of caffeine reduces symptoms of fibrocystic disease.[1,2] Caffeine is found in coffee, black and green tea, cola drinks, chocolate, and a number of over-the-counter drugs. The decrease in breast tenderness can take 6 months or more to occur after caffeine is eliminated. Breast lumpiness may not go away, but the pain often decreases.

Many doctors are confused about the effects of caffeine on breast tissue, because at first glance, the research appears contradictory. When researchers tell women to cut back or to eliminate caffeine for less than 6 months, results are unimpressive.[3,4] Moreover, for every study that says people with fibrocystic disease do not drink more coffee than other women,[5,6] there is a study that says otherwise.[7,8] More important, the original research did not claim that those with fibrocystic disease drink much coffee—only that they are especially sensitive to the coffee they do drink.

Twins with similar or identical genes should be affected similarly by caffeine. Research has been done studying the effects of caffeine on breast symptoms in twins. In that report, the twin with symptoms was more likely to be the coffee drinker.[9] This evidence clearly supports the idea that coffee drinking can affect breast symptoms in some women.

Fibrocystic disease has been linked to excess estrogen. When those with fibrocystic disease are put on a lowfat diet, their estrogen levels decrease.[10,11] After 3 to 6 months, the pain and lumpiness also decrease.[12,13] The link between fat and symptoms appears to be most strongly related to saturated fat.[14] Foods high in saturated fat include meat and dairy products. Fish, nonfat dairy, and tofu are possible replacements.

Lifestyle Changes That May Be Helpful

Exercise may decrease breast tenderness. In one study, women who ran 45 miles per menstrual cycle reported less breast tenderness as well as improvement in other symptoms, such as anxiety.[15]

Nutritional Supplements That May Be Helpful

Several studies report that 200–600 IU of **vitamin E** (p. 344) per day, taken for several months, reduces symptoms.[16,17] Most double-blind research has not found vitamin E to relieve fibrocystic breast disease symptoms, however.[18,19] Nonetheless, many women take 400 IU of vitamin E for 3 months to see if it helps.

As with vitamin E, the effectiveness of **vitamin B$_6$** (p. 340) remains unclear. Some,[20] but not all,[21] studies find that B$_6$ reduces symptoms. Women with **premenstrual syndrome** (p. 141) in addition to breast tenderness should discuss the use of vitamin B$_6$ with their nutritionally oriented doctor.

Some doctors of natural medicine use **iodine** (p. 303) for fibrocystic symptoms.[22] In animals, iodine deficiency can cause the equivalent of fibrocystic disease. What appears to be the most effective form— diatomic iodine[23]—is not readily available. Because some people are sensitive to iodine and high amounts can alter thyroid function, it should not be taken without a doctor's involvement.

In double-blind research, **evening primrose oil (EPO)** (p. 292) has reduced symptoms of fibrocystic disease.[24,25] However, the amount of improvement caused by EPO appears to be slight.[26] One group of researchers have reported that EPO normalizes blood levels of fatty acids in women with fibrocystic disease.[27] However, even these scientists had difficulty correlating the improvement in lab work with an actual reduction in symptoms. Nonetheless, most reports continue to show at least some reduction in symptoms resulting from EPO supplementation.[28,29] As a result, many nutritionally oriented doctors recommend a trial of 3 grams per day of EPO for at least 6 months to alleviate symptoms of fibrocystic breast disease.

Are There Any Side Effects or Interactions? Refer to the individual supplement for information about any side effects or interactions.

Herbs That May Be Helpful

Since many women with fibrocystic breast disease and cyclical breast tenderness also suffer from **premenstrual syndrome (PMS)** (p. 141), there is often an overlap in herbal recommendations for these two conditions despite a lack of research dealing directly with fibrocystic disease.

Vitex (p. 467) has been shown to help re-establish normal balance of estrogen and progesterone during a woman's menstrual cycle. This is important because some women may suffer from **PMS** (p. 141) and other menstrual irregularities due to underproduction of the hormone **progesterone** (p. 326) during the second half of their cycle. Vitex stimulates the pituitary gland to produce more luteinizing hormone, and this leads to a greater production of progesterone.[30] Studies have shown that using vitex once in the morning over a period of several months will help normalize hormone balance and alleviate symptoms of PMS.[31]

Doctors who use herbal medicine will typically suggest 40 drops of a liquid, concentrated vitex extract or one capsule of the equivalent dried, powdered extract to be taken once per day in the morning with some liquid. Vitex should be taken for at least four cycles to determine efficacy.

In traditional Chinese medicine, **Dong quai** (p. 417), or *Angelica sinensis*, is often referred to as the "female ginseng." Dong quai helps promote normal hormone balance and is particularly useful for women experiencing premenstrual cramping and pain.[32] Many doctors of natural medicine recommend 2 to 3 grams of dong quai capsules or tablets per day. Nonetheless, research has yet to link dong quai to a reduction in symptoms of fibrocystic disease.

Are There Any Side Effects or Interactions? Refer to the individual herb for information about any side effects or interactions.

Checklist for Fibrocystic Breast Disease

Ranking	Nutritional Supplements	Herbs
Secondary	Evening Primrose Oil (p. 292)	
Other	Iodine (p. 303) Vitamin B$_6$ (p. 340) Vitamin E (p. 344)	Dong Quai (p. 417) Vitex (p. 467)

Fibromyalgia

Fibromyalgia is a complex syndrome with no known cause or cure. Its predominant symptom is severe muscle pain, although other symptoms such as fatigue, chest pain, low-grade fever, swollen lymph nodes, **insomnia** (p. 105), frequent abdominal pain, **irritable bowel syndrome** (p. 109), and **depression** (p. 50), may accompany the muscle pain.[1]

Of the estimated three to six million people[2] afflicted with this disorder in the United States, the majority are women between 25 and 45 years of age.

Lifestyle Changes That May Be Helpful

Low-intensity exercise may improve fibromyalgia symptoms. People with fibromyalgia who exercise regularly have been reported to suffer less severe symptoms than those who remain sedentary.[3 4 5] Stress is believed by some researchers to be capable of exacerbating symptoms. Stress-reduction techniques such as meditation have also proven helpful in preliminary research.[6] Acupuncture has significantly improved symptoms in several trials studying people with fibromyalgia.[7,8]

Nutritional Supplements That May Be Helpful

A preliminary trial suggested that a combination of **magnesium** (p. 310) and **malic acid** (p. 311) might lessen muscle pain.[9] The amounts used in this preliminary trial were 300 to 600 mg of elemental magnesium and 1,200 to 2,400 mg of malic acid per day, taken for 8 weeks. A double-blind report by the same research group using 300 mg magnesium and 1,200 mg malic acid failed to show a reduction in symptoms.[10] Though these researchers claimed that magnesium and malic acid appeared to have some effect at higher levels (up to 600 mg magnesium and 2,400 mg malic acid), the positive effects were reported only in unblinded research. Therefore, the evidence supporting the use of these supplements for people with fibromyalgia remains weak and inconclusive.

Other studies have found people with fibromyalgia to have low **vitamin B$_1$** (p. 337) status and reduced activity of some thiamine-dependent enzymes.[11,12] What, if any, clinical role this marginal deficiency plays in fibromyalgia symptoms remains unknown.

One early preliminary study described the use of **vitamin E** (p. 344) supplements in the treatment of "fibrositis"—probably the rough equivalent of what is today called fibromyalgia. Several dozen individuals were treated with vitamin E in the range of 100 to 300 IU per day with positive and sometimes dramatic benefit.[13]

Some,[14,15] but not all,[16] double-blind trials using intravenous S-adenosylmethionine (**SAMe** [p. 330]) in people with fibromyalgia have led to a reduction in pain and depression. When 800 mg of SAMe was given orally to people with fibromyalgia for 6 weeks in a double-blind trial, pain and morning stiffness decreased significantly, but effects on other symptoms were equivocal.[17]

Individuals with fibromyalgia often have low serotonin levels in their blood.[18,19,20] Supplementation with 5-HTP (p. 295) may increase serotonin synthesis in these cases. Both preliminary[21] and double-blind studies[22] have reported that 5-HTP relieves some symptoms of fibromyalgia.

Are There Any Side Effects or Interactions? Refer to the individual supplement for information about any side effects or interactions.

Herbs That May Be Helpful

While no herbal supplements have been studied specifically for fibromyalgia, herbs used to relieve symptoms of **chronic fatigue syndrome (CFS)** (p. 36) might also be useful for fibromyalgia. These include the initial use of 2 grams of **licorice root** (p. 440) 3 times per day for 6 to 8 weeks, followed by the ongoing use of an adaptogenic herb, such as **Asian ginseng** (p. 394), 1 to 2 grams per day, or **eleuthero** (p. 419) (Siberian ginseng), 2 to 3 grams per day. Licorice needs to be used in its whole form; deglycyrrhizinated licorice (DGL) extracts will not work.

Are There Any Side Effects or Interactions? Refer to the individual herb for information about any side effects or interactions.

Checklist for Fibromyalgia

Ranking	Nutritional Supplements	Herbs
Secondary	5-HTP (p. 295)	
Other	Magnesium (p. 310) Malic acid (p. 311) SAMe (p. 330) Vitamin B₁ (p. 337) Vitamin E (p. 344)	Asian ginseng (p. 394) Eleuthero (p. 419) Licorice (p. 440)
See also: Homeopathic Remedies for **Fibromyalgia** (p. 538)		

Gallstones

Gallbladder attacks cause extreme pain in the upper-right quarter of the abdomen, often moving to the back. This pain can be accompanied by nausea and vomiting. The attacks frequently occur when gallstones block the bile duct.

Gallstones are formed in the gallbladder, primarily of cholesterol. They are commonly associated with bile that contains excessive cholesterol, a deficiency of other substances in bile (bile acids and lecithin), or a combination of these factors.

Dietary Changes That May Be Helpful

Cholesterol (p. 79) is the primary ingredient in most gallstones. Some,[1] but not all,[2] research links dietary cholesterol to the risk of gallstones. Some doctors of natural medicine suggest avoiding eggs, either due to their high cholesterol content or because eggs may be allergenic. (See the discussion about gallstones and allergies below.)

Most studies report that vegetarians are at low risk for gallstones.[3] In some trials, vegetarians have had only half the risk compared with gallstone risk in meat eaters.[4,5] Vegetarians often eat fewer calories and less cholesterol. They also tend to weigh less than meat eaters. All of these differences may reduce gallstone incidence. The specific factors in a vegetarian diet that associate with a low risk of gallstone formation remain somewhat unclear and may occur only in certain vegetarian diets and not others. For example, research from India found that vegetarians eating a high vegetable-fat diet have been reported to have elevated rather than reduced risks of gallstone formation.[6,7]

Constipation (p. 44) has been linked to the risk of forming gallstones.[8] When constipation is successfully resolved, it has reduced the risk of gallstone formation.[9] Wheat bran, commonly used to relieve constipation when combined with fluid, has been reported to reduce the relative amount of cholesterol in bile of a small group of people whose bile contained excessive cholesterol.[10] The same effect has been reported in people who already have gallstones.[11] Such a change in the relative constituents of bile should reduce the risk of gallstone formation. Nutritionally oriented doctors sometimes recommend starting with a quarter cup of bran per day, often eaten with cereal in the morning. Bran should always be accompanied by fluid. Adding more bran may cause gastrointestinal symptoms and should only be done with the guidance of a nutritionally oriented doctor.

Gallbladder attacks (though not the stones themselves) have been reported to result from **food allergies** (p. 8). The one study to examine this relationship found that all sixty-nine of the subjects with gallbladder problems showed relief from gallbladder pain when allergy-provoking foods were identified[12] and

Gallstones

eliminated from the diet. Egg, pork, and onions were reported to be the most common triggers. Pain returned when the problem foods were reintroduced into the diet. Nutritionally oriented doctors can help diagnose food allergies.

Lifestyle Changes That May Be Helpful

People with gallstones may consume too many calories[13] and are often overweight.[14] Obese women have seven times the risk of forming gallstones compared with women who are not overweight.[15] Even slightly overweight women have significantly higher risks.[16] Losing weight is likely to help,[17] but *rapid* weight loss might increase the risk of stone formation.[18] Any weight-loss program should be reviewed by a doctor. **Weight loss** (p. 165) plans generally entail reducing dietary fat, a change that itself correlates with protection against gallstone formation and attacks.[19,20]

Nutritional Supplements That May Be Helpful

Vitamin C (p. 341) is needed to convert cholesterol to bile acids. In theory, such a conversion should reduce gallstone risks. Vitamin C–deficient animals have a high incidence of gallstones. Vegetarians, who have a reduced risk of gallstones in most research, usually consume more vitamin C than do meat eaters. As a result of these pieces of evidence, some researchers speculate that vitamin C might help prevent gallstones.[21] One group of researchers reported that people who drink alcohol and take vitamin C supplements had only half the risk of gallstones when compared with other drinkers, though the apparent protective effect of vitamin C did not appear in nondrinkers.[22] In another trial, supplementation with vitamin C (500 mg taken 4 times per day for 2 weeks before gallbladder surgery) led to improvement in one parameter of gallstone risk ("nucleation time"), though there was no change in the relative level of cholesterol found in bile.[23] While many nutritionally oriented doctors recommend vitamin C supplementation to people with a history of gallstones, supportive evidence remains preliminary.

According to one older report, people with gallstones were likely to have insufficient stomach acid.[24] Some nutritionally oriented doctors assess adequacy of stomach acid in people with gallstones and, if appropriate, supplement with **betaine HCl** (p. 269). Nonetheless, no research has yet explored whether such supplementation reduces symptoms of gallbladder disease.

Phosphatidyl choline (PC) (p. 307), a purified extract from **lecithin** (p. 307), is one of the components of bile that helps protect against gallstone formation. Some preliminary studies suggest that 300 to 2,000 mg per day of PC is helpful.[25,26] Although not every study reports success,[27] some nutritionally oriented doctors suggest PC supplements as part of gallstone treatment.

Are There Any Side Effects or Interactions? Refer to the individual supplement for information about any side effects or interactions.

Herbs That May Be Helpful

Milk thistle (p. 445) extracts in capsules or tablets may be beneficial in preventing gallstones. In one study, silymarin (the active component of milk thistle) reduced cholesterol levels in bile,[28] which is one important way to avoid gallstones formation. The recommended amount to use is 600 mg of milk thistle extract (standardized to 70 to 80% silymarin) per day, which equates to 420 mg of silymarin per day.

A mixture of essential oils has been shown to occasionally dissolve gallstones when taken for several months in uncontrolled studies.[29] The greatest benefits occurred when the oils were combined with chenodeoxycholic acid, a prescription drug.[30] However, only about 10% of people with gallstones have shown significant dissolution as a result of taking essential oils. The closest available product to that which was used by these researchers is **peppermint** (p. 451) oil. Use of peppermint or any other essential oil to dissolve gallstones should only be attempted with close supervision of a doctor of natural medicine.

Numerous herbs known variously as cholagogues and choleretics have a reputation for helping prevent gallstones in traditional herbalism. Cholagogues are herbs that stimulate the gall bladder to contract, while choleretics stimulate the liver to secrete more bile. Both of these actions could potentially help reduce the risk of developing gallstones. No modern studies have been done to test these hypotheses. **Artichoke** (p. 393), **turmeric** (p. 465), fumitory (*Fumaria officinalis*), fringe tree (*Chionanthus virginicus*), greater celandine (*Chelidonium majus*), **dandelion** (p. 415) root, **barberry** (p. 395), and **Oregon grape** (p. 449) are cholagogues and choleretics. Greater celandine should only be used on the advice of a doctor of natural medicine. With the exception of fumitory, all of these herbs should be avoided during acute gallbladder attacks.

Are There Any Side Effects or Interactions? Refer to the individual herb for information about any side effects or interactions.

Checklist for Gallstones

Ranking	Nutritional Supplements	Herbs
Secondary	Phosphatidyl Choline (p. 307) Wheat bran	Peppermint oil (p. 451)
Other	Betaine HCl (p. 269) Vitamin C (p. 341)	Artichoke (p. 393) Barberry (p. 395) Dandelion (p. 415) (root) Fumitory Fringe tree, Greater celandine, Milk thistle (p. 445) Oregon grape (p. 449) Turmeric (p. 465)

See also: Homeopathic Remedies for **Gallstones** (p. 539)

Gastritis

Gastritis is a broad term for inflammation or irritation of the inner lining (mucosa) of the stomach. This condition can be caused by many factors and, in some cases, may lead to an ulcer (p. 158). For that reason, many of the same nutrients, herbs, and lifestyle changes that might benefit a person with a peptic ulcer might also help someone with gastritis. See the chapter on peptic ulcer for more information.

Bacterial infections, most notably *Helicobacter pylori,*[1] the same bug often responsible for peptic ulcers, is a major cause of gastritis. When addressing treatments for gastritis, many researchers now look for substances that eradicate *H. pylori,* including bismuth[2] and antibiotics.[3]

Other causes of gastritis include ingestion of caustic poisons, alcohol, and certain medications like aspirin or steroids as well as physical stress from the **flu** (p. 104), major surgery, severe burns, or injuries. For some, a drug allergy or food poisoning can prompt gastritis. Atrophic gastritis is a form of gastritis found particularly in the elderly, where stomach cells are destroyed, potentially leading to pernicious anemia.

Dietary Changes That May Be Helpful

Salt can irritate the stomach lining. Some research suggests that eating salty foods increases the risk of developing a *H. pylori* infection.[4] Researchers have speculated that increased salt intake may increase the risk of gastritis.[5]

Doctors commonly suggest that people with gastritis avoid spicy foods. However, one study found that capsaicin, the pungent ingredient in **cayenne** (p. 408) or chili, has protected against aspirin-induced gastritis in healthy persons. When eighteen people ate chili followed by 600 mg of aspirin, stomach injury was considerably less than in individuals who took only aspirin.[6] The researchers of this study speculate that chili helps by increasing blood flow to the stomach. Capsaicin has also been shown to protect against gastritis caused by excessive alcohol intake in rats,[7] though this has yet to be tested in humans.

Some researchers have suggested that **food allergies** (p. 8) or intolerance may be a causative factor in gastritis.[8] In one double-blind report, people with proven food sensitivities showed clear evidence of irritation of the stomach lining (including swelling, bleeding, and erosions) when challenged with foods to which they were known to react.[9] However, most of these people did not have abnormal results from standard blood tests for allergies. People suspecting food sensitivities or allergies should consider discussing an allergy elimination program with a nutritionally oriented doctor.

Lifestyle Changes That May Be Helpful

Gastritis is common among alcoholics.[10] Both heavy smoking and excessive alcohol consumption are known causes of acute gastritis.[11]

Many medications, such as aspirin and related drugs, can induce or aggravate stomach irritation.[12] People with a history of gastritis should never take aspirin or aspirin-like drugs without first discussing the matter with their doctor.

Caffeine found in coffee, black and **green tea** (p. 430), some soft drinks, chocolate, and many medications increases stomach acid,[13] though decaffeinated coffee does as well.[14] Avoiding these substances should therefore aid in the healing of gastritis.

Nutritional Supplements That May Be Helpful

When *Helicobacter* causes gastritis, free radical levels rise in the stomach lining.[15] These unstable molecules contribute to inflammation and gastric damage. **Vitamin C** (p. 336), an antioxidant that helps squelch free radical molecules, is low in the stomach juice of people with chronic gastritis. When people with gastritis took 500 mg of vitamin C twice a day, vitamin C levels in their gastric juice rose.[16] However, there is no direct evidence that taking vitamin C actually improves gastritis.

There is some evidence that the antioxidant **beta-carotene** (p. 268) may also reduce free radical damage in the stomach,[17] and eating foods high in beta-carotene has been linked to a decreased risk of developing chronic atrophic gastritis.[18] Moreover, people with active gastritis have been reported to have low levels of beta-carotene in their stomachs.[19] In preliminary research from Russia, giving 30,000 IU beta-carotene per day to people with **ulcers** (p. 158) or gastritis led to the disappearance of gastric erosions.[20] Combining vitamin C and beta-carotene also led to improvement in most people with chronic atrophic gastritis.[21]

Several amino acids have shown promise for people with gastritis. In a double-blind study, taking 200 mg of cysteine 4 times daily provided significant benefit for fifty-six individuals with bleeding gastritis caused by NSAIDs (nonsteroidal anti-inflammatory drugs, like aspirin) use.[22] Cysteine is a sulfur-containing amino acid that stimulates healing of gastritis. In another trial, preliminary findings showed that 1 to 4 grams of **N-acetyl cysteine** (p. 317) given to people with atrophic gastritis for 4 weeks appeared to increase healing.[23] **Glutamine** (p. 300) is a main energy source for cells in the stomach and may also increase blood flow to this region.[24] When burn victims were supplemented with the amino acid glutamine, they did not develop stress ulcers even after several operations.[25] It remains unclear to what extent glutamine supplementation might prevent or help existing gastritis. Preliminary evidence suggests that the amino acid **L-arginine** (p. 268) may both protect the stomach and increase its blood flow,[26] but research has yet to investigate the effects of arginine in people with gastritis.

Zinc (p. 346) and **vitamin A** (p. 336), nutrients that aid in healing, are commonly used to help people with peptic ulcers. For example, the ulcers of individuals taking 220 mg of zinc 3 times per day healed three times faster than those of people who took placebo.[27] While the research does not yet show that zinc specifically helps people with gastritis, taking it may nevertheless be useful. The amount of zinc used in this study is very high compared with what most people take (15 to 40 mg per day). Even at these levels, it is necessary to take 1 to 3 mg of **copper** (p. 285) per day to avoid a copper deficiency.

People who took 50,000 IU of vitamin A 3 times a day experienced a significant decrease in both ulcer size and pain.[28] Because this amount of vitamin A is very high and can be quite toxic, usage requires the guidance of a nutritionally oriented doctor. A safe amount for women of childbearing age is 10,000 IU per day and probably 25,000 IU for other adults. In preliminary research from Bulgaria, using vitamin A together with drugs and proper nutrition eliminated erosive gastritis after 3 weeks in three-quarters of affected individuals.[29]

People with pernicious anemia due to atrophic gastritis require very high amounts of **vitamin B$_{12}$** (p. 337). See a discussion of pernicious anemia in the vitamin B$_{12}$ chapter.

Several human trials suggest that **gamma oryzanol** (p. 298) might help people with gastritis and other gastrointestinal complaints. In one study, twenty-two individuals with chronic gastritis were given 300 mg of gamma oryzanol per day.[30] After 2 weeks, five of these people reported that gamma oryzanol was extremely effective and twelve said it was moderately effective. Overall, 87% experienced some benefit. Another study revealed similar results. Eighteen people with various types of gastritis also received 300 mg of gamma oryzanol per day.[31] After 2 weeks, more than 62% of those with superficial gastritis and over 87% with atrophic gastritis benefited; all individuals with erosive gastritis were helped.

In a large hospital study, approximately 2,000 people with various gastrointestinal complaints, including gastritis, were given gamma oryzanol in divided amounts of 100 mg 3 times per day.[32] In this study, some individuals required as much as 600 mg per day before their symptoms improved. While most took this supplement for less than a month, some took it longer, up to 275 days. People with gastritis wishing to take gamma oryzanol for long periods of time, or in amounts exceeding 300 mg per day, should first consult with a nutritionally oriented physician.

Herbs That May Be Helpful

Many of the same herbs that are helpful for peptic ulcers may also aid people with gastritis. **Licorice** (p. 440) root, for example, has been traditionally used to soothe inflammation and injury in the stomach. It also stalls the growth of *H. pylori*.[33] To avoid potential side effects, such as increasing blood pressure and water weight gain, many physicians use deglycyrrhizinated licorice (DGL). This form of licorice retains its healing qualities by removing the glycyrrhizin that causes problems in some people.

Goldenseal (p. 429) is noted as an herbal antibiotic and is used specifically for infections of the mucous membranes. While no specific research points to goldenseal as a treatment for gastritis, there is some evidence that berberine, an active ingredient in goldenseal, slows growth of *H. pylori*.[34]

Chamomile (p. 409), high in the bioflavonoid apigenin, can ease injured and inflamed mucous membranes. In addition, research has shown that apigenin inhibits *H. pylori*,[35] and chamazulene, another active ingredient in chamomile, reduces free radical activity,[36] both potential advantages for people with gastritis.

Demulcent herbs, such as **marshmallow** (p. 444) and **slippery elm** (p. 460), are high in mucilage. Mucilage might be advantageous for people with gastritis because its slippery nature soothes an irritated digestive tract. Marshmallow is utilized for mild inflammation of the gastric mucosa.[37]

Checklist for Gastritis

Ranking	Nutritional Supplements	Herbs
Primary	Gamma oryzanol (p. 298)	
Secondary	N-acetyl cysteine (p. 317)	
Other	L-arginine (p. 268) Beta-carotene (p. 268) Glutamine (p. 300) Vitamin A (p. 336) Vitamin C (p. 341) Zinc (p. 346)	Barberry (p. 395) Calendula (p. 406) Chamomile (p. 409) Goldenseal (p. 429) Licorice (p. 440) Marshmallow (p. 444) Slippery elm (p. 460)

Gingivitis (Periodontal Disease)

Gingivitis is an inflammation of the gums (gingivae). Periodontitis is an inflammation of both the gingivae and periodontal tissue that surrounds and supports the teeth. These common conditions are often progressive and can eventually result in loss of the underlying bone that supports the teeth. After age 30, periodontal disease is responsible for more tooth loss than are dental cavities. Severe periodontitis sometimes requires surgery to repair damaged gum tissue.

Nutritional Supplements That May Be Helpful

A 0.1% solution of **folic acid** (p. 297) used as a mouth rinse (5 ml taken twice a day for 30 to 60 days) has reduced gum inflammation and bleeding in people with gingivitis in double-blind studies.[1,2] Depending on the preparation, the folic acid solution is rinsed in the mouth for 1 to 5 minutes and then swallowed or spat out. Folic acid was also found effective when taken in capsule or tablet form (4 mg per day) in one report,[3] though in another trial studying pregnant women with gingivitis, only the mouthwash was effective—not folic acid in pill form.[4]

Dilantin therapy causes gum disease (gingival hyperplasia) in some people. A regular program of dental care has been reported to limit or prevent gum disease in people taking Dilantin.[5,6,7] Double-blind human research has shown that a daily oral rinse with a liquid folic acid preparation inhibited Dilantin-induced gum disease more than either folic acid in pill form or placebo.[8]

Preliminary evidence has linked gingivitis to a **coenzyme Q$_{10}$** (p. 283) deficiency.[9] Some researchers believe this deficiency could interfere with the body's ability to repair damaged gum tissue. In double-blind research, 50 mg per day of coenzyme Q$_{10}$ given for 3 weeks led to a significant reduction in symptoms of gingivitis.[10] Compared with conventional approaches alone, topical coenzyme Q$_{10}$ combined with conventional treatments resulted in better outcomes in a group of people with periodontal disease.[11]

People who are deficient in **vitamin C** (p. 341) have been reported to be at increased risk for periodontal disease.[12] When a group of people with periodontitis who normally consumed only 20 to 35 mg of vitamin C per day were given an additional 70 mg per day, objective improvement of periodontal tissue occurred in only 6 weeks.[13] It makes sense for those who are deficient to supplement with vitamin C in order to improve gingival health.

However, for people who consume adequate amounts of vitamin C in their diet, several studies have found supplemental vitamin C to have no additional therapeutic effect. Research,[14] including double-blind evidence,[15] shows that vitamin C fails to significantly reduce gingival inflammation in people who are not vitamin C deficient. In one study, administration of vitamin C plus **bioflavonoids** (p. 271) (300 mg per day of each) did improve gingival health in a group of individuals with gingivitis.[16] However, there was less improvement when vitamin C was given without bioflavonoids. Moreover, preliminary evidence has suggested that bioflavonoids by themselves may reduce inflammation of the gums.[17]

Some,[18] but not all,[19] research has found that giving 500 mg of **calcium** (p. 277) twice per day for 6 months to people with periodontal disease results in a reduction of symptoms (bleeding gums and loose

Glaucoma

teeth). Although some nutritionally oriented doctors recommend calcium supplementation to people with diseases of the gums, supportive scientific evidence remains weak.

Are There Any Side Effects or Interactions? Refer to the individual supplement for information about any side effects or interactions.

Checklist for Gingivitis (Periodontal Disease)

Ranking	Nutritional Supplements	Herbs
Primary	Folic acid (p. 297) (rinse only) Vitamin C (p. 341) (only if deficient)	
Secondary	Coenzyme Q$_{10}$ (p. 283)	Bloodroot (p. 399) Chamomile (p. 409) Clove, Echinacea (p. 417) Green tea (p. 430) Myrrh (p. 446) Peppermint (p. 451)
Other	Bioflavonoids (p. 271) Calcium (p. 277)	Rhatany Sage (p. 456)

See also: Homeopathic Remedies for **Gingivitis (Periodontal Disease)** (p. 532)

Herbs That May Be Helpful

A mouthwash combination that includes **sage** (p. 456) oil, **peppermint** (p. 451) oil, menthol, **chamomile** (p. 409) tincture, expressed juice from **echinacea** (p. 417), **myrrh** (p. 446) tincture, clove oil, and caraway oil has been used successfully to treat gingivitis.[20] In cases of acute gum inflammation, 0.5 ml of the herbal mixture in half a glass of water 3 times daily is recommended by some herbalists. This herbal preparation should be swished slowly in the mouth before spitting out. To prevent recurrences, slightly less of the mixture can be used less frequently.

A toothpaste containing sage oil, peppermint oil, chamomile tincture, expressed juice from *Echinacea purpurea*, myrrh tincture, and rhatany tincture has been used to accompany this mouthwash in managing gingivitis.[21]

Of the many herbs listed above, **chamomile** (p. 409), **echinacea** (p. 417), and **myrrh** (p. 446) should be priorities. These three herbs can provide anti-inflammatory and antimicrobial actions critical to successfully treating gingivitis.

Bloodroot (p. 399) contains alkaloids, principally sanguinarine, that are sometimes used in toothpaste

and other oral hygiene products because they inhibit oral bacteria.[22,23] Sanguinarine-containing toothpastes and mouth rinses can be used in the same way as other oral hygiene products. A 6-month, double-blind study found that use of a bloodroot and zinc toothpaste reduced gingivitis significantly better than placebo.[24] However, a similar study was unable to replicate these results.[25] Thus, at present, it is unknown who will respond to bloodroot toothpaste and who won't.

Are There Any Side Effects or Interactions? Refer to the individual herb for information about any side effects or interactions.

Glaucoma

The term glaucoma describes a group of eye conditions involving increased pressure within the eyeball. This pressure can ultimately cause blindness if left untreated. In many cases, the cause is unknown. In some cases, however, glaucoma is caused by an underlying condition that should be treated with conventional medicine. Therefore, it is important for people with glaucoma to be diagnosed by and under the care of an ophthalmologist; regular eye exams are especially important after age 40.

Dietary Changes That May Be Helpful

At least two older reports claim that **allergy** (p. 76) can exacerbate glaucoma.[1 2] If other approaches are not successful, it makes sense to consult a nutritionally oriented physician to diagnose and treat possible allergies.

Nutritional Supplements and Other Natural Therapies That May Be Helpful

Vitamin C (p. 341), according to six out of seven reports studying people with glaucoma, significantly reduces elevated pressure within the eye.[3] These studies used at least several grams per day of vitamin C, but the intake varied widely. Doctors of natural medicine often suggest that people with glaucoma take the amount of vitamin C causing loose stools, and then reduce this amount slightly—an amount called "bowel tolerance"—as a way to help people with glaucoma.[4] The amount of vitamin C needed to reach bowel tolerance varies considerably from person to person, ranging from about 5 to 20 or more grams per day. Vitamin C does not cure glaucoma and must be used continually to reduce ocular pressure.

Many years ago, the **bioflavonoid** (p. 271) rutin was used to reduce pressure within the eyes of people with glaucoma.[5] The amount used—20 mg 3 times per day—was quite moderate. Seventeen of twenty-six people showed clear improvement. The effects of rutin or other bioflavonoids in people with glaucoma have apparently not been studied since.

Less than 1 mg of **melatonin** (p. 312) has lowered pressure within the eyes of healthy people,[6] but studies have not yet been published on the effects of using melatonin with people who have glaucoma.

Magnesium (p. 310) can act as a dilator of blood vessels. One study looked at whether magnesium might improve vision in people with glaucoma by enhancing blood flow to the eyes. In that trial, people were given 245 mg of magnesium per day. Improvement in vision was noted after 4 weeks, but the change did not quite reach statistical significance.[7]

There is some evidence that **alpha lipoic acid** (p. 264), taken in the amount of 150 mg daily for 1 month improves visual function in people with both stage I and stage II glaucoma.[8]

Are There Any Side Effects or Interactions? Refer to the individual supplement for information about any side effects or interactions.

Checklist for Glaucoma

Ranking	Nutritional Supplements	Herbs
Primary	Vitamin C (p. 341)	
Other	Alpha lipoic acid (p. 264) Bioflavonoids (p. 271) Melatonin (p. 312) Magnesium (p. 310)	

Gout

Gout is a form of arthritis that occurs when crystals of uric acid accumulate in a joint, leading to the sudden development of pain and inflammation. Individuals with gout either overproduce uric acid or are less efficient at eliminating it. The big toe is the most commonly afflicted joint to accumulate uric acid crystals, although other joints may be affected.

Lifestyle Changes That May Be Helpful

Individuals who are **overweight** (p. 165) or have **high blood pressure** (p. 89) are at greater risk of developing gout.[1] Weight loss should not be rapid because restric-

tion of calories is known to increase uric acid levels temporarily.

Dietary Changes That May Be Helpful

There is a clear relationship between diet and gout. Foods that are high in a compound called purine raise uric acid levels in the body. Restricting purine intake can help control uric acid levels and in turn, the risk of an attack in individuals susceptible to gout. Foods high in purine are generally protein-rich foods, such as sweetbreads, anchovies, mackerel, sardines, chicken, dried beans and peas, liver and other organ meats, herring, scallops, red meat, and turkey.

Avoiding alcohol, particularly beer, or limiting alcohol intake to one drink per day or less can reduce the number of attacks of gout.[2,3] Refined sugars, including sucrose and fructose, should also be restricted, because they raise uric acid levels.[4]

According to a 1950 study of twelve individuals with gout, eating one-half pound of cherries or the equivalent amount of cherry juice prevented attacks of gout.[5] Black, sweet yellow, and red sour cherries were all effective. Since that study, there have been many anecdotal reports of cherry juice as an effective treatment of the pain and inflammation of gout. The active ingredient in cherry juice remains unknown.

Individuals with gout should not consume nutritional yeast or **brewer's yeast** (p. 275), as they can raise uric acid levels.

Nutritional Supplements That May Be Helpful

There is a limited number of studies indicating that large amounts of supplemental **folic acid** (p. 297) (up to 80 mg per day) reduces uric acid levels.[6] However, other research does not confirm the effectiveness of folic acid.[7]

In one small study, **vitamin C** (p. 341) was shown to increase urinary excretion of uric acid.[8] This enhanced excretion of uric acid from the body might be beneficial.

Quercetin (p. 328), a bioflavonoid, inhibits the enzyme xanthine oxidase, which makes uric acid.[9] Quercetin has shown anti-inflammatory effects in test tube studies.[10] Although human research is lacking, some doctors of natural medicine recommend 150 to 250 mg of quercetin 3 times per day (taken between meals).

Are There Any Side Effects or Interactions? Refer to the individual supplement for information about any side effects or interactions.

Herbs That May Be Helpful

Autumn crocus *(Colchicum autumnale)* is the herb from which the drug colchicine was originally isolated and is used as a conventional treatment for gout. The drug colchicine is much more commonly used than are herbal extracts of Autumn crocus. Both the herb and the drug have significant toxicity and for this reason should only be used under the guidance of a physician.

Are There Any Side Effects or Interactions? Refer to the individual herb for information about any side effects or interactions.

Checklist for Gout

Ranking	Nutritional Supplements	Herbs
Other	Folic acid (p. 297) Quercetin (p. 328) Vitamin C (p. 341)	
See also: Homeopathic Remedies for **Gout** (p. 540)		

Hay Fever

Hay fever is an **allergic condition** (p. 8) triggered by inhalant substances (frequently pollens), which leads to sneezing and inflammation of the nose and conjunctiva of the eyes.

Dietary Therapies That May Be Helpful

People with inhalant allergies are likely to also have food allergies.[1,2] A hypoallergenic diet has been reported to help people with **asthma** (p. 15) and allergic rhinitis,[3] but the effect of such a diet on hay fever symptoms has not been studied. People with hay fever interested in exploring the possible effects of a food allergy avoidance program should talk with a nutritionally oriented doctor. Discovering and eliminating offending food allergens is likely to improve overall health even if such an approach were to have no effect on hay fever symptoms.

Nutritional Supplements That May Be Helpful

Vitamin C (p. 341) has antihistamine activity. However, although vitamin C supplementation has been reported to help people with hay fever in preliminary research,[4,5] 2,000 mg of vitamin C per day did not reduce hay fever symptoms in a placebo-controlled trial.[6] Thus while some nutritionally oriented

doctors recommend that hay fever sufferers take 1,000 to 3,000 mg of vitamin C per day, supportive evidence remains weak.

In theory, bioflavonoids such as **quercetin** (p. 328) might act synergistically with vitamin C as both have antihistaminic activity. Although some doctors of natural medicine advise people with hay fever to take 400 mg of quercetin 2 to 3 times per day, only limited preliminary clinical research has yet suggested that quercetin benefits people with this condition.[7]

Are There Any Side Effects or Interactions? Refer to the individual supplement for information about any side effects or interactions.

Checklist for Hay Fever

Ranking	Nutritional Supplements	Herbs
Other	Bioflavonoids (p. 271) Quercetin (p. 328) Vitamin C (p. 341)	Elder Ephedra (p. 420) Eyebright (p. 422) Goldenrod Nettle (p. 447) Ragweed
See also: Homeopathic Remedies for **Hay Fever** (p. 541)		

Herbs That May Be Helpful

Nettle (p. 447) leaf led to a slight reduction in symptoms of hay fever—including sneezing and itchy eyes—according to an isolated double-blind study.[8] No other research has investigated this relationship. For help with hay fever symptoms, some herbally oriented doctors suggest taking 450 mg of nettle leaf capsules or tablets 2 to 3 times per day, or a 2 to 4 ml tincture 3 times per day.

Ephedra sinica (p. 420) (Ma huang) is a standard remedy for hay fever in traditional medicine.[9] Synthetic ephedrine and pseudoephedrine are popular over-the-counter drugs used for hay fever based on this tradition; however, whole ephedra appears to be safer than these isolated compounds.[10] Capsules of ephedra providing 20 mg of ephedrine per day are sometimes recommended by doctors of natural medicine.

In traditional medicine, some herbs whose pollen can cause symptoms of hay fever have been used as a way to reduce symptoms of hay fever. The most important of these are goldenrod and ragweed *(Ambrosia ambrosioides),* though **eyebright** (p. 422) and elder also have a reputation for use as hay fever remedies.[11] However, an individual allergic to one of these plants should avoid them unless under the care of a doctor of natural medicine. None of these herbs has been scientifically evaluated for effects in treating people with hay fever.

Are There Any Side Effects or Interactions? Refer to the individual herb for information about any side effects or interactions.

Hemorrhoids

Hemorrhoids are enlarged raised veins in the anus or rectum. They can bleed and become inflamed, often causing pain and itching. Common hemorrhoids are often linked to **diarrhea** (p. 58).[1]

Although the belief that hemorrhoids are caused by **constipation** (p. 44) is questioned by researchers,[2] most doctors feel that many hemorrhoids are triggered by the straining that accompanies chronic constipation.[3] Therefore, natural approaches to hemorrhoids sometimes focus on overcoming constipation.

Dietary Changes That May Be Helpful

Countries with high **fiber** (p. 293) intakes have a very low incidence of hemorrhoids. Double-blind research shows that increasing dietary fiber from **psyllium** (p. 452) seed powder (7 grams taken 3 times per day) reduces bleeding and pain from hemorrhoids.[4]

Insoluble **fiber** (p. 293)—kind found primarily in whole grains and vegetables—increases the bulk of stool. Drinking water with a high-fiber meal or supplement results in softer, bulkier stools, which can move more easily. People with hemorrhoids accompanied by constipation should read about fiber in the chapter on **constipation** (p. 44).

Psyllium (p. 452) husk has also been useful in the treatment of diarrhea.[5] People with hemorrhoids associated with chronic diarrhea should read the chapter on **diarrhea** (p. 58).

Herbs That May Be Helpful

Topical use of astringent herbs is a mainstay treatment for hemorrhoids. A leading herb for topical use is **witch hazel** (p. 470),[6] which is typically applied to hemorrhoids 3 to 4 times daily in an ointment base. Double-blind research suggests **horse chestnut** (p. 435) extracts are helpful for people with hemorrhoids.[7] Poor venous circulation, a component of hemorrhoids, can be helped by the internal use of horse chestnut or **butcher's broom** (p. 405) extracts. Some doctors of natural medicine recommend taking horse chestnut seed extracts standardized for aescin content

(16 to 21%) or isolated aescin preparations at an initial intake of 90 to 150 mg of aescin per day. Butcher's broom products can also be used in the amount of 1,000 mg 2 or 3 times per day. Witch hazel, butcher's broom, and **psyllium** (p. 452) are approved by the German government for people with hemorrhoids.[8]

Constipation (p. 44) may worsen hemorrhoid symptoms. Bulk-forming laxatives to alleviate constipation are often recommended for those with hemorrhoids. An excellent herbal product is **psyllium** (p. 452) seeds.[9] Take 7.5 grams of the seeds (2 teaspoons) or 1 teaspoon of the husks 1 to 2 times per day mixed with water or juice. It is important to maintain adequate fluid intake while using psyllium.

Are There Any Side Effects or Interactions? Refer to the individual herb for information about any side effects or interactions.

Checklist for Hemorrhoids

Ranking	Nutritional Supplements	Herbs
Primary		Psyllium (p. 452)
Secondary	Fiber (p. 293)	Horse chestnut (p. 435) Witch hazel (p. 470)
Other		Butcher's broom (p. 405)
See also: Homeopathic Remedies for **Hemorrhoids** (p. 542)		

Hepatitis

Hepatitis is a liver disease that can result from long-term alcohol abuse, infection, or exposure to various chemicals and drugs. Because hepatitis is potentially very dangerous, a health-care professional should be involved in its treatment.

Lifestyle Changes That May Be Helpful

Avoiding alcohol is the most obvious way to avoid the liver damage it causes.

Excessive intake of acetaminophen can damage the liver and should be avoided. Other painkillers may also have this effect; however, acetaminophen is the most common. People with hepatitis should ask their physician whether any medication they are taking poses a risk to the liver. A variety of other prescription drugs can damage the liver, as can **niacin** (p. 339) (vitamin B$_3$).

Good hygiene is necessary to avoid spreading the infection for individuals with hepatitis resulting from a viral infection. The hepatitis A virus can be spread very easily through food, so people with hepatitis should wash their hands very carefully after using the restroom and should not handle food at work. The hepatitis viruses B and C are both transmitted by blood and sexual contact.

Nutritional Supplements That May Be Helpful

Taking 3 grams per day of **phosphatidyl choline** (p. 307) (found in lecithin) was found to be beneficial in one investigation of people with chronic hepatitis B.[1] Signs of liver damage on biopsy were significantly reduced in this study when the participants took phosphatidyl choline.

Proteins from the thymus gland, an important part of the **immune system** (p. 94), have a beneficial effect in people with chronic hepatitis B. Initial studies done in Poland used injected thymus proteins with good results.[2] Further studies using a variety of thymus extracts by mouth have found that they can improve blood tests measuring liver damage as well as improve immune cell numbers.[3,4] Preliminary evidence also suggests these extracts can help people with hepatitis C.[5] The standard recommendation for supplementation is 200 mg 3 times each day of crude extracts or 40 mg 3 times each day of purified proteins.

Vitamin E (p. 344) levels have been shown to be low in people with hepatitis,[6] as well as in those who go on to develop liver cancer from long-standing infection.[7] Vitamin E levels in the liver may be decreased in some people with hepatitis.[8] A study in children with viral hepatitis using 300 IU per day did not find any benefit.[9] In adults, 1,200 IU per day has been shown to reduce liver damage to some extent.[10]

Vitamin C (p. 341) in the amount of 2 grams per day was reported in an uncontrolled study to prevent hepatitis infection by blood transfusion.[11] A repeat of the study comparing 2 grams vitamin C with placebo did not find any protective benefit.[12] An older study suggested that injections of vitamin C may be helpful in treating viral hepatitis.[13]

Vitamin B$_{12}$ (p. 337) has been reported in older investigations to help some people with hepatitis;[14][15] this has not been confirmed in modern studies. Vitamin B$_{12}$ injections are likely to be most beneficial, though 1,000 mcg (taken orally) each day can also be supplemented.

Catechin, a **bioflavonoid** (p. 271), has helped people with viral hepatitis,[16] though not all studies have found a benefit.[17] A typical amount used in successful trials is 500 to 750 mg 3 times each day. Although catechin is found in several plants, none contain sufficient amounts to reach the level used in the trial; thus, catechin supplements are needed.

Are There Any Side Effects or Interactions? Refer to the individual supplement for information about any side effects or interactions.

Herbs That May Be Helpful

Silymarin, the flavonoid extracted from **milk thistle** (p. 445), has been extensively studied for treating all types of liver disease. For acute hepatitis, double-blind studies have shown mixed results.[18,19] A combination of silymarin and **phosphatidyl choline** (p. 307) was reported to help sufferers of chronic viral hepatitis. One small pilot study found that at least 420 mg of silymarin was necessary each day.[20] A controlled investigation found that silymarin decreased liver damage.[21] Silymarin has generally been shown to treat hepatitis B and C equally well, though at least one study has not found silymarin effective for hepatitis C.[22]

For alcoholic hepatitis, use of 140 mg silymarin 3 times per day has been shown to prolong survival time compared with placebo in a double-blind trial.[23] Even when the damage from the alcohol has caused **diabetes** (p. 53), 140 mg 3 times per day of silymarin is beneficial.[24] Complete recovery in terms of signs of liver damage in biopsies has also been shown to occur when silymarin is given to those with alcohol-induced hepatitis.[25] More recently, the ability of silymarin to prolong survival in people with alcoholic cirrhosis has not been confirmed in a double-blind study.[26] However, there was a tendency for people in this study who were also infected with hepatitis C to do better on silymarin.

Phyllanthus (p. 452) *(Phyllanthus amarus),* an **Ayurvedic** herb, has been studied primarily in carriers of hepatitis viruses, as opposed to those with chronic active hepatitis. Up to 500 mg 4 times a day of powdered root has not rid people of the hepatitis B virus,[27] though other investigations have reported mixed results.[28,29] A West Indian species, *Phyllanthus urinaria* (not widely available in the United States or Europe), has achieved much better results than Indian *Phyllanthus amarus*.[30] Thus, the specific plant species used may be important for therapeutic effect.

One of the active constituents in **licorice** (p. 440), glycyrrhizin, is commonly used in Japan as an injected therapy for hepatitis B and C.[31][32] Glycyrrhizin also blocks hepatitis A virus from copying itself in test tubes.[33] It is unknown if oral licorice extracts high in glycyrrhizin are effective. Because glycyrrhizin can cause high blood pressure and other problems, it should only be taken on the advice of a doctor of natural medicine.

Preliminary human research demonstrates some efficacy for the mushroom **reishi** (p. 455) in treating chronic hepatitis B, although this use still needs to be confirmed.[34]

Shiitake (p. 460) formulations that contain the powdered mycelium of the mushroom before the cap and stem grow (called LEM) may help decrease chronic hepatitis B infectivity, as measured by specific liver and blood markers.[35]

Modern Chinese research suggests that compounds called lignans in **schisandra** (p. 458) regenerate liver tissue damaged by harmful influences, such as viral hepatitis and alcohol. These lignans lower blood levels of serum glutamic pyruvic transaminase (SGPT), a marker for infective hepatitis and other liver disorders.[36]

Are There Any Side Effects or Interactions? Refer to the individual herb for information about any side effects or interactions.

Checklist for Hepatitis

Ranking	Nutritional Supplements	Herbs
Primary	Bioflavonoids (p. 271) (silymarin)	Licorice (p. 440) (intravenous)
Secondary	Bioflavonoids (p. 271) (catechin) Thymus extracts	Milk thistle (p. 445) Phyllanthus (p. 452)
Other	Phosphatidyl choline (p. 307) Vitamin B$_{12}$ (p. 337) Vitamin C (p. 341) Vitamin E (p. 344)	Reishi (p. 455) Schisandra (p. 458) Shiitake (p. 460)

High Cholesterol
Section 1: Introduction

Although it is by no means the only major risk factor, elevated serum cholesterol is clearly associated with a high risk of heart disease. Most medical doctors suggest cholesterol levels should stay under 200 mg/dl (5.2 mmol/liter). Cholesterol levels lower than 200 are not without risk, however, as many people with levels below 200 have heart attacks. As levels fall below 200, heart disease risk continues to decline. Many

nutritionally oriented doctors consider cholesterol levels of no more than 180 to be optimal.

Medical laboratories now subdivide total cholesterol measurement into several components including LDL cholesterol (which is directly linked to heart disease) and HDL cholesterol (the so-called "good" cholesterol). The relative amount of HDL to LDL is more important than total cholesterol. For example, it is possible for someone with very high HDL to be at relatively low risk for heart disease even with total cholesterol above 200. Evaluation of changes in cholesterol requires consultation with a health-care professional and includes measurements of blood levels of total cholesterol as well as HDL and LDL cholesterol.

The discussion to follow is limited to information about the lowering of serum cholesterol levels using natural approaches. Because high cholesterol is linked to atherosclerosis and heart disease, people concerned about heart disease should also read the chapter on **Atherosclerosis** (p. 17).

Continue reading Section 2: **Dietary and Lifestyle Changes**.

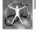

High Cholesterol
Section 2: Dietary and Lifestyle Changes

Dietary Changes That May Be Helpful

Eating animal foods containing saturated fat is linked to high serum cholesterol[1] and heart disease.[2] Significant amounts of animal-based saturated fat are found in beef, pork, veal, poultry (particularly in poultry skins and dark meat), cheese, butter, ice cream, and all other forms of dairy products not labeled "fat free." Avoiding consumption of these foods reduces cholesterol and has been reported to even reverse existing heart disease.[3] Unlike other dairy foods, skimmed milk, nonfat yogurt, and nonfat cheese are essentially fat-free. So-called "lowfat" dairy products, however, are not particularly low in fat. A full 25% of calories from 2% milk come from fat. (The "2%" refers to the fraction of volume filled by fat, not the more important percent of calories coming from fat.)

In addition to large amounts of saturated fat from animal-based foods, Americans eat small amounts of saturated fat from coconut and palm oils. Palm oil has been reported to elevate cholesterol.[4,5] Research regarding coconut oil is mixed, with some trials finding no link to heart disease[6] while other research reports that coconut oil elevates serum cholesterol.[7,8]

Despite the links between saturated fat intake and serum cholesterol levels, not every person responds to appropriate dietary changes with a drop in cholesterol. A subgroup of people with elevated cholesterol who have what researchers call "large LDL particles" have been reported to have no response to even dramatic reductions in dietary fat.[9] This phenomenon is not understood. People who significantly reduce intake of animal fats for several months and see no reduction in cholesterol levels should discuss other approaches to lowering cholesterol with a cardiologist and a nutritionally oriented doctor.

Yogurt and other fermented milk products have been reported to lower cholesterol in some[10] but not all research.[11] Until more is known, it makes sense for people with elevated cholesterol who consume these foods to select nonfat varieties.

Eating fish has been reported to increase HDL cholesterol[12] and is linked to a reduced risk of heart disease in most[13] but not all studies.[14] Fish contains very little saturated fat, and **fish oil** (p. 294) contains EPA and **DHA** (p. 287), omega-3 oils that appear to protect against heart disease.[15]

Vegetarians have lower cholesterol[16] and less heart disease[17] than meat eaters, in part because they avoid animal fat. Vegans (people who eat no meat, dairy, or eggs) have the lowest cholesterol levels,[18] and going on such a diet has reversed heart disease.[19]

Dietary cholesterol Most dietary cholesterol comes from egg yolks. Eating eggs increased serum cholesterol in most studies.[20] However, eating eggs does not increase serum cholesterol as much as eating foods high in saturated fat, and eating eggs may not increase serum cholesterol at all if the overall diet is low in fat.[21]

Egg consumption does not appear to be totally safe, however, even for people consuming a lowfat diet. When cholesterol from eggs is cooked or exposed to air, it oxidizes. Oxidized cholesterol is linked to increased risk of heart disease.[22] Eating eggs also makes LDL cholesterol more susceptible to damage, a change linked to heart disease.[23] Moreover, egg eaters are more likely to die from heart disease even when serum cholesterol levels are not elevated.[24] Therefore, the idea that egg consumption is unrelated to heart disease, a position taken by some doctors of natural medicine, is not supported by most scientific evidence.

Fiber Soluble **fiber** (p. 293) from beans,[25] **oats** (p. 448),[26] **psyllium** (p. 452) seed,[27] and fruit pectin[28] has lowered cholesterol levels in most trials.[29] Doctors of natural medicine often recommend that people with elevated cholesterol eat more of these high-soluble fiber foods. However, even grain fiber (which con-

tains *in*soluble fiber and does not lower cholesterol) has been linked to protection against heart disease, though the reason for the protection remains unclear.[30] It makes sense for people wishing to lower cholesterol levels and reduce their risk of heart disease to consume more of all types of fiber.

Flaxseed (p. 296), like other good sources of soluble fiber, has been reported to lower cholesterol.[31] A recent study found that partially defatted flaxseed containing 20 grams of fiber per day significantly lowered LDL cholesterol, suggesting that the cholesterol-lowering component in flaxseed is likely to be the fiber in this product and not the oil removed from it.[32] However, researchers and nutritionally oriented doctors are also interested in alpha-linolenic acid (ALA)—the special omega-3 oil found primarily in whole flaxseed and flaxseed oil. ALA is a precursor to EPA, a fish oil believed to protect against heart disease. To a limited extent, ALA can convert to EPA in the body.[33] However, ALA is not the same as EPA or DHA, and has been reported to not have the same effects on the cardiovascular system.[34] For example, EPA and DHA lower serum **triglyceride** (p. 85) levels (a risk factor for heart disease), but ALA does not.[35]

Moreover, preliminary research on the effects of ALA from flaxseed has produced results that appear somewhat contradictory. For example, ALA has improved parameters of arterial health that should protect people from heart disease, yet other data have implicated ALA as causing oxidation of LDL cholesterol.[36] Oxidation of LDL cholesterol is believed to be a precursor to atherosclerosis and heart disease. As a result of these preliminary disparate findings, it makes sense for people concerned about heart disease and attempting to lower their cholesterol to consider using partially defatted flaxseed as opposed to whole flaxseed or flaxseed oil until more is known.

Soy Tofu, tempeh, miso, and some protein powders in health food stores are derived from **soy beans** (p. 332). A meta-analysis of many studies has proven that soy protein reduces both total and LDL cholesterol.[37] Isoflavones from soy beans may also have this effect.[38] Trials showing statistically significant reductions in cholesterol have generally used more than 30 grams per day of soy protein.

Sugar Eating sugar has been reported to reduce protective HDL cholesterol[39] and increases other risk factors linked to heart disease.[40] However, higher sugar intake has been associated with only slightly higher risks of heart disease in most reports.[41] Although the exact relationship between sugar and heart disease remains somewhat unclear, many nutritionally oriented doctors recommend that people with high cholesterol reduce their sugar intake.

Coffee Drinking boiled or French press coffee increases cholesterol levels.[42] Modern paper coffee filters trap the offending chemicals and keep them from entering the cup. Therefore, drinking paper-filtered coffee generally does not increase cholesterol levels.[43,44] However, paper-filtered coffee does appear to significantly increase homocysteine—another risk factor for heart disease.[45] The effects of decaffeinated coffee on cholesterol levels remain in debate.[46]

Alcohol Moderate drinking (one to two drinks per day) increases protective HDL cholesterol.[47] This effect happens equally with different kinds of alcohol containing beverages.[48 49] Alcohol also acts as a blood thinner,[50] an effect that might lower heart disease. However, alcohol consumption can cause liver disease, cancer, high blood pressure, alcoholism, and, at high intake, an *increased* risk of heart disease. As a result, many doctors of natural medicine never recommend alcohol, even for people with high cholesterol. Nevertheless, those who have one to two drinks per day have been reported to live longer[51] and are clearly less likely to have heart disease.[52] Therefore, some people at very high risk of heart disease who are not alcoholics, have healthy livers and normal blood pressure, and are not at an especially high risk for cancer, may benefit from light drinking. In deciding whether light drinking might do more good than harm, people with high cholesterol should consult a nutritionally oriented doctor.

Olive oil Olive oil lowers LDL cholesterol,[53] especially when the olive oil replaces saturated fat in the diet.[54] People from countries that use significant amounts of olive oil appear to be at low risk for heart disease.[55] Authors of extremely lowfat diet approaches to heart disease recommending avoidance of olive oil are therefore not basing that decision of sound science. Although olive oil is clearly safe for people with elevated cholesterol, as with any fat or oil it very caloric, so its use should be limited in people who are overweight.

Trans Fatty Acids Trans fatty acids (TFAs) are found in many processed foods containing hydrogenated oils. The highest levels of TFAs occur in margarine. Margarine consumption is linked to increased risk of heart disease.[56] Eating TFAs increases the ratio of LDL-to-HDL.[57] Margarine and other processed foods containing partially hydrogenated oils should be avoided.

Garlic **Garlic** (p. 425) is available as a food, in powder as a spice, and as a supplement. Eating garlic helps lower cholesterol in some research,[58] though more recently, several double-blind studies have not found garlic to be effective.[59,60,61] Some of the negative reports have been criticized for flaws in their design.[62] Nonetheless, the relationship between garlic and cho-

lesterol lowering is no longer clear.[63] However, garlic is known to act as a blood thinner[64] and may reduce other risk factors for heart disease.[65] For these reasons, doctors of natural medicine typically recommend eating garlic as food, taking 900 mg of garlic powder from capsules, or using a tincture of 2 to 4 ml taken 3 times daily.

Number and Size of Meals The practice of eating many small meals rather than three large ones is sometimes called "grazing." When people eat more small meals, serum cholesterol levels fall compared with the effect of eating the same food in three big meals.[66,67] People with elevated cholesterol levels should probably avoid very large meals and eat more frequent but smaller meals.

Lifestyle Changes That May Be Helpful

Exercise increases protective HDL cholesterol,[68] an effect that occurs even from walking.[69] Exercisers have a relatively low risk of heart disease.[70] People over 40 years of age or who have heart disease should talk with their doctor before starting an exercise program; overdoing it can actually trigger heart attacks.[71]

Obesity increases the risk of heart disease,[72] in part because weight gain lowers HDL cholesterol.[73] **Weight loss** (p. 165) increases HDL and reduces **triglycerides** (p. 85), another risk factor for heart disease.[74]

Smoking is linked to a lowered level of HDL cholesterol[75] and is also known to cause heart disease.[76] Quitting smoking reduces the risk of having a heart attack.[77]

The combination of feelings of hostility, stress, and time urgency is called type A behavior. Men[78 79] (but not women[80]) with these traits are at high risk for heart disease in most, but not all, studies.[81] Stress[82] or type A behavior[83] may elevate cholesterol in men. Reducing stress and feelings of hostility has reduced the risk of heart disease.[84]

Continue reading Section 3: **Dietary Supplements and Herbs.**

High Cholesterol Section 3: Dietary Supplements and Herbs

Nutritional Supplements That May Be Helpful

High amounts (several grams per day) of niacin, a form of **vitamin B$_3$** (p. 339), lower cholesterol.[1] The other common form of B$_3$—niacinamide—does not.

Some cardiologists prescribe 3 grams of niacin per day or even higher amounts for people with high cholesterol levels. At such intakes, acute (flushing, headache, stomachache) and chronic (liver damage, diabetes, **gastritis** [p. 71], eye damage, possibly gout) toxicity may be severe. Many people are not able to continue taking these levels of niacin due to discomfort or danger to their health. Therefore, high intakes of niacin must only be taken under the supervision of a nutritionally oriented doctor or a cardiologist.

In an attempt to avoid the side effects of niacin, doctors of natural medicine increasingly use **inositol hexaniacinate** (p. 303), recommending 500 to 1,000 mg taken 3 times per day instead of niacin.[2,3] This special form of niacin has been reported to lower serum cholesterol but so far has not been found to cause significant toxicity.[4] Unfortunately, compared with niacin, far fewer investigations have studied the possible positive or negative effects of inositol hexaniacinate. As a result, people using inositol hexaniacinate should not take it without the supervision of a nutritionally oriented doctor, who will evaluate if it is helpful (by measuring cholesterol levels) and make sure toxicity is not occurring (by measuring liver enzymes, uric acid and glucose levels, and by taking medical history and doing physical examination).

In some,[5] but not all, studies[6] **vitamin E** (p. 344) has increased protective HDL cholesterol. Vitamin E is also known to protect LDL cholesterol from damage.[7] Most cardiologist believe that only damaged LDL increases the risk of heart disease. People who take at least 100 IU of vitamin E per day have been reported to have a much lower risk of heart disease.[8,9] Double-blind research has confirmed that vitamin E significantly reduces the risk of nonfatal heart disease.[10] Doctors of natural medicine often recommend that everyone supplement 400 IU of vitamin E per day to lessen the risk of having a heart attack, though the optimal intake remains in debate.

Like vitamin E, **vitamin C** (p. 341) protects LDL cholesterol from damage.[11] In some studies, cholesterol levels have fallen when people with elevated cholesterol supplement with vitamin C.[12] Reported decreases have selectively occurred in LDL cholesterol.[13] Nutritionally oriented doctors sometimes recommend 1 gram per day. A review of the disparate research with vitamin C and heart disease, however, has suggested that most protection against heart disease from vitamin C is likely to occur with as little as 100 mg per day.[14]

Pantethine (p. 340), a special form of vitamin B_5 (pantothenic acid), may help reduce the amount of cholesterol made by the body. Several studies have found that pantethine (300 mg taken 2 to 4 times per day) significantly lowers serum cholesterol levels and increases HDL.[15,16,17] Common pantothenic acid has not been reported to have this effect.

Vitamins B_6 (p. 340), B_{12} (p. 337), and **folic acid** (p. 297) lower homocysteine[18]—a substance linked to heart disease risk. Homocysteine may increase the rate at which LDL cholesterol is damaged.[19] Therefore, limiting homocysteine levels should help protect against heart disease, an idea supported by preliminary research. (See the chapter on **Atherosclerosis** [p. 17] for more information about vitamins B_6 and B_{12} and folic acid.)

Quercetin (p. 328) is a **bioflavonoid** (p. 271) that protects LDL cholesterol from damage.[20] Several studies have found that people who eat foods high in quercetin have a much lower risk of heart disease,[21,22,23] though research in this field has not been consistent.[24] Quercetin is found in apples, onions, and black tea, and as a supplement. Dietary amounts linked to protection from heart disease have been as low as 35 mg per day.

Chromium (p. 282) supplementation has reduced LDL cholesterol[25] and increased HDL cholesterol, in human studies.[26,27] **Brewer's yeast** (p. 275), which contains readily absorbable chromium, has also lowered serum cholesterol.[28] People with higher blood levels of chromium appear to be at lower risk of heart disease.[29] A reasonable and safe intake of supplemental chromium is 200 mcg per day. People wishing to use brewer's yeast as a source of chromium should look for products specifically labeled "from the brewing process" or "brewer's yeast" because most yeast found in health-food stores is not brewer's yeast and does not contain chromium. Optimally, true brewer's yeast contains up to 60 mcg of chromium per tablespoon, and a reasonable intake is 2 tablespoons per day.

Though even some nutritionally oriented doctors remain unaware of it, several studies have shown that supplemental **calcium** (p. 277) reduces cholesterol levels.[30,31] Possibly the calcium is binding with and preventing the absorption of dietary fat.[32] Reasonable supplemental levels are 800 to 1,000 mg per day.

Magnesium (p. 310) is needed by the heart to function properly. Although the mechanism is unclear, magnesium supplements (430 mg per day) lowered cholesterol in a South American study.[33] Others have reported that magnesium deficiency is associated with a low HDL cholesterol level.[34] Intravenous magnesium has reduced death following heart attacks in some, but not all, studies.[35] Though these outcomes would suggest that people with high cholesterol levels should take magnesium supplements, an isolated trial reported that people with a history of heart disease assigned to magnesium supplementation experienced an *increased* number of heart attacks.[36] More information is necessary before the scientific community can clearly evaluate the role magnesium should play for people with elevated cholesterol.

Carnitine (p. 279) is needed by heart muscle to utilize fat for energy. Some[37] but not all studies report that carnitine reduces serum cholesterol.[38] HDL cholesterol has also increased in response to carnitine supplementation.[39,40] People have been reported to stand a greater chance of surviving a heart attack if they are given carnitine supplements.[41] Most studies have used 1 to 4 grams of carnitine per day.

Soy (p. 332) protein lowers cholesterol in humans.[42] Section 2 on Dietary and Lifestyle Changes, provides more detail about the relationship between soy and cholesterol levels. Soy is available in foods (such as tofu, miso, and tempeh) and as supplemental protein powder. Soy contains phytosterols. One such molecule, **beta-sitosterol** (p. 270) is available as a supplement. **Beta-sitosterol** (p. 270), alone and in combination with similar plant sterols, has reduced blood levels of cholesterol.[43,44] This effect may occur because beta-sitosterol blocks absorption of cholesterol.[45] In one trial studying 0.8, 1.6, and 3.2 grams of plant sterols per day, the higher the intake, the greater the reduction in cholesterol, though the differences between the effects of these three amounts was not statistically significant and improvement in LDL/HDL ratios was just as good with 1.6 grams as with 3.2 grams.[46]

Chondroitin sulfate (p. 281) has lowered serum cholesterol levels in a preliminary trials.[47,48] Years ago, this supplement dramatically reduced the risk of heart attacks in a controlled 6-year follow-up of people with heart disease.[49] The few nutritionally oriented doctors aware of these older studies sometimes tell people with a history of heart disease or elevated cholesterol levels to take approximately 500 mg of chondroitin sulfate 3 times per day.

Octacosanol (p. 318), a substance found in wheat germ oil is sometimes available as a supplement. Small amounts (5–20 mg per day) of policosanol, an experimental supplement from Cuba consisting primarily of octacosanol, has led to large reductions in LDL cholesterol and/or increases in HDL.[50,51,52,53] Octacosanol may lower cholesterol by by inhibiting the liver's production of cholesterol.[54]

Although **lecithin** (p. 307) has been reported to increase HDL cholesterol and lower LDL cholesterol,[55] a review of the research found that the positive effect of lecithin was likely due to the polyunsaturated fat content of the lecithin.[56] If this were so, it would make more sense to use inexpensive vegetable oil rather than take lecithin supplements. However, a more recent animal study has challenged this view, finding that the cholesterol-lowering effect of lecithin is independent of polyunsaturate content.[57] Therefore, it remains unclear whether taking lecithin supplements is a useful way to lower cholesterol in people with elevated cholesterol levels.

The fiber-like supplement **chitosan** (p. 280) may lower blood cholesterol.[58] A preliminary trial reported that 3 to 6 grams per day of chitosan taken for 2 weeks resulted in a 6% drop in cholesterol and a 10% increase in protective HDL cholesterol.[59]

Royal jelly (p. 329) has prevented the cholesterol-elevating effect of nicotine[60] and has lowered serum cholesterol in animal studies.[61] Preliminary human trials have also found that royal jelly can lower cholesterol levels.[62,63] An analysis of cholesterol-lowering studies shows that 50 to 100 mg per day is the typical amount used in such research.[64]

Are There Any Side Effects or Interactions? Refer to the individual supplement for information about any side effects or interactions.

Herbs That May Be Helpful

Reports on all **garlic** (p. 425) studies performed until quite recently found cholesterol was lowered by an average of 9 to 12% over a 1- to 4-month period.[65,66] Most of these trials used 600 to 900 mg per day of garlic supplements. More recently, however, two double-blind studies have found garlic ineffective.[67,68] The negative studies have been criticized for flaws in their design,[69] but for the moment, the relationship between garlic and cholesterol lowering remains unclear.[70]

Part of the confusion may result from differing effects from dissimilar garlic products. In most but not all studies, aged garlic extracts and garlic oil (both containing no allicin) have not lowered cholesterol levels in humans.[71,72] Therefore both of these supplements cannot be recommended at this time for cholesterol lowering. Persons wishing to consume garlic and with no aversion to the odor can chew one whole clove of raw garlic daily. Odor-controlled, enteric-coated tablets standardized for allicin content are also available and in some trials appear more promising.[73] Doctors knowledgeable in the use of herbal medicine typically recommend 900 mg per day (providing 5,000 mcg of allicin), divided into 2 or 3 doses. For health maintenance, half of the therapeutic regimen may be adequate.

Guggul (p. 432), a mixture of substances taken from the plant *Commiphora mukul*, is an approved treatment for elevated cholesterol in India and has been a mainstay of the Ayurvedic approach to preventing atherosclerosis. One trial studying the effects of guggul reported that serum cholesterol dropped by 17.5%.[74] In another report comparing guggul to the drug clofibrate, the average fall in serum cholesterol was slightly greater in the guggul group; moreover, HDL cholesterol rose in 60% of people responding to guggul, while clofibrate did not elevate HDL.[75]

Checklist for High Cholesterol

Ranking	Nutritional Supplements	Herbs
Primary	Chromium (p. 282) Brewer's yeast (p. 275) Fiber (p. 293) Soy (p. 332) Vitamin B$_3$ (Niacin) (p. 339) (see toxicity warnings in text) Vitamin B$_5$ (Pantethine) (p. 340) Vitamin C (p. 341) (protection of LDL cholesterol) Vitamin E (p. 344) (protection of LDL cholesterol)	Guggul (p. 432) Psyllium (p. 452)
Secondary	Beta-sitosterol (p. 270) Calcium (p. 277) Inositol hexaniacinate (p. 303) Octacosanol (p. 318)	Artichoke (p. 393) Garlic (p. 425)
Other	Carnitine (p. 279) Chitosan (p. 280) Chondroitin sulfate (p. 281) Creatine monohydrate (p. 285) Folic acid (p. 297) (protection of LDL cholesterol) Lecithin (p. 307) Magnesium (p. 310) Quercetin (p. 328) Royal jelly (p. 329) Vitamin B$_6$ (p. 340) (protection of LDL cholesterol) Vitamin B$_{12}$ (p. 337) (protection of LDL cholesterol) Vitamin E (p. 344) (increasing HDL cholesterol)	Fo-ti (p. 425) Oats (p. 448) Wild yam (p. 469)

See also: **Atherosclerosis** (p. 17)

Daily intakes of guggul are based on the amount of guggulsterones in the extract. The recommended amount of guggulsterones is 25 mg taken 3 times per day. Most extracts contain 5 to 10% guggulsterones, and doctors familiar with its use usually recommend taking guggul for at least 12 weeks before evaluating its effect.

Fo-ti (p. 425) root has been shown to lower cholesterol levels, according to animal and human research, as well as to decrease atherosclerosis.[76,77] A tea can be made from processed roots by boiling 3 to 5 grams in a cup of water for 10 to 15 minutes. Three or more cups should be drunk each day. Fo-ti tablets containing 500 mg each are also available. Doctors who use herbal medicine may suggest taking five of these tablets 3 times per day.

Wild yam (p. 469) has been reported to raise HDL cholesterol in preliminary research.[78] Doctors familiar with its use sometimes recommend 2 to 3 ml of tincture taken 3 to 4 times per day, or 1 to 2 capsules or tablets of dried root taken 3 times per day.

Use of **psyllium** (p. 452) has been extensively studied as a way to reduce cholesterol levels. An analysis of all double-blind studies concluded that psyllium lowered cholesterol levels by 5% and LDL cholesterol by 9%.[79] Generally 5 to 10 grams of psyllium are added to the diet per day to lower cholesterol levels.

Artichoke (p. 393) has moderately lowered cholesterol and triglycerides in some,[80] but not all,[81] reports. Cholesterol lowering effects occurred when using 320 mg of standardized leaf extract taken 2 to 3 times per day for at least 6 weeks.

Are There Any Side Effects or Interactions? Refer to the individual herb for information about any side effects or interactions.

High Homocysteine

Homocysteine, a normal breakdown product of the essential amino acid methionine, is believed to exert a number of toxic effects in the body. A growing body of evidence suggests that an elevated homocysteine level is a risk factor for heart disease, independent of other known risk factors such as elevated serum **cholesterol** (p. 79) and **hypertension** (p. 89),[1] though, in some research the link has appeared only in women.[2]

While some scientists still have doubts,[3] this association may represent a cause-effect relationship, as homocysteine appears to be capable of promoting the development of **atherosclerosis** (p. 17) (hardening of the arteries). Increased homocysteine levels also appear to be a risk factor for the development of stroke,[4] and this compound may also play a role in the development of **osteoporosis** (p. 133).[5] Recently, elevated homocysteine levels have also been reported in people with inflammatory bowel disease (**Crohn's disease** [p. 48] and **ulcerative colitis** [p. 158])[6] and **Alzheimer's disease** (p. 11).[7]

Normally, the body detoxifies homocysteine by converting it back to methionine or by breaking it down further to a compound called cystathionine. However, the efficiency of these detoxification mechanisms may be impaired either by a genetic defect in one of the homocysteine-metabolizing enzymes or by a deficiency of one of the nutrients needed to activate these enzymes.

Lifestyle Changes That May Be Helpful

According to a recent study, both cigarette smoking and coffee consumption were associated with increased homocysteine levels.[8] These findings are consistent with studies that have found both smoking and caffeine consumption to be associated with an increased risk of both cardiovascular disease and osteoporosis.

Dietary Changes That May Be Helpful

Since homocysteine is produced from methionine, intake of large amounts of methionine would presumably increase homocysteine levels. Indeed, ingestion of supplemental methionine is sometimes used experimentally as a method of increasing homocysteine levels.[9] Foods high in methionine include meat, chicken, fish, and eggs. Although there is little research in this area, it seems logical that reducing one's intake of those foods might decrease homocysteine levels, thereby potentially reducing the risk of cardiovascular disease and osteoporosis.

Nutritional Supplements That May Be Helpful

Vitamin B$_6$ (p. 340), **folic acid** (p. 297), and **vitamin B$_{12}$** (p. 337) each function as cofactors for enzymes that can lower homocysteine levels. A number of studies have shown that supplementing with these nutrients can reduce homocysteine levels.[10,11,12] The amounts of these nutrients needed to reduce homocysteine levels is relatively low in cases where homocysteine is elevated as a result of dietary deficiencies (for example, 400 mcg of folic acid per day;

10 mg of vitamin B$_6$ per day; and 50 mcg of vitamin B$_{12}$ per day have been used in various studies). However, in individuals who have a genetic defect in homocysteine metabolism, considerably larger amounts of folic acid (such as 5 mg per day) or vitamin B$_6$ (such as 50 to 100 mg per day) have been used in studies. Now that blood tests for homocysteine are readily available, doctors can determine how much of these vitamins any particular individual needs in order to maintain homocysteine within the normal range.

Betaine (6 grams per day)[13] and choline (2 grams per day)[14] have each been shown to lower homocysteine levels. Supplementation with these nutrients is sometimes considered in cases in which folic acid, vitamin B$_6$, and vitamin B$_{12}$ do not reduce the levels sufficiently.

Are There Any Side Effects or Interactions Refer to the individual supplement for information about any side effects or interactions.

Checklist for High Homocysteine

Ranking	Nutritional Supplements	Herbs
Primary	Folic acid (p. 297) Vitamin B$_6$ (p. 340) Vitamin B$_{12}$ (p. 337)	
Secondary	Betaine (not HCl) (p. 269) Choline (p. 307)	

High Triglycerides (Hypertriglyceridemia)

Many people have elevated blood levels of triglycerides (TGs). TGs are composed of three fatty chains linked together. This is the way most fat exists in both food and the human body. People with diabetes often have elevated TG levels; see the chapter on **Diabetes** (p. 53) for further information. Successfully dealing with diabetes will, in some cases, lead to normalization of TG levels. Most studies indicate that people with elevated triglycerides are at higher risk of heart disease; see the chapters on **elevated cholesterol** (p. 79) and **atherosclerosis** (p. 17).

Dietary Changes That May Be Helpful

While moderate drinking does not affect TG levels, heavy drinking is believed to be the second most prevalent cause (after diabetes) of hypertriglyceridemia.[1]

Alcoholics with elevated TG levels should deal with the disease of alcoholism first.

Sugar increases TG levels as well.[2 3] It makes sense for people with elevated TGs to reduce intake of sugar, sweets, and other sugar-containing foods.

Diets high in **fiber** (p. 293) have lowered TGs in several studies,[4] although many researchers have not seen this effect.[5] Water-soluble fibers, such as pectin found in fruit, guar gum and other gums found in beans, and beta-glucan found in **oats** (p. 448), may be particularly helpful in lowering triglycerides.

Lowfat, high-carbohydrate diets have lowered TGs in some,[6] but not all, studies.[7] Suddenly switching to a high-carbohydrate, lowfat diet will generally increase TGs temporarily, but making the switch gradually protects against this short-term problem.[8] Cardiologists and most nutritionally oriented doctors recommend a diet low in saturated fat (meaning avoidance of red meat and all dairy except nonfat dairy) to reduce TGs and the risk of heart disease.[9]

Some,[10,11] but not all, studies[12] report that fish eaters have a lower risk of heart disease. Significant amounts of TG-lowering omega-3 oils EPA and **DHA** (p. 287) can be found in the **fish oil** (p. 294) of salmon, herring, mackerel, sardines, anchovies, albacore tuna, and black cod. Many doctors of natural medicine recommend that people with elevated TGs increase their intake of these fatty fish.

Lifestyle Changes That May Be Helpful

Exercise lowers TG levels.[13] People who have diabetes, heart disease, or are over the age of 40, should talk with a doctor before beginning an exercise program.

Smoking has been linked to elevated TG levels.[14] As always, it makes sense for smokers to quit.

Obesity (p. 165) increases TG levels.[15] Maintaining ideal body weight helps protect against elevated TG levels. Many nutritionally oriented doctors encourage people who have elevated TGs and who are overweight to lose the extra weight.

Nutritional Supplements That May Be Helpful

Many double-blind studies consistently demonstrate that the **fish oils** (p. 294) EPA and DHA, mentioned above, lower TG levels.[16] The amount used in much of the research is 3,000 mg per day of omega-3 fatty acid. To calculate how much omega-3 fatty acid is in a supplement, add together the amounts of EPA and **DHA** (p. 287). For example, if a given fish oil capsule contains 1,000 mg of fish oil, of which 180 mg is EPA and 120 mg is DHA, then the total omega-3 oil content is 300 mg. At this level, 10 capsules per day would be required to reach 3,000 mg. Other forms of omega-3 oil, such as **flaxseed oil** (p. 296), do not lower TGs; while they have other benefits, they should not be used for this purpose.

Cod liver oil will also lower TGs.[17] Cod liver oil is less expensive than omega-3 fish oil. However, most cod liver oil contains large amounts of **vitamin A** (p. 336) and **vitamin D** (p. 343); too much of either can cause side effects. Doctors will often order blood work for people who take high doses of vitamins A or D, and the cost of the blood work may exceed the savings in using cod liver oil. Those wishing to use cod liver oil instead of omega-3 fish oil should consult a nutritionally oriented doctor.

Omega-3 oil from fish oil and cod liver oil has been reported to affect blood in many other ways which might lower the risk of heart disease.[18] However, it sometimes increases LDL—the bad form of cholesterol. A doctor can check to see if fish oil has this effect on an individual. Research shows that when 900 mg of **garlic** (p. 425) extract is added to fish oil, the combination still dramatically lowers TG levels but no longer increases LDL.[19] Therefore, it appears that taking garlic supplements may be a way to avoid the increase in LDL cholesterol sometimes associated with taking fish oil. People who take omega-3 fish oil may also need to take **vitamin E** (p. 344) to protect the oil from oxidative damage in the body.[20]

Carnitine (p. 279) is another supplement that has lowered TGs in several studies.[21,22] Some nutritionally oriented doctors recommend 1 to 3 grams of carnitine per day.

Pantethine (p. 340) is a special form of the B vitamin pantothenic acid. Several studies show that 300 mg of pantethine taken 3 times per day will lower TG levels.[23,24,25] The form found in most B vitamins—pantothenic acid—does not have this effect. Some nutritionally oriented doctors recommend supplementing with pantethine to reduce TG levels.

The **niacin** (p. 339) form of vitamin B_3 is used by both cardiologists and nutritionally oriented doctors to lower cholesterol levels, but niacin also lowers TG levels.[26] The amount of niacin needed to lower cholesterol and TGs is several grams per day. Such quantities often have side effects and should not be taken without the supervision of a cardiologist or nutritionally oriented doctor. Rather than using niacin (and risking side effects), doctors of natural medicine increasingly use **inositol hexaniacinate** (p. 303) in the amount of 500 mg 3 times per day.[27,28]

Are There Any Side Effects or Interactions? Refer to the individual supplement for information about any side effects or interactions.

Checklist for High Triglycerides

Ranking	Nutritional Supplements	Herbs
Primary	Fish oil (p. 294) (EPA/DHA [p. 287]) Pantethine (p. 340) Niacin/inositol hexaniacinate (p. 339)	Fenugreek (p. 424) Garlic (p. 425) Guggul (p. 432) Oats (p. 448) Psyllium (p. 452)
Secondary	Carnitine (p. 279)	
Other	Creatine monohydrate (p. 285) Fiber (p. 293)	Green tea (p. 430) Reishi (p. 455) Wild yam (p. 469)

Herbs That May Be Helpful

More than thirty-two human studies, mostly double blind, have demonstrated **garlic's** (p. 425) ability to lower serum triglycerides levels. Common garlic intakes in these studies range from 600 to 900 mg per day for 4 to 16 weeks. Reports that have analyzed the results of all studies performed to date on the TG-lowering effect indicate that over a 1- to 4-month period, garlic supplements reduce triglyceride levels by 8 to 27%.[29,30]

People with no aversion to the odor can chew one whole clove of raw garlic daily. Otherwise, odor-controlled, enteric-coated tablets standardized for allicin content can be taken in the amount of 900 mg daily (providing 5,000 mcg of allicin), divided into two daily doses. For health maintenance, half of the therapeutic regimen is adequate.

Guggul (p. 432), the mixture of ketonic steroids from the gum oleoresin of *Commiphora mukul,* is an approved treatment of hyperlipidemia in India and has been a mainstay of Ayurvedic herbal approaches to preventing atherosclerosis. Clinical studies indicate that guggul is effective in the treatment of high triglycerides; one study found total serum triglycerides to drop by 30.3%.[31]

Daily intake of guggul is typically based on the amount of guggulsterones in the extract. The recommended amount of guggulsterones is 25 mg 3 times per day. Most extracts contain 5 to 10% guggulsterones, and nutritionally oriented doctors often recommend taking it for 12 to 20 weeks.

Wild yam (p. 469) has been shown to lower blood triglycerides in humans.[32] Typical amounts used are 2–3 ml of tincture 3 to 4 times per day or 1 or 2 capsules or tablets of the dried root 3 times each day.

Reishi (p. 455), a type of mushroom, contains several constituents that seem to help decrease triglyceride levels based on preliminary reports.

Other herbal supplements that may help lower serum triglycerides include **psyllium** (p. 452), **fenugreek** (p. 424), and **green tea** (p. 430).

Are There Any Side Effects or Interactions? Refer to the individual herb for information about any side effects or interactions.

HIV Support

Acquired immunodeficiency syndrome (AIDS) is a condition in which the immune system becomes severely weakened and loses its ability to fight infections. Most scientists believe that the disease results from infection with the human immunodeficiency virus (HIV). AIDS is an extremely complex disorder, and no cure is currently available. Certain pharmaceuticals appear to be capable of slowing the progression of the disease. In addition, various nutritional factors may be helpful. However, because of the complicated nature of this disorder, medical supervision is strongly recommended with regard to dietary changes and nutritional supplements.

Dietary Changes That May Be Helpful

Individuals with AIDS often lose significant amounts of weight or suffer from recurrent **diarrhea** (p. 58). A diet high in protein and total calories may help a person maintain his or her body weight. In addition, whole foods are preferable to refined and processed foods. Whole foods contain larger amounts of many vitamins and minerals, and individuals with HIV infection tend to suffer from multiple nutritional deficiencies. Nonetheless, no evidence currently suggests that dietary changes are curative for people with AIDS or even that they significantly impact the course of the disease.

Nutritional Supplements That May Be Helpful

Because individuals with HIV infection or AIDS often have multiple nutritional deficiencies, a broad-spectrum nutritional supplement may be beneficial. In one study, HIV-infected men who took a **multivitamin supplement** (p. 314) had slower disease progression, compared with men who did not take a supplement.[1]

Vitamin A (p. 336) deficiency appears to be very common in people with HIV infection. Low levels of vitamin A are associated with greater disease severity[2] and increased transmission of the virus from a pregnant mother to her infant.[3] However, little research has explored whether vitamin A supplements are helpful. In one trial, giving people an extremely high (300,000 IU) amount of vitamin A one time only did not improve short-term measures of immunity in women with HIV.[4]

Beta-carotene (p. 268) levels have also been found to be low in HIV-infected individuals, particularly those with more advanced disease.[5] However, studies on the effect of beta-carotene supplements have produced conflicting results. In one double-blind study, supplementing with 300,000 IU per day of beta-carotene significantly increased the number of CD4+ cells (an infection-fighting type of white blood cell that is low in people with AIDS).[6] In another study, the same amount of beta-carotene had no effect on CD4+ cell counts or various other measures of immune function.[7]

Thiamine (vitamin B$_1$ [p. 337]) deficiency has been identified in nearly one-quarter of people with AIDS.[8] It has been suggested that a deficiency of this vitamin may contribute to some of the neurological abnormalities that are associated with AIDS. In another study, vitamin B$_6$ (p. 340) deficiency was found in more than one-third of HIV-positive men, and a deficiency of this vitamin was associated with decreased immune function.[9] Low blood levels of folic acid (p. 297) and vitamin B$_{12}$ (p. 337) are also common in HIV-infected individuals.[10]

Vitamin C (p. 341) has been shown to inhibit HIV replication in test tubes.[11] Some doctors recommend large amounts of vitamin C for people with AIDS. Reported benefits in vitamin C preliminary research include greater resistance against infection and an improvement in overall well-being.[12] In test tube studies, vitamin E (p. 344) improved the effectiveness of the anti-HIV drug zidovudine (AZT) while reducing its toxicity.[13]

Blood levels of coenzyme Q$_{10}$ (p. 283) were also found to be low in individuals with HIV infection or AIDS. Six people with HIV infection received 200 mg per day of coenzyme Q$_{10}$. Five of these individuals experienced no further infections for up to 7 months, and the white blood cell count improved in three cases.[14]

In the category of minerals, both zinc (p. 346)[15] and selenium (p. 331)[16] levels are frequently low in people with HIV infection, and iron (p. 304) deficiency is often present in HIV-infected children.[17] Zinc supplements have been shown to reduce the number of infections in individuals with AIDS.[18] HIV-infected people who received selenium supplements experienced fewer infections, better intestinal function, improved appetite, and improved heart function (which had been impaired by the disease).[19]

The amino acid N-acetyl cysteine (NAC) (p. 317) has been shown to inhibit the replication of HIV in the test tube.[20] In a double-blind study, supplementing with 800 mg per day of NAC slowed the rate of decline in immune function. NAC may work better when glutamine (p. 300) (another amino acid) is also supplied. In combination, these two amino acids promote the synthesis of glutathione, a naturally occurring antioxidant that is believed to be protective in people with HIV infection.[21]

The nonpathogenic yeast Saccharomyces boulardii in the amount of 1 gram 3 times per day has been shown to help stop diarrhea (p. 58) in HIV-positive people in double-blind research.[22]

Are There Any Side Effects or Interactions? Refer to the individual supplement for information about any side effects or interactions.

Herbs That May Be Helpful

Many different herbs have been shown in test tube studies to inhibit the function or replication of HIV. Few of these studies have been followed up with any kind of investigation in infected humans. Some notable exceptions to this rule are discussed below.

One double-blind study has found that 990 mg per day of an extract of boxwood (Buxus sempervirens) leaves and stems could delay progression of HIV infection as measured by decline in CD4 cell counts.[23] No adverse effects were reported due directly to the extract. Taking twice the dose of boxwood extract did not lead to further benefits and may have actually decreased its usefulness.

Garlic (p. 425) may be helpful. In one study, administration of an aged garlic extract reduced the number of infections and relieved diarrhea in a group of people with AIDS.[24]

Licorice (p. 440) has shown the ability to inhibit reproduction of HIV in test tubes.[25] Studies on injections of glycyrrhizin isolated from licorice show it could have a beneficial effect on AIDS.[26] Preliminary evidence on orally administered licorice has also found it to be safe and effective for long-term treatment of HIV infection.[27] A physician should monitor the blood pressure of anyone taking licorice or glycyrrhizin long term. Deglycyrrhizinated licorice (DGL) will not inhibit HIV. Approximately 2 grams of licorice root should be taken per day in capsules or as tea.

Immune-modulating plants often used by doctors of herbal medicine include Asian ginseng (p. 394), eleuthero (Siberian ginseng) (p. 419), ashwagandha (p. 393), and the medicinal mushrooms shiitake (p. 460) and reishi (p. 455).

Maitake (p. 443) mushrooms contain polysaccharides, including beta-D-glucan, which is currently under review as a supportive tool for HIV infection.[28,29]

Bitter melon (p. 397) contains two proteins—alpha- and beta-momorcharin—that inhibit the AIDS virus in test tubes. Very early reports indicate bitter melon juice or enemas may be beneficial for people infected with HIV,[30] but much more research is necessary before the effect of bitter melon is known for certain.

An open trial of a combination naturopathic protocol (consisting of multiple nutrients, **licorice** [p. 440], **lomatium** [p. 443], a combination Chinese herbal product, **lecithin** [p. 307], calf thymus extract, lauric acid monoglycerol ester, and **St. John's wort** [p. 461]) found that it could possibly slow progression of mild HIV infection and reduce some symptoms.[31] These results can be seen as preliminary at best and need to be repeated in controlled studies. It does begin to suggest that using several natural products in combination can be safe and potentially helpful.

Are There Any Side Effects or Interactions? Refer to the individual herb for information about any side effects or interactions.

Checklist for HIV Support

Ranking	Nutritional Supplements	Herbs
Secondary	Saccharomyces boulardii Multiple vitamin/mineral (p. 314) N-acetyl cysteine (NAC) (p. 317)	Boxwood, Licorice (p. 440)
Other	Beta-carotene (p. 268) Coenzyme Q$_{10}$ (p. 283) Folic acid (p. 297) Glutamine (p. 300) Iron (p. 304) Methionine (p. 313) Selenium (p. 331) Vitamin A (p. 336) Vitamin B$_1$ (p. 337) Vitamin B$_6$ (p. 340) Vitamin B$_{12}$ (p. 337) Vitamin C (p. 341) Vitamin E (p. 344) Zinc (p. 346)	Ashwagandha (p. 393) Asian ginseng (p. 394) Bitter melon (p. 397) Eleuthero (p. 419) Garlic (p. 425) Maitake (p. 443) Reishi (p. 455) Shiitake (p. 460)

Hypertension (High Blood Pressure)

Hypertension is the medical term for high blood pressure, a condition with many causes. Approximately 90% of people with high blood pressure have "essen-tial" or "idiopathic" hypertension, for which the cause is poorly understood. The terms "hypertension" and "high blood pressure" as used here refer only to this most common form and not to high blood pressure either associated with pregnancy or clearly linked to a known cause, such as Cushing's syndrome, pheochromocytoma, or kidney disease. Hypertension must always be evaluated by a health-care professional.

Extremely high blood pressure (malignant hypertension) or rapidly worsening blood pressure (accelerated hypertension) almost always require treatment with conventional medicine. People with mild to moderate high blood pressure should work with a nutritionally oriented doctor before attempting to use the information contained here, as blood pressure requires monitoring and in some cases the use of blood pressure–lowering drugs.

As with conventional drugs, the use of natural substances sometimes controls blood pressure if taken consistently but does not lead to a cure for high blood pressure. Thus, someone whose blood pressure is successfully reduced by **weight loss** (p. 165), avoidance of salt, and increased intake of fruit and vegetables would need to maintain these changes permanently in order to maintain control of blood pressure.

Dietary Changes That May Be Helpful

Primitive societies exposed to very little salt suffer from little or no hypertension.[1] Salt intake has also been definitively linked to hypertension in western societies.[2] Eliminating salt from the diet lowers blood pressure in most people.[3] An overview of the best studies found that the more salt is restricted, the greater the blood pressure–lowering effect.[4] Individual studies sometimes come to differing conclusions about the relationship between salt intake and blood pressure, in part because blood pressure–lowering effects of salt restriction vary from person to person, and small to moderate reductions in salt intake often have minimal effects on blood pressure. Nonetheless, dramatic reductions in salt intake are generally effective for many people with hypertension.

With the prevalence of salted processed and restaurant food, simply avoiding the salt shaker no longer leads to large decreases in salt intake for most people. Totally eliminating salt is more effective, but is also quite difficult to achieve. Moreover, whereas an overview of the research has reported "There is no evidence that sodium reduction as achieved in these trials presents any safety hazards,"[5] reports of short-term paradoxical *increases* in blood pressure in response to salt restriction have occasionally appeared.[6] Therefore, people wishing to use salt

High Blood Pressure (Hypertension)

restriction to lower their blood pressure should consult with a nutritionally oriented doctor.

Vegetarian diets have been reported to significantly lower blood pressure.[7] This occurs partly because fruits and vegetables contain **potassium** (p. 323)—a known blood pressure–lowering mineral.[8] The best way to supplement potassium is with fruit, which contains more of the mineral than amounts found in potassium supplements. However, fruit contains so much potassium that people taking "potassium sparing" drugs (as some hypertensives do) can end up with too much potassium by eating several pieces of fruit per day. Therefore, people taking potassium-sparing diuretics should consult the prescribing doctor before increasing fruit intake. The **fiber** (p. 293) provided by vegetarian diets may also help reduce high blood pressure.[9]

In the Dietary Approaches to Stop Hypertension (DASH) trial, increasing intake of fruits and vegetables (and therefore fiber) and reducing cholesterol and dairy fat led to large reductions in blood pressure (in medical terms, 11.4 systolic and 5.5 diastolic) in just 8 weeks.[10] Even though it did not employ a vegetarian diet itself, the outcome of the DASH trial supports the usefulness of vegetarian diets because diets employed by DASH researchers were related to what many vegetarians eat. The DASH trial also showed that blood pressure can be significantly reduced in hypertensive people (most dramatically in African Americans) with diet alone without weight loss or even restriction of salt.[11]

Sugar has been reported to increase blood pressure in both animals[12] and humans.[13] Though the real importance of this experimental effect remains somewhat unclear,[14] some nutritionally oriented doctors recommend that people with high blood pressure cut back on their intake of sugar.

Shortly after consuming caffeine, blood pressure increases.[15] In a review of eleven trials lasting almost 2 months on average, coffee drinking led to increased blood pressure, though these increases were typically small to moderate.[16] Nonetheless, the effects of long-term avoidance of caffeine (from coffee, tea, chocolate, cola drinks, and some medications) on blood pressure remain unclear. In fact, a few reports claim that long-term coffee drinkers have *lower* blood pressure than those who avoid coffee.[17] On the basis of the 2-month intervention trials, many nutritionally oriented doctors tell people with high blood pressure to avoid caffeine-containing food and drink despite the lack of clarity in published research.

Food allergy (p. 8) was reported to contribute to high blood pressure in a study of people who had **migraine** (p. 121) headaches.[18] In that report, all fifteen people who also had high blood pressure experienced a significant drop in blood pressure when put on a hypoallergenic diet. People suspecting food allergies should check with a nutritionally oriented doctor.

Exposure to lead and other heavy metals has also been linked to high blood pressure in some,[19] but not all, research.[20] If other approaches to high blood pressure prove unsuccessful, it makes sense for people with hypertension to have their body's burden of lead evaluated by a health-care professional.

Lifestyle Changes That May Be Helpful

Smoking is particularly injurious for people with hypertension.[21] The combination of hypertension and smoking greatly increases the risk of heart disease–related sickness and death. All people with high blood pressure need to quit smoking.

Many studies have found a relationship between alcohol consumption and blood pressure. A recent review of the research reported that above the equivalent of approximately three drinks per day, blood pressure increases in proportion to the amount of alcohol consumed.[22] Whether one or two drinks per day meaningfully increases blood pressure remains unclear.

Daily exercise can lower blood pressure significantly.[23] People over 40 years of age should consult with their doctor before starting an exercise regime. A 12-week program of Chinese T'ai Chi was reported to be almost as effective as aerobic exercise in lowering blood pressure in sedentary elderly people with high blood pressure.[24]

Many people with high blood pressure are overweight. **Weight loss** (p. 165) can lower blood pressure significantly in those who are both overweight and hypertensive.[25] People with hypertension who are overweight should talk with a nutritionally oriented doctor about a weight-loss program.

Anxiety (p. 14) in men (but not women) has been linked to eventual hypertension in a respected long-term study.[26] Several research groups have shown a relationship between job strain and high blood pressure in men.[27,28,29] Some researchers have tied blood pressure specifically to suppressed aggression.[30]

Although some kind of relationship between stress and high blood pressure appears to exist, the effects of treatment for stress remains controversial. A meta-analysis of twenty-six trials reported that reductions in blood pressure caused by biofeedback or meditation were no greater than those seen with placebo.[31] Though some stress management interventions have not been at all helpful in reducing blood pressure,[32,33] the more promising trials have used combinations of yoga, biofeedback, and/or meditation.[34,35,36] Despite the lack of consensus in published research, most doctors who utilize natural medicine continue to recommend a variety of stress-reducing measures, sometimes tailoring them to the person seeking help.

Nutritional Supplements That May Be Helpful

Calcium (p. 277) supplementation—typically 800–1,500 mg per day—lowers blood pressure. However, while an analysis of forty-two trials reported that calcium supplementation led to an average drop in blood pressure that was highly *statistically* significant, the decrease was not large enough to meaningfully improve health (in medical terms, a drop of 1.4 systolic over 0.8 diastolic pressure).[37] Results would likely be better were analysis limited only to studies of hypertensive people, because calcium has little if any effect on those with normal blood pressure. In the analysis of forty-two trials, effects were seen both with dietary calcium and with use of calcium supplements. Although average decreases in blood pressure from calcium are clearly small, each person responds differently. Some evidence suggests that people with hypertension whose blood pressure is affected most by changes in salt intake respond best to calcium supplementation.[38] A 12-week trial of 1,000 mg per day of calcium accompanied by blood pressure monitoring is a reasonable way to assess efficacy in a given individual.

Some,[39] but not all,[40] studies show that **magnesium** (p. 310) supplements—typically 350–500 mg per day—lower blood pressure. Magnesium appears to be particularly effective in people who are taking potassium-depleting diuretics.[41] As so-called "potassium depleting" diuretics also deplete magnesium, the drop in blood pressure resulting from magnesium supplementation in people taking these drugs may result from overcoming a mild magnesium deficiency.

Vitamin C (p. 341) plays an important role in maintaining the health of arteries.[42] A review of vitamin C research reported that most studies linked increased blood and dietary levels of the vitamin to reduced blood pressure.[43] However, these links might result from diets high in fruit and vegetables rather than from vitamin C itself. The same review reported that blood pressure was reduced in all four double-blind trials examining the effects of vitamin C, but the reduction was statistically significant in only two of the four, and in some cases reductions were quite modest. Nonetheless, some nutritionally oriented doctors recommend that people with elevated blood pressure supplement with 1,000 mg vitamin C per day.

Coenzyme Q$_{10}$ (CoQ$_{10}$) (p. 283) has been reported to affect blood vessels in a way that should cause a decrease in blood pressure.[44] Both uncontrolled[45,46,47]

and controlled trials have reported that CoQ$_{10}$ significantly lowers blood pressure in people with hypertension.[48] All trials used at least 50 mg of CoQ$_{10}$ taken twice per day, and most trials lasted for at least 10 weeks.

EPA and **DHA** (p. 287), the omega-3 fatty acids found in **fish oil** (p. 294), lower blood pressure, according to a meta-analysis of thirty-one trials.[49] That analysis found the effect was dependent on the amount of omega-3 oil used, with the best results occurring in studies using extremely high intakes (15 grams per day). To obtain 15 grams of omega-3 typically requires consumption of 50 grams of fish oil—an unsustainably high amount. Although results with lower intakes were not as impressive, studies using over 3 grams of omega-3 (generally requiring at least 10 grams of fish oil, or ten 1,000 mg pills per day) also reported significant reduction in blood pressure.

A deficiency of the amino acid **taurine** (p. 334) is thought by some researchers to play an important role in elevating blood pressure in people with hypertension.[50] Limited taurine research has found that supplementation lowers blood pressure in animals[51] and people (at 6 grams per day),[52] possibly by reducing levels of the hormone epinephrine (adrenaline).

Animal and preliminary human research has suggested that the fiber-like supplement **chitosan** (p. 280) may prevent blood pressure-elevating effects of salt, possibly by reducing absorption of chloride. A small study showed that 5 grams of chitosan taken by men with a highly salted meal resulted in no elevation in blood pressure, while the same meal without chitosan significantly elevated systolic blood pressure.[53]

The amino acid **arginine** (p. 268) is needed by the body to make nitric oxide, a substance that allows blood vessels to dilate, thus leading to reduced blood pressure. As a result, intravenous administration of arginine has reduced blood pressure in humans in some reports.[54] Most research has not used oral arginine, but in one such trial, the combination of arginine (2 grams taken 3 times per day) plus conventional drugs used to treat hypertension was significantly more effective than placebo alone in people who previously did not respond to the same drugs taken without arginine.[55]

Are There Any Side Effects or Interactions? Refer to the individual supplement for information about any side effects or interactions.

Herbs That May Be Helpful

Garlic (p. 425) lowers blood pressure, according to a meta-analysis that included ten double-blind studies.[56] All of these trials administered garlic for at least

4 weeks, typically using 600–900 mg of garlic extract per day. In those trials limited to people with hypertension, the average blood pressure–lowering effect was highly clinically significant.

Rauwolfia *(Rauwolfia serpentina)* and European mistletoe *(Viscum album)* have potent blood pressure–lowering effects. However, neither herb should be used except under the careful supervision of a physician highly trained in their use, because each can cause serious side effects.

Are There Any Side Effects or Interactions? Refer to the individual herb for information about any side effects or interactions.

Checklist for High Blood Pressure

Ranking	Nutritional Supplements	Herbs
Primary	Fish oil (p. 294) (EPA/DHA [p. 287]) Potassium (p. 323) (for people *not* taking potassium-sparing diuretics)	Garlic (p. 425)
Secondary	Coenzyme Q$_{10}$ (p. 283) Calcium (p. 277) Fiber (p. 293) Magnesium (p. 310) (for people taking potassium-depleting diuretics)	
Other	Arginine (p. 268) Chitosan (p. 280) Taurine (p. 334) Vitamin C (p. 341)	European mistletoe, Rauwolfia

See also: Homeopathic Remedies for **High Blood Pressure** (p. 544)

Hypoglycemia

The technical meaning of hypoglycemia is low blood sugar. Occasionally, hypoglycemia can be a potentially dangerous problem (for example, when caused by a tumor of the pancreas, liver disease, or from injecting too much insulin). More often, however, when people say they have hypoglycemia, they are describing a group of symptoms that occur when the body reacts to increasing blood sugar levels after eating and may overdo its efforts to bring blood sugar back down. Common symptoms are fatigue, **anxiety** (p. 14), headaches, difficulty concentrating, sweaty palms, shakiness, excessive hunger, drowsiness, abdominal pain, and **depression** (p. 50). This condition is sometimes called reactive hypoglycemia.

Many people with reactive hypoglycemia do not literally have low blood sugar levels,[1] and many people who do have low blood sugar levels do not have any symptoms of reactive hypoglycemia.[2] Some evidence suggests that reactive hypoglycemia may partially be a psychological condition.[3] As a result of this confusion, some medical doctors have decided that reactive hypoglycemia essentially does not exist.[4]

Nonetheless, when they are monitored continuously, people with reactive hypoglycemia have been found to have large surges in blood levels of the hormone epinephrine at the moment they suffer their symptoms.[5]

Dietary Changes That May Be Helpful

Doctors of natural medicine generally find that individuals with hypoglycemia usually improve when they eliminate refined sugars, caffeine, and alcohol from their diet; eat foods high in **fiber** (p. 293) (such as whole grains, fruits, vegetables, legumes, and nuts); and eat small, frequent meals. Few studies have investigated the effects of these changes, but the meager amount of research is generally supportive.[6,7,8,9] Some symptoms of low blood sugar may be related to or made worse by **food allergies** (p. 8).[10]

Some people claim to have fewer symptoms when eating a high-protein, low-carbohydrate diet. However, research shows that increasing protein intake can actually impair the body's ability to process sugar,[11] probably because protein increases insulin levels[12] (insulin reduces blood sugar levels). Despite these facts, on the basis of anecdotes from people with hypoglycemia, some nutritionally oriented doctors continue to try high-protein diets when the usual high-fiber/high-carbohydrate diets do not seem to reduce symptoms.

Nutritional Supplements That May Be Helpful

Research has shown that supplementing with **chromium** (p. 282) (200 mcg per day)[13] or **magnesium** (p. 310) (340 mg per day)[14] can prevent blood sugar levels from falling excessively in people with hypoglycemia. **Niacinamide** (p. 339) (vitamin B$_3$) has also been found to be helpful for hypoglycemic individuals.[15] Other nutrients, including **vitamin C** (p. 341), **vitamin E** (p. 344), **zinc** (p. 346), **copper** (p. 285), **manganese** (p. 311), and **vitamin B$_6$** (p. 340), help control blood sugar levels in diabetics.[16] Since the body regulates high and low blood sugar in similar ways, these nutrients might be helpful for hypoglycemia as well.

Are There Any Side Effects or Interactions? Refer to the individual supplement for information about any side effects or interactions.

Checklist for Hypoglycemia

Ranking	Nutritional Supplements	Herbs
Primary	Chromium (p. 282)	
Other	Copper (p. 285) Manganese (p. 311) Magnesium (p. 310) Vitamin B₃ (Niacinamide) (p. 339) Vitamin B₆ (p. 340) Vitamin C (p. 341) Vitamin E (p. 344) Zinc (p. 346)	

Hypothyroidism

Hypothyroidism is a condition in which the thyroid gland fails to function adequately, resulting in reduced levels of thyroid hormone in the body. Cretinism is a type of hypothyroidism that occurs at birth and results in both stunted physical growth and mental development. Severe hypothyroidism is called myxedema.

There are many causes of hypothyroidism. Hashimoto's thyroiditis, an autoimmune disease of the thyroid gland, may lead to hypothyroidism. Some medical treatments, such as surgery or radiation to the thyroid gland, or certain drugs like lithium and phenylbutazone, may also induce this condition. Extreme **iodine** (p. 303) deficiency, which is rare in the United States, is another possible cause. Failure of the pituitary gland or hypothalamus to stimulate the thyroid gland properly can cause a condition known as secondary hypothyroidism.

Some people with goiter (an enlargement of the thyroid gland) also have hypothyroidism. Goiter can be caused by iodine deficiency, by eating foods that contain goitrogens (goiter-causing substances), or by other disorders that interfere with thyroid hormone production. In many cases the cause of goiter cannot be determined. While natural therapies may help to some extent, thyroid hormone replacement is necessary for most people with hypothyroidism.

Dietary Changes That May Be Helpful

Some foods, such as rapeseed (used to make canola oil) and Brassica vegetables (cabbage, Brussels sprouts, broccoli, and cauliflower), contain natural goitrogens that appear to act by interfering with thyroid hormone synthesis.[1] Cooking has been reported to inactivate this effect in Brussels sprouts.[2] Cassava, a starchy root that is the source of tapioca, has also been identified as a goitrogenic food.[3] Other goitrogens include maize, sweet potatoes, lima beans, and pearl millet.[4]

Lifestyle Changes That May Be Helpful

Preliminary studies have found an association between multiple chemical sensitivities and hypothyroidism.[5] One study found a correlation between high blood levels of lead, a toxic substance, and low thyroid hormone levels in people working in a brass foundry.[6] Of the forty-seven workers tested, twelve were considered hypothyroid; many of these individuals also complained of depression, fatigue, constipation, and poor memory (symptoms of hypothyroidism). Occupational exposure to polybrominated biphenyls and carbon disulfide has also been associated with decreased thyroid function.

Nutritional Supplements That May Be Helpful

The relationship between **iodine** (p. 303) and thyroid function is complex. Iodine is required by the body to form thyroid hormones, and iodine deficiency can lead to goiter and hypothyroidism.[7] Severe and prolonged iodine deficiency can potentially lead to serious types of hypothyroidism, such as myxedema or cretinism. It is estimated that one and a half billion people living in 118 countries around the world are at risk of developing iodine deficiency.[8]

Today, most cases of iodine deficiency occur in developing nations. In industrialized countries where iodized salt is used, iodine deficiency has become extremely rare. On the other hand, iodine toxicity has become a concern in some of these countries.[9] Excessive iodine intake can result in either hypothyroidism[10] or hyperthyroidism (overactive thyroid).[11] Sources of iodine include foods (iodized salt, milk, water, seaweed, ground beef), dietary supplements (**multiple vitamin/mineral formulas** [p. 314], seaweed extracts), drugs (potassium iodide, amiodarone, topical antiseptics), and iodine-containing solutions used in certain laboratory tests. Many nutritional supplements contain 150 mcg of iodine. While that amount of iodine should prevent a deficiency, it is not clear whether supplementing with iodine is necessary or desirable for most individuals. People wishing to take a nutritional supplement containing iodine should consult a nutritionally oriented doctor.

Experimental animals with severe **zinc** (p. 346) deficiency developed hypothyroidism, whereas moderate zinc deficiency did not affect thyroid function.[12] In a study of fourteen healthy people with primarily high or low serum zinc levels, thyroid hormone (thyroxine) levels tended to be lower in those with lower serum zinc. In those individuals with low serum zinc, supplementing with zinc increased thyroxine levels.[13] One case has been reported of a woman with severe zinc deficiency (caused by the combination of alcoholism and malabsorption) who developed hypothyroidism that was corrected by supplementing with zinc.[14] Although the typical Western diet is marginally low in zinc,[15] additional research is needed to determine whether zinc supplementation would be effective for preventing or correcting hypothyroidism.

Selenium (p. 331) also plays a role in thyroid hormone metabolism. Recently, severe selenium deficiency has also been implicated as a possible cause of goiter.[16] In one study, it was reported that giving 50 mcg of selenium per day to people who were deficient in both selenium and iodine decreased thyroid function in those who were already hypothyroid.[17] Other researchers have suggested that selenium should not be given to people who are deficient in both selenium and iodine, without first giving them iodine or thyroid hormone supplementation.[18] There is no research demonstrating that selenium supplementation helps people with hypothyroidism who are not selenium-deficient.

Preliminary data indicate that **nicotinic acid** (p. 339) (a form of vitamin B₃) may decrease thyroid hormone levels. In one small study, five people were given an average of 2.6 grams of nicotinic acid per day to help lower blood fat levels.[19] After a year or more, thyroid hormone levels had fallen significantly in each person, although none experienced symptoms of hypothyroidism. In another case report, thyroid hormone levels decreased in two individuals who were taking nicotinic acid for **high cholesterol** (p. 79) and **triglycerides** (p. 85); one of these individuals was diagnosed with hypothyroidism.[20] When the nicotinic acid was discontinued for 1 month, thyroid hormone levels returned to normal.

Desiccated thyroid, also called thyroid extract, is used by some doctors as an alternative to synthetic thyroid hormones (such as thyroxine and Synthroid) for people with hypothyroidism. Thyroid extract contains two biologically active hormones (thyroxine and triiodothyronine), whereas the most commonly prescribed thyroid-hormone preparations contain only thyroxine. One study has shown that the combination of the two hormones contained in desiccated thyroid

is more effective than thyroxine alone for individuals with hypothyroidism.[21] One doctor reported that in his experience, thyroid extract works better than standard thyroid preparations for some people with hypothyroidism.[22] Glandular thyroid products, which are available from health-food stores, have had most of the thyroid hormone removed and would therefore not be expected to be effective for individuals with hypothyroidism. Intact desiccated thyroid is available only by prescription. People with hypothyroidism who want to use desiccated thyroid must first consult with a nutritionally oriented physician.

Are There Any Side Effects or Interactions? Refer to the individual supplement for information about any side effects or interactions.

Herbs That May Be Helpful

Chinese herbs show some promise for people with hypothyroidism. In one study, thirty-two people with hypothyroidism were given a combination of Chinese herbs.[23] After 1 year, symptoms of hypothyroidism were markedly improved and blood levels of thyroid hormones had significantly increased. In an animal study, administration of certain Chinese herbs raised thyroid hormone levels in the blood.[24] Neither study listed the specific herbs used. People with hypothyroidism who wish to use Chinese herbs should consult with a physician skilled in their use.

Are There Any Side Effects or Interactions? Refer to the individual herb for information about any side effects or interactions.

Checklist for Hypothyroidism

Ranking	Nutritional Supplements	Herbs
Secondary	Desiccated thyroid, Iodine (p. 303) Selenium (p. 331)	
Other	Vitamin B₃ (p. 339) (nicotinic acid) Zinc (p. 346)	

Immune Function

The immune system is an intricate network of specialized tissues, organs, cells, and chemicals. The lymph nodes, spleen, bone marrow, thymus gland, and tonsils all play a role, as do lymphocytes (specialized white blood cells), antibodies, and interferon.

Two types of immunity protect the body: innate and adaptive. Innate immunity is present at birth and provides the first barrier against microorganisms. The skin, mucus secretions, and the acidity of the stomach are examples of innate immunity that act as a barriers to keep unwanted germs away from more vulnerable tissues.

Adaptive immunity is the second barrier to infection. It is acquired later in life, for example after an immunization or successfully fighting off an infection. The adaptive immune system retains a memory of all the invaders it has faced. This is why people usually get the measles only once although they may be repeatedly exposed to the disease. Unfortunately some bugs—such as the viruses that cause the **common cold** (p. 41)—"disguise" themselves and must be fought off time and again by the immune system.

Dietary Changes That May Be Helpful

Both excessive thinness and severe obesity are associated with impaired immune responses,[1] and obesity increases the risk of infection, at least in hospitalized patients, according to preliminary research.[2] However, these effects may not occur with mild to moderate obesity in otherwise healthy people, and attempts to lose weight through dietary restriction may actually be harmful to the immune system.[3] The detrimental effects of both excess weight and weight-loss diets appear to be offset when people regularly perform aerobic exercise.[4,5]

All forms of sugar (including honey) interfere with the ability of white blood cells to destroy bacteria.[6,7] Animal studies suggest diets high in sucrose (table sugar) impair some aspects of immune function.[8,9] The importance of these effects in the prevention of infections in humans remains unclear.

Alcohol intake, including single episodes of moderate consumption, interferes with a wide variety of immune defenses.[10,11] Alcohol's immune-suppressive effect may be one mechanism for the association between alcohol intake and certain cancers[12] and infections.[13,14] However, moderate alcohol consumption (up to three to four drinks per day) has been associated with either no risk[15] or a *decreased* risk for upper respiratory infections in young non-smokers.[16]

The effect of fats on the immune system is complex and only partially understood. Excessive intake of total dietary fat impairs immune response, but some types of fat may be neutral or even beneficial.[17] For example, monounsaturated fats, as found in in olive oil, appear to have no detrimental effect on the immune system in humans at reasonable dietary levels.[18]

Research on the effect of the omega-3 fats abundant in some fish, **fish oils** (p. 294), and **flaxseed oil** (p. 296) is conflicting. Liquid diets containing omega-3 oils used in hospitals for critically ill people have been shown to improve immune function and reduce infections.[19,20] However, in one controlled study in healthy people, a lowfat diet improved or maintained immune function, but when fish was added to increase omega-3 fatty acid intake, immune function was significantly *inhibited*.[21] Some studies suggest that increased oxidative damage might be the reason for the negative effects on the immune system sometimes caused by fish oil, and that increased intake of antioxidants such as **vitamin** E (p. 344) could correct the problem.[22]

As with omega-3 oils, omega-6 fatty acids (as found in vegetable oils) have also produced conflicting effects on the immune system. Enriching a lowfat diet with omega-6 fatty acids did not impair immunity.[23] However, diets high in omega-6 oils have suppressed immunity in other reports.[24,25]

In summary, lowfat diets with moderate levels of monounsaturated fat from olive oil appear least likely to compromise immune function and may provide small benefits. Conclusions about the desirability of diets high in either omega-3 or omega-6 fatty acid supplementation await further research.

Allergy (p. 76) has been suggested to predispose people to recurrent infection,[26] and many doctors of natural medicine consider allergy treatment for people with recurrent infections. The links between allergy and **ear infections** (p. 63),[27,28] **urinary tract infections** (p. 160) in children,[29] and **yeast vaginitis** (p. 169) in women[30,31] have been documented.

Lifestyle Changes That May Be Helpful

The immune system is suppressed during times of stress, while optimal nutrition may help maintain a strong immune system and combat the harmful effects of stress. Chronic mental and emotional stress can reduce immune function, but whether this effect is sufficient to increase the risk of infection or cancer is less clear.[32,33] Nevertheless, immune function has been increased by stress-reducing techniques such as relaxation exercises, biofeedback, and other approaches,[34,35] although not all studies have shown a significant effect.[36]

The effects of exercise on immune function depend on many factors, including frequency and intensity of exercise.[37] Regular moderate physical activity has positive effects, at least on some immunity parameters, and has been shown to reduce risk of upper respiratory infection. However, vigorous exercise appears to be detrimental to the immune system, and may actually increase the risk of infections.[38] The positive effects of moderate exercise on immunity may also partly explain the reduced susceptibility to cancer of physically active people.[39]

Nutritional Supplements That May Be Helpful

Zinc (p. 346) supplements have been reported to increase immune function.[40,41] This effect may be especially important in the elderly.[42,43] Some nutritionally oriented doctors recommend zinc supplements for people with recurrent infections, suggesting 25 mg per day for adults and lower amounts for children (depending on body weight). However, too much zinc (300 mg per day) has been reported to impair immune function.[44]

While zinc lozenges have been shown to be effective for reducing the symptoms and duration of the common cold in some controlled studies, it is not clear whether this effect is due to an enhancement of immune function or to the direct effect of zinc on the viruses themselves.[45]

Vitamin A (p. 336) plays an important role in immune system function and helps mucous membranes, including those in the lungs, resist invasion by microorganisms.[46] However, most research shows that while vitamin A supplementation helps people prevent or treat infections in third-world countries where deficiencies are common,[47] little to no positive effect, and even slight *adverse* effects, have resulted from giving vitamin A supplements to people in countries where most people consume adequate amounts of vitamin A.[48,49,50,51,52,53]

Beta-carotene (p. 268) and other carotenoids have increased immune cell numbers and activity in animal and human research, an effect that appears to be separate from their role as precursors to vitamin A.[54,55] Placebo-controlled research has shown positive benefits of beta-carotene supplements in increasing numbers of some white blood cells and enhancing cancer-fighting immune functions in healthy people at 25,000–100,000 IU/day.[56,57] In the elderly, supplementation with 40,000 to 150,000 IU/day of beta-carotene has increased natural killer cell activity,[58] but not several other measures of immunity.[59]

Controlled research has found 50,000 IU per day supplementation with beta-carotene boosted immunity in people with colon cancer but not those with precancerous conditions in the colon.[60] Beta-carotene has also prevented immune suppression from ultraviolet light exposure.[61] Effects on immunodeficiency in **HIV**-positive people (p. 87) have been inconsistent using beta-carotene.[62,63]

Vitamin C (p. 341) stimulates the immune system by elevating interferon levels[64] and enhancing the activity of certain immune cells.[65,66] Two studies came to opposite conclusions about the ability of vitamin C to improve immune function in the elderly,[67,68] and two other studies did not agree on whether vitamin C could protect people from hepatitis.[69,70] However, a review of twenty double-blind studies concluded that while vitamin C up to several grams per day has only a small effect in *preventing* colds (p. 41), when taken at the onset of a cold it does significantly reduce the duration of a cold.[71] In controlled reports studying people doing heavy exercise, cold frequency was reduced an average of 50% with vitamin C supplements ranging from 600–1,000 mg per day.[72]

Vitamin E (p. 344) enhances some measures of immune cell activity in the elderly.[73] This effect is broader with 200 IU per day compared to either lower (60 IU per day) or higher (800 IU per day) amounts according to double-blind research.[74] Intakes under 200 IU per day have not boosted immune function in some reports.[75]

A combination of antioxidant **vitamins A** (p. 336), **C** (p. 341), and **E** (p. 344) significantly improved immune cell number and activity compared to placebo in a group of hospitalized elderly people.[76] Daily intake of a 1,000 mg vitamin C plus 200 IU vitamin E for 4 months improved several measures of immune function in an uncontrolled study.[77] To what extent immune boosting combinations of antioxidants actually reduce the risk of infection remains unknown.

Most,[78,79] but not all,[80] double-blind studies find that elderly people have better immune function and reduced infection rates when taking a **multiple vitamin/mineral** (p. 314) formula. In one double-blind trial, supplements of 100 mcg per day of **selenium** (p. 331) and 20 mg per day of **zinc** (p. 346), with or without additional **vitamins C** (p. 341), **E** (p. 344), and **beta-carotene** (p. 268), reduced infections in elderly people, though vitamins without minerals had no effect.[81] Burn victims have also experienced fewer infections after receiving trace mineral supplements in double-blind research.[82] These studies suggest that trace minerals may be the most important micronutrients for enhancing immunity and preventing infections in the elderly.

The effects of eating fish and other dietary sources of **omega-3 oils** (p. 294) is discussed above in the nutritional section. In terms of **EPA** (p. 294) supplements, except for effects in hospitalized patients, most studies have reported that additional omega-3 intake decreases immune function.[83,84,85,86] Antioxidants may correct this problem, according to preliminary research.[87]

The amino acid **glutamine** (p. 300) is important for immune system function. Liquid diets high in glutamine have been reported to be more helpful to critically ill people than other diets.[88,89] Endurance athletes are susceptible to upper respiratory tract infections after heavy exercise, which depletes glutamine levels in blood.[90] Although the effects of glutamine supplementation on immune function after exercise have been inconsistent,[91,92] a double-blind study giving athletes glutamine (2.5 grams after exercise and again 2 hours later) reported 81% without subsequent infection compared to 49% in the placebo group.[93]

Supplements of **Lactobacillus acidophilus** (p. 325), other friendly bacteria, or the growth factors that encourage their development in the gastrointestinal tract may help protect the body from harmful organisms in the intestine that cause local or systemic infection.[94,95] Infectious **diarrhea** (p. 58) in children has been successfully reduced with supplements of friendly bacteria.[96,97]

Liquid diets containing supplemental **arginine** (p. 268), omega-3 fatty acids, and nucleotides such as ribonucleic acid (RNA) have been more effective in maintaining immune function, reducing infections than other liquid diets in treating the critically ill and in post-surgical patients in hospitals in most,[98,99,100,101] but not all double-blind trials.[102,103] No research has studied the effects of these supplements in people with less severe health problems.

Are There Any Side Effects or Interactions? Refer to the individual supplement for information about any side effects or interactions.

Herbs That May Be Helpful

In general, human studies have found that **echinacea** (p. 417) taken orally stimulates the function of a variety of immune cells, particularly natural killer cells.[104] The balance of evidence currently available from studies suggests echinacea speeds recovery from the **common cold** (p. 41), apparently via immune stimulation (as opposed to killing the cold virus directly).[105] Evidence on preventing the common cold with echinacea is mixed, suggesting its immune activity may be mild in generally healthy persons. Refer to the **echinacea** (p. 417) chapter for more discussion of this issue. Other studies on oral echinacea have not found that it stimulates activity of white blood cells known as neutrophils.[106] Many doctors of natural medicine recommend 3–5 ml of tincture 3 times per day to improve immune function. Echinacea in capsule form is also commonly available.

Asian ginseng (p. 394) has a long history of use for preventing and fighting conditions related to the immune system. A double-blind study found that taking 100 mg of a standardized extract of Asian ginseng twice per day improved immune function.[107] A nonstandardized extract in the same amount had milder beneficial effects.

Eleuthero (p. 419) or Siberian ginseng has also historically been used to stimulate the immune system. Preliminary Russian research has supported this traditional use.[108] A double-blind study has shown that healthy people who take 10 ml of eleuthero tincture 3 times per day develop elevated levels of beneficial T-lymphocytes.[109] Although no side effects were seen in this study, the amount of eleuthero used in this trial is exceptionally high.

Complex polysaccharides present in **astragalus** (p. 395), and **maitake** (p. 443) and coriolus mushrooms have the unique ability to act as "immunomodulators" and, as such, are being researched for their potential role in **AIDS** (p. 87) and cancer. Presently the only human studies on astragalus are in Chinese, though they indicate that at the very least astragalus can prevent white blood cell numbers from falling in persons given chemotherapy and radiotherapy, and can elevate antibody levels in healthy persons.[110] Maitake has only been studied in animals as a way to increase immune function.[111] The primary immunoactivating polysaccharide, beta-D-glucan, is well absorbed when taken orally[112] and is currently under investigation as a supportive tool for HIV infection.

Oxyindole alkaloids, substances found in **cat's claw** (p. 408), have been shown to stimulate the immune system.[113] However, little is known about whether this effect is sufficient to help fight infection.

Green tea (p. 430) has stimulated production of immune cells and has anti-bacterial properties in animal studies.[114,115,116] More research is needed to evaluate the effectiveness of green tea in protecting against infection.

Preliminary research suggests that **fo-ti** (p. 425) plays a role in a strong immune system and has anti-bacterial action.[117]

Ashwagandha (p. 393) is considered a general stimulate of the immune system,[118] as well as being considered as a tonic or adaptogen[119]—an herb with multiple, nonspecific actions that counteract the effects of stress and generally promote wellness.

The main active compound in **ligustrum** (p. 442) is ligustrin (oleanolic acid). Studies, mostly conducted in China, suggest that ligustrum stimulates the immune system.[120]

Are There Any Side Effects or Interactions? Refer to the individual herb for information about any side effects or interactions.

Impotence

Checklist for Immune Function

Ranking	Nutritional Supplements	Herbs
Primary	Beta-carotene (p. 268) (for elderly people) Multiple vitamin/mineral (p. 314) (for elderly people) Vitamin E (p. 344) (for elderly people)	Echinacea (p. 417) Eleuthero (p. 419) Asian ginseng (p. 394)
Secondary	Acidophilus (p. 325) Glutamine (p. 300) (for post-exercise infection in performance athletes) Vitamin A (p. 336) Vitamin C (p. 341)	Ashwagandha (p. 393) Ligustrum (p. 442)
Other	Zinc (p. 346)	Astragalus (p. 395) Cat's Claw (p. 408) Fo-ti (p. 425) Green Tea (p. 430) Maitake (p. 443)

Impotence

Impotence, or erectile dysfunction, is the inability of a male to attain or sustain an erection sufficient for intercourse. It can be a persistent condition; however, almost half of all men experience impotence occasionally. Impotence can have either physical or psychological (or both) causes. Although some doctors used to believe differently, most researchers and doctors now believe that a majority of men suffering from impotence have physical causes. Psychological counseling can be helpful, however, if the impotence is related to emotional factors. There are several physical contributors to impotence, including **atherosclerosis** (p. 17), **diabetes** (p. 53), **hypothyroidism** (p. 93), **multiple sclerosis** (p. 127), chronic alcohol use, or what doctors sometimes call "venous leakage" of blood. Certain medications can also be the culprit.

Lifestyle Changes That May Be Helpful

Impotence that cannot be linked to physical causes has been successfully treated by hypnosis.[1] In this trial, 3 hypnosis sessions per week were used initially, later decreasing to 1 per month during a 6-month period. Three out of every four men in the trial were helped.

Nutritional Supplements and Other Natural Therapies That May Be Helpful

Dilation of blood vessels necessary for a normal erection depends on a substance called nitric oxide. In turn, the amino acid **arginine** (p. 268) is needed for nitric oxide formation. In aging rats, arginine supplementation increases nitric oxide levels and improves erectile response.[2] In a group of fifteen men with erectile dysfunction given 2,800 mg arginine per day for 2 weeks, six were helped, though none improved while taking placebo.[3] Although little is known about how effective arginine will be for men with erectile dysfunction or which subset of these men would be helped, available research looks promising and suggests that at least some men are likely to benefit.

Low blood levels of the hormone dehydroepiandrosterone (**DHEA** [p. 288]) have been reported in some men with erectile dysfunction. In one double-blind trial, forty men with low DHEA levels and impotence were given 50 mg DHEA per day for 6 months.[4] Significant improvement in both erectile function and interest in sex occurred in the men assigned to DHEA but not in those assigned to placebo. No significant change occurred in testosterone levels or in factors that could affect the prostate gland. Experts have concerns about the safe use of DHEA, particularly because long-term safety data do not exist. See the **DHEA** (p. 288) chapter for more information about the safety concerns.

Are There Any Side Effects or Interactions? Refer to the individual supplement for information about any side effects or interactions.

Herbs That May Be Helpful

Yohimbe (p. 472) dilates blood vessels, making this herb useful for treating male impotence. Yohimbine (the primary active constituent in yohimbe) has been shown in several double-blind studies to help treat men with impotence;[5,6] negative studies have also been reported.[7,8] Somewhat surprisingly, yohimbe appears to help regardless of the cause of impotence. A tincture of yohimbe bark is often used in the amount of 5–10 drops 3 times per day. There are also standardized yohimbe products available for the treatment of impotence. A typical daily amount of yohimbine is 15–30 mg. It is best to use yohimbine under the supervision of a physician.

Damiana (p. 415) is a traditional herb for men with impotence. However, no modern studies have confirmed its effectiveness.

Ginkgo biloba (p. 427), by increasing arterial blood flow, may help some impotent men.[9] One unblinded study, involving thirty men who were experiencing erectile dysfunction as a result of medication use (selective serotonin reuptake inhibitors and other medications), found that approximately 200 mg per day of ginkgo had a positive effect on sexual function in 76% of the men.[10]

Asian ginseng (p. 394) has traditionally been used as a supportive herb for male potency, although there are no studies to support this usage.

Are There Any Side Effects or Interactions? Refer to the individual herb for information about any side effects or interactions.

Checklist for Impotence

Ranking	Nutritional Supplements	Herbs
Primary		Yohimbe (p. 472)
Secondary	DHEA (p. 288)	Asian ginseng (p. 394) *Ginkgo biloba* (p. 427) (for impotence of vascular origin)
Other	Arginine (p. 268)	Damiana (p. 415)

See also: Homeopathic Remedies for **Impotence** (p. 546)

Indigestion, Heartburn, and Low Stomach Acidity

Indigestion refers to any number of gastrointestinal complaints, which can include gas or wind and upset stomach. Heartburn is a burning feeling caused by stomach acid regurgitating into the esophagus from the stomach. If the burning is in the stomach, the problem is not heartburn but indigestion or perhaps **gastritis** (p. 71) or even a **stomach ulcer** (p. 138).

Heartburn One cause of heartburn is a condition called hiatal hernia. With this condition, a small portion of the stomach gets caught in the sphincter that separates the esophagus from the stomach. A hiatal hernia usually does not require any specific therapy, but any accompanying gastroesophageal reflux should get treatment. This same condition can occur if there is a defective sphincter between the esophagus and the stomach.

According to Jonathan Wright, M.D., and some other doctors of natural medicine, another cause of heartburn can be too *little* stomach acid.[1] This may seem to be a paradox, but based on the clinical experience of doctors such as Dr. Wright, supplementing with **betaine HCl** (p. 269) relieves the symptoms of heartburn and improves digestion.

Low Stomach Acidity Medical researchers since the 1930s have been concerned with the consequences of too little stomach acid (hypochlorhydria). While all the health consequences are still not entirely clear, some have been well documented.

Many minerals and vitamins require proper stomach acid to be absorbed optimally—examples are **iron** (p. 304),[2] **calcium** (p. 277),[3,4] **zinc** (p. 346),[5] and **B-complex vitamins** (p. 341),[6] including **folic acid** (p. 297).[7] People with achlorhydria (no stomach acid) or hypochlorhydria (low stomach acid) may be at risk for developing certain mineral deficiencies. Since minerals are important not only for body structure (as in bones and teeth) but also to activate enzymes (such as superoxide dismutase) and hormones (such as insulin), deficiencies can lead to health problems.

One of the major tasks of stomach acid is to break proteins down to the point that pancreatic **proteolytic enzymes** (p. 289) can easily work. If this does not occur, these proteins might be absorbed in more complicated chains. This malabsorption has been suggested by some researchers to be a major cause of immunological stress and food allergies.[8,9]

In addition, partially digested protein provides a favorable environment for "unfriendly" bacteria that live in the colon.[10,11] Some of these bacteria produce toxic substances that can be absorbed by the body.

Some researchers have found that people with certain diseases sometimes have an inability to produce enough stomach acid. This does not mean the diseases are caused by too little stomach acid, only that there is a correlation. Jonathan Wright, M.D., will usually test stomach acid if people suffer from food allergies, arthritis (both **rheumatoid arthritis** [p. 151] and **osteoarthritis** [p. 130]), pernicious anemia (too little **vitamin B$_{12}$** [p. 337]), **asthma** (p. 151), **diabetes** (p. 53), **vitiligo** (p. 164), **eczema** (p. 64), tic douloureux, Addison's disease, celiac disease, **lupus erythematosus** (p. 115), or **thyroid disease** (p. 93).[12]

Antacids To relieve heartburn, some people try antacids, which often provide symptomatic relief. Antacids can have their own side effects as well, since they can interfere with the absorption of some vitamins and minerals.

Nutrients That Might Be Helpful

Lactose intolerance (p. 114) can cause many digestive problems, including gas, cramps, and **diarrhea** (p. 58); in such cases, the **lactase** (p. 306) enzyme can be helpful when taken before consuming dairy products. Pancreatic enzymes, which include **lipase** (p. 307), aids in the digestion of fats and acts as a digestive aid.

Probiotics (p. 325), such as acidophilus, promote healthy digestion. Enzymes secreted by probiotic bacteria also aid digestion. Acidophilus is a source of lactase enzyme, which is needed to digest milk but is lacking in lactose-intolerant individuals.

Double-blind research suggests that bismuth subcitrate can relieve indigestion.[13] However, not all studies

Indigestion

agree.[14] Usually 1 teaspoon of liquid bismuth preparations are used 2 to 3 times per day, or two 120 mg tablets twice per day.

Are There Any Side Effects or Interactions? Refer to the individual supplement for information about any side effects or interactions.

Herbs That May Be Helpful

Chamomile (p. 409) is effective in relieving inflamed or irritated mucous membranes of the digestive tract. Since heartburn sometimes involves reflux of stomach acid into the esophagus, the anti-inflammatory properties of chamomile are also useful.[15] In addition, chamomile promotes normal digestion.[16] However, modern studies are lacking to prove chamomile beneficial.

Chamomile is typically taken in tea form 3 to 4 times per day, between meals. Boiling water is poured over dried flowers and allowed to steep. Other options are to mix 3–5 ml of chamomile tincture with hot water or to take 2–3 grams of chamomile in capsule or tablet form.

Various herbs known as carminatives have been used to relieve symptoms of indigestion, particularly when there is excessive gas. Among the most notable and well-studied of these are **peppermint** (p. 451), **fennel** (p. 423), and caraway. Double-blind studies have shown that combinations of peppermint and caraway oil and a combination of peppermint, fennel, caraway, and **wormwood** (p. 470) could help people with indigestion.[17,18] It is believed that carminative agents work, at least in part, by relieving spasms in the intestinal tract.[19] Generally 3–5 drops of natural essential oils or 3–5 ml tincture of any of these herbs taken in water 2 to 3 times per day can be helpful. Alternately, a tea can be made by grinding 2–3 teaspoons of the seeds of these plants then simmering them in a cup of water for 10 minutes covered. Drink 3 or more cups per day just after meals.

Lemon balm (p. 440) is another carminative herb used traditionally for indigestion,[20] though it has not been as well studied as peppermint or fennel.[21] Lemon balm is usually taken as tea, steeping 2–3 teaspoons of leaves in hot water for 10 to 15 minutes in a covered container. Drink 3 or more cups per day just after meals. Tincture can also be used in the amount of 3–5 ml 3 times per day.

There are numerous other carminative herbs, including European angelica *(Angelica archangelica)* root, anise, cardamom, cinnamon, cloves, coriander, dill, **ginger** (p. 427), **rosemary** (p. 455), and **sage** (p. 456).[22] Many of these are common kitchen herbs

and thus are easily available for making tea to calm an upset stomach.

Checklist for Indigestion, Heartburn, and Low Stomach Acidity

Ranking	Nutritional Supplements	Herbs
Primary	Lactase (p. 306) (for lactose intolerance only) Lipase (p. 307) (for pancreatic insufficiency only)	Artichoke (p. 393) Peppermint (p. 451)
Secondary	Bismuth	Boldo (p. 401) (indigestion) Caraway Fennel (p. 423) Turmeric (p. 465) Wormwood (p. 470)
Other	Betaine HCl (p. 269) Proteolytic Enzymes (p. 289) Lactobacillus acidophilus (p. 325)	Barberry (p. 395) Blessed Thistle (p. 399) Boldo (p. 401) (heartburn) Chamomile (p. 409) Chaparral (p. 410) Cinnamon (p. 411) Dandelion (leaves and root) (p. 415) Devil's Claw (p. 416) Elecampane (p. 418) Fennel (p. 423) Horehound (p. 434) Lavender (p. 439) Lemon Balm (p. 440) Licorice (DGL) (p. 440) Oregon Grape (p. 449) Yarrow (p. 471) Yellow Dock (p. 472)

See also: Homeopathic Remedies for **Indigestion, Heartburn, and Low Stomach Acidity** (p. 547)

Another potentially beneficial category of herbs for people with indigestion and/or low stomach acid are bitters. **Wormwood** (p. 470) has already been mentioned above as being used in combination with carminative herbs for people with indigestion.[23] Other important bitters are **gentian** (p. 426), **dandelion** (p. 415), **blessed thistle** (p. 399), **yarrow** (p. 471), **devil's claw** (p. 416), bitter orange, and centaury.[24] These are thought to stimulate digestive function by increasing saliva production and promoting both stomach acid and digestive enzyme production.[25] Bitters are taken either by mixing 1–3 ml tincture into water and sipping slowly 10 to 15 minutes before eating, or making tea, which is also sipped slowly before eating.

Some bitters widely used in traditional medicine in North America include yarrow, **yellow dock** (p. 472), **goldenseal** (p. 429), and **Oregon grape** (p. 449). Oregon grape's European cousin **barberry** (p. 395) is also used as a bitter traditionally. Besides stimulating digestion like other bitters, animal studies indicate yarrow, barberry, and Oregon grape may relieve spasms in the intestinal tract.[26]

Horehound (p. 434) contains a number of constituents, including alkaloids, flavonoids, diterpenes (e.g., marrubiin), and trace amount of volatile oils.[27] The major active constituent marrubium and possibly its precursor, premarrubiim, are herbal bitters that increase the flow of saliva and gastric juice, thereby stimulating the appetite.[28]

Artichoke (p. 393) is a mildly bitter plant and healthy food. Extracts of it have been repeatedly shown in double-blind research to be beneficial for people with indigestion.[29] Artichoke is particularly useful when the problem is lack of bile production by the liver.[30] Extracts providing 500–1,000 mg per day of cynarin, the main active constituent of artichoke, are recommended by doctors of natural medicine.

The bright yellow herb **turmeric** (p. 465) relieved indigestion problems in a double-blind study conducted in Thailand.[31] Two capsules containing 250 mg turmeric powder were given 4 times per day.

Licorice (p. 440) protects the mucous membranes lining the digestive tract by increasing production of mucin, a substance that protects against stomach acid and other harmful substances.[32] Licorice root in its deglycyrrhizinated form (DGL) has the glycyrrhizic acid removed (glycyrrhizic acid is the portion of licorice root associated with increasing blood pressure and water retention in some persons). The mucous membrane-healing part of the root, however, remains in DGL. One to two chewable tablets of DGL (250–500 mg) can be taken 15 minutes before meals and 1 to 2 hours before bedtime and may provide relief.[33]

Boldo (p. 401) was used for a variety of digestive conditions in South America, although this may have stemmed from its impact on intestinal infections or liver function. Studies specifically showing a benefit from taking boldo in persons with indigestion and heartburn have not been performed. A physician knowledgeable in botanicals should be consulted before using boldo to ensure safe use.

People in the southwestern United States and northern Mexico have long turned to a tea made from **chaparral** (p. 410) to help calm an upset stomach. The strong-tasting tea was used in only small amounts. Modern research has not confirmed the usefulness of chaparral for indigestion, and there are serious concerns about the safe use of this herb internally.

Traditionally, **elecampane** (p. 418) has been used to treat poor digestion and general complaints of the intestinal tract.

Are There Any Side Effects or Interactions? Refer to the individual herb for information about any side effects or interactions.

Infection

Infections are caused by microorganisms, usually bacteria or viruses. Not all microorganisms cause infections in the body, and exposure to a disease-causing microorganism does not always result in symptoms. The body's immune system plays a large role in determining whether the body will fight off infection.

Refer to the **immune function** (p. 94) chapter for more detailed information about the role of the immune system in infection. Other useful topics to refer to are **common cold/sore throat** (p. 41), **influenza** (p. 104), **cough** (p. 47), **recurrent ear infections** (p. 63), **urinary tract infection** (p. 160), **yeast infection** (p. 169), **athlete's foot** (p. 20), **cold sores** (p. 39), **HIV support** (p. 87), **shingles** (p. 155), and **parasites** (p. 137).

Lifestyle Changes That May Be Helpful

Stress can depress the immune system, thus increasing the body's susceptibility to infection. Coping more effectively with stress is important.[1] Exercise increases natural killer cell activity, which may help prevent infections.[2]

Dietary Changes That May Be Helpful

Nutrition is a major contributor to the functioning of the immune system, which in turn influences whether or not the body is resistant to infection. Specifically, it makes sense to restrict sugar, because sugar interferes with the ability of white blood cells to destroy bacteria.[3] Alcohol interferes with a wide variety of immune defenses.[4] Excessive dietary fat reduces natural killer cell activity.[5]

Nutritional Supplements That May Be Helpful

The nutrients discussed in the immune function chapter are also applicable for preventing infections. The skin and mucous membranes act as barriers to microorganisms; without adequate amounts of **vitamin A** (p. 336), infections are more likely.[6] **Zinc** (p. 346) supplements taken in moderate amounts may increase immune function.[7 8] Some nutritionally oriented doctors recommend zinc supplements for individuals experiencing recurrent infections, suggesting 25 mg per day for adults and lower amounts for children (depending on body weight).

Vitamin C (p. 341) has antiviral activity, helping to prevent virus infections or, in the case of the common cold, reducing the severity and duration of an infection.[9 10] **Lactobacillus acidophilus** (p. 325) (the friendly bacteria found in yogurt) produces acids that kill invading bacteria.[11]

Are There Any Side Effects or Interactions? Refer to the individual supplement for information about any side effects or interactions.

Checklist for Infection

Ranking	Nutritional Supplements	Herbs
Primary	Vitamin A (p. 336) Vitamin C (p. 341)	Echinacea (p. 417)
Secondary	Lactobacillus acidophilus (p. 325) Zinc (p. 346)	Elderberry (p. 418)
Other		American ginseng (p. 392) Ashwagandha (p. 393) Asian ginseng (p. 394) Astragalus (p. 395) Blue Flag (p. 400) Eleuthero (p. 419) Garlic (p. 425) Green tea (p. 430) Ligustrum (p. 442) Lomatium (p. 443) Maitake (p. 443) Oregon grape (p. 449) Pau d'arco (p. 450) (for fungal infection only) Rosemary (p. 455) Sandalwood (p. 456) Schisandra (p. 458) Usnea (p. 465)

See also: Homeopathic Remedies for **Infection** (p. 548)

Herbs That May Be Helpful

Echinacea (p. 417) promotes healthy short-term immune response and may thereby shorten the duration of infection.[12] **Garlic** (p. 425) has natural antibiotic abilities.

Complex polysaccharides present in **astragalus** (p. 395) and the **maitake** (p. 443) mushroom have the unique ability to act as immunomodulators. **Pau**

d'arco (p. 450), according to laboratory tests, has antifungal properties to prevent fungus infections.[13] **Sandalwood** (p. 456), as an essential oil applied topically, possesses antibacterial properties.[14]

Many herbs have a traditional role in boosting resistance to infection, including **elderberry** (p. 418), **green tea** (p. 430), **American ginseng** (p. 392), **Asian ginseng** (p. 394), **eleuthero** (p. 419), **ligustrum** (p. 442), **ashwagandha** (p. 393), **schisandra** (p. 458), **lomatium** (p. 443), **Oregon grape** (p. 449), **rosemary** (p. 455), **usnea** (p. 465), and **blue flag** (p. 400).

Are There Any Side Effects or Interactions? Refer to the individual herb for information about any side effects or interactions.

Infertility (Female)

Infertility is defined by doctors as the failure to become pregnant after a year of unprotected intercourse. It can be caused by sex-hormone abnormalities, low thyroid function, endometriosis, scarring of the tubes connecting the ovaries with the uterus, or a host of other causes. Some of the causes of infertility readily respond to natural medicine, while others do not. The specific cause of infertility should always be diagnosed by a physician before considering possible solutions.

Dietary Changes That May Be Helpful

Caffeine consumption equivalent to more than 2 cups of coffee per day has been linked to tubal disease and endometriosis—both of which can cause female infertility.[1] As little as 1 to 1½ cups of coffee per day appears to delay conception in women trying to get pregnant.[2] Some studies find 1 cup of coffee per day cuts fertility in half,[3] although others report that it takes 2[4] or 3[5] cups to have detrimental effects.

Caffeine is found in regular coffee, black and **green tea** (p. 430), some soft drinks, chocolate, cocoa, and many over-the-counter pharmaceuticals. While not every study finds that caffeine reduces female fertility,[6] most doctors of natural medicine recommend that women trying to get pregnant avoid caffeine.

Decaffeinated coffee has been linked to spontaneous abortion.[7] Some researchers suspect that the tannic acid found in any kind of coffee and black tea may contribute to infertility.[8]

Lifestyle Changes That May Be Helpful

The more women smoke, the less likely they are to conceive.[9] In fact, women whose mothers smoked during *their* pregnancy are only half as likely to conceive as those whose mothers were non-smokers.[10] It's important to quit smoking.

Even moderate drinking in women is linked to an increased risk of infertility in some,[11] although not all, research.[12] Until more is known, women wishing to conceive should probably avoid alcohol.

Excessive or insufficient weight can also be causes of female infertility.[13] Infertile women who are overweight or underweight should consult a nutritionally oriented physician.

Some conventional medications can interfere with fertility. If in doubt, individuals taking prescription drugs should consult their physician.

Nutritional Supplements That May Be Helpful

Gross deficiencies of many nutrients, including **iron** (p. 304) and the **B vitamins** (p. 341), reduce female fertility, but not much is known about the specific role most nutrients play.[14] Nonetheless, double-blind research has shown that taking a **multivitamin/mineral** (p. 314) supplement increases female fertility.[15]

Vitamin E (p. 344) deficiency in animals leads to infertility.[16] In a preliminary human trial, 100–200 IU of vitamin E given to each man and woman of infertile couples led to a significant increase in fertility.[17]

Women who are infertile should rule out the possibility of **iron** (p. 304) deficiency with the help of a doctor. A preliminary report found that women sometimes regain their fertility when given iron supplements.[18]

PABA (p. 319) appears to enhance the effects of cortisone,[19] estrogen, and possibly other hormones by delaying their breakdown in the liver. Some infertile women have increased their ability to become pregnant after taking PABA.[20]

Are There Any Side Effects or Interactions? Refer to the individual supplement for information about any side effects or interactions.

Herbs That May Be Helpful

Vitex (p. 467) is sometimes used as an herbal treatment for infertility—particularly in cases with established luteal phase defect (shortened second half of the menstrual cycle) and high prolactin levels. In one study, forty-eight women diagnosed with infertility (ages 23 to 39) took vitex once daily for 3 months.[21] Forty-five women completed the study, with successful treatment reported in thirty-nine women. Seven women became pregnant during the study, while in twenty-five of the women, progesterone levels normalized—which may increase the chances for pregnancy. Many doctors of natural medicine recommend

taking 40 drops of a liquid extract of vitex each morning with some liquid. Encapsulated powdered vitex provides a similar amount of the product, with one capsule taken in the morning.

Are There Any Side Effects or Interactions? Refer to the individual herb for information about any side effects or interactions.

Checklist for Infertility (Female)

Ranking	Nutritional Supplements	Herbs
Secondary		Vitex (p. 467)
Other	B-complex vitamins (p. 341) Iron (p. 304) (for deficiency) Multivitamin/mineral (p. 314) PABA (p. 319) Vitamin E (p. 344)	

Infertility (Male)

Infertility is defined by doctors as the failure of a couple to achieve pregnancy after a year of unprotected intercourse. In men, infertility is usually associated with a decrease in the number or quality of sperm. There are multiple possible underlying causes for this. Some of the causes of infertility readily respond to natural medicine, while others do not. The specific cause of infertility should always be diagnosed by a physician before considering possible solutions.

Lifestyle Changes That May Be Helpful

Some conventional medications can interfere with fertility. If in doubt, individuals taking prescription drugs should consult their physician.

Nutritional Supplements That May Be Helpful

Vitamin C (p. 341) protects sperm from oxidative damage.[1] Supplementing vitamin C improves the quality of sperm in smokers.[2] When sperm stick together (a condition called agglutination), fertility is reduced. Vitamin C reduces sperm agglutination,[3] increasing the fertility of men with this condition.[4] Many doctors of natural medicine recommend 1 gram of vitamin C per day for infertile men, particularly those diagnosed with sperm agglutination.

A lack of **zinc** (p. 346) can reduce testosterone levels.[5] For men with low testosterone levels, zinc supplementation raises testosterone and also increases fertility.[6] For men with low semen zinc levels, zinc supplements may increase both sperm counts and fertility.[7] Most studies have infertile men take zinc supplements for at least several months. The ideal amount of supplemental zinc remains unknown, but some doctors of natural medicine recommend 25 mg 3 times per day.

Checklist for Infertility (Male)

Ranking	Nutritional Supplements	Herbs
Primary	Vitamin C (p. 341) (for sperm agglutination) Zinc (p. 346) (for deficiency)	
Secondary	Arginine (p. 268) Carnitine (p. 279) Vitamin B$_{12}$ (p. 337) (shots)	
Other	Coenzyme Q$_{10}$ (p. 283) SAMe (p. 330) Vitamin E (p. 344)	
See also: Homeopathic Remedies for **Infertility (Male)** (p. 546)		

Arginine (p. 268) is an amino acid found in many foods; it is needed to produce sperm. Most research shows that several months of arginine supplementation increases sperm count and quality[8 9] and also fertility.[10 11] However, some studies have reported that arginine helps few,[12] if any, infertile men.[13] Nonetheless, many doctors of natural medicine suggest 4 grams of arginine per day for several months to see if it will help infertile men.

Coenzyme Q$_{10}$ (p. 283) is a nutrient used by the body in the production of energy. While its exact role in the formation of sperm is unknown, there is evidence that as little as 10 mg per day (over a 2-week period) will increase sperm count and motility.[14]

Vitamin E (p. 344) deficiency in animals leads to infertility.[15] In a preliminary human trial, 100–200 IU of vitamin E given to each man and woman of infertile couples led to a significant increase in fertility.[16]

Vitamin B$_{12}$ (p. 337) is needed to maintain fertility. Vitamin B$_{12}$ injections have increased sperm counts for men with low numbers of sperm.[17] These results have been duplicated in double-blind research.[18] Men seeking B$_{12}$ injections should consult a nutritionally oriented physician.

Carnitine (p. 279) is a substance made in the body and also found in supplements. It appears to be necessary for normal functioning of sperm cells. In studies,

supplementing with 3–4 grams per day for 4 months has helped to normalize sperm motility in men with low sperm quality.[19 20]

Preliminary research suggests oral **SAMe (S-adenosyl-L-methionine)** (p. 330) may increase sperm activity in infertile men.[21]

Are There Any Side Effects or Interactions? Refer to the individual supplement for information about any side effects or interactions.

Influenza

Influenza is the name of a virus and the infection it causes. Symptoms of infection include fever, muscle aches, and fatigue. Although for most people the infection is mild, it can be severe and even deadly in people with compromised immune systems, including infants, the elderly, and people with diseases such as cancer and **AIDS** (p. 87). In the past, huge epidemics of influenza have caused millions of deaths. This information specifically covers the flu; the general nutritional and herbal support for the immune system that is discussed in the chapter on **immune function** (p. 94) can also be helpful.

Lifestyle Changes That May Be Helpful

Because family stress has been shown to increase the risk of influenza infection,[1] measures to relieve stressful situations may be beneficial.

Nutritional Supplements That May Be Helpful

Dockworkers given 100 mg of **vitamin C** (p. 341) each day for 10 months caught influenza 28% less than their coworkers not taking vitamins; the average infection was 10% shorter in those taking vitamin C.[2] Numerous older studies have reported that vitamin C in high doses (2 grams every hour for 12 hours) can lead to rapid improvement of influenza infections.[3 4] Such high amounts should only be used under medical supervision.

Are There Any Side Effects or Interactions? Refer to the individual supplement for information about any side effects or interactions.

Herbs That May Be Helpful

Echinacea (p. 417) has long been used for colds and flu. Double-blind studies in Germany have shown that infections with flu-like symptoms clear more rapidly when taking echinacea.[5] Echinacea appears to work by stimulating the immune system. Taking 3–5 ml of tincture or 300 mg of dried root powder 3 times per day is usually recommended.

Elderberry (p. 418) has been studied in a small double-blind trial for treatment of influenza.[6] People with influenza recovered three times faster when they took one capsule of elderberry extract 4 times daily compared with those taking placebo.

Although **garlic** (p. 425) is known to kill influenza virus in test tubes,[7] it has not been studied for use in treating influenza. Doctors of natural medicine often recommend taking several cloves of raw garlic per day during an infection.

Asian ginseng (p. 394) and **eleuthero** (p. 419) have immune-enhancing properties, which play a potential role in preventing infection with influenza. **Boneset** (p. 402) has been shown in test tube and other studies to stimulate immune cell function.[8] This may explain boneset's traditional use to help fight off minor viral infections, such as the flu.

According to test tube experiments, **wild indigo** (p. 469) contains polysaccharides and proteins that are believed to stimulate the immune system, which might account for its role in herbal medicine traditionally to fight the flu.[9] However, wild indigo is rarely used alone and is instead used in combination with herbs such as **echinacea** (p. 417), **goldenseal** (p. 429), or thuja.

Are There Any Side Effects or Interactions? Refer to the individual herb for information about any side effects or interactions.

Checklist for Influenza

Ranking	Nutritional Supplements	Herbs
Primary		Echinacea (p. 417)
Secondary	Vitamin C (p. 341)	Elderberry (p. 418)
Other		Asian ginseng (p. 394) Boneset (p. 402) Eleuthero (p. 419) Garlic (p. 425) Goldenseal (p. 429) Wild indigo (p. 469)
See also: Homeopathic Remedies for **Influenza** (p. 549)		

Insomnia

The inability to get a good night's sleep can result from waking up in the middle of the night and having trouble getting back to sleep. It also occurs when people have a hard time getting to sleep in the first place.

Insomnia can be a temporary, occasional, or chronic problem.

Dietary Changes That May Be Helpful

Caffeine is a stimulant.[1] The effects of caffeine can last up to 20 hours,[2] so some people will have disturbed sleep patterns even when their last cup of coffee was in the morning. Besides regular coffee, black and green tea, cocoa, chocolate, some soft drinks, and many over-the-counter pharmaceuticals also contain caffeine.

Doctors of natural medicine will sometimes recommend eating a high-carbohydrate food before bedtime, such as a slice of bread or some crackers. Eating carbohydrates can significantly increase serotonin levels in the body,[3] and the hormone serotonin is known to reduce **anxiety** (p. 14) and promote sleep.

Lifestyle Changes That May Be Helpful

Insomnia can be triggered by psychological stress. Dealing with that stress, through counseling or other techniques, may be the key to a better night's rest. Psychological intervention has helped in many studies.[4]

A steady sleeping and eating schedule combined with caffeine avoidance and counseling sessions using behavioral therapy has reduced insomnia for some people, as has listening to relaxation tapes.[5]

Only scant research explores the effect of exercise on sleep, yet some doctors of natural medicine recommend daily exercise as a way to reduce stress, which in turn can help with insomnia.

A naturopathic therapy for insomnia is to precede sleep with a 15- to 20-minute hot Epsom-salts bath. One or two cups of Epsom salts (magnesium sulfate) in a hot bath acts as a muscle relaxant.

Smokers are more likely to have insomnia than nonsmokers.[6] As with many other health conditions, it's important for people with insomnia to quit smoking.

Nutritional Supplements and Other Natural Therapies That May Be Helpful

Melatonin (p. 312) is a natural hormone that regulates the human biological clock. The body produces less melatonin with advancing age, which may explain why elderly people often have difficulty sleeping[7] and why melatonin supplements improve sleep in the elderly.[8]

Other adults with insomnia also have lower melatonin levels.[9] Double-blind research with young adults shows that melatonin facilitates sleep.[10]

Insomnia

Normally, the body makes melatonin for several hours per night—an effect best duplicated with time-release supplements. Studies using time-release melatonin have reported good results.[11] Many doctors of natural medicine suggest 1–3 mg of melatonin taken 1½ to 2 hours before bedtime.

Insomnia has been associated with tryptophan deficiency in the tissues of the brain,[12] in which case 5-HTP (p. 295) may provide a remedy for the deficiency.

Are There Any Side Effects or Interactions? Refer to the individual supplement for information about any side effects or interactions.

Herbs That May Be Helpful

Herbal remedies have been used safely for centuries for insomnia. In modern herbal medicine, the leading herb for insomnia is **valerian** (p. 467). Valerian root makes getting to sleep easier and increases deep sleep and dreaming. Valerian does not cause a morning "hangover," a side effect common to prescription sleep drugs and melatonin in some individuals.[13][14] A concentrated valerian root supplement in the amount of 300–400 mg can be taken 30 minutes before bedtime.

One German study compared the effect of a combination product containing an extract of valerian root (320 mg at bedtime) and extract of **lemon balm** (p. 440), *Melissa officinalis*, with the sleeping drug Halcion.[15] After monitored sleep for nine nights, the herbal duo matched Halcion in boosting the ability to get to sleep as well as in the quality of sleep. However, the Halcion group felt hung over and had trouble concentrating the next day, while those taking the valerian/lemon balm combination reported no negative effect.

Combining valerian root with other mildly sedating herbs is common both in Europe and the U.S. **Chamomile** (p. 409), **hops** (p. 434), **passion flower** (p. 449), **lemon balm** (p. 440), **scullcap** (p. 459), and **catnip** (p. 407) are commonly recommended by doctors of natural medicine.[16] These herbs can also be used alone as mild sedatives for those suffering from insomnia or nervous exhaustion. Chamomile is a particularly good choice for younger children whose insomnia may be related to gastrointestinal upset. Hops and lemon balm are approved by the German government for relieving sleep disturbances.[17]

Historically, **wild oats** (p. 448) have been used to ease insomnia; oat alkaloids are believed to account for this herb's relaxing effect. However, some European experts do not endorse this herb as a sedative.

The volatile or essential oil of **lavender** (p. 439) contains many medicinal components, including perillyl alcohol, linalool, and geraniol. The oil is calming[18] and thus can be helpful in some cases of insomnia. One study of elderly persons with sleeping troubles found that inhaling lavender oil was as effective as tranquilizers.[19] Lavender is approved by the German government for people with insomnia.[20]

Are There Any Side Effects or Interactions? Refer to the individual herb for information about any side effects or interactions.

Checklist for Insomnia

Ranking	Nutritional Supplements	Herbs
Primary		Valerian (p. 467)
Secondary	Melatonin (p. 312)	
Other	5-HTP (p. 295)	Catnip (p. 407) Chamomile (p. 409) Hops (p. 434) Lavender (p. 439) Lemon balm (p. 440) Oats (p. 448) Passion flower (p. 449) Scullcap (p. 459)

See also: Homeopathic Remedies for **Insomnia** (p. 573)

Intermittent Claudication

Intermittent claudication requires a diagnosis from a health-care practitioner. People with this condition experience leg pain when they walk due to a decreased blood supply. A lack of blood decreases the amount of oxygen reaching the legs, and the lack of oxygen indirectly triggers the leg pain. The cause of intermittent claudication is **atherosclerosis** (p. 17) (hardening of the arteries) that in turn is linked to **high cholesterol** (p. 79), dietary and lifestyle factors that influence heart disease, and heart disease itself. Therefore, the basic natural approaches to intermittent claudication are generally the same as for atherosclerosis.

After reading this chapter, go to the **atherosclerosis** (p. 17) chapter for more information about dietary changes necessary to reduce hardening of the arteries or the risk of heart disease associated with it. What follows is a discussion limited to those aspects of lifestyle and natural medicine that have been studied specifically in relation to intermittent claudication.

Lifestyle Changes That May Be Helpful

Smoking is directly linked to intermittent claudication. Quitting smoking is a critical step in the process of disease prevention.

Although exercise may be helpful in the treatment of intermittent claudication, it is important for all people with this condition to consult a health-care practitioner before beginning an exercise program.

Dietary Changes That May Be Helpful

Important dietary changes in protecting arteries from intermittent claudication include avoiding meat and dairy fat, increasing **fiber** (p. 293), and possibly avoiding foods containing trans fatty acids. More details are provided in the **atherosclerosis** (p. 17) chapter.

Nutritional Supplements That May Be Helpful

Inositol hexaniacinate (p. 339), a special form of vitamin B₃, has been used to successfully treat intermittent claudication. The advantage of inositol hexaniacinate over niacin (another form of vitamin B₃) is a lower risk of toxicity. A double-blind study explored the effect of 2 grams of inositol hexaniacinate taken twice per day for 3 months.[1] After a month, people assigned to inositol hexaniacinate reported a 71% improvement in walking distance, compared with a 45% improvement in the placebo group. Although the overall increase in walking distance was similar in both groups, when smokers who continued to smoke the same number of cigarettes were studied, there was no improvement in the placebo group compared with a 45% increase in walking distance in the inositol hexaniacinate group. Other double-blind research has confirmed inositol hexaniacinate's ability to improve symptoms of intermittent claudication compared with placebo.[2]

Vitamin E (p. 344) supplementation has been shown in controlled trials to increase both walking distance in people with intermittent claudication and blood flow through arteries of the lower legs.[3 4] Dietary vitamin E also correlates with better blood flow to the legs.[5] Some early studies did not find vitamin E useful; possibly this failure was due to the short duration of these studies.[6] A review shows that a minimum of 4 to 6 months of vitamin E supplementation is necessary before significant improvement can be seen.[7]

Magnesium (p. 310) can increase blood supply by acting as a vasodilator. At least one trial found that magnesium supplementation can increase walking distance in people with intermittent claudication.[8] Many doctors of natural medicine suggest that people with atherosclerosis (including intermittent claudication) take approximately 250 mg of magnesium per day.

Double-blind research has found that supplements of **evening primrose oil** (p. 292) led to a 10% increase in exercise tolerance in people with intermittent claudication.[9]

Double-blind research has found that both **carnitine** (p. 279) and propionyl-L-carnitine increase walking distance in people with intermittent claudication. Walking distance increased 75% after 3 weeks of carnitine supplementation (2 grams taken twice per day for a total of 4 grams per day).[10] In the propionyl-L-carnitine study, significant improvement was limited to those who could not walk 250 meters to begin with. In that group, maximum walking distance increased 78% compared with only 44% with placebo.[11] The amount used was 1 gram per day, increasing to 2 grams per day after 2 months and 3 grams per day after an additional 2 months if needed. The results of both studies were statistically significant.

Are There Any Side Effects or Interactions? Refer to the individual supplement for information about any side effects or interactions.

Herbs That May Be Helpful

Extensive studies have been done with **Ginkgo biloba** (p. 427) extracts (GBE) for treatment of intermittent claudication.[12] Two double-blind placebo-controlled studies with 139 people with intermittent claudication found that 120 mg of GBE was effective for increasing pain-free and total walking distance.[13 14]

Garlic (p. 425) has been tested for treatment of intermittent claudication. Capsules of garlic extract, 400 mg twice per day, were found to improve walking distance significantly compared with placebo.[15]

Are There Any Side Effects or Interactions? Refer to the individual herb for information about any side effects or interactions.

Checklist for Intermittent Claudication

Ranking	Nutritional Supplements	Herbs
Primary		Garlic (p. 425) *Ginkgo biloba* (p. 427)
Secondary	Carnitine (p. 279) Vitamin B₃ (niacin— inositol hexaniacinate) (p. 339) Vitamin E (p. 344)	
Other	Evening primrose oil (p. 292) Magnesium (p. 310)	

Iron-Deficiency Anemia

Anemia is a reduction in the number of red blood cells (RBCs), in the amount of hemoglobin in those cells,

Iron-Deficiency Anemia

Iron-Deficiency Anemia

and in another related index called "hematocrit." All three are measured on a complete blood count, which doctors shorten to "CBC." As opposed to all other common causes for anemia, iron-deficiency anemia also causes RBCs to be abnormally small.

Since RBCs are needed to carry oxygen to tissues, anemia impairs oxygen supply to the body. Some common symptoms of anemia include fatigue, lethargy, weakness, poor concentration, and impaired **immune function** (p. 94). In iron-deficiency anemia, fatigue also occurs because **iron** (p. 304) is needed to make optimal amounts of ATP—the energy source the body runs on. This fatigue usually begins long *before* a person is anemic. Said another way, a lack of anemia does not rule out iron deficiency in tired people.

To rule out an iron deficiency in the absence of anemia, a doctor needs to run common lab tests (either serum ferritin or the combination of total iron binding capacity and serum iron). People should never be told their body has sufficient iron simply because they are not anemic. Iron deficiency, whether it is severe enough to lead to anemia or not, can have many non-nutritional causes (such as excessive menstrual bleeding, bleeding **ulcers** [p. 158], **hemorrhoids** [p. 77], gastrointestinal bleeding caused by aspirin or related drugs, frequent blood donations, or colon cancer) or can be caused by a lack of dietary iron. Menstrual bleeding is probably the leading cause of iron deficiency. However, despite common beliefs to the contrary, only about one premenopausal women in ten is iron deficient.[1] Deficiency of **vitamin B**$_{12}$ (p. 337), **folic acid** (p. 297), **vitamin B**$_6$ (p. 340), or **copper** (p. 285) can cause other forms of nutrition anemias; many non-nutritional anemias exist, but this chapter will only cover iron-deficiency anemia.

Dietary Changes That May Be Helpful

Iron (p. 304) deficiency is rarely caused by a lack of dietary iron alone. Nonetheless, a lack of iron in the diet is often part of the problem, so ensuring an adequate supply of iron is important. The most absorbable form of iron, called "heme" iron, is found in meat, poultry, and fish. Non-heme iron is also found in these foods, as well as in dried fruit, molasses, leafy green vegetables, wine, and most iron supplements. Acidic foods (such as tomato sauce) cooked in an iron pan can also be a source of dietary iron.

Vegetarians eat less iron than non-vegetarians, and the iron they eat is somewhat less absorbable. As a result, vegetarians are more likely to have reduced iron stores.[2] Vegetarians can increase their iron intake by emphasizing iron-containing foods within their

diet (see above) or in some cases by supplementing iron if needed.

Coffee interferes with the absorption of iron.[3] However, moderate intake of coffee (4 cups per day) may not adversely affect risk of iron-deficiency anemia when the diet contains adequate amounts of iron and **vitamin C** (p. 341).[4] Black tea contains tannins that strongly inhibit the absorption of non-heme iron. In fact, this iron-blocking effect is so effective that drinking black tea can help treat hemochromotosis, a disease of iron overload.[5] Consequently, individuals who are iron deficient should avoid drinking tea.

Fiber (p. 293) is another dietary component that can impact the absorption of iron from foods. Foods high in bran fiber can reduce the absorption of iron from foods consumed at the same meal by half.[6] Therefore, it makes sense for people needing to take iron supplements to avoid doing so during mealtime if the meal contains significant amounts of fiber.

Nutritional Supplements That May Be Helpful

Before iron deficiency can be treated, it must be diagnosed and the cause must be found by a doctor. In addition to dealing with the cause when possible (avoiding aspirin, treating a bleeding **ulcer** [p. 138], etc.), supplementation with iron is the primary way to resolve iron-deficiency anemia. People who are not diagnosed with iron deficiency should not supplement iron because taking iron when it isn't needed does no good and may do some harm.

If a doctor diagnoses iron deficiency, iron supplementation is essential. Though some doctors use higher amounts, a common adult level is 100 mg per day. Even though symptoms of deficiency should disappear much sooner, iron-deficient people usually need to keep supplementing with iron for 6 months to 1 year, until the blood test "serum ferritin" is completely normal. Even after taking enough iron to overcome the deficiency, some people with recurrent iron deficiency—particularly some premenopausal women—need to continue to supplement with smaller levels of iron such as the 18 mg present in most multiple-vitamin/mineral supplements. This need for continual iron supplementation even after deficiency has been overcome should be determined by a doctor.

Taking **vitamin A** (p. 336) and iron together has been reported to help overcome iron deficiency more effectively than iron supplements alone.[7] Although the optimal amount of vitamin A needed to help people with iron deficiency has yet to be established, some doctors of natural medicine recommend 10,000 IU per day.

Vitamin C (p. 341) increases the absorption of iron.[8] Although many nutritionally oriented doctors tell iron-deficient people to supplement with vitamin C (sometimes 500 mg per day), the actual increase in iron absorption caused by vitamin C supplementation appears to be quite small.[9]

Are There Any Side Effects or Interactions? Refer to the individual supplement for information about any side effects or interactions.

Checklist for Iron-Deficiency Anemia

Ranking	Nutritional Supplements	Herbs
Primary	Iron (p. 304)	
Secondary	Vitamin A (p. 336) (as an adjunct to supplemental iron) Vitamin C (p. 341) (as an adjunct to supplemental iron)	

Irritable Bowel Syndrome (IBS)

Irritable bowel syndrome (IBS) is a very common gastrointestinal disorder that sometimes causes significant discomfort even though it is not a serious health threat. Typical symptoms include abdominal bloating and soreness, gas, and alternating **diarrhea** (p. 58) and **constipation** (p. 44). People with IBS are more likely than others to have backaches, fatigue, and several other seemingly unrelated problems. The cause of IBS remains unknown.

Dietary Changes That May Be Helpful

Several studies report that **food sensitivities** (p. 8) occur in only a small percentage of people with IBS.[1,2,3] Research outcomes are much less clear regarding what percentage of IBS sufferers are truly sensitive to foods. However, some studies find that most IBS sufferers have food sensitivities and that gas production and IBS symptoms diminish when these foods are discovered and avoided.[4,5,6,7] According to a leading researcher in the field, at least 3.5 ounces of the offending food are frequently needed to provoke symptoms of IBS.[8] Others have reported that the offending foods need to be eaten at each meal for at least 2 days to evaluate the potential of food sensitivity.[9] The amount of test food used in studies reporting food sensitivity in only a small proportion of IBS sufferers was less than 3.5 ounces. The inadequate quantities of food may have affected the outcome of these studies.

Preliminary evidence suggests that some people with IBS malabsorb the sugars lactose (as found in milk), fructose (as found in high concentration in fruit juice and dried fruit), and sorbitol (as found in some dietetic candy).[10] Lactose is frequently malabsorbed, and fructose and sorbitol absorb more slowly and less completely than regular table sugar, even in healthy people. As a result, most people in the study, including those who were healthy, showed evidence of malabsorption of at least one of these sugars. However, unlike healthy people, those with IBS-like symptoms had greater symptoms when consuming high concentrations of lactose or the combination of fructose and sorbitol. In this report, restricting intake of these sugars led to reduction in symptoms in 40% of those people with IBS-like symptoms. Therefore, when attempting to uncover food sensitivities, people with IBS should consider the possibility that milk, fruit juice, and dried fruit might cause problems.

Researchers have found that standard blood tests used to evaluate allergies do not help uncover food sensitivities associated with IBS, because IBS food sensitivities are not true allergies.[11,12] The only practical way to evaluate which foods might trigger IBS symptoms is to avoid the foods and then reintroduce them. Such a procedure requires the guidance of a nutritionally oriented doctor. Attempts to find and avoid offending foods without professional help may well fail or exacerbate symptoms.

Limited research has suggested that **fiber** (p. 293) might help people with IBS.[13,14] However, most studies find that IBS sufferers do not benefit by adding wheat bran to their diets.[15,16,17,18] In fact, some people with IBS actually feel worse as a result of wheat bran supplementation.[19] It has been suggested that the lack of positive response to wheat bran may result from a wheat sensitivity,[20] which is one of the most common triggers for food sensitivity in people with IBS.[21] Rye, brown rice, oatmeal, barley vegetables, and **psyllium** (p. 452) husk are good sources of fiber and less likely to trigger food sensitivities than is wheat bran. However, except for psyllium (see below), little is known about the effects of these other fibers in people with IBS.

Lifestyle Changes That May Be Helpful

IBS sufferers have increased rectal pain sensitivity linked to psychological factors.[22] Stress is known to increase symptoms of IBS.[23] Reducing stress or practicing stress management skills have been reported to be beneficial. In one trial, psychotherapy and relaxation combined with conventional treatment were more effective than conventional treatment alone in two-thirds of people with IBS.[24] Hypnosis for relaxation has dramatically relieved symptoms of IBS in some people.[25,26,27]

Nutritional Supplements That May Be Helpful

In one trial, young women with IBS who experienced worsening symptoms before and during their menstrual period were helped by taking enough **evening primrose oil (EPO)** (p. 292) to provide 360–400 mg of gamma linolenic acid (GLA) per day.[28] In that trial more than half reported improvement with EPO, but none was helped in the placebo group. The effects of EPO in other groups of IBS sufferers has not been explored. Double-blind research has shown that avoidance of lactose in people with IBS who are also **lactose intolerant** (p. 114) will relieve IBS symptoms.[29] Alternatively, **lactase** (p. 306) enzyme may be used prior to consuming milk.

Are There Any Side Effects or Interactions? Refer to the individual supplement for information about any side effects or interactions.

Herbs That May Be Helpful

Enteric-coated **peppermint** (p. 451) oil has relieved symptoms of IBS in double-blind research.[30] In one double-blind trial, four out of every five IBS sufferers studied experienced reduced symptoms when given enteric-coated peppermint oil.[31] In another of the double-blind trials reporting significant improvement, 3 to 6 capsules providing 0.2 ml of peppermint oil per pill were taken per day.[32] The combination of 90 mg of peppermint oil plus 50 mg of caraway oil in enteric-coated capsules taken 3 times per day led to significant reduction in IBS symptoms in yet another controlled trial.[33] The combination of **peppermint** (p. 451), caraway seeds, and two other carminitive (gas relieving) herbs, **fennel** (p. 423) seeds and **wormwood** (p. 470), was reported to be an effective treatment for upper abdominal complaints, including IBS, according to another double-blind study.[34]

Enteric coating appears to protect peppermint oil while it is passing through the acid environment of the stomach. In the intestinal tract, peppermint oil reduces gas production, eases intestinal cramping, and soothes irritation. In preliminary research, peppermint oil has also reduced spasms of intestinal musculature.[35] Caraway oil is believed to have similar effects to peppermint oil.

A few studies have not found peppermint oil to be helpful. However, the negative trials are either very short (2 weeks)[36] or, in one case where peppermint oil *increased* symptoms, did not administer the oil by

mouth.[37] Besides the use of enteric-coated capsules, herbalists sometimes suggest that peppermint may also be taken as a tincture (2–3 ml 3 times daily) or even as pure essential oil in liquid form (1–2 drops with symptoms up to 3 to 4 times per day). Pure food grade essential oil of peppermint is extremely strong and must never be consumed except in 1–2 drop amounts.

Chamomile (p. 409) acts as a carminative as well as soothing and toning agent for the digestive tract. Chamomile's essential oils have also eased intestinal cramping and irritation in animals.[38] It is sometimes used by herbalists for those with IBS experiencing alternating bouts of diarrhea and constipation, though research has yet to investigate these effects.

Chamomile is typically taken 3 times per day, between meals, in a tea form by dissolving 2–3 grams of powdered chamomile or by adding 3–5 ml of herbal extract tincture to hot water.

Some people with IBS may benefit from bulk-forming laxatives. **Psyllium** (p. 452) seeds (3.25 g taken 3 times per day) have helped regulate normal bowel activity in some people with IBS.[39] Psyllium has improved some symptoms of IBS in double-blind trials.[40,41]

Comfrey (p. 413) has a long, consistent history of use as a topical agent for improving **healing of wounds** (p. 167), skin ulcers, thrombophlebitis, strains, and sprains.[42,43] It was also used for persons with gastrointestinal problems, such as stomach **ulcers** (p. 138) and inflammatory bowel syndrome, and for lung problems.

Are There Any Side Effects or Interactions? Refer to the individual herb for information about any side effects or interactions.

Checklist for Irritable Bowel Syndrome

Ranking	Nutritional Supplements	Herbs
Primary	Lactase (p. 306) (for lactose-intolerant people)	Psyllium (p. 452)
Secondary		Peppermint (p. 451)
Other	Evening Primrose Oil (p. 292) (for premenstrual IBS) Fiber (p. 293) (other than wheat)	Caraway, Chamomile (p. 409) Fennel (p. 423) Wormwood (p. 470)

See also: Homeopathic Remedies for **Irritable Bowel Syndrome** (p. 545)

Jet Lag

Jet lag is a disturbance of the sleep-wake cycle triggered by travel across time zones. The symptoms of jet lag include difficulty falling asleep at the new sleep time, sleepiness during the day, poor concentration, and fatigue. The symptoms can last from a day to a week or longer, depending on the individual and number of time zones crossed.

Nutritional Supplements and Other Natural Therapies That May Be Helpful

Melatonin (p. 312) is a natural hormone that regulates the human biological clock and appears to be helpful in relieving symptoms of jet lag. One double-blind trial, involving fifty-two international flight crew members taking either melatonin or a placebo for 3 days before and 5 days after an international flight, found that melatonin significantly reduced symptoms of jet lag and resulted in a quicker recovery of pre-flight energy levels and alertness.[1]

Another double-blind study compared various amounts of melatonin in 234 individuals who traveled through six to eight time zones.[2] Either fast-release or controlled-release melatonin formulations were taken at bedtime for 4 days after the flight. The fast-release products were found to be more effective than the controlled-release. The 5 mg and 0.5 mg fast-release melatonin were almost equally effective for improving sleep quality, time it took to fall asleep, and daytime sleepiness.

Are There Any Side Effects or Interactions? Refer to the individual supplement for information about any side effects or interactions.

Checklist for Jet Lag

Ranking	Nutritional Supplements	Herbs
Primary	Melatonin (p. 312)	

Kidney Stones

Kidney stones are hard masses that can grow from crystals forming within the kidneys. The medical term for kidney stone formation is nephrolithiasis. The stones themselves are called renal calculi. Kidney stones often cause severe pain, sometimes accompa-

nied by gastrointestinal symptoms, chills, fever, and blood in urine.

Most kidney stones are made of calcium oxalate. People with a history of kidney stone formation should talk with their doctor to learn what type of stones they have—approximately one stone in three is made of something other than calcium oxalate and one in five contains little if any calcium (p. 277) in any form. **Note:** The information included in this chapter pertains to prevention of calcium oxalate kidney stone recurrence only—not to other kidney stones or to the treatment of acute disease. The term "kidney stone" as used in this chapter refers only to calcium oxalate stones. However, information regarding how natural substances affect urinary calcium levels may also be important for people with a history of calcium phosphate stones.

Calcium oxalate stone formation is rare in primitive societies, suggesting that this condition is preventable.[1] People who have formed a calcium oxalate stone are at high risk of forming another kidney stone.

Dietary Changes That May Be Helpful

Increasing dietary oxalate can lead to an increase in urinary oxalate excretion. Increased urinary oxalate increases the risk of stone formation. As a result, most doctors agree that kidney stone formers should reduce their intake of oxalate from food as a way to reduce urinary oxalate.[2] Many foods contain oxalate; however, only a few—spinach, rhubarb, beet greens, nuts, chocolate, tea, bran, almonds, peanuts, and strawberries—appear to significantly increase urinary oxalate levels.[3 4]

Increased levels of urinary calcium also increases the risk of stone formation. Consumption of animal protein from meat, dairy, poultry, or fish increases urinary calcium. Perhaps for this reason, animal protein has been linked to an increased risk of forming stones,[5,6] and vegetarians have been reported to be at lower risk for stone formation.[7] As a result, some nutritionally oriented doctors recommend reducing intake of foods containing animal protein. One isolated report paradoxically found an *increase* in kidney stone recurrences following the restriction of animal protein while at the same time increasing dietary fiber.[8] However, other researchers find such a diet appears to reduce the risk of forming stones,[9] and most researchers continue to find links between kidney stone risk and animal protein intake.[10,11]

Salt increases urinary calcium excretion in stone formers.[12,13,14] In theory, this should increase the risk of forming a stone. As a result, some researchers have suggested that reducing dietary salt may be a useful way to decrease the chance of forming additional stones.[15,16] Increasing dietary salt has also affected a variety of other risk factors in ways that suggest an increased chance of kidney stone formation.[17] Nutritionally oriented doctors generally recommend that people with a history of kidney stones reduce salt intake. To what extent such a dietary change would reduce the risk of stone recurrence remains unclear.

Potassium (p. 323) reduces urinary calcium excretion,[18] and people who eat high amounts of dietary potassium appear to be at low risk of forming kidney stones.[19] Most kidney stone research involving potassium uses the form potassium citrate, although citrate itself may lower the risk of stone recurrence. However, in some potassium research, a significant decrease in urinary calcium occurs even in the absence of added citrate.[20] This outcome suggests that increasing potassium itself may reduce the risk of kidney stone recurrence. The best way to increase potassium is to eat fruits and vegetables. The level of potassium in food is much higher than the small amounts found in supplements.

Most citrate research conducted with people who have a history of kidney stones involves supplementation with potassium citrate or magnesium citrate. In one double-blind trial, recurrence of kidney stone formation dropped from 64% to 13% for those receiving high amounts of both supplements.[21] In that trial, people were instructed to take 6 pills per day—enough potassium citrate to provide 1,600 mg of potassium and enough magnesium citrate to provide 500 mg of magnesium. Both placebo and citrate groups were also advised to restrict salt, sugar, animal protein, and foods rich in oxalate. Several similar trials have proven that potassium and magnesium citrate supplementation reduces kidney stone recurrences.[22]

Citric acid is found in many foods and may also protect against kidney stone formation.[23,24] The best food source commonly available is citrus fruits, particularly lemons. One preliminary study found that drinking 2 liters (approximately 2 quarts) of lemonade per day improved the quality of the urine in ways that are associated with stone prevention.[25] Lemonade was far more effective than orange juice. The lemonade was made by mixing 4 ounces of lemon juice with enough water to make 2 liters. The smallest amount of sweetener possible should be added to make the taste acceptable. Further study is necessary, however, to determine whether lemonade can prevent recurrence of kidney stones.

Drinking grapefruit juice has actually been linked to an increased risk of kidney stones in two large studies.[26,27] Whether grapefruit juice actually causes kidney stone recurrence or is merely associated with something else that increases risks remains unclear; some nutritionally oriented doctors suggest that people with a history of stones should restrict grapefruit juice intake until more is known.

Bran, a rich source of insoluble fiber (p. 293), reduces the absorption of calcium, which in turn causes urinary calcium to fall.[28] In one trial, risk of forming kidney stones was significantly reduced simply by adding one-half ounce of rice bran per day to the diet.[29] Oat and wheat bran are also good sources of insoluble fiber and are available in natural food stores and supermarkets. Before supplementing with bran, people should check with a nutritionally oriented doctor because some people—even a few with kidney stones—don't absorb enough calcium. For those people, supplementing with bran might deprive them of much-needed calcium.

People who form kidney stones have been reported to process sugar abnormally.[30] Sugar has also been reported to increase urinary oxalate,[31] and in some reports, urinary calcium as well.[32] As a result, some nutritionally oriented doctors recommend that people who form stones avoid sugar.[33,34] To what extent, if any, such a dietary change decreased the risk of stone recurrence has not been studied and remains unclear.

Drinking water increases the volume of urine. In the process, substances that form kidney stones are diluted, reducing the risk of kidney stone recurrence. For this reason, people with a history of kidney stones should drink at least 2 quarts per day. It is particularly important that people in hot climates increase their fluid intake to reduce their risk.[35]

Drinking coffee or other caffeine-containing beverages increases urinary calcium.[36] Long-term caffeine consumers are reported to have an increased risk of osteoporosis (p. 133),[37] suggesting that the increase in urinary calcium caused by caffeine consumption may be significant. However, coffee consists mostly of water, and increasing water consumption is known to reduce the risk of forming a kidney stone. While many nutritionally oriented doctors are concerned about the possible negative effects of caffeine consumption in people with a history of kidney stones, preliminary studies in both men[38,39] and women[40] have found that coffee and tea consumption is actually associated with a *reduced* risk of forming a kidney stone. These reports suggest that the helpful effect of consuming more water by drinking coffee or tea may compensate for the theoretically harmful effect that caffeine has in elevating urinary calcium. Therefore, the bulk of current research suggests that it is not important for kidney stone formers to avoid coffee and tea.

Similarly, some nutritionally oriented doctors have been concerned about a reported link between drinking soft drinks and risk of kidney stones[41] that was followed by a study showing that men who refrained from drinking soft drinks (especially drinks containing phosphoric acid) reduced their risk of stone recurrences compared with men permitted to consume soft drinks.[42] Phosphoric acid is thought to affect calcium metabolism in ways that might increase kidney stone recurrence risk. Research in this area remains somewhat inconsistent, however. In one large trial, people who consumed more soft drinks were not at increased risk.[43]

Nutritional Supplements That May Be Helpful

In the past, medical doctors commonly recommended that people with a history of kidney stones restrict **calcium** (p. 277) intake because a higher calcium intake increases the amount of calcium in the urine. However, calcium (from supplements or food) binds to oxalate in the gut before either can be absorbed, thus interfering with the absorption of oxalate. When oxalate is not absorbed, it cannot be excreted in urine. The resulting decrease in urinary oxalate actually *reduces* the risk of stone formation.[44] The question is, which effect of supplemental calcium is more important—the increase in urinary calcium, which should increase risk of stone recurrence, or the reduction in urinary oxalate, which should reduce the risk? According to an editorial in the *New England Journal of Medicine*, the oxalate binding is more important than increases in urinary calcium;[45] therefore it makes sense that, for most people, calcium might reduce rather than increase the risk of kidney stone formation.

According to research published in the *New England Journal of Medicine*, people who eat more calcium have a lower risk of forming kidney stones than people who consume less calcium.[46] Most studies have also reported that people who consume more calcium have a lower, not higher, risk of forming kidney stones.[47,48]

However, while *dietary* calcium has been linked to reduction in the risk of forming stones, calcium supplements have been associated with an *increased* risk in a large study of American nurses.[49] The researchers who conducted this trial speculate that the difference in effects between dietary and supplemental calcium resulted from differences in timing of calcium consumption. All *dietary* calcium is eaten with food, and so it can then block absorption of oxalates that may be present at the same meal. In the study of American nurses, however, most *supplemental* calcium was consumed apart from food.[50] Calcium taken without food

will increase urinary calcium, thus increasing the risk of forming stones; but calcium taken without food cannot reduce the absorption of oxalate from food consumed at a different time. For this reason, these researchers speculate that calcium supplements were linked to *increased* risk because they were taken between meals. Thus, calcium supplements may be beneficial for many stone formers, as dietary calcium appears to be, but only if taken with meals. Taken between meals, calcium supplements may *increase* the risk of stone formation.

When nutritionally oriented doctors recommend **calcium** (p. 277) supplements to stone formers, they usually suggest 800 mg per day in the form of calcium citrate, taken with meals. Citrate helps reduce the risk of forming a stone (see Dietary section for more information).[51] Calcium citrate has been shown to increase urinary citrate in stone formers, which should act as protection against any increase in urinary calcium.[52]

Despite the fact that calcium supplementation taken with meals may be helpful for some, people with a history of kidney stone formation should not take calcium supplements without the supervision of a health-care professional. Although the increase in urinary calcium caused by calcium supplements can be mild or even temporary,[53] some stone formers show a potentially dangerous increase in urinary calcium following calcium supplementation; this may, in turn, increase the risk of stone formation.[54] People who are "hyperabsorbers" of calcium should not take supplemental calcium until more is known. Using a protocol established years ago in the *Journal of Urology*, 24-hour urinary calcium studies conducted both with and without calcium supplementation determine which stone formers are calcium "hyperabsorbers."[55] Any health-care practitioner can order this simple test.

Increased blood levels of activated vitamin D are found in some kidney stone formers, according to some,[56] but not all, research.[57] Until more is known, kidney stone formers should avoid taking **vitamin D** (p. 343) supplements without consulting a nutritionally oriented doctor.[58]

Both **magnesium** (p. 310) and **vitamin B_6** (p. 340) are used by the body to convert oxalate into other substances. Vitamin B_6 deficiency leads to an increase in kidney stones as a function of elevated urinary oxalate.[59] Vitamin B_6 is also known to reduce elevated urinary oxalate in some stone formers who are not necessarily B_6 deficient.[60,61] Years ago, the *Merck Manual* recommended 100–200 mg vitamin B_6 and 200 mg magnesium per day for some kidney stone formers with elevated urinary oxalate.[62] Most studies have shown that supplementing with magnesium and/or vitamin B$_6$ significantly lowers the risk of forming kidney stones.[63,64][65] Results have varied from only a slight reduction in recurrences[66] to a greater than 90% decrease in recurrences.[67]

Optimal supplemental levels of vitamin B$_6$ and magnesium remain unknown. Many nutritionally oriented doctors advise 200–400 mg per day of magnesium. While the effective intake of vitamin B$_6$ appears to be as low as 10–50 mg per day, certain people with elevated urinary oxalate may require much higher amounts, and therefore require medical supervision. In some cases, as much as 1,000 mg of vitamin B$_6$ per day (a potentially toxic level) has been used successfully.[68]

Nutritionally oriented doctors who do advocate use of **magnesium** (p. 310) for people with a history of stone formation generally suggest the use of magnesium citrate because citrate itself reduces kidney stone recurrences. As with calcium supplementation, it appears important to take magnesium with meals in order for it to reduce kidney stone risk by lowering urinary oxalate.[69]

It has been suggested that people who form kidney stones should avoid **vitamin C** (p. 341) supplements, because vitamin C can convert into oxalate and increase urinary oxalate.[70,71] Initially, these concerns were questioned because the vitamin C had been converting to oxalate *after* urine had left the body.[72,73] However, using newer methodology that rules out this problem, recent evidence shows that as little as 1 gram of vitamin C per day can increase the urinary oxalate levels in some people, even those without a history of kidney stones.[74,75] In one case, 8 grams per day of vitamin C led to dramatic increases in urinary oxalate excretion and kidney stone crystal formation, which causes bloody urine.[76] Until more is known, people with kidney stones or a history of stone formation should not take large amounts (1 gram per day) of supplemental vitamin C. Amounts significantly lower (100–200 mg per day) appear to be safe.

Glucosamine sulfate (p. 299) and **chondroitin sulfate** (p. 281) may play a role in reducing the risk of kidney stone formation. One study found 60 mg per day of such supplements significantly lowered urinary oxalate levels in stone formers.[77] Such a decrease should reduce the risk of stone formation.

Are There Any Side Effects or Interactions? Refer to the individual supplement for information about any side effects or interactions.

Herbs That May Be Helpful

Highly trained practitioners of botanical medicine use several herbs to help facilitate passage of small kidney stones and to help prevent their formation.

The efficacy of these herbs has not been documented scientifically for people with kidney stones. Because the risks associated with acute kidney stones are high, it is essential to consult with a trained practitioner before attempting to use any herb to help pass kidney stones.

The German government has approved a number of herbs that increase urine volume (herbal diuretics) as a way to help prevent kidney stone formation.[78] These herbs include asparagus root, birch leaf, couch grass, goldenrod, **horsetail** (p. 436), Java tea (*Orthosiphon stamineus*), lovage, parsley, spiny restharrow, and **stinging nettle** (p. 444). Generally they are given as teas to further increase water intake as well as deliver the medicinal herbs.

Checklist for Calcium Oxalate Kidney Stones

Ranking	Nutritional Supplements	Herbs
Primary	Magnesium citrate/ potassium citrate Vitamin B$_6$ (p. 340) (in the presence of elevated urinary oxalate)	
Secondary	Vitamin B$_6$ (p. 340) (in the absence of elevated urinary oxalate)	
Other	Calcium (p. 277) Chondroitin sulfate (p. 281) Fiber (p. 293) Glucosamine sulfate (p. 299) Lemonade (citric acid)	Asparagus root Birch leaf Couch grass Goldenrod Horsetail (p. 436) Java tea (*Orthosiphon stamineus*) Lovage Parsley Spiny restharrow Stinging nettle (p. 447)

Lactose Intolerance

Lactose intolerance is the impaired ability to digest lactose (the naturally occurring sugar in milk). The enzyme **lactase** (p. 306) is needed to digest lactose, and a few children and many adults do not produce sufficient lactase to digest the milk sugar; the condition is rare in infants. In people with lactose intolerance, consuming foods containing lactose results in cramps, gas, and **diarrhea** (p. 58).

Only one-third of the population worldwide retains the ability to digest lactose into adulthood. Most adults of Asian, African, Middle Eastern, and Native American descent are lactose intolerant. In addition, half of Hispanics and about 20% of Caucasians do not produce lactase as adults.[1]

A simple test for lactose intolerance is to drink at least 2 glasses of milk on an empty stomach and note any gastrointestinal symptoms that develop in the next 4 hours; the test should then be repeated using several ounces of cheese (which does not contain much lactose). If symptoms result from milk but not cheese, then the person has lactose intolerance. If symptoms occur with both milk and cheese, the person may be allergic to dairy (very rarely can lactose intolerance be so severe that even eating cheese will cause symptoms).

In addition to gastrointestinal problems, one study has reported a correlation in women between lactose intolerance and a higher risk of **depression** (p. 50) and **PMS** (p. 141).[2] However, this study is only preliminary and does not establish a cause-and-effect relationship.

Dietary Changes That May Be Helpful

Although symptoms of lactose intolerance are triggered by the lactose in some dairy products, few lactose-intolerant individuals need to avoid all dairy. Dairy products have varying levels of lactose, which affects how much lactase is required for proper digestion. Milk, ice cream, and yogurt contain significant amounts of lactose—although for complex reasons yogurt often doesn't trigger symptoms in lactose-intolerant people. In addition, lactose-reduced milk is available in some supermarkets and can be used by lactose-intolerant people.

Nutritional Supplements That May Be Helpful

Supplemental sources of the enzyme **lactase** (p. 306) can be used to prevent symptoms of lactose intolerance when consuming lactose-containing dairy products. Lactase drops can be added to regular milk 24 hours before drinking to reduce lactose levels. Lactase drops, capsules, and tablets can also be taken directly, as needed, immediately before a meal containing dairy products. The degree of lactose intolerance varies by individual, so a greater or lesser amount of lactase may be needed to eliminate symptoms of lactose intolerance.

Researchers have yet to clearly determine whether lactose-intolerant individuals absorb less **calcium** (p. 277). As dairy products are a rich source of calci-

um and some individuals with lactose intolerance avoid some forms of dairy, alternative sources of calcium (foods or supplements) might be necessary. A typical amount of supplemental calcium is 1,000 mg per day.

Are There Any Side Effects or Interactions? Refer to the individual supplement for information about any side effects or interactions.

Checklist for Lactose Intolerance

Ranking	Nutritional Supplements	Herbs
Primary	Lactase (p. 306)	

Lupus (Systemic Lupus Erythematosus)

Systemic lupus erythematosus (SLE) is an autoimmune illness that causes a characteristic rash accompanied by inflammation of connective tissue, particularly joints, throughout the body. In autoimmune diseases, the **immune system** (p. 94) attacks the body instead of protecting it. Kidney, lung, and vascular damage are potential problems resulting from SLE.

The cause of SLE is unknown, though 90% of cases occur in women of childbearing age. Several drugs, such as procainamide, hydralazine, methyldopa, and chlorpromazine, can create SLE-like symptoms. Similarly, environmental pollution and industrial emissions may also trigger SLE-like symptoms in some people.[1] In one reported case, **zinc** (p. 346) supplementation appears to have aggravated drug-induced SLE.[2]

Risk factors include a family history of SLE, other collagen diseases or **asthma** (p. 15),[3] menstrual irregularity,[4] beginning menstruation at age 15 or later,[5] exposure to toxic chemicals,[6] and low blood levels of **antioxidant** (p. 267) nutrients, such as **vitamins A** (p. 336) and **E** (p. 344), or **beta-carotene** (p. 268).[7] Free radicals are thought to promote SLE.[8]

Discoid lupus erythematosus (DLE) is a milder form of lupus that affects the skin. Like SLE, it is not known what causes DLE, though sun exposure can trigger the first outbreak. DLE is most common among women in their 30s.

Dietary Changes That May Be Helpful

An isolated case of someone with SLE improving significantly after the introduction of a vegetarian diet has been reported.[9] In Japan, women who frequently ate fatty meats, such as beef and pork, were reported to be at higher risk for SLE compared with women eating little of these foods.[10] Consuming fewer calories, less fat, and foods low in **phenylalanine** (p. 320) and **tyrosine** (p. 335) (prevalent in high protein foods, such as meat and dairy) might be helpful, according to animal and preliminary human studies.[11]

Foods high in omega-3 fats, such as fish and **flaxseed** (p. 296), may decrease lupus-induced inflammation. In one trial, nine people with kidney damage due to SLE were fed increasing amounts of flaxseed for a total of 12 weeks.[12] After examining the results, researchers concluded that 30 grams per day was the optimal intake for improving kidney function, decreasing inflammation, and reducing **atherosclerotic** (p. 17) development. Flaxseeds also contain antioxidants, potentially helpful to those with SLE.[13]

To date, all studies on **fish oil** (p. 298) have used supplements and not fish (see below). Nonetheless, many nutritionally oriented doctors recommend people with SLE eat several servings of fatty fish each week.

Spanish researchers discovered that individuals with SLE tend to have more **allergies** (p. 8), including food allergies, than do healthy people or even people with other autoimmune diseases.[14] While one study reported that drinking milk was associated with a decrease in SLE risk,[15] other investigations point to both beef[16] and dairy[17] as foods that might trigger allergic reactions in some people with SLE. Casein, the main protein in cow's milk, has immune-stimulating properties.[18] This might explain why some people with SLE have been reported to be intolerant of milk products. Researchers and doctors still do not know whether avoidance of allergens will significantly help people with SLE. People wishing to explore the effects of discovering and avoiding foods they might be sensitive to should consult a nutritionally oriented doctor.

Alfalfa (p. 391) seeds and sprouts contain the amino acid L-canavanine, which provokes a lupus-like condition in monkeys[19] and possibly humans.[20] For this reason, some nutritionally oriented doctors recommend that people with SLE should avoid these foods. Cooking alfalfa seeds has been reported to erase this effect.[21]

Lifestyle Changes That May Be Helpful

In preliminary research, smoking has been linked to significantly increased risk of developing SLE, while drinking alcohol has been associated with a decrease in risk.[22] The importance of these associations remains

unclear, though an increased risk for many other diseases has been definitively linked to excessive consumption of alcohol.

Nutritional Supplements and Other Natural Therapies That May Be Helpful

The omega-3 fatty acids in **fish oil** (p. 298)—eicosapentaenoic acid (EPA) and docosahexaenoic acid (**DHA** [p. 287])—decrease inflammation. Supplementation with EPA and DHA has prevented autoimmune lupus in animal research.[23] In a double-blind study, 20 grams of fish oil daily combined with a lowfat diet led to improvement in fourteen of seventeen people with SLE in 12 weeks.[24] Smaller amounts of fish oil have led to only temporary improvement in other double-blind research.[25] People wishing to take such a large amount of fish oil should first consult with a nutritionally oriented doctor.

Antioxidant (p. 267) levels have been reported to be low in people with SLE, though this finding was not statistically significant in one trial.[26] When animals are fed antioxidant-deficient diets, they develop a condition similar to SLE; supplementation with antioxidants such as **vitamins C** (p. 341) and **E** (p. 344), **beta-carotene** (p. 268), and **selenium** (p. 331) has helped animals with existing SLE.[27] It remains unclear whether antioxidant supplementation would have a positive effect on people with SLE.

Some preliminary evidence suggests that **vitamin E** (p. 344) might help people with DLE. Two doctors reported good to excellent results by giving 800–2,000 IU of vitamin E per day to eight people with DLE.[28,29] According to these researchers, lower amounts of vitamin E did not work as well. In another small trial, vitamin E, also given in high amounts, had no effect.[30] Unlike with DLE, there appears to be no reports on the effects of vitamin E in people with SLE.

In one report, 250,000 IU **beta-carotene** (p. 268) per day cleared up all facial rashes in as little as 1 week for three people with DLE.[31] However, another study involving twenty-six people (nineteen with DLE and seven with SLE) found that using an even higher intake (400,000 IU per day) for an average of 5½ months was ineffective.[32] Research has not yet supported the use of beta-carotene for people with SLE.

Preliminary data suggest that **pantothenic acid** (p. 340) may help those with DLE. In one study, taking 10–15 grams of pantothenic acid per day with 1,500–3,000 IU of **vitamin E** (p. 344) for as long as 19 months, helped sixty-seven people with DLE.[33] Pantothenic acid by itself for shorter periods of time in lower amounts has been reported to fail.[34] The amounts of pantothenic acid and vitamin E used in the first study are very high and should not be taken without the supervision of a nutritionally oriented physician.

In a double-blind trial, twenty-seven women with mild to moderate SLE were given 200 mg of **DHEA** (p. 288) per day or placebo.[35] Three months later, those assigned to DHEA were significantly better and were able to decrease prednisone use more than those taking placebo. Other studies have also supported the use of DHEA in people with SLE.[36,37] Low blood levels of DHEA and DHEA-sulfate have been associated with more severe symptoms in people with SLE.[38] Two hundred milligrams per day is an extremely high and potentially toxic amount of DHEA. No one should take such amounts without medical supervision. Experts have concerns about the use of DHEA, particularly because long-term safety data do not exist. Side effects at high intakes (50–200 mg per day) appear to be acne (in over 50% of people), increased facial hair (18%), and increased perspiration (8%). Less common problems caused by DHEA have been reported to be breast tenderness, weight gain, mood alteration, headache, oily skin, and menstrual irregularity.[39] Because this trial was not controlled, it is possible that some of the less common "side effects" were unrelated to DHEA and might have occurred even with placebo.

High amounts of DHEA have caused cancer in animals.[40 41] Although *anti*cancer effects of DHEA have also been reported,[42] they involve trials using animals that do not process DHEA the way humans do, so these positive effects may have no relevance for people. Links have begun to appear between higher DHEA levels and risks of prostate cancer in humans.[43] At least one person with prostate cancer has been reported to have had a worsening of his cancer despite feeling better while taking very high amounts (up to 700 mg per day) of DHEA.[44] While younger women with breast cancer may have low levels of DHEA, postmenopausal women with breast cancer appear to have high levels of DHEA, which has researchers concerned.[45] These cancer concerns make sense because DHEA is a precursor to testosterone (linked to prostate cancer) and estrogen (linked to breast cancer). Until more is known, it would be prudent for individuals with breast or prostate cancer or a family history of these conditions to avoid supplementing with DHEA. Preliminary evidence has also linked higher DHEA levels to ovarian cancer in women.[46]

Some doctors recommend that people taking DHEA have liver enzymes measured routinely. Anecdotes of DHEA supplementation (of at least 25 mg per day) leading to heart arrhythmias have appeared.[47] At only 25 mg per day, DHEA has lowered HDL cholesterol while increasing insulin-like growth factor (IGF).[48] Decreasing HDL could increase the risk of heart disease. Increasing IGF might increase the risk of breast cancer.

Are There Any Side Effects or Interactions? Refer to the individual supplement for information about any side effects or interactions.

Herbs That May Be Helpful

Preliminary evidence indicates that some Chinese herbs may help those with SLE. In one trial, a formula composed of seventeen Chinese herbs was given to 306 people with SLE.[49] Of the 230 individuals who were also taking cortisone, 92% improved, but 85% of those taking the herbs alone also benefited. Forty-one people with SLE-induced kidney damage given a combination of conventional drugs plus a Chinese herbal formula for 6 months did significantly better than thirty-rive individuals given the drugs alone.[50] Various Chinese herbs have prolonged survival in animals with SLE.[51]

One of these Chinese herbs, *Tripterygium wilfordi*, is thought to benefit those with SLE or DLE by both suppressing immunity and acting as an anti-inflammatory agent. When twenty-six people with DLE took 30–60 grams of Tripterygium per day for 2 weeks, most experienced some degree of improvement.[52] Skin rashes in eight people completely cleared up, while in ten over 50% of the rash improved. Tripterygium (30–45 grams per day) was also given to 103 people with SLE. After 1 month, 54% experienced relief from symptoms such as joint pain and malaise. Because of potential side effects, people with SLE should consult with a doctor experienced in Chinese herbal medicine before using this herb.

Two separate trials have reported that people taking Tripterygium may experience side effects.[53] In less than 8% of women with DLE, amenorrhea (cessation of menstruation) occurred; approximately one-third of women with SLE experienced amenorrhea. Other side effects ranged from stomach upset or pain, to nausea, loss of appetite, dizziness, and increased facial coloring. Both studies found that these effects subsided with time once individuals stopped using the herb.

Alfalfa (p. 391) tablets have been reported to worsen SLE,[54] though this association has been disputed.[55] Some nutritionally oriented doctors suggest that until more is known, people with SLE should avoid alfalfa seeds and supplements.

Are There Any Side Effects or Interactions? Refer to the individual herb for information about any side effects or interactions.

Macular Degeneration *(sidebar)*

Checklist for SLE

Ranking	Nutritional Supplements	Herbs
Primary		Tripterygium
Secondary	DHEA (p. 288) Fish oil (p. 298) (EPA/DHA [p. 287])	
Other	Pantothenic acid (p. 340) Vitamin E (p. 344)	

Macular Degeneration

The macula is a portion of the retina in the back of the eye. Degeneration of the macula is the leading cause of blindness in elderly Americans.[1]

Lifestyle Changes That May Be Helpful

Smoking has been linked to macular degeneration. Quitting smoking may reduce the risk of developing macular degeneration.

Nutritional Supplements That May Be Helpful

Sunlight triggers oxidative damage in the eye, which in turn can cause macular degeneration.[2] Animals given **antioxidants** (p. 267)—which protect against oxidative damage—have a lower risk of this vision problem.[3] People with high blood levels of antioxidants also have a lower risk.[4] Those with the highest levels of the antioxidants **selenium** (p. 331), **vitamin C** (p. 341), and **vitamin E** (p. 344) may have a 70% lower risk of developing macular degeneration.[5] People who eat fruits and vegetables high in **beta-carotene** (p. 268), another antioxidant, are also at low risk.[6] Some doctors of natural medicine recommend antioxidant supplements to reduce the risk of macular degeneration; reasonable adult levels include 200 mcg of selenium, 1,000 mg vitamin C, 400 IU of vitamin E, and 25,000 IU of natural beta-carotene per day.

Lutein (p. 308) and zeaxanthin are antioxidants in the carotenoid family. These carotenoids, found in high concentrations in spinach and kale, concentrate in the part of the retina where macular degeneration strikes. Once there, they protect the retina from damage caused by sunlight.[7] As expected, spinach and kale eaters have a lower risk of macular degeneration, although blood levels of lutein have not correlated with risk of macular degeneration in one trial.[8,9]

Harvard researchers report that people eating the most lutein and zeaxanthin—a total of 5.8 mg per day—have a 57% decreased risk of macular degeneration, compared with people eating the least.[10] Lutein and zeaxanthin can be taken as supplements; 6 mg or more per day of lutein may be a useful amount.

Two important enzymes needed for vision in the retina require **zinc** (p. 346). Double-blind research using 80 mg of zinc or placebo for 2 years found that zinc prevented vision loss by 42% in people with macular degeneration;[11] other double-blind research did not confirm these results.[12]

Are There Any Side Effects or Interactions? Refer to the individual supplement for information about any side effects or interactions.

Herbs That May Be Helpful

Ginkgo biloba (p. 427) may help treat early-stage macular degeneration, according to double-blind research.[13] Many doctors of natural medicine recommend 120–240 mg of standardized extract in capsules or tablets per day or a tincture of 0.5 ml 3 times daily for support of healthy vision.

Bilberry's (p. 396) active bioflavonoid compounds, anthocyanosides, act as an antioxidant in the retina of the eye. This makes it a potential preventive measure against macular degeneration.[14] Bilberry has also been shown to strengthen capillaries and reduce hemorrhaging in the retina.[15] A typical amount used in studies is 240–480 mg per day of bilberry extract in capsules or tablets standardized to 25% anthocyanosides.

Are There Any Side Effects or Interactions? Refer to the individual herb for information about any side effects or interactions.

Checklist for Macular Degeneration

Ranking	Nutritional Supplements	Herbs
Secondary	Lutein/zeaxanthin (p. 308)	Bilberry (p. 396) *Ginkgo biloba* (p. 427)
Other	Beta-Carotene (p. 268) Selenium (p. 331) Vitamin C (p. 341) Vitamin E (p. 344) Zinc (p. 346)	

Menopause

Menopause is the cessation of the monthly female menstrual cycle. Women who have not had a period for a year are considered postmenopausal. Most commonly, menopause takes place when a women is in her late 40s or early 50s. Women who have gone through menopause are no longer fertile. Menopause is not a disease and cannot be prevented.

Many hormonal changes occur during menopause. Primarily as a result of decreases in estrogen, postmenopausal women are at higher risk of heart disease and **osteoporosis** (p. 133). A number of unpleasant symptoms may also accompany menopause. Some, such as vaginal dryness, result from the lack of estrogen. Others, such as hot flashes and decreased libido are caused by more complex hormonal changes.

Dietary and Other Natural Therapies That May Be Helpful

Soybeans (p. 332) contain compounds called phytoestrogens that are related in structure to estrogen, though in some reports, the estrogenic activity of soy is quite weak.[1] Soy is known to affect the menstrual cycle in premenopausal women.[2] Researchers have linked societies with high consumption of soy products to a low incidence of hot flashes during menopause.[3] In one double-blind trial, 60 grams of soy protein caused a 33% decrease in the number of hot flashes after 4 weeks and a 45% reduction after 12 weeks.[4] Other double-blind research has reported significant reduction in the number of hot flashes.[5]

In one randomized trial, high intake of phytoestrogens from soy and **flaxseed** (p. 296) reduced both hot flashes and vaginal dryness, but much (though not all) of the benefit was also seen in the control group.[6] As a result of these studies, doctors of natural medicine often recommend that women experiencing menopausal symptoms eat tofu, soy milk, tempeh, roasted soy nuts, and other soy-based sources of phytoestrogens. Soy sauce contains very little phytoestrogen content, and many processed foods made from soybean concentrates have low levels of phytoestrogens. Supplements containing isoflavones extracted from soy are commercially available, and flaxseed (as opposed to flaxseed oil) is also a good source of phytoestrogens.

Although natural **progesterone** (p. 326) has been anecdotally linked to reduction in symptoms of menopause,[7,8,9] clinical research has not yet supported the use of natural progesterone for this purpose. In one trial, natural progesterone was found to have no independent effect on symptoms, and synthetic progestins were found to increase breast tenderness.[10] In trials reporting that synthetic progestins reduced symptoms of menopause, natural progesterone has not been tested.[11,12,13]

Lifestyle Changes That May Be Helpful

Sedentary women are more likely to have moderate or severe hot flashes compared with women who exercise.[14,15] In one trial, menopausal symptoms were reduced immediately after aerobic exercise.[16]

Nutritional Supplements That May Be Helpful

Many years ago, researchers studied the effects of **vitamin E** (p. 344) in reducing symptoms of menopause. Most,[17,18,19,20,21] but not all,[22] studies found vitamin E to be helpful. Many nutritionally oriented doctors suggest that women going through menopause take 800 IU per day of vitamin E for a trial period of at least 3 months to see if symptoms are reduced. If helpful, this amount may be continued. Using lower amounts for less time has led to statistically significant changes, but only marginal clinical improvement.[23]

In 1964, a preliminary trial reported that 1,200 mg each of **vitamin C** (p. 341) and the **bioflavonoid** (p. 271) hesperidin, taken over the course of the day, helped relieve hot flashes.[24] Although placebo effects are strong in women with hot flashes, other treatments used in that trial failed to act as effectively as the bioflavonoid/vitamin C combination. Since then, researchers have not explored the effects of bioflavonoids or vitamin C in women with menopausal symptoms.

Are There Any Side Effects or Interactions? Refer to the individual supplement for information about any side effects or interactions.

Herbs That May Be Helpful

Double-blind studies support the usefulness of **black cohosh** (p. 391) for women with hot flashes associated with menopause.[25] A review of eight trials concluded black cohosh to be both safe and effective.[26] Many doctors of natural medicine recommend 20 mg of a highly concentrated extract taken twice per day; 2–4 ml of tincture 3 times per day may also be used.

Sage (p. 456) may be of some benefit for women who are sweating excessively due to menopausal hot flashes during the day or at night.[27] It is believed this is because sage directly decreases production of sweat. This is based on traditional herbal prescribing and has not been evaluated in clinical studies.

A variety of herbs with weak estrogen-like actions similar to the effects of soy such as **licorice** (p. 440), **alfalfa** (p. 391), and **red clover** (p. 453) have traditionally been used for women with menopausal symptoms.[28] Modern research has not attempted to confirm the potential benefit of these phytoestrogens.

Contrary to popular belief, **wild yam** (p. 469) is not a natural source of progesterone nor has it been shown to reduce symptoms of menopause. Although a pharmaceutical conversion process can produce progesterone from wild yam, the body cannot duplicate this conversion.

Are There Any Side Effects or Interactions? Refer to the individual herb for information about any side effects or interactions.

Checklist for Menopause

Ranking	Nutritional Supplements	Herbs
Primary	Soy (p. 332)	Black cohosh (p. 391)
Other	Bioflavonoids (hesperidin) (p. 271) Progesterone (p. 326) Vitamin C (p. 341) Vitamin E (p. 344)	Alfalfa (p. 391) Licorice (p. 440) Red clover (p. 453) Sage (p. 456) Wild Yam (p. 469)
See also: Homeopathic Remedies for **Menopause** (p. 553)		

Menorrhagia (Heavy Menstruation)

Doctors call heavy menstrual blood loss menorrhagia. It needs to be diagnosed by a doctor to rule out a variety of potentially serious underlying conditions that sometimes cause increased menstrual bleeding.

Nutritional Supplements That May Be Helpful

Once women with menorrhagia have had serious underlying causes ruled out, they need to be tested for **iron** (p. 304) deficiency—a condition diagnosed with simple blood tests. Since blood is rich in iron, blood loss can lead to iron depletion. If an iron deficiency is diagnosed, many doctors will recommend 100–200 mg of iron per day, although recommendations vary widely.

The relationship between iron deficiency and menorrhagia is complicated. Not only can the condition lead to iron deficiency, but iron deficiency can lead to menorrhagia. Supplementing with iron decreases excess menstrual blood loss in women who have no other underlying cause for their condition.[1,2] Iron sup-

plements should only be taken by individuals with iron deficiency.

Women with menorrhagia may be deficient in **vitamin A** (p. 336). Women taking 25,000 IU of vitamin A twice per day for 15 days have been reported to show significant improvements and a complete normalization of menstrual blood loss.[3] However, women who are or could become pregnant should not supplement with more than 10,000 IU (3,000 mcg) per day of vitamin A.

Research reports that some women with menorrhagia caused by using intrauterine devices (IUD) for birth control, found relief from taking **vitamin E** (p. 344) at 100 IU per day for 2 weeks.[4] The cause of IUD-induced menstrual blood loss is different from other menorrhagia; therefore, it's possible that vitamin E supplements might not help with menorrhagia not associated with IUD use.

Both **vitamin C** (p. 341) and **bioflavonoids** (p. 271) protect capillaries (small blood vessels) from damage. In so doing, they might protect against the blood loss of menorrhagia. In one report, fourteen of sixteen women with menorrhagia improved when given 200 mg vitamin C and 200 mg bioflavonoids 3 times per day.[5]

Are There Any Side Effects or Interactions? Refer to the individual supplement for information about any side effects or interactions.

Herbs That May Be Helpful

With its emphasis on long-term balancing of a woman's hormonal system, **vitex** (p. 467) is not a fast-acting herb. For **premenstrual syndrome** (p. 141) or frequent or heavy periods, vitex can be used continuously for 4 to 6 months. Women with amenorrhea (lack of menstruation) and **infertility** (p. 102) can remain on vitex for 12 to 18 months, unless pregnancy occurs during treatment.

Forty drops of the concentrated liquid herbal extract of vitex can be added to a glass of water and drunk in the morning. Vitex is also available in powdered form in tablets and capsules, again to be taken in the morning.

Cinnamon (p. 411) has been used historically for the treatment of various menstrual disorders, including heavy menstruation.[6] This is also the case with shepherd's purse *(Capsella bursa-pastoris)*.[7]

The medicinal use of **false unicorn** (p. 423) root is based in Native American tradition, where it was recommended for a large number of women's health conditions, including amenorrhea, **painful menstruation** (p. 61), and other irregularities of menstruation, as well as to prevent miscarriages.[8] Steroidal saponins are generally credited with providing false unicorn root's activity. Modern investigations have not confirmed this, and there is no research yet about the medical applications of this herb.

Are There Any Side Effects or Interactions? Refer to the individual herb for information about any side effects or interactions.

Checklist for Menorrhagia (Heavy Menstruation)

Ranking	Nutritional Supplements	Herbs
Primary	Iron (p. 304) (with deficiency)	
Secondary	Vitamin A (p. 336)	
Other	Bioflavonoids (p. 271) Vitamin C (p. 341) Vitamin E (p. 344)	Cinnamon (p. 411) False Unicorn (p. 423) Shepherd's purse Vitex (p. 467)
See also: Homeopathic Remedies for **Heavy Menstruation** (p. 554)		

Migraine Headaches

Migraines are very painful headaches sometimes involving nausea, vomiting, and changes in vision. They usually begin on only one side of the head and may become worse with exposure to light.

Potential Role of Allergies

Migraines can be triggered by **allergies** (p. 8) and may be relieved by identifying and avoiding the problem foods.[1,2,3,4] Uncovering these foods with the help of a nutritionally oriented doctor is often a useful way to treat migraines. In children suffering migraines who also have epilepsy, there is evidence that eliminating offending foods will also reduce seizures.[5]

Some people who suffer from migraines also react to salt, and eliminating salt is helpful for some of these people.[6] **Lactose-intolerant** (p. 114) individuals may benefit from avoiding milk and ice cream.[7] In addition, some migraine sufferers are unable to break down tyramine, a substance found in many foods.[8] This can lead to the absorption of intact tyramine,[9] which in turn may trigger a migraine.[10]

Tryptophan, an amino acid found in protein-rich foods, is converted to serotonin, a substance that might worsen some migraines. As a result, low-protein diets have been used with some success to reduce migraine attacks.[11] [12] Some doctors have found reac-

tions to smoking and birth control pills to be additional contributing factors in migraines.

Nutritional Supplements That May Be Helpful

Fish oil (p. 224) containing EPA and **DHA** (p. 287) may reduce the symptoms of migraine headaches.[13,14] One study used 1 gram of fish oil per 10 pounds of body weight. Fish oil probably helps because of its effects in modifying prostaglandins, hormone-like substances made by the body.

On average, people with migraine have lower levels of **magnesium** (p. 310) than other people.[15] Preliminary research shows that premenopausal women with migraines benefit from magnesium supplements.[16] Intravenous magnesium can relieve some migraines in a matter of minutes.[17] Double-blind research shows that 360 mg of magnesium per day decreases premenstrual migraines.[18] Most of the benefit of supplemental magnesium seems to be with younger women.

High doses of **calcium** (p. 277) and **vitamin D** (p. 343) have also been useful in treating several cases of migraines.[19,20] Some nutritionally oriented doctors may recommend that people take 800 mg of calcium and 400 IU of vitamin D per day.

One group of researchers using high (400 mg per day) amounts of **vitamin B$_2$** (p. 338) in treating forty-nine people who had migraine found beneficial results in most of the migraine sufferers.[21]

Preliminary research also suggests that oral supplements of **SAMe (S-adenosyl-L-methionine)** (p. 330) are helpful in the treatment of migraine headaches.[22]

The cause of migraine headaches is related to abnormal serotonin function in blood vessels,[23] and **5-HTP** (p. 295) may help correct this abnormality.

Are There Any Side Effects or Interactions? Refer to the individual supplement for information about any side effects or interactions.

Herbs That May Be Helpful

The most frequently used herb for the long-term treatment and prevention of migraines is **feverfew** (p. 424). Feverfew inhibits both hyperaggregation of platelets and the release of serotonin and some inflammatory mediators.[24] Double-blind studies have shown that continuous use of feverfew leads to a reduction in the severity, duration, and frequency of migraine headaches.[25,26,27]

Studies suggest that taking standardized feverfew leaf extracts that supply a minimum of 250 mcg of parthenolide (the active constituent) per day is best. Results may not be evident for at least 4 to 6 weeks.

One case report suggested success using 4–6 grams per day of powdered **ginger** (p. 427) for migraines and the nausea that accompanies them.[28] Ginger may also be taken as a tincture in the amount of 1.5–3 ml 3 times daily. *Ginkgo biloba* (p. 427) extract may also help because it reduces the formation of a substance known as platelet-activating factor,[29] which may contribute to migraines.

There is preliminary evidence that capsaicin, the active constituent of **cayenne** (p. 408), can be used in the treatment of migraines.[30]

Are There Any Side Effects or Interactions? Refer to the individual herb for information about any side effects or interactions.

Checklist for Migraine Headaches

Ranking	Nutritional Supplements	Herbs
Primary	Vitamin B$_2$ (p. 338)	Feverfew (p. 424)
Secondary	Magnesium (p. 310)	
Other	5-HTP (p. 295) Calcium (p. 277) Fish oil (p. 294) (EPA/DHA [p. 287]) SAMe (p. 330) Vitamin D (p. 343)	Cayenne (p. 408) Ginger (p. 427) *Ginkgo biloba* (p. 427)
See also: Homeopathic Remedies for **Migraine Headaches** (p. 558)		

Minor Injuries
Sprains, Strains, and Skin Wounds

The healing of minor injuries, such as sprains, strains, and **skin wounds** (p. 122), requires the involvement of many body systems, including the circulatory system, the immune system, and the cellular mechanisms needed to repair and grow new tissues. Also refer to the chapters on **immune function** (p. 94), **bruising** (p. 28), **minor burns** (p. 29), **bursitis** (p. 30), and **carpal tunnel syndrome** (p. 33) for more information about minor injuries.

Dietary Changes That May Be Helpful

The body repairs and builds new tissues in a process called anabolism. Adequate amounts of calories and protein are required for anabolism, as the skin and underlying tissues are comprised of protein and ener-

gy is needed to fuel repair mechanisms. While major injuries requiring hospitalization raise protein and calorie requirements significantly, minor injuries should not necessitate changes from a typical, healthful diet.[1]

Nutritional Supplements That May Be Helpful

Many vitamins and minerals have essential roles in tissue repair, and deficiencies of one or more of these nutrients have been demonstrated in animal studies to impair the healing process.[2] This could argue for the use of **multiple vitamin/mineral** (p. 314) supplements by people with minor injuries who might have deficiencies due to poor diets or other problems, but controlled human research is lacking to support this.

Antioxidant (p. 267) supplements, including **vitamin C** (p. 341) and **vitamin E** (p. 344), may help prevent exercise-related muscle injuries by neutralizing free radicals produced during strenuous activities.[3] Placebo-controlled research, some of it double-blind, has shown that 400–3,000 mg per day of vitamin C may reduce pain and speed up muscle strength recovery after intense exercise.[4,5] Reductions in blood indicators of muscle damage and free radical activity have also been reported for supplementation with 400–1,200 IU per day of vitamin E in most studies,[6,7,8] but no measurable benefits in exercise recovery have been reported.[9] A combination of 90 mg per day of **coenzyme Q$_{10}$** (p. 283) and a very small amount of **vitamin E** (p. 344) did not produce any protective effects in one double-blind study.[10]

Antioxidants may also protect the skin from sunburn due to free-radical producing ultraviolet rays.[11] Combinations of 1,000–2,000 IU per day of **vitamin E** (p. 344) and 2,000–3,000 mg per day of **vitamin C** (p. 341), but not either one given alone, have a significant protective effect against ultraviolet rays, according to double-blind studies.[12,13,14] Oral **beta-carotene** (p. 268) alone was not found to provide effective protection in a recent double-blind study,[15] but it has been suggested that other carotenoids such as **lycopene** (p. 308) may be more important for ultraviolet protection.[16] Double-blind research has also shown that topical application of antioxidants protects against sunburn if used before,[17] but not after,[18] exposure.

Vitamin A (p. 336) supplements have been shown to improve healing in animal studies,[19] and may be especially useful in a topical ointment for skin injuries in people taking corticosteroid medications.[20] Although vitamin A plays a central role in wound healing,[21] the effect of supplemental vitamin A in people who are not vitamin A-deficient but who have suffered a minor injury remains unclear.

A combination of vitamins B$_1$ (p. 337), B$_6$ (p. 340), and B$_{12}$ (p. 337) has proved useful for preventing a relapse of a common type of back pain linked to vertebral syndromes,[22] as well as reducing the amount of anti-inflammatory medications needed to control back pain, according to double-blind studies.[23] Typical amounts used have been 100 mg each of vitamins B$_1$ and B$_6$, and 500 mcg of vitamin B$_{12}$, all taken 3 times per day.[24] Such high amounts of vitamin B$_6$ require supervision by a nutritionally oriented doctor.

Vitamin C (p. 341) is needed to make collagen, the "glue" that strengthens skin, muscles, and blood vessels, and to ensure proper wound healing. Injury, at least when severe, appears to increase vitamin C requirements,[25] and vitamin C deficiency causes delayed healing.[26] Preliminary human studies have suggested that vitamin C supplementation in nondeficient people can speed healing of various types of wounds and trauma, including surgery, minor injuries, herniated intervertebral discs, and skin ulcers.[27,28] Double-blind research has not confirmed these effects for skin ulcers[29] or athletic injuries,[30] but a combination of 1–3 grams per day of vitamin C and 200–900 mg per day of **pantothenic acid** (p. 340) has produced minor improvements in the strength of healing skin tissue.[31,32]

Bioflavonoids (p. 271) have anti-inflammatory activity and can limit swelling after injury.[33,34] Two placebo-controlled studies (one double-blind) found that athletes who were taking 900–1,800 mg per day of citrus bioflavonoids, with or without the addition of vitamin C, had reduced healing times from injuries compared to those taking placebo.[35,36]

Topical application of **vitamin E** (p. 344) is sometimes recommended for preventing or treating post-injury scars; however, only three placebo-controlled studies have been reported. Two of these trials found no effect on scar prevention after surgery,[37,38] and one trial found vitamin E improved the effect of silicon bandages on large scars called keloids.[39]

Zinc (p. 346) is a component of many enzymes, including some that are needed to repair wounds. Even a marginal deficiency of zinc can interfere with optimal recovery from everyday tissue damage as well as more serious trauma.[40,41] Topical zinc-containing treatments have improved healing of skin wounds even when there is no deficiency,[42] but oral zinc has helped tissue healing only when an actual deficiency exists.[43]

Other trace minerals, such as **manganese** (p. 311), **copper** (p. 285), and **silicon** (p. 331) are known to be important in the biochemistry of tissue healing.[44,45,46,47] However, neither the effect of deficiencies of these minerals nor the results of oral supplementation have been explored in controlled studies of people with minor injuries.

Glucosamine sulfate (p. 299) and **chondroitin sulfate** (p. 281) may both play a role in wound healing by providing the raw material needed by the body to manufacture molecules called glycosaminoglycans found in skin, tendons, ligaments, and joints.[48] Test tube and animal studies have found these substances, and others like them, can promote improved tissue healing.[49,50,51,52,53] One controlled human study found that wounds healed with greater strength when they were treated topically with a chondroitin sulfate-containing powder.[54] Injectable forms of chondroitin sulfate have been used in Europe for various types of sports-related injuries to tendons and joints,[55,56,57,58] and one uncontrolled study reported reduced pain and good healing in young athletes with chondromalacia patella (a chronic knee irritation) who were given 750–1,500 mg per day of glucosamine sulfate.[59]

Improved healing from major trauma and surgery has been demonstrated with oral supplements of several grams per day of either **arginine** (p. 268) and/or **glutamine** (p. 300),[60,61] and **ornithine alpha-ketoglutarate** (p. 319).[62] Two placebo-controlled studies have shown increased tissue synthesis in surgical wounds in people given 17–25 grams of oral arginine per day.[63,64]

Proteolytic enzymes (p. 289), including **bromelain** (p. 276), trypsin, and chymotrypsin, may be helpful in healing minor injuries because they have anti-inflammatory activity and are capable of being partially absorbed from the gastrointestinal tract.[65,66,67] Several uncontrolled studies have reported reduced pain and swelling, and/or faster healing in people with a variety of conditions using either bromelain,[68,69,70] papain from papaya,[71,72,73] or a combination of trypsin and chymotrypsin.[74]

Double-blind trials have reported faster recovery from athletic injuries and earlier return to activity using eight tablets daily of trypsin/chymotrypsin,[75,76,77,78,79] four to eight tablets daily of papain,[80] eight tablets of bromelain (single-blind only),[81] or a combination of these enzymes.[82] However, one double-blind study using eight tablets per day of trypsin/chymotrypsin to treat sprained ankles found no significant effect on swelling, bruising, or overall function.[83]

Bromelain is measured in MCUs (milk clotting units) or GDUs (gelatin dissolving units). One GDU equals 1.5 MCU. Strong products contain at least 2,000 MCU (1,333 GDU) per gram (1,000 mg). A supplement containing 500 mg labeled "2,000 MCU per gram" would have 1,000 MCU of activity, because 500 mg is half a gram. Some doctors of natural medicine recommend 3,000 MCU taken 3 times per day for several days, followed by 2,000 MCU 3 times per day. Some of the research, however, uses smaller amounts, such as 2,000 MCU taken in divided amounts in the course of a day (500 MCU taken 4 times per day). Other enzyme preparations, such as trypsin/chymotrypsin, have different measuring units. Recommended use is typically 2 tablets 4 times per day on an empty stomach, but as with bromelain, the strength of trypsin/chymotrypsin tablets can vary significantly from product to product.

The use of **DMSO** (p. 291), a colorless, oily liquid primarily used as an industrial solvent, for therapeutic applications is controversial. However, some evidence indicates that when applied directly to the skin, DMSO has anti-inflammatory properties and inhibits the transmission of pain messages by nerves, and in this way might ease the pain of minor injuries.[84,85,86] Two double-blind studies successfully used topical DMSO to reduce pain and improve movement in people with tendinitis of the shoulder or elbow.[87,88]

L-carnitine (p. 279) is required for normal energy production from fats in muscle and other tissues. One placebo-controlled study showed that individuals who supplement with 3 grams per day L-carnitine for 3 weeks before engaging in an exercise regimen are less likely to experience muscle soreness.[89]

Are There Any Side Effects or Interactions? Refer to the individual supplement for information about any side effects or interactions.

Herbs That May Be Helpful

Aloe (p. 391) has been historically used for minor cuts and burns and continues to be recommended by herbalists for minor skin injuries.[90] Topical aloe vera has facilitated wound healing in some controlled research.[91] However, in one controlled trial, topical aloe vera gel was inferior to conventional management of surgical wounds.[92]

Australian Aboriginals used the leaves of tea tree to treat cuts and skin infections, crushing and applying them to the affected area. Modern herbalists recommend **tea tree oil** (p. 463) (at a strength of 70–100%) applied moderately in small areas at least twice per day to the affected areas of skin.[93] For a variety of reasons, some researchers have suggested that tea tree oil should not be used to treat burns.[94]

Checklist for Minor Injuries

Ranking	Nutritional Supplements	Herbs
Primary	Bioflavonoids (p. 271) (for prevention only) Bromelain (p. 276) DMSO (p. 291) (topical) Proteolytic enzymes (p. 289) Vitamin C (p. 341) (oral and topical, for sunburn protection) Vitamin E (p. 344) (oral and topical, for sunburn protection) Zinc (p. 346) (for deficiency only)	
Secondary	Arginine (p. 268) L-carnitine (p. 279) (for exercise-related muscle injury) Vitamin A (p. 336) (for deficiency only) Vitamin C (p. 341) Zinc (p. 346) (topical for skin wounds)	Aloe (p. 391) Gotu kola (p. 430) Horse chestnut (p. 435)
Other	Chondroitin sulfate (p. 281) Copper (p. 285) Glucosamine sulfate (p. 299) Manganese (p. 311) Multiple vitamin/ mineral (p. 314) Silicon (p. 331) Vitamin B$_1$ (p. 337) Vitamin B$_6$ (p. 340) Vitamin B$_{12}$ (p. 337) Vitamin E (p. 344) (for exercise-related muscle strain) Vitamin E (p. 344) (topical for scars)	Autumn crocus, Calendula (p. 406) Cat's claw (p. 408) Comfrey (p. 413) (topical) Meadowsweet (p. 444) St. John's wort (p. 461) Tea tree (p. 463) Witch hazel (p. 470) Yarrow (p. 471)

See also: Homeopathic Remedies for **Minor Injuries** (p. 550)

Echinacea (p. 417) is widely used in Europe to promote wound healing[95] and is approved by the German government for this use.[96] Creams or ointments are applied several times a day to minor wounds.

Calendula (p. 406) flowers were historically considered beneficial for wound healing, reducing inflammation, and as an antiseptic.[97] Like echinacea, calendula is approved in Germany for use in treating poorly healing wounds.[98] Generally 1 tablespoon of calendula flowers is steeped in hot water for 15 minutes. Then cloths are dipped into the liquid to make compresses. These should be applied for at least 15 minutes several times per day initially, then tapering off as the wound improves.

Arnica is considered by some practitioners to be among the best vulnerary (wound-healing) herbs available.[99] Some doctors of natural medicine recommend mixing 1 tablespoon of arnica tincture in 500 ml water, then soaking thin cloth or gauze in the liquid and applying it to the wound for at least 15 minutes 4 to 5 times per day. Arnica is approved by the German government for improving wound healing.[100]

Comfrey (p. 413) is also widely used in traditional medicine as a topical application to help heal wounds.[101] Native Americans used poultices of **witch hazel** (p. 470) leaves and bark to treat wounds, insect bites, and ulcers.[102]

Colchicine (p. 125) is a remedy derived from the autumn crocus that may be helpful for chronic back pain caused by herniated discs. A review reports that colchicine can provide relief from pain, muscle spasm, and weakness associated with disc disease.[103] The author of this study suggests that colchicine leads to dramatic improvement in four out of ten cases of disc disease. In most studies, colchicine has been given intravenously.[104] However, the oral administration of this herb-based remedy may also have moderate effectiveness. A physician expert in the use of herbal medicine should be consulted for the administration of colchicine.

Although **St. John's wort** (p. 461) is best known for treating depression, it has many other uses. The oil was used in Europe and by Native Americans for wound healing. Preliminary Russian research has confirmed the benefit of St. John's wort for wound healing.[105] Another herb, **yarrow** (p. 471), has wound healing and anti-inflammatory properties and was used to help heal wounds in traditional herbal medicine.

Horse chestnut (p. 435) contains a compound called aescin that acts as an anti-inflammatory and reduces edema (swelling with fluid) following trauma, particularly those following sports injuries, surgery, and head injury.[106] A topical aescin preparation is popular in Europe for the treatment of acute sprains during sporting events.

Cat's claw (p. 408) is a South American remedy traditionally used to promote wound healing and reduce the inflammation of minor injuries.

One uncontrolled study in humans found that a **gotu kola** (p. 430) extract helped heal infected wounds (unless the infection had reached bone).[107]

Meadowsweet (p. 444) was used historically for a wide variety of conditions, including treating rheumatic complaints of the joints and muscles.[108] While not as potent as **white willow** (p. 468), which has a higher salicin content, the salicylates in meadowsweet do give it a mild anti-inflammatory effect and the potential to reduce fevers during a cold or flu. However, this role is based on historical use and knowledge of the chemistry of meadowsweet's constituents; to date, no human studies have been completed with meadowsweet.

Are There Any Side Effects or Interactions? Refer to the individual herb for information about any side effects or interactions.

Mitral Valve Prolapse

The mitral valve is one of the four valves of the heart. Normally, stringlike cords keep the mitral valve from opening too far. Sometimes these cords are too long, allowing the valve to open excessively when the heart beats. Most people with mitral valve prolapse (MVP) never have any symptoms. Some develop dull chest pain, palpitations, anxiety, and other symptoms associated with the sympathetic ("fight or flight") response. When MVP causes these symptoms, it is referred to as "dysautonomia" syndrome.

Lifestyle Changes That May Be Helpful

People with dysautonomia symptoms should avoid stressful situations and work on techniques for coping with stress.

Dietary Changes That May Be Helpful

In people who have dysautonomia, low salt intake may be part of the problem. Therefore, unless there is another health problem (such as **high blood pressure** [p. 89]) that is worsened by high salt intake, people with MVP should not restrict the amount of salt in the diet.[1]

Nutritional Supplements That May Be Helpful

Magnesium (p. 310) deficiency has been proposed as one cause of MVP.[2] A large study found that many people who have MVP are low in magnesium, and taking 600 mg of magnesium 1 to 3 times each day improved symptoms and the underlying problems in MVP compared with placebo.[3] Anyone taking more than 600 mg of magnesium per day should first talk to a nutritionally oriented doctor.

Coenzyme Q$_{10}$ (Co Q$_{10}$) (p. 283) has been used for MVP as well. A study in children found that Coenzyme Q10 supplementation could improve one measure of MVP.[4] An investigation of adults with MVP used 60 mg of Coenzyme Q$_{10}$ 3 to 4 times per day and found an improvement in symptoms and a reduction in heart wall thickness[5] (increased heart wall thickness is a sign that the heart is working too hard).

Are There Any Side Effects or Interactions? Refer to the individual supplement for information about any side effects or interactions.

Checklist for Mitral Valve Prolapse

Ranking	Nutritional Supplements	Herbs
Primary	Magnesium (p. 310)	
Secondary	Coenzyme Q$_{10}$ (p. 283)	

Morning Sickness

Morning sickness is the common but poorly understood nausea that frequently accompanies early pregnancy. It is generally not serious, although it can be quite unpleasant. Hyperemesis gravidarum is a severe form of morning sickness that can cause dehydration and electrolyte imbalance, and can lead to hospitalization.

Dietary Changes That May Be Helpful

Some obstetricians recommend that women with morning sickness eat dry crackers upon arising and drink liquids and eat solid foods at separate times.

Women with a high intake of saturated fat (from meat and dairy) may have a much higher risk of severe morning sickness than women eating less saturated fat. A Harvard study found that the equivalent of one cheeseburger or 3 cups of milk more than tripled the risk of developing morning sickness.[1]

Nutritional Supplements That May Be Helpful

Vitamin K (p. 345) and **vitamin C** (p. 341), taken together, may provide remarkable relief of symptoms for some women. In one study, women who took 5 mg of vitamin K and 25 mg of vitamin C per day reported the complete disappearance of morning sickness within 3 days;[2] however, most nutritionally oriented doctors use higher amounts of vitamin C (500–1,000 mg).

Vitamin B$_6$ (p. 340), at an intake of 10–25 mg 3 times per day, may also help relieve morning sickness.[3,4]

Are There Any Side Effects or Interactions? Refer to the individual supplement for information about any side effects or interactions.

Herbs That May Be Helpful

Ginger (p. 427) is well-known for alleviating nausea and improving digestion. It has also been used to reduce vomiting in hyperemesis gravidarum.[5] Women with hyperemesis gravidarum should consult their doctor before pursuing any course of treatment.

To reduce nausea, 250 mg of ginger (in capsule, tablet, or tea form) is taken 4 times per day.[6] It may also be taken as a tincture in the amount of 1.5–3 ml 3 times daily. Ginger should only be used for short periods of time, and the amount taken daily should not exceed 1 gram per day.

Horehound (p. 434) *(Marrubium vulgare)* has been used in traditional medicine to relieve morning sickness. Consult with a doctor expert in botanical medicine before using horehound during pregnancy.

Are There Any Side Effects or Interactions? Refer to the individual herb for information about any side effects or interactions.

Checklist for Morning Sickness

Ranking	Nutritional Supplements	Herbs
Primary	Vitamin B$_6$ (p. 340)	Ginger (p. 427)
Other	Vitamin C (p. 341) Vitamin K (p. 345)	Horehound (p. 434)
See also: Homeopathic Remedies for **Morning Sickness** (p. 559)		

Motion Sickness

Nausea, dizziness, and overall malaise that is triggered by travel in a boat, car, train, or plane all fall into the category of motion sickness.

Herbs That May Be Helpful

A double-blind clinical trial of thirty-six men and women susceptible to motion sickness found that those taking 940 mg of powdered **ginger** (p. 427) in capsules experienced less gastrointestinal distress than those who took Dramamine.[1] Another double-blind study reported that 1 gram of powdered ginger root, compared with placebo, lessened seasickness by 38% and vomiting by 72% in a group of eighty naval cadets sailing in heavy seas.[2] Ginger's beneficial effect on motion sickness appears to be related to its action on the gastrointestinal tract rather than the central nervous system.[3,4]

Multiple Sclerosis

Are There Any Side Effects or Interactions? Refer to the individual herb for information about any side effects or interactions.

Checklist for Motion Sickness

Ranking	Nutritional Supplements	Herbs
Primary		Ginger (p. 427)

See also: Homeopathic Remedies for **Motion Sickness** (p. 560)

Multiple Sclerosis

Multiple sclerosis (MS) is a chronic progressive condition that affects the nervous system. Indirect evidence suggests that it may be an autoimmune disease wherein the **immune system** (p. 94) attacks the central nervous system. The many neurological symptoms of this condition are caused by a loss of the protective covering, or myelin, in the brain and spinal cord.

MS is more common among people who live in temperate climates compared with people in tropical climates who receive greater exposure to the sun. Possible causes for MS may include genetic susceptibility, diet, environmental toxins, exposure to dogs, cats, or caged birds,[1] and viral infections. Epstein-Barr virus has also been named as a risk factor,[2] though the real cause or causes of MS remain unclear.

Dietary Changes That May Be Helpful

The amount and type of fat eaten may affect both the likelihood of getting the disease for people who are healthy and the outcome of the disease for those already diagnosed with MS. For many years, the leading researcher linking dietary fat to MS risk and progression has been Dr. Roy Swank. In one of his reports, a lowfat diet was recommended to 150 people with MS.[3] Although hydrogenated oils, peanut butter, and animal fat (including fat from dairy) were dramatically reduced or eliminated, 5 grams per day of cod liver oil were added and linoleic acid from vegetable oil (see below) was used. After 34 years, 31% of individuals consuming an average of 17 grams of fat per day died compared with 79% of those who ate an average of 25 grams of fat per day. People who began to follow the lowfat diet early in the disease did better than those who changed their eating habits after the disease had progressed.

A survey of people in thirty-six different countries also suggests that the types of fat people eat might impact MS.[4] In that report, people with MS who ate foods high in polyunsaturated and monounsaturated fatty acids had less chance of dying from MS than those who ate more saturated fats.[5] In another survey, researchers gathered information from nearly 400 individuals (half with MS) over 3 years.[6] They found that people who ate more fish had less risk of developing MS, while those who ate pork, hot dogs, and other foods high in animal (saturated) fats were at greater risk. This same report found consumption of vegetable protein, fruit juice, and foods rich in **vitamin C** (p. 341), **thiamine** (p. 337), **riboflavin** (p. 338), **calcium** (p. 277), and **potassium** (p. 323) correlated with a decreased MS risk; eating sweets was linked to an increased risk.

Despite research showing improvement with a low-animal-fat diet in some people with MS, the link between foods containing animal fat and MS risk may not necessarily be due to the fat itself. Preliminary evidence from one report revealed an association between eating dairy foods (cow's milk, butter, and cream) and an increased prevalence of MS, yet in the same report, no link was found between (high fat) cheese and MS.[7]

MS has been associated with a variety of dietary components apparently unrelated to fat intake,[8] and the link between MS and diet remains poorly understood. Nonetheless, the most consistent links to date appear to involve certain foods containing animal fat. People with MS wishing to pursue a nutritional approach that incorporates an understanding of this research should consult with a nutritionally oriented doctor familiar with the "Swank diet."

Some people with MS avoid gluten (a protein found in wheat, rye, and barley) in hopes of diminishing symptoms, because a preliminary study reported that consumption of grain (bread and pasta) was linked to development of MS.[9] However, another trial found an association between eating cereals and breads and reduced MS risk.[10] Other researchers have found gluten sensitivity to be no more common among individuals with MS than among healthy people.[11] Therefore, it does not make sense for people to avoid gluten-containing foods with the expectation that doing so will reduce symptoms of MS.

Lifestyle Changes That May Be Helpful

While some studies dispute it,[12,13] there is preliminary evidence that exposure to organic solvents,[14] insecticides,[15] and X-rays[16] may cause or aggravate MS. This may explain why clusters of multiple sclerosis cases occasionally occur in certain geographical areas, or even work sites.[17]

Swiss researchers found that nicotine temporarily impairs arm movement in people with MS.[18] When

Multiple Sclerosis

twenty-one individuals with MS smoked cigarettes, movement for sixteen was diminished for 10 minutes.

While the outcome of some research disputes the connection between MS and mercury,[19] other investigations have reported an association between dental amalgams and this disease. One study reports that mercury levels in the hair of people with MS are higher than hair mercury levels in healthy individuals.[20] This same report found that people with MS who had their amalgam fillings removed experienced one-third fewer relapses than individuals who kept their fillings. Another preliminary trial found that people with a large number of fillings that had been in place for a long time appeared to be at increased risk for MS compared with those with fewer fillings.[21] Preliminary evidence has also identified an association between tooth decay—as opposed to fillings—and multiple sclerosis.[22] The importance of the reported links between mercury, tooth decay, and risk of MS remains poorly understood.

Nutritional Supplements That May Be Helpful

Although some nutritionally oriented doctors recommend **fish oil** (p. 294) capsules for people with MS, few investigations have explored the effects of this supplement. In one trial, twelve people with MS were given approximately 20 grams of fish oil in capsules per day.[23] After 1 to 4 months, five of these people received slight, but significant benefits, including less urinary incontinence and improved eyesight. However, a longer double-blind study involving over 300 people with MS found that half this amount of fish oil given per day did not help.[24]

In another preliminary report, ten people with MS were given 20 grams of cod liver oil, as well as approximately 680 mg of **magnesium** (p. 310) and 1,100 mg of **calcium** (p. 277) per day in the form of dolomite tablets.[25] After 1 year, the average number of MS attacks decreased significantly for each individual. Unlike fish oil capsules, the cod liver oil in this trial contained not only eicosapentaenoic acid (EPA) and docosahexaenoic acid (**DHA** [p. 287]), but 5,000 IU of **vitamin D** (p. 343). Therefore, it is not known whether the vitamin D or fatty acids were responsible for the cod liver oil's effects. One preliminary study found that giving vitamin D-like drugs to animals with MS was helpful.[26] It's also possible that the magnesium and/or calcium given to these individuals reduced MS attacks. Magnesium[27] and calcium[28] levels have been reported to be lower in the nerve tissue of people with MS compared with healthy individuals.

Checklist for Multiple Sclerosis

Ranking	Nutritional Supplements	Herbs
Other	Calcium (p. 277) Evening primrose oil (p. 292) Fish oil (p. 294) Linoleic acid, Magnesium (p. 310) Niacin (p. 339) Thiamine (p. 337)	

The omega-six fatty acids, found in such oils as **evening primrose oil** (p. 292) (EPO) and sunflower seed oil, may also be beneficial. When sixteen people with MS were given 4 grams of EPO for 3 weeks, hand grip improved.[29] In a review of three double-blind studies, approximately 17–23 grams of linoleic acid (from sunflower seed oil) per day were given to people with MS.[30] Two of the trials reported that linoleic acid reduced the severity and length of relapses. When the data were reexamined, it was found that taking linoleic acid decreased disability due to MS in all three trials. According to these researchers, taking linoleic acid while following a low-animal-fat/high-polyunsaturated-fat diet may be even more beneficial.

Deficiency of **thiamine** (p. 337) (vitamin B$_1$) may contribute to nerve damage.[31] Many years ago, researchers found that injecting thiamine[32] into the spinal cord or using intravenous thiamine combined with **niacin** (p. 339)[33] in people with MS led to a reduction in symptoms. Using injectable vitamins requires medical supervision. No research has yet studied the effects of oral supplementation with B vitamins in people with MS.

Are There Any Side Effects or Interactions? Refer to the individual supplement for information about any side effects or interactions.

Herbs That May Be Helpful

Padma 28, a commercial product containing twenty-eight herbs and based on an traditional Tibetan formula, was given to 100 people with MS.[34] After taking two pills 3 times per day, 44% of these people experienced increased muscle strength and general overall improvement.

Inflammation of the nervous tissue is partly responsible for the breakdown of myelin in people with MS. When injections of *ginkgo* (p. 427) were given to ten people with MS for 5 days, eight were reported to improve.[35] People wishing to explore the intravenous use of ginkgo should first consult with a physician skilled in herbal medicine.

Are There Any Side Effects or Interactions? Refer to the individual herb for information about any side effects or interactions.

MSG Sensitivity
(Chinese Restaurant Syndrome)

MSG sensitivity, also known as Chinese restaurant syndrome, is a group of symptoms that occur in some people after consuming monosodium glutamate (MSG). Although some Chinese (and other) restaurants now avoid the use of MSG, many still use significant amounts of this flavor enhancer. The symptoms of Chinese restaurant syndrome commonly include headache, flushing, tingling, weakness, and stomachache.

Dietary Changes That May Be Helpful

Simply avoiding MSG will prevent the symptoms caused by its exposure in sensitive individuals. MSG is found in some Chinese and Japanese food (as Aji no Moto) and is also used as a meat tenderizer (as Accent). Often MSG is difficult to avoid, as it also occurs in hydrolyzed vegetable protein, textured vegetable protein, gelatin, yeast extracts, calcium and sodium caseinate, vegetable broth, whey, smoke flavoring, malt extracts, and several other food ingredients—without appearing on the label.

Checklist for MSG Sensitivity

Ranking	Nutritional Supplements	Herbs
Secondary	Vitamin B$_6$ (p. 340)	

Nutritional Supplements That May Be Helpful

Years ago, researchers discovered that animals who were deficient in **vitamin B$_6$** (p. 340) could not properly process MSG.[1] Typical reactions to MSG have also been linked to vitamin B$_6$ deficiency in people.[2] In one study, eight out of nine such people stopped reacting to MSG when given 50 mg of vitamin B$_6$ per day for at least 12 weeks. The actual percentage of people with MSG sensitivity who are vitamin B$_6$ deficient and who respond to B$_6$ supplementation remains unknown. Nonetheless, many doctors of natural medicine suggest that people who have these symptoms try supplementing with vitamin B$_6$ for 3 months as a trial.

Are There Any Side Effects or Interactions? Refer to the individual supplement for information about any side effects or interactions.

Night Blindness

People with night blindness see poorly at night but see normally during the day. The condition does not actually involve true blindness, even at night.

Nutritional Supplements That May Be Helpful

Night blindness can be an early sign of **vitamin A** (p. 336) deficiency, often the result of a diet lacking in vegetables containing **beta-carotene** (p. 268), which the body can make into vitamin A.

Most people don't get enough **zinc** (p. 346) in their diets, and a lack of zinc can reduce retinol dehydrogenase, an enzyme needed to help vitamin A work in the eye. Zinc helps night blindness in those who are zinc-deficient;[1] therefore, many nutritionally oriented physicians suggest 15–30 mg of zinc per day to support healthy vision. Because long-term zinc supplementation reduces **copper** (p. 285) levels, 1–3 mg of copper should accompany zinc supplementation lasting more than a few weeks.

Are There Any Side Effects or Interactions? Refer to the individual supplement for information about any side effects or interactions.

Herbs That May Be Helpful

Bilberries (p. 396), a close relative of blueberries, are high in a bioflavonoid complex known as anthocyanosides. Anthocyanosides speed the regeneration of rhodopsin, the purple pigment that is used by the rods in the eye for night vision.[2] This makes bilberry a possible first line of defense for those with poor night vision.[3] Bilberry extract standardized to 25% anthocyanosides can be taken at 240–480 mg per day in capsules or tablets.

Are There Any Side Effects or Interactions? Refer to the individual herb for information about any side effects or interactions.

Checklist for Night Blindness

Ranking	Nutritional Supplements	Herbs
Primary	Beta-carotene (p. 268) Vitamin A (p. 336) Zinc (p. 346)	
Other		Bilberry (p. 396)

Osgood-Schlatter Disease

Osgood-Schlatter disease (a form of osteochondrosis) occurs in adolescence and is often the result of a combination of rapid growth and competitive sports that overstress the knee joint. The patellar tendon, which normally attaches to the tibial tuberosity, is sometimes strained by the powerful quadriceps muscles. This tearing or avulsion can be extremely painful and is sometimes disabling. It may occur in both knees. The knee is usually sore to pressure at the point where the large tendon from the kneecap attaches to the prominence below.

Nutritional Supplements That May Be Helpful

Based on the personal experience of a doctor who reported his findings,[1] some nutritionally oriented physicians recommend **vitamin E** (p. 344) at 400 IU per day and **selenium** (p. 331) at 50 mcg 3 times per day. Jonathan Wright, M.D., reports anecdotally that he has had considerable success with this regimen and often sees results in 2 to 6 weeks.[2]

Are There Any Side Effects or Interactions?
(Refer to the individual supplement for complete information.)

Checklist for Osgood-Schlatter Disease

Ranking	Nutritional Supplements	Herbs
Other	Selenium (p. 331) Vitamin E (p. 344)	

Osteoarthritis

Osteoarthritis is a common disease that develops when linings of joints fail to maintain normal structure, leading to pain and decreased mobility. It is associated with aging and injury (it used to be called "wear-and-tear" arthritis), and can occur secondary to many other conditions. However, in most cases its true cause remains unknown.

Dietary Changes That May Be Helpful

In the 1950s through the 1970s, Dr. Max Warmbrand used a diet free of meat, poultry, dairy, chemicals, sugar, eggs, and processed foods for those with **rheumatoid arthritis** (p. 151) and osteoarthritis,

claiming significant anecdotal success.[1] He reported that clinical results took at least 6 months to develop. The Warmbrand diet has never been properly tested in clinical research. Moreover, although the diet is healthful and should reduce the risk of being diagnosed with many other diseases, it is difficult for most people to follow. This difficulty plus the lack of published research, leads many nutritionally oriented doctors who are aware of the Warmbrand diet to use it only if other approaches have not proven successful.

Solanine is a substance found in nightshade plants, including tomatoes, white potatoes, all peppers (except black pepper), and eggplant. In theory, if not destroyed in the intestine, solanine could be toxic. A horticulturist, Dr. Norman Childers, hypothesized that some people with osteoarthritis may not be able to destroy solanine in the gut, leading to solanine absorption resulting in osteoarthritis. Eliminating solanine from the diet has been reported to bring relief to some arthritis sufferers in preliminary research.[2,3] An uncontrolled survey of people avoiding nightshade plants revealed that 28% claimed to have a "marked positive response" and another 44% a "positive response." Researchers have never put this diet to a strict clinical test; however, the treatment continues to be used by some nutritionally oriented doctors in people who have osteoarthritis. As with the Warmbrand diet, proponents claim exclusion of solanine requires up to 6 months before potential effects can be seen. Totally eliminating tomatoes and peppers requires complex dietary changes for most people. In addition, even proponents of the diet acknowledge that many arthritis sufferers are not helped by using this approach. Therefore, nutritionally oriented doctors tend to prescribe a long-term trial avoidance of solanine-containing foods only for people with severe cases of osteoarthritis that have not responded to other natural treatments.

Most of the studies linking **allergies** (p. 8) to joint disease have focused on rheumatoid arthritis, although mention of what was called rheumatism (some of which may have been osteoarthritis) in older reports suggests a possible link between food reactions and exacerbations of osteoarthritis symptoms.[4] If other therapies are unsuccessful in relieving symptoms, people with osteoarthritis might choose to discuss food allergy identification and elimination with a nutritionally oriented physician.

Lifestyle Changes That May Be Helpful

Obesity is a risk factor for osteoarthritis of weight-bearing joints. Weight loss is thought by arthritis experts to be of potential benefit, at least in reducing pain levels.[5]

Nutritional Supplements That May Be Helpful

Glucosamine sulfate (GS) (p. 299), a nutrient derived from sea shells, contains a building block needed for the repair of joint cartilage. GS has significantly reduced symptoms of osteoarthritis in uncontrolled,[6,7] and single-blind trials.[8,9] Many double-blind studies have also reported efficacy.[10,11,12,13,14] All published clinical investigations on the effects of GS in people with osteoarthritis report statistically significant improvement. Most research trials use 500 mg GS taken 3 times per day. Benefits from GS generally become evident after 3 to 8 weeks of treatment. Continued supplementation is needed in order to maintain benefits.

Several criticisms of GS research have been raised, including criticisms about the methods used in certain research trials or the small number of subjects in each study.[15,16] Regardless of the number of subjects in individual trials, the research has shown—in many controlled and several double-blind scientific studies—that GS has a statistically significant effect on reducing symptoms of osteoarthritis.

Chondroitin sulfate (CS) (p. 281) is a major component of the lining of joints. In structure, CS is related to several molecules of GS attached to each other. Levels of chondroitin sulfate have been reported to be reduced in joint cartilage affected by osteoarthritis. Possibly as a result, CS may help restore joint function in people with osteoarthritis.[17] On the basis of preliminary evidence, researchers had believed that CS did not absorb in humans.[18] As a result, double-blind CS research showing reduced symptoms in people with osteoarthritis had been done mostly by injection.[19,20] It now appears, however, that a significant amount of CS is absorbable in humans,[21] though dissolving CS in water leads to better absorption than swallowing whole pills.[22]

The importance of absorbability issues has recently been overridden by strong clinical evidence supporting the use of orally administered CS. With consistency, many double-blind trials have all shown that CS reduces pain, increases joint mobility, and/or shows objective evidence (including X-ray changes) of healing within joints of people with osteoarthritis.[23,24,25,26,27,28,29,30,31,32] Most studies have used 400 mg of CS taken 2 to 3 times per day. One study found that taking the full daily amount (1,200 mg) at one time was as effective as taking 400 mg 3 times per day.[33] Reduction in symptoms typically occurs within several months.

Due to the similarity in structure, nutritionally oriented doctors have wondered whether people with osteoarthritis need to take both GS and CS. To date, no studies have compared GS versus CS versus the combination of both. The popular idea that GS is clinically "preferred" over CS, or that CS is "not necessary,"[34] has not been examined (let alone supported) by appropriate comparative research. An opposite theory, also popular, posits that GS and CS in combination have stronger effects than either supplement alone.[35] This idea is based only on anecdotes and hypotheses.

S-adenosyl methionine (**SAMe** [p. 330]) possesses anti-inflammatory, pain-relieving, and tissue-healing properties that may help protect the health of joints,[36,37] though the primary way in which SAMe reduces osteoarthritis symptoms remains unclear. Double-blind reports studying effects in people with osteoarthritis have consistently shown that SAMe increases the formation of healthy tissue[38] and reduces pain, stiffness, and swelling better than placebo and equal to drugs such as ibuprofen and naproxen.[39,40,41,42,43,44,45,46] On the basis of outcomes reported in published research, 400 mg taken 3 times per day appears to be the optimal intake of SAMe.

Beginning years ago, researchers reported that supplemental **niacinamide** (p. 339) increased joint mobility, improved muscle strength, and decreased fatigue in people with osteoarthritis.[47,48,49] These preliminary trials were followed by a more recent double-blind study confirming reduction in symptoms within 12 weeks.[50] Although amounts used have varied from study to study, many nutritionally oriented doctors recommend 250 mg of niacinamide 4 or more times per day (with higher amounts reserved for people with more advanced arthritis). The mechanism by which niacinamide reduces symptoms remains unknown.

People who have osteoarthritis and eat high levels of **antioxidants** (p. 267) from food have been reported to exhibit a much slower rate of joint deterioration, particularly in the knees, compared with people eating foods containing lower levels of antioxidants.[51] Of the individual antioxidants, only vitamin E has been studied in controlled trials. **Vitamin E** (p. 344) has reduced

Osteoarthritis

Osteoarthritis

symptoms of osteoarthritis in both single-[52] and double-blind research.[53,54] In these trials, 400–600 IU of vitamin E per day has been used. Results have been reported to occur within several weeks.

Boron (p. 273) affects calcium metabolism, and a link between boron deficiency and arthritis has been suggested.[55] Although boron levels in bones associated with osteoarthritis joints have been reported to be lower than boron in other bones, several other minerals also are deficient in the osteoarthritis bones.[56] An isolated double-blind study reported that 6 mg of boron per day, taken for 2 months, relieved symptoms of osteoarthritis in five of ten people compared with improvement in only one of the ten people assigned to placebo.[57]

The omega-3 fatty acids, EPA and **DHA** (p. 287), in **fish oil** (p. 294) have been used primarily for rheumatoid arthritis (RA) because RA involves significant inflammation and EPA and DHA have anti-inflammatory effects. However, osteoarthritis also includes some element of inflammation.[58] In a 24-week controlled but preliminary trial studying people with osteoarthritis, EPA led to "strikingly lower" pain scores than observed in the placebo group.[59] No further research has yet explored the effects of EPA and DHA in people with osteoarthritis.

D-phenylalanine (p. 320), a synthetic variation of the amino acid L-phenylalanine, has reduced chronic pain due to osteoarthritis in an uncontrolled study.[60] In that report, 250 mg was given 3 to 4 times per day, with pain relief beginning in 4 to 5 weeks. Others have confirmed the effect of D-phenylalanine in pain control in preliminary human research.[61] D-phenylalanine inhibits the enzyme that breaks down some of the body's natural pain killers, substances called enkephalins. By inhibiting this enzyme, enkephalins might be better able to decrease pain levels. Phenylalanine should be taken between meals, because protein found in food can compete for uptake of phenylalanine into the brain, potentially reducing its effect.[62] D-phenylalanine is available in combination with L-phenylalanine in products labeled "DL-phenylalanine" or "DLPA."

Several studies have suggested that individuals with osteoarthritis may benefit from supplementation with bovine **cartilage** (p. 279). In one uncontrolled trial, use of injected and topical bovine cartilage led to relief of symptoms in most people studied.[63] A 10-year European study confirmed improvement with long-term use of bovine cartilage.[64] Optimal intake of bovine cartilage remains unknown.

The use of **DMSO** (p. 291) for therapeutic applications is controversial, but some research shows that DMSO applied directly to the skin has anti-inflammatory properties and alleviates pain, including pain associated with osteoarthritis.[65,66] DMSO appears to reduce pain by inhibiting the transmission of pain messages by nerves[67] rather than through a process of healing damaged joints.

Are There Any Side Effects or Interactions? Refer to the individual supplement for information about any side effects or interactions.

Herbs That May Be Helpful

Boswellia (p. 403) has unique anti-inflammatory action, much like the conventional non-steroidal anti-inflammatory drugs (NSAIDs) used by many for inflammatory conditions.[68] Clinical studies in humans are lacking, so use of this herb for people with osteoarthritis is theoretical. Unlike NSAIDs, however, long-term use of boswellia does not lead to irritation or ulceration of the stomach.

The silicon content of **horsetail** (p. 436) is believed to exert a connective tissue strengthening and anti-arthritic action in traditional medicine. Research has yet to investigate the effects of horsetail extracts in people with osteoarthritis.

White willow (p. 468) has anti-inflammatory and pain-relieving effects. Although the analgesic actions of willow are typically slow-acting, they tend to last longer than aspirin. One double-blind study found that a product featuring white willow (though also containing **black cohosh** [p. 397], guaiac [*Guaiacum officinale*], **sarsaparilla** [p. 457], and aspen bark) effectively reduced osteoarthritis pain compared to placebo.[69] White willow products providing approximately 100 mg salicin per day are generally recommended by doctors of natural medicine.

Capsaicin, the "burning" substance in **cayenne** (p. 408) creams, has been used topically to relieve pain from osteoarthritis. The benefit from cayenne creams, generally containing 0.025–0.075% of the active ingredient capsaicin, has been confirmed in double-blind research.[70]

According to arthritis research, saponins found in the herb **yucca** (p. 473) appear to block the release of toxins from the intestines that inhibit normal formation of cartilage. A double-blind but preliminary study suggested yucca might reduce symptoms of osteoarthritis.[71] Only limited evidence currently supports the use of yucca for people with osteoarthritis.

Are There Any Side Effects or Interactions? Refer to the individual herb for information about any side effects or interactions.

Checklist for Osteoarthritis

Ranking	Nutritional Supplements	Herbs
Primary	Chondroitin sulfate (p. 281) Glucosamine sulfate (p. 299) SAMe (p. 330) Vitamin E (p. 344)	Cayenne (p. 408) (topical, for pain only)
Secondary	DMSO (p. 291) Vitamin B$_3$ (Niacinamide) (p. 339)	Boswellia (p. 403) White willow (p. 468)
Other	Boron (p. 273) Cartilage (p. 279) D-phenylalanine (p. 320) Fish oil (p. 294) (EPA/DHA [p. 287])	Horsetail (p. 436) Yucca (p. 473)

See also: Homeopathic Remedies for **Osteoarthritis** (p. 562)

Osteoporosis

People with osteoporosis have brittle bones, which increases the risk of bone fracture, particularly in the hip, spine, and wrist. Although the risk of becoming osteoporotic is tied to many dietary and lifestyle issues, the true cause of this condition remains somewhat unclear. Osteoporosis is most common in postmenopausal Oriental and white women. Premenopausal women are partially protected against bone loss by the hormone estrogen. Black women often have slightly greater bone mass in early adulthood compared with other women, which helps protect against bone fractures even though postmenopausal black women lose bone mass just as other women do. In men, testosterone partially protects against bone loss even after middle age. Beyond issues of race, age, and gender, incidence varies widely from society to society, suggesting that osteoporosis is largely preventable.

Dietary and Other Natural Therapies That May Be Helpful

When over 85,000 American women were followed for 12 years, those who ate the most animal protein (meat, poultry, and dairy) had a significantly higher risk of osteoporotic fractures.[1] Similarly, higher protein intake correlates with increased hip fracture in studies comparing different cultures.[2] When dietary protein increases, so does the loss of **calcium**

(p. 277) in urine,[3,4] (though this extra calcium loss is not always statistically significant).[5] Many nutritionally oriented doctors recommend a move toward vegetarian diets for people wishing to avoid osteoporosis or those already diagnosed with it.

However, bone formation requires protein and therefore people can eat too little protein as well as too much. In one trial of older women (average age 82) who had suffered an osteoporotic fracture, those given a 20-gram-per-day protein supplement had fewer complications, were less likely to die, and had much shorter hospital stays compared with women not assigned to receive extra protein.[6] Similarly, in a 3-year study of American women aged 50 to 69 funded by the National Diary Council, those eating more animal protein had a *lower* risk of osteoporotic hip fracture compared with those eating less.[7] A related double-blind trial in older women who had recently suffered an osteoporotic hip fracture found that a 20-gram-per-day protein supplement reduced bone loss compared with those not receiving protein.[8]

Pending further research, these conflicting reports show that drawing the line between too much protein and too little remains elusive. Nonetheless, most studies currently suggest that a life-long intake of high animal protein correlates with an increased risk of osteoporosis; however, protein supplementation following a fracture in elderly people appears to result in better bone and overall health compared with no protein supplementation.

Short-term increases in dietary salt result in increased urinary calcium loss, which suggests that over time, salt intake may cause significant bone loss.[9] Researchers have shown that increasing dietary salt increases markers of bone loss in post- (though not pre-) menopausal women.[10,11,12] Although a definitive link between salt intake and osteoporosis has yet to be proven, most nutritionally oriented doctors recommend that people wishing to protect themselves against bone loss use less salt and less highly salted processed and restaurant foods.

Caffeine has also been linked to fracture of the hip in a large study following American women for 6 years.[13] Like salt, caffeine increases urinary loss of calcium.[14] In one trial, caffeine was linked with lower bone mass but only in women who consumed relatively little calcium.[15] The authors of this report concluded that 2 to 3 cups of coffee per day might speed bone loss in women with calcium intakes of less than 800 mg per day. Most nutritionally oriented doctors recommend decreasing caffeine intake from caffeinated coffee, black tea, and cola drinks as a way to improve bone mass.

The relationship between soft drinks and bone mass is controversial. In some reports, young cola drinkers have an increased incidence of bone fractures,[16] though *short*-term consumption of carbonated beverages has not affected markers of bone health.[17] The problem, if one exists, may be linked to phosphoric acid, a substance found in many soft drinks. In one trial, children consuming at least six glasses of soft drinks containing phosphoric acid had more than five times the risk of developing low blood levels of calcium compared with other children.[18] Avoidance of phosphoric acid-containing soft drinks has also reduced **kidney stone** (p. 111) recurrence, again incriminating soda pop as a cause of abnormal calcium metabolism.[19] Although a few studies have not linked soft drinks to bone loss,[20] the preponderance of evidence now suggests that a problem may exist, and there is certainly no harm in decreasing drinks filled with sugar and chemicals, a dietary change that may reduce urinary loss of calcium.

Soy (p. 332) foods such as tofu, soy milk, roasted soy beans, and soy extract powders may be beneficial in preventing osteoporosis. Isoflavones from soy protect animals from bone loss.[21] Taking 40 grams of soy protein powder containing 90 mg isoflavones increased bone mineral density of the spine in a double-blind trial.[22] However, lower intakes (providing 56 mg isoflavones) did not improve bone density in this report. A synthetic isoflavone, ipriflavone, has reduced osteoporotic bone fractures in several reports.[23] Although the use of soy in the prevention of osteoporosis looks hopeful, knowing to what extent soy reduces bone loss will require further research.

Preliminary evidence suggests that **progesterone** (p. 326) might play a role in bone metabolism that, in theory, could reduce the risk of osteoporosis.[24] An uncontrolled preliminary study using topically applied natural progesterone cream in combination with diet, exercise, vitamin and calcium supplementation, and estrogen therapy, reported consistent gains in bone density over a 3-year period in postmenopausal women, but no comparison was made to the same protocol without progesterone.[25] However, at least one trial has found that adding natural progesterone to estrogen therapy does not improve the bone-sparing effects of estrogen when taken alone.[26] Because so few studies have investigated the effects of progesterone on bone mass and results from those limited reports are not consistent, the true effects of progesterone on bone mass remain unclear.

Progesterone is a hormone, and as such there are concerns about its inappropriate use. Women considering the use of natural progesterone should consult a doctor familiar with its use before using this hormone.

Lifestyle Changes That May Be Helpful

Smoking leads to increased bone loss.[27] For this and many other health reasons, smoking should be avoided.

Exercise is known to help protect against bone loss.[28] The more weight-bearing exercise done by men and postmenopausal women, the greater their bone mass and the lower the risk of osteoporosis. Walking is sometimes considered the perfect weight-bearing exercise. For premenopausal women, exercise is also important, but taken to extreme, it can be overdone. Exercise so excessive that it leads to cessation of the menstrual cycle actually *contributes* to osteoporosis.[29]

Nutritional Supplements That May Be Helpful

Many trials have investigated the effects of calcium on bone mass. Although insufficient when used as the only intervention, **calcium** (p. 277) supplements have helped to prevent osteoporosis.[30] Though some of the research remains controversial, the protective effect of calcium on bone mass is one of very few health claims permitted by the U.S. Food and Drug Administration.

In several studies, calcium intake has not correlated with protection—for example in men[31] or in women shortly after becoming menopausal.[32] Moreover, even most positive studies focusing on the effects of isolated calcium supplementation on bone mass show only minor effects. Nonetheless, a review of the research shows that calcium supplementation plus hormone replacement therapy is much more effective than hormone replacement therapy without calcium.[33] Double-blind research has found that increasing calcium intakes results in greater bone mass in girls.[34] A meta-analysis of many studies investigating the effects of calcium supplementation in premenopausal women has also shown a significant positive effect.[35] Most nutritionally oriented doctors, as well as most conventional medical doctors, recommend calcium supplementation as a way to partially reduce the risk of osteoporosis and to help people already diagnosed with the condition. In order to achieve the 1,500-mg-per-day calcium intake many researchers deem optimal, 800–1,000 mg of supplemental calcium are generally added to diets that commonly contain between 500–700 mg calcium.

Osteoporosis

Vitamin D (p. 343) increases calcium absorption, but surprisingly the effect of vitamin D on osteoporosis risk remains somewhat unclear,[36],[37] with some studies reporting little if any benefit.[38] Commonly, trials reporting reduced risk of fracture have used the combination of vitamin D and calcium compared with placebo, making it impossible to assess the specific benefit of vitamin D.[39] Nonetheless, vitamin D does appear partially protective, at least in certain circumstances. Double-blind research indicates that vitamin D supplementation reduces bone loss in women who consume insufficient amounts of vitamin D from food.[40] A double-blind trial also supports the use of higher (700 IU per day) supplemental intakes of vitamin D, particularly as a way to reduce bone loss in women during winter and spring, when vitamin D levels are typically at their lowest.[41]

While people who get outdoors regularly and live in sunny climates are unlikely to need vitamin D supplementation (particularly during the summer), nutritionally oriented doctors generally recommend vitamin D to most other people as a way to help protect bone mass despite remaining inconsistencies in the research. Typical supplemental amounts are between 400–800 IU per day, depending upon dietary intake and exposure to sunlight.

In a preliminary study, people with osteoporosis were reported to be at high risk for **magnesium** (p. 310) malabsorption.[42] Both bone[43] and blood levels of magnesium have also been reported to be low in people with osteoporosis.[44] Supplemental magnesium has reduced markers of bone loss in men.[45] Supplementing 250 (up to 750) mg per day of magnesium has also arrested bone loss or increased bone mass in twenty-seven of thirty-one people with osteoporosis in a 2-year controlled trial.[46] As a result of this research, most nutritionally oriented doctors recommend that people with osteoporosis supplement 250–350 mg of magnesium per day.

The idea that magnesium supplementation should be used *instead of* calcium[47] remains theoretical at best. No study has yet compared the effects of calcium versus magnesium versus the combination of the two, nor has any trial uncovered the optimal ratio of calcium to magnesium for the purpose of maintaining bone mass.

Levels of **zinc** (p. 346) in both blood and bone have been reported to be low in people with osteoporosis.[48] Urinary loss of zinc may be high in osteoporotic people according to preliminary research.[49] In one trial, men consuming only 10 mg of zinc per day had almost twice the risk of osteoporotic fractures compared with those eating significantly more zinc from their diets.[50] Whether zinc supplementation protects against bone loss has not yet been proven, though in one trial, combining minerals including zinc with calcium supplementation was more effective than calcium supplementation by itself.[51] Many nutritionally oriented doctors recommend that people with osteoporosis and those trying to protect themselves from this condition supplement 10–30 mg of zinc per day.

Copper (p. 285) is needed for normal bone synthesis. A recent controlled 2-year study reported that 3 mg of copper per day prevented bone loss.[52] Although evaluation of the importance of copper for people with osteoporosis requires further research, many nutritionally oriented doctors recommend 2–3 mg per day, particularly if **zinc** (p. 346) is supplemented. (Supplemental zinc significantly depletes copper nutriture, thus people taking zinc supplements for more than a few weeks generally need to supplement copper.) All minerals discussed so far—**calcium** (p. 277), **magnesium** (p. 310), **zinc** (p. 346), and **copper** (p. 285)—sometimes found at appropriate levels in high potency **multi-vitamin/minerals** (p. 314).

A preliminary trail found that supplementation with 3 mg per day of the trace mineral **boron** (p. 273) reduced urinary loss of both calcium and magnesium,[53] but both outcomes have been contradicted by more recent research.[54] Moreover, there is evidence that people taking magnesium supplements see no further calcium-sparing effect when adding supplemental boron.[55] Finally, in the original report claiming that boron reduced loss of calcium,[56] the effect was achieved by significantly increasing estrogen and testosterone levels, hormones that have been linked to cancer risks. Therefore, until evidence appears suggesting that the combination of boron plus magnesium has any advantage over magnesium supplementation without boron, it makes sense for people with osteoporosis to supplement with magnesium *instead of* rather than in addition to boron.

Interest in the effect of **manganese** (p. 311) and bone health began when famed basketball player Bill Walton's repeated fractures were prevented with manganese supplementation.[57] A subsequent unpublished trial reported manganese deficiency in a small group of osteoporotic women.[58] Since that time, although a combination of minerals including manganese was reported to halt bone loss,[59] no human trial has investigated the effect of isolated manganese supplementation on bone mass. Nonetheless, some nutritionally oriented doctors recommend 10–20 mg of manganese per day to people concerned with maintenance of bone mass.

Silicon (p. 331) plays a significant role in bone formation.[60] Supplementation with silicon has increased bone formation in animal research.[61] In preliminary human research, supplementation with silicon increased bone mineral density in a group of eight women with osteoporosis.[62] Optimal levels remain unknown, though some multi-vitamin/mineral supplements now contain small amounts of this trace mineral.

Strontium (p. 333) is also believed to play a role in bone formation and preliminary evidence suggests that women with osteoporosis may have reduced absorption of this trace mineral.[63] (The supplement considered here, sometimes called "stable strontium," is not the dangerous radioactive form of strontium people are more familiar with.) Many years ago in a preliminary uncontrolled trial, thirty-two people with osteoporosis given 1.7 grams of stable strontium for between 3 months and 3 years reported significant reduction in bone pain, supported by x-rays suggesting an increase in bone mass.[64] Increased bone formation and decreased bone pain were also reported in a group of six people with osteoporosis given 600–700 mg of stable strontium per day.[65] Although levels used in preliminary research have been quite high, optimal intakes remain unknown. Some nutritionally oriented doctors recommend a few milligrams per day (1–3 mg)—less than many people currently consume from their diets, but an amount that has begun to appear in some mineral formulas geared toward bone health.

Folic acid (p. 297), **vitamin B$_6$** (p. 340), and **vitamin B$_{12}$** (p. 337) are known to reduce blood levels of the amino acid homocysteine in the body, while homocysteinuria, a condition associated with high homocysteine levels, frequently causes osteoporosis. Although some doctors of natural medicine have suggested these B vitamins might help prevent osteoporosis by lowering homocysteine,[66] no research has yet explored this relationship. For the purpose of lowering homocysteine, amounts of folic acid and vitamins B$_6$ and B$_{12}$ found in high-potency **B-complex** (p. 341) supplements and **multi-vitamins** (p. 314) should be adequate.

Vitamin K (p. 345) is needed for bone formation. Those with osteoporosis have been reported to have both low blood levels[67,68] and low dietary levels of vitamin K.[69] One study found that post- (though not pre-) menopausal women have reduced urinary loss of calcium after taking 1 mg per day of vitamin K after just 2 weeks.[70] In controlled trials, people with osteoporosis given large amounts of vitamin K$_2$ (45 mg per day)

showed an increase in bone density after 6 months[71] and decreased bone loss after 1 year.[72] In a group of eight young women, those with estrogen deficiency (but not those with a normal menstrual cycle) showed evidence of increased bone formation when given 10 mg of vitamin K per day for 1 month.[73] Nutritionally oriented doctors frequently recommend 1 mg vitamin K$_1$ to postmenopausal women as a way to help maintain bone mass, though optimal intake remains unknown.

Are There Any Side Effects or Interactions? Refer to the individual supplement for information about any side effects or interactions.

Herbs That May Be Helpful

Horsetail (p. 436) is a rich source of **silicon** (p. 331), and preliminary research suggests that this trace mineral may help maintain bone mass (see *Diet and Other Natural Therapies* section above). Effects of horsetail on bone mass have not yet been studied.

Black cohosh (p. 397) has been shown to improve bone mineral density in animals fed a low **calcium** (p. 277) diet[74] but have not yet been studied for this purpose in humans.

Are There Any Side Effects or Interactions? Refer to the individual herb for information about any side effects or interactions.

Checklist for Osteoporosis

Ranking	Nutritional Supplements	Herbs
Primary	Calcium (p. 277)	
Secondary	Magnesium (p. 310) Soy (p. 332) Vitamin D (p. 343) Vitamin K (p. 345)	
Other	Boron (p. 273) Folic Acid (p. 297) Progesterone (p. 326)	Black cohosh (p. 397) Horsetail (p. 436)
See also: Homeopathic Remedies for **Osteoporosis** (p. 563)		

Pap Smear (Abnormal)

Women are advised to have periodic Pap smears because cancer of the cervix is a fairly common and sometimes fatal disease. A Pap smear checks cells from the cervix for any evidence of pre-cancerous or cancerous changes. If an abnormality is detected early, the doctor can prescribe effective treatment before the problem becomes more serious. Cervical dysplasia is a term used to describe abnormal cervical cells. Cervical dysplasia is usually graded according to its severity, which can range from mild inflammation to pre-cancerous changes to localized cancer. It is now known that the human papillomavirus (HPV), also the cause of genital warts, is the major cause of cervical dysplasia.

Nutritional Supplements That May Be Helpful

Women with cervical dysplasia may have lower blood levels of **beta-carotene** (p. 268) and **vitamin E** (p. 344) compared to healthy women.[1] Low levels of **selenium** (p. 331)[2] and low dietary intake of **vitamin C** (p. 341)[3] have also been observed in women with cervical dysplasia. Women with a low intake of **vitamin A** (p. 336) have an increased risk of abnormal Pap smear.[4] These dietary associations do not necesarily indicate that these nutrients would be helpful if used as supplements. Rather, it is possible that women consuming more of these nutrients from their diets are eating more produce, and other substances in produce might account for protection. In a double-blind trial, when women with cervical abnormalities were given 500 mg of vitamin C and or 50,000 IU beta-carotene per day for 2 years, no significant evidence of improvement was seen, and those assigned to both supplements experienced a statistically insignificant worsening of their condition.[5] Although the apparent association between these supplements and deterioration of the condition of the cervix appears to have been due to chance, there is currently no sound evidence supporting the use of vitamin C or beta-carotene supplements for people with cervical dysplasia.

Large amounts of **folic acid** (p. 297)—10 mg per day—have been shown to improve the abnormal Pap smears of women who are taking birth control pills.[6] Folic acid does not improve the Pap smears of women who are not taking oral contraceptives.[7,8] High blood levels of folic acid have been linked to protecting against the development of cervical dysplasia.[9]

Are There Any Side Effects or Interactions? Refer to the individual supplement for information about any side effects or interactions.

Herbs That May Be Helpful

Several herbs have been used by naturopathic physicians and other practitioners of natural medicine as part of an approach for women with mild cervical dysplasia. These include **myrrh** (p. 446), **echinacea** (p. 417), **usnea** (p. 465), **goldenseal** (p. 429), **marshmallow** (p. 444), geranium, and **yarrow** (p. 471).[10] These are used for their anti-viral actions as well as to stimulate tissue healing. These are generally administered in a suppository preparation. A doctor of natural medicine should be consulted to discuss the use and availability of these herbs.

Checklist for Abnormal Pap Smear

Ranking	Nutritional Supplements	Herbs
Primary	Folic acid (p. 297) (for women using oral contraceptives)	
Other	Selenium (p. 331) Vitamin A (p. 336) Vitamin E (p. 344)	Echinacea (p. 417) Geranium Goldenseal (p. 429) Marshmallow (p. 444) Myrrh (p. 446) Usnea (p. 465) Yarrow (p. 471)

Parasites

A number of organisms known collectively as parasites can cause infections in humans. Parasites differ from bacteria in that they are more complex and larger (although still too small to see with the naked eye, in many cases). The most common parasites are giardia (*Giardia lamblia*), amoeba (*Entamoeba histolytica*), cryptosporidium (*Cryptosporidium* spp.), roundworm (*Ascarias lumbricoides*), hookworm (*Ancylostoma duodenale* and *Necator americanus*), pinworm (*Enterobius vermicularus*), and tapeworm (*Taenia* spp.). Parasites can lead to a variety of symptoms, including gas, **diarrhea** (p. 58), weight loss, and abdominal cramping and pain. Amoebas and all types of parasites in people with poorly functioning immune systems can cause lethal infections. Therefore, individuals should consult a physician if parasites are suspected.

Dietary Changes That May Be Helpful

When traveling outside the United States, people should avoid drinking tap water and eating uncooked foods, foods prepared by street vendors, ice, and fruits that cannot be peeled. All of these are potential sources of parasitic infection. People should not drink untreated stream water while camping, as it is frequently contaminated with giardia, even in the United States. Undercooked meats, poultry, and fish can also contain parasites.

Herbs That May Be Helpful

Garlic (p. 425) has been demonstrated to kill parasites, including amoeba[1] and hookworm,[2] in test tubes and in animals. Older studies in humans support the use of garlic to treat roundworm, pinworm, and hookworm.[3] Garlic on its own is not sufficient to treat parasites; however, its safety makes it an excellent adjunct to other treatments for parasites.

Checklist for Parasites

Ranking	Nutritional Supplements	Herbs
Primary		Berberine
Other		Black walnut Chaparral (p. 410) Cloves Garlic (p. 425) Goldenseal (p. 429) Male fern Oregon grape (p. 449) Pumpkin seed Sweet Annie (p. 463) Tansy Wormseed Wormwood (p. 470)

Berberine is derived from several plants, including **Oregon grape** (p. 449) and **goldenseal** (p. 429). Berberine has been successfully used to treat giardia infections,[4][5] and test tube studies show that it kills amoeba.[6] The amount required is approximately 200 mg 3 times per day for an adult—a high enough level to potentially cause side effects. Therefore, berberine should not be used without consulting a knowledgeable health-care provider.

A traditional remedy for worms is wormseed *(Chenopodium ambrosioides).* However, a study in Mexico did not find the powdered herb beneficial for treatment of hookworm, roundworm, or whipworm.[7]

Pumpkin seeds *(Curcurbita pepo)* have purported effects against tapeworms. Given their safety, they are often recommended as an addition to other, more reliable therapies. In Germany, 200–400 grams are ground and taken with milk and honey, followed by castor oil 2 hours later.[8] Tapeworms can cause severe illness and should not be treated without professional medical assistance.

Several other herbs are traditionally used for treatment of parasites, including male fern *(Dryopteris filix-mas),* tansy *(Tanacetum vulgare),* **wormwood** (p. 470), black walnut *(Juglans nigra),* and cloves *(Syzygium aromaticum).* It is important to note that anything potent enough to kill parasites could potentially harm the person taking it. Although some of these herbs have antiparasitic actions in test tubes,[9] none has been tested in scientific studies for efficacy or safety. Their use requires the skills of an experienced herbal practitioner.

In some cultures, it was customary to bathe in **chaparral** (p. 410) once per year to eliminate skin parasites and detoxify; however, there is no modern research to confirm this use of chaparral.

Are There Any Side Effects or Interactions? Refer to the individual herb for information about any side effects or interactions.

Peptic Ulcer

The term "peptic" ulcer distinguishes this condition from ulcerations that affect other parts of the body. Peptic ulcers are erosions in the stomach or duodenum (the first part of the small intestine). These ulcers often bleed and may cause sharp burning pain in the area of the stomach or just below it. Peptic ulcer should never be treated without proper diagnosis.

Peptic ulcer is often caused by infection from *Helicobacter pylori.* People with peptic ulcer due to infection should discuss conventional treatment directed toward eradicating the infection—a combination of antibiotics and bismuth—with a medical doctor. Ulcers can also be caused or exacerbated by stress, alcohol, smoking, and dietary factors.

Dietary Changes That May Be Helpful

People with ulcers have been reported to eat more sugar than people without ulcers,[1] though this link may only occur in those with a genetic susceptibility toward ulcer formation.[2] Sugar has also been reported to increase stomach acidity,[3] which could exacerbate ulcer symptoms. Salt is a stomach and intestinal irritant. Higher intakes of salt have been linked to higher risk of stomach (though not duodenal) ulcer.[4] As a result of these reports, some nutritionally oriented doctors suggest that people with ulcers should restrict the use of both sugar and salt. However, the amount of benefit obtained by making such dietary changes remains unknown.

Many years ago, researchers reported that cabbage juice accelerated healing of peptic ulcers.[5,6,7,8] Drinking a quart of cabbage juice per day was necessary for symptom relief in some reports. Although only preliminary modern research supports this approach,[9] many nutritionally oriented doctors claim considerable success using 1 quart per day for 10 to 14 days, with ulcer symptoms frequently decreasing in only a few days. Carrot juice may be added to improve the flavor.

Fiber (p. 293) slows the movement of food and acidic fluid from the stomach to the intestines, which should help those with duodenal though not stomach ulcers.[10] When people with recently healed duodenal ulcers were put on a long-term (6-month) high-fiber diet, the rate of ulcer recurrence was dramatically reduced in one controlled study,[11] though short-term (4-week) use of fiber in people with active duodenal ulcers led to only negligible improvement.[12]

Ayurvedic doctors in India have traditionally used dried banana powder to treat ulcers. In animal studies, banana powder protects the lining of the stomach from acid.[13] A human trial has also found dried banana helpful in those with peptic ulcer. In that report, 2 capsules of dried raw banana powder taken 4 times per day for 8 weeks led to significant improvement.[14] Bananas and unsweetened banana chips may be good substitutes, although ideal intake remains unknown.

Years ago, **food allergies** (p. 8) were linked to peptic ulcer.[15] Exposing the lining of the stomach to foods a person was known to be allergic to has caused bleeding in the stomach.[16] If not triggered by *Helicobacter* infection nor helped by other natural approaches, peptic ulcer may respond to avoidance of allergens. Consultation with a nutritionally oriented doctor is needed to discover to which foods a person is sensitive.

Lifestyle Changes That May Be Helpful

Aspirin and related drugs,[17] alcohol,[18] coffee[19] (including decaf),[20] and tea[21] are known to increase stomach acidity, which can interfere with the healing of an ulcer. Smoking is known to slow ulcer healing.[22] Whether or not an ulcer is caused by infection, people with peptic ulcer should avoid use of these substances.

Nutritional Supplements That May Be Helpful

Vitamin A (p. 336) is needed in the healing of mucosal tissue, including linings of the stomach and intestines. In one controlled trial, vitamin A facilitated healing in a small group of people with stomach ulcer.[23] The amount used in that report—50,000 IU taken 3 times per day—is highly toxic, can cause birth defects, and should never be taken by a woman who is or could become pregnant, nor by anyone else without careful supervision from a nutritionally oriented doctor. Objective evidence of healing from taking vitamin A has been reported by the same research group.[24] The effect of lower amounts of vitamin A has not been studied in people with peptic ulcer.

Zinc (p. 346) is also needed in the repair of damaged tissue and has protected rats from stomach ulceration.[25] In Europe, zinc combined with acexamic acid,

an anti-inflammatory substance, is used as a drug in the treatment of peptic ulcers.[26] In an isolated controlled trial that used 88 mg of zinc taken 3 times per day, the speed of healing tripled compared with placebo.[27] Some nutritionally oriented doctors suspect that such an exceptionally high intake of zinc may be unnecessary, suggesting instead that people with ulcers wishing to take zinc supplements have only 25–50 mg of zinc per day. Even at these lower levels, 1–3 mg of **copper** (p. 285) per day must be taken to avoid copper deficiency that would otherwise be induced by the zinc supplementation.

Glutamine (p. 300), an amino acid, is the principal source of energy for cells that line the small intestine and stomach. Years ago, glutamine was reported to help people with peptic ulcer in a preliminary trial.[28] Glutamine has also prevented stress ulcers triggered by severe burns in another preliminary report.[29] Despite the limited amount of published research, some nutritionally oriented doctors suggest 500–1,000 mg of glutamine taken 2 to 3 times per day to help people overcome peptic ulcers.

Research has shown that **bioflavonoids** (p. 271)—such as **quercetin** (p. 328), catechin, and apigenin, which is found in **chamomile** (p. 409)—inhibit the growth of *Helicobacter pylori*, the microorganism that frequently causes peptic ulcer.[30] Bioflavonoids have also been used for ulcers because of their anti-inflammatory activity,[31] though most published research has studied leg ulcers—not peptic ulcer. Some nutritionally oriented doctors recommend 500 mg of quercetin taken 2 to 3 times per day, though optimal intake remains unknown.

A study from Malaysia reports that oral dimethyl sulfoxide (**DMSO** [p. 291]) reduced relapse rates for peptic ulcer significantly better than placebo or the ulcer drug cimetidine.[32] Previous research showed that DMSO in combination with cimetidine was more effective than cimetidine alone.[33] These trials used 500 mg of DMSO taken 4 times per day. The authors of these trials believe the antioxidant activity of DMSO may have a protective effect.

Are There Any Side Effects or Interactions? Refer to the individual supplement for information about any side effects or interactions.

Herbs That May Be Helpful

Licorice (p. 440) root has a long history of use for soothing inflamed and injured mucous membranes in the digestive tract. Licorice may protect the stomach and duodenum by increasing production of mucin, a substance that protects the lining of these organs against stomach acid and other harmful substances.[34]

Bioflavonoids in licorice also appear to inhibit *Helicobacter pylori*, according to laboratory research.[35]

For people with peptic ulcer, many doctors who use herbal medicine use the deglycyrrhizinated form of licorice (DGL). In making DGL, the portion of licorice root that can increase blood pressure and cause water retention is removed, while the mucous membrane-healing part of the root is retained. In some reports, DGL has compared favorably to the popular drug cimetidine (Tagamet) for treatment of peptic ulcer,[36] while in other trials cimetidine has appeared to be initially more effective.[37] However, after DGL and cimetidine were discontinued, one study reported fewer recurrences in the former DGL group compared with the former cimetidine group.[38] Though not every trial has reported efficacy,[39] most studies find DGL to facilitate healing of peptic ulcer. A review of the DGL research shows that the studies not reporting efficacy used capsules, and the trials finding DGL to be helpful used chewable tablets.[40] Doctors typically suggest taking 1 to 2 chewable tablets of DGL (250–500 mg) 15 minutes before meals and 1 to 2 hours before bedtime.

The gummy extract of *Pistachia lentiscus*, also known as mastic, has been shown in two double-blind studies to heal peptic ulcers.[41,42] This may be related to its ability to kill *Helicobacter pylori* in test tubes.[43] This herbal preparation is not yet available in the U.S.

Chamomile (p. 409) has a soothing effect on inflamed and irritated mucous membranes. It is also high in the bioflavonoid apigenin. Many doctors of natural medicine recommend drinking 2 to 3 cups of strong chamomile tea each day. The tea can be made by combining 3–5 ml of chamomile tincture with hot water or by steeping 2–3 teaspoons of chamomile flowers in the water, covered, for 10 to 15 minutes. Chamomile is also available in capsules; 2 can be taken 3 times per day. **Calendula** (p. 406) is another plant with anti-inflammatory and healing activity used as part of the approach to people with peptic ulcers in traditional medicine. The same amount as chamomile can be used.

Marshmallow (p. 444) is high in mucilage. High-mucilage-containing herbs have a long history of use for irritated or inflamed mucous membranes in the digestive system, though no clinical research has yet investigated effects in people with peptic ulcer.

Garlic (p. 425),[44] **thyme** (p. 464) tea, and **cinnamon** (p. 411) tincture have all been reported to have anti-*Helicobacter* activity in test tube studies.[45] Whether garlic, thyme, or cinnamon would be effective in humans with peptic ulcers caused by this bacterium has yet to be explored in clinical research.

Comfrey (p. 413) has a long, traditional history of use as a topical agent for improving healing of **wounds** (p. 167) and skin ulcers.[46,47] It was also used for people with gastrointestinal problems, including stomach **ulcers** (p. 138), though these traditional uses have yet to be tested in scientific studies.

Are There Any Side Effects or Interactions? Refer to the individual herb for information about any side effects or interactions.

Checklist for Peptic Ulcer

Ranking	Nutritional Supplements	Herbs
Primary		Deglycyrrhizinated Licorice (p. 440) (chewable) Mastic
Secondary	Banana powder, Vitamin A (p. 336) Zinc (p. 346)	
Other	Bioflavonoids (p. 271) (Quercetin [p. 328], catechin, apigenin) DMSO (p. 291) Fiber (p. 293) (for duodenal ulcer) Glutamine (p. 300)	Calendus (p. 406) Chamomile (p. 409) Cinnamon (p. 411) Comfrey (p. 413) Garlic (p. 425) Marshmallow (p. 444) Thyme (p. 464)

Photosensitivity

Several conditions, such as erythropoietic protoporphyria and polymorphous light eruption, share the common symptom of hypersensitivity to light—typically sunlight. People taking certain prescription drugs (sulfonamides, tetracycline, and thiazide diuretics) and those diagnosed with **systemic lupus erythematosis** (p. 115) are more likely to overreact to sun exposure. People with photosensitivities typically break out in a rash when exposed to sunlight; how much exposure causes a reaction varies from person to person.

Dietary Changes That May Be Helpful

One of the conditions that can trigger photosensitivity—porphyria cutanea tarda—has been linked to alcohol consumption.[1] People with this form of porphyria should avoid alcohol.

Lifestyle Changes That May Be Helpful

People with photosensitivities need to protect themselves from the sun by using sunscreen, wearing protective clothing (such as long-sleeved shirts), and avoiding excess exposure to the sun.

Checklist for Photosensitivity

Ranking	Nutritional Supplements	Herbs
Primary	Beta-carotene (p. 268)	
Other	Adenosine mono-phosphate (p. 263) Vitamin B₃ (Niacina-mide) (p. 339) Vitamin B₆ (p. 340) Vitamin E (p. 344)	

See also: Homeopathic Remedies for **Photosensitivity** (p. 564)

Nutritional Supplements That May Be Helpful

Beta-carotene (p. 268) collects primarily in the skin. Years ago, researchers theorized that beta-carotene in skin might help protect against sensitivity to ultraviolet light from the sun. Large amounts of beta-carotene (up to 150,000 IU per day for at least several months) have allowed people with photosensitivities to stay out in the sun several times longer than they otherwise could tolerate.[2,3,4] The protective effect appears to result from beta-carotene's ability to protect against free radical damage caused by sunlight.[5]

Less is known about the effects of other **antioxidants** (p. 267). Research with **vitamin E** (p. 344) has been limited and has not yielded consistent results.[6,7]

Cases have been reported of people with photosensitivities who respond to **vitamin B₆** (p. 340) supplements.[8,9] Amounts of vitamin B₆ used to successfully reduce reactions to sunlight have varied considerably. Some nutritionally oriented doctors suggest a trial of 100–200 mg per day for 3 months.

Niacinamide (p. 317), a form of vitamin B₃, can reduce the formation of a kynurenic acid—a substance that has been linked to photosensitivities. One trial studied the effects of niacinamide in people who had polymorphous light eruption, one of the photosensitivity diseases.[10] Taking 1 gram 3 times per day, most people remained free of problems despite exposure to the sun.

Adenosine monophosphate (AMP) (p. 263) is a substance made in the body and is also found as a supplement, although it is not widely available. Nineteen out of twenty-one people with porphyria cutanea tarda responded well to 160–200 mg of AMP per day taken for at least 1 month, reports one group of researchers.[11] Partial and even complete alleviation of

photosensitivity associated with this condition occurred in several people.

Are There Any Side Effects or Interactions? Refer to the individual supplement for information about any side effects or interactions.

PMS (Premenstrual Syndrome)

Many premenopausal women suffer from symptoms of premenstrual syndrome (PMS). These symptoms typically begin at the end of each monthly cycle and resolve with the start of menstruation. PMS is also known as premenstrual tension (PMT). Specific problems—cramping, bloating, mood changes, and breast tenderness—may vary from woman to woman. Women with breast tenderness should see the chapter on **fibrocystic breast disease** (p. 66).

Dietary and Other Natural Therapies That May Be Helpful

Women who eat more sugary foods appear to have an increased risk of PMS.[1] Alcohol can affect hormone metabolism, and alcoholic women are more likely to suffer PMS than are non-alcoholic women.[2] In a study of Chinese women, increasing tea consumption was associated with increasing prevalence of PMS.[3] Among a group of college students in the United States, consumption of caffeine-containing beverages was associated with increases in both the prevalence and severity of PMS.[4] Moreover, the more caffeine women consumed, the more likely they were to suffer from PMS.[5] Therefore, many nutritionally oriented doctors recommend that women with PMS avoid sugar, alcohol, and caffeine.

Several studies suggest that diets low in fat or **high in fiber** (p. 293) may help to reduce symptoms of PMS.[6] Many nutritionally oriented doctors recommend diets very low in meat and dairy fat and high in fruit, vegetables, and whole grains.

Most well-controlled studies have not found vaginally applied natural **progesterone** (p. 326) to be effective against the symptoms of premenstrual syndrome.[7] However, some doctors of natural medicine report that orally or rectally administered progesterone may be effective.[8]

Progesterone is a hormone, and as such there are concerns about its inappropriate use. A nutritionally oriented physician should be consulted before using this hormone. Few side effects have been associated with use of topical progesterone creams, but skin reactions may occur. The effect of natural

PMS (Premenstrual Syndrome)

progesterone on breast cancer risk remains unclear; some research suggests the possibility of increased risk, whereas other research points to a possible reduction in risk.

Lifestyle Changes That May Be Helpful

Women with PMS who jogged an average of about 12 miles a week for 6 months experienced a reduction in breast tenderness, fluid retention, depression, and stress.[9] Nutritionally oriented doctors frequently recommend regular exercise as a way to reduce symptoms of PMS.

Nutritional Supplements That May Be Helpful

Vitamin B$_6$ (p. 340) can reduce some of the effects of estrogen in animals, and excess estrogen may be responsible for PMS symptoms. A number of studies show that taking 50–400 mg of vitamin B$_6$ per day for several months can relieve symptoms of PMS.[10,11,12,13,14]

Although some studies have not found vitamin B$_6$ to be helpful,[15] most nutritionally oriented doctors feel that vitamin B$_6$ is worth a try and suggest 50–400 mg per day for at least 3 months. However, intakes greater than 200 mg per day can cause side effects.

Many years ago, research linked B vitamin deficiencies to PMS.[16,17] Based on that early work, some nutritionally oriented doctors recommend the **B-complex** (p. 341) vitamins for women with PMS.[18]

Women with PMS have been shown to have impaired conversion of linoleic acid (an essential fatty acid) to gamma linolenic acid (GLA).[19] Because a deficiency of GLA might, in theory, be a factor in PMS and because **evening primrose oil (EPO)** (p. 292) contains significant amounts of GLA, researchers have studied EPO as a potential way to reduce symptoms of PMS. In several double-blind studies, EPO was found to be beneficial,[20,21,22,23] whereas in other studies it was no more effective than placebo.[24,25]

Despite these conflicting results, many nutritionally oriented doctors consider EPO to be worth a try; the usual amount recommended is 3–4 grams per day. EPO seems to work best when used over several menstrual cycles and may be more helpful in women with PMS who also experience breast tenderness or **fibrocystic breast disease** (p. 66).[26]

Women with PMS are often deficient in **magnesium** (p. 310).[27,28] Supplementing with magnesium may help reduce symptoms.[29,30] While the ideal amount of magnesium has yet to be determined, some doctors recommend 400 mg per day.[31]

Women who consume more **calcium** (p. 277) from their diets are less likely to suffer severe PMS.[32] Double-blind research has shown that supplementing 1,000 mg of calcium per day relieves symptoms in women with PMS.[33,34]

Progesterone may relieve some symptoms of PMS, and **vitamin A** (p. 336) appears to increase progesterone levels.[35] Very high amounts of vitamin A—100,000 IU per day or more—have reduced symptoms of PMS,[36,37] but such an amount can cause serious side effects with long-term use. Women who are or who could become pregnant should not supplement with more than 10,000 IU (3,000 mcg) per day of vitamin A. Other people should not take more than 25,000 IU per day without the supervision of their nutritionally oriented doctor.

Although women with PMS do not appear to be deficient in **vitamin E** (p. 344),[38] double-blind research shows that 300 IU of vitamin E per day may decrease symptoms of PMS.[39]

Some of the nutrients mentioned above appear together in **multivitamin/mineral** (p. 314) supplements. One double-blind trial used a multivitamin/mineral supplement containing vitamin B$_6$ (600 mg per day), magnesium (500 mg per day), vitamin E (200 IU per day), vitamin A (25,000 IU per day), B-complex vitamins, and various other vitamins and minerals.[40] This supplement was found to relieve each of the four different categories of symptoms that have been associated wtih PMS. Similar results were reported in another study.[41]

Are There Any Side Effects or Interactions? Refer to the individual supplement for information about any side effects or interactions.

Herbs That May Be Helpful

Vitex (p. 467) has been shown to help re-establish normal balance of estrogen and progesterone during a woman's menstrual cycle. This is important because some women suffer from PMS and other menstrual irregularities due to underproduction of the hormone progesterone during the second half of their cycle. Vitex stimulates the pituitary gland to produce more luteinizing hormone, and this leads to greater production of progesterone.[42] Studies have shown that using vitex once in the morning over a period of several months helps normalize hormone balance to alleviate the symptoms of PMS.[43] Vitex has been shown to be as effective as 200 mg **vitamin B$_6$** (p. 340) in a double-blind study of women with PMS.[44]

Use 40 drops of a liquid, concentrated vitex extract or one capsule of the equivalent dried, powdered extract once per day in the morning with some liquid.

Vitex should be taken for at least four cycles to determine efficacy.

In traditional Chinese medicine, **dong quai** (p. 417) *(Angelica sinensis)* is often referred to as the "female ginseng." Dong quai helps promote normal hormone balance and is particularly useful for women experiencing premenstrual cramping and pain.[45] Many women take 2–3 grams of dong quai capsules or tablets per day.

The medicinal use of **false unicorn** (p. 423) root is based in Native American tradition, where it was recommended for a large number of women's health conditions, including lack of menstruation (amenorrhea), **painful menstruation** (p. 61), and other irregularities of menstruation, as well as to prevent miscarriages.[46] Steroidal saponins are generally credited with providing false unicorn root's activity. Modern investigations have not confirmed this, and there is no research yet about the medical applications of this herb.

Black cohosh (p. 397) is approved in Germany for use in women with PMS.[47] However, most modern use centers on symptomatic relief of hot flashes during menopause, not PMS relief.

Yarrow (p. 471) tea, taken internally or used as a sitz bath, has been used by European doctors practicing herbal medicine when the main symptom of PMS is spastic pain.[48] Combine 2–3 teaspoons of yarrow flowers with 1 cup of hot water, then cover and steep for 15 minutes. Drink 3 to 5 cups per day beginning 2 days before PMS symptoms usually commence. In addition, 1–3 cups of the tea added to hot or cold water can be used as a sitz bath.

Are There Any Side Effects or Interactions? Refer to the individual herb for information about any side effects or interactions.

Checklist for PMS (Premenstrual Syndrome)

Ranking	Nutritional Supplements	Herbs
Secondary	Calcium (p. 277) Evening Primrose Oil (p. 292) Magnesium (p. 310) Multiple Vitamin/ Mineral (p. 314) Vitamin B$_6$ (p. 340) Vitamin E (p. 344)	Vitex (p. 467)
Other	B-complex (p. 341) Fiber (p. 293) Progesterone (p. 326) Vitamin A (p. 336) (see dosage warnings)	Dong quai (p. 417) False unicorn root (p. 423) Yarrow (p. 471)

See also: Homeopathic Remedies for **PMS** (p. 554)

Pregnancy and Postpartum Support

Pregnancy lasts an average of 40 weeks from the date of the last menstrual period to delivery. In the first trimester, many pregnant women experience nausea. Usually these women report that they feel best during the second trimester. During the third (final) trimester, the increasing size of the fetus begins to pose mechanical strains on the woman, often causing back pain, leg swelling, and other health problems.

Dietary Changes That May Be Helpful

Nearly all pregnant women can benefit from good nutritional habits prior to and during pregnancy. The increased number of birth defects during times of famine attest to the adverse effects of poor nutrition during pregnancy.[1]

Women who consume a standard Western diet (high in fat and sugar and low in complex carbohydrates) during pregnancy and breastfeeding may not be obtaining adequate amounts of essential vitamins and minerals; this can result in health problems for the newborn.[2]

Pregnant women should choose a well-balanced and varied diet that includes fresh fruits and vegetables, whole grains, legumes, beans, and fish. Refined sugars, white flour, fried foods, processed foods, and chemical additives should be avoided.

Lifestyle Changes That May Be Helpful

A woman can reduce her risk of complications during pregnancy and delivery by avoiding harmful substances, such as alcohol, caffeine, nicotine, recreational drugs, and some prescription or over-the-counter drugs.

Even minimal alcohol ingestion during pregnancy can increase the risk of hyperactivity, short attention span, and emotional problems in the child.[3] Pregnant women should, therefore, avoid alcohol completely.

Cigarette smoking during pregnancy causes lower birth weights and smaller-sized newborns. The rate of miscarriage in smokers is twice as high as that in nonsmokers,[4] and babies born to mothers who smoke have more than twice the risk of dying from sudden infant death syndrome (SIDS).[5]

Research also links excessive caffeine ingestion during pregnancy to growth-retardation or low birth weight in infants.[6] Pregnant women should limit their caffeine intake to a maximum of 300 mg per day; this is equivalent to approximately 3 cups of coffee per day.

Nutritional Supplements That May Be Helpful

The requirement for the B vitamin **folic acid** (p. 297) doubles during pregnancy.[7] Deficiencies of folic acid during pregnancy have been linked to low birth weight and to an increased incidence of neural tube defects in infants. In one study, women who were at high risk of giving birth to babies with neural tube defects were able to lower their risk by 72% by taking folic acid supplements prior to and during pregnancy.[8] In another study, women who took folic acid supplements during pregnancy had fewer infections and gave birth to babies with higher birth weights and better Apgar scores.[9] The recommended daily intake of folic acid during pregnancy is 600 mcg.

The requirement for **iron** (p. 304) is increased during pregnancy. In one study, fifteen of twenty-three women who were not given extra iron developed iron deficiency during pregnancy, compared with none of twenty-two women who received an iron supplement[10] However, supplementation with large amounts of iron has been shown to reduce blood levels of zinc.[11] Although the significance of that finding is not clear, low blood levels of **zinc** (p. 346) have been associated with an increased risk of complications in both the mother and fetus.[12] In addition, iron supplementation was associated in one study with an increased incidence of birth defects,[13] possibly as a result of an iron-induced deficiency of zinc. Although additional research needs to be done, the evidence suggests that women who are supplementing with iron during pregnancy should also take a **multiple vitamin/mineral** (p. 314) formula that contains adequate amounts of zinc. To be on the safe side, pregnant women should discuss their supplement program with a nutritionally oriented doctor.

Supplementation with **niacin** (p. 339) (a form of vitamin B$_3$) during the first trimester has been correlated with higher birth weights, longer length, and larger head circumference (all signs of healthier infants).[14]

Calcium (p. 277) needs double during pregnancy.[15] Low dietary intake of this mineral is associated with increased risk of pre-eclampsia, a potentially dangerous (but preventable) condition characterized by high blood pressure and swelling. Supplementation with calcium may reduce the risk of pre-term delivery, which is often associated with pre-eclampsia. Calcium may also reduce the risk of **hypertensive** (p. 89) disorders of pregnancy.[16] Pregnant women should consume

1,500 mg of calcium per day. Food sources of calcium include milk products, dark green leafy vegetables, tofu, sardines (canned with edible bones), salmon (canned with edible bones), peas, and beans.

Since a 1995 report from the *New England Journal of Medicine*,[17] women who are or could become pregnant have been told by doctors to take less than 10,000 IU (3,000 mcg) per day of **vitamin A** (p. 336) to avoid the risk of birth defects. A recent report studied several hundred women exposed to 10,000–300,000 IU (median exposure of 50,000 IU) per day.[18] Three major malformations occurred in this study, but all could have happened in the absence of vitamin A supplementation. Surprisingly, no congenital malformations happened in any of the 120 infants exposed to maternal intakes of vitamin A that exceeded 50,000 IU per day. In fact, when compared with infants not exposed to vitamin A, there was a 50% decreased risk for malformations in this high-exposure group. The authors note that previous trials either based the link to birth defects on very few cases, didn't measure vitamin A intake, or found no link to birth defects whatsoever. A closer look at the recent study reveals a 32% higher than expected risk of birth defects in infants exposed to 10,000–40,000 IU of vitamin A per day, but paradoxically a 37% decreased risk for those exposed to even higher levels, suggesting that both "higher" and "lower" risks may have been due to chance. At present, the level at which birth defects might be caused by vitamin A supplementation is not known, though it may well be higher than 10,000 IU per day. Nevertheless, women who are pregnant should talk with a nutritionally oriented doctor before supplementing with more than 10,000 IU per day.

Are There Any Side Effects or Interactions? Refer to the individual supplement for information about any side effects or interactions.

Herbs That May Be Helpful

Tonic herbs, which nourish and tone the system, can be taken safely every day during pregnancy. Examples of these tonic herbs include **dandelion** (p. 415) leaf and root, **red raspberry** (p. 454) leaf, and **nettles** (p. 447). Dandelion leaf and root are rich sources of vitamins and minerals, including beta-carotene, calcium, potassium, and iron. Dandelion leaf is mildly diuretic; it also stimulates bile flow and helps with the common digestive complaints of pregnancy. Dandelion root tones the liver.[19]

Red raspberry leaf is the most often mentioned traditional herbal tonic for general support of pregnancy and breastfeeding. Rich in vitamins and minerals (especially iron), it tones the uterus, increases milk flow, and restores the mother's system after childbirth.[20]

Nettle leaf provides the minerals calcium and iron, is mildly diuretic, and aids in the elimination of excess water from tissues. Nettle enriches and increases the flow of breast milk and restores the mother's energy following childbirth.[21]

In one study, addition of **lavender** (p. 439) oil to a bath was more effective than a placebo in relieving perineal pain after childbirth.[22] However, the improvement was not statistically significant, so more research is needed to determine whether lavender oil is truly effective.

Numerous herbs are used in traditional herbal medicine systems around the world to promote production of breast milk.[23] These are known as lactagogues or galactagogues. **Vitex** (p. 467) is one of the best recognized herbs in Europe for promoting lactation. A double-blind study found that 15 drops of a vitex tincture three times per day could increase the amount of milk produced by mothers with or without pregnancy complications compared with mothers given **vitamin B$_1$** (p. 337) or nothing.[24]

Goat's rue *(Galega officinanlis)* also has a history of use in Europe for supporting breastfeeding. Taking 1 teaspoon of goat's rue tincture is considered by European practitioners to be helpful in increasing milk volume.[25] Studies are as yet lacking to support the use of goat's rue as a lactagogue.

Sage (p. 456) has been used traditionally to dry up milk production when a woman is no longer wishing to breastfeed.[26]

Are There Any Side Effects or Interactions? Refer to the individual herb for information about any side effects or interactions.

Checklist for Pregnancy and Postpartum Support

Ranking	Nutritional Supplements	Herbs
Primary	Folic acid (p. 297)	
Secondary		Lavender (p. 439)
Other	Calcium (p. 277) Vitamin B$_3$ (Niacin) (p. 339)	Dandelion (leaves and root) (p. 415) Goat's rue Nettle (p. 447) Red raspberry (p. 454) Sage (p. 456)
See also: Homeopathic Remedies for **Pregnancy and Postpartum Support** (p. 565)		

Prostatic Hyperplasia, Benign

The prostate is a small gland that surrounds the neck of the bladder and urethra. Its major function is to contribute to seminal fluid. If the prostate enlarges or swells, it can put pressure on the urethra, acting a bit like a clamp. This condition is known as benign prostatic hyperplasia (BPH). Half of all 50-year-old men have BPH. A man with BPH has to urinate more often and experiences less force and caliber while urinating, often dribbling. If the prostate enlarges too much, urination is difficult or impossible and the risk of **urinary tract infection** (p. 160) and kidney damage increases. The name "benign prostatic hyperplasia" has replaced the older term "benign prostatic hypertrophy"; both terms refer to the same condition.

Drugs are available that can decrease urinary symptoms in about half of people with BPH, although it is not clear whether these drugs slow the progression of the condition. However, one of these drugs (finasteride) causes erectile dysfunction (**impotence** [p. 98]) in about 5% of men who take it. Doctors often recommend surgery when symptoms are severe or when there is a high risk of urinary obstruction. Although prostate surgery has a high success rate, it also has a higher rate of complications than drug therapy.

Nutritional Supplements That May Be Helpful

In a 1941 report, nineteen men with BPH were given an essential-fatty-acid (EFA) supplement.[1] In every case, the amount of retained urine was reduced, and nighttime urination problems stopped in 69% of cases. Dribbling was eliminated in eighteen of the nineteen men. All men also reported improved libido and a reduction in the size of the enlarged prostate (as determined by physical examination). Because this study did not include a control group, the possibility of a placebo effect cannot be ruled out. In addition, the amount of EFAs used in this study was much smaller (only about one-sixth of a teaspoon daily for maintenance) than the amount recommended by most nutritionists. One might, therefore, question whether the improvements reported in this study could have been due to a placebo effect.

Despite the lack of good published research, most nutritionally oriented doctors have been impressed with the effectiveness of EFAs in cases of BPH. A typical recommendation is 1 tablespoon of **flaxseed oil** (p. 296) per day, perhaps reduced to 1 or

Prostatic Hyperplasia, Benign

2 teaspoons per day after several months. Because taking EFAs increases the requirement for **vitamin E** (p. 344), most nutritionally oriented doctors recommend taking a vitamin E supplement along with EFAs.

Prostatic secretions are known to contain a high concentration of **zinc** (p. 346); that observation suggests that zinc plays a role in normal prostate function. In one study, nineteen men with benign prostatic hyperplasia took 150 mg of zinc daily for 2 months, and then 50–100 mg daily. In fourteen of the nineteen men (74%), the prostate became smaller.[2] Because this study did not include a control group, the possibility of a placebo effect cannot be ruled out. Zinc also reduced prostatic size in an animal study, but only when given by local injection.[3] Although the research supporting the use of zinc is weak, many doctors of natural medicine recommend its use.

Because supplementing with large amounts of zinc (such as 30 mg per day or more) can potentially lead to **copper** (p. 285) deficiency, most doctors recommend taking 2–3 mg of copper per day along with zinc.

In another study, forty-five men with BPH received a supplement containing three amino acids (**glycine** [p. 300], **alanine** [p. 264], and **glutamic acid** [p. 299]), while forty other men with BPH were given placebo. After 3 months, 66% of those receiving the amino acid mixture showed reduced urinary urgency; 50% had less delay in starting urine flow; 46% had less difficulty in maintaining flow; and 43% had reduced frequency. In contrast, these improvements were reported by less than 15% of the men who received a placebo. No side effects were observed.[4] Although it is not known how the amino acid combination works, it is believed to reduce the amount of swelling in prostate tissue.

Beta-sitosterol (p. 270), a compound found in many edible plants, has also been found to be helpful for men with BPH. In one double-blind study, 200 men with BPH received 20 mg of beta-sitosterol 3 times a day or a placebo for 6 months. Men receiving beta-sitosterol had a significant improvement in urinary flow and an improvement in symptoms, whereas no change was reported in men receiving the placebo.[5]

Flower pollen (p. 322) has been reported to improve symptoms of BPH, possibly through an anti-inflammatory effect.[6] (Flower pollen is not the same as bee pollen.)

Are There Any Side Effects or Interactions? Refer to the individual supplement for information about any side effects or interactions.

Herbs That May Be Helpful

In many parts of Europe, herbal supplements are considered standard medical treatment for BPH.

Although herbs for BPH are available without prescription, men wishing to take them should be monitored by a physician.

The fat-soluble (liposterolic) extract of the **saw palmetto** (p. 457) berry has become the leading natural treatment for BPH. This extract, when used regularly, has been shown to help keep symptoms in check.[7] Saw palmetto appears to inhibit 5-alpha-reductase, the enzyme that converts testosterone to its more active form, dihydrotestosterone (DHT). Saw palmetto also blocks DHT from binding in the prostate.[8] Studies have used 320 mg per day of saw palmetto extract that is standardized to contain approximately 85% fatty acids.

A 3-year study in Germany found that 160 mg of saw palmetto extract taken twice daily reduced nighttime urination in 73% of people in the study group and improved urinary flow rates signficantly.[9] In a multicenter study at various sites in Europe, 160 mg of saw palmetto extract taken twice per day treated BPH as effectively as finasteride (Proscar) without side effects, such as loss of libido.[10] A 1-year study found that 320 mg once per day was as effective as 160 mg twice per day in the treatment of BPH.[11] A review of all available double-blind studies has concluded that saw palmetto is effective for treatment of men with BPH and is just as effective as, with fewer side effects than, the drug finasteride.[12]

Pygeum (p. 453), an extract from the bark of the African tree, has been approved in Germany, France, and Italy as a remedy for BPH. Controlled studies published over the past 25 years have shown that pygeum is safe and effective for individuals with BPH of mild or moderate severity.[13] These studies have used 50–100 mg of pygeum extract (standardized to contain 14% triterpenes) twice per day. Pygeum relieves the symptoms of BPH; this herb contains three compounds that might help the prostate: pentacyclic triterpenoids, which have a diuretic action; phytosterols, which have anti-inflammatory activity; and ferulic esters, which help rid the prostate of any cholesterol deposits that accompany BPH.

Another herb for BPH is a concentrated extract made from the roots of the **nettle** (p. 447) plant. This extract may increase urinary volume and the maximum flow rate of urine in men with early-stage BPH.[14] It has been successfully combined with both saw palmetto and pygeum to treat BPH.[15] An appropriate amount appears to be 120 mg of nettle root extract (in capsules or tablets) twice per day or 2–4 ml of tincture 3 times per day.

Although no studies are published, pumpkin *(Cucurbita pepo)* seeds are frequently recommended by doctors of natural medicine for men with BPH. This therapy is approved in Germany.[16] Approximately 10 grams (one small handful) of seeds need to be eaten each day.

Are There Any Side Effects or Interactions? Refer to the individual herb for information about any side effects or interactions.

Checklist for Benign Prostatic Hyperplasia

Ranking	Nutritional Supplements	Herbs
Primary	Beta-sitosterol (p. 270)	Pygeum (p. 453) Saw palmetto (p. 457)
	Flower Pollen (p. 322) (not bee pollen)	
Secondary	Amino acids (p. 265) (alanine [p. 264], glutamic acid [p. 299], glycine [p. 300])	Nettle (p. 447)
Other	Copper (p. 285) Flaxseed oil (p. 296) Zinc (p. 346)	Pumpkin seeds

See also: Homeopathic Remedies for **Benign Prostatic Hyperplasia** (p. 567)

Psoriasis

Psoriasis is a common disease that produces silvery, scaly plaques on the skin. A dermatologist should be consulted to confirm the diagnosis of psoriasis.

Dietary Changes That May Be Helpful

Ingestion of alcohol appears to be a risk factor for psoriasis in men but not women.[1,2] It would therefore be prudent for men with psoriasis to drink moderately, if at all.

Anecdotal evidence suggests that people with psoriasis may improve on a hypoallergenic diet.[3] One study reported that eliminating gluten (found in wheat, oats, rye, and barley) improved psoriasis for some people.[4] A nutritionally oriented doctor can help individuals with psoriasis determine whether gluten or other foods are contributing to their skin condition.

Nutritional Supplements That May Be Helpful

In a double-blind study, **fish oil** (p. 294) (10 grams per day) was found to improve the skin lesions of psoriasis.[5] In another study, supplementing with 3.6 grams per day of purified eicosapentaenoic acid (EPA, one of the fatty acids found in fish oil) reduced the severity of psoriasis after 2 to 3 months.[6,7]

That amount of EPA is contained in about 20 grams of fish oil. However, when purified EPA was used in combination with purified docosahexaenoic acid (**DHA** [p. 287], another fatty acid contained in fish oil), no improvement was observed.[8] Additional research is needed to determine whether fish oil itself or some of its components are more effective for individuals with psoriasis. One study showed that applying a preparation containing 10% fish oil directly to psoriatic lesions twice daily resulted in improvement after 7 weeks.[9]

Supplementing with fish oil also may help prevent the increase in blood levels of triglycerides that occurs as a side effect of certain drugs used to treat psoriasis (e.g., etretinate and acetretin).[10]

Some nutritionally oriented doctors have been impressed with the effectiveness of **flaxseed oil** (p. 296) (usually 1–3 tablespoons per day) against psoriasis, although there have been no published studies to support that observation.

The **vitamin D** (p. 343) that is present in food or manufactured by sunlight is converted in the body into a powerful hormone-like molecule called 1,25-dihydroxyvitamin D. That compound and a related naturally occurring molecule (1 alpha-hydroxyvitamin D3) have been found to be helpful when given orally to people with psoriasis.[11] Topical application of these compounds has worked well in some,[12,13,14,15] but not all, studies.[16,17] These activated forms of vitamin D are believed to work by preventing the excessive proliferation of cells that occurs in the skin of people with psoriasis. Because these potent forms of vitamin D can cause potentially dangerous increases in blood levels of **calcium** (p. 277), they are available only by prescription. The use of these compounds (under the supervision of a qualified dermatologist) may be considered in difficult cases of psoriasis. The form of vitamin D that is available without a prescription is unlikely to be effective against psoriasis.

Fumaric acid (p. 298), in the chemically bound form known as fumaric acid esters, has been shown in some studies to be effective against psoriasis.[18,19] However, because fumaric acid esters can cause significant side effects, they should be taken only under the supervision of a doctor familiar with their use.

Herbs That May Be Helpful

Cayenne (p. 408) contains a resinous and pungent substance known as capsaicin. This chemical relieves pain and itching by depleting certain neurotransmitters from sensory nerves. In a double-blind study, application of a capsaicin cream to the skin relieved both the itching and the skin lesions in people with psoriasis.[20]

Creams containing 0.025–0.075% capsaicin are generally used. There may be a burning sensation the first several times the cream is applied, but this should gradually become less pronounced with each use. The hands must be carefully and thoroughly washed after use, or gloves should be worn, to prevent the cream from accidentally reaching the eyes, nose, or mouth and causing a burning sensation. Do not apply the cream to areas of broken skin.

In traditional herbal texts, **burdock root** (p. 405) is described as a blood purifier or alterative.[21] Burdock root was believed to clear the bloodstream of toxins. It was used both internally and externally for psoriasis. Traditional herbalists recommend 2–4 ml of burdock root tincture per day. For the dried root preparation in tablet or capsule form, the common amount to take is 1–2 grams 3 times per day. Many herbal preparations will combine burdock root with other alterative herbs, such as **yellow dock** (p. 472), **red clover** (p. 453), or **cleavers** (p. 412).

Some nutritionally oriented doctors believe that "sluggish" liver function is a contributing factor in psoriasis, possibly explaining why **milk thistle** (p. 445) seeds, which promote normal liver function, can be beneficial. Milk thistle can be taken in an amount that provides 420 mg of silymarin per day. Milk thistle is available in capsules, tablets, or an extract that is standardized to contain 70–80% silymarin. Once improvement occurs, intake is often reduced to 280 mg of silymarin per day. This lower amount may also be used for preventive purposes.

Psyllium (p. 452) husk powder is sometimes used by psoriasis sufferers, since maintaining normal bowel health is believed to be important for managing psoriasis. Psyllium acts as a bulk-forming laxative to cleanse the bowel and encourage normal elimination. Some doctors of natural medicine suggest 7.5 grams of the seeds or 5 grams of the husks to be taken 1 to 2 times per day, with water or juice. It's important to maintain adequate fluid intake when using psyllium.

Sarsaparilla (p. 457) may be beneficial as an anti-inflammatory agent. Capsules or tablets should provide at least 9 grams of the dried root per day, usually taken in divided doses. Tincture is used in the amount of 3 ml 3 times per day.

An ointment containing **Oregon grape** (p. 449) has been shown in a double-blind study to be effective against psoriasis.[22] Whole Oregon grape extracts were shown in one laboratory study to reduce inflammation (often associated with psoriasis) and to stimulate the white blood cells known as macrophages.[23] In this study, isolated alkaloids from Oregon grape did not have these effects. This suggests that there are other active ingredients besides alkaloids in Oregon grape. **Barberry** (p. 395), which is very similar to Oregon grape, is believed to have similar effects. An ointment made from a 10% extract of Oregon grape or barberry can be applied topically 3 times per day.

Are There Any Side Effects or Interactions? Refer to the individual herb for information about any side effects or interactions.

Checklist for Psoriasis

Ranking	Nutritional Supplements	Herbs
Primary		Cayenne (p. 408) (topical)
Secondary	Fish oil (p. 294) (EPA/DHA [p. 287])	
Other	Fumaric acid esters (p. 298)	Barberry (p. 395) Burdock (p. 405) Milk thistle (p. 445) Oregon grape (p. 449) Psyllium (p. 452) Sarsaparilla (p. 457)

See also: Homeopathic Remedies for **Psoriasis** (p. 567)

Raynaud's Disease

Raynaud's disease is caused by constriction and spasms of small arteries in the extremities after exposure to cold. In the person with Raynaud's disease, the hands (and sometimes the toes, cheeks, nose, and ears) turn white or bluish and become painful. Its cause is unknown. A condition called Raynaud's phenomenon causes similar symptoms, but it is the result of connective tissue disease or exposure to certain chemicals. The same natural remedies are used for both disorders.

Lifestyle Changes That May Be Helpful

Dressing warmly and wearing gloves or mittens are important for preventing attacks of Raynaud's disease. Individuals with Raynaud's disease should not smoke, because nicotine decreases blood flow to the extremities. Women with Raynaud's disease should not use birth control pills, as this method of contraception affects circulation.

Nutritional Supplements That May Be Helpful

Inositol hexaniacinate (p. 303)—a variation on the B vitamin niacin—has been used with some success for relieving symptoms of Raynaud's disease.[1] In one study, thirty individuals with Raynaud's disease taking 4 grams of inositol hexaniacinate each day for 3 months showed less spasm of their arteries.[2] Another study, involving six individuals taking 3 grams per day of inositol hexaniacinate, showed that this supplement improved peripheral circulation.[3]

Evening primrose oil (p. 292) inhibits the prostaglandins that may otherwise promote blood vessel constriction. A double-blind study of twenty-one individuals with Raynaud's disease found that, compared with placebo, evening primrose oil reduced the number and severity of attacks despite the fact that blood flow did not appear to increase.[4] Researchers often use 3,000–6,000 mg of evening primrose oil per day.

Abnormalities of **magnesium** (p. 310) metabolism have been found in individuals with Raynaud's disease.[5] Symptoms similar to those seen with Raynaud's disease occur in individuals with magnesium deficiency,[6] probably because a deficiency of this mineral results in spasm of blood vessels.[7] Some nutritionally oriented doctors recommend that individuals with Raynaud's disease supplement with 200–600 mg of magnesium per day; however, no clinical studies support this treatment.

In one study, twelve people with Raynaud's disease were given **L-carnitine** (p. 279) (1 gram 3 times a day) for 20 days.[8] After receiving L-carnitine, these individuals showed less blood-vessel spasm in their fingers in response to cold exposure. This study suggests that supplementing with L-carnitine may be useful for people with Raynaud's disease.

In a double-blind study, supplementation with 12 large capsules of **fish oil** (p. 294) per day (providing 3.96 grams of eicosapentaenoic acid per day) for 6 or 12 weeks reduced the severity of blood-vessel spasm in five of eleven individuals with Raynaud's phenomenon.[9] Fish oil was effective in people with primary Raynaud's disease, but not in those whose symptoms were secondary to another disorder.

Are There Any Side Effects or Interactions? Refer to the individual supplement for information about any side effects or interactions.

Herbs That May Be Helpful

Ginkgo biloba (p. 427) appears to improve the circulation in small blood vessels.[10] For that reason, some doctors of natural medicine recommend ginkgo for individuals with Raynaud's disease. However, no studies have been published on the use of ginkgo for this purpose. Ginkgo is often used as a standard extract (containing 24% ginkgo heterosides) in the amount of 40 mg 3 times per day. **Garlic** (p. 425),

which is known to improve circulation, is also recommended by some doctors of natural medicine as a supportive nutrient for people with Raynaud's disease. For those who do not mind the taste, one whole clove of raw garlic can be chewed per day. Otherwise, odor-controlled, enteric-coated tablets or capsules with standardized allicin potential can be taken in amounts of 400–500 mg once or twice per day (providing up to 5,000 mcg of allicin). As an alternative, 2 to 4 ml of a tincture can be taken 3 times daily.

Are There Any Side Effects or Interactions? Refer to the individual herb for information about any side effects or interactions.

Checklist for Raynaud's Disease

Ranking	Nutritional Supplements	Herbs
Secondary	Fish oil (p. 294) Vitamin B$_3$ (niacin—inositol hexaniacinate) (p. 339)	
Other	Evening primrose oil (p. 292) L-carnitine (p. 279) Magnesium (p. 310)	Garlic (p. 425) *Ginkgo biloba* (p. 427)

See also: Homeopathic Remedies for **Raynaud's Disease** (p. 569)

Restless Legs Syndrome

An uncomfortable feeling of needing to move the legs is known as restless legs syndrome. Occasionally the condition may also involve the arms. It can cause sudden jerking motions of the legs and can also occur during sleep, leading to **insomnia** (p. 105). It is most common in middle-aged women, **pregnant** (p. 143) women, and people with severe kidney disease, **rheumatoid arthritis** (p. 151), and nerve diseases (neuropathy). Restless legs have also been reported to occur in persons with varicose veins and to be relieved when the varicose veins are treated.[1] Refer to the **varicose veins** (p. 163) chapter for information about treatment of that disorder.

Lifestyle Changes That May Be Helpful

One study reports that restless legs syndrome resolved in a 70-year-old woman after she stopped smoking.[2] Although additional research is needed to confirm this report, a trial of smoking cessation seems prudent for people who suffer from restless legs.

Dietary Changes That May Be Helpful

In a study of 131 people with reactive hypoglycemia, 8% were found to have restless legs. The symptoms usually improved following dietary modifications designed to regulate blood-sugar levels.[3] For people with reactive hypoglycemia, nutritionally oriented doctors usually recommend elimination of sugar, refined flour, caffeine, and alcohol from the diet; eating small, frequent meals; and eating whole grains, nuts and seeds, fresh fruits and vegetables, and fish. Another study confirmed the relationship between caffeine ingestion and restless legs.[4]

Nutritional Supplements That May Be Helpful

Mild **iron** (p. 304) deficiency has been shown to exist in many people, particularly the elderly, who have restless legs syndrome.[5] Iron deficiency may be present even in individuals who are not anemic; the deficiency may be detected by a blood test called "serum ferritin." When iron deficiency is the cause of restless legs syndrome, supplementation with iron will reduce the severity of the symptoms.

In a subset of individuals with restless legs syndrome, the condition is familial (that is, it runs in the family). Individuals with familial restless legs syndrome appear to have inherited an unusually high requirement for **folic acid** (p. 297). In one report, forty-five people were identified to be from families with folic acid–responsive restless legs syndrome. The amount of folic acid required to relieve their symptoms ranged from 5 to 30 mg per day,[6] which is considerably more than the amount found in the diets or in nutritional supplements.

One study has also found **vitamin E** (p. 344) to improve restless legs syndrome.[3] At least 400 IU of vitamin E per day are recommended.

Are There Any Side Effects or Interactions? Refer to the individual supplement for information about any side effects or interactions.

Checklist for Restless Legs Syndrome

Ranking	Nutritional Supplements	Herbs
Other	Folic acid (p. 297) Iron (p. 304) (for deficiency) Vitamin E (p. 344)	

See also: Homeopathic Remedies for **Restless Legs Syndrome** (p. 570)

Retinopathy

Several conditions can cause damage to the retina of the eye. Long-term **diabetes** (p. 53) and **high blood pressure** (p. 99) are the most common causes of retinopathy. Partial or total blindness may indicate the presence of retinopathy.

Lifestyle Changes That May Be Helpful

In a study of 181 diabetics, cigarette smoking was found to be a risk factor for the development of retinopathy.[1] In a study of type 1 (juvenile-onset) diabetics, those who maintained their blood-sugar levels closer to the normal range had less severe retinopathy, compared with those whose blood-sugar levels were higher.[2] Tighter control of blood-sugar levels can be achieved with a medically supervised program of diet, exercise, and, when appropriate, medication.

Dietary Changes That May Be Helpful

Animal studies suggest that dietary fructose may contribute to the development of retinopathy.[3] Although such an association has not been demonstrated in humans, some nutritionally oriented doctors advise people with diabetes to avoid foods containing added fructose or high-fructose corn syrup. On the other hand, the fructose that occurs naturally in some fruits has not been found to be harmful.[4]

Nutritional Supplements That May Be Helpful

Free radicals (p. 267) have been implicated in the development and progression of many forms of retinopathy.[5] This is primarily the case in premature infants and anyone exposed to high levels of oxygen. Large amounts of **vitamin E** (p. 344) have been shown to prevent the retinopathy that sometimes occurs in premature infants.[6] However, the administration of vitamin E was associated with a higher incidence of infections and other problems in these infants. Additional research is needed to determine whether supplementation with large amounts of vitamin E is appropriate for premature infants. Vitamin E has also been found to prevent retinopathy in individuals with a rare genetic disease known as abetalipoproteinemia.[7] People with this disorder are lacking a protein that transports fat-soluble nutrients, and can therefore develop deficiencies of vitamin E and other nutrients. However, vitamin E (600 IU per day for 3 months, followed by 300 IU per day for 1 year) did not improve visual acuity or ocular status in twelve individuals with diabetic retinopathy.[8]

Because oxidation damage is believed to play a role in the development of retinopathy, antioxidant nutrients would, in theory, be protective. One doctor has administered a daily regimen of 500 mcg **selenium** (p. 331), 800 IU vitamin E, 10,000 IU **vitamin A** (p. 336), and 1,000 mg **vitamin C** (p. 341) for several years to twenty people with diabetic retinopathy. During that time, nineteen of the twenty showed either improvement or no progression of their retinopathy.[9]

Low blood levels of **magnesium** (p. 310) have been found to be a risk factor for retinopathy in white people with diabetes,[10,11] but not in black people with diabetes.[12] So far, no studies have determined whether supplementing with magnesium would help prevent the development of retinopathy.

In a preliminary study, one group of researchers proposed that supplementation with **vitamin B**$_6$ (p. 340) could prevent diabetic retinopathy.[13] However, this study did not include a control group, and additional research is needed to confirm this hypothesis.

One study investigated the effect of adding 100 mcg per day of **vitamin B**$_{12}$ (p. 337) to the insulin injections of fifteen children with diabetic retinopathy.[14] After 1 year, signs of retinopathy disappeared in seven of fifteen cases; after 2 years, eight of fifteen were free of retinopathy. Adults with diabetic retinopathy did not benefit from vitamin B$_{12}$ injections. Consultation with a physician is necessary before adding injectable vitamin B$_{12}$ to insulin.

Quercetin (p. 328) (a **bioflavonoid** [p. 271]) has been shown to inhibit the enzyme aldose reductase.[15] This enzyme appears to contribute to worsening of diabetic retinopathy. However, because the absorption of quercetin is limited, it is questionable whether supplementing with quercetin can produce the tissue levels that are needed to inhibit aldose reductase. Although human studies have not been done using quercetin to treat retinopathy, many doctors of natural medicine prescribe 400 mg of quercetin 3 times per day.

Are There Any Side Effects or Interactions? Refer to the individual supplement for information about any side effects or interactions.

Herbs That May Be Helpful

Bilberry (p. 396) extracts standardized to contain 25% anthocyanosides have been recommended for **diabetic** (p. 53) and **hypertensive** (p. 89) retinopathy. Such an extract, when taken in the amount of 200 mg

3 times per day, was found to benefit people with retinopathy in one non-controlled study.[16]

A standardized extract of **ginkgo** (p. 427) has been shown to improve impaired color vision in people with mild diabetic retinopathy in a double-blind study.[17] Most often, 60 mg of an extract is taken twice daily.

Are There Any Side Effects or Interactions? Refer to the individual herb for information about any side effects or interactions.

Checklist for Retinopathy

Ranking	Nutritional Supplements	Herbs
Secondary	Vitamin E (p. 344) (for retrolental fibroplasia)	Bilberry (p. 396) *Ginkgo biloba* (p. 427)
Other	Vitamin E (p. 344) (associated with abetalipoproteinemia) Following associated with diabetic retinopathy: Magnesium (p. 310) Quercetin (p. 328) Selenium (p. 331) Vitamin A (p. 336) and Vitamin E (p. 344) (combined) Vitamin C (p. 341) Vitamin B$_6$ (p. 340) Vitamin B$_{12}$ (p. 337)	

Rheumatoid Arthritis (RA)

Rheumatoid arthritis (RA) is a chronic inflammatory condition; it is an autoimmune disease, in which the immune system attacks the joints and sometimes other parts of the body.

Dietary Changes That May Be Helpful

The role of dietary fats in rheumatoid arthritis is complex, but potentially important. In experimental animals that are susceptible to autoimmune disease, feeding a high-fat diet increases the severity of the disease.[1]

There is evidence that people with RA eat more fat, particularly animal fat, than those without RA.[2] In short-term studies, diets completely free of fat reportedly helped people with RA;[3] however, since at least some dietary fat is essential for humans, the significance of this finding is not clear. Strict vegetarian diets

Rheumatoid Arthritis (RA)

that were very low in fat have also been found to be helpful.[4][5] In one trial, 14 weeks of a gluten-free (no wheat, rye, or barley) pure vegetarian diet gradually changed to a lactovegetarian diet (permitting dairy), which led to significant improvement in symptoms and objective laboratory measures of disease.[6]

In the 1950s through the 1970s, Max Warmbrand, a naturopathic doctor, used a very lowfat diet for individuals with both rheumatoid arthritis and **osteoarthritis** (p. 130). He recommended a diet free of meat, dairy, chemicals, sugar, eggs, and processed foods.[7] Dr. Warmbrand claimed that his diet took at least 6 months to achieve noticeable results; a short-term (10-week) study with a similar approach failed to produce beneficial effects.[8]

Rheumatoid arthritis may be linked to **food allergies** (p. 8) and sensitivities.[10] In many people, RA is made worse when they eat foods to which they are allergic or sensitive, and made better by avoiding these foods.[11,12,13,14] English researchers suggest that one-third of people with RA can control the disease completely through allergy elimination.[15] Finding and eliminating foods that trigger symptoms should be done with the help of a nutritionally oriented physician.

Lifestyle Changes That May Be Helpful

Although exercise may increase pain initially, gentle exercises help people with RA.[16,17] Many doctors recommend swimming, stretching, or walking.

Nutritional Supplements That May Be Helpful

The concentration of **vitamin E** (p. 344) has been found to be low in the joint fluid of individuals with rheumatoid arthritis.[18] This reduction in vitamin E levels is believed to be caused by consumption of the vitamin during the inflammatory process. In a double-blind study, approximately 1,800 IU per day of vitamin E was found to have a beneficial effect in people with rheumatoid arthritis.[19]

Research suggests that people with RA may be partially deficient in **pantothenic acid** (p. 340) (vitamin B$_5$).[20] In one trial, those with RA had less morning stiffness, disability, and pain when they took 2,000 mg of pantothenic acid per day.[21] Many nutritionally oriented doctors suggest **pantothenic acid** (p. 340) (sometimes in lower amounts such as 1,000 mg) to people with RA.

Zinc (p. 346) metabolism is altered in RA. Some studies have found zinc helpful,[22] whereas others have not.[23][24] It has been suggested that zinc might help only those who are deficient.[25] Although there is no univer-

sally accepted test for zinc deficiency, some doctors check white blood cell zinc levels.

The relationship of **copper** (p. 285) to RA is complex. Copper acts as an anti-inflammatory agent, because it is needed to activate superoxide dismutase, an enzyme that protects joints from inflammation. People with RA tend toward copper deficiency.[26] The *Journal of the American Medical Association* quoted one researcher as saying that while "Regular aspirin had 6% the anti-inflammatory activity of [cortisone] . . . copper [added to aspirin] had 130% the activity."[27]

Several copper compounds have been used successfully with RA,[28] and a single-blind trial using copper bracelets reported surprisingly effective results.[29] However, under certain circumstances, copper might actually increase inflammation in rheumatoid joints.[30] Moreover, the most consistently effective form of copper, copper aspirinate (a combination of copper and aspirin), is not readily available. A reasonable amount of copper might be 1–3 mg per day.

Many double-blind trials have shown that omega-3 fatty acids in **fish oil** (p. 294), called EPA and **DHA** (p. 287), help relieve symptoms of RA.[31,32,33,34,35,36] The effect results from the anti-inflammatory activity of fish oil.[37] Many doctors recommend 3 grams per day of EPA and DHA. This amount is commonly found in 10 grams of fish oil. Positive results can take 3 months to become evident.

Oils containing the omega-6 fatty acid gamma liolenic acid (GLA), such as **borage** (p. 402) oil,[38,39] black currant seed oil,[40] and **evening primrose oil (EPO)** (p. 292),[41,42] have also been reported to be effective in the treatment of RA. The most pronounced effects were seen with borage oil; however, that may have been due to the fact that larger amounts of GLA were used (such as 1.4 grams per day). The results with EPO were conflicting and somewhat confusing, possibly because the placebo used in these studies (olive oil) appeared to have an anti-inflammatory effect of its own. In a double-blind study, positive results were seen when EPO was used in combination with fish oil.[43] GLA appears to be effective because it is converted in part to prostaglandin E1, a compound known to have anti-inflammatory activity.

Preliminary research suggests that **boron** (p. 273) supplementation at 3–9 mg per day may be beneficial, particularly in juvenile RA.[44] However, more research on this is needed.

The DL form of **phenylalanine (DLPA)** (p. 320) has been used to treat chronic pain, including rheumatoid arthritis, with mixed effectiveness.[45] Some doctors of natural medicine suggest that individuals with arthritis may benefit from **cartilage** (p. 279); however, well-designed research is lacking, and many experts question the use of cartilage in this regard.

Some individuals with rheumatoid arthritis have low levels of the amino acid **histidine** (p. 301); taking histidine supplements may improve arthritis symptoms in some of these individuals.

The use of **DMSO** (p. 291) for therapeutic applications is controversial; but there is some evidence that when applied directly to the skin, DMSO has anti-inflammatory properties and alleviates pain, such as that associated with rheumatoid arthritis.[46,47] DMSO appears to reduce pain by inhibiting the transmission of pain messages by nerves.[48]

There is limited evidence that some individuals with RA may have inadequate stomach acid.[49] Some doctors of natural medicine believe that when stomach acid is low, supplementing with **betaine HCl** (p. 269) can reduce food-allergy reactions by improving digestion.

Bromelain (p. 276) has significant anti-inflammatory activity. Preliminary evidence in people with rheumatoid arthritis shows that bromelain might help reduce symptoms, such as joint swelling and impaired joint mobility.[50]

Are There Any Side Effects or Interactions? Refer to the individual supplement for information about any side effects or interactions.

Herbs That May Be Helpful

Boswellia (p. 403), a traditional herbal remedy from the Indian system of Ayurvedic medicine, has been investigated for its effects on arthritis. A double-blind study using boswellia found a beneficial effect on pain and stiffness, as well as improved joint function.[51] Boswellia showed no negative effects in this study. The herb has a unique anti-inflammatory action, much like the conventional non-steroidal anti-inflammatory drugs (NSAIDs) used by many for inflammatory conditions. But unlike NSAIDs, long-term use of boswellia is generally considered safe and does not lead to irritation or ulceration of the stomach. Some doctors of natural medicine suggest using 400 to 800 mg of gum resin extract in capsules or tablets 3 times per day.

Turmeric (p. 465) is a yellow spice that is often used to make brightly colored curry dishes. The active principle is curcumin, a potent anti-inflammatory compound, which protects the body against the ravages of **free radicals** (p. 267).[52] A preliminary double-blind study found that 400 mg curcumin 3 times per day was as effective as the drug phenylbutazone for people with rheumatoid arthritis.[53] Many doctors of

natural medicine recommend 400 mg of curcumin in capsules or tablets 3 times per day.

Ginger (p. 427) has been used in Ayurvedic medicine as an anti-inflammatory. Several published case studies of people with rheumatoid arthritis taking 6–50 grams of fresh or powdered ginger per day indicated that ginger might be helpful.[54]

A cream containing small amounts of capsaicin, a compound found in **cayenne** (p. 408) peppers, can help relieve pain when rubbed onto arthritic joints, according to the results of a double-blind study.[55] It does this by depleting the nerves of a pain-mediating neurotransmitter known as substance P. Although application of capsaicin cream may initially cause a burning feeling, the burning will lessen with each application and soon disappear for most people. A cream containing 0.025–0.075% of capsaicin can be applied to the affected joints 3 to 5 times a day.

Yucca (p. 473), a traditional remedy, is a desert plant that contains soap-like components known as saponins. Yucca tea (7 or 8 grams of the root simmered in a pint of water for 15minutes) is often drunk for symptom relief 3 to 5 times per day.

Burdock root (p. 405) has been used historically both internally and externally to treat painful joints. **Horsetail** (p. 436) is thought in traditional medicine to exert a connective tissue strengthening and anti-arthritic action, possibly because of the high silicon content of this herb.

Devil's claw (p. 416) has anti-inflammatory and analgesic actions. Several open and double-blind studies have been conducted on the anti-arthritic effects of devil's claw.[56] The results of these studies have been mixed, so it is unclear if devil's claw lives up to its reputation in traditional herbal medicine for people with rheumatoid arthritis. A typical amount used is 800 mg of encapsulated extracts or 2 to 4 ml of tincture 3 times per day.

Sarsaparilla (p. 457) has anti-inflammatory properties that may be helpful for people with rheumatoid arthritis. **White willow** (p. 468) bark has anti-inflammatory and pain-relieving effects. Extracts providing 60–120 mg salicin per day are approved for people with rheumatoid arthritis by the German government.[57] Although the analgesic actions of willow are typically slow-acting, they last longer than aspirin.

Topical applications of several botanical oils are approved by the German government for relieving symptoms of rheumatoid arthritis.[58] These include primarily cajeput (*Melaleuca leucodendra*) oil, camphor oil, **eucalyptus** (p. 421) oil, fir (*Abies alba* and *Picea abies*) needle oil, pine (*Pinus* spp.) needle oil, and **rosemary** (p. 455) oil. A few drops of oil or more can be applied to painful joints several times a day as needed.

Southwestern Native American and Hispanic herbalists have long recommended use of **chaparral** (p. 410) topically on people's joints affected by rheumatoid arthritis. The anti-inflammatory effects of chaparral found in the test tube suggests this practice could have value, though studies have not yet confirmed chaparral's usefulness in humans. Chaparral should not be used internally for this purpose.

Are There Any Side Effects or Interactions? Refer to the individual herb for information about any side effects or interactions.

Checklist for Rheumatoid Arthritis

Ranking	Nutritional Supplements	Herbs
Primary	Evening Primrose Oil (p. 292) Fish oil (p. 294) (EPA/DHA [p. 287])	Cayenne (p. 408) (topical)
Secondary	DMSO (p. 291) Boswellia (p. 403) Vitamin B₅ (Pantothenic acid) (p. 340) Vitamin E (p. 344)	Borage (p. 402) Devil's claw (p. 416) Turmeric (p. 465)
Other	Betaine HCl (p. 269) Boron (p. 273) Bromelain (p. 276) Cartilage (p. 279) Copper (p. 285) D, L-phenylalanine (DLPA) (p. 320) Histidine (p. 301) Zinc (p. 346)	Burdock (p. 405) Cajeput oil Camphor oil Chaparral (p. 410) (topical) Eucalyptus oil (p. 421) Fir needle oil (topical) Ginger (p. 427) Horsetail (p. 436) Pine needle oil (topical) Rosemary oil (p. 455) (topical) Sarsaparilla (p. 457) White willow (p. 468) Yucca (p. 473)

See also: Homeopathic Remedies for **Rheumatoid Arthritis** (p. 571)

Rickets/Osteomalacia

Children with rickets have abnormal bone formation resulting from inadequate **calcium** (p. 277) in their bones. This lack of calcium can result from inadequate exposure to sunshine (needed to make vitamin D) or from not eating enough **vitamin D** (p. 343)—a nutrient needed for calcium absorption. Rickets is worsened by a lack of dietary calcium.

Rickets can also be caused by conditions that impair absorption of vitamin D and/or calcium, even when these nutrients are consumed in appropriate amounts. Activation of vitamin D in the body requires normal liver and kidney function. Damage to either organ can cause rickets. Some variations of rickets do not respond well to supplementation with vitamin D and calcium. Proper diagnosis must be made by a health-care professional.

Osteomalacia is an adult version of rickets. Although this condition does not result in leg bowing, it is similar to rickets and treated in a similar fashion.

Dietary Changes That May Be Helpful

Dietary changes should only be considered if a medical professional has diagnosed rickets and determined that the cause is a simple nutritional deficiency. Rickets caused by a simple deficiency is more likely in a child with a pure vegetarian diet (that does not include vitamin D) or with dark skin and/or a lack of sunlight exposure (which reduces the amount of vitamin D made in the skin).

The few foods that contain vitamin D include egg yolks, butter, vitamin D–fortified milk, fish liver oil, breast milk, and infant formula. Calcium, in addition to being present in breast milk and formula, is found in dairy products, sardines, salmon (canned with edible bones), green leafy vegetables, and tofu. Pure vegetarians may use supplements instead of eggs and dairy as sources for both calcium and vitamin D.

Lifestyle Changes That May Be Helpful

Direct exposure of the skin (that is, hands, face, arms, etc.) to sunlight stimulates the body to manufacture vitamin D. However, both clothing and use of a sunscreen prevent the ultraviolet light that triggers the formation of vitamin D from reaching the skin. Depending on latitude, sunlight during the winter may not provide enough ultraviolet light to promote adequate vitamin D production. At other times during the year, even 30 minutes of exposure per day will usually lead to large increases in the amount of vitamin D made. If it is difficult to get sunlight exposure, full-spectrum lighting can be used to stimulate vitamin D production.

Nutritional Supplements That May Be Helpful

Vitamin D (p. 343) and **calcium** (p. 277) supplements should be used to treat rickets only if a medical professional has diagnosed rickets and also determined that the cause is a nutritional deficiency. Amounts needed to treat rickets should be determined by a nutritionally oriented doctor, and will depend on the age, weight, and condition of the child. For *prevention* of rickets, 400 IU of vitamin D per day is considered reasonable. Doctors often suggest 1,600 IU per day for *treating* rickets caused by a lack of dietary vitamin D.

The National Institutes of Health in the United States has recommended that the following amounts of total calcium intake per day are useful to *prevent* rickets:

- 400 mg until 6 months of age
- 600 mg from 6 to 12 months
- 800 mg from 1 year through age 5
- 800–1,200 mg from age 6 until age 10

Are There Any Side Effects or Interactions? Refer to the individual supplement for information about any side effects or interactions.

Checklist for Rickets

Ranking	Nutritional Supplements	Herbs
Primary	Calcium (p. 277) Vitamin D (p. 343) (rickets)	
Other	Vitamin D (p. 343) (osteomalacia)	

Shingles (Herpes Zoster) and Postherpetic Neuralgia

Shingles consists of a very painful rash that most often appears on one side of the body in a narrow band. Shingles usually affects the elderly or people with compromised **immune systems** (p. 94). The same virus (varicella zoster) that causes chicken pox also causes shingles. Nerve pain that persists after the rash has cleared is called postherpetic neuralgia.

Nutritional Supplements That May Be Helpful

Some doctors have observed that intramuscular injections of **vitamin B**$_{12}$ (p. 337) appear to relieve the symptoms of postherpetic neuralgia.[1,2] However, since these studies did not include a control group, the possibility of a placebo effect cannot be ruled out. Oral vitamin B$_{12}$ supplements have not been tested, but they are not likely to be effective against postherpetic neuralgia.

Some doctors have found **vitamin E** (p. 344) to be effective for individuals with postherpetic neuralgia—

even people who have had the problem for many years.[3,4] The recommended amount of vitamin E by mouth is 1,200–1,600 IU per day. In addition, vitamin E at a concentration of 30 IU per gram can be applied to the skin. Several months of continuous vitamin E use may be needed in order to see an improvement. Not all studies have found a beneficial effect of vitamin E.[5] However, in the study that produced negative results, vitamin E may not have been used for a long enough period of time.

Adenosine monophosphate (AMP) (p. 263), a compound that occurs naturally in the body, has been found to be effective against shingles outbreaks. In one double-blind study, thirty-two individuals with an outbreak of herpes zoster were given either 100 mg of AMP intramuscularly 3 times a week or a placebo for 4 weeks. Compared with the placebo, AMP promoted faster healing and reduced the duration of pain.[6] Most important, AMP appeared to prevent the development of postherpetic neuralgia, a chronic, painful, and difficult-to-treat condition that often follows an episode of shingles.[7,8]

Are There Any Side Effects or Interactions? Refer to the individual supplement for information about any side effects or interactions.

Checklist for Shingles and Postherpetic Neuralgia

Ranking	Nutritional Supplements	Herbs
Primary		Cayenne (p. 408) (topical, for pain only)
Other	Adenosine monophosphate (p. 263) (injection) Vitamin B$_{12}$ (p. 337) (injection)	Licorice (p. 440) (topical)

See also: Homeopathic Remedies for **Shingles and Postherpetic Neuralgia** (p. 572)

Herbs That May Be Helpful

The hot principal in **cayenne** (p. 408) peppers, known as capsaicin, is used for many painful conditions, including shingles and postherpetic neuralgia. In a double-blind trial, a cream containing 0.075% capsaicin, applied 3 to 4 times per day to the painful area, greatly reduced pain.[9] In another study, a lower concentration of capsaicin (0.025%) was also effective.[10] Two or more weeks of treatment may be required to get the full benefit of the cream.

Licorice (p. 440) has also been used by doctors of natural medicine as a topical agent for shingles and postherpetic neuralgia; however, no clinical trials support its use for this purpose. Glycyrrhizin, one of the active components of licorice, has been shown to block the replication of varicella zoster, the virus that causes shingles.[11] Licorice gel is usually applied 3 or more times per day. Licorice gel is not widely available, but may be obtained through a doctor who practices herbal medicine.

Are There Any Side Effects or Interactions? Refer to the individual herb for information about any side effects or interactions.

Sinusitis

Sinusitis, an upper respiratory condition, involves inflammation of the sinus passages. There are four pairs of sinuses in the human skull that help circulate moist air throughout the nasal passages. The **common cold** (p. 41) is the most prevalent predisposing factor to sinusitis. Acute sinusitis typically causes symptoms of nasal congestion and a thick yellow or green discharge. Other symptoms include tenderness and pain over the sinuses, frontal headaches, and sometimes chills, fever, and pressure in the area of the sinuses. Chronic sinusitis differs slightly, in that symptoms can be milder and may only include postnasal drip, bad breath, and an irritating dry cough. **Hay fever** (p. 76), environmental triggers unrelated to hay fever, food allergens, and dental infections can also lead to sinusitis.

Dietary and Lifestyle Changes That May Be Helpful

According to some studies, 25–70% of people with sinusitis have environmental **allergies** (p. 8).[1] Although food allergies may also contribute to the problem, some researchers believe food allergies only rarely cause sinusitis.[2,3] If other treatment approaches are unsuccessful, people with sinusitis may choose to work with a nutritionally oriented doctor to evaluate what, if any, effect elimination of food and other allergens might have on reducing their symptoms.

Nutritional Supplements That May Be Helpful

In a preliminary trial, supplementation with 250 mg of **pantothenic acid** (p. 340) 2 times a day was demonstrated to help most people suffering from allergic rhinitis, a significant predisposing factor for sinusitis.[4] However, research has yet to investigate the effects of pantothenic acid supplementation with people who have sinusitis.

Histamine is associated with increased nasal and sinus congestion. In one study, **vitamin C** (p. 341) supplementation (1,000 mg 3 times per day) reduced histamine levels in people with either high histamine levels or low blood levels of vitamin C.[5] Another study found that 2,000 mg of vitamin C helped protect individuals exposed to a histamine challenge.[6] Not every study has reported reductions in histamine.[7] Although preliminary evidence supports the use of vitamin C when injected into the sinuses of people suffering with acute sinusitis, the effect of oral vitamin C on symptoms of sinusitis has yet to be formally studied.[8]

Bromelain (p. 276), an enzyme derived from pineapple, has been reported to relieve symptoms of acute sinusitis. In a double-blind study comparing the use of bromelain with placebo, 87% of those who took bromelain reported good to excellent results compared with 68% of the placebo group.[9] Other double-blind research has shown that bromelain reduces symptoms of sinusitis.[10,11]

Studies conducted in the past have used bromelain compounds with therapeutic strengths measured in Rorer units. Potency of contemporary bromelain compounds are quantified in either MCUs (milk clotting units) or GDUs (gelatin dissolving units); one GDU equals 1.5 MCU. A supplement containing 500 mg with a labeled potency of 2,000 MCU per gram (1,000 mg) would have 1,000 MCU of activity. Nutritionally oriented physicians sometimes use 3,000 MCU taken 3 times per day for several days, followed up by 2,000 MCU per day.[12] Much of the research conducted has used smaller amounts likely to be the equivalent (in modern units of activity) of approximately 500 MCU taken 4 times a day.

Checklist for Sinusitis

Ranking	Nutritional Supplements	Herbs
Primary	Bromelain (p. 276)	
Secondary		Stinging nettle (p. 447)
Other	Pantothenic acid (p. 340) Vitamin C (p. 341)	Eucalyptus (p. 421)

Herbs That May Be Helpful

An isolated double-blind study compared the use of freeze-dried **stinging nettles** (p. 447) with placebo. In that 1-week trial, 300 mg of stinging nettles taken twice per day led to moderate effectiveness among 58% of those in the treatment group compared with only 37% in the placebo group.[13]

Eucalyptus (p. 421) oil is often used in a steam inhalation to help clear nasal and sinus congestion. Eucalyptus oil is said to function in a fashion similar to that of menthol by acting on receptors in the nasal mucosa, leading to a reduction in the symptoms of, for example, nasal stuffiness.[14]

Tardive Dyskinesia

Long-term use of so-called "neuroleptic drugs" (antipsychotic medications), which are used to treat schizophrenia and related psychiatric disorders, often causes as a side effect a disorder known as tardive dyskinesia. The term tardive (which means "late") is used because the condition appears only after chronic use of drugs such as chlorpromazine (Thorazine), thioridazine (Mellaril), and trifluoperazine (Stelazine). Dyskinesia means "abnormal movement." Individuals with tardive dyskinesia suffer from repetitive and uncontrollable movements (such as smacking their lips or moving their legs back and forth) that can interfere greatly with their quality of life. Tardive dyskinesia may gradually diminish in severity after the medication is discontinued, but all too often the problem persists after drug withdrawal and becomes permanent. Conventional treatment for tardive dyskinesia is unsatisfactory, so prevention is considered crucial. It is important that individuals requiring neuroleptic drugs be given the lowest effective dose and that treatment be discontinued as soon as it is feasible.

Nutritional Supplements That May Be Helpful

During a 10-year period, doctors at the North Nassau Mental Health Center in New York treated approximately 11,000 schizophrenics with a megavitamin regimen that included **vitamin C** (p. 341) (up to 4 grams per day), **vitamin B$_3$** (p. 339)—sometimes in the form of niacinamide (up to 4 grams per day), **vitamin B$_6$** (p. 340) (up to 800 mg per day), and **vitamin E** (p. 344) (up to 1,200 IU per day). During that time, not a single new case of tardive dyskinesia was seen, even though many of the people were taking neuroleptic drugs.[1] Another psychiatrist who routinely used niacinamide, vitamin C, and vitamin **B-complex** (p. 341) over a 28-year period, rarely saw tardive dyskinesia develop in her patients.[2] Further research is needed to determine which nutrients or combinations of nutrients were most important for preventing tardive dyskinesia. Levels of niacinamide and vitamin B$_6$ used in this research may cause significant side effects

and require monitoring by a nutritionally oriented doctor.

Checklist for Tardive Dyskinesia

Ranking	Nutritional Supplements	Herbs
Primary	Vitamin E (p. 344)	
Secondary	Choline (p. 307) Lecithin (p. 307) Manganese (p. 311)	
Other	Evening primrose oil (p. 292) Vitamin B-complex (p. 341) Vitamin B$_3$ (p. 339) (niacin or niacinamide) Vitamin B$_6$ (p. 340) Vitamin C (p. 341)	

Vitamin E (p. 344) has been found in a number of studies to reduce the severity of tardive dyskinesia. In a double-blind study, twenty-eight individuals with tardive dyskinesia were randomly assigned to receive vitamin E (800 IU per day for 2 weeks and 1,600 IU per day thereafter) or a placebo. Vitamin E was significantly more effective than placebo in reducing involuntary movements.[3] Other studies have also found that vitamin E supplements reduce the severity of tardive dyskinesia.[4,5,6] Two studies failed to show a beneficial effect of vitamin E.[7,8] However, the people in those studies had been receiving neuroleptics for at least 10 years, and research has shown that vitamin E is most effective when started within the first 5 years of neuroleptic treatment.[9,10]

Although it is not known how vitamin E works, some doctors believe that it prevents neuroleptic-induced oxidation damage of certain parts of the brain.

One doctor has found that administering the trace mineral **manganese** (p. 311) (15 mg per day) can prevent the development of tardive dyskinesia and that higher amounts (up to 60 mg per day) can reverse tardive dyskinesia that has already developed.[11] Others have reported similar improvements with manganese.[12]

Several individuals have experienced an improvement in tardive dyskinesia while taking **evening primrose oil** (p. 292).[13] However, in a double-blind study, supplementing with evening primrose oil (12 capsules per day) resulted only in a minor, clinically insignificant improvement.[14]

Choline (p. 307) and **lecithin** (p. 307), a dietary source of choline, have both been used for individuals with tardive dyskinesia. While some studies have shown a beneficial effect,[15,16] others have failed to find any improvement.[17] Nutritionally oriented doctors do not often recommend choline or lecithin for individuals taking neuroleptic medications, because it could, on occasion, trigger **depression** (p. 50).

Are There Any Side Effects or Interactions? Refer to the individual supplement for information about any side effects or interactions.

Tinnitus (Ringing in the Ears)

Tinnitus is the medical term for ringing in the ears. Rarely, tinnitus is due to an actual sound such as blood rushing through an enlarged vein—a problem that requires medical treatment. More commonly the problem is due to nerve irritation from an unknown source or an underlying ear problem often induced by noise damage. The cause of tinnitus should be diagnosed by a doctor.

Dietary Changes and Other Natural Therapies That May Be Helpful

Ménière's disease (a condition characterized by tinnitus, vertigo, and hearing loss) is reportedly associated with various metabolic abnormalities, including elevations of serum cholesterol and/or triglycerides and abnormal regulation of blood sugar. Among individuals with Ménière's disease who replaced refined carbohydrates in their diet with high-fiber, complex carbohydrates, tinnitus frequently improved or disappeared.[1]

Nutritional Supplements and Other Natural Therapies That May Be Helpful

Vitamin B$_{12}$ (p. 337) deficiency has been reported to be common in people exposed to loud noise on the job who developed tinnitus and hearing loss.[2] Intramuscular injections of vitamin B$_{12}$ reduced the severity of tinnitus in some of these people. Injectable vitamin B$_{12}$ is available only by prescription. The effect of oral vitamin B$_{12}$ on tinnitus has not been studied.

Zinc (p. 346) supplements have been used to treat individuals who had both tinnitus and hearing loss (usually age-related). Of those who had initially low serum levels of zinc, about 25% experienced an improvement in tinnitus after taking zinc for 3 to 6 months.[3] In another study, zinc was not more effective than placebo at relieving tinnitus. However, the participants in that study did not have low serum zinc levels.[4]

In a double-blind study of people who had difficulty sleeping because of tinnitus, supplementation with 3 mg of **melatonin** (p. 312) per night for 1 month resulted in improved sleep.[5] Although melatonin did not reduce overall symptom scores for tinnitus, people in this trial with higher symptom scores did appear to obtain some benefit.

Are There Any Side Effects or Interactions? Refer to the individual supplement for information about any side effects or interactions.

Herbs That May Be Helpful

Ginkgo biloba (p. 427) has been used to treat tinnitus. Two studies have found an extract of ginkgo standardized to contain 24% flavone glycosides and 6% terpene lactones in the amount of 120 mg per day useful for tinnitus sufferers,[6,7] although other studies have failed to find ginkgo beneficial.[8]

The lesser periwinkle, *Vinca minor,* contains a compound known as vincamine. Extracts containing vincamine have been used in Germany to help decrease tinnitus.[9] Because these extracts are not widely available outside of Germany, consult with a doctor knowledgeable in botanical medicine about obtaining them.

Are There Any Side Effects or Interactions? Refer to the individual herb for information about any side effects or interactions.

Checklist for Tinnitus (Ringing in the Ears)

Ranking	Nutritional Supplements	Herbs
Secondary	Melatonin (p. 312)	
Other	Vitamin B$_{12}$ (p. 337) (injection)	*Ginkgo biloba* (p. 427) Lesser periwinkle

See also: Homeopathic Remedies for **Tinnitus** (p. 576)

Ulcerative Colitis

Ulcerative colitis (UC) is a chronic disease characterized by bloody diarrhea and an inflamed colon. UC is relatively common but remains poorly understood. Diagnosis must be made by a health-care practitioner—typically a gastroenterologist. **Irritable bowel syn-**

drome (p. 109), a completely unrelated and less serious condition, was sometimes called mucous colitis in the past. As a result, the general term "colitis" is still sometimes used inappropriately to refer to irritable bowel syndrome. It is critical that people who are diagnosed with "colitis" find out whether they have irritable bowel syndrome or ulcerative colitis.

Conventional treatment for UC is often essential in emergency circumstances. However, conventional treatments for UC frequently offer only a partial solution and in some cases are accompanied by significant side effects. Because of the limitations of conventional therapy, many people with UC look to natural medicine in an attempt to deal with their condition. All people with UC wishing to use natural approaches should work with a nutritionally oriented doctor.

Lifestyle Changes That May Be Helpful

Smokers have a lower risk of UC for unknown reasons. The nicotine patch has actually been used to induce remissions in people with UC,[1] although this treatment has been ineffective in preventing relapses.[2] On the other hand, **Crohn's disease** (p. 48), which is in many ways similar to UC, is made *worse* by smoking.[3] Despite the possible protective effect of smoking in individuals with UC, a strong case can be made that the risks of smoking outweigh the benefits. Even the use of nicotine patches remains experimental and carries its own side effects.

Dietary Changes That May Be Helpful

Although one study showed that high sugar intake was associated with a nearly threefold increase in risk for UC,[4] other research failed to find any association with sugar intake.[5][6] In an Israeli study, individuals with a high intake of animal fat and cholesterol had a fourfold increase in risk, compared with people who consumed less of these fats.[7] A study from Japan also found that ingestion of certain high-fat foods (particularly margarine) was associated with increased risk.[8] Although these associations do not prove cause-and-effect, reducing one's intake of refined sugar and animal fats is often recommended as a means of improving overall health.

More than a half-century ago, several doctors reported that **food allergies** (p. 8) play an important role in some cases of UC.[9][10] Since that time, many nutritionally oriented doctors have observed that avoidance of allergenic foods will often reduce the severity of UC and can sometimes completely control the condition. However, the relationship between food allergies and UC remains controversial[11] and is not generally accepted by the conventional medical community. People who wish to explore the possibility that food sensitivities might trigger their symptoms should see a nutritionally oriented doctor.

Nutritional Supplements That May Be Helpful

UC is linked to an increased risk of colon cancer. Studies have found that people with ulcerative colitis who have been taking **folic acid** (p. 297) supplements or who have high blood levels of folic acid have a reduced risk of colon cancer compared with other individuals who have UC.[12][13][14] Although these associations do not prove that folic acid was responsible for the reduction in risk, this vitamin has been shown to prevent experimentally induced colon cancer in animals.[15] Low folic acid levels have been found in more than half of people with UC.[16] Individuals with UC who are taking the drug sulfasalazine, which inhibits the absorption of folic acid,[17] are at particularly high risk of developing folic acid deficiency. Folic acid supplementation may therefore be important for many people with UC. However, since taking folic acid may mask the diagnosis of **vitamin B$_{12}$** (p. 337) deficiency, individuals with UC who wish to take folic acid should be monitored by a physician.

Ingestion of alcohol, which is known to promote folic acid deficiency, has also been linked to an increased risk of colon cancer.[18] Consequently, people with UC should keep alcohol intake to a minimum.

Because UC is an inflammatory condition and **fish oil** (p. 294) has anti-inflammatory activity, fish oil has been tested as a potential remedy for people with UC. In a 4-month, double-blind study, people with UC who were given fish oil (containing 3.2 grams of EPA and 2.2 grams of DHA [p. 287] per day—the two important fatty acids found in fish oil) required lower levels of prescription anti-inflammatory drugs.[19] Fish oil supplementation also resulted in other improvements, such as weight gain and reduced intestinal inflammation. In another study, fish oil reduced the need for steroid medication in people with active UC, but did not prevent relapses in people whose disease was in remission.[20] Other research shows at least some positive effects from the use of fish oil for people with UC.[21][22]

A fatty acid called butyrate, which is synthesized by intestinal bacteria, serves as fuel for the cells that line the small intestine. Administration of butyrate by enema has been found to produce marked improvement in some individuals with UC.[23] Orally administered butyrate is not likely to be beneficial, as suffi-

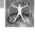

Urinary Tract Infection (UTI)

cient quantities would not reach the colon after oral administration. Although butyrate enemas are not widely available, they can be obtained by prescription through a compounding pharmacist.

Are There Any Side Effects or Interactions? Refer to the individual supplement for information about any side effects or interactions.

Herbs That May Be Helpful

One study has been done using the gum resin of **Boswellia serrata** (p. 103), an Ayurvedic herb.[24] Administration of boswellia (350 mg 3 times per day for 6 weeks) was found to be as effective as the standard drug sulfasalazine.

Aloe vera (p. 391) juice has been used by some doctors of natural medicine for people with UC. Although aloe is known to have anti-inflammatory activity, it has not been studied specifically in people with UC. The same is true of other traditional anti-inflammatory and demulcent herbs, including **calendula** (p. 406), **flaxseed** (p. 296), **licorice** (p. 440), **marshmallow** (p. 444), **myrrh** (p. 446), and **yarrow** (p. 471). Many of these herbs are most effective, according to clinical experience, if taken internally as well as in enema form.[25] Enemas should be avoided during acute flare-ups, but are useful for mild and chronic inflammation. It is best to consult with a doctor experienced with botanical medicine to learn more about herbal enemas before using them. However, more research needs to be done to determine the effectiveness of these herbs.

Checklist for Ulcerative Colitis

Ranking	Nutritional Supplements	Herbs
Primary	Fish oil (p. 294)	
Secondary	Folic acid (p. 297)	Boswellia (p. 403)
Other	Glutamine (p. 300)	Aloe (p. 391) Calendula (p. 406) Chamomile (p. 409) Flaxseed Licorice (p. 440) Marshmallow (p. 444) Myrrh (p. 446) St. John's wort (p. 461) Yarrow (p. 471)

German doctors practicing phytotherapy (herbal medicine) have recommended **chamomile** (p. 409) for individuals with colitis.[26] A cup of strong tea drunk 3 times per day is standard, along with enemas. Enemas of oil of **St. John's wort** (p. 461) may also be

beneficial.[27] Consult with a doctor of natural medicine before using St. John's wort oil enemas.

Are There Any Side Effects or Interactions? Refer to the individual herb for information about any side effects or interactions.

Urinary Tract Infection (UTI)

Urinary tract infections (UTIs) are infections of the kidney, bladder, and urethra. They are generally triggered by bacteria and are more common with any partial blockage of the urinary tract. In some people, UTIs tend to recur.

Dietary Changes That May Be Helpful

When healthy volunteers ingested a large amount (100 grams) of refined sugar, the ability of their white blood cells to destroy bacteria was impaired for at least 5 hours.[1] Ingestion of excessive amounts of alcohol has also been shown to suppress the **immune system** (p. 94),[2] whereas reducing the intake of dietary fat stimulates immunity.[3] For these reasons, many nutritionally oriented doctors recommend a reduced intake of sugar, alcohol, and fat during an acute infection and for prevention of recurrences.

People who have recurrent or chronic **infections** (p. 101) should discuss with a nutritionally oriented doctor the possible role of **allergies** (p. 8). Chronic infections have been linked to allergies in many reports.[4,5,6,7] Identifying and eliminating the foods that trigger problems may help reduce the number of infections.

Nutritional Supplements That May Be Helpful

Many nutritionally oriented doctors recommend 5,000 mg or more of **vitamin C** (p. 341) per day for an acute UTI, as well as long-term supplementation for individuals who are prone to recurrent UTIs. Although no controlled studies have demonstrated the effectiveness of vitamin C for this purpose, this vitamin has been shown to inhibit the growth of *E. coli*, the most common bacterial cause of UTIs.[8] In addition, ingestion of 4,000 mg or more of vitamin C per day results in a slight acidization of the urine,[9] creating an "unfriendly" environment for certain bacteria.

Vitamin A (p. 336) deficiency increases the risk of many infections. Although much of the promising research with vitamin A supplements and infections has focused on measles,[10] vitamin A is also thought to be helpful in other infections. Some doctors of natural medicine recommend that people with urinary tract infections take vitamin A.

The **proteolytic enzyme** (p. 289) **bromelain** (p. 276) (from pineapple) appears to be effective for people with a UTI. In one double-blind study, twenty-eight individuals with a UTI received antibiotics plus either bromelain or a placebo. Signs of infection resolved in all of those who received bromelain, compared with only 46% of those given placebo.[11]

Since the immune system requires many nutrients in order to function properly, many people take a **multivitamin/mineral** (p. 314) supplement for "insurance." In one double-blind study, healthy elderly people using such a supplement for 1 year showed improvements in certain measures of immune function, as well as a significant reduction in the total number of infections (including non-urinary-tract infections).[12]

Are There Any Side Effects or Interactions? Refer to the individual supplement for information about any side effects or interactions.

Herbs That May Be Helpful

Modern research has confirmed the benefits of **cranberry** (p. 414) for the prevention of urinary tract infections. In a double-blind study, elderly women who drank 300 ml (10 ounces) of cranberry juice per day had a decrease in the amount of bacteria in their urine.[13] In another study, elderly residents of a nursing home consumed either 4 ounces of cranberry juice or 6 capsules containing concentrated cranberry daily for 13 months. During that time, the number of UTIs decreased by 25%.[14] Researchers have suggested two possible ways in which cranberry is effective against UTIs. First, cranberry prevents *E. coli*, the bacteria that causes most urinary tract infections, from attaching to the walls of the bladder.[15] Second, cranberry contains hippuric acid, a compound that has been found to have antibiotic activity.[16] However, cranberry is not a substitute for antibiotics in the treatment of acute UTIs.

Drinking 300–500 ml (10–16 ounces) unsweetened or lightly sweetened cranberry juice is recommended by many doctors of natural medicine for prevention and as part of the treatment of urinary tract infections. Alternately, 400 mg of concentrated cranberry extracts twice per day can be used.

Goldenseal (p. 429) is reputed to help treat many types of **infections** (p. 101). It contains berberine, an alkaloid that may prevent UTIs by inhibiting bacteria from adhering to the wall of the urinary bladder.[17] Goldenseal and other plants containing berberine (such as **Oregon grape** [p. 449]) may help in the treatment of urinary tract infections.

Many doctors of natural medicine recommend taking goldenseal root for UTIs. The usual recommendation is 250–500 mg 3 times per day of an extract standardized to contain 10% berberine. Goldenseal root capsules, tablets, or tinctures that are not standardized can be used in amounts of 3–4 grams per day. Goldenseal is not a substitute for antibiotic treatment during an acute UTI.

An extract of **uva ursi** (p. 466) is widely used in Europe as a treatment for UTI.[18] This herb is approved in Germany for treatment of bladder infections.[19] The active constituent in uva ursi is arbutin. In the alkaline environment of the urine, arbutin is converted into another chemical, called hydroquinone, which kills bacteria. A generally useful amount of uva ursi tincture is 3–5 ml 3 times per day. Otherwise, 100–250 mg of arbutin in herbal extract capsules or tablets 3 times per day can be used.

Asparagus (*Asparagus officinalis*), birch (*Betula* spp.), couch grass (*Galium aparine*), goldenrod (*Solidago virgaurea*), **horsetail** (p. 436), Java tea (*Orthosiphon stamineus*), lovage (*Levisticum officinale*), parsley (*Petroselinum crispum*), spiny restharrow (*Ononis spinosa*), and **nettle** (p. 447) are approved in Germany as part of the therapy of people with UTIs. These herbs appear to work by increasing urinary volume, thereby helping to flush bacteria out of the urinary tract.[20] **Juniper** (p. 437) is used in a similar fashion by many doctors knowledgeable in botanical medicine. Generally, these plants are taken as tea. Mix 1–3 teaspoons (5–15 grams) of herb in each cup of water and allow to steep for 15 minutes in the case of birch, couch grass, goldenrod, horsetail, Java tea, lovage, and nettle. Use ¼ teaspoon (2 grams) in the case of parsley herb. Mix 1–3 teaspoons (5–15 grams) of asparagus and spiny restharrow and simmer for 10 minutes and allow to cool. Drink 3 or more cups of tea per day.

Buchu (p. 404) leaf preparations have a history of use in traditional herbal medicine as a urinary tract disinfectant and diuretic;[21] however, the German Commission E monograph on buchu concludes that insufficient evidence supports the modern use of buchu for the treatment of urinary tract infections or inflammation.[22]

The essential oil of **horseradish** (p. 436) has been shown to kill bacteria that can cause urinary tract infections.[23] The concentration that is required to kill these bacteria can be attained in human urine after oral ingestion of the oil. One early study found that horseradish extract may help people with urinary tract infections.[24] Further studies are necessary to confirm this report.

Cleavers (p. 412) is one of numerous plants considered diuretic in ancient times.[25] It was therefore used to relieve **edema** (p. 65) and to promote urine formation during bladder infections.

Are There Any Side Effects or Interactions? Refer to the individual herb for information about any side effects or interactions.

Checklist for Urinary Tract Infection (UTI)

Ranking	Nutritional Supplements	Herbs
Secondary	Bromelain (p. 276)	Cranberry (p. 414)
Other	Multivitamin/mineral (p. 314) Vitamin A (p. 336) Vitamin C (p. 341)	Asparagus Birch Buchu (p. 404) Cleavers (p. 412) Couch grass Goldenrod Goldenseal (p. 429) Horseradish (p. 436) Horsetail (p. 436) Java tea Juniper (p. 437) Lovage Nettle (p. 447) Oregon grape (p. 449) Parsley Spiny restharrow Uva ursi (p. 466)

See also: Homeopathic Remedies for **Urinary Tract Infection** (p. 577)

Vaginitis

Vaginitis, inflammation of the vagina, is responsible for an estimated 10% of all visits by women to their health-care practitioners. The three general causes of vaginitis are hormonal imbalance, irritation, and infection. Hormone-related vaginitis includes the atrophic vaginitis generally found in **postmenopausal** (p. 553) or postpartum women, and occasionally in young girls before puberty. Irritant vaginitis can result from allergies or irritating substances. Infectious vaginitis is most common in reproductive-age women and is generally caused by one of three types of infections: bacterial vaginosis (BV), candidiasis (**yeast infection** [p. 169]), or trichomoniasis. A health-care professional should be consulted for the diagnosis and treatment of any vaginal infection.

Lifestyle Changes That May Be Helpful

Yeast infections are three times more common in women who wear nylon underwear or tights than in those who wear cotton underwear.[1] Additional predisposing factors for candida infection include the use of antibiotics, oral contraceptives, or adrenal corticosteroids (such as prednisone).

Underlying health conditions that may predispose someone to candida overgrowth include **pregnancy** (p. 143), **diabetes** (p. 53), and **HIV** (p. 87) infection. **Allergies** (p. 8) have also been reported to promote the development of recurrent yeast vaginitis. When the allergens are avoided and the allergies treated, often the chronic recurring yeast infections resolve.[2] In most cases, sexual transmission is not thought to play a role in candida vaginitis. However, in persistent cases, sexual transmission should be considered, and the sexual partner should be examined and treated.

For irritant vaginitis, minimizing friction and reducing exposure to perfumes, chemicals, and irritating lubricants and spermicides can be beneficial.

Dietary Changes That May Be Helpful

Some nutritionally oriented doctors believe that a well-balanced diet low in fats, sugars, and refined foods is important for preventing vaginal infections caused by candida. In one uncontrolled study, avoidance of sugar, dairy products, and artificial sweeteners resulted in a sharp reduction in the incidence and severity of candida vaginitis.[3] Many nutritionally oriented doctors advise women who have a **yeast infection** (p. 169) (or are predisposed to such infections) to limit their intake of sugar, fruit juices, and refined carbohydrates. For persistent or recurrent infections, some doctors recommend that fruit also be avoided. **Food allergies** (p. 8) are believed to be a contributory factor in some cases of recurrent irritant vaginitis.

In a controlled study, women who consumed 8 ounces of **acidophilus** (p. 325) yogurt per day had a threefold decrease in the incidence of vaginal yeast infections and a reduction in the frequency of candida colonization in the vagina.[4]

In another study, women who ingested 45 grams of **soy** (p. 332) flour or 25 grams of **flaxseeds** (p. 296) per day showed an improvement in the estrogen effect on their vaginal epithelial tissue.[5] That observation suggests that supplementing with either of these foods may be helpful for preventing or reversing atrophic vaginitis.

Nutritional Supplements That May Be Helpful

Lactobacillus acidophilus (p. 325) is a strain of friendly bacteria that is an integral part of normal vaginal flora. Lactobacilli help maintain the vaginal microflora by preventing overgrowth of unfriendly bacteria and candida. Lactobacilli produce lactic acid, which acts like a natural antibiotic; these friendly bacteria also compete with other organisms for the utilization of glucose. The production of lactic acid and hydrogen peroxide by lactobacilli also helps to maintain the acidic pH that is needed for healthy vaginal flora to thrive. Most of the research has used yogurt containing live cultures of *Lactobacillus acidophilus* or the topical application of such yogurt or *Lactobacillus acidophilus* into the vagina.

Some doctors of natural medicine recommend **vitamin E** (p. 344), either orally, topically, or intravaginally, for certain types of vaginitis. Vitamin E as a suppository in the vagina or vitamin E oil can be used once or twice per day for 3 to 14 days to soothe the mucous membranes of the vagina and vulva. Some doctors of natural medicine recommend intravaginal administration of **vitamin A** (p. 336) to improve the integrity of the vaginal tissue and to enhance the function of local immune cells. Vitamin A can be administered intravaginally by inserting a vitamin A capsule or using a prepared vitamin A suppository. Vitamin A used this way can be irritating to local tissue, so it should not be used more than once per day for up to 7 consecutive days.

Boric acid (p. 272) capsules inserted in the vagina have been used successfully to treat yeast vaginitis. One study demonstrated that 98% of women who used boric acid capsules were cured of chronic recurring yeast vaginitis.[6]

Are There Any Side Effects or Interactions? Refer to the individual supplement for information about any side effects or interactions.

Herbs That May Be Helpful

Topically applied **tea tree** (p. 463) oil has been studied and used successfully as a topical treatment for *Trichomonas, Candida albicans,* and other vaginal infections.[7] Some nutritionally oriented physicians suggest using tea tree oil by mixing the full-strength oil with vitamin E oil in the proportion of one-third tea tree oil to two-thirds **vitamin E** (p. 344) oil. Saturate a tampon with this mixture or put the mixture in a capsule to be inserted in the vagina each day for a maximum of 6 weeks.

The growth of *Candida albicans* is inhibited by **garlic** (p. 425).[8] Although no scientific studies demonstrate its effectiveness in humans, some doctors recommend that women with candida vaginitis supplement with garlic capsules orally or insert garlic capsules or a raw peeled clove of garlic into the vagina daily for several days. Eating one clove of uncooked garlic per day or taking a supplement containing 5,000 mcg of allicin

is also recommended in order to increase the effectiveness of the intravaginal remedy.

Teas of **goldenseal** (p. 429), **barberry** (p. 395), and **echinacea** (p. 417) are also sometimes used to treat infectious vaginitis. Although all three plants are known to be antibacterial in the test tube, the effectiveness of these herbs against vaginal infections has not been tested in humans. The usual approach is to douche with one of these teas twice each day, using 1–2 tablespoons of herb per pint of water. One to two pints are usually enough for each douching session. Echinacea is also known to improve **immune function** (p. 94) in humans.[9] In order to increase resistance against infection, many doctors of natural medicine recommend oral use of the tincture or alcohol-preserved fresh juice of echinacea in the amount of 1 teaspoon (5 ml) 3 or more times per day—during all types of infection—to improve resistance.

Are There Any Side Effects or Interactions? Refer to the individual herb for information about any side effects or interactions.

Checklist for Vaginitis

Ranking	Nutritional Supplements	Herbs
Primary	*Lactobacillus acidophilus* (p. 325)	
Other	Boric acid (p. 272) (topical) Flaxseed (p. 296) Soy (p. 332) Vitamin A (p. 336) Vitamin E (p. 344)	Barberry (p. 395) Echinacea (p. 94) Garlic (p. 425) Goldenseal (p. 429) Tea tree (p. 463)

Varicose Veins

Veins contain valves that keep blood from flowing backward as a result of gravity. When these valves become too weak, blood pools in the veins and causes them to bulge. These enlarged vessels are called varicose veins. Standing and sitting for long periods of time, lack of exercise, **obesity** (p. 165), and **pregnancy** (p. 143) all tend to promote the formation of varicose veins. Sometimes varicose veins are painful. Elevating the affected leg usually brings significant relief.

Lifestyle Changes That May Be Helpful

Keeping the legs elevated relieves pain. People with varicose veins should avoid sitting or standing for prolonged periods of time and should walk regularly.

Vitiligo

Herbs That May Be Helpful

The treatment of varicose veins is essentially the same as for **chronic venous insufficiency** (p. 38). Refer to that chapter for further information.

Although **witch hazel** (p. 470) is known primarily for combatting hemorrhoids, it may also be useful for varicose veins.[1,2] Application of a witch hazel ointment 3 or more times per day for 2 or more weeks is necessary before results can be expected.

Horse chestnut (p. 435) can be used both internally and as an external application for disorders of venous circulation, including varicose veins.[3] Preliminary studies in humans have shown that 300 mg 3 times per day of a standardized extract of horse chestnut can produce some benefit on one aspect of varicose veins.[4]

Bilberry (p. 396) supports normal formation of connective tissue and strengthens capillaries; these effects might be expected to be of value for the prevention of varicose veins. **Butcher's broom** (p. 405) and **gotu kola** (p. 430) are additional herbs that can be helpful for varicose veins.

Are There Any Side Effects or Interactions? Refer to the individual herb for information about any side effects or interactions.

Checklist for Varicose Veins

Ranking	Nutritional Supplements	Herbs
Primary		Horse chestnut (p. 435)
Other		Bilberry (p. 396) Butcher's broom (p. 405) Gotu kola (p. 430) Witch hazel (p. 470)

See also: Homeopathic Remedies for **Varicose Veins** (p. 579)

Vitiligo

Vitiligo is a disorder of skin pigmentation characterized by progressively widening areas of depigmented (very white) skin. The phenomenon is associated with the local destruction of melanocytes, the cells that produce melanin pigment to darken the skin. It affects 1–4% of the world's population.[1]

Nutritional Supplements That May Be Helpful

A clinical report describes the use of vitamin supplements in the treatment of vitiligo.[2] **Folic acid** (p. 297) and/or **vitamin B$_{12}$** (p. 337) and **vitamin C** (p. 341) levels were abnormally low in most of the fifteen people studied. Supplementation with large amounts of folic acid (1–10 mg per day), along with vitamin C (1 gram per day) and intramuscular vitamin B$_{12}$ injections (1,000 mcg every 2 weeks), produced marked repigmentation in eight people. These improvements became apparent after 3 months, but complete repigmentation required 1 to 2 years of continuous supplementation. In another study of 100 individuals with vitiligo, oral supplementation with folic acid (10 mg per day) and vitamin B$_{12}$ (2,000 mcg per day), combined with sun exposure, resulted in some repigmentation after 3 to 6 months in fifty-two cases.[3] This combined regimen was more effective than either vitamin supplementation or sun exposure alone.

Supplementation with the amino acid **L-phenylalanine** (p. 320) may have value when combined with ultraviolet (UVA) radiation therapy. Several clinical trials, including one double-blind trial, indicated that L-phenylalanine given in amounts of 50 mg per kilogram body weight per day (3,500 mg per day for a 154-pound person) or less, increased the extent of repigmentation induced by UVA therapy. L-phenylalanine alone also produced a more modest repigmentation in some people.[4] Another study of vitiligo in children reported that L-phenylalanine plus UVA was an effective treatment in the majority of children.[5] Recently, a group of Spanish doctors reported on their experience using L-phenylalanine over a 6-year period. Some of the 171 people with vitiligo received L-phenylalanine (50 or 100 mg per kg body weight per day) for up to 3 years. Between April and October of each year, those people also applied a 10% L-phenylalanine gel, prior to exposing their skin to the sun for 30 minutes. Some improvement was seen in 83% of the people treated, and in 57% the results were rated as good (75% improvement or better).[6]

In one early report, lack of stomach acid (achlorhydria) was found to be associated with vitiligo. Administration of dilute hydrochloric acid after meals resulted in gradual repigmentation of the skin (after 1 year or more).[7] Hydrochloric acid, or its more modern counterpart **betaine hydrochloride (HCl)** (p. 269), should be taken only under the supervision of a nutritionally oriented doctor.

Another early report described the use of **PABA** (p. 319) (para-aminobenzoic acid)—a compound that is commonly associated with **B-complex** (p. 391) vitamins. Persistent use of 100 mg of PABA 3 or 4 times per day along with an injectable form of PABA and a variety of hormones tailored to individual needs, resulted, in many cases, in repigmentation of areas affected by vitiligo.[8]

Are There Any Side Effects or Interactions? Refer to the individual supplement for information about any side effects or interactions.

Herbs That May Be Helpful

An extract from khella *(Ammi visnaga)* may be useful in repigmenting the skin of those with vitiligo. Khellin, the active constituent, appears to work like psoralen drugs—it stimulates repigmentation of the skin by increasing sensitivity of remaining pigment-containing cells (melanocytes) to sunlight. Studies have used 120–160 mg of khellin per day.[9]

Another herb that may prove useful for vitiligo is St. John's wort (p. 461).[10] As with khella, it increases the response of the skin to sunlight. However, to date no studies have demonstrated the effectiveness of St. John's wort for vitiligo.

Are There Any Side Effects or Interactions? Refer to the individual herb for information about any side effects or interactions.

Checklist for Vitiligo

Ranking	Nutritional Supplements	Herbs
Secondary		Khella
Other	B-Complex (p. 341) Betaine HCl (p. 269) Folic acid (p. 297) L-phenylalanine (p. 320) PABA (p. 319) Vitamin B₁₂ (p. 337) Vitamin C (p. 341)	St. John's wort (p. 461)

Weight Loss and Obesity

About one-third of the U.S. population is overweight. Because excess body weight is implicated as a risk factor for many different diseases (including heart disease, **diabetes** [p. 53], several cancers, and **gallstones** [p. 69]), maintaining a healthy body weight seems prudent. Unfortunately, losing weight—and keeping it off—is very difficult for most people.

Dietary Changes That May Be Helpful

Societies in which very little fat is eaten have virtually no obesity. Reducing fat in the diet is an important component of weight-loss efforts. Foods with a high proportion of calories from fat should be eliminated or limited in the diet; these include red meat, poultry skins, dark poultry meat, fried foods, butter, mar-

garine, cheese, milk (except skim milk), junk foods, and most processed foods. Vegetable oils should also be restricted, as should nuts, seeds, and avocados (although these foods are healthful for people who have no weight problem). Instead, the diet should be based on fruits, vegetables, whole grains, and nonfat dairy products (and lowfat fish for non-vegetarians).

Eating adequate amounts of **fiber** (p. 293) is believed to be important for individuals wishing to lose weight. Fiber contains bulk and tends to produce a sense of fullness, which allows people to consume fewer calories.[1] However, research on the effect of fiber intake on weight loss is conflicting. Some studies have shown that supplementation with a source of fiber accelerated weight loss in individuals who were following a low-calorie diet.[2,3] In another study, supplementation with a bulking agent called glucomannan (1.5 grams before breakfast and dinner) promoted weight loss in overweight individuals who were not following a special diet.[4] However, other researchers found that increasing fiber intake had no effect on body weight, even though it resulted in a reduction in food intake.[5] Different types of dietary fiber are available from a variety of sources, and the amount recommended depends on the kind being used. Individuals wishing to use a fiber supplement should consult with a nutritionally oriented doctor.

Although the relationship between **food sensitivities** (p. 8) and body weight remains uncertain, according to one researcher, chronic food allergy may lead to overeating and obesity.[6]

People who go on and off diets frequently complain that fewer calories result in weight gain with each weight fluctuation. Evidence now clearly demonstrates that the body gets "stingier" in its use of calories after each diet.[7] This means it becomes easier to gain weight and harder to lose it the next time. Therefore, dietary changes need to be long term.

Lifestyle Changes That May Be Helpful

Exercise is usually recommended to enhance the effectiveness of a low-calorie diet. In addition, studies have shown that exercise alone (without dietary restriction) can promote weight loss in obese individuals.[8] Moreover, a study of overweight women found that engaging in an exercise program helped the women adhere to a low-calorie diet.[9]

Nutritional Supplements That May Be Helpful

Diets that are low in total calories may not contain adequate amounts of various vitamins and minerals. For that reason, proponents of most weight-loss programs advocate taking a **multiple vitamin/mineral** (p. 314) supplement.

The mineral **chromium** (p. 282) plays an essential role in the metabolism of carbohydrates and fats and in the action of insulin. Chromium, in a form called chromium picolinate, has been studied for its potential role in altering body composition. Preliminary research in animals[10] and humans[11][12] suggested that supplementation with chromium picolinate promoted a loss of body fat and an increase in muscle mass. However, follow-up research in humans found that chromium picolinate had no effect on body composition.[13]

Hydroxycitric acid (HCA) (p. 302), extracted from the rind of the Garcinia cambogia fruit grown in Southeast Asia, has a chemical composition similar to that of citric acid (the primary acid in oranges and other citrus fruits). Preliminary studies in animals suggest that HCA may be a useful weight-loss aid.[14][15] HCA has been demonstrated in the laboratory (but not yet in clinical trials with people) to reduce the conversion of carbohydrates into stored fat by inhibiting certain enzyme processes.[16][17]Animal research indicates that HCA suppresses appetite and induces weight loss.[18][19][20][21] In one case report, an individual who ate 1 gram of the fruit containing HCA before each meal lost 1 pound per day.[22] However, much more research in humans is needed to determine the effectiveness of HCA as a weight-loss aid.

Pyruvate (p. 328), a compound that occurs naturally in the body, might aid weight-loss efforts.[23] A clinical trial found that pyruvate supplements (22–44 grams per day), compared with placebo, enhanced weight loss and resulted in a greater reduction of body fat in overweight adults consuming a lowfat diet.[24] Animal studies suggest that pyruvate leads to weight loss by increasing the resting metabolic rate.[25] However, additional research is needed to determine the long-term effectiveness and safety of pyruvate as a weight-loss aid.

Spirulina (p. 333), a type of algae, is a rich source of protein, vitamins, minerals, and essential fatty acids. In one double-blind study of sixteen overweight individuals, ingestion of 2.8 grams of spirulina 3 times per day for 4 weeks resulted in a small but statistically significant weight loss.[26]

5-Hydroxytryptophan (5-HTP) (p. 295), the precursor to the neurotransmitter serotonin, has been shown in two short-term controlled studies to reduce appetite and to promote weight loss.[27][28] In one of these studies, a 12-week double-blind trial, overweight women who took 600–900 mg of 5-HTP per day lost significantly more weight than did women who received placebo.

Are There Any Side Effects or Interactions? Refer to the individual supplement for information about any side effects or interactions.

Herbs That May Be Helpful

The herb **guaraná** (p. 431) contains guaranine (which is nearly identical to caffeine) and the closely related alkaloids theobromine and theophylline; these compounds may curb appetite and increase weight loss. Caffeine's effects (and hence those of guaranine) are well known and include stimulating the central nervous system, increasing metabolic rate, and producing a mild diuretic effect.[29] Because of concerns about potential adverse effects, many doctors of natural medicine do not advocate using caffeine or caffeine-like substances to reduce weight.

Ephedra sinica (p. 420), commonly known as ma huang, is a central nervous system stimulant. Double-blind studies have shown that ephedra, particularly when combined with caffeine, promotes weight loss. However, many nutritionally oriented doctors discourage the use of ephedra as a weight-loss aid because of the many side effects that can occur with its use, especially since many of the side effects are intensified when ephedra is combined with caffeine.[30][31]

Are There Any Side Effects or Interactions? Refer to the individual herb for information about any side effects or interactions.

Checklist for Weight Loss and Obesity

Ranking	Nutritional Supplements	Herbs
Primary	Fiber (p. 293)	
Secondary	Pyruvate (p. 328)	Ephedra (p. 420) Psyllium (p. 452)
Other	5-HTP (p. 295) Chromium (p. 282) Hydroxycitric acid (HCA) (p. 302) Spirulina (p. 333)	Guaraná (p. 431)

Wilson's Disease

Wilson's disease is a genetic disorder that results in excessive accumulation of **copper** (p. 285) in many parts of the body. If left untreated, this condition can be fatal, but fortunately it is readily treatable.

Dietary Changes That May Be Helpful

Most foods contain at least some copper, so it is not possible to avoid the metal completely. Foods high in copper, such as organ meats and oysters, should be eliminated from the diet. Some foods are relatively high in copper but are quite nutritious (nuts and legumes, for example)—these foods should be eaten in moderation by people with Wilson's disease. Grains contain significant amounts of copper but are important components of a healthful diet, and dietary restriction may be neither wise nor necessary, particularly if zinc is supplemented.

Nutritional Supplements That May Be Helpful

Zinc (p. 346) is known for its ability to reduce copper absorption and has been used successfully in people with Wilson's disease,[1] with some trials lasting up to 7 years.[2] Researchers have called zinc a "remarkably effective and nontoxic therapy for Wilson's disease."[3]

Zinc has also been used to keep normal copper levels from rising in people with Wilson's disease who had been successfully treated with prescription drugs.[4] Zinc in the amount of 50 mg taken 3 times per day has been used for this type of maintenance therapy,[5] although some researchers have used the same amount of zinc successfully with people who have untreated Wilson's disease.[6]

Zinc is so effective in lessening the body's burden of copper that a copper deficiency was reported in someone with Wilson's disease who took too much (480 mg per day) zinc.[7] Nonetheless, zinc does not help everyone with Wilson's disease. Sometimes increased copper levels can occur in the liver after zinc supplementation;[8] however, leading researchers believe this increase is both temporary and not harmful.[9]

Copper is present in several dietary supplements, especially multimineral and **multivitamin/mineral** (p. 314) preparations. Copper-containing supplements should be avoided.

Are There Any Side Effects or Interactions? Refer to the individual supplement for information about any side effects or interactions.

Checklist for Wilson's Disease

Ranking	Nutritional Supplements	Herbs
Primary	Zinc (p. 346)	

Wound Healing

Wound healing is the process of repair that follows injury to the skin and other soft tissues. Wounds may result from trauma or from a surgical incision. In addition, pressure ulcers (also known as decubitus ulcers or pressure sores), which develop on areas of the body where the blood supply has been reduced because of prolonged pressure, might also be considered wounds. The capacity of a wound to heal depends in part on its depth, as well as on the overall health and nutritional status of the individual.

Following injury, an inflammatory response occurs and the cells below the dermal layer begin to increase collagen production. Later, the epithelial tissue (the outer skin layer) is regenerated. Dietary modifications and nutritional and herbal supplements may improve the quality of wound healing by influencing inflammatory or reparative processes.

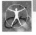

Dietary Changes That May Be Helpful

Pressure ulcers and **diabetic** (p. 53) ulcers frequently develop in malnourished and/or institutionalized individuals. In a 21-day double-blind study, malnourished people applied to their skin 20 ml of a solution containing either essential fatty acids (linoleic acid extracted from sunflower oil) plus **vitamins A** (p. 336) and **E** (p. 344), or the same solution without the essential fatty acids (control solution). Each solution was applied to the skin 3 times per day. Compared with the control solution, the solution containing essential fatty acids significantly reduced the incidence of pressure ulcers and improved the hydration and elasticity of the skin.[1]

In a study of twenty-eight malnourished people with pressure ulcers, those who were given a diet containing 24% protein showed a significant reduction in the size of the ulcer, whereas those given a diet containing 14% protein had no significant improvement.[2] This study suggests that increasing dietary protein in malnourished individuals can improve wound healing. It is not known whether the same benefit would be observed in well-nourished people.

Nutritional Supplements That May Be Helpful

Vitamin C (p. 341) participates in the process of wound healing by promoting the synthesis of collagen. In a study of dental students, supplementation with vitamin C (1–2 grams per day) increased the rate of healing of experimental **gingival** (p. 73) wounds.[3] In a double-blind study of surgical patients with decubitus ulcers, supplementation with 500 mg of vitamin C twice a day accelerated ulcer healing.[4]

The mineral **zinc** (p. 346) plays a role in cell division and cell proliferation, both of which are involved in the process of wound healing. Zinc deficiency is associated with impaired wound healing.[5] The healing time of a surgical wound was reduced by 43% following oral supplementation with zinc sulfate in the amount of 50 mg 3 times per day.[6] Zinc supplementation also improved healing in elderly people suffering from chronic leg ulcers[7] and pressure sores.[8] In another study, intravenous administration of zinc significantly reduced the number of post-operative complications in surgical patients.[9]

In a study of people deficient in zinc, topically applied zinc oxide (as an additive to a gauze bandage) enhanced the regeneration of epithelial tissue on leg ulcers. In addition, inflammation and bacterial growth were reduced.[10] In a study of thirty-seven elderly individuals with leg ulcers, application of zinc oxide compresses promoted ulcer healing.[11] Although zinc oxide produced beneficial effects in these studies, topically applied zinc sulfate was ineffective.

Rats fed a vitamin A–supplemented diet showed enhanced wound healing, compared with those fed a standard diet.[12] The beneficial effect of vitamin A on wound healing may be due to an increase in collagen synthesis.[13] Supplementation with vitamin A also reversed the impairment of wound healing seen in rats with experimentally induced diabetes.[14]

Animal studies have shown that supplementing with vitamin E can decrease the formation of unwanted adhesions following a surgical wound. In addition, wound healing was more rapid in animals fed a vitamin E–rich diet than in those fed a standard diet.[15] However, in another study, wound healing was inhibited by supplementation with a massive amount of vitamin E (equivalent to about 35,000 IU).[16] This adverse effect of vitamin E was prevented by supplementation with vitamin A. Although the relevance of these studies to human is not clear, many doctors of natural medicine recommend supplementing with both vitamins A and E in order to enhance wound healing and prevent adhesion formation.

Copper (p. 285) is a required cofactor for the enzyme lysyl oxidase, which plays a role in the cross-linking (and strengthening) of connective tissue.[17] Doctors of natural medicine often recommend a copper supplement as part of a comprehensive nutritional program to promote wound healing.

Thiamine (p. 337) (vitamin B$_1$),[18] **pantothenic acid** (p. 340) (vitamin B$_5$),[19] and other B vitamins[20] have each been shown to play a role in wound healing. For this reason, doctors of natural medicine often recommend a B vitamin supplement to promote wound healing.

Ingestion of **bromelain** (p. 276), an enzyme derived from pineapple, prior to and following a surgical procedure has been shown to reduce swelling, bruising, healing time, and pain.[21] Supplementation with bromelain has also been shown to accelerate the healing of soft-tissue injuries in men following a boxing match.[22]

Are There Any Side Effects or Interactions? Refer to the individual supplement for information about any side effects or interactions.

Checklist for Wound Healing

Ranking	Nutritional Supplements	Herbs
Primary	B-complex vitamins (p. 341) Bromelain (p. 276) Vitamin C (p. 341) Zinc (p. 346) Zinc (p. 346) (topical)	
Secondary	Copper (p. 285) Vitamin A (p. 336) Vitamin E (p. 344)	Aloe vera (p. 391) Aloe vera (p. 391) (topical) Calendula (topical) (p. 406) Gotu kola (p. 430)
Other	Arginine (p. 268) Glucosamine sulfate (p. 299) Ornithine alpha-ketoglutarate (OKG) (p. 319)	Chamomile (p. 409) Chaparral (p. 410) Comfrey (p. 413) *Equiseti herba* (topical) Essential fatty acids (topical) Plantain, St. John's wort (p. 461) Witch hazel (p. 470)

Herbs That May Be Helpful

Calendula (p. 406) is used by herbalists in a topical dressing to assist in wound healing. Studies indicate a potent anti-inflammatory effect.[23,24]

Traditional herbalists frequently recommend a combination of herbs for wound healing in order to achieve a desired effect. The herbs **St. John's wort** (p. 461), calendula, **chamomile** (p. 409), and plantain *(Plantaginis lanceolatae)* have all been shown to exert anti-inflammatory effects in a rat model.[25] It is unknown whether a synergistic effect may be achieved by using the combination of these herbs rather than single herbs. These herbs have shown beneficial actions; for example, plantain acts as an anti-inflammatory when used externally,[26] and St. John's wort in a topical application demonstrates an anti-inflammatory action.[27]

In addition, **comfrey** (p. 413) is an external anti-inflammatory that may decrease bruising.[28] **Witch hazel** (p. 470) can be used both internally and externally to decrease inflammation and stop bleeding.[29] **Horsetail** (p. 436) can be used both internally and externally to decrease inflammation and promote wound healing.[30] In a rat model of skin inflammation, both topical and oral **aloe vera** (p. 391) have proven beneficial in decreasing inflammation and promoting cellular repair.[31,32]

Are There Any Side Effects or Interactions? Refer to the individual herb for information about any side effects or interactions.

Yeast Infection

Yeast infections are one of the most common reasons that women consult health-care professionals. Yeast infections result from an overgrowth of a species of fungus called Candida albicans. The hallmark symptom of **vaginitis** (p. 162) caused by a yeast infection is itching of the external and internal genitalia, which is often associated with a white discharge that can be thick, curdy, or like cottage cheese. Severe infections lead to inflammation of the tissue and subsequent redness, swelling, and even pinpoint bleeding.

Dietary Changes That May Be Helpful

Some nutritionally oriented doctors believe that a well-balanced diet low in fats, sugars, and refined foods is important for preventing vaginal infections caused by candida. In one controlled study, avoidance of sugar, dairy products, and artificial sweeteners resulted in a sharp reduction in the incidence and severity of candida vaginitis.[1] Many nutritionally oriented doctors advise women who have a yeast infection (or are predisposed to such infections) to limit their intake of sugar, fruit juices, and refined carbohydrates.

Lifestyle Changes That May Be Helpful

Yeast infections are three times more common in women who wear nylon underwear or tights than in those who wear cotton underwear.[2] Additional predisposing factors for candida infection include the use of antibiotics, oral contraceptives, or adrenal corticosteroids (such as prednisone).

Underlying health conditions that may predispose someone to candida overgrowth include **pregnancy** (p. 143), **diabetes** (p. 53) mellitus, or **HIV** (p. 87) infection. **Allergies** (p. 8) have also been reported to promote the development of recurrent yeast vaginitis. In one study, when the allergens were avoided and the allergies treated, the chronic recurrent yeast infections frequently resolved.[3] In most cases, sexual transmission does not play a role in yeast infection. However, in extremely persistent cases, sexual transmission should be considered, and the sexual partner should be examined and treated.

Nutritional Supplements That May Be Helpful

Lactobacillus acidophilus (p. 325) is a species of friendly bacteria that is an integral part of normal vaginal flora. Lactobacilli help to maintain the vaginal ecosystem by preventing the overgrowth of unfriendly bacteria and candida. Lactobacilli produce lactic acid which acts like a natural antibiotic; these friendly bacteria also compete with other organisms for the utilization of glucose.

Lactobacillus acidophilus can be taken orally in the form of acidophilus yogurt,[4] or in capsules or powder; it can also be administered intravaginally. Many women find relief using an acidophilus-yogurt douche daily for a few days or weeks, depending on the severity of the infection.[5] Three capsules of acidophilus or one-quarter teaspoon of powder can be taken 1 to 3 times daily. Acidophilus can also be taken preventively during antibiotic use to reduce the risk of candida vaginitis.[6,7]

Boric acid (p. 272) capsules inserted into the vagina have been used with great success as a treatment for yeast vaginitis. In one study of 100 women with chronic yeast vaginitis who had failed to respond to various over-the-counter or prescription antifungal medicines, 98% successfully treated their infections with boric acid capsules, inserted into the vagina twice per day for 2 to 4 weeks.[8]

Are There Any Side Effects or Interactions? Refer to the individual supplement for information about any side effects or interactions.

Herbs That May Be Helpful

Topically applied **tea tree oil** (p. 463) may be useful for some women with vaginal yeast infections. It can be diluted and used as a douche or used as part of a coconut oil-based suppository (with 2% tea tree oil).[9] For more serious or persistent infections of the cervix or vagina, however, a health-care professional should be consulted. Concentrations of tea tree oil as strong as 40% may be used with caution as a vaginal douche.

Checklist for Yeast Infection

Ranking	Nutritional Supplements	Herbs
Primary	Lactobacillus acidophilus (p. 325)	
Secondary	Boric acid (p. 272)	
Other		Cinnamon (p. 411) Echinacea (p. 417) Garlic (p. 425) Pau d'arco (p. 450) Tea tree oil (p. 463)
See also: Homeopathic Remedies for **Yeast Infection** (p. 579)		

Garlic (p. 425) has been shown to inhibit the growth of *Candida albicans*.[10] Although controlled studies in humans have not been done, many doctors of natural medicine recommend garlic for individuals with yeast infections. For people who have no aversion to the odor, one whole clove of raw garlic can be chewed daily. Otherwise, odor-controlled, enteric-coated tablets standardized for allicin content can be taken in the amount of 900 mg per day (providing 5,000 mcg of allicin), preferably divided into two equal doses. As an alternative, 2–4 ml of a tincture may be taken 3 times per day. For health maintenance, one-half of the therapeutic amount is adequate.

Another herb recommended for yeast infections is **pau d'arco** (p. 450). This South American herb's active constituents have powerful anti-yeast actions.[11] However, these compounds are also somewhat toxic, and the amount needed to kill yeast is apparently greater than the amount contained in most herbal supplements.

Many doctors of natural medicine recommend that individuals with recurrent yeast infections take measures to support their immune system. **Echinacea** (p. 417), which has the capacity to enhance immune function, is often used by people who suffer from recurrent infections. In one study, women who took echinacea experienced a 43% decline in the recurrence rate of yeast infections.[12] However, echinacea is not a substitute for anti-yeast medication. The essential oil of **cinnamon** (p. 411) contains various terpenoids that are believed to be responsible for cinnamon's medicinal effects. Important among these compounds are eugenol and cinnamaldehyde. Cinnamaldehyde and cinnamon oil vapors are extremely potent antifungal compounds.[13] In a preliminary study in individuals with **AIDS** (p. 87), topical application of cinnamon oil was effective against oral candida infections (thrush).[14]

Are There Any Side Effects or Interactions? Refer to the individual herb for information about any side effects or interactions.

Yellow Nail Syndrome

People with yellow nail syndrome have thickened nails with yellow or greenish discoloration, often accompanied by stunted growth and swelling of the ankles and sometimes other parts of the body.

Nutritional Supplements That May Be Helpful

Vitamin E (p. 344) has been used successfully with people who have yellow nail syndrome.[1,2,3] Although topical use of the vitamin is helpful,[4] taking vitamin E supplements is much easier and less messy. A typical amount is 800 IU per day, with results beginning to appear after several months.

Checklist for Yellow Nail Syndrome

Ranking	Nutritional Supplements	Herbs
Primary	Vitamin E (p. 344)	

Part One: References

Acne

1. Fulton JE Jr, Plewig G, Kligman AM. Effect of chocolate on acne vulgaris. *JAMA* 1969; 210: 2071–74.

2. Anderson PC. Foods as the cause of acne. *Am Family Phys* 1971; 3: 102–3.

3. Gaby A. Commentary. *Nutr Healing* Feb 1997; 1,10,11.

4. Hillstrom L et al. Comparison of oral treatment with zinc sulfate and placebo in acne vulgaris. *Br J Dermatol* 1977; 97: 679–84.

5. Michaelsson G et al. A double blind study of the effect of zinc and oxytetracycline in acne vulgaris. *Br J Dermatol* 1977; 97: 561–66.

6. Kligman AM et al. Oral vitamin A in acne vulgaris. *Int J Dermatol* 1981; 20: 278–85.

7. Leung LH. Pantothenic acid deficiency as the pathogenesis of acne vulgaris. *Med Hypoth* 1995; 44: 490–92.

8. Shality AR, Smith JR, Parish LC, et al. Topical nicotinamide compared with clindamycin gel in the treatment of inflammatory acne vulgaris. *Internat J Dermatol* 1995; 34: 434–37.

9. Snider B, Dietman DF. Pyridoxine therapy for premenstrual acne flare. *Arch Dermatol* 1974; 110: 130–31.

10. Bassett IB, Pannowitz DL, Barnetson RS. A comparative study of tea-tree oil versus benzoyl peroxide in the treatment of acne. *Med J Austral* 1990; 53: 455–58.

11. Hoffman D. *The Herbal Handbook: A User's Guide to Medical Herbalism*. Rochester, VT: Healing Arts Press, 1988, 23–24.

12. Amann W. Improvement of acne vulgaris with *Agnus castus* (Agnolyt). *Ther Gegenw.* 1967; 106: 124–26 [in German].

13. Amann W. Acne vulgaris and *Agnus castus* (Agnolyt) . *Z Allgemeinmed* 1975; 51: 1645–58 [in German].

Alcohol Withdrawal

1. Guenther RM. Role of nutritional therapy in alcoholism treatment. *Int J Biosoc Res* 1983; 4: 5–18.

2. Werbach MR. Alcohol craving. *Internat J Alternative Complementary Med* Jul 1993: 32.

3. Biery JR, Williford JH, McMullen EA. Alcohol craving in rehabilitation: assessment of nutrition therapy. *J Am Dietet Assoc* 1991; 91: 463–66.

4. Cleary JP. The NAD deficiency diseases. *J Orthomol Med* 1986; 1: 149–57.

5. Cleary JP. Etiology and biological treatment of alcohol addiction. *J Neuro Ortho Med Surg* 1985; 6: 75–77.

6. Smith RF. A five-year field trial of massive nicotinic acid therapy of alcoholics in Michigan. *J Orthomol Psychiatr* 1974; 3: 327–31.

7. O'Halloren P. Pyridine nucleotides in the prevention, diagnosis and treatment of problem drinkers. *West J Surg Obstet Gynecol* 1961; 69: 101–104.

8. Eriksson CJP. Increase in hepatic NAD level—its effect on the redox state and on ethanol and acetaldehyde metabolism. *Fed Europ Biochem Soc* 1974; 40: 3117–20.

9. Baker H. A vitamin profile of alcoholism. *Internat J Vit Nutr Res* 1983(suppl 24): 179.

10. Schuckit MA. Alcohol and Alcoholism. *Harrison's Principles of Internal Medicine, 14th Edition.* Fauci AS, Braunwald E, Isselbacher KJ, et al, eds. New York: McGraw-Hill, 1998, 2503–08.

11. Norton VP. Interrelationships of nutrition and voluntary alcohol consumption in experimental animals. *Brit J Addiction* 1977; 72: 205–12.

12. Replogle WH, Eicke FJ. Megavitamin therapy in the reduction of anxiety and depression among alcoholics. *J Orthomol Med* 1988; 4: 221–24.

13. Morgan MY, Levine JA. Alcohol and nutrition. *Proc Natl Acad Sci* 1988; 47: 85–98.

14. Chapman K, Prabhudesai M, Erdman JW. Vitamin A status of alcoholics upon admission and after two weeks of hospitalization. *J Am Coll Nutr* 1993; 12: 77–83.

15. Chen M, Boyce W, Hsu JM. Effect of ascorbic acid on plasma alcohol clearance. *J Am Coll Nutr* 1990; 9: 185–89.

16. Blum K. A commentary on neurotransmitter restoration as a common mode of treatment for alcohol, cocaine and opiate abuse. *Integr Psychiatr* 1986; 6: 199–204.

17. Rogers LL, Pelton RB. Glutamine in the treatment of alcoholism. *Quarterly J Stud Alcohol* 1957; 18: 581–87.

18. Embry CK, Lippmann S. Use of magnesium sulfate in alcohol withdrawal. *Am Fam Phys* 1987; 35: 167–70.

19. Horrobin DF. Essential fatty acids, prostaglandins, and alcoholism: an overview. *Alcoholism: Clin Exper Res* 1987; 11: 2–9.

20. Glen AIM, Glen EMT, MacDonnell LEF, et al. Essential fatty

acids in the management of withdrawal symptoms and tissue damage in alcoholics. Presented at the 2nd International Congress on Essential Fatty Acids, Prostaglandins and Leukotrienes, London, Zoological Society. March 24–27, 1985 [abstract 53].

21. Keung W, Vallee B. Daidzin and daidzein suppress free-choice ethanol intake by Syrian golden hamsters. *Proc Natl Acad Sci USA* 1993; 90: 10,008–12.

22. Leng-Peschlowe. Alcohol-related liver diseases-use of Legalon. *Z Klin Med* 1994; 2: 22–27.

23. Faulstich H, Jahn W, Wieland T. Silibinin inhibition of amatoxin uptake in the perfused rat liver. *Arzneim-Forsch Drug Res* 1980; 30: 452–54.

24. Tuchweber B, Sieck R, Trost W. Prevention by silibinin of phalloidin induced hepatotoxicity. *Toxicol Appl Pharmacol* 1979; 51: 265–75.

25. Feher J, Lang I et al. Free radicals in tissue damage in liver diseases and therapeutic approach. *Tokai J Exp Clin Med* 1986; 11: 121–34.

26. Sonnenbichler J, Zetl I. Stimulating influence of a flavonolignan derivative on proliferation, RNA synthesis and protein synthesis in liver cells. In *Assessment and Management of Hepatobiliary Disease.* L Okolicsanyi, G Csomos, G Crepaldi, eds. Berlin: Springer-Verlag, 1987, 265–72.

Allergies and Sensitivities (Food and Chemical)

1. Breneman JC. *Basics of Food Allergy.* Springfield, IL: Charles C Thomas, 1978, 45–53.

2. Gaby A. Commentary. *Nutr Healing* Feb; 1997: 1, 10, 11.

3. Darlington LG, Ramsey NW, Mansfield JR. Placebo-controlled, blind study of dietary manipulation therapy in rheumatoid arthritis. *Lancet* 1986; i: 236–38.

4. Beri D et al. Effect of dietary restrictions on disease activity in rheumatoid arthritis. *Ann Rheum Dis* 1988; 47: 69–72.

5. Panush RS. Possible role of food sensitivity in arthritis. *Ann Allerg* 1988; 61(part 2): 31–35.

6. Taylor MR. Food allergy as an etiological factor in arthropathies: a survey. *J Internat Acad Prev Med* 1983; 8: 28–38 [review].

7. Darlington LG, Ramsey NW. Diets for rheumatoid arthritis. *Lancet* 1991; 338: 1209 [letter].

8. Rowe AH, Young EJ. Bronchial asthma due to food allergy alone in ninety-five patients. *JAMA* 1959; 169: 1158.

9. Bock SA, Lee W-Y, Remigio LK, May CD. Studies of hypersensitivity reactions to foods in infants and children. *J Allerg Clin Immunol* 1978; 62: 327–34.

10. Allen DH, Delohery J, Baker G. Monosodium L-glutamate–induced asthma. *J Allerg Clin Immunol* 1987; 80: 530–37.

11. Sampson HA, Mendelson L, Rosen JP. Fatal and near-fatal anaphylactic reactions to food in children and adolescents. *N Engl J Med* 1992; 327: 380.

12. O'Shea JA, Porter SF. *J Learning Disabilities* 1981; 14(4): 189–91.

13. Salzman LK. Allergy testing, psychological assessment and dietary treatment of the hyperactive child syndrome. *Med J Australia* 1976; Aug 14: 248–51.

14. Crook WG. Food and chemical allergies: relationship to behavior. *J Applied Nutr* 1983; 35(1): 47–53.

15. Allergies may lead to minimal brain dysfunction in children. *JAMA* 1970; 212(1): 33–34.

16. Levy F, Dumbrell S, Hobbes G, et al. Hyperkinesis and diet: A double-blind crossover trial with a tartrazine challenge. *Med J Aust* 1978; 1: 61–64.

17. Boris M, Mandel FS. Foods and additives are common causes of the attention deficit hyperactive disorder in children. *Ann Allergy* 1994; 72: 462–68.

18. Carter CM, Urbanowicz M, Hemsley R, et al. Effects of a few food diet in attention deficit disorder. *Arch Dis Child* 1993; 69: 564–68.

19. Rowe KS, Rowe KJ. Synthetic food coloring and behavior: A dose response effect in a double-blind, placebo-controlled, repeated-meas-

ures study. *J Pediatr* 1994; 125: 691–98.

20. Harley JP, Ray RS, Tomasi L, et al. Hyperkinesis and food additives: Testing the Feingold hypothesis. *Pediatr* 1978; 61: 818–21.

21. Egger J, Stolla A, McEwen LM. Controlled trial of hyposensitisation in children with food-induced hyperkinetic syndrome. *Lancet* 1992; 339: 1150–53.

22. Breneman JC. Allergic cystitis: the cause of nocturnal enuresis. *General Practice* 1959; 20: 85–98.

23. Zaleski A, Shokeir MK, Garrard JW. Enuresis: familial incidence and relationship to allergic disorders. *Can Med Assoc J* 1972; 106: 30–31.

24. Horesh AJ. Allergy and infection. *J Asthma Res* 1967; 4: 269.

25. Rudolph JA. Allergy as a cause of frequent recurring colds and coughs in children. *Dis Chest* 1940; 6: 138.

26. Berman BA. Pseudomononucleosis of allergic origin: a new clinical entity. *Ann Allerg* 1964; 22: 403.

27. Randolph TG, Hettig RA. The coincidence of allergic disease, unexplained fatigue, and lymphadenopathy: possible diagnostic confusion with infectious mononucleosis. *Am J Med Sci* 1945; 209: 306.

28. Kudelco N. Allergy in chronic monilial vaginitis. *Ann Allerg* 1971; 29: 266–67.

29. Hay KD, Reade PC. The use of an elimination diet in the treatment of recurrent aphthous ulceration of the oral cavity. *Oral Surg Oral Med Oral Pathol* 1984; 57: 504–507.

30. Wray D. Gluten-sensitive recurrent aphthous stomatitis. *Dig Dis Sci* 1981; 26: 737–40.

31. Wright A et al. Food allergy or intolerance in severe recurrent aphthous ulceration of the mouth. *BMJ* 1986; 292: 1237.

32. Wray D et al. Food allergens and basophil histamine release in recurrent aphthous stomatitis. *Oral Surg Oral Med Oral Pathol* 1982; 54: 338–95.

33. Hill DJ, Hudson IL, Sheffield LJ, et al. A low allergen diet is a significant intervention in infantile colic:

results of a community-based study. *Clin Immunol* 1995; 96: 886–92.

34. Iacono G, Cavataio F, Montalto G, et al. Intolerance of cow's milk and chronic constipation in children. *N Engl J Med* 1998; 339: 1100–104.

35. Riordan AM, Hunter JO, Cowan RE, et al. Treatment of active Crohn's disease by exclusion diet: East Anglian Multicentre Controlled Trial. *Lancet* 1993; 342: 1131–34.

36. Alun Jones V, Dickinson RJ, Workman E, et al. Crohn's disease: maintenance of remission by diet. *Lancet* 1985; ii: 177–80.

37. Gettis A. Food sensitivities and psychological disturbance: a review. *Nutr Health* 1989; 6: 135–46.

38. King DS. Can allergic exposure provoke psychological symptoms? A double-blind test. *Biol Psychiatr* 1981; 16: 3–19.

39. Brown M, Gibney M, Husband PR, Radcliffe M. Food allergy in polysymptomatic patients. *Practitioner* 1981; 225: 1651–54.

40. James JM, Burks AW. Food-associated gastrointestinal disease. *Curr Opin Pediatr* 1996; 8: 471–75 [review].

41. McMahan JT, Calenoff E, Croft J, et al. Chronic otitis media with effusion and allergy: modified RAST analysis of 119 cases. *Otolaryngol Head Neck Surg* 1981; 89: 427–31.

42. Nsouli TM, Nsouli SM, Linde RE, et al. Role of food allergy in serous otitis media. *Ann Allerg* 1994; 73: 215–19.

43. McGovern JP, Haywood TH, Fernandez AA. Allergy and secretory otitis media. *JAMA* 1967; 200: 134–38.

44. Roukonen J, Pagnaus A, Lehti H. Elimination diets in the treatment of secretory otitis media. *Internat J Pediatr Otorhinolaryngol* 1982; 4: 39–46.

45. Sampson HA, Scanlon SM. Natural history of food hypersensitivity in children with atopic dermatitis. *J Pediatr* 1989; 115: 23–27.

46. Burks AW, Mallory SB, Williams LW, Shirrell MA. Atopic dermatitis: clinical relevance of food hypersensitivity. *J Pediatr* 1988; 113: 447–51.

47. Atherton DJ. Diet and atopic eczema. *Clin Allerg* 1988; 18: 215–28 [review].

48. Breneman JC. Allergy elimination diet as the most effective gallbladder diet. *Ann Allerg* 1968; 26: 83.

49. Pelto L, Salminen PL, Lilius E-M, et al. Milk hypersensitivity—key to poorly defined gastrointestinal symptoms in adults. *Allergy* 1998; 53: 307–10.

50. Berens C et al. Allergy in glaucoma. Manifestations of allergy in three glaucoma patients as determined by the pulse-diet method of Coca. *Ann Allerg* 1947; 5: 526.

51. Raymond LF. Allergy and chronic simple glaucoma. *Ann Allerg* 1996; 22: 146.

52. Eriksson NE. Food sensitivity reported by patients with asthma and hay fever. *Allergy* 1978; 25: 189–196.

53. Grant ECG. Food allergies and migraine. *Lancet* 1979; i: 966–69.

54. Rippere V. A little something between meals: masked addiction not low blood-sugar. *Lancet* 1979; Jun 23: 1349 [letter].

55. Bentley SJ, Pearson DJ, Rix KJ. Food hypersensitivity in irritable bowel syndrome. *Lancet* 1983; ii: 295–97.

56. Alun Jones V, McLaughlan P, Shorthouse M, et al. Food intolerance: a major factor in the pathogenesis of irritable bowel syndrome. *Lancet* 1982; ii: 1115–17.

57. Henz BM, Zuberbier T. Most chronic urticaria is food-dependent, and not idiopathic. *Exp Dermatol* 1998; 7: 139–42.

58. Grant EC. Food allergies and migraine. *Lancet* 1979; i: 966–69.

59. Monro J, Brostoff J, Carini C, Zilkha K. Food allergy in migraine. *Lancet* 1980; ii: 1–4.

60. Egger J, Carter CM, Wilson J, et al. Is migraine food allergy? A double-blind controlled trial of oligoantigenic diet treatment. *Lancet* 1983; ii: 865–69.

61. Hughs EC, Gott PS, Weinstein RC, Binggeli R. Migraine: a diagnostic test for etiology of food sensitivity by a nutritionally support-ed fast and confirmed by long-term report. *Ann Allerg* 1985; 55: 28–32.

62. Egger J, Carter CM, Soothill JF, Wilson J. Oligoantigenic diet treatment of children with epilepsy and migraine. *J Pediatr* 1989; 114: 51–58.

63. Kaufman W. Food-induced, allergic musculoskeletal syndromes. *Ann Allerg* 1953; Mar/Apr: 179–84.

64. Gaboardi F, Perlett L, Mihansch MJ. Dermatitis herpetiformis and nephrotic syndrome. *Clin Nephrol* 1983; 20: 49.

65. Meadow SR, Sarsfield JK. Steroid-responsive nephrotic syndrome and allergy: clinical studies. *Arch Dis Childhood* 1981; 56: 509–16.

66. Randolph TG. Masked food allergy as a factor in the development and persistence of obesity. *J Lab Clin Med* 1947; 32: 1547.

67. Douglas JM. Psoriasis and diet. *Western J Med* 1980; 133: 450 [letter].

68. Michaelsson G, Gerden B. How common is gluten intolerance among patients with psoriasis? *Acta Derm Venereol* 1991; 71: 90.

69. Rowe AH, Rowe A. Perennial nasal allergy due to food sensitization. *J Asthma Res* 1965; 3(2): 141–54.

70. Gerrard JW. Familiar recurrent thiorrhea and bronchitis due to cow's milk. *JAMA* 1966; 198(6): 137.

71. Eriksson NE. Food sensitivity reported by patients with asthma and hay fever. *Allergy* 1978; 25: 189–96.

72. Kern RA, Stewart G. Allergy in duodenal ulcer: incidence and significance of food hypersensitivities as observed in 32 patients. *J Allergy* 1931; 3: 51.

73. Reimann HJ, Lewin J. Gastric mucosal reactions in patients with food allergy. *Am J Gastroenterol* 1988; 83: 1212–19.

74. Horesh AJ. Allergy and infection. *J Asthma Res* 1967; 4: 269.

75. Rudolph JA. Allergy as a cause of frequent recurring colds and coughs in children. *Dis Chest* 1940; 6: 138.

76. Berman BA. Pseudomononucleosis of allergic origin: a new clinical entity. *Ann Allerg* 1964; 22: 403.

77. Randolph TG, Hettig RA. The coincidence of allergic disease, unexplained fatigue, and lymphadenopathy: possible diagnostic confusion with infectious mononucleosis. *Am J Med Sci* 1945; 209: 306.

78. Am Academy of Allergy. Position statements: controversial techniques. *J Allergy Clin Immunol* 1981: 333–8.

79. Gleich G, Yunginger J. The radioallergosorbent test: its present place and likely future in the practice of allergy. *Adv Asthma Allergy* 1975(Spring): 1.

80. Wraith DG. Recognition of food-allergic patients and their allergens by the RAST technique and clinical investigation. *Clin Allergy* 1979: 25–36.

81. Lieberman P et al. Controlled study of the cytotoxic food test. *JAMA* 1975: 728–30.

82. Miller JB. A double-blind study of food extract injection therapy: a preliminary report. *Ann Allerg* 1977: 185–91.

83. Hosen H. Provocative testing for food allergy diagnosis. *J Asthma Res* 1976: 45–51.

84. Jewett DL, Fein G, Greenberg MH. A double-blind study of symptom provocation to determine food sensitivity. *New Engl J Med* 1990; 323: 429–33.

85. Mandell M. *Dr. Mandell's 5-Day Allergy Relief System.* Pocket Books, New York, 1979.

86. Zamm AV, Gannon R. *Why Your House May Endanger Your Health.* Touchstone, New York, 1980.

87. Randolph TG. *Human Ecology and Susceptibility to the Chemical Environment.* Springfield, IL: Charles C Thomas, 1978.

Alzheimer's Disease

1. Priest ND. Satellite symposium on Alzheimer's disease and dietary aluminium. *Proc Nutr Soc* 1993; 52: 231–40.

2. Munoz DG. Is exposure to aluminum a risk factor for the development of Alzheimer disease?—No. *Arch Neurol* 1998; 55: 737–39 [review].

3. Munoz DG. Is exposure to aluminum a risk factor for the development of Alzheimer disease?—No. *Arch Neurol* 1998; 55: 737–39.

4. Forbes WF, Hill GB. Is exposure to aluminum a risk factor for the development of Alzheimer disease?—Yes. *Arch Neurol* 1998; 55: 740–41.

5. Grant WB. Dietary links to Alzheimer's disease. *Alz Dis Rev* 1997; 2: 42–55.

6. Smith MA, Petot GJ, Perry G. Diet and oxidative stress: a novel synthesis of epidemiological data on Alzheimer's disease. *Alz Dis Rev* 1997; 2: 58–59.

7. Kalmijn S, Lauher LJ, Ott A, et al. Dietary fat intake and the risk of incident dementia in the Rotterdam study. *Ann Neurol* 1997; 42: 776–82.

8. Crook T et al. Effects of phosphatidylserine in Alzheimer's disease. *Psychopharmacol Bull* 1992; 28: 61–66.

9. Gindin J, Novickov M, Kedar D, et al. The effect of plant phosphatidylserine on age-associated memory impairment and mood in the functioning elderly. Rehovot, Israel: Geriatric Institute for Education and Research, and Department of Geriatrics, Kaplan Hospital, 1995.

10. Sano M, Ernesto C, Thomas RG, et al. A controlled trial of selegiline, alpha-tocopherol, or both as treatment for Alzheimer's disease. *N Engl J Med* 1997; 336: 1216–22.

11. Morris MC, Beckett LA, Scherr PA, et al. Vitamin E and vitamin C supplement use and risk of incident Alzheimer disease. *Alz Dis Assoc Disorders* 1998; 12: 121–26.

12. Schmidt R, Hayn M, Reinhart B, et al. Plasma antioxidants and cognitive performance in middle-aged and older adults: results of the Austrian Stroke Prevention Study. *J Am Geriatr Soc* 1998; 46: 1407–10.

13. Lethem R, Orrell M. Antioxidants and dementia. *Lancet* 1997; 349: 1189–90 [commentary].

14. Ferris SH, Sathananthan G, Gershon S, et al. Senile dementia. Treatment with Deanol. *J Am Ger Soc* 1977; 25: 241–44.

15. Fisman M, Mersky H, Helmes E. Double-blind trial of 2-dimethylaminoethanol in Alzheimer's disease. *Am J Psych* 1981; 138: 970–72.

16. Pettegrew JW, Klunk WE, Panchalingam K, et al. Clinical and neurochemical effects of acetyl-L-carnitine in Alzheimer's disease. *Neurobio Aging* 1995; 16: 1–4.

17. Salvioli G, Neri M. L-acetyl-carnitine treatment of mental decline in the elderly. *Drugs Exp Clin Res* 1994; 20: 169–76.

18. Cucinotta D et al. Multicenter clinical placebo-controlled study with acetyl-L-carnitine (LAC) in the treatment of mildly demented elderly patients. *Drug Development Res* 1988; 14: 213–16.

19. Thal LJ, Carta A, Clarke WR, et al. A 1-year multi-center placebo-controlled study of aceyl-L-carnitine in patients with Alzheimer's disease. *Neurol* 1996; 47: 705–11.

20. Calvani M, Carta A, Caruso G, et al. Action of acetyl-L-carnitine in neurodegeneration and Alzheimer's disease. *Ann NY Acad Sci* 1992; 663: 483–86.

21. Xu SS, Gao ZX, Weng Z, et al. Efficacy of tablet huperzine-A on memory, cognition, and behavior in Alzheimer's disease. *Chung Kuo Yao Li Hsueh Pao* 1995; 16: 391–95.

22. Zhang RW, Tang XC, Han YY, et al. Drug evaluation of huperzine A in the treatment of senile memory disorders. *Chung Kuo Yao Li Hsueh Pao* 1991; 12: 250–52 [in Chinese].

23. Imagawa M, Naruse S, Tsuji S, et al. Coenzyme Q_{10}, iron, and vitamin B_6 in genetically-confirmed Alzheimer's disease. *Lancet* 1992; 340: 671 [letter].

24. Bush AI, Pettingell WH, Multhaup G, et al. Rapid induction of Alzheimer A8 amyloid formation by zinc. *Science* 1994; 265: 1464–65.

25. Potocnik FCV, van Rensburg SJ, Park C, et al. Zinc and platelet membrane microviscosity in Alzheimer's disease. *S Afr Med J* 1997; 87: 1116–19.

26. Prasad AS. Zinc in human health: an update. *J Trace Elements Exper Med* 1998; 11: 63–87.

27. Birkmayer JGD. Coenzyme nicotinamide adenine dinucleotide: New therapeutic approach for improving dementia of the Alzheimer type. *Ann Clin Lab Sci* 1996; 26: 1–9.

28. Clarke R, Smith D, Jobst KA, et al. Foate, vitamin B$_{12}$, and serum total homocysteine levels in confirmed Alzheimer disease. *Arch Neurol* 1998; 55: 1449–55.

29. Joosten E, Lesaffre E, Riezler R, et al. Is metabolic evidence for vitamin B-12 and folate deficiency more frequent in elderly patients with Alzheimer's disease? *J Gastroenterol* 1997; 52A: M76–M79.

30. Le Bars PL, Katz MM, Berman N, et al. A placebo-controlled, double-blind, randomized trial of an extract of *Ginkgo biloba* for dementia. North American EGb Study Group. *JAMA* 1997; 278: 1327–32.

31. Hofferberth B. The efficacy of EGb 761 in patients with senile dementia of the Alzheimer type, a double-blind, placebo-controlled study on different levels of investigation. *Human Psychopharmacol* 1994; 9: 215–22.

32. Kanowski S, Herrmann W, Stephan K, et al. Proof of efficacy of the *Ginkgo biloba* special extract EGb 761 in outpatients suffering from mild to moderate primary degenerative dementia of the Alzheimer type or multi-infarct dementia. *Pharmacopsychiatry* 1996; 29: 47–56.

33. Bhattacharya SK, Kumar A, Ghosal S. Effects of glycowithanolides from *Withania somnifera* on an animal model of Alzheimer's disease and perturbed central cholinergic markers of cognition in rats. *Phytother Res* 1995; 9: 110–13.

34. D'Angelo L, Grimaldi R, et al. A double-blind, placebo-controlled clinical study of a standardized ginseng extract on psychomotor performance in healthy volunteers. *J Ethnopharmacol* 1986; 16: 15–22.

35. Owen RT. Ginseng—a pharmacological profile. *Drugs Today* 1981; 17: 343–51.

Angina

1. Deanfield J, Wright C, Krikler S, et al. Cigarette smoking and the treatment of angina with propranolol, atenolol, and nifedipine. *N Engl J Med* 1984; 310: 951–54.

2. Glantz SA, Parmley WW. Passive smoking and heart disease. *JAMA* 1995; 273: 1047–53 [review].

3. Todd IC, Ballantyne D. Antianginal efficacy of exercise training: A comparison with beta blockade. *Br Heart J* 1990; 64: 14–19.

4. LaCroix AZ, Mead LA, Liang KY, et al. Coffee consumption and the incidence of coronary heart disease. *N Engl J Med* 1986; 315: 977–82.

5. Cherchi A, Lai C, Angelino F, et al. Effects of L-carnitine on exercise tolerance in chronic stable angina: A multicenter, double-blind, randomized, placebo-controlled crossover study. *Int J Clin Pharm Ther Toxicol* 1985; 23: 569–72.

6. Canale C, Terrachini V, Biagini A, et al. Bicycle ergometer and echocardiographic study in healthy subjects and patients with angina pectoris after administration of L-carnitine: Semiautomatic computerized analysis of M-mode tracing. *Int J Clin Pharmacol Ther Toxicol* 1988; 26: 221–24.

7. Cacciatore L, Cerio R, et al. The therapeutic effect of L-carnitine in patients with exercise-induced stable angina: A controlled study. *Drugs Exp Clin Res* 1991; 17: 225–35.

8. Kamikawa T, Kobayashi A, Yamashita T, et al. Effects of coenzyme Q$_{10}$ on exercise tolerance in chronic stable angina pectoris. *Am J Cardiol* 1985; 56: 247.

9. Mortensen SA. Perspectives on therapy of cardiovascular diseases with coenzyme Q$_{10}$ (ubiquinone). *Clin Invest* 1993; 71: S116–23 [review].

10. Riemersma RA, Wood DA, Macintyre CC, et al. Risk of angina pectoris and plasma concentrations of vitamins A, C, and E and carotene. *Lancet* 1991; 337: 1–5.

11. Rinzler SH, Bakst H, Benjamin ZH, et al. Failure of alpha-tocopherol to influence chest pain in patients with heart disease. *Circulation* 1950; 1: 288–90.

12. Rapola RM, Virtamo J, Haukka JK, et al. Effect of vitamin E and beta carotene on the incidence of angina pectoris. A randomized, double-blind, controlled trial. *JAMA* 1996; 275: 693–98.

13. Miwa K, Miyagi Y, Igawa A, et al. Vitamin E deficiency in variant angina. *Circulation* 1996; 94: 14–18.

14. Saynor R, Verel D, Gillott T. The long-term effect of dietary supplementation with fish lipid concentrate on serum lipids, bleeding time, platelets and angina. *Atheroscl* 1984; 50: 3–10.

15. Mehta JL, Lopez LM, Lawson D, et al. Dietary supplementation with omega-3 polyunsaturated fatty acids in patients with stable coronary heart disease. Effects on indices of platelet and neutrophil function and exercise performance. *Am J Med* 1988; 84: 45–52.

16. Wander RC, Du SH, Ketchum SO, Rowe KE. Alpha-tocopherol influences in vivo indices of lipid peroxidation in postmenopausal women given fish oil. *J Nutr* 1996; 126: 643–52.

17. Turlapaty P, Altura B. Magnesium deficiency produces spasms of coronary arteries: Relationship to etiology of sudden death ischemic heart disease. *Science* 1980; 208: 199–200.

18. Goto K, Yasue H, Okumura K, et al. Magnesium deficiency detected by intravenous loading test in variant angina pectoris. *Am J Cardiol* 1990; 65: 709–12.

19. Cohen L, Kitzes R. Magnesium sulfate in the treatment of variant angina. *Magnesium* 1984; 3: 46–49.

20. Cohen L, Kitzes R. Prompt termination and/or prevention of cold-pressor-stimulus-induced vasoconstriction of different vascular beds by magnesium sulfate in patients with Prinzmetal's angina. *Magnesium* 1986; 5: 144–49.

21. Mollace V, Romeo F, Martuscelli E, et al. Low formation of nitric oxide in polymorphonuclear cells in unstable angina pectoris. *Am J Cardiol* 1994; 74: 65–68.

22. Ceremuzynski L, Chamiec T, Herbaczynska-Cedro K. Effect of supplemental oral L-arginine on exercise capacity in patients with stable angina pectoris. *Am J Cardiol* 1997; 80: 331–33.

23. Egashira K, Hirooka Y, Kuga T, et al. Effects of L-arginine supplementation on endothelium-dependent coronary vasodilation in patients with angina pectoris and normal coronary

Part One: References

arteriograms. *Circulation* 1996; 94: 130–34.

24. Heinicke R, van der Wal L, Yokoyama M. Effect of bromelain (Ananase) on human platelet aggregation. *Experientia* 1972; 28: 844–45.

25. Nieper HA. Effect of bromelain on coronary heart disease and angina pectoris. *Acta Med Empirica* 1978; 5: 274–78.

26. Seligman B. Oral bromelains as adjuncts in the treatment of acute thrombophlebitis. *Angiology* 1969; 20: 22–26.

27. Hanack T, Bruckel MH. The treatment of mild stable forms of angina pectoris using Crataegutt novo. *Therapiewoche* 1983; 33: 4331–33 [in German].

Anxiety

1. Miler JJ, Fletcher K, Kabat-Zinn J, et al. Three-year follow-up and clinical implications of a mindfulness meditation-based stress reduction intervention in the treatment of anxiety disorders. *Gen Hosp Psychiatry* 1995; 17: 192–200.

2. Bruce M et al. Anxiogenic effects of caffeine in patients with anxiety disorders. *Arch Gen Psychiatry* 1992; 49: 867–69.

3. Weston PG et al. Magnesium sulfate as a sedative. *Am J Med Sci* 1923; 165: 431–33.

4. Benjamin J, Levine J, Fux M, et al. Double-blind, placebo-controlled, crossover trial of inositol treatment for panic disorder. *Am J Psychiatry* 1995; 152: 1084–86.

5. Mohler H, Polc P, Cumin R, et al. Niacinamide is a brain constituent with benzodiazepine-like actions. *Nature* 1979; 278: 563–65.

6. Vescovi PP et al. Nicotinic acid effectiveness in the treatment of benzodiazepine withdrawal. *Curr Ther Res* 1987; 41: 1017.

7. Piscopo G. Kava kava: Gift of the islands. *Alt Med Rev* 1997; 2: 355–81 [review].

8. Lehmann EE, Kinzler J, Friedmann J. Efficacy of a special kava extract (*Piper methysticum*) in patients with states of anxiety, tension and excitedness of non-mental origin. A double-blind placebo-controlled study of four weeks treatment. *Phytomedicine* 1996; 3: 113–19.

9. Volz HP, Kieser M. Kava-kava extract WS 1490 versus placebo in anxiety disorders. A randomized placebo-controlled 25-week outpatient trial. *Pharmacopsychiatry* 1997; 30: 1–5.

10. Warnecke G. Psychosomatic dysfunctions in the female climacteric. Clinical effectiveness and tolerance of kava extract WS 1490. *Fortscher Med* 1991; 119–22 [in German].

11. Almeida JC, Grimsley EW. Coma from the health food store: Interaction between kava and alprazolam. *Arch Intern Med* 1996; 125: 940–41.

12. Woelk H, Kapoula S, Lehrl S, et al. Treatment of patients suffering from anxiety—double-blind study: Kava special extract versus benzodiazepines. *Z Allegemeinmed* 1993; 69: 271–77 [in German].

13. Volz HP, Kieser M. Kava-kava extract WS 1490 vs. placebo in anxiety disorders—A randomized placebo-controlled 25-week outpatient trial. *Pharmacopsychiatry* 1997; 30: 1–5.

14. Witte B, Harrer G, Kaptan T, et al. Treatment of depressive symptoms with a high concentration Hypericum preparation. A multicenter placebo-controlled double-blind study. *Fortschr Med* 1995; 113: 404–408 [in German].

15. Baureithel KH, Buter KB, Engesser A, et al. Inhibition of benzodiazepine binding in vitro by amentoflavone, a constituent of various species of Hypericum. *Pharm Acta Helv* 1997; 72: 153–57.

16. Viola H, de Stein ML, et al. Apigenin, a component of *Matricaria recutita* flowers, is a central benzodiazpine receptors-ligand with anxiolytic effects. *Planta Med* 1995; 61: 213–16.

17. Yamada K, Miura T, Mimaki Y, Sashida Y. Effect of inhalation of chamomile oil vapour on plasma ACTH level in ovariectomized rats under restriction stress. *Biol Pharm Bull* 1996; 19: 1244–46.

18. Brown D. Valerian root: Non-addictive alternative for insomnia and anxiety. *Quart Rev Nat Med* 1994; Fall: 221–24 [review].

Asthma

1. Lindahl O, Lindwall L, Spangberg A, et al. Vegan regimen with reduced medication in the treatment of bronchial asthma. *J Asthma* 1985; 22: 45–55.

2. Chiaramonte LT, Altman D. Food sensitivity in asthma: perception and reality. *J Asthma* 1991; 28: 5–9.

3. Rowe AH, Young EJ. Bronchial asthma due to food allergy alone in ninety-five patients. *JAMA* 1959; 169: 1158.

4. Sampson HA, Mendelson L, Rosen JP. Fatal and near-fatal anaphylactic reactions to food in children and adolescents. *N Engl J Med* 1992; 327: 380.

5. Genton C, Frie PC, Pecoud A. Value of oral provocation tests to aspirin and food additives in the routine investigation of asthma and chronic urticaria. *J Asthma* 1985; 76: 40–45.

6. Townes SJ, Mellis CM. Role of acetyl salicylic acid and sodium metabisulfite in chronic childhood asthma. *Pediatr* 1984; 73: 631–37.

7. Soyka F, Edmonds A. *The Ion Effect*. New York: Bantam, 1977.

8. Bowler SD, Green A, Mitchell CA. Buteyko breathing techniques in asthma: a blinded randomised controlled trial. *Med J Austral* 1998; 169: 575–78.

9. Collipp PJ et al. Tryptophane metabolism in bronchial asthma. *Ann Allergy* 1975; 35: 153–58.

10. Weir MR et al. Depression of vitamin B_6 levels due to theophylline. *Ann Allergy* 1990; 65: 59–62.

11. Collipp PJ et al. Pyridoxine treatment of childhood bronchial asthma. *Ann Allergy* 1975; 35: 93–97.

12. Reynolds RD, Natta CL. Depressed plasma pyridoxal phosphate concentrations in adult asthmatics. *Am J Clin Nutr* 1985; 41: 684–88.

13. Sur S, Camara M, Buchmeier A, et al. Double-blind trial of pyridoxine (vitamin B_6) in the treatment of steroid-dependent asthma. *Ann Allerg* 1993; 70: 141–52.

14. Haury VG. Blood serum magnesium in bronchial asthma and its treatment by the administration of magnesium sulfate. *J Lab Clin Med* 1940; 26: 340–44.

15. Skobeloff EM et al. Intravenous magnesium sulfate for the treatment of acute asthma in the emergency department. *JAMA* 1989; 262: 1210–13.

16. Zuskin E et al. Byssinosis and airway responses due to exposure to textile dust. *Lung* 1976; 154: 17–24.

17. Bucca C, Rolla G, Oliva A, Farina J-C. Effect of vitamin C on histamine bronchial responsiveness of patients with allergic rhinitis. *Ann Allerg* 1990; 65: 311–14.

18. Ruskin SL. Sodium ascorbate in the treatment of allergic disturbances. The role of adrenal cortical hormone-sodium-vitamin C. *Am J Dig Dis* 1947; 14: 302–306.

19. Anibarro B et al. Asthma with sulfite intolerance in children: A blocking study with cyanocobalamin. *J Allerg Clin Immunol* 1992; 90: 103–109.

20. Johnson JL et al. Molybdenum cofactor deficiency in a patient previously characterized as deficient in sulfite oxidase. *Biochem Med Metabol Biol* 1988; 40: 86–93.

21. Stone J, Hinks LJ, Beasley R, et al. Reduced selenium status of patients with asthma. *Clin Sci* 1989; 77: 495–500.

22. Flatt A, Pearce N, Thomson CD, et al. Reduced selenium in asthmatic subjects in New Zealand. *Thorax* 1990; 45: 95–99.

23. Owen S, Pearson D, Suarez-Mendez V, et al. Evidence of free-radical activity in asthma. *N Engl J Med* 1991; 325: 586–87 [letter].

24. Hasselmark L, Malmgren R, Zetterstrom O, Unge G. Selenium supplementation in intrinsic asthma. *Allerg* 1993; 48: 30–36.

25. Arm JP, Horton CE, Eiser NM, et al. The effects of dietary supplementation with fish oil on asthmatic responses to antigen. *Allerg Clin Immunol* 1988; 81: 183 [abstract #57].

26. Broughton KS, Johnson CS, Pace BK, et al. Reduced asthma symptoms with n-3 fatty acid ingestion are related to 5-series leukotriene production. *Am J Clin Nutr* 1997; 65: 1011–17.

27. Dry J, Vincent D. Effect of a fish oil diet on asthma: results of a 1-year double-blind study. *Int Arch Allerg Appl Immunol* 1991; 95: 156–57.

28. Thien FCK, Woods RK, Waters EH. Oily fish and asthma—a fishy story? *Med J Austral* 1996; 164: 135–36 [editorial].

29. Hodge L, Salome CM, Peat JK, et al. Consumption of oily fish and childhood asthma risk. *Med J Austral* 1996; 164: 137–40.

30. Bray GW. The hypochlorhydria of asthma in childhood. *Quart J Med* 1931; 24: 181–97.

31. Welton AF, Tobias LD, Fiedler-Nagy C, et al. Effect of flavonoids on arachidonic acid metabolism. *Prog Clin Biol Res* 1986; 213: 231–42.

32. Schafer A, Adelman B. Plasma inhibition of platelet function and of arachidonic acid metabolism. *J Clin Invest* 1985; 75: 456–61.

33. Leung AY, Foster S. *Encyclopedia of Common Natural Ingredients Used in Foods, Drugs, and Cosmetics,* 2d ed. New York: John Wiley & Sons, 1996, 227–29.

34. Guinot P, Brambilla Dunchier J, et al. Effect of BN 52063, a specific PAF-ascether antagonist, on bronchial provocation test to allergens in asthmatic patients—a preliminary study. *Prostaglandins* 1987; 34(5): 723–31.

35. Li M, Yang B, Yu H, Zhang H. Clinical observation of the therapeutic effect of ginkgo leaf concentrated oral liquor on bronchial asthma. *Chinese J Integrative & Western Med* 1997; 3: 264–67.

36. Felter HW, Lloyd JU. *King's American Dispensatory,* 18th ed. Sandy, OR: Eclectic Medical Publications, 1898, 1983, 1199–1205.

37. Ellingwood F. *American Materia Medica, Therapeutics and Pharmacognosy,* 11th ed. Sandy, OR: Eclectic Medical Publications, 1919, 1998, 235–42.

Atherosclerosis (Hardening of the Arteries)

1. Nelson GJ. Dietary fat, *trans* fatty acids, and risk of coronary heart disease. *Nutr Rev* 1998; 250–52.

2. Brown L, Rosner B, Willett WW, Sacks FM. Cholesterol-lowering effects of dietary fiber: a meta-analysis. *Am J Clin Nutr* 1999; 69: 30–42.

3. Ascherio A, Willett WC. Health effects of trans fatty acids. *Am J Clin Nutr* 1997; 66(suppl): 1006S–10S [review].

4. Raloff J. Oxidized lipids: a key to heart disease? *Sci News* 1985; 127: 278.

5. Ornish D, Brown SE, Scherwitz LW, et al. Can lifestyle changes reverse coronary heart disease? *Lancet* 1990; 336: 129–33.

6. Belcher JD, Balla J, Balla G, et al. Vitamin E, LDL, and endothelium: Brief oral vitamin supplementation prevents oxidized LDL-mediated vascular injury in vitro. *Arterioscler Thromb* 1993; 13: 1779–89.

7. Stephens NG, Parsons A, Schofield PM, et al. Randomised controlled trial of vitamin E in patients with coronary disease: Cambridge Heart Antioxidant Study (CHAOS). *Lancet* 1996; 347: 781–86.

8. Rimm E. Micronutrients, Coronary Heart disease and cancer: Should we all be on supplements? Presented at the 60th Annual Biology Colloquium, Oregon State University, Corvallis, OR, February 25, 1999.

9. Salonen JT et al. Association between cardiovascular death and myocardial infarction and serum selenium in a matched-pair longitudinal study. *Lancet* 1982; ii: 175.

10. Shamberger RJ, Willis CE. Epidemiological studies on selenium and heart disease. *Fed Proc* 1976; 35: 578 [abstract #2061].

11. Korpela H, Kumpulainen J, Jussila E, et al. Effect of selenium supplementation after acute myocardial infarction. *Res Comm Chem Pathol Pharmacol* 1989; 65: 249–52.

12. Ronzio RA. Antioxidants, nutraceuticals and functional foods. *Townsend Letter for Doctors and Patients* Oct 1996: 34–35 [review].

Part One: References

13. Hertog MGL, Feskens EJM, Hollman PCH, et al. Dietary antioxidant flavonoids and risk of coronary heart disease: the Zutphen Elderly Study. *Lancet* 1993; 342: 1007–11.

14. Hertog MGL, Kromhout D, Aravanis C, et al. Flavonoid intake and long-term risk of coronary heart disease and cancer in the Seven Countries Study. *Arch Intern Med* 1995; 155: 381–86.

15. Knekt P, Jarvinen R, Reunanen A, Maatela J. Flavonoid intake and coronary mortality in Finland: a cohort study. *BMJ* 1996; 312: 478–81.

16. Rimm EB, Katan MB, Ascherio A, et al. Relation between intake of flavonoids and risk for coronary heart disease in male health professionals. *Ann Intern Med 1996*; 125: 384–89.

17. Hertog MGL, Sweetnam PM, Fehily AM, et al. Antioxidant flavonols and ischemic heart disease in a Welsh population of men: the Caerphilly Study. *Am J Clin Nutr* 1997; 65: 1489–94.

18. Stampfer MJ, Malinow R, Willett WC, et al. A prospective study of plasma homocyst(e)ine and risk of myocardial infarction in U.S. physicians. *JAMA* 1992; 268: 877–81.

19. Folsom AR, Nieto FJ, McGovern PG, et al. Prospective study of coronary heart disease incidence in relation to fasting total homocysteine, related genetic polymorphisms, and B vitamins. *Circulation* 1998; 98: 204–10.

20. Kuller LH, Evans RW. Homocysteine, vitamins, and cardiovascular disease. *Circulation* 1998; 98: 196–99 [editorial/review].

21. Stolzenberg-Solomon RZ, Miller ER III, Maguire MG, et al. Association of dietary protein intake and coffee consumption with serum homocysteine concentrations in an older population. *Am J Clin Nutr* 1999; 69: 467–75.

22. Selhub J, Jacques PF, Wilson PW, et al. Vitamin status and intake as primary determinants of homocysteinemia in an elderly population. *JAMA* 1993; 270: 2693–98.

23. Ubbink JB, Hayward WJ, van der Merwe A, et al. Vitamin require-ments for the treatment of hyperho-mocysteinemia in humans. *J Nutr* 1994; 124: 1927–33.

24. Manson JB, Miller JW. The effects of vitamin B_{12}, B_6, and folate on blood homocysteine levels. *Ann NY Acad Sci* 1992; 669: 197–204 [review].

25. Franken DG, Boers GHJ, Blom HJ, et al. Treatment of mild hyperhomocysteinemia in vascular disease patients. *Arterioscler Thromb* 1994; 14: 465–70.

26. Ubbink JB, Vermaak WJH, van der Merwe A, et al. Vitamin requirements for the treatment of hyperhomocysteinemia in humans. *J Nutr* 1994; 124: 1927–33.

27. Ubbink JB, van der Merwe A, Vermaak WJH, Delport R. Hyperhomocysteinemia and the response to vitamin supplementation. *Clin Investig* 1993; 71: 993–98.

28. Folsom AR, Nieto FJ, McGovern PG, et al. Prospective study of coronary heart disease incidence in relation to fasting total homocysteine, related genetic polymorphisms, and B vitamins. *Circulation* 1998; 98: 204–10.

29. Chambers JC, McGregor A, Jean-Marie J, et al. Demonstration of rapid onset vascular endothelial dysfunction after hyperhomocysteinemia. An effect reversible with vitamin C therapy. *Circulation* 1999; 99: 1156–60.

30. Frei B. Ascorbic acid protects lipids in human plasma and low-density lipoprotein against oxidative damage. *Am J Clin Nutr* 1991; 54: 1113S–18S.

31. Balz F. Antioxidant Vitamins and Heart Disease. Presented at the 60th Annual Biology Colloquium, Oregon State University, Corvallis, OR, February 25, 1999.

32. Boberg M, Vessby B, Selinus I. Effects of dietary supplementation with n-6 and n-3 long-chain polyunsaturated fatty acids on serum lipoproteins and platelet function in hypertriglceridaemic patients. *Acta Med Scand* 1986; 220: 153–60.

33. Horrobin DF, Manku MS. How do polyunsaturated fatty acids lower plasma cholesterol levels? *Lipids* 1983; 558–62.

34. Morrison LM, Branwood AW, Ershoff BH, et al. The prevention of coronary arteriosclerotic heart disease with chondroitin sulfate A: Preliminary report. *Exp Med Surg* 1969; 27: 278–89.

35. Morrison LM, Enrick NL. Coronary heart disease: Reduction of death rate by chondroitin sulfate A. *Angiology* 1973; 24: 269–82.

36. Bertelli AA, Giovanninni L, Bernini W, et al. Antiplatelet activity of cis-resveratrol. *Drugs Exp Clin Res* 1996; 22(2): 61–63.

37. Chen CK, Pace-Asciak CR. Vasorelaxing activity of resveratrol and quercetin in isolated rat aorta. *Gen Pharm* 1996; 27(2): 363–66.

38. Pace-Asciak CR, Rounova O, Hahn SE, et al. Wines and grape juices as modulators of platelet aggregation in healthy human subjects. *Clin Chim Acta* 1996; 246(1–2): 163–82.

39. Batista J, Stusser R, Penichet M, Uguet E. Doppler-ultrasound pilot study of the effects of long-term policosanol therapy on carotid-vertebral atherosclerosis. *Curr Ther Res* 1995; 56: 906–8.

40. Salonen JT, Nyssönen K, Korpela H, et al. High stored iron levels are associated with excess risk of myocardial infarction in Eastern Finnish men. *Circulation* 1992; 86: 803–11.

41. Van Asperen IA, Feskens EJM, Bowles CH, Kromhout D. Body iron stores and mortality due to cancer and ischaemic heart disease: a 17-year follow-up study of elderly men and women. *Int J Epidemiol* 1995; 24: 665–70.

42. Iribarren C, Sempos CT, Eckfeldt JH, Folsom AR. Lack of association between ferritin level and measures of LDL oxidation: the ARIC study. *Atherosclerosis* 1998; 139: 189–95.

43. Corti M-C, Guralnik JM, Salive ME, et al. Serum iron level, coronary artery disease, and all-cause mortality in older men and women. *Am J Cardiol* 1997; 79: 120–27.

44. Tzonou A, Lagiou P, Trichopoulou A, et al. Dietary iron and coronary heart disease risk: a study from Greece. *Am J Epidemiol* 1998; 147: 161–66.

45. Kiechl S, Willeit J, Egger G, et al. Body iron stores and the risk of carotid atherosclerosis. *Circulation* 1997; 96: 3300–307.

46. Danesh J, Appleby P. Coronary heart disease and iron status. Meta-analyses of prospective studies. *Circulation* 1999; 99: 852–54.

47. Olson BH, Anderson SM, Becker MP, et al. Psyllium-enriched cereals lower blood total cholesterol and LDL cholesterol, but not HDL cholesterol, in hypercholesterolemic adults: Results of a meta-analysis. *J Nutr* 1997; 127: 1973–80.

48. Neil HAW, Silagy CA, Lancaster T, et al. Garlic powder in the treatment of moderate hyperlipidaemia: A controlled trial and a meta-analysis. *J R Coll Phys* 1996; 30: 329–34.

49. McCrindle BW, Helden E, Conner WT. Garlic extract therapy in children with hypercholesterolemia. *Arch Pediatr Adolesc Med* 1998; 152: 1089–94.

50. Isaacsohn JL, Moser M, Stein EA, et al. Garlic powder and plasma lipids and lipoproteins. *Arch Intern Med* 1998; 158: 1189–94.

51. Berthold HK, Sudhop T, von Bergmann K. Effect of a garlic oil preparation on serum lipoproteins and cholesterol metabolism. *JAMA* 1998; 279: 1900–902.

52. Lawson L. Garlic oil for hypercholesterolemia–negative results. *Quart Rev Natural Med* 1998; Fall: 185–86.

53. Garlic powder for hyperlipidemia–analysis of recent negative results. *Quart Rev Natural Med* 1998; Fall: 187–89.

54. Kiesewetter H et al. Effect of garlic on thrombocyte aggregation, microcirculation and other risk factors. *Int J Pharm Ther Toxicol* 1991; 29(4): 151–54.

55. Srivastava KC, Tyagi OD. Effect of a garlic derived principle (ajoene) on aggregation and arachidonic acid metabolism in human blood platelets. *Prostagl Leukotr Ess Fatty Acids* 1993; 49: 587–95.

56. Braquet P, Touqui L, Shen TS, Vargaftig BB. Perspectives in platelet activating factor research. *Pharmacol Rev* 1987; 39: 97–210.

57. Brown DJ. *Herbal Prescriptions for Better Health.* Rocklin, CA: Prima Publishing, 1996, 119–28.

58. Kiesewetter H, Jung F, Mrowietz C, et al. Effects of garlic on blood fluidity and fibrinolytic activity: A randomised, placebo-controlled, double-blind study. *Br J Clin Pract Suppl* 1990; 69: 24–29.

59. Jung F, Mrowietz C, Kiesewetter H, Wenzel E. Effect of *Ginkgo biloba* on fluidity of blood and peripheral microcirculation in volunteers. *Arzneim Forsch Drug Res* 1990; 40: 589–93.

60. Brown D, Austin S. *Hyperlipidemia and Prevention of Coronary Heart Disease.* Seattle: Natural Product Research Consultants, 1997, 4–6.

61. Phelps S, Harris WS. Garlic supplementation and lipoprotein oxidation susceptibility. *Lipids* 1993; 28(5): 475–77.

62. Yan LJ, Droy-Lefaix MT, Packer L. *Ginkgo biloba* extract (EGb 761) protects human low density lipoproteins against oxidative modification mediated by copper. *Biochem Biophys Res Comm* 1995; 212: 360–66.

63. Singh K, Chander R, Kapoor NK. Guggulsterone, a potent hypolipidaemic, prevents oxidation of low density lipoprotein. *Phytother Res* 1997; 11: 291–94.

64. Sharma RD, Raghuram TC, Dayasagar Rao V. Hypolipidaemic effect of fenugreek seeds. A clinical study. *Phytother Res* 1991; 5: 145–47.

65. Foster A, Chongxi Y. *Herbal Emissaries.* Rochester, VT: Healing Arts Press, 1992, 79–85.

66. Bordia A, Verma SK, Srivastava KC. Effect of ginger (*Zingiber officinale* Rosc) and fenugreek (*Trigonella foenumgraceum* L) on blood lipids, blood sugar, and platelet aggregation in patients with coronary artery disease. *Prostagland Leukotrienes Essential Fatty Acids* 1997; 56: 379–84.

67. Lumb AB. Effect of dried ginger on human platelet function. *Thromb Haemost* 1994; 7: 110–11.

68. Janssen PLTMK, Meyboom S, van Staveren WA, de Vegt F, Katan MB. Consumption of ginger (*Zingiber officinale* Roscoe) does not affect ex vivo platelet thromboxane production in humans. *Eur J Clin Nutr* 1996; 50: 772–74.

69. Srivastava R, Dikshit M, Srimal RC, Dhawan BN. Anti-thrombotic action of curcumin. *Throm Res* 1985; 404: 413–17.

70. Srivastava KC, Bordia A, Verma SK. Curcumin, a major component of food spice turmeric (*Curcuma longa*) inhibits aggregation and alters eicosanoid metabolism in human blood platelets. *Prost Leuk Essen Fat Acids.* 1995; 52: 223–27.

71. Pulliero G, Montin S, et al. Ex vivo study of the inhibitory effects of *Vaccinium myrtillus* (bilberry) anthocyanosides on human platelet aggregation. *Fitoterapia* 1989; 60: 69–75.

72. Mavers VWH, Hensel H. Changes in local myocardial blood flow following oral administration to a *Crataegus* extract to non-anesthetized dogs. *Arzneim Forsch* 1974; 24: 783–85.

73. Felix W, Schmidt Y, Nieberle J. Protective effect of *Ruscus* extract against injury of vascular endothelium and vascular smooth muscle caused by ethracrynic acid. *Int Angiol* 1983; 3: 77.

Athlete's Foot

1. Tong MM, Altman PM, Barnetson RS. Tea tree oil in the treatment of tinea pedis. *Aust J Dermatol* 1992; 33: 145–49.

2. Ledezma E, DeSousa L, Jorquera A, et al. Efficacy of ajoene, an organosulphur derived from garlic, in the short-term therapy of tinea pedis. *Mycoses* 1996; 39: 393–95.

Athletic Performance

1. American Dietetic Association: Position of the American Dietetic Association and the Canadian Dietetic Association: Nutrition for physical fitness and athletic performance for adults. *J Am Diet Assoc* 1993; 93: 691–96.

2. McArdle WD, Katch FI, Katch VL. *Sports & exercise nutrition.*

Chapter 12, Body composition assessment and sport-specific observations. Philadelphia, PA: Lippincott, Williams & Wilkins, 1999.

3. Wilmore JH, Costill DL. *Physiology of sport and exercise.* Champaign, IL: Human Kinetics, 1994, 110–14.

4. Grandjean AC. *Sports nutrition.* In: Mellion MB, Walsh WM, Shelton GL, eds. The team physician's handbook. Philadelphia, PA: Hanley & Belfus, 1990,78–91.

5. Thornton JS. Feast or famine: eating disorders in athletes. *Phys Sportsmed* 1990; 18: 116–22 [review].

6. Thornton JS. How can you tell when an athlete is too thin? *Phys Sportsmed* 1990; 18: 124–33 [review].

7. Walberg-Rankin J. Dietary carbohydrate as an ergogenic aid for prolonged and brief competitions in sport. *Int J Sport Nutr* 1995; 5: S13–38 [review].

8. Jacobs KA, Sherman WM. The efficacy of carbohydrate supplementation and chronic high-carbohydrate diets for improving endurance performance. *Int J Sport Nutr* 1999; 9: 92–115 [review].

9. Costill DL. Carbohydrates for exercise: dietary demands for optimal performance. *Int J Sports Med* 1988; 9: 1–18 [review].

10. Walberg-Rankin J. Dietary carbohydrate as an ergogenic aid for prolonged and brief competitions in sport. *Int J Sport Nutr* 1995; 5: S13–28 [review].

11. Ivy JL. Glycogen resynthesis after exercise: effect of carbohydrate intake. *Int J Sports Med* 1998; 19: S142–45 [review].

12. Cade JR, Reese RH, Privette RM, et al. Dietary intervention and training in swimmers. *Eur J Appl Physiol* 1991; 63: 210–15.

13. Kraemer WJ, Volek JS, Bush JA, et al. Hormonal responses to consecutive days of heavy-resistance exercise with or without nutritional supplementation. *J Appl Physiol* 1998; 85: 1544–55.

14. Chandler RM, Byrne HK, Patterson JG, et al. Dietary supplements affect the anabolic hormones after weight-training exercise. *J Appl Physiol* 1994; 76: 839–45.

15. Hawley JA, Schabort EJ, Noakes TD, et al. Carbohydrate-loading and exercise performance. An update. *Sports Med* 1997; 24: 73–81 [review].

16. Costill DL. Carbohydrates for exercise: dietary demands for optimal performance. *Int J Sports Med* 1988; 9: 1–18 [review].

17. Lemon PW. Effects of exercise on dietary protein requirements. *Int J Sport Nutr* 1998; 8: 426–47 [review].

18. Lemon PW. Is increased dietary protein necessary or beneficial for individuals with a physically active lifestyle? *Nutr Rev* 1996; 54: S169–75 [review].

19. Hawley JA, Brouns F, Jeukendrup A. Strategies to enhance fat utilisation during exercise. *Sports Med* 1998; 25: 241–57 [review].

20. Jeukendrup AE, Saris WH, Wagenmakers AJ. Fat metabolism during exercise: a review—part III: effects of nutritional interventions. *Int J Sports Med* 1998 Aug; 19(6): 371–79 [review].

21. Whitley HA, Humphreys SM, Campbell IT, et al. Metabolic and performance responses during endurance exercise after high-fat and high-carbohydrate meals. *J Appl Physiol* 1998; 85: 418–24.

22. Helge JW, Wulff B, Kiens B. Impact of a fat-rich diet on endurance in man: role of the dietary period. *Med Sci Sports Exerc* 1998; 30: 456–61.

23. Pivarnik JM, Palmer JM. Water and electrolyte balance during rest and exercise. In: Wolinsky I, Hickson JF, eds. Nutrition in exercise and sport, 2nd ed. Boca Raton: CRC Press, 1994, 245–63 [review].

24. Convertino VA, Armstrong LE, Coyle EF, et al. American College of Sports Medicine position stand. Exercise and fluid replacement. *Med Sci Sports Exerc* 1996; 28(1): i–vii [review].

25. Short SH. Surveys of dietary intake and nutrition knowledge of athletes and their coaches. In Wolinsky I, Hickson JF, eds., *Nutrition in Exercise and Sport,* 2nd ed. Boca Raton, FL: CRC Press, 1994, 367–416.

26. Clarkson PM, Haymes EM. Exercise and mineral status of ath-

letes: calcium, magnesium, phosphorus, and iron. *Med Sci Sports Exerc* 1995 Jun; 27(6): 831–43 [review].

27. Lukaski HC. Micronutrients (magnesium, zinc, and copper): are mineral supplements needed for athletes? *Int J Sport Nutr* 1995; 5: S74–83 [review].

28. Van der Beek EJ. Vitamin supplementation and physical exercise performance. *J Sports Sci* 1991; 9: 77–90 [review].

29. McDonald R, Keen CL. Iron, zinc and magnesium nutrition and athletic performance. *Sports Med* 1988; 5: 171–84 [review].

30. Telford RD, Catchpole EA, Deakin V, et al. The effect of 7 to 8 months of vitamin/mineral supplementation on athletic performance. *Int J Sport Nutr* 1992; 2: 135–53.

31. Singh A, Moses FM, Deuster PA. Chronic multivitamin-mineral supplementation does not enhance physical performance. *Med Sci Sports Exerc* 1992; 24: 726–32.

32. Weight LM, Myburgh KH, Noakes TD. Vitamin and mineral supplementation: effect on the running performance of trained athletes. *Am J Clin Nutr* 1988; 47: 192–95.

33. Pivarnik JM, Palmer JM. Water and electrolyte balance during rest and exercise. In: Wolinsky I, Hickson JF, eds. Nutrition in exercise and sport, 2nd ed. Boca Raton: CRC Press, 1994: 245–63 [review].

34. Convertino VA, Armstrong LE, Coyle EF, et al. American College of Sports Medicine position stand. Exercise and fluid replacement. *Med Sci Sports Exerc* 1996; 28(1): i–vii [review].

35. Kanter M. Free radicals, exercise and antioxidant supplementation. *Proc Nutr Soc* 1998; 57: 9–13 [review].

36. Dekkers JC, van Doornen LJ, Kemper HC. The role of antioxidant vitamins and enzymes in the prevention of exercise-induced muscle damage. *Sports Med* 1996; 21(3): 213–38 [review].

37. Jakeman P, Maxwell S. Effect of antioxidant vitamin supplementation on muscle function after eccentric exercise. *Eur J Appl Physiol* 1993; 67: 426–30.

Part One: References

38. Kaminski M, Boal R. An effect of ascorbic acid on delayed-onset muscle soreness. *Pain* 1992; 50: 317–21.

39. McBride JM, Kraemer WJ, Triplett-McBride T, et al. Effect of resistance exercise on free radical production. *Med Sci Sports Exerc* 1998; 30: 67–72.

40. Rokitzki L, Logemann E, Huber G, et al. Alpha-Tocopherol supplementation in racing cyclists during extreme endurance training. *Int J Sport Nutr* 1994; 4: 253–64.

41. Meydani M, Evans WJ, Handelman, et al. Protective effect of vitamin E on exercise-induced oxidative damage in young and older adults. *Am J Physiol* 1993; 264: R992–98.

42. Tiidus PM, Houston ME. Vitamin E status and response to exercise training. *Sports Med* 1995; 20: 12–23 [review].

43. Kaikkonen J, Kosonen L, Nyyssonen K, et al. Effect of combined coenzyme Q_{10} and d-alpha-tocopheryl acetate supplementaion on exercise-induced lipid peroxidation and muscular damage: a placebo-controlled double-blind study in marathon runners. *Free Radic Res* 1998; 29: 85–92.

44. Singh A, Failla ML, Deuster PA. Exercise-induced changes in immune function: effects of zinc supplementation. *J Appl Physiol* 1994; 76: 2298–303.

45. Johnston CS, Swan PD, Corte C. Substrate utilization and work efficiency during submaximal exercise in vitamin C depleted-repleted adults. *Int J Vitam Nutr Res* 1999; 69: 41–44.

46. Gerster H. The role of vitamin C in athletic performance. *J Am Coll Nutr* 1989; 8: 636–43 [review].

47. Tiidus PM, Houston ME. Vitamin E status and response to exercise training. *Sports Med* 1995; 20: 12–23 [review].

48. Simon-Schnass I, Pabst H. Influence of vitamin E on physical performance. *Int J Vitam Nutr Res* 1988; 58: 49–54.

49. Shepard RJ. Vitamin E and athletic performance. *J Sports Med* 1983; 23: 461–70 [review].

50. Keith R, Alt L. Riboflavin status of female athletes consuming normal diets. *Nutr Res* 1991; 11(7): 727–34.

51. Van der Beek EJ, van Dokkum W, Wedel M, et al. Thiamin, riboflavin and vitamin B_6: impact of restricted intake on physical performance in man. *J Am Coll Nutr* 1994; 13: 629–40.

52. Van der Beek EJ. Vitamin supplementation and physical exercise performance. *J Sports Sci* 1991; 9: 77–90 [review].

53. Winters LR, Yoon JS, Kalkwarf HJ, et al. Riboflavin requirements and exercise adaptation in older women. *Am J Clin Nutr* 1992; 56: 526–32.

54. Trembly A et al. The effects of riboflavin supplementation on the nutritional status and performance of elite swimmers. *Nutr Res* 1984; 4: 201.

55. Murray R, Bartoli WP, Eddy DE, et al. Physiological and performance responses to nicotinic-acid ingestion during exercise. *Med Sci Sports Exerc* 1995; 27: 1057–62.

56. Manore MM. Vitamin B_6 and exercise. *Int J Sport Nutr* 1994; 4: 89–103.

57. P. TG, Ward TL, Southern LL. Effect of chromium picolinate on growth and carcass characteristics of growing-finishing pigs. *J Animal Sci* 1991; 69: 356.

58. Lefavi R, Anderson R, Keith R, et al. Efficacy of chromium supplementation in athletes: Emphasis on anabolism. *Int J Sport Nutr* 1992; 2: 111–22.

59. McCarty MF. The case for supplemental chromium and a survey of clinical studies with chromium picolinate. *J Appl Nutr* 1991; 43: 59–66.

60. Campbell WW, Joseph LJ, Davey SL, et al. Effects of resistance training and chromium picolinate on body composition and skeletal muscle in older men. *J Appl Physiol* 1999; 86: 29–39.

61. Walker LS, Bemben MG, Bemben DA, et al. Chromium picolinate effects on body composition and muscular performance in wrestlers. *Med Sci Sports Exerc* 1998; 30: 1730–37.

62. Anderson RA. Effects of chromium on body composition and weight loss. *Nutr Rev* 1998; 56: 266–70 [review].

63. Kaats GR, Blum K, Fisher JA, Adelman JA. Effects of chromium picolinate supplementation on body composition: a randomized, double-masked, placebo-controlled study. *Curr Ther Res* 1996; 57: 747–56.

64. Kaats GR, Blum K, Pullin D, et al. A randomized, double-masked, placebo-controlled study of the effects of chromium picolinate supplementation on body composition: a replication and extension of a previous study. *Curr Ther Res* 1998; 59: 379–88.

65. Mechrefe A, Wexler B, Feller E. Sports anemia and gastrointestinal bleeding in endurance athletes. *Med Health R I* 1997; 80: 216–18.

66. Clarkson PM. Micronutrients and exercise: anti-oxidants and minerals. *J Sports Sci* 1995; 13: S11–24.

67. Smith JA. Exercise, training and red blood cell turnover. *Sports Med* 1995; 19: 9–31.

68. Nielsen P, Nachtigall D. Iron supplementation in athletes. Current recommendations. *Sports Med* 1998; 26: 207–16.

69. Smith JA. Exercise, training and red blood cell turnover. *Sports Med* 1995; 19: 9–31 [review].

70. McDonald R, Keen CL. Iron, zinc and magnesium nutrition and athletic performance. *Sports Med* 1988; 5: 171–84 [review].

71. Weller E, Bachert P, Meinck HM, et al. Lack of effect of oral Mg-supplementation on Mg in serum, blood cells, and calf muscle. *Med Sci Sports Exerc* 1998; 30: 1584–91.

72. Brilla LR, Haley TF. Effect of magnesium supplementation on strength training in humans. *J Am Coll Nutr* 1992; 11: 326–29.

73. Golf SW, Bender S, Gruttner J. On the significance of magnesium in extreme physical stress. *Cardiovasc Drugs Ther* 1998; 12(suppl 2): 197–202.

74. Margaritis I, Tessier F, Prou E, et al. Effects of endurance training on skeletal muscle oxidative capacities with and without selenium supplementation. *J Trace Elem Med Biol* 1997; 11: 37–43.

Part One: References

75. Fawcett JP, Farquhar SJ, Walker RJ, et al. The effect of oral vanadyl sulfate on body composition and performance in weight-training athletes. *Int J Sport Nutr* 1996; 6: 382–90.

76. Kreider RB, Miriel V, Bertun E. Amino acid supplementation and exercise performance. Analysis of the proposed ergogenic value. *Sports Med* 1993; 16: 190–209 [review].

77. Kelly GS. Sports nutrition: A review of selected nutritional supplements for bodybuilders and strength athletes. *Alt Med Rev* 1997; 2: 184–201.

78. Van Hall G, Raaymakers JSH, Saris WHM, Wagenmakers AJM. Supplementation with branched-chain amino acids (BCAA) and tryptophan has no effect on performance during prolonged exercise. *Clin Sci* 1994; 87: 52 [abstract #75].

79. Blomstrand E, Hassmen P, Ek S, et al. Influence of ingesting a solution of branched-chain amino acids on perceived exertion during exercise. *Acta Physiol Scand* 1997; 159: 41–49.

80. Van Hall G, Raaymakers JSH, Saris WHM, Wagenmakers AJM. Supplementation with branched-chain amino acids (BCAA) and tryptophan has no effect on performance during prolonged exercise. *Clin Sci* 1994; 87: 52 [abstract #75].

81. Madsen K, MacLean DA, Kiens B, et al. Effects of glucose, glucose plus branched-chain amino acids, or placebo on bike performance over 100 km. *J Appl Physiol* 1996; 81: 2644–50.

82. Vukovich MD, Sharp RL, Kesl LD, et al. Effects of a low-dose amino acid supplement on adaptations to cycling training in untrained individuals. *Int J Sport Nutr* 1997; 7: 298–309.

83. Freyssenet D, Berthon P, Denis C, et al. Effect of a 6-week endurance training programme and branched-chain amino acid supplementation on histomorphometric characteristics of aged human muscle. *Arch Physiol Biochem* 1996; 104: 157–62.

84. Schena F, Guerrini F, Tregnaghi P, et al. Branched-chain amino acid supplementation during trekking at high altitude. The effects on loss of body mass, body composition, and muscle power. *Eur J Appl Physiol* 1992; 65: 394–98.

85. Mittleman KD, Ricci MR, Bailey SP. Branched-chain amino acids prolong exercise during heat stress in men and women. *Med Sci Sports Exerc* 1998; 30: 83–91.

86. Hassmén P, Blomstrand E, Ekblom B, Newsholme EA. Branched-chain amino acid supplementation during 30-km competitive run: mood and cognitive performance. *Nutrition* 1994; 10: 405–10.

87. Blomstrand E, Hassmen P, Ek S, et al. Influence of ingesting a solution of branched-chain amino acids on perceived exertion during exercise. *Acta Physiol Scand* 1997; 159: 41–49.

88. Blomstrand E, Hassmen P, Ekblom B, et al. Administration of branched-chain amino acids during sustained exercise-effects on performance and on plasma concentration of some amino acids. *Eur J Appl Physiol* 1991; 63: 83–88.

89. Cerretelli P, Marconi C. L-carnitine supplementation in humans. The effects on physical performance. *Int J Sports Med* 1990; 11: 1–14 [review].

90. Heinonen OJ. Carnitine and physical exercise. *Sports Med* 1996; 22: 109–32 [review].

91. Bucci LR. Nutrients as ergogenic aids for sports and exercise. Boca Raton, FL: CRC Press, 1993, 47–52 [review].

92. Colombani P, Wenk C, Kunz I, et al. Effects of L-carnitine supplementation on physical performance and energy metabolism of endurance-trained athletes: a double blind crossover field study. *Eur J Appl Physiol* 1996; 73: 434–39.

93. Decombaz J, Deriaz O, Acheson K, et al. Effect of L-carnitine on submaximal exercise metabolism after depletion of muscle glycogen. *Med Sci Sports Exerc* 1993; 25: 733–40.

94. Trappe SW, Costill DL, Goodpaster B, et al. The effects of L-carnitine supplementation on performance during interval swimming. *Int J Sports Med* 1994; 15: 181–85.

95. Green RE, Levine AM, Gunning MJ. The effect of L-carnitine supplementation on lean body mass in male amateur body builders. *J Am Dietet Assoc* 1997; (suppl): A–72 [abstract].

96. Besset A, Bonardet A, Rondouin G, et al. Increase in sleep related GH and Prl secretion after chronic arginine aspartate administration in man. *Acta Endocrinologica* 1982; 99: 18–23.

97. Bucci L, Hickson JF, Pivarnik JF, et al. Ornithine ingestion and growth hormone release in bodybuilders. *Nutr Res* 1990; 10: 239–45.

98. Gater DR, Gater DA, Uribe JM, et al. Effects of arginine/lysine supplementation and resistance training on glucose tolerance. *J Appl Physiol* 1992; 72: 1279–84.

99. Bucci LR, Hickson JF Jr, Wolinsky I, et al. Ornithine supplementation and insulin release in bodybuilders. *Int J Sport Nutr* 1992; 2: 287–91.

100. Suminski RR, Robertson RJ, Goss FL, et al. Acute effect of amino acid ingestion and resistance exercise on plasma growth hormone concentration in young men. *Int J Sport Nutr* 1997; 7: 48–60.

101. Fogelholm GM, Naveri HK, Kiilavuori KT, et al. Low-dose amino acid supplementation: no effects on serum human growth hormone and insulin in male weightlifters. *Int J Sport Nutr* 1993; 3: 290–97.

102. Elam RP. Morphological changes in adult males from resistance exercise and amino acid supplementation. *J Sports Med Phys Fitness* 1988; 28: 35–39.

103. Elam RP, Hardin DH, Sutton RA, et al. Effects of arginine and ornithine on strength, lean body mass and urinary hydroxyproline in adult males. *J Sports Med Phys Fitness* 1989; 29: 52–56.

104. Antonio J, Street C. Glutamine: a potentially useful supplement for athletes. *Can J Appl Physiol* 1999; 24: 1–14 [review].

105. Rowbottom DG, Keast D, Morton AR. The emerging role of glutamine as an indicator of exercise stress and overtraining. *Sports Med* 1996; 21: 80–97 [review].

106. Welbourne TC. Increased plasma bicarbonate and growth hormone after an oral glutamine load. *Am J Clin Nutr* 1995; 61: 1058–61.

107. Varnier M, Leese GP, Thompson J, et al. Stimulatory effect of glutamine on glycogen accumulation in human skeletal muscle. *Am J Physiol* 1995; 269: E309–15.

108. Haub MD, Potteiger JA, Nau KL, et al. Acute L-glutamine ingestion does not improve maximal effort exercise. *J Sports Med Phys Fitness* 1998; 38: 240–44.

109. Rohde T, MacLean DA, Pedersen BK. Effect of glutamine supplementation on changes in the immune system induced by repeated exercise. *Med Sci Sports Exerc* 1998; 30: 856–62.

110. Castell LM, Newsholme EA. Glutamine and the effects of exhaustive exercise upon the immune response. *Can J Physiol Pharmacol* 1998; 76: 524–32 [review].

111. Castell LM, Poortmans JR, Newsholme EA. Does glutamine have a role in reducing infections in athletes? *Eur J Appl Physiol* 1996; 73: 488–90.

112. Kaikkonen J, Nyyssonen K, Tuomainen TP, et al. Determinants of plasma coenzyme Q_{10} in humans. *FEBS Lett* 1999; 443: 163–66 [review].

113. Overvad OK, Diamant B, Holm L, et al. Efficacy and safety of dietary supplementation containing Q_{10}. *Ugeskr Laeger* 1997; 159: 7309–15 [review][in Danish].

114. Zuliani U, Bonetti A, Campana M, et al. The influence of ubiquinone (Co Q_{10}) on the metabolic response to work. *J Sports Med Phys Fitness* 1989; 29: 57–62 [review].

115. Bucci L. *Nutrients as ergogenic aids for sports and exercise.* Boca Raton: CRC Press, 1993, 54–57 [review].

116. Snider IP, Bazzarre TL, Murdoch SD, et al. Effects of coenzyme athletic performance system as an ergogenic aid on endurance performance to exhaustion. *Int J Sport Nutr* 1992; 2: 272–86.

117. Malm C, Svensson M, Ekblom B, et al. Effects of ubiquinone-10 supplementation and high intensity training on physical performance in humans. *Acta Physiol Scand* 1997; 161: 379–84.

118. Laaksonen R, Fogelholm M, Himberg JJ, et al. Ubiquinone supplementation and exercise capacity in trained young and older men. *Eur J Appl Physiol* 1995; 72: 95–100.

119. Stanko RT, Robertson RJ, Galbreath RW, et al. Enhanced leg exercise endurance with a high-carbohydrate diet and dihyroxyacetone and pyruvate. *J Appl Phys* 1990; 69(5): 1651–56.

120. Stanko RT, Robertson RJ, Spina RJ, et al. Enhancement of arm exercise endurance capacity with dihydroxyacetone and pyruvate. *J Appl Phys* 1990; 68(1): 119–24.

121. Bucci LR. *Nutrients as ergogenic aids for sports and exercise.* Boca Raton, FL: CRC Press, 1993, 45–47 [review].

122. Wesson M, McNaughton L, Davies P, et al. Effects of oral administration of aspartic acid salts on the endurance capacity of trained subjects. *Res Quart Exer Sport* 1988; 59: 234–36.

123. Maughan RJ, Sadler DJ. The effects of oral administration of salts of aspartic acid on the metabolic response to prolonged exhausting exercise in man. *Int J Sports Med* 1983; 4: 119–23.

124. Hagan RD, Upton SJ, Duncan JJ, et al. Absence of effect of potassium-magnesium aspartate on physiologic responses to prolonged work in aerobically trained men. *Int J Sports Med* 1982; 3: 177–81.

125. Tuttle JL, Potteiger JA, Evans BW, et al. Effect of acute potassium-magnesium aspartate supplementation on ammonia concentrations during and after resistance training. *Int J Sport Nutr* 1995; 5: 102–9.

126. De Haan A, van Doorn JE, Westra HG. Effects of potassium + magnesium aspartate on muscle metabolism and force development during short intensive static exercise. *Int J Sports Med* 1985; 6: 44–49.

127. Le Boucher J, Cynober LA. Ornithine alpha-ketoglutarate: the puzzle. *Nutrition* 1998; 14: 870–73 [review].

128. Brocker P, Vellas B, Albarede J, et al. A two-centre, randomized, double blind trial of ornithine oxoglutarate in 194 elderly, ambulatory, convalescent subjects. *Age Aging* 1994; 23: 303–6.

129. Greenhaff PL, Bodin K, Soderlund K, et al. Effect of oral creatine supplementation on skeletal muscle phosphocreatine resynthesis. *Am J Physiol* 1994; 266: E725–30.

130. Greenhaff PL. Creatine and its application as an ergogenic aid. *Int J Sport Nutr* 1995; 5: 94–101.

131. Harris RC, Soderlund K, Hultman E. Elevation of creatine in resting and exercised muscle of normal subjects by creatine supplementation. *Clin Sci* 1992; 83: 367–74.

132. Green AL, Simpson EJ, Littlewood JJ, et al. Carbohydrate ingestion augments creatine retention during creatine feeding in humans. *Acta Physiol Scand* 1996; 158: 195–202.

133. Kreider RB, Ferreira M, Wilson M, et al. Effects of creatine supplementation on body composition, strength, and sprint performance. *Med Sci Sports Exerc* 1998; 30: 73–82.

134. Toler SM. Creatine is an ergogen for anaerobic exercise. *Nutr Rev* 1997; 55: 21–25.

135. Greenhaff PL. The nutritional biochemistry of creatine. *J Nutr Biochem* 1997; 8: 610–18.

136. Mujika I, Padilla S. Creatine supplementation as an ergogenic aid for sports performance in highly trained athletes: a critical review. *Int J Sports Med* 1997; 18: 491–96 [review].

137. Grindstaff PD, Kreider R, Bishop R, et al. Effects of creatine supplementation on repetitive sprint performance and body composition in competitive swimmers. *Int J Sports Nutr* 1997; 7: 330–46.

138. Peyrebrune MC, Nevill ME, Donaldson FJ, et al. The effects of oral creatine supplementation on performance in single and repeated sprint swimming. *J Sports Sci* 1998; 16: 271–79.

Part One: References

Part One: References

139. Balsom PD, Harridge SDR, Soderlund K, et al. Creatine supplementation per se does not enhance endurance exercise performance. *Acta Physiol Scand* 1993; 149: 521–23.

140. Stout JR, Eckerson J, Noonan D, et al. The effects of a supplement designed to augment creatine uptake on exercise performance and fat-free mass in football players. *Med Sci Sports Exerc* 1997; 29: 251.

141. Wheeler KB, Garleb KA. Gamma oryzanol-plant sterol supplementation: metabolic, endocrine, and physiologic effects. *Int J Sport Nutr* 1991; 1: 170–77 [review].

142. Fry AC, Bonner E, Lewis DL, et al. The effects of gamma-oryzanol supplementation during resistance exercise training. *Int J Sport Nutr* 1997; 7: 318–29.

143. Bucci LR, Blackman G, Defoyd W, et al. Effect of ferulate on strength and body composition of weightlifters. *J Appl Sport Sci Res* 1990; 4: 110 [abstract].

144. Jeukendrup AE, Saris WHM, van Diesen RAJ, et al. Exogenous MCT oxidation from carbohydrate-medium chain triglyceride supplements during moderate intensity exercise. *Clin Sci* 1994; 87: 33.

145. Berning JR. The role of medium-chain triglycerides in exercise. *Int J Sport Nutr* 1996; 6: 121–33 [review].

146. Goedecke JH, Elmer-English R, Dennis SC, et al. Effects of medium-chain triaclyglycerol ingested with carbohydrate on metabolism and exercise performance. *Int J Sport Nutr* 1999; 9: 35–47.

147. Van Zyl CG, Lambert EV, Hawley JA, et al. Effects of medium-chain triglyceride ingestion on carbohydrate metabolism and cycling performance. *J Appl Physiol* 1996; 80: 2217–25.

148. Jeukendrup AE, Thielen JJ, Wagenmakers AJ, et al. Effect of medium-chain triacylglycerol and carbohydrate ingestion during exercise on substrate utilization and subsequent cycling performance. *Am J Clin Nutr* 1998; 67: 397–404.

148. Cureton TK. The physiological effects of wheat germ oil on humans. In *Exercise*. Springfield, IL: Charles C Thomas, 1972, 296–300.

149. Saint-John M, McNaughton L. Octacosanol ingestion and its effects on metabolic responses to submaximal cycle ergometry, reaction time and chest and grip strength. *Int Clin Nutr Rev* 1986; 6(2): 81–87.

150. Saint-John M, McNaughton L. Octacosanol ingestion and its effects on metabolic responses to submaximal cycle ergometry, reation time and chest and grip strength. *Int Clin Nutr Rev* 1986; 6(2): 81–87.

151. Nissen SL, Morrical D, Fuller JC. Effects of the leucine catabolite beta-hydroxy-beta-methyl-butyrate (HMB) on the growth and health of growing lambs. *J Animal Sci* 1994; 77: 243.

152. Nissen S, Panton L, Wilhelm R, et al. Effect of beta-hydroxy-beta-methylbutyrate (HMB) supplementation on strength and body composition of trained and untrained males undergoing intense resistance training. *FASEB J* 1996; 10: A287 [abstract].

153. Nissen S, Sharp R, Ray M, et al. Effect of leucine metabolite beta-hydroxy-beta-methylbutyrate on muscle metabolism during resistive-exercise training. *J Appl Phys* 1996; 81: 2095–104.

154. Horswill CA. Effects of bicarbonate, citrate, and phosphate loading on performance. *Int J Sport Nutr* 1995; 5: S111–19 [review].

155. Linderman JK, Gosselink KL. The effects of sodium bicarbonate ingestion on exercise performance. *Sports Med* 1994; 18: 75–80 [review].

156. Linossier MT, Dormois D, Bregere P, et al. Effect of sodium citrate on performance and metabolism of human skeletal muscle during supramaximal cycling exercise. *Eur J Appl Physiol* 1997; 76: 48–54.

157. Potteiger JA, Nickel GL, Webster MJ, et al. Sodium citrate ingestion enhances 30 km cycling performance. *Int J Sports Med* 1996; 17: 7–11.

158. Hausswirth C, Bigard AX, Lepers R, et al. Sodium citrate ingestion and muscle performance in acute hypobaric hypoxia. *Eur J Appl Physiol* 1995; 71: 362–68.

159. Horswill CA. Effects of bicarbonate, citrate, and phosphate loading on performance. *Int J Sport Nutr* 1995; 5: S111–19 [review].

160. Van Someren K, Fulcher K, McCarthy J, et al. An investigation into the effects of sodium citrate ingestion on high-intensity exercise performance. *Int J Sport Nutr* 1998; 8: 356–63.

161. Cox G, Jenkins DG. The physiological and ventilatory responses to repeated 60 s sprints following sodium citrate ingestion. *J Sports Sci* 1994; 12: 469–75.

162. McNaughton L, Cedaro R. Sodium citrate ingestion and its effects on maximal anaerobic exercise of different durations. *Eur J Appl Physiol* 1992; 64: 36–41.

163. Potteiger JA, Webster MJ, Nickel GL, et al. The effects of buffer ingestion on metabolic factors related to distance running performance. *Eur J Appl Physiol* 1996; 72: 365–71.

164. Tiryaki GR, Atterbom HA. The effects of sodium bicarbonate and sodium citrate on 600 m running time of trained females. *J Sports Med Phys Fitness* 1995; 35: 194–98.

165. McNaughton LR. Sodium citrate and anaerobic performance: implications of dosage. *Eur J Appl Physiol* 1990; 61: 392–97.

166. Galloway SD, Tremblay MS, Sexsmith JR, et al. The effects of acute phosphate supplementation in subjects of different aerobic fitness levels. *Eur J Appl Physiol* 1996; 72: 224–30.

167. Williams MH. Ergogenic and ergolytic substances. *Med Sci Sports Exer* 1992; 24: S344–48 [review].

168. Bucci LR. *Nutrients as ergogenic aids for sports and exercise*. Boca Raton, FL: CRC Press, 1993, 61–62 [review].

169. Williams MH, Kreider RB, Hunter DW, et al. Effect of inosine supplementation on 3-mile treadmill run performances and VO2 peak. *Med Sci Sports Exerc* 1990; 22: 517–22.

170. Starling RD, Trappe TA, Short KR, et al. Effect of inosine supplementation on aerobic and anaerobic cycling performance. *Med Sci Sports Exerc* 1996; 28: 1193–98.

171. Spriet LL. Caffeine and performance. *Int J Sport Nutr* 1995; 5: S84–99 [review].

172. Greer F, McLean C, Graham TE. Caffeine, performance, and metabolism during repeated Wingate exercise tests. *J Appl Physiol* 1998; 85: 1502–8.

173. Williams JH. Caffeine, neuromuscular function and high-intensity exercise performance. *J Sports Med Phys Fitness* 1991 Sep; 31(3): 481–89 [review].

174. Doherty M. The effects of caffeine on the maximal accumulated oxygen deficit and short-term running performance. *Int J Sport Nutr* 1998; 8: 95–104.

175. Jackman M, Wendling P, Friars D, et al. Metabolic catecholamine, and endurance responses to caffeine during intense exercise. *J Appl Physiol* 1996; 81: 1658–63.

176. Van Soeren MH, Graham TE. Effect of caffeine on metabolism, exercise endurance, and catecholamine responses after withdrawal. *J Appl Physiol* 1998; 85: 1493–501.

177. Kovacs EMR, Stegen JHCH, Brouns F. Effect of caffeinated drinks on substrate metabolism, caffeine excretion, and performance. *J Appl Physiol* 1998; 85: 709–15.

178. MacIntosh BR, Wright BM. Caffeine ingestion and performance of a 1,500-metre swim. *Can J Appl Physiol* 1995; 20: 168–77.

179. Pasman WJ, van Baak MA, Jeukendrup AE, et al. The effect of different dosages of caffeine on endurance performance time. *Int J Sports Med* 1995; 16: 225–30.

180. Cohen BS, Nelson AG, Prevost MC, et al. Effects of caffeine ingestion on endurance racing in heat and humidity. *Eur J Appl Physiol* 1996; 73: 358–63.

181. Tarnopolsky MA. Caffeine and endurance performance. *Sports Med* 1994; 18: 109–25 [review].

182. Graham TE, Hibbert E, Sathasivam P. Metabolic and exercise endurance effects of coffee and caffeine ingestion. *J Appl Physiol* 1998; 85: 883–89.

183. Pasman WJ, van Baak MA, Jeukendrup AE, et al. The effect of different dosages of caffeine on endurance performance time. *Int J Sports Med* 1995; 16: 225–30.

184. Mahesh VB, Greenblatt RB. The in vivo conversion of dehydroepiandrosterone and androstenedione to testosterone in the human. *Acta Endocrinologica* 1962; 41: 400–6.

185. German patent number DE 42 14953 A1.

186. Kelly GS. Sports nutrition: A review of selected nutritional supplements for endurance athletes. *Alt Med Rev* 1997; 2: 282–95 [review].

187. Pieralisi G, Ripari P, Vecchiet L. Effects of a standardized ginseng extract combined with dimethylaminoethanol bitartrate, vitamins, minerals and trace elements on physical performance during exercise. *Clin Ther* 1991: 12(3): 373–82.

188. Allen JD, McLung J, Nelson AG, Welsch M. Ginseng supplementation does not enhance healthy young adults' peak aerobic exercise performance. *J Am Coll Nutr* 1998; 17: 462–66.

189. Morris AC, Jacobs I, McLellan TM, et al. No ergogenic effect of ginseng ingestion. *Int J Sport Nutr* 1996; 6: 263–71.

190. Kelly GS. Sports nutrition: A review of selected nutritional supplements for endurance athletes. *Alt Med Rev* 1997; 2: 282–95 [review].

191. McNaughton L. A comparison of Chinese and Russian ginseng as ergogenic aids to improve various facets of physical fitness. *Int Clin Nutr Rev* 1989; 9: 32–35.

192. Dowling EA, Redondo DR, Branch JD, et al. Effect of *Eleutherococcus senticosus* on submaximal and maximal exercise performance. *Med Sci Sports Exer* 1996; 28: 482–89.

Attention Deficit–Hyperactivity Disorder

1. Milberger S, Biederman J, Faraone SV, et al. Is maternal smoking during pregnancy a risk factor for attention deficit hyperactivity disorder in children? *Am J Psych* 1996; 153: 1138–42.

2. Tuthill RW. Hair lead levels related to children's classroom attention-deficit behavior. *Arch Environ Health* 1996; 51: 214–20.

3. Krigman MR, Bouldin TW, Mushak P. Metal toxicity in the nervous system. *Monogr Pathol* 1985; (26): 58–100.

4. Harley JP, Ray RS, Tomasi L, et al. Hyperkinesis and food additives: Testing the Feingold hypothesis. *Pediatr* 1978; 61: 818–21.

5. Levy F, Dumbrell S, Hobbes G, et al. Hyperkinesis and diet: A double-blind crossover trial with a tartrazine challenge. *Med J Aust* 1978; 1: 61–64.

6. Williams JI, Cram DM. Diet in the management of hyperkinesis: A review of the tests of Feingold's hypotheses. *Can Psychiatr Assoc J* 1978; 23: 241–48 [review].

7. Rowe KS, Rowe KJ. Synthetic food coloring and behavior: A dose response effect in a double-blind, placebo-controlled, repeated-measures study. *J Pediatr* 1994; 125: 691–98.

8. Boris M, Mandel FS. Foods and additives are common causes of the attention deficit hyperactive disorder in children. *Ann Allergy* 1994; 72: 462–68.

9. Carter CM, Urbanowicz M, Hemsley R, et al. Effects of a few food diet in attention deficit disorder. *Arch Dis Child* 1993; 69: 564–68.

10. Egger J, Stolla A, McEwen LM. Controlled trial of hyposensitisation in children with food-induced hyperkinetic syndrome. *Lancet* 1992; 339: 1150–53.

11. Prinz RJ, Roberts WA, Hantman E. Dietary correlates of hyperactive behavior in children. *J Consult Clin Psychol* 1980; 48: 760–69.

12. Rosen LA, Booth SR, Bender ME, et al. Effects of sugar (sucrose) on children's behavior. *J Consult Clin Psychol* 1988; 56: 583–89.

13. Wolraich ML, Lindgren SD, Stumbo PJ, et al. Effects of diets high in sucrose or aspartame on the behavior and cognitive performance of children. *N Engl J Med* 1994; 330: 301–307.

Part One: References

14. Wolraich ML, Wilson DB, White JW. The effect of sugar on behavior or cognition in children. A meta-analysis. *JAMA* 1995; 274: 1617–21.

15. Mitchell EA, Aman MG, Turbott SH, Manku M. Clinical characteristics and serum essential fatty acid levels in hyperactive children. *Clin Pediatr* 1987; 26: 406–11.

16. Stevens LJ, Zentall SS, Deck JL, et al. Essential fatty acid metabolism in boys with attention-deficit hyperactivity disorder. *Am J Clin Nutr* 1995; 62: 761–68.

17. Aman MG, Mitchell EA, Turbott SH. The effects of essential fatty acid supplementation by Efamol in hyperactive children. *J Abnorm Child Psychol* 1987; 15: 75–90.

18. Bhagavan HN, Coleman M, Coursin DB. The effect of pyridoxine hydrochloride on blood serotonin and pyridoxal phosphate contents in hyperactive children. *Pediatrics* 1975; 55: 437–41.

19. Coleman M, Steinberg G, Tippett J, et al. A preliminary study of the effect of pyridoxine administration in a subgroup of hyperkinetic children: A double-blind crossover comparison with methylphenidate. *Biol Psych* 1979; 14: 741–51.

20. Brenner A. The effects of megadoses of selected B complex vitamins on children with hyperkinesis: Controlled studies with long term followup. *J Learning Dis* 1982; 15: 258–64.

21. Haslam RHA. Is there a role for megavitamin therapy in the treatment of attention deficit hyperactivity disorder? *Adv Neurol* 1992; 58: 303–310.

22. Starobrat-Hermelin B, Kozielec T. The effects of magnesium physiological supplementation on hyperactivity in children with attention deficit hyperactivity disorder (ADHD). Positive response to magnesium oral loading test. *Magnes Res* 1997; 10: 149–56.

Autism

1. Reichelt K-L, Ekrem J, Scott H. Gluten, milk proteins and autism: dietary intervention effects on behav-ior and peptide section. *J Appl Nutr* 1990; 42: 1–11.

2. Werbach M. Autism. *Int J Alternative Complementary Med* 1996; Oct: 8.

3. Martineau J, Garreau B, Barthelemy C, et al. Effects of vitamin B_6 on averaged evoked potentials in infantile autism. *Biol Psychiatr* 1981; 16: 627–39.

4. Lelord G, Muh JP, Barthelemy C, et al. Effects of pyridoxine and magnesium on autistic symptoms: Initial observations. *J Autism Developmental Disorders* 1981; 11: 219–29.

5. Rimland B, Callaway E, Dreyfus P. The effect of high doses of vitamin B_6 on autistic children: a double-blind crossover study. *Am J Psychiatr* 1978; 135: 472–75.

6. Rimland B. Vitamin B_6 versus Fenfluramine: a case-study in medical bias. *J Nutr Med* 1991; 2: 321–22.

7. Martineau J, Barthelemy C, Garreau B, Lelord G. Vitamin B_6, magnesium, and combined B_6-Mg: Therapeutic effects in childhood autism. *Biol Psychiatr* 1985; 20: 467–78.

8. Dolske MC, Spollen J, McKay S, et al. A preliminary trial of ascorbic acid as supplemental therapy for autism. *Prog Neuropsycholpharmacol Biol Psychiatry* 1993; 17: 765–74.

Brittle Nails

1. Bates B. *A guide to physical examination*, 2d ed. Philadelphia: J. B. Lippincott, 1979, 51.

2. Pfeiffer CC. *Mental and Elemental Nutrients*. New Canaan, CT: Keats Publishing, 1975, 229.

3. Yang G, Wang S, Zhou R, Sun S. Endemic selenium intoxication of humans in China. *Am J Clin Nutr* 1983; 37: 872–81.

4. Colombo VE, Gerber F, Bronhofer M, Floersheim GL. Treatment of brittle fingernails and onychoschizia with biotin: Scanning electron microscopy. *J Am Acad Dermatol* 1990; 23: 1127–32.

5. Hochman LG, Scher RK, Meyerson MS. Brittle nails: Response to daily biotin supplementation. *Cutis* 1993; 51: 303–305.

Bruising

1. Shamrai EF. Vitamin P. Its chemical nature and mechanism of physiologic action. *Uspekhi Sovremennoi Biologii* 1968; 65: 186–201.

2. Calabrese C, Preston P. Report of the results of a double-blind, randomized, single-dose trial of a topical 2% escin gel versus placebo in the acute treatment of experimentally-induced hematoma in volunteers. *Planta Med* 1993; 59: 394–97.

3. Moore M. *Medicinal Plants of the Mountain West*. Santa Fe: Museum of New Mexico Press, 1979, 152.

4. Gruenwald J, Brendler T, Jaenicke C (eds). *PDR for Herbal Medicines*. Montvale, NJ: Medical Economics Co, 1998, 966–67.

5. Mills SY. *Out of the Earth: The Essential Book of Herbal Medicine*. New York: Viking Arkana, 1991, 544–47.

6. Weiss RF. *Herbal Medicine*. Gothenburg, Sweden: Ab Arcanum and Beaconsfield, UK: Beaconsfield Publishers Ltd, 1988, 334–35.

Burns, Minor

1. Della Loggia R, Tubaro A, Sosa S, et al. The role of triterpenoids in the topical anti-inflammatory activity of *Calendula officinalis* flowers. *Planta Medica* 1994; 60: 516–20.

2. Patrick KFM, Kumar S, Edwardson PAD, Hutchinson JJ. Induction of vascularisation by an aqueous extract of the flowers of *Calendula officinalis* L the European marigold. *Phytomedicine* 1996; 3: 11–18.

Bursitis

1. Klemes IS. Vitamin B_{12} in acute subdeltoid bursitis. *Indust Med Surg* 1957; 26: 290–92.

2. Kellman M. Bursitis: a new chemotherapeutic approach. *J Am Osteopathic Assoc* 1962; 61: 896–903.

Canker Sores (Mouth Ulcers)

1. Chanine L, Sempson N, Wagoner C. The effect of sodium lau-

ryl sulfate on recurrent aphthous ulcers: a clinical study. *Compend Contin Educ Dent* 1997; 18: 1238–40.

2. Herlosfson BB, Barkvoll P. Sodium lauryl sulfate and recurrent aphthous ulcers. A preliminary trial. *Acta Odontol Scand* 1994; 52: 257–59.

3. Herlosfson BB, Barkvoll P. The effect of tow toothpaste detergents on the frequency of recurrent aphthous ulcers. *Acta Odontol Scand* 1996; 54: 150–53.

4. Hay KD, Reade PC. The use of an elimination diet in the treatment of recurrent aphthous ulceration of the oral cavity. *Oral Surg Oral Med Oral Pathol* 1984; 57: 504–507.

5. Wray D. Gluten-sensitive recurrent aphthous stomatitis. *Dig Dis Sci* 1981; 26: 737–40.

6. Wright A et al. Food allergy or intolerance in severe recurrent aphthous ulceration of the mouth. *BMJ* 1986; 292: 1237.

7. Wray D et al. Food allergens and basophil histamine release in recurrent aphthous stomatitis. *Oral Surg Oral Med Oral Pathol* 1982; 54: 338–95.

8. Porter SR et al. Hematologic status in recurrent aphthous stomatitis compared to other oral disease. *Oral Surg Oral Med Oral Pathol* 1988; 66: 41–44.

9. Palopoli J, Waxman J. Recurrent aphthous stomatitis and vitamin B_{12} deficiency. *South Med J* 1990; 83: 475–77.

10. Wray D et al. Nutritional deficiencies in recurrent aphthae. *J Oral Pathol* 1978; 7: 418–23.

11. Nolan A et al. Recurrent aphthous ulceration. *J Oral Pathol Med* 1991; 20: 389–91.

12. Haisraeli-Shalish M, Livneh A, Katz J, et al. Recurrent aphthous stomatitis and thiamine deficiency. *Oral Surg Oral Med Oral Pathol Oral Radiol Endod* 1996; 82: 634–36.

13. James APR. Common dermatologic disorders. *CIBA Clin Symposia* 1967; 19: 38–64.

14. Werbach MR. *Nutritional Influences on Illness*, 2d ed; Tarzana,

CA: Third Line Press, 1993, 56 [review].

15. Gerenrich RL, Hart RW. Treatment of oral ulcerations with Bacid (Lactobacillus acidophilus). *Oral Surg* 1970; 30: 196–200.

16. Das SK, Gulati AK, Singh VP. Deglycyrrhizinated licorice in aphthous ulcers. *J Assoc Physicians India* 1989; 37: 647.

17. Nasemann T: Kamillosan therapy in dermatology. *Z Allgemeinmed* 1975; 25: 1105–106.

18. Plemons JM, Reps TD, Binnie WH, et al. Evaluation of acemannan in the treatment of recurrent aphthous stomatitis. *Wounds* 1994; 6: 40–45.

Capillary Fragility

1. Tomson CR, Channon SM, Parkinson IS. Correction of subclinical ascorbate deficiency in patients receiving dialysis: Effects on plasma oxalate, serum cholesterol, and capillary fragility. *Clin Chem Acta* 1989; 180: 255–64.

2. Borisov IM, Sluka PP. Use of artificially ionized air and vitamins C and P for preventing increased capillary fragility in student athletes. *Gig Sanit* 1973; 38: 105–107 [in Russian].

3. Cox BD, Butterfield WJ. Vitamin C supplements and diabetic cutaneous capillary fragility. *Br Med J* 1975; 3: 205.

4. Schlebusch H, Kern D. Stabilization of collagen by polyphenols. *Angiologica* 1972; 9: 248–56 [in German].

5. Monboisse J, Braquet P, Randoux A, Borel J. Non-enzymatic degradation of acid-soluble calf skin collagen by superoxide ion: Protective effect of flavonoids. *Biochem Pharmacol* 1983; 32: 53–58.

6. Bruneton J. *Pharmacognosy Phytochemistry Medicinal Plants.* Andover: Intercept Ltd., 1995, 277.

Cardiovascular Disease Overview

1. Kannel WB. Hazards, risks, and threats of heart disease from the early stages to symptomatic coronary heart disease and cardiac failure. *Cardiovasc Drugs Ther* 1997; 11(suppl): 199–212 [review].

2. Kinosian B, Glick H, Garland G. Cholesterol and coronary heart disease: predicting risks by levels and ratios. *Ann Intern Med* 1994; 121: 641–7.

3. Kwiterovich PO Jr. The antiatherogenic role of high-density lipoprotein cholesterol. *Am J Cardiol* 1998; 82: 13Q–21Q [review].

4. Gotto AM Jr. Triglyceride as a risk factor for coronary artery disease. *Am J Cardiol* 1998; 82: 22Q–25Q [review].

5. Seman LJ, McNamara JR, Schaefer EJ. Lipoprotein(a), homocysteine, and remnantlike particles: emerging risk factors. *Curr Opin Cardiol* 1999; 14: 186–91.

6. Kannel WB. Office assessment of coronary candidates and risk factor insights from the Framingham study. *J Hypertens Suppl* 1991; 9: S13–19.

7. Megnien JL, Denarie N, Cocaul M, et al. Predictive value of waist-to-hip ratio on cardiovascular risk events. *Int J Obes Relat Metab Disord* 1999; 23: 90–7.

8. Freund KM, Belanger AJ, D'Agostino RB, Kannel WB. The health risks of smoking. The Framingham Study: 34 years of follow-up. *Ann Epidemiol* 1993; 3: 417–24.

9. Law MR, Morris JK, Wald NJ. Environmental tobacco smoke exposure and ischaemic heart disease: an evaluation of the evidence. *BMJ* 1997; 315: 973–80.

10. Schaefer FJ, Lamon-Fava S, Ordovas JM, et al. Factors associated with low and elevated plasma high density lipoprotein cholesterol and apolipoprotein A-1 levels in the Framingham Offspring Study. *J Lipid Res* 1994; 35: 871–82.

11. Lee CD, Blair SN, Jackson AS. Cardiorespiratory fitness, body composition, and all-cause and cardiovascular disease mortality in men. *Am J Clin Nutr* 1999; 69: 373–80.

12. Law MR, Morris JK. By how much does fruit and vegetable consumption reduce the risk of ischaemic heart disease? *Eur J Clin Nutr* 1998; 52: 549–56.

13. Pietinen P, Rimm EB, Korhonen P, et al. Intake of dietary

Part One: References

fiber and risk of coronary heart disease in a cohort of Finnish men. The Alpha-Tocopherol, Beta-Carotene Cancer Prevention Study. *Circulation* 1996; 94: 2720–7.

14. Albert Cm, Hennekens CH, O'Donnell CJ, et al. Fish consumption and risk of sudden cardiac death. *JAMA* 1998; 279: 23–8.

15. Hu FB, Stampfer MJ, Rimm E, et al. Dietary fat and coronary heart disease: a comparison of approaches for adjusting for total energy intake and modeling repeated dietary measurements. *Am J Epidemiol* 1999; 149: 531–40.

Carpal Tunnel Syndrome

1. Fuhr JF, Farrow A, Nelson HS. Vitamin B_6 levels in patients with carpal tunnel syndrome. *Arch Surg* 1989; 124: 1329–30.

2. Keniston RC, Nathan PA, Leklem JE, Lockwood RS. Vitamin B_6, vitamin C, and carpal tunnel syndrome. *J Occup Environ Med* 1997; 39: 949–59.

3. Franzblau A, Rock CL, Werner RA, et al. The relationship of vitamin B_6 status to median nerve function and carpal tunnel syndrome among active industrial workers. *J Occup Environ Med* 1996; 38: 485–91.

4. Smith GP, Rudge PJ, Peters TJ. Biochemical studies of pyridoxal and pyridoxal phosphate status and therapeutic trial of pyridoxine in patients with carpal tunnel syndrome. *Ann Neurol* 1984; 15: 104–107.

5. Ellis JM, Azuma J, Watanbe T, Folkers K. Survey and new data on treatment with pyridoxine of patients having a clinical syndrome including the carpal tunnel and other defects. *Res Comm Chem Path Pharm* 1977; 17(1): 165–77.

6. Ellis JM. Vitamin B_6 deficiency in patients with a clinical syndrome including the carpal tunnel defect. Biochemical and clinical response to therapy with pyridoxine. *Res Comm Chem Path Pharm* 1976; 13(4): 743–57.

7. D'Souza M. Carpal tunnel syndrome: clinical or neurophysiological diagnosis. *Lancet* 1985; i: 1104–105.

8. Driskell JA, Wesley RL, Hess IE. Effectiveness of pyridoxine hydrochloride treatment on carpal tunnel syndrome patients. *Nutr Rep Internat* 1986; 34(4): 1031–39.

9. Ellis JM. Treatment of carpal tunnel syndrome with vitamin B_6. *Southern Med J* 1987; 80(7): 882–84.

10. Browning DM. Carpal tunnel syndrome: clinical or neurophysiological diagnosis? *Lancet* 1985; i: 1104–105 [letter].

11. Smith GP et al. Biochemical studies of pyridoxal and pyridoxal phosphate status and therapeutic trial of pyridoxine in patients with carpal tunnel syndrome. *Ann Neurol* 1984; 15: 104–107.

12. Amadio PC. Pyridoxine as an adjunct in the treatment of carpal tunnel syndrome. *J Hand Surg* 1985; 10A(2): 237–41.

13. Stransky M et al. Treatment of carpal tunnel syndrome with vitamin B_6: a double-blind study. *Southern Med J* 1989; 82(7): 841–42.

14. Bernstein AL, Dinesen JS. Brief communication: effect of pharmacologic doses of vitamin B_6 on carpal tunnel syndrome, electronencephalographic results, and pain. *J Am Coll Nutri* 1993; 12: 73–76.

15. Gaby AR. Literature review & commentary. *Townsend Letter for Doctors and Patients.* 1990; Jun: 338–39.

16. Parry G, Bredesen DE. Sensory neuropath with low-dose pyridoxine. *Neurology* 1985; 35: 1466–68.

17. Schaumburg H, Kaplan J, Windebank A, et al. Sensory neuropathy from pyridoxine abuse. *N Engl J Med* 1983; 309(8): 445–48.

Cataracts

1. Kahn HA, Leibowitz HM, Ganley JP, et al. The Framingham Eye Study: I. Outline and major prevalence findings. *Am J Epidemiol* 1977; 106: 17–32.

2. Schocket SS, Esterson J, Bradford B, et al. induction of cataracts in mice by exposure to oxygen. *Isr J Med Sci* 1972; 8: 1596–1601.

3. Palmquist B, Phillipson B, Barr P. Nuclear cataract and myopia during hyperbaric oxygen therapy. *Br J Ophthalmol* 1984; 68: 113–17.

4. Jacques PF, Chylack LT Jr. Epidemiologic evidence of a role for the antioxidant vitamins and carotenoids in cataract prevention. *Am J Clin Nutr* 1991; 53: 352S–55S.

5. Knekt P, Heliovaara M, Rissanen A, et al. Serum antioxidant vitamins and risk of cataract. *BMJ* 1992; 305: 1392–94.

6. Taylor A, Jacques PF, Nadler D, et al. Relationship in humans between ascorbic acid consumption and levels of total and reduce ascorbic acid in lens, aqueous humor, and plasma. *Curr Eye Res* 1991; 10: 751–59.

7. Reddy VN. Glutathione and its function in the lens—An overview. *Exp Eye Res* 1990; 150: 771–78.

8. Packer JE, Slater TF, Wilson RL. Direct observation of a free radical interaction between vitamin E and vitamin C. *Nature* 1979; 278: 737–38.

9. Taylor A. Cataract: relationship between nutrition and oxidation. *J Am Coll Nutr* 1993; 12: 138–46 [review].

10. Taylor A, Jacques PF, Nadler D, et al. Relationship in humans between ascorbic acid consumption and levels of total and reduced ascorbic acid in lens, aqueous humor, and plasma. *Curr Eye Res* 1991; 10: 751–59.

11. Jacques PF, Chylack LT Jr. Epidemiologic evidence of a role for the antioxidant vitamins and carotenoids in cataract prevention. *Am J Clin Nutr* 1991; 53: 352S–55S.

12. Jacques PF, Chylack LT, McGandy RB, Hartz SC. Antioxidant status in persons with and without senile cataract. *Arch Ophthalmol* 1988; 106: 337–40.

13. Robertson JMD, Donner AP, Trevithick JR. Vitamin E intake and risk of cataracts in humans. *Ann NY Acad Sci* 1989; 570: 372–82.

14. Seddon JM, Christen WG, Manson JE, et al. The use of vitamin supplements and the risk of cataract

among U.S. male physicians. *Am J Public Health* 1994; 84: 788–92.

15. Robertson JMD, Donner AP, Trevithick JR. A possible role for vitamins C and E in cataract prevention. *Am J Clin Nutr* 1991; 53: 346S–51S.

16. Hankinson SE, Stampfer MJ, Seddon JM, et al. Nutrient intake and cataract extraction in women: a prospective study. *BMJ* 1992; 305: 335–39.

17. Jacques PF, Taylor A, Hankinson SE, et al. Long-term vitamin C supplement use and prevalence of early age-related lens opacities. *Am J Clin Nutr* 1997; 66: 911–16.

18. Rouhiainen P, Rouhiainen H, Salonen JT. Association between low plasma vitamin E concentration and progression of early cortical lens opacities. *Am J Epidemiol* 1996; 144: 496–500.

19. Trevithick JR, Creighton MO, et al. Modelling cortical cataractogenesis: 2. *In vitro* effects on the lens of agents preventing glucose- and sorbitol-induced cataracts. *Can J Ophthalmol* 1981; 16: 32–38.

20. Robertson JMD, Donner AP, Trevithick JR. A possible role for vitamins C and E in cataract prevention. *Am J Clin Nutr* 1991; 53: 346S–51S.

21. Seddon JM, Christen WG, Manson JE, et al. The use of vitamin supplements and the risk of cataract among U.S. male physicians. *Am J Public Health* 1994; 84: 788–92.

22. Leske MC, Chylack LT Jr, He Q, et al. Antioxidant vitamins and nuclear opacities. The Longitudinal Study of Cataract. *Ophthalmology* 1998; 105: 831–36.

23. Teikari JM, Virtamo J, Rautalahti M, et al. Long-term supplementation with alpha-tocopherol and beta-carotene and age-related cataract. *Acta Ophthalmol Scand* 1997; 75: 634–40.

24. Hankinson SE, Stampfer MJ, Seddon JM, et al. Nutrient intake and cataract extraction in women: a prospective study. *BMJ* 1992; 305: 335–39.

25. Teikari JM, Virtamo J, Rautalahti M, et al. Long-term supplementation with alpha-tocopherol and

beta-carotene and age-related cataract. *Acta Ophthalmol Scand* 1997; 75: 634–40.

26. Hankinson SE, Stampfer MJ, Seddon JM, et al. Nutrient intake and cataract extraction in women: a prospective study. *BMJ* 1992; 305: 335–39.

27. Yeum K-J, Taylor A, Tang G, Russell RM. Measurement of carotenoids, retinoids, and tocopherols in human lenses. *Ophthalmol Vis Sci* 1995; 36: 2756–61.

28. Bhat KS. Nutritional status of thiamine, riboflavin and pyridoxine in cataract patients. *Nutr Rep Internat* 1987; 36: 685–92.

29. Prchal JT, Conrad ME, Skalka HW. Association of presenile cataracts with heterozygosity for galactosaemic states and with riboflavin deficiency. *Lancet* 1978; i: 12–13.

30. Sperduto RD, Hu TS, Milton RC, et al. The Linxian cataract studies. *Arch Ophthalmol* 1993; 111: 1246–53.

31. Varma SD et al. Diabetic cataracts and flavonoids. *Science* 1977; 195: 205.

32. van Acker SA, van den Berg DJ, Tromp MN, et al. Structural aspects of antioxidant activity of flavonoids. *Free Rad Biol Med* 1996; 20: 331–42.

33. Salvayre R, Braquet P, et al. Comparison of the scavenger effect of bilberry anthocyanosides with various flavonoids. *Proceed Intl Bioflavonoids Symposium*, Munich 1981,437–42.

34. Bravetti G. Preventive medical treatment of senile cataract with vitamin E and anthocyanosides: clinical evaluation. *Ann Ottamol Clin Ocul* 1989; 115: 109.

Celiac Disease

1. Auricchio S, Follo D, de Ritis G, et al. Does breast feeding protect against the development of clinical symptoms of celiac disease in children? *J Pediatr Gastroenterol Nutr* 1983; 2: 428–33.

2. Udall JN, Colony P, Fritze L, et al. Development of gastrointestinal

mucosal barrier. II. The effect of natural versus artificial feeding on intestinal permeability to macromolecules. *Pediatr Res* 1981; 15: 245–49.

3. Janatuinen EK, Pikkarainen PH, Kemppainen TA, et al. A comparison of diets with and without oats in adults with celiac disease. *N Engl J Med* 1995; 333: 1033–37

4. Srinivassan U, Leonard N, Jones E, et al. Absence of oats toxicity in adult coeliac disease. *BMJ* 1996; 313: 1300–1.

5. Jantauinen EK, Pikkarainen PH, Kemppainen TA, et al. A comparison of diets with and without oats in adults with celiac disease. *N Engl J Med* 1995; 333: 1033–37.

6. Greenberger JN, Isselbacher KJ. Disorders of absorption. In Fauci AS, Braunwald E, Isselbacher KJ, et al. (eds). *Harrison's Principles of Internal Medicine*, 14th Edition. New York: McGraw-Hill, 1998, chapter 285.

7. Holmes GKT, Prior P, Lane MR, et al. Malignancy in coeliac disease—effect of a gluten free diet. *Gut* 1989; 30: 333–38.

8. Mora S, Barera G, Ricotti A, et al. Reversal of low bone density with a gluten-free diet in children and adolescents with celiac disease. *Am J Clin Nutr* 1998; 67: 477–81.

9. McFarlane XA, Bhalla AK, Robertson DAF. Effect of a gluten free diet on osteopenia in adults with newly diagnosed coeliac disease. *Gut* 1996; 39: 180–84.

10. Baker PG, Read AE. Reversible infertility in male coeliac patients. *Br Med J* 1975; 2: 316–17.

11. Sewell P, Cooke WT, Cox EV, Meynell MJ. Milk intolerance in gastrointestinal disorders. *Lancet* 1963; 2: 1132–35.

12. Haeney MR, Goodwin BJF, Barratt MEJ, et al. Soya protein antibodies in man: their occurrence and possible relevance in coeliac disease. *J Clin Pathol* 1982; 35: 319–22.

13. Mike N, Haeney M, Asquith P. Soya protein hypersensitivity in coeliac disease: evidence for cell mediated immunity. *Gut* 1983; 24: A990.

14. Ament ME, Rubin CE. Soy protein—another cause of the flat

intestinal lesion. *Gastroenterology* 1972; 62: 227—34.

15. Connon JJ. Celiac disease. In Shils ME, Olson JA, Shike M (eds). *Modern Nutrition in Health and Disease*, Eighth Edition. Philadelphia: Lea & Febiger, 1994, 1062.

16. Crofton RW, Glover SC, Ewen SWB, et al. Zinc absorption in celiac disease and dermatitis herpetiformis: a test of small intestinal function. *Am J Clin Nutr* 1983; 38: 706–12.

17. Solomons NW, Rosenberg IH, Sandstead HH. Zinc nutrition in celiac sprue. *Am J Clin Nutr* 1976; 29: 371—75.

18. Rude RK, Olerich M. Magnesium deficiency: possible role in osteoporosis associated with glutensensitive enteropathy. *Osteoporos Int* 1996; 6: 453–61.

19. Russell RM, Smith VC, Multak R, et al. Dark-adaptation testing for diagnosis of subclinical vitamin-A deficiency and evaluation of therapy. *Lancet* 1973; 2: 1161–64.

20. Hallert C, Astrom J, Walan A. Reversal of psychopathology in adult celiac disease with the aid of pyridoxine (vitamin B$_6$). *Scand J Gastroenterol* 1983; 18: 299–304.

Chronic Fatigue Syndrome

1. Fulcher KY, White PD. Randomised controlled trial of graded exercise in patients with the chronic fatigue syndrome. *Br Med J* 1997; 314: 1647–52.

2. McCully KK, Sisto SA, Natelson BH. Use of exercise for treatment of chronic fatigue syndrome. *Sports Med* 1996; 21: 35–48 [review].

3. Sharpe M, Hawton K, Simkin S, et al. Cognitive behaviour therapy for the chronic fatigue syndrome: A randomized controlled trial. *Br Med J* 1996; 312: 22–26.

4. De Lorenzo F, Hargreaves J, Kakkar VV. Pathogenesis and management of delayed orthostatic hypotension in patients with chronic fatigue syndrome. *Clin Auton Res* 1997; 7: 185–90.

5. Shaw DL et al. Management of fatigue: A physiologic approach. *Am J Med Sci* 1962; 243: 758.

6. Crescente FJ. Treatment of fatigue in a surgical practice. *J Abdom Surg* 1962; 4: 73.

7. Cox IM, Campbell MJ, Dowson D. Red blood cell magnesium and chronic fatigue syndrome. *Lancet* 1991; 337: 757–60.

8. Howard JM, Davies S, Hunnisett A. Magnesium and chronic fatigue syndrome. *Lancet* 1992; 340: 426.

9. Clague JE, Edwards RH, Jackson MJ. Intravenous magnesium loading in chronic fatigue syndrome. *Lancet* 1992; 340: 124–25.

10. Gantz NM. Magnesium and chronic fatigue. *Lancet* 1991; 338: 66 [letter].

11. Hinds G, Bell NP, McMaster D, McCluskey DR. Normal red cell magnesium concentrations and magnesium loading tests in patients with chronic fatigue syndrome. *Ann Clin Biochem* 1994; 31(Pt. 5): 459–61.

12. Kaufman W. The use of vitamin therapy to reverse certain concomitants of aging. *J Am Geriatr Soc* 1955; 3: 927–36.

13. Ellis FR, Nasser S. A pilot study of vitamin B$_{12}$ in the treatment of tiredness. *Br J Nutr* 1973; 30: 277–83.

14. Lawhorne L, Rindgahl D. Cyanocobalamin injections for patients without documented deficiency. *JAMA* 1989; 261: 1920–23.

15. AR. Literature Review & Commentary. *Townsend Letter for Doctors & Patients* Feb/Mar 1997, 27 [review].

16. Lapp CW, Cheney PR. The rationale for using high-dose cobalamin (vitamin B$_{12}$). *CFIDS Chronicle Physicians' Forum*, Fall 1993, 19–20.

17. Kuratsune H, Yamaguti K, Takahashi M, et al. Acylcarnitine deficiency in chronic fatigue syndrome. *Clin Infect Dis* 1994; 18(suppl 1): S62–67.

18. Plioplys AV, Plioplys S. Amantadine and L-carnitine treatment of chronic fatigue syndrome. *Neuropsycholbiol* 1997; 35: 16–23.

19. Forsyth LM, MacDowell-Carnciro AL, Birkmayer GD, et al. The use of NADH as a new therapeutic approach in chronic fatigue syndrome. Presented at the annual meeting of the American College of Allergy, Asthma & Immunology, 1998.

20. Bou-Holaigah I, Rowe PC, Kan J, Calkins H. The relationship between neurally mediated hypotension and the chronic fatigue syndrome. *JAMA* 1995; 274: 961–67.

21. Baschetti R. Chronic fatigue syndrome and liquorice. *New Z Med J* 1995; 108: 156–57.

22. Brown D. Licorice root—potential early intervention for chronic fatigue syndrome. *Quart Rev Natural Med* 1996; Summer: 95–97.

Chronic Venous Insufficiency

1. Rehn D, Brunnauer H, Diebschlag W, Lehmacher W. Investigation of the therapeutic equivalence of different galenical preparations of O-(s-hydroxyethyl)-rutosides following multiple dose per oral administration. *Arzneim Forsch* 1996; 46: 488–92.

2. Bergqvist D, Hallbook T, Lindblad B, Lindhagen A. A double-blind trial of O-(s-hydroxyethyl)-rutoside in patients with chronic venous insufficiency. *Vasa* 1981; 10: 253–60.

3. Unkauf M, Rehn D, Klinger J, et al. Investigation of the efficacy of oxerutins compared to placebo in patients with chronic venous insufficiency treated with compression stockings. *Arzneim Forsch Drug Res* 1996; 46: 478–82.

4. Stegmann W, Hubner K, Deichmann B, Muller B. Efficacy of O-(s-hydroxyethyl)-rutosides in the treatment of venous leg ulcers. *Phlebologie* 1987; 40: 149–56 [in French].

5. Diehm C, Trampisch JH, Lange S, Schmidt C. Comparison of leg compression stocking and oral horse-chestnut seed extract therapy in patients with chronic venous insufficiency. *Lancet* 1996; 347: 292–94.

6. Diehm C, Vollbrecht D, Amendt K, Comberg HU. Medical oedema protection—clinical benefits in patients with chronic deep vein incompetence. A placebo controlled double blind study. *Vasa* 1992; 21: 188–92.

7. Bisler H, Pfeifer R, Klüken, Pauschinger P. Wirkung von Ro βkastaniensamenextrakt auf die Transkapilläre Filtration bei chronishcer venöser Insuffizienz. *Deutche Med Wochenschr* 1986; 111: 1321–29 [in German].

8. Dartenuc JY, Marache P, Choussat H. Resistance Capillaire en Geriatrie Etude d'un Microangioprotecteur. *Bordeax Médical* 1980; 13: 903–907 [in French].

9. Delacroix P. Etude en double avengle de l'Endotelon dans l'insuffisance veineuse chronique. *Therapeutique, la Revue de Medicine* 1981; Sept 27–28: 1793–1802 [in French].

10. Thebaut JF, Thebaut P, Vin F. Study of Endotelon in functional manifestations of peripheral venous insufficiency. *Gazette Medicale* 1985; 92: 96–100 [in French].

11. Cappelli R, Nicora M, Di Perri T. Use of extract of *Ruscus aculeatus* in venous disease in the lower limbs. *Drugs Exp Clin Res* 1988; 14: 277–83.

Cold Sores

1. Algert SJ, Stubblefield NE, Grasse BJ, et al. Assessment of dietary intake of lysine and arginine in patients with herpes simplex. *J Am Diet Assoc* 1987: 87: 1560–61.

2. Tankersley RW Jr. Amino acid requirements of herpes simplex virus in human cells. *J Bacteriol* 1964; 87: 609–13.

3. Flodin NW. The metabolic roles, pharmacology, and toxicology of lysine. *J Am Coll Nutr* 1997; 16(1): 7–21.

4. Flodin NW. The metabolic roles, pharmacology, and toxicology of lysine. *J Am Coll Nutri* 1997; 16: 7–21 [review].

5. Flodin NW. The metabolic roles, pharmacology, and toxicology of lysine. *J Am Coll Nutr* 1997; 16(1): 7–21.

6. Griffith RS, Norins AL, Kagan C. A multicentered study of lysine therapy in herpes simplex infection. *Dermatologica* 1978; 156: 257–67.

7. Kagan C. Lysine therapy for herpes simplex. *Lancet* 1974; i: 137 [letter].

8. Griffith RS, Walsh DE, Myrmel KH, et al. Success of L-lysine therapy in frequently recurrent herpes simplex infection. *Dermatologica* 1987; 175: 183–90.

9. Milman N, Scheibel J, Jessen O. Lysine prophylaxis in recurrent herpes simplex labialis: a double blind, controlled crossover study. *Acta Derm Venereol* 1980; 60: 85–87.

10. DiGiovanna JJ, Blank H. Failure of lysine in frequently recurrent herpes simplex infection. Treatment and prophylaxis. *Arch Dermatol* 1984; 120: 48–51.

11. Milman N, Scheibel J, Jessen O. Failure of lysine treatment in recurrent herpes simplex labialis. *Lancet* 1978; ii: 942 [letter].

12. Eby GA, Halcomb WW. Use of topical zinc to prevent recurrent herpes simplex infection: Review of literature and suggested protocols. *Med Hypoth* 1985; 17: 157–65.

13. Brody I. Topical treatment of recurrent herpes simplex and post-herpetic erythema multiforme with low concentrations of zinc sulphate solution. *Br J Derm* 1981; 104: 191–94.

14. Apisariyakulm A, Buddhasukh D, Apisariyakul S, et al. Zinc monoglycerolate is effective against oral herpetic sores. *Med J Aust* 1990; 152: 54.

15. Nead DE. Effective vitamin E treatment for ulcerative herpetic lesions. *Dental Survey* 1976; 52: 50–51.

16. Fink M, Fink J. Treatment of herpes simplex by alpha-tocopherol (vitamin E). *Br Dent J* 1980; 148: 246 [letter].

17. Skinner GRB, Hartley CE, Millar D, Bishop E. Possible treatment for cold sores. *BMJ* 1979; 2(6192): 704.

18. Wöhlbling RH, Leonhardt K. Local therapy of herpes simplex with dried extract of Melissa officinalis. *Phytomedicine* 1994; 1(1): 25–31.

19. Serkedjieva J, Manolova N, Zgorniak-Nowosielska I, et al. Antiviral activity of the infusion (SHS-174) from flowers of *Sambucus nigra* L., aerial parts of *Hypericum perforatum* L., and roots of *Saponaria officinalis* L. against influenza and herpes simplex viruses. *Phytother Res* 1990; 4: 97–100.

Colic

1. Taubman B. Clinical trial of the treatment of colic by modification of parent-infant interaction. *Pediatr* 1984; 74: 998–1003.

2. Sampson HA. Infantile colic and food allergy: Fact or fiction? *J Pediatr* 1989; 115: 583–84.

3. Lothe L, Lindberg T. Cow's milk whey protein elicits symptoms of infantile colic in colicky formula-fed infants: A double-blind crossover study. *Pediatr* 1989; 83(2): 262–66.

4. Lothe L, Lindberg T, Jakobsson I. Cow's milk formula as a cause of infantile colic: A double-blind study. *Pediatr* 1982; 70(1): 7–10.

5. Jakobsson I, Lindberg T. Cow's milk proteins cause infantile colic in breast-fed infants: A double-blind crossover study. *Pediatr* 1983; 71(2): 268–71.

6. Evans RW, Fergusson DM, Allardyce RA, et al. Maternal diet and infantile colic in breast-fed infants. *Lancet* 1981; 49: 1340–42.

7. Clyne PS, Kulczycki A. Human breast milk contains bovine IgG. Relationship to infant colic? *Pediatr* 1991; 87: 439–44.

8. Hill DJ, Hudson IL, Sheffield LJ, et al. A low allergen diet is a significant intervention in infantile colic: Results of a community-based study. *J Allergy Clin Immunol* 1995; 96: 886–92.

9. Weizman Z, Alkrinawi S, Goldfarb D, Bitran C. Efficacy of herbal tea preparation in infantile colic. *J Pediatr* 1993; 122: 650–52.

10. Weizman Z, Alkrinawi S, Goldfarb D, Bitran C. Efficacy of herbal tea preparation in infantile colic. *J Pediatr* 1993; 122: 650–52.

11. Schilcher H. *Phytotherapy in Paediatrics*. Stuttgart: Medpharm Scientific Publishers, 1997, 80.

Common Cold/Sore Throat

1. Hemilä H. Does vitamin C alleviate the symptoms of the common

cold?—A review of current evidence. *Scand J Infect Dis* 1994; 26: 1–6.

2. Macknin ML. Zinc lozenges for the common cold. *Cleveland Clin J Med* 1999; 66: 27–32 [review].

3. Eby G, Davis DR, Halcomb WW. Reduction in duration of common colds by zinc gluconate lozenges in a double-blind study. *Antimicrobial Agents Chemotherapy* 1984; 25: 20–24.

4. Al-Nakib W, Higgins PG, Barrow I, et al. Prophylaxis and treatment of rhinovirus colds with zinc gluconate lozenges. *J Antimicrobial Chemotherapy* 1987; 20: 893–901.

5. Macknin ML, Piedmonte M, Calendine C, et al. Zinc gluconate lozenges for treating the common cold in children. A randomized controlled trial. *JAMA* 1998; 279: 1962–67.

6. Jackson JL, Peterson C, Lesho E. A meta-analysis of zinc salts lozenges and the common cold. *Arch Intern Med* 1997; 157: 2373–76.

7. Macknin ML. Zinc lozenges for the common cold. *Cleveland Clin J Med* 1999; 66: 27–32 [review].

8. Eby G. Where's the bias? *Ann Intern Med* 1998; 128: 75 [letter].

9. Garland ML, Hagmeyer KO. The role of zinc lozenges in treatment of the common cold. *Ann Pharmacother* 1998; 32: 63–69 [review].

10. Petrus EJ, Lawson KA, Bucci LR, Blum K. Randomized, double-masked, placebo-controlled clinical study of the effectiveness of zinc acetate lozenges on common cold symptoms in allergy-tested subjects. *Curr Ther Res* 1998; 59: 595–607.

11. Weismann K, Jakobsen JP, Weismann JE, et al. Zinc gluconate lozenges for common cold. A double-blind clinical trial. *Dan Med Bull* 1990; 37: 279–81.

12. Melchart D, Linde K, Worku F, et al. Immunomodulation with echinacea—a systematic review of controlled clinical trials. *Phytomedicine* 1994; 1: 245–54 [review].

13. Melchart D, Linde K, Worku F, et al. Immunomodulation with echinacea—a systematic review of controlled clinical trials. *Phytomedicine* 1994; 1: 245–54 [review].

14. Schilcher H. *Phytotheraphy in Paediatrics: Handbook for Physicians and Pharmacists*. Stuttgart: Medpharm Scientific Publishers, 1997, 43–45.

15. Dorn M, et al. Placebo-controlled, double-blind study of *Echinacea pallidae* radix in upper respiratory tract infections. *Compl Ther Med* 1997; 5: 40–42.

16. Melchart D, Walther E, Linde K, et al. Echinacea root extracts for the prevention of upper respiratory tract infections. *Arch Fam Med* 1998; 7: 541–45.

17. Grimm W, Mueller HH. A randomized controlled clinical trial of the effect of fluid extract of *Echinacea purpurea* on the incidence and severity of colds and respiratory infections. *Am J Med* 1999; 106: 138–43.

18. Murray MT. *The Healing Power of Herbs*. Rocklin, CA: Prima Publishing, 1995, 162–72.

19. Bradley PR, ed. *British Herbal Compendium*, Vol. 1. Bounemouth, Dorset, UK: British Herbal Medicine Association, 1992, 119–20.

20. Schilcher H. *Phytotherapy in Paediatrics*. Stuttgart, Germany: Medpharm Scientific Publishers, 1997, 126–27.

21. Beuscher N, Kopanski L. Stimulation of immunity by the contents of *Baptisia tinctoria*. *Planta Med* 1985; 5: 381–84.

22. Schulz V, Hansel R, Tyler VE. *Rational Phytotherapy*, 3rd ed. Berlin, Germany: Springer Verlag, 1998, 146–47.

23. Zeylstra H. *Filipendila ulmaria*. *Br J Phytotherapy* 1998; 5: 8–12.

Congestive Heart Failure (CHF)

1. Coats AJS. Effects of physical training in chronic heart failure. *Lancet* 1990; 335: 63–66.

2. Belardinelli R, Georgiou D, Cianci G, Purcaro A. Randomized, controlled trial of long-term moderate exercise training in chronic heart failure. *Circulation* 1999; 99: 1173–82.

3. Mortensen SA, Vadhanavikit S, Baandrup U, Folkers K. Long-term coenzyme Q_{10} therapy: a major advance in the management of resistant myocardial failure. *Drug Exptl Clin Res* 1985; 11: 581–93.

4. Morisco C, Trimarco B, Condorelli M. Effect of coenzyme Q_{10} in patients with congestive heart failure: a long-term multicenter randomized study. *Clin Invest* 1993; 71: S134–36.

5. Mortensen SA, Vadhanavikit S, Baandrup U, Folkers K. Long-term coenzyme Q_{10} therapy: a major advance in the management of resistant myocardial failure. *Drug Exptl Clin Res* 1985; 11: 581–93.

6. Bartels GL, Remme WJ, Pillay M, et al. Effects of L-propionylcarnitine on ischemia-induced myocardial dysfunction in men with angina pectoris. *Am J Cardiol* 1994; 74: 125–30.

7. Suzuki Y, Masumura Y, Kobayashi A, et al. Myocardial carnitine deficiency in chronic heart failure. *Lancet* 1982; i: 116 [letter].

8. Mancini M, Rengo F, Lingetti M, Sorrentino GP, Nolfe G. Controlled study on the therapeutic efficacy of propionyl-L-carnitine in patients with congestive heart failure. *Arzneimittelforschung* 1992; 42: 1101–104.

9. Pucciarelli G, Mastursi M, Latte S, et al. The clinical and hemodynamic effects of propionyl-L-carnitine in the treatment of congestive heart failure. *Clin Ther* 1992; 141: 379–84.

10. Kobayashi A, Masumura Y, Yamazaki N. L-carnitine treatment for congestive heart failure—experimental and clinical study. *Jpn Circ J* 1992; 56: 86–94.

11. Bashir Y, Sneddon JF, Staunton A, et al. Effects of long-term oral magnesium chloride replacement in congestive heart failure secondary to coronary artery disease. *Am J Cardiol* 1993; 72: 1156–62.

12. Packer M, Gottlieb SS, Kessler PD. Hormone-electrolyte interactions in the pathogenesis of lethal cardiac arrhythmias in patients with congestive heart failure. *Am J Med* 1986; 80(suppl 4A): 23–29.

13. Azuma J, Sawamura A, Awata N, et al. Double-blind random-

ized crossover trial of taurine in congestive heart failure. *Curr Ther Res* 1983; 34(4): 543–57.

14. Azuma J, Hasegawa H, Sawamura N, et al. Taurine for treatment of congestive heart failure. *Int J Cardiol* 1982; 2: 303–304.

15. Azuma J, Hasegawa H, Sawamura A, et al. Therapy of congestive heart failure with orally administered taurine. *Clin Ther* 1983; 5(4): 398–408.

16. Azuma J, Takihara K, Awata N, et al. Taurine and failing heart: experimental and clinical aspects. *Prog Clin Biol Res* 1985; 179: 195–213.

17. Rector TS, Bank A, Mullen KA, et al. Randomized, double-blind, placebo controlled study of supplemental oral L-arginine in patients with heart failure. *Circulation* 1996; 93: 2135–41.

18. Leuchtgens H. *Crataegus* special extract (WS 1442) in cardiac insufficiency. *Fortschr Med* 1993; 111: 352–54.

19. Schmidt U, Kuhn U, et al. Efficacy of the hawthorn (*Crataegus*) preparation LI 132 in 78 patients with chronic congestive heart failure defined as NYHA functional class II. *Phytomed* 1994; 1: 17–24.

20. Maevers VW, Hensel H. Changes in local myocardial blood flow following oral administration of a *Crataegus* extract to non-anesthetized dogs. *Arzneim-Forsch Drug Res* 1974; 24: 783–85.

21. Weikl A, Noh HS. The influence of *Crataegus* on global cardiac insufficiency. *Herz Gerfässe* 1992; 11: 516–24.

22. Bahorun T, Trotin F, et al. Antioxidant activities of *Crataegus monogyna* extracts. *Planta Med* 1994; 60: 323–28.

Conjunctivitis (Pinkeye) and Blepharitis

1. Rankov BG. Vitamin A and carotene concentration in serum in persons with chronic conjunctivitis and pterygium. *Int J Vitam Nutr Res* 1976; 46: 454–7 [in German].

2. Chan E. Displacement of bilirubin from albumin by berberine. *Biol Neonate* 1993; 63: 201–8.

Constipation

1. Müller-Lissner SA. Effect of wheat bran on weight of stool and gastrointestinal transit time: a meta analysis. *BMJ* 1988; 296: 615–17.

2. Marcus SN, Heaton KW. Effects of a new, concentrated wheat fibre preparation on intestinal transit, deoxycholic acid metabolism and the composition of bile. *Gut* 1986; 27: 893–900.

3. Iacono G, Cavataio F, Montalto G, et al. Intolerance of cow's milk and chronic constipation in children. *N Engl J Med* 1998; 339: 1100–104.

4. Oettl GJ. Effect of moderate exercise on bowel habit. *Gut* 1991; 32: 941–44.

5. Bingham SA, Cummings JH. Effect of exercise and physical fitness on large intestinal function. *Gastroenterology* 1989; 97: 1389–99.

6. Young RW, Beregi JS Jr. Use of chlorophyllin in the care of geriatric patients. *J Am Geriatr Soc* 1980; 28: 46–47.

7. Passmore AP, Wilson-Davies K, et al. Chronic constipation in long stay elderly patients: A comparison of lactulose and senna-fiber combination. *BMJ* 1993; 307: 769–71.

Chronic Obstructive Pulmonary Disease

1. Pingleton SK, Harmon GS. Nutritional management in acute respiratory failure. *JAMA* 1987; 257(22): 3094–99.

2. Fiaccadori E, Del Canale S, Coffrini E, et al. Hypercapnic-hypoxemic chronic obstructive pulmonary disease (COPD): influence of severity of COPD on nutritional status. *Am J Clin Nutr* 1988; 48: 680–85.

3. Efthimiou J, Mounsey PJ, Bensen DN, et al. Effect of carbohydrate rich versus fat rich loads on gas exchange and walking performance in patients with chronic obstructive lung disease. *Thorax* 1992; 47: 451–56.

4. Miedema I, Feskens EJM, Heederik D, et al. Dietary determi-

nants of long-term incidence of chronic nonspecific lung diseases. *Am J Epidemiol* 1993; 138: 37–45.

5. Businco L, Businco E. Allergic pathogenesis in chronic bronchitis. *Allergol Immunopathol* (Madr) 1975; 3: 1–8.

6. Krawczyk Z. Role of allergy of the immediate type in the pathogenesis of chronic bronchitis in adults. *Pneumonol Pol* 1976; 44: 829–36 [in Polish].

7. No author listed. Preliminary study on the relation between allergy and chronic bronchitis. *Chin Med J* 1976; 2: 63–68.

8. Rowe AH, Rowe A Jr, Sinclair C. Food allergy: its role in the symptoms of obstructive emphysema and chronic bronchitis. *J Asthma Res* 1967; 5: 11–20.

9. Gualtierotti R, Solimene U, Tonoli D. Ionized air respiratory rehabilitation technics. *Minerva Medica* 1977; 68: 3383–9.

10. Jones DP, O'Connor SA, Collins JV, et al. Effect of long-term ionized air treatment on patients with bronchial asthma. *Thorax* 1976; 31(4): 428–32.

11. Van Schayck CP, Dekhuijzen PNR, Gorgels WJMJ, et al. Are antioxidant and anti-inflammatory treatments effective in different subgroups of COPD? A hypothesis. *Respir Med* 1998; 92: 1259–64.

12. Boman G, Bäcker U, Larsson S, et al. Oral acetylcysteine reduces exacerbation rate in chronic bronchitis: a report of a trial organized by the Swedish Society for Pulmonary Diseases. *Eur J Respir Dis* 1983; 64: 405–15.

13. Multicenter Study Group. Long-term oral acetylcysteine in chronic bronchitis. A double-blind controlled study. *Eur J Respir Dis* 1980; 61: 111: 93–108.

14. Sridhar MK. Nutrition and lung health. *BMJ* 1995; 310: 75–76.

15. Rautalahti M, Virtamo J, Haukka J, et al. The effect of alpha-tocopherol and beta-carotene supplementation on COPD symptoms. *Am J Respir Crit Care Med* 1997; 156: 1447–52.

Part One: References

16. Shahar E, Folsom AR, Melnick SL, et al. Dietary n-3 polyunsaturated fatty acids and smoking-related chronic obstructive pulmonary disease. Atherosclerosis Risk in Communities Study Investigators. *N Engl J Med* 1994; 331: 228–33.

17. Rolla G, Bucca C, Bugiani M, et al. Hypomagnesiumia in chronic obstructive lung disease: effect of therapy. *Magnesium Trace Elem* 1990; 9: 132–36.

18. Fiaccadori E, Del Canale S, Coffrini E, et al. Muscle and serum magnesium in pulmonary intensive care unit patients. *Crit Care Med* 1988; 16: 751–60.

19. Skorodin MS, Tenholder MF, Yetter B, et al. Magnesium sulfate in exacerbations of chronic obstructive pulmonary disease. *Arch Intern Med* 1995; 155: 496–500.

20. Okayama H, Aikawa T, Okayama M, et al. Bronchodilating effect of intravenous magnesium sulfate in bronchial asthma. *JAMA* 1987; 257: 1076–78.

21. Dal Negro R, Pomari G, et al. L-carnitine and rehabilitative respiratory physiokinesitherapy: metabolic and ventilatory response in chronic respiratory insufficiency. *Int J Clin Pharmacol Ther Toxicol* 1986; 24: 453–56.

22. Dal Negro R, Turco P, Pomari C, De Conti F. Effects of L-carnitine on physical performance in chronic respiratory insufficiency. *Int J Clin Pharmacol Ther Toxicol* 1988; 26: 269–72.

23. Fujimoto S, Kurihara N, Hirata K, Takeda T. Effects of coenzyme Q_{10} administration on pulmonary function and exercise performance in patients with chronic lung diseases. *Clin Investig* 1993; 71(8 suppl): S162–66.

24. Hoffman D. *The Herbal Handbook: A User's Guide to Medical Herbalism*. Rochester VT: Healing Arts Press, 1988, 67.

25. Boyd EM. Expectorants and respiratory tract fluid. *Pharmacol Rev* 1954; 6: 521–42 [review].

Cough

1. Nosal'ova G, Strapkova A, Kardosova A, et al. Antitussive action of extracts and polysaccharides of marshmallow (*Althea officinalis* L, var robusta). *Pharmazie* 1992; 47: 224–26 [in German].

2. Schilcher H. *Phytotherapy in Paediatrics*. Stuttgart: Medpharm Scientific Publishers, 1997, 38.

3. Wichtl M, Bisset N, eds. *Herbal Drugs and Phytopharmaceuticals*. Stuttgart: Medpharm Scientific Publishers and Boca Raton, FL: CRC Press, 1994.

4. Muller-Limmroth W, Frohlich HH. Effect of various phytotherapeutic expectorants on mucocililary transport. *Fortschr Med* 1980; 98: 95–101 [in German].

5. Boatto G et al. Composition and antibacterial activity of *Inula helenium* and *Rosmarinus officinalis* essential oils. *Fitoterapia* 1994; 6: 279–80.

6. Zgorniak-Nowosielska I et al. Antiviral activity of flos verbasci infusion against influenza and herpes simplex viruses. *Arch Immunol Ther Exp* 1991; 39: 103–108.

7. Castleman M. *The Healing Herbs*. Emmaus, PA: Rodale Press, 1991, 162–63.

8. Leung AY, Foster S. *Encyclopedia of Common Natural Ingredients Used in Food, Drugs, and Cosmetics*. New York: John Wiley & Sons, 1996, 492–95.

9. Gruenwald J, Brendler T, Jaenicke C. *PDR for Herbal Medicines*. Montvale, NJ: Medical Economics, 1998, 1184–85.

10. Weiss RF. *Herbal Medicine*. Gothenburg, Sweden: Ab Arcanum and Beaconsfield, UK: Beaconsfield Publishers Ltd, 1988, 208–209.

Crohn's Disease

1. Mayberry JF, Rhodes J. Epidemiological aspects of Crohn's disease: a review of the literature. *Gut* 1984; 886–99.

2. Heaton KW, Thornton JR, Emmett PM. Treatment of Crohn's disease with an unrefined-carbohydrate, fibre-rich diet. *BMJ* 1979; 2(6193): 764–66.

3. Brandes JW, Lorenz-Meyer H. Sugar free diet: a new perspective in the treatment of Crohn disease? Randomized, control study. *Z Gastroneterol* 1981; 19: 1–12.

4. Shoda R, Masueda K, Yamato S, Umeda N. Epidemiologic analysis of Crohn's disease in Japan: increased dietary intake of n-6 polyunsaturated fatty acids and animal protein relates to the increased incidence of Crohn's disease in Japan. *Am J Clin Nutr* 1996; 63: 741–5.

5. Riordan AM, Hunter JO, Cowan RE, et al. Treatment of active Crohn's disease by exclusion diet: East Anglian Multicentre Controlled Trial. *Lancet* 1993; 342: 1131–4.

6. Wantke F, Gotz M, Jarisch R. *Lancet* 1994; 343: 113 [letter].

7. McDonald PJ, Fazio VW. What can Crohn's patients eat? *Eur J Clin Nutr* 1988; 42: 703–708.

8. Gaby AR. Commentary. *Nutr Healing* January 1998; 1, 10–11; [review].

9. Cottone M, Rosselli M, Orlando A, et al. Smoking habits and recurrence in Crohn's disease. *Gastroenterol* 1994; 106: 643–8.

10. Imes S, Plinchbeck BR, Dinwoodie A, et al. Iron, folate, vitamin B-12, zinc, and copper status in out-patients with Crohn's disease: effect of diet counseling. *J Am Dietet Assoc* 1987; 87: 928–30.

11. Sandstead HH. Zinc deficiency in Crohn's disease. *Nutr Rev* 1982; 40: 109–12.

12. Dvorak AM. Vitamin A in Crohn's disease. *Lancet* 1980; i: 1303–4.

13. Skogh M, Sundquist T, Tagesson C. Vitamin A in Crohn's disease. *Lancet* 1980; i: 766 [letter].

14. Dvorak AM. Vitamin A in Crohn's Disease. *Lancet* 1980; i: 1303–304 [letter].

15. Wright JP, Mee AS, Parfitt A, et al. Vitamin A therapy inpatients with Crohn's disease. *Gastroenterology* 1985; 88: 512–14.

16. Leichtmann GA, Bengoa JM, Bolt MJG, Sitrin MD. Intestinal absorption of cholecalciferol and 25-hydrocycholecalciferol in patients with both Crohn's disease and intestinal resection. *Am J Clin Nutr* 1991; 54: 548–52.

17. Harris AD, Brown R, Heatley RV, et al. Vitamin D status in Crohn's

disease: association with nutrition and disease activity. *Gut* 1985; 26: 1197–1203.

18. Driscoll RH, Meredith SC, Sitrin M, Rosenberg IH. Vitamin D deficiency and bone disease in patients with Crohn's disease. *Gastroenterol* 1982; 83: 1252–8.

19. Mate J, Castanos R, Garcia-Samaniego J, Pajares JM. Does dietary fish oil maintain the remission of Crohn's disease: a case control study. *Gastroenterology* 1991; 100: A228 [abstract].

20. Belluzzi A, Brignola C, Campieri M, et al. Effect of an enteric-coated fish-oil preparation on relapses in Crohn's disease. *N Engl J Med* 1996; 334: 1557–60.

21. Lorenz R, Weber PC, Szimnau P, et al. Supplemenation with n-3 fatty acids from fish oil in chronic inflammatory bowel disease—a randomized, placebo-controlled, double-blind cross-over trial. *J Intern Med Suppl* 1989; 225: 225–32.

22. Ref: Lorenz-Meyer H, Bauer P Nicolay C, et al. Omega-3 fatty acids and low carbohydrate diet for maintenance of remission in Crohn's disease. A randomized controlled multicenter trial. German Crohn's Disease Study Group Members. *Scand J Gastroenterol* 1996; 31: 778–85.

23. Belluzzi A, Brignola C, Campieri M, et al. Effects of new fish oil derivative on fatty acid phospholipid-membrane pattern in a group of Crohn's disease patients. *Dig Dis Sci* 1994; 39: 2589–94.

24. Plein K, Hotz J. Therapeutic effects of *Saccharomyces boulardii* on mild residual symptoms in a stable phase of Crohn's disease with special respect to chronic diarrhea—a pilot study. *Z Gastroenterol* 1993; 31: 129–34.

25. Bleichner G, Blehaut H, Mentec H, Moyse D. *Saccharomyces boulardii* prevents diarrhea in critically ill tube-fed patients. A muticenter, randomized, double-blind placebo-controlled trial. *Intensive Care Med* 1997; 23: 517–23.

26. Hegnhoj J, Hansen CP, Rannem T, et al. Pancreatic function in Crohn's disease. *Gut* 1990; 31: 1076–79.

27. Plein K, Burkard G, Hotz J. [Treatment of chronic diarrhea in Crohn disease. A pilot study of the clinical effect of tannin albuminate and ethacridine lactate.] *Fortschr Med* 1993; (Mar 10)111(7): 114–18 [in German].

Depression

1. Gettis A. Food sensitivities and psychological disturbance: a review. *Nutr Health* 1989; 6: 135–46.

2. King DS. Can allergic exposure provoke psychological symptoms? A double-blind test. *Biol Psychiatr* 1981; 16: 3–19.

3. Brown M, Gibney M, Husband PR, Radcliffe M. Food allergy in polysymptomatic patients. *Practitioner* 1981; 225: 1651–54.

4. Christensen L. Psychological distress and diet-effects of sucrose and caffeine. *J Applied Nutr* 1988; 40: 44–50.

5. Greden JF, Fontaine P, Lubetsky M, Chamberlin K. Anxiety and depression associated with caffeinism among psychiatric inpatients. *Am J Psychiatry* 1978; 135: 963–66.

6. Kawachi I, Willett WC, Colditz GA, Stampfer MJ, Speizer FE. A prospective study of coffee drinking and suicide in women. *Arch Intern Med* 1996; 156: 521–25.

7. Gilliland K, Bullock W. Caffeine: a potential drug of abuse. *Adv Alcohol Subst Abuse* 1983-84; 3: 53–73.

8. Martinsen EW. Benefits of exercise for the treatment of depression. *Sports Med* 1990; 9: 380–89.

9. Martinsen EW, Medhus A, Sandivik L. Effects of aerobic exercise on depression: a controlled study. *BMJ* 1985; 291: 109.

10. Adams PW, Wynn V, Rose DP, et al. Effect of pyridoxine hydrochloride (Vitamin B$_6$) upon depression associated with oral contraception. *Lancet* 1973; I: 897–904.

11. Russ CS, Hendricks TA, Chrisley BM, et al. Vitamin B$_6$ status of depressed and obsessive-compulsive patients. *Nutr Rep Internat* 1983; 27: 867–73.

12. Gunn ADG. Vitamin B$_6$ and the premenstrual syndrome (PMS). *Int*

J Vitam Nutr Res 1985; (suppl 27): 213–24 [review].

13. Kleijnen J, Riet GT, Knipschild P. Vitamin B$_6$ in the treatment of the premenstrual syndrome—a review. *Brit J Obstet Gynaecol* 1990; 97: 847–52.

14. Lindenbaum J, Healton EB, Savage DG, et al. Neuropsychiatric disorders caused by cobalamin deficiency in the absence of anemia or macrocytosis. *N Engl J Med* 1988; 318: 1720–28.

15. Holmes JM. Cerebral manifestations of vitamin B$_{12}$ deficiency. *J Nutr Med* 1991; 2: 89–90.

16. Ellis FR, Nasser S. A pilot study of vitamin B$_{12}$ in the treatment of tiredness. *Br J Nutr* 1973; 30: 277–83.

17. Reynolds E et al. Folate deficiency in depressive illness. *Br J Psychiatr* 1970; 117: 287–92.

18. Coppen A, Chaudrhy S, Swade C. Folic acid enhances lithium prophylaxis. *J Affective Disorders* 1986; 10: 9–13.

19. Di Palma C, Urani R, Agricola R, et al. Is methylfolate effective in relieving major depression in chronic alcoholics? A hypothesis of treatment. *Curr Ther Res* 1994; 55: 559–67.

20. Edwards R, Peet M, Shay J, Horrobin D. Omega-3 polyunsaturated fatty acid levels in the diet and in red blood cell membranes of depressed patients. *J Affect Disord* 1998; 48: 149–55.

21. Adams PB, Lawson S, Sanigorski A, Sinclair AJ. Arachidonic acid to eicosapentaenoic acid ratio in blood correlates positively with clinical symptoms of depression. *Lipids* 1996; 31: S-157–S-161.

22. Rose DP, Cramp DG. Reduction of plasma tyrosine by oral contraceptives and oestrogens: a possible consequence of tyrosine amino-transferase induction. *Clin Chem Acta* 1970; 29: 49–53.

23. Moller SE. Tryptophan and tyrosine availability and oral contraceptives. *Lancet* 1979; ii: 472 [letter].

24. Kishimoto H, Hama Y. The level and diurnal rhythm of plasma tryptophan and tyrosine in manic-

depressive patients. *Yokohama Med Bull* 1976; 27: 89–97.

25. Gelenberg AJ, Wojcik JD, Growdon JH, et al. Tyrosine for the treatment of depression. *Am J Psychiatr* 1980; 137: 622–23.

26. Sabelli HC, Fawcett J, Gustovsky F, et al. Clinical studies on the phenylethylamine hypothesis of affective disorder: urine and blood phenylacetic acid and phenylalanine dietary supplements. *J Clin Psychiatr* 1986; 47: 66–70.

27. Sabelli HC, Fawcett J, Gustovsky F, et al. Clinical studies on the phenylethylamine hypothesis of affective disorder: urine and blood phenylacetic acid and phenylalanine dietary supplements. *J Clin Psychiatr* 1986; 47: 66–70.

28. Beckmann H, Strauss MA, Ludolph E. DL-Phenylalanine in depressed patients: an open study. *J Neural Transmission* 1977; 41: 123–34.

29. Beckmann H, Athen D, Olteanu M, Zimmer R. DL-phenylalanine versus imipramine: a double-blind controlled study. *Arch Psychiatr Nervenkr* 1979; 227: 49–58.

30. Maggioni M, Picotti GB, Bondiolotti GP, et al. Effects of phosphatidylserine therapy in geriatric patients with depressive disorders. *Acta Psychiatr Scand* 1990; 81: 265–70.

31. Wolkowitz OM, et al. Dehydroepiandrosterone (DHEA) treatment of depression. *Biol Psychiatr* 1997; 41: 311–18.

32. Wolkowitz OW, Reus VI, Keebler A, et al. Double-blind treatment of major depression with dehydroepiandrosterone. *Am J Psychiatry* 1999; 156: 646–49.

33. Barkai AI, Dunner DL, Gross HA, et al. Reduced myo-inositol levels in cerebrospinal fluid from patients with affective disorder. *Biol Psych* 1978; 13: 65–72.

34. Birkmayer JGD, Birkmayer W. The coenzyme nicotinamide adenine dinucleotide (NADH) as biological antidepressive agent: Experience with 205 patients. *New Trends Clin Neuropharmacol* 1991; 5: 19–25.

35. Bell KM, Potkin SG, Carreon D, Plon L. S-adenosylmethionine blood levels in major depression: changes with drug treatment. *Acta Neurol Scand* 1994; 154(suppl): 15–18.

36. Bressa GM. S-adenosyl-l-methionine (SAMe) as antidepressant: Meta-analysis of clinical studies. *Acta Neurol Scand* 1994; 154(suppl): 7–14.

37. Salmaggi P, Bressa GM, Nicchia G, et al. Double-blind, placebo-controlled study of s-adenosyl-methionine in depressed postmenopausal women. *Psychotherapy & Psychosomatics* 1993; 59: 34–40.

38. Kagan BL, Sultzer DL, Rosenlicht N, et al. Oral S-adenosyl-methionine in depression: A randomized, double-blind, placebo-controlled trial. *Am J Psychiatr* 1990; 147: 591–95.

39. Fava M, Rosenbaum JF, Birnbaum R, et al. The thyrotropin-releasing hormone as a predictor of response to treatment in depressed outpatients. *Acta Psychiatr Scand* 1992; 86: 42–45.

40. De Vanna M, Rigamonti R. Oral S-adenosyl-L-methionine in depression. *Curr Ther Res* 1992; 52: 478–85.

41. Van Praag HM, Lemus C. Monoamine precursors in the treatment of psychiatric disorders. In *Nutrition and the Brain*, vol. 7. eds. RJ Wurtman, JJ Wurtman. New York: Raven Press, 1986 [review].

42. Van Praag H, de Hann S. Depression vulnerability and 5-hydroxytryptophan prophylaxis. *Psychiatry Res* 1980; 3: 75–83.

43. Angst J, Woggon B, Schoepf J. The treatment of depression with L-5-hydroxytryptophan versus imipramine. Results of two open and one double-blind study. *Arch Psychiatr Nervenkr* 1977; 224: 175–86.

44. Nolen WA, van de Putte JJ, Dijken WA, et al. Treatment strategy in depression. II. MAO inhibitors in depression resistant to cyclic antidepressants: two controlled crossover studies with tranylcypromine versus L-5-hydroxytryptophan and nimifensine. *Acta Psychiatr Scand* 1988; 78: 676–83.

45. Nolen WA, van de Putte JJ, Dijken WA, Kamp JS. L-5-HTP in depression resistant to re-uptake inhibitors. An open comparative study with tranylcypromine. *Br J Psychiatry* 1985; 147: 16–22.

46. D'Elia G, Hanson L, Raotma H. L-tryptophan and 5-hydroxytryptophan in the treatment of depression. A review. *Acta Psychiatr Scand* 1978; 57: 239–52 [review].

47. Harrer G, Sommer H. Treatment of mild/moderate depressions with *Hypericum*. *Phytomedicine* 1994; 1: 3–8.

48. Ernst E. St. John's wort, an antidepressant? A systemic, criteria-based review. *Phytomedicine* 1995; 2: 67–71.

49. Vorbach EU, Hübner WD, Arnoldt KH. Effectiveness and tolerance of the *Hypericum* extract LI 160 in comparison with imipramine: Randomized double-blind study with 135 outpatients. *J Ger Psychiatr Neurol* 1994; 7(suppl): S19–S23.

50. Wheatley D. LI 160, an extract of St. John's wort versus amitriptyline in mildly to moderately depressed outpatients—controlled six week clinical trial. *Pharmacopsychiatry* 1997; 30(suppl): 77–80.

51. Harrer G, Hübner WD, Poduzweit H. Effectiveness and tolerance of the *Hypericum* extract LI 160 compared to maprotiline: A multicenter double-blind study. *J Ger Psychiatr Neurol* 1994; 7(suppl 1); S24–S28.

52. Vorbach EU, Arnoldt KH, Hübner WD. Efficacy and tolerability of St. John's wort extract LI 160 versus imipramine in patients with severe depressive episodes according to ICD-10. *Pharmacopsychiatry* 1997; 30(suppl): 81–85.

53. Blumenthal M, Busse WR, Goldberg A, et al. (eds). *The Complete Commission E Monographs: Therapeutic Guide to Herbal Medicines*. Boston, MA: Integrative Medicine Communications, 1998, 214–215.

54. Chatterjee SS, Bhattacharya SK, Wonnemann M, et al. Hyperforin as a possible antidepressant components of hypericum extracts. *Life Sci* 1998; 63: 499–510.

55. Schubert H, Halama P. Depressive episode primarily unresponsive to therapy in elderly patients; efficacy of *Ginkgo biloba* extract (EGb 761) in combination with antidepressants. *Geriatr Forsch* 1993; 3: 45–53.

Diabetes: Section 2: Dietary and Lifestyle Changes

1. Colagiuri S, Miller JJ, Edwards RA. Metabolic effects of adding sucrose and aspartame to the diet of subjects with noninsulin-dependent diabetes mellitus. *Am J Clin Nutr* 1989; 50: 474–78.

2. Abraira C, Derler J. Large variations of sucrose in constant carbohydrate diets in type II diabetes. *Am J Med* 1988; 84: 193–200.

3. Loghmani E, Rickard K, Washburne L, et al. Glycemic response to sucrose-containing mixed meals in diets of children with insulin-dependent diabetes mellitus. *J Pediatr* 1991; 119: 531–37.

4. Wright DW, Hansen RI, Mondon CE, Reaven GM. Sucrose-induced insulin resistance in the rat: modulation by exercise and diet. *Am J Clin Nutr* 1983; 38: 879–83.

5. Lettle GJ, Emmett PM, Heaton KW. Glucose and insulin responses to manufactured and whole-food snacks. *Am J Clin Nutr* 1987; 45: 86–91.

6. Florholmen J, Arvidsson-Lenner R, Jorde R, Burhol PG. The effect of Metamucil on postprandial blood glucose and plasma gastric inhibitory peptide in insulin-dependent diabetics. *Acta Med Scand* 1982; 212: 237–39.

7. Rodríguez-Morán M, Guerrero-Romero F, Lazcano-Burciaga G. Lipid- and glucose-lowering efficacy of plantago psyllium in type II diabetes. *Diabetes Its Complications* 1998; 12: 273–78.

8. Landin K, Holm G, Tengborn L, Smith U. Guar gum improves insulin sensitivity, blood lipids, blood pressure, and fibrinolysis in healthy men. *Am J Clin Nutr* 1992; 56: 1061–65.

9. Schwartz SE, Levine RA, Weinstock RS, et al. Sustained pectin ingestion: effect on gastric emptying and glucose tolerance in non-insulin-dependent diabetic patients. *Am J Clin Nutr* 1988; 48: 1413–17.

10. Hallfrisch J, Scholfield DJ, Behall KM. Diets containing soluble oat extracts improve glucose and insulin responses of moderately hypercholesterolemic men and women. *Am J Clin Nutr* 1995; 61: 379–84.

11. Doi K, Matsuura M, Kawara A, Baba S. Treatment of diabetes with glucomannan (konjac mannan). *Lancet* 1979; i: 987–88 [letter].

12. Sharma RD, Raghuram TC. Hypoglycaemic effect of fenugreek seeds in non-insulin dependent diabetic subjects. *Nutr Res* 1990; 10: 731–39.

13. Raghuram TC, Sharma RD, et al. Effect of fenugreek seeds on intravenous glucose disposition in non-insulin dependent diabetic patients. *Phytother Res* 1994; 8: 83–86.

14. Nuttall FW. Dietary fiber in the management of diabetes. *Diabetes* 1993; 42: 503–8.

15. Feskens EJM, Bowles CH, Kromhout D. Inverse association between fish intake and risk of glucose intolerance in normoglycemic elderly men and women. *Diabetes Care* 1991; 14: 935–41.

16. Snowdon DA, Phillips RL. Does a vegetarian diet reduce the occurrence of diabetes? *Am J Publ Health* 1985; 75: 507–12.

17. Crane MG, Sample CJ. Regression of diabetic neuropathy with vegan diet. *Am J Clin Nutr* 1988; 48: 926 [abstract #P28].

18. Crane MG, Sample C. Regression of diabetic neuropathy with total vegetarian (vegan) diet. *J Nutr Med* 1994; 4: 431–39.

19. Cohen D, Dodds R, Viberti G. Effect of protein restriction in insulin dependent diabetics at risk of nephropathy. *BMJ* 1987; 294: 795–98.

20. Evanoff G, Thompson C, Bretown J, Weinman E. Prolonged dietary protein restriction in diabetic nephropathy. *Arch Intern Med* 1989; 149: 1129–33.

21. Gin H, Aparicio M, Potauz L, et al. Low-protein, low-phosphorus diet and tissue insulin sensitivity in insulin-dependent diabetic patients with chronic renal failure. *Nephron* 1991; 57: 411–15.

22. Garg A, Bananome A, Grundy SM, et al. Comparison of a high-carbohydrate diet with a high-monounsaturated-fat diet in patients with non-insulin dependent diabetes mellitus. *N Engl J Med* 1988; 319: 829–34.

23. Dahl-Jorgensen K, Joner G, Hanssen KF. Relationship between cows' milk consumption and incidence of IDDM in childhood. *Diabetes Care* 1991; 14: 1081–83.

24. Coleman DL, Kuzava JE, Leiter EH. Effect of diet on incidence of diabetes in nonobese diabetic mice. *Diabetes* 1990; 39: 432–36.

25. Gerstein H. Cow milk exposure and type I diabetes mellitus. *Diabetes Care* 1994; 17: 13–19.

26. Karajalainen J, Martin JM, Knip M, et al. A bovine albumin peptide as a possible trigger of insulin-dependent diabetes mellitus. *N Engl J Med* 1992; 327: 302–7.

27. Scott FWE, Norris JM, Kolb H. Milk and type I diabetes. *Diabetes Care* 1996; 19: 379–83 [review].

28. Atkinson MA, Bowman MA, Kao K-J, et al. Lack of immune responsiveness to bovine serum albumin in insulin-dependent diabetes. *N Engl J Med* 1993; 329: 1853–58.

29. Pettit DJ, Forman MR, Hanson RL, et al. Breast feeding and incidence of non-insulin-dependent diabetes mellitus in Pima Indians. *Lancet* 1997; 350: 166–68.

30. Isida K, Mizuno A, Murakami T, Shima K. Obesity is necessary but not sufficient for the development of diabetes mellitus. *Metabolism* 1996; 45: 1288–95.

31. Casassus P, Fontbonne A, Thibult N, et al. Upper-body fat distribution: a hyperinsulinemia-independent predictor of coronary heart disease mortality. *Arterioscler Thromb* 1992; 1387–92.

32. Karter AJ, Mayer-Davis EJ, Selby JV, et al. Insulin sensitivity and abdominal obesity in African-American, Hispanic, and non-Hispanic

white men and women. *Diabetes* 1996; 45: 1547–55.

33. Park KS, Hree BD, Lee K-U, et al. Intra-abdominal fat is associated with decreased insulin sensitivity in healthy young men. *Metabolism* 1991; 40: 600–3.

34. Long SD, Swanson MS, O'Brien K, et al. Weight loss in severely obese subjects prevents the progression of impaired glucose tolerance to type II diabetes. *Diabetes Care* 1994; 17: 372.

35. Pi-Sunyer FX. Weight and non-insulin-dependent diabetes mellitus. *Am J Clin Nutr* 1996; 63(suppl): 426S–9S.

36. Wing RR, Marcuse MD, Blair EH, et al. Caloric restriction per se is a significant factor in improvements in glycemic control and insulin sensitivity during weight loss in obese NIDDM patients. *Diabetes Care* 1994; 17: 30.

37. Henry RR, Gumbiner B. Benefits and limitations of very-low-calorie diet therapy in obese NIDDM. *Diabetes Care* 1991; 14: 802–23.

38. Hersey III WC, Graves JE, Pollack ML, et al. Endurance exercise training improves body composition and plasma insulin responses in 70- to 79-year-old men and women. *Metabol* 1994; 43: 847–54.

39. Rasmussen OW, Lauszus FF, Hermansen K. Effects of postprandial exercise on glycemic response in IDDM subjects. *Diabetes Care* 1994; 17: 1203.

40. Helmrich SP, Ragland DR, Leung RW, Paffenbarger RS. Physical activity and reduced occurrence of non-insulin-dependent diabetes mellitus. *N Engl J Med* 1991; 325: 147–52.

41. Grimm J-J, Muchnick S. Type I diabetes and marathon running. *Diabetes Care* 1993; 16: 1624 [letter].

42. Bell DSH. Exercise for patients with diabetes—benefits, risks, precautions. *Postgrad Med* 1992; 92: 183–96 [review].

43. Kiechl S, Willeit J, Poewe W, et al. Insulin sensitivity and regular alcohol consumption: large, prospective, cross sectional population study Bruneck study. *BMJ* 1996; 313: 1040–44.

44. Facchini F, Chen Y-DI, Reaven GM. Light-to-moderate alco-

hol intake is associated with enhanced insulin sensitivity. *Diabetes Care* 1994; 17: 115.

45. Rimm EB, Chan J, Stampfer MJ, et al. Prospective study of cigarette smoking, alcohol use, and the risk of diabetes in men. *BMJ* 1995; 310: 555–59.

46. Stampfer MJ, Colditz GA, Willett WC, et al. A prospective study of moderate alcohol drinking and risk of diabetes in women. *Am J Epidemiol* 1988; 128: 549–58.

47. Goden G, Chen X, Desantis R, et al. Effects of ethanol on carbohydrate metabolism in the elderly. *Diabetes* 1993; 42: 28–34.

48. Ben G, Gnudi L, Maran A, et al. Effects of chronic alcohol intake on carbohydrate and lipid metabolism in subjects with type II (non-insulin-dependent) diabetes. *Am J Med* 1991; 90: 70.

49. Young RJ, McCulloch DK, Prescott RJ, Clarke PF. Alcohol: another risk factor for diabetic retinopathy? *BMJ* 1984; 288: 1035.

50. Connor H, Marks V. Alcohol and diabetes. A position paper prepared by the Nutrition Subcommittee of the British Diabetic Association's Medical Advisory Committee and approved by the Executive Council of the British Diabetic Association. *Human Nutr Appl Nutr* 1985; 39A: 393–99.

51. Stegmayr B, Lithner F. Tobacco and end stage diabetic nephropathy. *BMJ* 1987; 295: 581–82.

52. Scala C, LaPorte RE, Dorman JS, et al. Insulin-dependent diabetes mellitus mortality—the risk of cigarette smoking. *Circulation* 1990; 82: 37–43.

53. Rimm EB, Manson JE, Stampfer MJ, et al. Cigarette smoking and the risk of diabetes in women. *Am J Public Health* 1993; 83: 211–14.

Diabetes: Section 3: Dietary Supplements and Herbs

1. Salonen JT, Nyssonen K, Tuomainen T-P, et al. Increased risk of non-insulin dependent diabetes mellitus at low plasma vitamin E concentrations: a four year follow up study in men. *BMJ* 1995; 311: 1124–27.

2. Bierenbaum ML, Noonan FJ, Machlin LJ, et al. The effect of supplemental vitamin E on serum parameters in diabetics, post coronary and normal subjects. *Nutr Rep Internat* 1985; 31: 1171–80.

3. Paolisso G, D'Amore A, Giugliano D, et al. Pharmacologic doses of vitamin E improve insulin action in healthy subjects and non-insulin dependent diabetic patients. *Am J Clin Nutr* 1993; 57: 650–56.

4. Paolisso G, D'Amore A, Galzerano D, et al. Daily vitamin E supplements improve metabolic control but not insulin secretion in elderly type II diabetic patients. *Diabetes Care* 1993; 16: 1433–37.

5. Tütüncü NB, Bayraktar M, Varli K. Reversal of defective nerve condition with vitamin E supplementation in type 2 diabetes. *Diabetes Care* 1998; 21: 1915–18.

6. Paolisso G, Di Maro G, Galzerano D, et al. Pharmacological doses of vitamin E and insulin action in elderly subjects. *Am J Clin Nutr* 1994; 59: 1291–96.

7. Paolisso G, Gambardella A, Galzerano D, et al. Antioxidants in adipose tissue and risk of myocardial infarction. *Lancet* 1994; 343: 596 [letter].

8. Tütüncü NB, Bayraktar M, Varli K. Reversal of defective nerve condition with vitamin E supplementation in type 2 diabetes. *Diabetes Care* 1998; 21: 1915–18.

9. Colette C, Pares-Herbute N, Monnier LH, Cartry E. Platelet function in type I diabetes: effects of supplementation with large doses of vitamin E. *Am J Clin Nutr* 1988; 47: 256–61.

10. Gisnger C, Jeremy J, Speiser P, et al. Effect of vitamin E supplementation on platelet thromboxane A2 production in type I diabetic patients: Double-blind crossover trial. *Diabetes* 1988; 37: 1260–64.

11. Ross WM, Creighton MO, Stewart-DeHaan PJ, et al. Modelling cortical cataractogenesis: 3. In vivo effects of vitamin E on cataractogenesis in diabetic rats. *Can J Ophthalmol* 1982; 17: 61.

12. Knekt P Reunanen A, Marniumi J, et al. Low vitamin E sta-

tus is a potential risk factor for insulin-dependent diabetes mellitus. *J Intern Med* 1999; 245: 99–102.

13. Ceriello A, Giugliano D, Quatraro A, et al. Vitamin E reduction of protein glycosylation in diabetes. *Diabetes Care* 1991; 14: 68–72.

14. Duntas L, Kemmer TP, Vorberg B, Scherbaum W. Administration of d-alpha-tocopherol in patients with insulin-dependent diabetes mellitus. *Curr Ther Res* 1996; 57: 682–90.

15. Reaven PD, Barnett J, Herold DA, Edelman S. Effect of vitamin E on susceptibility of low-density lipoprotein and low-density lipoprotein subfractions to oxidation and on protein glycation in NIDDM. *Diabetes Care* 1995; 18: 807.

16. Cunningham JJ, Ellis SL, McVeigh KL, et al. Reduced mononuclear leukocyte ascorbic acid content in adults with insulin-dependent diabetes mellitus consuming adequate dietary vitamin C. *Metabol* 1991; 40: 146–49.

17. Davie SJ, Gould BJ, Yudkin JS. Effect of vitamin C on glycosylation of proteins. *Diabetes* 1992; 41: 167–73.

18. Will JC, Tyers T. Does diabetes mellitus increase the requirement for vitamin C? *Nutr Rev* 1996; 54: 193–202 [review].

19. Eriksson J, Kohvakka A. Magnesium and ascorbic acid supplementation in diabetes mellitus. *Ann Nutr Metabol* 1995; 39: 217–23.

20. Paolisso G, Balbi V, Volpe C, et al. Metabolic benefits deriving from chronic vitamin C supplementation in aged non-insulin dependent diabetics. *J Am Coll Nutr* 1995; 14: 387–92.

21. Will JC, Tyers T. Does diabetes mellitus increase the requirement for vitamin C? *Nutr Rev* 1996; 54: 193–202 [review].

22. Mayer-Davis E, Bell RA, Reboussin BA, et al. Antioxidant nutrient intake and diabetic retinopathy. The San Luis Valley Diabetes Study. *Ophthalmology* 1998; 105: 2264–70.

23. Wilson RG, Davis RE. Serum pyridoxal concentrations in children with diabetes mellitus. *Pathol* 1977; 9: 95–99.

24. Davis RE, Calder JS, Curnow DH. Serum pyridoxal and folate concentrations in diabetics. *Pathol* 1976; 8: 151–56.

25. McCann VJ, Davis RE. Serum pyridoxal concentrations in patients with diabetic neuropathy. *Austral NZ Med* 1978; 8: 259–61.

26. Spellacy WN, Buhi WC, Birk SA. Vitamin B₆ treatment of gestational diabetes mellitus. *Am J Obstet Gynecol* 1977; 127: 599–602.

27. Coelingh HJT, Schreurs WHP. Improvement of oral glucose tolerance in gestational diabetes by pyridoxine. *BMJ* 1975; 3: 13–15.

28. Spellacy WN, Buhi WC, Birk SA. The effects of vitamin B₆ on carbohydrate metabolism in women taking steroid contraceptives: preliminary report. *Contraception* 1972; 6: 265–73.

29. Passariello N, Fici F, Giugliano D, et al. Effects of pyridoxine alpha-ketoglutarate on blood glucose and lactate in type I and II diabetics. *Internat J Clin Pharmacol Ther Toxicol* 1983; 21: 252–56.

30. Solomon LR, Cohen K. Erythrocyte O2 transport and metabolism and effects of vitamin B₆ therapy in type II diabetes mellitus. *Diabetes* 1989; 38: 881–86.

31. Rao RH, Vigg BL, Rao KSJ. Failure of pyridoxine to improve glucose tolerance in diabetics. *J Clin Endocrinol Metabol* 1980; 50: 198–200.

32. Yamane K, Usui T, Yamamoto T, et al. Clinical efficacy of intravenous plus oral mecobalamin in patients with peripheral neuropathy using vibration perception thresholds as an indicator of improvement. *Curr Ther Res* 1995; 56: 656–70 [review].

33. Coggeshall JC, Heggers JP, Robson MC, Baker H. Biotin status and plasma glucose in diabetics. *Ann NY Acad Sci* 1985; 447: 389–92.

34. Maebashi M, Makino Y, Furukawa Y, et al. Therapeutic evaluation of the effect of biotin on hyperglycemia in patients with non-insulin dependent diabetes mellitus. *J Clin Biochem Nutr* 1993; 14: 211–18.

35. Koutsikos D, Agroyannis B, Tzanatos-Exarchou H. Biotin for dia-

betic peripheral neuropathy. *Biomed Pharmacother* 1990; 44: 511–14.

36. Molnar GD, Berge KG, Rosevear JW, et al. The effect of nicotinic acid in diabetes mellitus. *Metabol* 1964; 13: 181–89.

37. Gaut ZN, Pocelinko R, Solomon HM, Thomas GB. Oral glucose tolerance, plasma insulin, and uric acid excretion in man during chronic administration in nicotinic acid. *Metabol* 1971: 1031–35.

38. Clearly JP. The importance of oxidant injury as a cause of impaired mitochondrial oxidation in diabetes. *J Orthomol Med* 1988; 3: 164–74.

39. Clearly JP. Vitamin B₃ in the treatment of diabetes mellitus: case reports and review of the literature. *J Nutr Med* 1990; 1: 217–25.

40. Lewis CM, Canafax DM, Sprafka JM, Bazrbosa JJ. Double-blind randomized trail of nicotinamide on early-onset diabetes. *Diabetes Care* 1992; 15: 121–23.

41. Chase HP, Butler-Simon N, Garg S, et al. A trial of nicotinamide in newly diagnosed patients with type 1 (insulin-dependent) diabetes mellitus. *Diabetologia* 1990; 33: 444–46.

42. Mendola G, Casamitjana R, Gomis R. Effect of nicotinamide therapy upon B-cell function in newly diagnosed type 1 (insulin-dependent) diabetic patients. *Diabetologia* 1989; 32: 160–62.

43. Elliott RB, Picher CC, Fergusson DM, Stewart AWAD. A population based strategy to prevent insulin-dependent diabetes using nicotinamide. *J Pediatr Endocrinol Metabol* 1996; 9: 501–9.

44. Lampeter EF, Klinghammer A, Scherbaum WA, et al. The Deutsche Nicotinamide Intervention Study. An attempt to prevent type 1 diabetes. *Diabetes* 1998; 47: 980–84.

45. Haugen HN. The blood concentration of thiamine in diabetes. *Scand J Clin Lab Invest* 1964; 16: 260–66.

46. Vorhaus MG, Williams RR, Waterman RE. Studies on crystalline vitamin B₁: observations in diabetes. *Am J Dig Dis* 1935; 2: 541–57.

47. Abbas ZG, Swai ABM. Evaluation of the efficacy of thiamine and pyridoxine in the treatment of

symptomatic diabetic peripheral neuropathy. *East African Med J* 1997; 74: 804–8.

48. Stracke H, Lindemann A, Federlin K. A benfotiamine-vitamin B combination in treatment of diabetic polyneuropathy. *Exp Clin Endocrinol Diabetes* 1996; 104: 311–16.

49. Ref: Labriji-Mestaghanmi H, Billaudel B, Garnier PE, Sutter BCJ. Vitamin D and pancreatic islet function. 2. Time course for changes in insulin secretion and content during vitamin deprivation and repletion. *J Endocrine Invest* 1988; 11: 577–87.

50. Boucher BJ. Inadequate vitamin D status: does it contribute to the disorders comprising syndrome 'X'? *Br J Nutr* 1998; 79: 315–27 [review].

51. Schroeder HA. Serum cholesterol and glucose levels in rats fed refined and less refined sugars and chromium. *J Nutr* 1969; 97: 237–42.

52. Herepath WB. *Journal Provincial Med Surg Soc* Apr 28, 1854: 374.

53. Offenbacher EG, Li-Sunyer FX. Improvement of glucose tolerance and blood lipids in elderly subjects. *Am J Clin Nutr* 1980; 33: 916 [abstract].

54. Evans GW. The effect of chromium picolinate on insulin controlled parameters in humans. *Int J Biosocial Med Res* 1989; 11: 163–80.

55. Gaby AR, Wright JV. Diabetes. In *Nutritional Therapy in Medical Practice: Reference Manual and Study Guide.* Kent, WA: Wright/Gaby Seminars, 1996, 54–64 [review].

56. Anderson RA, Polansky MM, Bryden NA, Canary JJ. Supplemental-chromium effects on glucose, insulin, glucagon, and urinary chromium losses in subjects consuming controlled low-chromium diets. *Am J Clin Nutr* 1991; 54: 909–16.

57. Jovanovic-Peterson L, Gutierrez M, Peterson CM. Chromium supplementation for gestational diabetic women improves glucose tolerance and decreases hyperinsulinemia. *J Am Coll Nutr* 1995; 14: 530 [abstract #26].

58. Anderson RA, Polansky MM, Bryden NA, et al. Chromium supplementation of human subjects: effects on glucose, insulin, and lipid variables. *Metabol* 1983; 32: 894–99.

59. Urberg M, Zemel MB. Evidence for synergism between chromium and nicotinic acid in the control of glucose tolerance in elderly humans. *Metabol* 1987; 36: 896–99.

60. Lee NA, Reasner CA. Beneficial effect of chromium supplementation on serum triglyceride levels in NIDDM. *Diabetes Care* 1994; 17: 1449–52.

61. Gaby AR, Wright JV. Nutritional protocols: diabetes mellitus. In *Nutritional Therapy in Medical Practice: Protocols and Supporting Information.* Kent, WA: Wright/Gaby Seminars, 1996, 10.

62. Paolisso G, Scheen A, D'Onofrio FD, Lefebvre P. Magnesium and glucose homeostasis. *Diabetologia* 1990; 33: 511–14 [review].

63. Eibl NL, Schnack CJ, Kopp H-P, et al. Hypomagnesemia in type II diabetes: effect of a 3-month replacement therapy. *Diabetes Care* 1995; 18: 188.

64. Paolisso G, Sgambato S, Pizza G, et al. Improved insulin response and action by chronic magnesium administration in aged NIDDM subjects. *Diabetes Care* 1989; 12: 265–69.

65. Paolisso G, Sgambato S, Gambardella A, et al. Daily magnesium supplements improve glucose handling in elderly subjects. *Am J Clin Nutr* 1992; 55: 1161–67.

66. Smellie WS, O'Reilly D St J, Martin BJ, Santamaria J. Magnesium replacement and glucose tolerance in elderly subjects. *Am J Clin Nutr* 1993; 57: 594–95 [letter].

67. Sjorgren A, Floren CH, Nilsson A. Oral administration of magnesium hydroxide to subjects with insulin dependent diabetes mellitus. *Magnesium* 1988; 121: 16–20.

68. de Valk HW, Verkaaik R, van Rijn HJM, et al. Oral magnesium supplementation in insulin-requiring type 2 diabetic patients. *Diabet Med* 1998; 15: 503–7.

69. McNair P, Christiansen C, Madsbad S, et al. Hypomagnesemia, a risk factor in diabetic retinopathy. *Diabetes* 1978; 27: 1075–77.

70. Mimouni F, Miodovnik M, Tsang RC, et al. Decreased maternal serum magnesium concentration and adverse fetal outcome in insulin-dependent diabetic women. *Obstet Gynecol* 1987; 70: 85–89.

71. American Diabetes Association. Magnesium supplementation in the treatment of diabetes. *Diabetes Care* 1992; 15: 1065–67.

72. Nakamura T, Higashi A, Nishiyama S, et al. Kinetics of zinc status in children with IDDM. *Diabetes Care* 1991; 14: 553–57.

73. Mocchegiani E, Boemi M, Fumelli P, Fabris N. Zinc-dependent low thymic hormone level in type I diabetes. *Diabetes* 1989; 12: 932–37.

74. Rao KVR, Seshiah V, Kumar TV. Effect of zinc sulfate therapy on control and lipids in type I diabetes. *JAPI* 1987; 35: 52 [abstract].

75. Niewoehner CB, Allen JI, Boosalis M, et al. Role of zinc supplementation in type II diabetes mellitus. *Am J Med* 1986; 81: 63–68.

76. Pidduck HG, Wren PJJ, Price Evans DA. Hyperzincuria of diabetes mellitus and possible genetic implications of this observation. *Diabetes* 1970; 19: 240–47.

77. Cunningham JJ, Fu A, Mearkle PL, Brown RG. Hyerzincuria in individuals with insulin-dependent diabetes mellitus: concurrent zinc status and the effect of high-dose zinc supplementation. *Metabolism* 1994; 43: 1558–62.

78. Shigeta Y, Izumi K, Abe H. Effect of coenzyme Q7 treatment on blood sugar and ketone bodies of diabetics. *J Vitaminol (Kyoto)* 1966; 12: 293–98.

79. Henriksen JE, Bruun Andersen C, Hother-Nielsen O, et al. Impact of ubiquinone (coenzyme Q_{10}) treament on glycaemic control, insulin requirement and well-being in patients with Type 1 diabetes mellitus. *Diaabetic Med* 1999; 16: 312–18.

80. Salway JG, Whitehead L, Finnegan JA, et al. Effect of *myo*-inositol on peripheral-nerve function in diabetes. *Lancet* 1978; II: 1282–84.

81. Packer L, Witt EH, Tartschler HJ. Alpha-lipoic acid as a biological antioxidant. *Free Radical Biol Med* 1995; 19: 227–50.

Part One: References

82. Abdel-Aziz MT, Abdou MS, Soliman K, et al. Effect of carnitine on blood lipid pattern in diabetic patients. *Nutr Rep Internat* 1984; 29: 1071–79.

83. Onofrj M, Fulgente T, Mechionda D, et al. L-acetylcarnitine as a new therapeutic approach for peripheral neuropathies with pain. *Int J Clin Pharmacol Res* 1995; 15: 9–15.

84. Franconi F, Bennardini F, Mattana A, et al. Plasma and platelet taurine are reduced in subjects with insulin-dependent diabetes mellitus: effects of taurine supplementation. *Am J Clin Nutr* 1995; 61: 1115–19.

85. Zak A, Zeman M, Hrabak P, et al. Changes in the glucose tolerance and insulin secretion in hypertriglyceridemia: effects of dietary n-3 fatty acids. *Nutr Rep Internat* 1989; 39: 235–42.

86. Popp-Snijders C, Schouten J, et al. Dietary supplementation of omega-3 fatty acids improves insulin sensitivity in non-insulin dependent diabetes. *Neth J Med* 1985; 28: 531–32.

87. Popp-Snijders C, Schouten JA, Heine RJ, et al. Dietary supplementation of omega-3 polyunsaturated fatty acids improves insulin sensitivity in non-insulin-dependent diabetes. *Diabetes Res* 1987; 4: 141–47.

88. Albrink MJ, Ullrich IH, Blehschmidt NG, et al. The beneficial effect of fish oil supplements on serum lipids and clotting function of patients with type II diabetes mellitus. *Diabetes* 1986; 35 (suppl 1): 43A (abstract #172).

89. Wei I, Ulchaker M, Sheehan J. Effect of omega-3 fatty acids (FA) in non-obese non-insulin dependent diabetes (NIDDM). *Am Clin Nutr* 1988; 47: 775 (abstract #70).

90. Vandongen R, Mori TA, Codde JP, et al. Hypercholesterolaemic effect of fish oil in insulin-dependent diabetic patients. *Med J Austral* 1988; 148: 141–43.

91. Schectman G, Kaul S, Kissebah AH. Effect of fish oil concentrate on lipoprotein composition in NIDDM. *Diabetes* 1988; 37: 1567–73.

92. Stackpoole PW, Alig J, Kilgore LL, et al. Lipodystrophic diabetes mellitus. Investigations of lipoprotein metabolism and the effects of omega-3 fatty acid administration in two patients. *Metabol* 1988; 37: 944–51.

93 Glauber H, Wallace P, Griver K, Brechtel G. Adverse metabolic effect of omega-3 fatty acids in non-insulin-dependent diabetes mellitus. *Ann Intern Med* 1988; 108: 663–68.

94. Okuda Y, Mizutani M, Ogawa M, et al. Long-term effects of eicosapentaenoic acid on diabetic peripheral neuropathy and serum lipids in patients with type II diabetes mellitus. *J Diabetes Complications* 1996; 10: 280–87.

95. Reichert R. Evening primrose oil and diabetic neuropathy. *Quarterly Rev Natural Med* Summer 1995: 129–33 [review].

96. Gaby A. Preventing complications of diabetes *Townsend Letter* 1985; #32: 307 [editorial].

97. Halberstam M, Cohen N, Schlimovich P, et al. Oral vanadyl sulfate improves insulin sensitivity in NIDDM but not in obese nondiabetic subjects. *Diabetes* 1996; 45: 659–66.

98. Boden G, Chen X, Ruiz J, et al. Effects of vanadyl sulfate on carbohydrate and lipid metabolism in patients with non-insulin dependent diabetes mellitus. *Metabolism* 1996; 45: 1130–35.

99. Aharon Y, Mevorach M, Shamoon H. Vanadyl sulfate does not enhance insulin action in patients with type 1 diabetes. *Diabetes Care* 1998; 21: 2194 [letter].

100. Baskaran K, Ahmath BK, Shanmugasundaram KR, Shanmugasundaram ERB. Antidiabetic effect of a leaf extract from *Gymnema sylvestre* in non-insulin-dependent diabetes mellitus patients. *J Ethnopharmacol* 1990; 30: 295–305.

101. Shanmugasundaram ERB, Rajeswari G, Baskaran K, et al. Use of *Gymnema sylvestre* leaf extract in the control of blood glucose insulin-dependent diabetes mellitus. *J Ethnopharmacol* 1990; 30: 281–94.

102. Zhang T, Hoshino M, et al. Ginseng root: Evidence for numerous regulatory peptides and insulinotropic activity. *Biomed Res* 1990; 11: 49–54.

103. Suzuki Y, Hikino H. Mechanisms of hypoglycemic activity of panaxans A and B, glycans of *Panax ginseng* roots: Effects on plasma levels, secretion, sensitivity and binding of insulin in mice. *Phytother Res* 1989; 3: 20–24.

104. Waki I, Kyo H, et al. Effects of a hypoglycemic component of ginseng radix on insulin biosynthesis in normal and diabetic animals. *J Pharm Dyn* 1982; 5: 547–54.

105. Sotaniemi EA, Haapakoski E, Rautio A. Ginseng therapy in non-insulin-dependent diabetic patients. *Diabetes Care* 1995; 18: 1373–75.

106. Scharrer A, Ober M. Anthocyanoside in der Behandlung von Retinopathien. *Klin Monatsblatt Augenheilk* 1981; 178: 386–89.

107. Bunyapraphatsara N, Yongchaiyudha S, Rungpitarangsi V, Chokechaijaroenporn O. Antidiabetic activity of *Aloe vera* L juice II. Clinical trial in diabetes mellitus patients in combination with glibdenclamide. *Phytomed* 1996; 3: 245–48.

108. Yongchaiyudha S, Rungpitarangsi V, Bunyapraphatsara N, Chokeshaijaroenporn O. Antidiabetic activity of *Aloe vera* L juice I. Clinical trial in new cases of diabetes mellitus. *Phytomed* 1996; 3: 241–43.

109. Leatherdale BA, Panesar RK, Singh G, et al. Improvement of glucose tolerance due to *Momordica charantia* (karela). *BMJ* 1981; 282: 1823–24.

110. Srivastava Y, Venkatakrishna-bhatt H, Verma Y, et al. Antidiabetic and adaptogenic properties of *Momordica charantia* extract: An experimental and clinical evaluation. *Phytother Res* 1993; 7: 285–89.

111. Welihinda J, Karunanaya E, Sheriff MHB, Jayasinghe K. Effect of *Momordica charantia* on the glucose tolerance in maturity onset diabetes. *J Ethnopharm* 1986; 17: 277–82.

112. Capsaicin study group. Treatment of painful diabetic neuropathy with topical capsaicin. A multicenter, double-blind, vehicle-controlled study. The capsaicin study group. *Arch Int Med* 1991; 151: 2225–29.

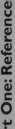

113. Capsaicin study group. Effect of treatment with capsaicin on daily activities of patients with painful diabetic neuropathy. The capsaicin study group. *Diabet Care* 1992; 15: 159–65.

Diarrhea

1. Hyams JS, Etienne NL, Leichtner AM, Theuer RC. Carbohydrate malabsorption following fruit juice ingestion in young children. *Pediatr* 1988; 82: 64–68.

2. Barness LA. Safety considerations with high ascorbic acid dosage. *Ann NY Acad Sci* 1975; 258: 523–28 [review].

3. Babb RR. Coffee, sugars and chronic diarrhea. *Postgrad Med* 1984; 75: 82,86–87.

4. James JM, Burks AW. Food-associated gastrointestinal disease. *Curr Opin Pediatr* 1996; 8: 471–75 [review].

5. Bowie MD, Hill ID, Mann MD. Response of severe infantile diarrhea to soya-based feeds. *S Afr Med J* 1988; 73: 343–45.

6. Haffejee IE. Effect of oral folate on duration of acute infantile diarrhoea. *Lancet* 1988; ii: 334–35 [letter].

7. Ashraf H, Rahman MM, Fuchs GJ, Mahalanabis D. Folic acid in the treatment of acute watery diarrhoea in children: a double-blind, randomized, controlled trial. *Acta Pædiatr* 1998; 87: 1113–15.

8. Schellenberg D, Bonington A, Champion C, et al. Treatment of Clostridium difficile diarrhea with brewer's yeast. *Lancet* 1994; 343: 171–72 [letter].

9. Izadnia F, Wong CT, Kocoshis SA. Brewer's yeast and Saccharomyces boulardii both attenuate Clostridium difficile-induced colonic secretion in the rat. *Dig Dis Sci* 1998; 43: 2055–60.

10. Pothoulakis C, Kelly CP, Joshi MA, et al. *Saccharomyces boulardii* inhibits *Clostridium difficile* toxin A binding and enterotoxicity in rat ileum. *Gastroenterology* 1993; 104: 1108–15.

11. Surzwicz CM, Elmer GW, Speelman P, et al. Prevention of antibi-otic-associated diarrhea by *Saccharomyces boulardii*: a prospective study. *Gastroenterology* 1989; 96: 981–88.

12. Bleichner G, Blehaut H, Mentec H, Moyse D. *Saccharomyces boulardii* prevents diarrhea in critically ill tube-fed patients. A muticenter, randomized, double-blind placebo-controlled trial. *Intensive Care Med* 1997; 23: 517–23.

13. Kollaritsch H, Holst H, Grobara P, Widermann G. Prevention of traveler's diarrhea with *Saccharomyces boulardii*. Results of a placebo controlled double-blind study. *Fortschr Med* 1993; 111: 152–56 [in German].

14. Kirchelle A, Fruhwein N, Toburen D. Treatment of persistent diarrhea with *S. boulardii* in returning travelers. Results of a prospective study. *Forstchr Med* 1996; 114: 136–40 [in German].

15. Plein K, Hotz J. Therapeutic effects of Saccharomyces on mild residual symptoms in a stable phase of Crohn's disease with special respect to chronic diarrhea—a pilot study. *Z Gastroenterol* 1993; 31: 129–34.

16. Lewis SJ, Potts LF, Barry RE. The lack of therapeutic effect of *Saccharomyces boulardii* in the prevention of antibiotic-related diarrhoea in elderly patients. *J Infect* 1998; 36: 171–74.

17. Poupard JA, Hussain J, Norris RF. Biology of the bifidobacteria. *Bact Rev* 1973; 37: 136–65.

18. Saavedra JM, Bauman NA, Oung I, et al. Feeding of *Bifidobacterium bifidum* and *Streptococcus thermophilus* to infants in hospital for prevention of diarrhoea and shedding of rotavirus. *Lancet* 1994; 344: 1046–49.

19. Colombel JF, Cortot A, Neut C, Romond C. Yogurt with *Bifidobacterium longum* reduces erythromycin-induced gastrointestinal effects. *Lancet* 1987; ii: 43 [letter].

20. Montes RG, Perman JA. Lactose intolerance. *Postgrad Med* 1991; 89: 175–84 [review].

21. Werbach MR. *Nutritional influences on Illness*, 2d ed. Tarzana, CA: Third Line Press, 1993, 256–61 [review].

22. Bhan J, Bhandari N. The role of zinc and viatmin A in persistent diarrhea among infants and young children. *J Pediatr Gastroenterol Nutri* 1998; 26: 446–53 [review].

23. Eherer AH, Santa Ana CA, Porter J, Fordtran JS. Effect of psyllium, calcium polycarbophil, and wheat bran on secretory diarrhea induced by phenolphthalein. *Gastroenterol* 1993; 104: 1007–12.

24. Loeb H, Vandenplas Y, et al. Tannin-rich pod for treatment of acute-onset diarrhea. *J Pediatr Gastroenterol Nutr* 1989; 8: 480–85.

25. Achterrath-Tuckerman U, Kunde R, et al. Pharmacological investigations with compounds of chamomile. V. Investigations on the spasmolytic effect of compounds of chamomile and Kamillosan on isolated guinea pig ileum. *Planta Med* 1980; 39: 38–50.

26. Tyler VE. *Herbs of Choice: The Therapeutic Use of Phytomedicinals*. New York: Pharmaceutical Products Press, 1994, 51–54.

27. Weiss RF. *Herbal Medicine*. Gothenburg, Sweden: Ab Arcanum and Beaconsfield, UK: Beaconsfield Publishers Ltd, 1988, 101–102.

28. Duke JA. *CRC Handbook of Medicinal Plants*. Boca Raton, FL: CRC Press, 1985, 209.

29. Konig M, Scholz E, Hartmann R, Lehmann W, Rimpler H. Ellagitannins and complex tannins from *Quercus petraea* bark. *J Nat Prod* 1994; 57(10): 1411–15.

30. Schilcher H. *Phytotherapy in Paediatrics*. Stuttgart, Germany: Medpharm Scientific Publishers, 1997, 49–50.

31. Khin-Maung U, Myo-Khin, Nyunt-Nyunt-Wai, et al. Clinical trial of berberine in acute watery diarrhoea. *Br Med J* 1985; 291: 1601–605.

Dupuytren's Contracture

1. Thomson GR. Treatment of Dupuytren's contracture with vitamin E. *BMJ* 1949; Dec 17: 1382–83.

2. Richards HJ. Dupuytren's contracture treated with vitamin E. *BMJ* 1952; June 21: 1328.

3. Kirk JE, Chieffi M. Tocopherol administration to patients with Dupuytren's contracture: effect on plasma tocopherol levels and degree of contracture. *Pro Soc Exp Biol Med* 1952; 80: 565 [review].

4. Jacob SW, Wood DC. Dimethyl sulfoxide (DMSO). Toxicology, pharmacology, and clinical experience. *Am J Surg* 1967; 114: 414–26.

Dysmenorrhea (Painful Menstruation)

1. Galeao R. La dysmenorrhee, syndrome multiforme. *Gynecologie* 1974; 25: 125 [in French].

2. Metheny WP, Smith RP. The relationship among exercise, stress, and primary dysmenorrhea. *J Behav Med* 1989; 12: 569–86.

3. Bolomb LM, Solidmum AA, Warren MP. Primary dysmenorrhea and physical activity. *Med Sci Sports Exerc* 1998; 30: 906–909 [review].

4. Ben-Menachem M. Treatment of dysmenorrhea: A relaxation therapy program. *Int J Gynaecol Obstet* 1980; 17: 340–42.

5. Jarrett M, Heitkemper MM, Shaver JF. Symptoms and self-care strategies in women with and without dysmenorrhea. *Health Care Women Int* 1995; 16: 167–78.

6. Parazzini F, Tozzi L, Mezzopane R, et al. Cigarette smoking, alcohol consumption, and risk of primary dysmenorrhea. *Epidemiology* 1994; 5: 469–72.

7. Teperi J, Rimpela M. Menstrual pain, health and behaviour in girls. *Soc Sci Med* 1989; 29: 163–69.

8. Hudgins, AP. *Am Practice Digest Treat* 1952; 3: 892–93.

9. Hudgins AP. Vitamins P, C and niacin for dysmenorrhea therapy. *West J Surg* 1954; Dec: 610–11.

10. Penland J, Johnson P. Dietary calcium and manganese effects on menstrual cycle symptoms. *Am J Obstet Gynecol* 1993; 168: 1417–23.

11. Thys-Jacobs S, Starkey P, Bernstein D, et al. Calcium carbonate and the premenstrual syndrome: effects on premenstrual and menstrual symptoms. *Am J Obstet Gyencol* 1998; 179: 444–52.

12. Harel Z, Biro FM, Kottenhahn RK, Rosenthal SL. Supplementation with omega-3 polyunsaturated fatty acids in the management of dysmenorrhea in adolescents. *Am J Obstet Gynecol* 1996; 174: 1335–38.

13. Nicholson JA, Darby TD, Jarobe CH. Viopudial, a hypotensive and smooth muscle antispasmotic from Viburnum opulus. *Proc Soc Exp Biol Med* 1972; 40: 457–61.

14. Hoffmann D. *The Holistic Herbal*. Forres, Scotland: The Findhorn Press, 1986, 88.

15. Murray MT. *The Healing Power of Herbs*. Rocklin, CA: Prima Publishing, 1995, 376.

16. Bradley PR, ed. *British Herbal Compendium*, vol 1. Bournemouth, Dorset, UK: British Herbal Medicine Association, 1992, 34–36.

17. Blumenthal M, Busse WR, Goldberg A, et al. (eds). *The Complete Commission E Monographs: Therapeutic Guide to Herbal Medicines*. Boston, MA: Integrative Medicine Communications, 1998, 90.

18. Jones TK, Lawson BM. Profound neonatal congestive heart failure caused by maternal consumption of blue cohosh herbal medication. *J Pediatr* 1998; 132: 550–52.

19. Blumenthal M, Busse WR, Goldberg A, et al. (eds). *The Complete Commission E Monographs: Therapeutic Guide to Herbal Medicines*. Boston, MA: Integrative Medicine Communications, 1998, 233–34.

Ear Infections, Recurrent

1. Del Mar C, Glasziou P, Hayem M. Are antibiotics indicated as initial treatment for children with acute otitis media? A meta-analysis. *BMJ* 1997; 314: 1526–29.

2. Kozyrskyj AL, Hildes-Ripstein GE, Longstaffe SE, et al. Treatment of acute otitis media with a shortened course of antibiotics: a meta-analysis. *JAMA* 1998; 279: 1736–42.

3. Le CT, Freeman DW, Fireman BH. Evaluation of ventilating tubes and myringotomy in the treatment of recurrent or persistent otitis media. *Pediatr Infect Dis J* 1991; 10: 2–11.

4. McMahan JT, Calenoff E, Croft J, et al. Chronic otitis media with effusion and allergy: modified RAST analysis of 119 cases. *Otolaryngol Head Neck Surg* 1981; 89: 427–31.

5. Nsouli TM, Nsouli SM, Linde RE, et al. Role of food allergy in serous otitis media. *Ann Allerg* 1994; 73: 215–19.

6. McGovern JP, Haywood TH, Fernandez AA. Allergy and secretory otitis media. *JAMA* 1967; 200: 134–38.

7. Roukonen J, Pagnaus A, Lehti H. Elimination diets in the treatment of secretory otitis media. *Internat J Pediatr Otorhinolaryngol* 1982; 4: 39–46.

8. Sanchez A, JL, Reassure JL, Al HS, et al. Role of sugars in human neutrophilic phagocytosis. *Am J Clin Nutr* 1973; 26: 1180–84.

9. Bernstein J, Alert S, Anus KM, Suspend R. Depression of lymphocyte transformation following oral glucose ingestion. *Am J Clin Nutr* 1977; 30: 613 [abstract].

10. Uhari M, et al. Xylitol chewing gum in prevention of acute otitis media: double blind randomised trial. *BMJ* 1996; 313: 1180–84.

11. Uhari M, Kontiokari T, Niemela M. A novel use of xylitol sugar in preventing acute otitis media. *Pediatr* 1998; 102: 879–84.

12. Ethel RA, Pattishall EN, Haley NJ, et al. Passive smoking and middle ear effusion among children in day care. *Pediatr* 1992; 90: 228–32.

13. Ross A, Collins M, Sanders C. Upper respiratory tract infection in children, domestic temperatures, and humidity. *J Epidemiol Community Health* 1990; 44: 142–46.

14. Leibovitz B, Siegel BV. Ascorbic acid, neutrophil function, and the immune response. *Int J Vitam Nutr Res* 1978; 48: 159–64.

15. Vojdani A, Ghoneum M. In vivo effect of ascorbic acid on enhancement of human natural killer cell activity. *Nutr Res* 1993; 13: 753–64.

16. Duchateau J, Delespesse G, Vereecke P. Influence of oral zinc supplementation on the lymphocyte

response to mitogens of normal subjects. *Am J Clin Nutr* 1981; 34: 88–93.

17. Fraker PJ, Gershwin ME, Good RA, Prasad A. Interrelationships between zinc and immune function. *Fed Proc* 1986; 45: 1474–79.

18. Brown DJ. *Herbal Prescriptions for Better Health.* Rocklin, CA: Prima Publishing, 1996, 213–14 [review].

19. Schilcher H. *Phytotherapy in Paediatrics: Handbook for Physicians and Pharmacists.* Stuttgart: Medpharm Scientific Publishers, 1997, 43–45.

Eczema

1. Sampson HA, Scanlon SM. Natural history of food hypersensitivity in children with atopic dermatitis. *J Pediatr* 1989; 115: 23–27.

2. Burks AW, Mallory SB, Williams LW, Shirrell MA. Atopic dermatitis: clinical relevance of food hypersensitivity. *J Pediatr* 1988; 113: 447–51.

3. Niggemann B, Sielaff B, Beyer K, et al. Outcome of double-blind, placebo-controlled food challenge tests in 107 children with atopic dermatitis. *Clin Exp Allergy* 1999; 29: 91–96.

4. Atherton DJ. Diet and atopic eczema. *Clin Allerg* 1988; 18: 215–28 [review].

5. Veien NK, Hattel T, Justesen O, et al. Dermatoses in coffee drinkers. *Cutis* 1987; 40: 421–22.

6. Manku MS, Horrobin DF, Morse NL, et al. Essential fatty acids in the plasma phospholipids of patients with atopic eczema. *Br J Dermatol* 1984; 110: 643–48.

7. Schalin-Karrila M, Mattila L, Jansen CT, et al. Evening primrose oil in the treatment of atopic eczema: effect on clinical status, plasma phospholipid fatty acids and circulating blood prostaglandis. *Br J Dermatol* 1987; 117: 11–19.

8. Lovell CR, Burton JL, Horrobin DF. Treatment of atopic eczema with evening primrose oil. *Lancet* 1981; I: 278 [letter].

9. Wright S, Burton JL. Oral evening-primrose oil improves atopic eczema. *Lancet* 1982; ii: 1120–22.

10. Morse PF, Horrobin DF, Manku MS, et al. Meta-analysis of placebo-controlled studies of the efficacy of Epogam in the treatment of atopic eczema. Relationship between plasma essential fatty acid changes and clinical response. *Br J Dermatol* 1989; 121: 75–90.

11. Berth-Jones J, Graham-Brown RAC. Placebo-controlled trial of essential fatty acid supplementation in atopic dermatitis. *Lancet* 1993; 341: 1557–60.

12. Bamford JTM, Gibson RW, Renier CM. Atopic eczema unresponsive to evening primrose oil (linoleic and gamma-linolenic acids). *J Am Acad Dermatol* 1985; 13: 959–65.

13. Horrobin DF, Stewart C. Evening primrose oil in atopic eczema. *Lancet* 1990; I: 864–65.

14. Landi G. Oral administration of borage oil in atopic dermatitis. *J Appl Cosmetology* 1993; 11: 115–20.

15. Borreck S, Hildebrandt A, Forster J. Borage seed oil and atopic dermatitis. *Klinische Pediatrie* 1997; 203: 100–4.

16. Cornbleet T. Use of maize oil (unsaturated fatty acids) in the treatment of eczema. *Arch Dermatol Syph* 1935; 31: 224–34.

17. Hansen AE, Knott EM, Wiese HF, et al. Eczema and essential fatty acids. *Am J Dis Child* 1947; 73: 1–18.

18. Bjørneboe A, Søyland E, Bjørneboe G-E A, et al. Effect of dietary supplementation with eicosapentaenoic acid in the treatment of atopic dermatitis. *Br J Dermatol* 1987; 117: 463–69.

19. Bjørnboe A, Søyland E, Bjørnboe GE, et al. Effect of n-3 fatty acid supplement to patients with atopic dermatitis. *J Intern Med Suppl* 1989; 225: 233–36.

20. Søyland E, Rajka G, Bjørneboe A, et al. The effect of eicosapentaenoic acid in the treatment of atopic dermatitis. A clinical Study. *Acta Derm Venereol* (Stockh) 1989; 144(suppl): 139.

21. Berth-Jones J, Graham-Brown RAC. Placebo-controlled trial

of essential fatty acid supplementation in atopic dermatitis. *Lancet* 1993; 341: 1557–60.

22. Søyland E, Funk J, Rajka G, et al. Dietary supplementation with very long-chain n-3 fatty acids in patients with atopic dermatitis. A double-blind multicentre study. *Br J Dermatol* 1994; 130: 757–64.

23. Olsen PE, Torp EC, Mahon RT, et al. Oral vitamin E for refractory hand dermatitis. *Lancet* 1994; 343: 672–73 [letter].

24. Fairris GM, Perkins PJ, Lloyd B, et al. The effect on atopic dermatitis of supplementation with selenium and vitamin E. *Acta Derm Vernereol* 1989; 69: 359–62.

25. Manzano D, Aguirre A, Gardeazabal J, et al. Allergic contact dermatitis from tocopheryl acetate (vitamin E) and retinol palmitate (vitamin A) in a moisturizing cream. *Contact Dermatitis* 1994; 31: 324.

26. Anonymous. Severe atopic dermatitis responds to ascorbic acid. *Med World News* 1989; April 24: 41.

27. Sheehan MP, Atherton DJ. One-year follow up of children treated with Chinese medical herbs for atopic eczema. *Br J Dermatol* 1994; 130: 488–93.

28. Sheehan MP, Rustin MHA, et al. Efficacy of traditional Chinese herbal therapy in adult atopic dermatitis. *Lancet* 1992; 340: 13–17.

29. Evans FQ. The rational use of glycyrrhetinic acid in dermatology. *Br J Clin Pract* 1958; 12: 269–79.

30. Laux P, Oschmann R. Witch hazel–*Hamamelis virgincia* L. *Zeitschrift Phytother* 1993; 14: 155–66.

31. Weiss RF. *Herbal Medicine.* Gothenberg, Sweden: Ab Arcanum and Beaconsfield: Beaconsfield Publishers Ltd, 1988, 328–29.

Edema (Water Retention)

1. Piller NB. A comparison of the effectiveness of some anti-inflammatory drugs on thermal oedema. *Br J Exp Pathol* 1975; 56: 554–59.

2. Becker HM, Niedermaier G, Orend KH. Benzopyrone in the therapy of postreconstructive edema. A

clinical double-blind study. *Fortschr Med* 1985; 103: 593–96 [in German].

3. Loprinzi CL, Kugler JW, Sloan JA, et al. Lack of effect of coumarin in women with lymphedema after treatment for breast cancer. *New Engl J Med* 1999; 340: 346–50.

4. Piller NB, Morgan RG, Casley-Smith JR. A double-blind cross over trial of o-beta-hydroxyethyl-rutosides (benzopyrones) in the treatment of lymphoedema of the arms and legs. *Br J Plast Surg* 1988; 41: 20–27.

5. Tyler V. *Herbs of Choice: The Therapeutic Use of Phytomedicinals.* New York: Pharmaceutical Products Press, 1994, 74 [review].

6. Racz-Kotilla E, Racz G, Solomon A. The action of *Taraxacum officinale* extracts on the body weight and diuresis of laboratory animals. *Planta Medica* 1974; 26: 212–17.

7. Doan DD, Nguyen NH, Doan HK, et al. Studies on the individual and combined diuretic effects of four Vietnamese traditional herbal remedies (*Zea mays, Imperata cylindrica, Plantago major* and *Orthosiphon stamineus*). *J Ethnopharm* 1994; 36: 225–31.

8. Dini D, Bianchini M, Massa T, Fassio T. Treatment of upper limb lymphedema after mastectomy with escine and levo-thyroxine. *Minerva Med* 1981; 72: 2319–22 [in Italian].

9. Wilhelm K, Feldmeier C. Thermometric investigations about the efficacy of beta-escin to reduce postoperative edema. *Med Klin* 1977; 72: 128–34 [in German].

10. Tyler V. *Herbs of Choice: The Therapeutic Use of Phytomedicinals.* New York: Pharmaceutical Products Press, 1994, 76–77 [review].

11. Mills SY. *Out of the Earth: The Essential Book of Herbal Medicine.* London: Viking Arkana, 1991, 493–94.

Fibrocystic Breast Disease

1. Minton JP, Foecking MK, Webster DJT, Matthew RH. Caffeine, cyclic nucleotides, and breast disease. *Surgery* 1979; 86: 105–108.

2. Minton JP, Abou-Issa H, Reiches N, et al. Clinical and bio-chemical studies on methylxanthine-related fibrocystic breast disease. *Surgery* 1981; 90: 299–304.

3. Ernster VL, Mason L, Goodson WH, et al. Effects of a caffeine-free diet on benign breast disease: a randomized trial. *Surgery* 1982; 91: 263.

4. Allen S, Froberg DG. The effect of decreased caffeine consumption on benign proliferative breast disease: a randomized clinical trial. *Surgery* 1987; 101: 720–30.

5. Marshall JM, Graham S, Swanson M. Caffeine consumption and benign breast disease: a case-control comparison. *Am J Publ Health* 1982; 72(6): 610–12.

6. Lubin F, Ron E, Wax Y, et al. A case-control study of caffeine and methylxanthines in benign breast disease. *JAMA* 1985; 253(16): 2388–92.

7. Boyle CA, Berkowitz GS, LiVoisi VA, et al. Caffeine consumption and fibrocystic breast disease: a case-control epidemiologic study. *J Natl Cancer Inst* 1984; 72: 1015–19.

8. Vecchia C, Franceschi S, Parazzini F, et al. Benign breast disease and consumption of beverages containing methylxanthines. *J Natl Cancer Inst* 1985; 74: 995–1000.

9. Odenheimer DJ, Zunzunegui MV, King MC, et al. Risk factors for benign breast disease: A case-control study of discordant twins. *Am J Epidemiol* 1984; 120: 565–71.

10. Rose DP, Boyar AP, Cohen C, Strong LE. Effect of a low-fat diet on hormone levels in women with cystic breast disease. I. Serum steroids and gonadotropins. *J Natl Cancer Inst* 1987; 78: 623–26.

11. Woods MN, Gorbach S, Longcope C, et al. Low-fat, high-fiber diet and serum estrone sulfate in premenopausal women. *Am J Clin Nutr* 1989; 49: 1179–83.

12. Rose DP, Boyar A, Haley N, et al. Low fat diet in fibrocystic disease of the breast with cyclic mastalgia: a feasibility study. *Am J Clin Nutr* 1985; 41(4): 856 [abstract].

13. Boyd NF, McGuire V, Shannon P, et al. Effect of a low-fat high-carbohydrate diet on symptoms of cyclical mastopathy. *Lancet* 1988; ii: 128–32.

14. Lubin F, Wax Y, Ron E, et al. Nutritional factors associated with benign breast disease etiology: a case-control study. *Am J Clin Nutr* 1989; 50: 551–56.

15. Prior JC, Vigna Y, Sciarretta D, et al. Conditioning exercise decreases premenstrual symptoms: a prospective, controlled 6-month trial. *Fertil Steril* 1987; 47(3): 402–408.

16. Abrams AA. Use of vitamin E in chronic cystic mastitis. *N Engl J Med* 1965; 272(20): 1080–81.

17. London RS, Sundaram GS, Schultz M, et al. Endocrine parameters and alpha-tocopherol therapy of patients with mammary dysplasia. *Cancer Res* 1981; 41: 3811–13.

18. Ernster VL, Goodson WH, Hunt TK, et al. Vitamin E and benign breast "disease": a double-blind, randomized clinical trial. *Surgery* 1985; 97: 490–94.

19. London RS, Sundaram GS, Murphy L, et al. The effect of vitamin E on mammary dysplasia: a double-blind study. *Obstet Gynecol* 1985; 65: 104–106.

20. Brush MG, Perry M. Pyridoxine and the premenstrual syndrome. *Lancet* 1985; i: 1399.

21. Smallwood J, Ah-Kye D, Taylor I. Vitamin B_6 in the treatment of pre-menstrual mastalgia. *Br J Clin Pract* 1986; 40: 532–33.

22. Krouse TB, Eskin BA, Mobini J. Age-related changes resembling fibrocystic disease in iodine-blocked rat breasts. *Arch Pathol Lab Med* 1979; 103: 631–34.

23. Ghent WR, Eskin BA, Low DA, Hill L. Iodine replacement in fibrocystic disease of the breast. *Can J Surg* 1993; 36: 453–60.

24. Mansel RE, Pye JK, Hughes LE. Effects of Essential fatty acids on cyclical mastalgia and noncyclical breast disorders. In *Omega-6 essential fatty acids: Pathophysiology and roles in clinical medicine.* Alan R Liss, New York, 1990, 557–66.

25. Preece PE, Hanslip JI, Gilbert L, et al. Evening primrose oil (EFAMOL) for mastalgia. In: *Clinical Uses of Essential Fatty Acids,* ed. DF

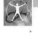

Horrobin, Montreal: Eden Press, 1982, 147–54.

26. Mansel RE, Harrison BJ, Melhuish J, et al. A randomized trial of dietary intervention with essential fatty acids in patients with categorized cysts. *Ann NY Acad Sci* 1990; 586: 288–94.

27. Gateley CA, Maddox PR, Pritchard GA, et al. Plasma fatty acid profiles in benign breast disorders. *Br J Surg* 1992; 79: 407–409.

28. Harding C, Harvey J, Kirkman R, Bundred N. Hormone replacement therapy-induced mastalgia responds to evening primrose oil. *Br J Surg* 1996; 83(suppl 1): 24 [abstr # Breast 012].

29. Pye JK, Mansel RE, Hughes LE. Clinical experience of drug treatments for mastalgia. *Lancet* 1985; ii: 373–77.

30. Böhnert KJ, Hahn G. Phytotherapy in gynecology and obstetrics—*Vitex agnus castus. Erfahrungsheilkunde* 1990; 39: 494–502.

31. Dittmar FW, Böhnert KJ, et al. Pre-menstrual syndrome: Treatment with a phytopharmaceutical. *Therapiwoche Gynäkol* 1992; 5: 60–68.

32. Qi-bing M, Jing-yi T, Bo C. Advance in the pharmacological studies of radix *Angelica sisnensis* (oliv) diels (Chinese danggui). *Chin Med J* 1991; 104: 776–81.

Fibromyalgia

1. Wolfe F, Ross K, Anderson J, Russell J. Aspects of fibromyalgia in the general population: Sex, pain threshold, and FM symptoms. *J Rheumatol* 1995; 22(1): 151–55.

2. Anonymous. Is fibromyalgia caused by a glycolysis impairment? *Nutr Rev* 1994; 52(7): 248–250.

3. Wilke W. Fibromyalgia: Recognizing and addressing the multiple interrelated factors. *Postgrad Med* 1996; 100(1): 153–170.

4. Carette S. Fibromyalgia 20 years later: What have we really accomplished? *J Rheumatol* 1995; 22(4): 590–94.

5. Mengshail AM, Komnaes HB, Forre O. The effects of 20 weeks of

physical fitness training in female patients with fibromyalgia. *Clin Exp Rheumatol* 1992; 10: 345–49.

6. Kaplan KH, Goldberg DL, Galvin-Naduea M. The impact of a meditation-based stress reduction program on fibromyalgia. *Gen Hosp Psychiatry* 1993; 15: 284–89.

7. Deluze C. Bosia L, Zirbs A, et al. Electroacupuncture in fibromyalgia: results of a controlled trial. *BMJ* 1992; 305: 1249–1252.

8. Sprott H, Frankle S, Kluge H, Hein G. Pain treatment of fibromyalgia by acupuncture. *Rheumatol Int* 1998; 18: 35–36.

9. Abraham G. Flechas J. Management of fibromyalgia: Rationale for the use of magnesium and malic acid. *J Nutr Med* 1992; 3: 49–59.

10. Russell J, Michalek J, Flechas J, et al. Treatment of fibromyalgia syndrome with SuperMalic: A randomized, double-blind, placebo-controlled, crossover pilot study. *J Rheumatol* 1995; 22(5): 953–57.

11. Eisinger J, Zakarian H, Plantamura A, et al. Studies of transketolase in chronic pain. *J Adv Med* 1992; 5: 105–113.

12. Eisinger J, Bagneres D, Arroyo P, et al. Effects of magnesium, high energy phosphates, piracetam, and thiamin on erythrocyte transketolase. *Magnesium Res* 1994; 7(1): 59–61.

13. Steinberg CL. The tocopherols (vitamin E) in the treatment of primary fibrositis. *J Bone Joint Surg* 1942; 24: 411–23.

14. Tavoni A, Jeracitano G, Cirigliano G. Evaluation of S-adenosylmethionine in secondary fibromyalgia: A double-blind study. *Clin Exp Rheumatol* 1998; 16: 106–107 [letter].

15. Tavoni A, Vitali C, Bombardieri S, et al. Evaluation of S-adenosylmethionine in primary fibromyalgia: A double-blind crossover study. *Am J Med* 1987; 83(suppl 5A): 107–110.

16. Volkmann H, Norregaard J, Jacobsen S, et al. Double-blind, placebo-controlled cross-over study of intravenous S-adenosyl-L-methionine

in patients with fibromyalgia. *Scand J Rheumatol* 1997; 26: 206–211.

17. Jacobsen S, Danneskiold-Samsoe B, Andersen RB. Oral S-adenosylmethionine in primary fibromyalgia: Double-blind clinical evaluation. *Scand J Rheumatol* 1991; 20: 294–302.

18. Fava M, Rosenbaum JF, MacLaughlin R, et al. Neuroendocrine effects of S-adenosyl-L-methionine, a novel putative antidepressant. *J Psychiatr Res* 1990; 24: 177–84.

19. Bell KM, Potkin SG, Carreon D, Plon L. S-adenosylmethionine blood levels in major depression: Changes with drug treatment. *Acta Neurol Scand* 1994; 154(suppl): 15–18.

20. Bell KM, Potkin SG, Carreon D, Plon L. S-adenosylmethionine blood levels in major depression: changes with drug treatment. *Acta Neurol Scand* 1994; 154(suppl): 15–18.

21. Puttini PS, Caruso I. Primary fibromyalgia syndrome and 5-hydroxy-L-tryptophan: a 90-day open study. *J Int Med Res* 1992; 20: 182–89.

22. Caruso I, Sarzi Puttini P, Cazzola M, Azzolini V. Double-blind study of 5-hydroxytryptophan versus placebo in the treatment of primary fibromyalgia syndrome. *J Int Med Res* 1990; 18: 201–209.

Gallstones

1. Lee DWT, Gilmore CJ, Bonorris G, et al. Effect of dietary cholesterol on biliary lipids in patients with gallstones and normal subjects. *Am J Clin Nutr* 1985; 42: 414.

2. Andersen E, Hellstrom K. The effect of cholesterol feeding on bile acid kinetics and biliary lipids in normolipidemic and hypertriglyceridemic subjects. *J Lipid Res* 1979; 20: 1020–27.

3. Kratzer W, Kachele V, Mason RA, et al. Gallstone prevalence in relation to smoking, alcohol, coffee consumption, and nutrition. The Ulm Gallstone Study. *Scand J Gastroenterol* 1997; 32: 953–58.

4. Pixley F, Mann J. Dietary factors in the aetiology of gall stones: a case control study. *Gut* 1988; 29: 1511–15.

5. Pixley F, Wilson D, McPherson K, Mann J. Effect of vegetarianism on development of gall stones in women. *BMJ* 1985; 291: 11–12.

6. Singh A, Bagga SP, Jindal VP, et al. Gall bladder disease: an analytical report of 250 cases. *J Indian Med Assoc* 1989; 87: 253–56.

7. Jayanthi V, Malathi S, Ramathilakam B, et al. Is vegetarianism a precipitating factor for gallstones in cirrhotics? *Trop Gastroenterol* 1998; 19: 21–23.

8. Heaton KW, Emmett PM, Symes CL, Braddon FEM. An explanation for gallstones in normal-weight women: slow intestinal transit. *Lancet* 1993; 341: 8–10.

9. Marcus SN, Heaton KW. Intestinal transit, deoxycholic acid and the cholesterol saturation of bile—three interrelated factors. *Gut* 1986; 27: 550.

10. Watts JM, Jablonski P, Toouli J. The effect of added bran to the diet on the saturation of bile in people without gallstones. *Am J Surg* 1978; 135: 321–24.

11. McDougall RM, Kakymyshyn L, Walker K, Thurston OG. Effect of wheat bran on serum lipoproteins and biliary lipids. *Can J Surg* 1978; 21: 433–35.

12. Breneman JC. Allergy elimination diet as the most effective gallbladder diet. *Ann Allerg* 1968; 26: 83–87.

13. Sarles H, Gerolami A, Cros RC. Diet and cholesterol gallstones. *Digestion* 1978; 17: 121–27.

14. Kern F Jr. Epidemiology and natural history of gallstones. *Semin Liver Dis* 1983; 3: 87–96.

15. Stampfer MJ, Maclure KM, Colditz GA, et al. Risk of symptomatic gallstones in women with severe obesity. *Am J Clin Nutr* 1992; 55: 652–58.

16. Maclure KM, Hayes KC, Colditz GA, et al. Weight, diet, and the risk of symptomatic gallstones in middle-aged women. *N Engl J Med* 1989; 321: 563–69.

17. Thornton JR. Gallstone disappearance associated with weight loss. *Lancet* 1979; ii: 478 [letter].

18. Everhart JE. Contributions of obesity and weight loss to gallstone disease. *Ann Intern Med* 1993; 119: 1029–35.

19. Scragg RKR. Diet, alcohol, and relative weight in gall stone disease: a case-control study. *BMJ* 1984; 288: 1113–19.

20. Morrison LM. The effects of a low fat diet on the incidence of gallbladder disease. *Am J Gastroenterol* 1956; 25: 158–63.

21. Simon JA. Ascorbic acid and cholesterol gallstones. *Med Hypotheses* 1993; 40: 81–84.

22. Simon JA, Grady D, Snabes MC, et al. Ascorbic acid supplement use and the prevalence of gallbladder disease. *J Clin Epidemiol* 1998; 51: 257–65.

23. Gustafsson U, Wang F-H, Axelson M, et al. The effect of vitamin C in high doses on plasma and biliary lipid composition in patients with cholesterol gallstones: prolongation of the nucleation time. *Eur J Clin Invest* 1997; 27: 387–91.

24. Capper WM, et al. Gallstones, gastric secretion and flatulent dyspepsia. *Lancet* 1967; i: 413–15.

25. Toouli J, Jablonski P, Watts J McK Gallstone dissolution in man using cholic acid and lecithin. *Lancet* 1975; ii: 1124–26.

26. Tuzhilin SA, Dreiling D, Narodetskaja RV, Lukahs LK. The treatment of patients with gallstones by lecithin. *Am J Gastroenterol* 1976; 165: 231–35.

27. Holan KR, Holzbach T, Hsieh JYK, et al. Effect of oral administration of 'essential' phospholipid, 8-glycerophosphate, and linoleic acid on biliary lipids in patients with cholelithiasis. *Digestion* 1979; 19: 251–58.

28. Nassuato G, Iemmolo RM, et al. Effect of silibinin on biliary lipid composition. Experimental and clinical study. *J Hepatol* 1991; 12: 290–95.

29. Somerville KW, Ellis WR, Whitten BH, et al. Stones in the common bile duct: Experience with medical dissolution therapy *Postgrad Med J* 1985; 61: 313–16.

30. Werbach MR, Murray MT. *Botanical Influences on Illness: A Sourcebook of Clinical Research.* Tarzana, CA: Third Line Press, 1994, 166–68 [review].

Gastritis

1. Kelly DJ. The physiology and metabolism of the human gastric pathogen Helicobacter pylori. *Adv Micro Physiol* 1998; 40: 137–89 [review].

2. Kumar M, Yachha SK, Aggarwal R, et al. Healing of chronic antral gastritis: effect of sucralfate and colloidal bismuth subcitrate. *Indian J Gastroenterol* 1996; 15(3): 90–93.

3. Lieber CS. Gastric ethanol metabolism and gastritis: interactions with other drugs, Helicobacter pylori, and antibiotic therapy (1957–1997)—a review. *Alcohol Clin Exp Res* 1997; 21(8): 1360–66.

4. Tsugane S, Tei Y, Takahashi T, et al. Salty food intake and risk of Helicobacter pylori infection. *Jpn J Cancer Res* 1994; 85(5): 474–78.

5. Jooseens JV, Geboers, J. Nutrition and gastric cancer. *Nutr Cancer* 1981; 2: 250–61.

6. Yeoh KG, Kang JY, Yap I, et al. Chili protects against aspirin-induced gastroduodenal mucosal injury in humans. *Dig Dis Sci* 1995; 40(3): 580–83.

7. Yeoh KG, Kang JY, Yap I, et al. Chili protects against aspirin-induced gastroduodenal mucosal injury in humans. *Dig Dis Sci* 1995; 40(3): 580–83.

8. Aiuti F, Paganelli R. Food allergy and gastrointestinal diseases. *Ann Allergy* 1983; 51(two Pt 2): 275–80 [review].

9. Reimann H-J, Lewin J. Gastric mucosal reactions in patients with food allergy. *Am J Gastroenterol* 1988; 83: 1212–19.

10. Altman C, Ladouch A, Briantais MJ, et al. Antral gastritis in chronic alcoholism. Role of cirrhosis and Helicobacter pylori. *Presse Med* 1995; 24(15): 708–10 [in French].

11. Robbins SL, Cotran RS, Kumar V. *Pathologic Basis of Disease*

3rd ed. Philadelphia, PA: WB Saunders Co, 1984, 809–14.

12. Scheiman JM. NSAIDs, gastrointestinal injury, and cytoprotection. *Gastroenterology Clinics of North America* 1996; 25(2): 279–98 [review].

13. Chou T. Wake up and smell the coffee. Caffeine, coffee, and the medical consequences. *West J Med* 1992; 157(5): 544–53 [review].

14. Elta GH, Behler EM, Colturi TJ. Comparison of coffee intake and coffee-induced symptoms in patients with duodenal ulcer, nonulcer dyspepsia, and normal controls. *Am J Gastroenterol* 1990; 85(10): 1339–42.

15. Drake IM, Mapstone NP, Schorah CJ, et al. Reactive oxygen species activity and lipid peroxidation in *Helicobacter pylori* associated gastritis: relation to gastric mucosal ascorbic acid concentrations and effect of *H pylori* eradication. *Gut* 1998; 42(6): 768–71.

16. Waring AJ, Drake IM, Schorah CJ, et al. Ascorbic acid and total vitamin C concentrations in plasma, gastric juice, and gastrointestinal mucosa: effects of gastritis and oral supplementation. *Gut* 1996; 38(2): 171–76.

17. Spirichev VB, Levachev MM, Rymarenko TV, et al. The effect of administration of beta-carotene in an oil solution on its blood serum level and antioxidant status of patients with duodenal ulcer and erosive gastritis. *Vopr Med Khim* 1992; 38(6): 44–47 [in Russian].

18. Palli D, Decarli A, Cipriani F, et al. Plasma pepsinogens, nutrients, and diet in areas of Italy at varying gastric cancer risk. *Cancer Epidemiol Biomarkers Prev* 1991; 1(1): 45–50.

19. Zhang ZW, Patchett SE, Perrett D, et al. Gastric mucosal and luminal beta-carotene concentrations in patients with chronic *H pylori* infection. *Gut* 1996; 38(suppl 1): A5 [abstr #W11].

20. Spirichev VB, Levachev MM, Rymarenko TV, et al. The effect of administration of beta-carotene in an oil solution on its blood serum level and antioxidant status of patients with

duodenal ulcer and erosive gastritis. *Vopr Med Khim* 1992; 38: 44–47 [in Russian].

21. Tsubono Y, Okubo S, Hayashi M, et al. A randomized controlled trial for chemoprevention of gastric cancer in high-risk Japanese population; study design, feasibility and protocol modification. *Jpn J Cancer Res* 1997; 88: 344–49.

22. Salim AS. Sulfhydryl-containing agents in the treatment of gastric bleeding induced by nonsteroidal antiinflammatory drugs. *Can J Surg* 1993; 36(1): 53–58.

23. Farinati F, Cardin R, Della Libera G, et al. Effects of N-acetyl-L-cysteine in patients with chronic atrophic gastritis and nonulcer dyspepsia: a phase III pilot study. *Curr Ther Res* 1997; 58: 724–33.

24. Houdijk AP, Van Leeuwen PA, Boermeester MA, et al. Glutamine-enriched enteral diet increases splanchnic blood flow in the rat. *Am J Physiol* 1994; 267(6 Pt 1): G1035–40.

25. Yan R, Sun Y, Sun R. Early enteral feeding and supplement of glutamine prevent occurrence of stress ulcer following severe thermal injury. *Chung Hua Cheng Hsing Shao Shang Wai Ko Tsa Chih* 1995; 11(3): 189–92.

26. Brzozowski T, Konturek SJ, Sliwowski Z, et al. Role of L-arginine, a substrate for nitric oxide-synthase, in gastroprotection and ulcer healing. *J Gastroenterol* 1997; 32(4): 442–52.

27. Frommer DJ. The healing of gastric ulcers by zinc sulphate. *Med J Aust* 1975; 22(21): 793–96.

28. Mozsik G, Hunyady B, Garamszegi M, et al. Dynamism of cytoprotective and antisecretory drugs in patients with unhealed gastric and duodenal ulcers. *J Gastroenterol Hepatol* 1994; 9(suppl 1): S88–92.

29. Kolarski V, Petrova-Shopova K, Vasileva E, et al. Erosive gastritis and gastroduodenitis—clinical, diagnostic and therapeutic studies. *Vutr Boles* 1987; 26(3): 56–59.

30. Maruyama K et al. Usefulness of Hi-Z fine granule (gamma-Oryzanol) for the treatment of autonomic instability in gastrointestinal

system. *Shinyaku To Rinsho* 1976; 25: 124 [in Japanese].

31. Kamiji M, et al. Practical usage of gamma-oryzanol on indefinite complaints of digestive system. *Shinyaku To Rinsho* 1976; 25: 136 [in Japanese].

32. Takemoto T, et al. Clinical trial of Hi-Z fine granules (gamma-oryzanol) on gastrointestinal symptoms at 375 hospitals (Japan). *Shinyaku To Rinsho* 1977; 26 [in Japanese].

33. Beil W, Birkholz W, Sewing KF. Effects of flavonoids on parietal cell acid secretion, gastric mucosal prostaglandin production and *Helicobacter pylori* growth. *Arzneim Forsch* 1995; 45: 697–700.

34. Bae EA, Han MJ, Kim NJ, Kim DH. Anti–*Helicobacter pylori* activity of herbal medicines. *Biol Pharm Bull* 1998; 21(9): 990–92.

35. Beil W, Birkholz W, Sewing KF. Effects of flavonoids on parietal cell acid secretion, gastric mucosal prostaglandin production and *Helicobacter pylori* growth. *Arzneim Forsch* 1995; 45: 697–700.

36. Rekka EA, Kourounakis AP, Kourounakis PN. Investigation of the effect of chamazulene on lipid peroxidation and free radical processes. *Res Commun Mol Pathol Pharmacol* 1996; 92(3): 361–64.

37. Blumenthal M, Busse WR, Goldberg A, et al. (eds). *The Complete German Commission E Monographs: Therapeutic Guide to Herbal Medicines.* Austin: American Botanical Council and Boston: Integrative Medicine Communications, 1998, 167.

Gingivitis (Periodontal Disease)

1. Pack ARC. Folate mouthwash: effects on established gingivitis in periodontal patients. *J Clin Periodontol* 1984; 11: 619–28.

2. Vogel RI, et al. The effect of topical application of folic acid on gingival health. *J Oral Med* 1978; 33(1): 20–22.

3. Vogel RI, et al. The effect of folic acid on gingival health. *J Periodontol* 1976; 47: 667–68.

4. Pack ARC, Thomson ME. Effects of topical and systemic folic acid supplementation on gingivitis in pregnancy. *J Clin Periodontol* 1980; 7: 402–14.

5. Francetti L, Maggiore E, Marchesi A, et al. Oral hygiene in subjects treated with diphenylhydantoin: effects of a professional program. *Prev Assist Dent* 1991; 17(30): 40–43 [in Italian].

6. Fitchie JG, Comer RW, Hanes PJ, Reeves GW. The reduction of phenytoin-induced gingival overgrowth in a severely disabled patient: a case report. *Compendium* 1989; 10(6): 314.

7. Steinberg SC, Steinberg AD. Phenytoin-induced gingival overgrowth control in severely retarded children. *J Periodontol* 1982; 53(7)429–33.

8. Drew HJ et al. Effect of folate on phenytoin hyperplasia. *J Clin Periodontol* 1987; 14: 350–56.

9. Nakamura R, Littarru GP, Folkers K. Deficiency of coenzyme Q in gingiva of patients with periodontal disease. *Int J Vitam Nutr Res* 1973; 43: 84–92.

10. Wilkinson EG, et al. Bioenergetics in clinical medicine. VI. Adjunctive treatment of periodontal disease with coenzyme Q_{10}. *Res Commun Chem Pathol Pharmacol* 1976; 14: 715–19.

11. Ref: Hanioka T, Tanaka M, Ojima M, et al. Effect of topical application of coenzyme Q10 on adult periodontitis. *Mol Aspects Med* 1994; 15(suppl): S241–48.

12. Vaananen MK, Markkanen HA, Tuovinen VJ, et al. Periodontal health related to plasma ascorbic acid. *Proc Finn Dent Soc* 1993; 89: 51–59.

13. Aurer-Kozelj J, Kralj-Klobucar N, Buzina R, Bacic M. The effect of ascorbic acid supplementation on periodontal tissue ulstructure in subjects with progressive periodontitis. *Int J Vitam Nutr Res* 1982; 52: 333–41.

14. Woolfe SN, Kenney EB, Hume WR, Carranza FA Jr. Relationship of ascorbic acid levels of blood and gingival tissue with response to periodontal therapy. *J Clin Periodontol* 1984; 11: 159–65.

15. Vogel RI, Lamster IB, Wechsler SA, et al,. The effects of megadoses of ascorbic acid on PMN chemotaxis and experimental gingivitis. *J Periodontol* 1986; 57: 472–79.

16. El-Ashiry GM, Ringsdorf WM, Cheraskin E. Local and systemic influences in periodontal disease. II. Effect of prophylaxis and natural versus synthetic vitamin C upon gingivitis. *J Periodontol* 1964; 35: 250–259.

17. Carvel I, Halperin V. Therapeutic effect of water soluble bioflavonoids in gingival inflammatory conditions. *Oral Surg Oral Med Oral Pathol* 1961; 14: 847–55.

18. Krook L, et al. Human periodontal disease. Morphology and response calcium therapy. *Cornell Vet* 1972; 62: 32–53.

19. Uhrbom E, Jacobson L. Calcium and periodontitis: a clinical effect of calcium medication. *J Clin Periodontol* 1984; 11: 230–41.

20. Serfaty R, Itic J. Comparative trial with natural herbal mouthwash versus chlorhexidine in gingivitis. *J Clin Dentistry* 1988; 1: A34.

21. Yamnkell S, Emling RC. Two-month evaluation of Parodontax dentifrice. *J Clin Dentistry* 1988; 1: A41.

22. Dzink JL, Socransky SS. Comparative in vitro activity of sanguinarine against oral microbial isolates. *Antimicrob Agents Chemother* 1985; 27(4): 663–65.

23. Hannah JJ, Johnson JD, Kuftinec MM. Long-term clinical evaluation of toothpaste and oral rinse containing sanguinaria extract in controlling plaque, gingival inflammation, and sulcular bleeding during orthodontic treatment. *Am J Orthod Dentofacial Orthop* 1989; 96(3): 199–207.

24. Harper DS, Mueller LJ, Fine JB, et al. Clinical efficacy of a dentifrice and oral rinse containing sanguinaria extract and zinc chloride during 6 months of use. *J Periodontol* 1990; 61(6): 352–58.

25. Mauriello SM, Bader JD Six-month effects of a sanguinarine dentifrice on plaque and gingivitis. *J Periodontol* 1988; 59(4): 238–43.

Glaucoma

1. Berens C, et al. Allergy in glaucoma. Manifestations of allergy in three glaucoma patients as determined by the pulse-diet method of Coca. *Ann Allerg* 1947; 5: 526.

2. Raymond LF. Allergy and chronic simple glaucoma. *Ann Allerg* 1996; 22: 146.

3. Ringsdorf WM Jr, Cheraskin E. Ascorbic acid and glaucoma: a review. *J Holistic Med* 1981; 3: 167–72.

4. Boyd HH. Eye pressure lowering effect of vitamin C. *J Orthomol Med* 1995; 10: 165–68.

5. Stocker FW. New ways of influencing the intraocular pressure. *NY State J Med* 1949; 49: 58–63.

6. Samples RJ, et al. Effect of melatonin on intraocular pressure. *Curr Eye Res* 1988; 7: 649–53.

7. Gaspar AZ, et al. The influence of magnesium on visual field and peripheral vasospasm in glaucoma. *Ophthalmologica* 1995; 209: 11–13.

8. Filina AA, Davydova NG, Endrikhovskii SN, et al. Lipoic acid as a means of metabolic therapy of open-angle glaucoma. *Vestn Oftalmol* 1995; 111: 6–8.

Gout

1. Loenen H, Eshuis H, Lowik M, et al. Serum uric acid correlates in elderly men and women with special reference to body composition and dietary intake (Dutch Nutrition Surveillance System). *J Clin Epidemiol* 1990; 43(12): 1297–1303.

2. Ralston SH, Capell HA, and Sturrock RD. Alcohol and response to treatment of gout. *BMJ* 1988; 296: 1641–42.

3. Scott JT. Alcohol and Gout. *BMJ* 1989; 298: 1054.

4. Emmerson BT. Effect of oral fructose on urate production. *Ann Rheuma Dis* 1974; 33: 276.

5. Blau LW. Cherry diet control for gout and arthritis. *Tex Rep Biol Med* 1950; 8: 309–11.

6. Oster KA. Xanthine oxidase and folic acid. *Ann Intern Med* 1977; 87: 252–53.

7. Boss GR, Ragsdale RA, Zettner A, et al. Failure of folic acid

Part One: References

(pteroylglutamic acid) to affect hyper-uricemia. *J Lab Clin Med* 1980; 96: 783–89.

8. Stein HB, et al. Ascorbic acid-induced uricosuria: a consequence of megavitamin therapy. *Ann Intern Med* 1976; 84: 385–88.

9. Bindoli A, Valente M, Cavallini L. Inhibitory action of quercetin on xanthine oxidase and xanthine dehydrogenase activity. *Pharm Res Comm* 1985; 17: 831–39.

10. Busse W, Kopp D, Middleton E. Flavonoid modulation of human neutrophil function. *J Allerg Clin Immunol* 1984; 73: 801–809

Hay Fever

1. Speer F. Multiple food allergy. *Ann Allerg* 1975; 34: 71–76.

2. Buczylko K, Kowalczyk J, Zeman K, et al. Allergy to food in children with pollinosis. *Rocz Akad Med Bialymst* 1995; 40: 568–72.

3. Ogle KA, Bullock JD. Children with allergic rhinitis and/or bronchial asthma treated with elimination diet. *Ann Allergy* 1977; 39: 8–11.

4. Holmes, HM, Alexander W: Hay fever and vitamin C. *Science* 1942: 96: 497.

5. Ruskin SL. High dose vitamin C in allergy. *Am J Dig Dis* 1945; 12: 281.

6. Fortner BR Jr, Danziger RE, Rabinowitz PS, Nelson HS. The effect of ascorbic acid on cutaneous and nasal response to histamine and allergen. *J Allergy Clin Immunol* 1982; 69: 484–88.

7. Balabolkin II, Gordeeva GF, Fuseva ED, et al. Use of vitamins in allergic illnesses in children. *Vopr Med Khim* 1992; 38: 36–40.

8. Mittman P. Randomized double-blind study of freeze-dried Urtica diocia in the treatment of allergic rhinitis. *Planta Med* 1990; 56: 44–47.

9. Weiss RF. *Herbal Medicine.* Gothenburg, Sweden: Ab Arcanum and Beaconsfield, UK: Beaconsfield Publishers Ltd, 1988, 219 [review].

10. Weiss RF. *Herbal Medicine.* Gothenburg, Sweden: Ab Arcanum and Beaconsfield, UK: Beaconsfield Publishers Ltd, 1988, 219 [review].

11. Meserole L, Yarnell E. Botanical prevention and treatment for hay fever. *Alt Compl Ther* 1996; 2: 83–86 [review].

Hemorrhoids

1. Johanson JF, Sonnenberg A. Constipation is not a risk factor for hemorrhoids: a case-control study of potential etiological agents. *Am J Gastroenterol* 1994; 89: 1981–86.

2. Johanson JF, Sonnenberg A. The prevalence of hemorrhoids and chronic constipation. *Gastroenterol* 1990; 98: 380–86.

3. Deutsch AA, Kaufman Z, Reiss R. Hemorrhoids: a plea for nonsurgical treatment. *Isr J Med Sci* 1980; 16: 649–54.

4. Moesgaard F, Nielsen ML, Hansen JB, Knudsen JT. High-fiber diet reduces bleeding and pain in patients with hemorrhoids. *Dis Colon Rectum* 1982; 25: 454–56.

5. Eherer AJ, Santa Ana CA, Porter J, Fordtran JS. Effect of psyllium, calcium polycarbophil, and wheat bran on secretory diarrhea induced by phenolphthalein. *Gastroenterol* 1993; 104: 1007–12.

6. Wichtl M. *Herbal Drugs and Phytopharmaceuticals.* Boca Raton, FL: CRC Press, 1994, 268–70.

7. Nini G, Di Cicco CO. Controlled clinical evaluation of a new anti-hemorrhoid drug, using a completely randomized experimental plan. *Clin Ther* 1978; 86(6): 545–59 [in Italian].

8. Blumenthal M, Busse WR, Goldberg A, et al. (eds). *The Complete German Commission E Monographs: Therapeutic Guide to Herbal Medicines.* Austin: American Botanical Council and Boston: Integrative Medicine Communications, 1998, 428.

9. Leung AY, Foster S. *Encyclopedia of Common Natural Ingredients Used in Food, Drugs and Cosmetics.* New York: John Wiley & Sons, 1996, 427–29.

Hepatitis

1. Jenkins PJ, Portmann BP, Eddleston AL, Williams R. Use of

polyunsaturated phosphatidyl choline in HBsAg negative chronic active hepatitis: Results of prospective double-blind controlled trial. *Liver* 1982; 2: 77–81.

2. Skotnicki AB. Therapeutic application of calf thymus extract (TFX). *Med Oncol Tumor Pharmacother* 1989; 6: 31–43 [review].

3. Galli M, Crocchiolo P, Negri C, et al. Attempt to treat acute type B hepatitis with an orally administered thymic extract (thymomodulin): Preliminary results. *Drugs Exp Clin Res* 1985; 11: 665–69.

4. Bortolotti F et al. Effect of an orally administered thymic derivative, thymomodulin, in chronic type B hepatitis in children. *Curr Ther Res* 1988; 43: 67–72.

5. Civeira MP, Castilla A, Morte S, et al. A pilot study of thymus extract in chronic non-A, non-B hepatitis. *Aliment Pharmacol Ther* 1989; 3: 395–401.

6. Von Herbay A, Stahl W, Niederau C, et al. Diminished plasma levels of vitamin E in patients with severe viral hepatitis. *Free Radic Res* 1996; 25: 461–66.

7. Pan WH, Wang CY, Huang SM, et al. Vitamin A, Vitamin E or beta-carotene status and hepatitis B-related hepatocellular carcinoma. *Ann Epidemiol* 1993; 3: 217–24.

8. Mezes M, Par A, Nemeth P, Javor T. Studies of the blood lipid peroxide status and vitamin E levels in patients with chronic active hepatitis and alcoholic liver disease. *Int J Clin Pharmacol Res* 1986; 6: 333–38.

9. Yurdakok M, Kanra G. Vitamin E therapy in viral hepatitis. *Mikrobiyol Bul* 1986; 20: 91–94 [in Turkish].

10. Houglum K, Venkataramani A, Lyche K, Chojkier M. A pilot study of the effects of d-alpha-tocopherol on hepatic stellate cell activation in chronic hepatitis C. *Gastroenterology* 1997; 113: 1069–73.

11. Morishige F, Murata A. Vitamin C for prophylaxis of viral hepatitis B in transfused patients. *J Int Acad Prev Med* 1978; 5: 54.

12. Knodell RG, Tate MA, Akl BF, Wilson JW. Vitamin C prophylaxis

for posttransfusion hepatitis: lack of effect in a controlled trial. *Am J Clin Nutr* 1981; 34: 20–23.

13. Baur H, Staub H. Treatment of hepatitis with infusions of ascorbic acid: Comparison with other therapies. *JAMA* 1954; 156: 565 [abstract].

14. Campbell RE, Pruitt FW. Vitamin B$_{12}$ in the treatment of viral hepatitis. *Am J Med Sci* 1952; 224: 252–62.

15. Campbell RE, Pruitt FW. The effect of vitamin B$_{12}$ and folic acid in the treatment of viral hepatitis. *Am J Med Sci* 1955; 229: 8.

16. Suzuki H, Yamamoto S, Hirayama C, et al. Cianidanol therapy for HBs-antigen-positive chronic hepatitis: A multicentre, double-blind study. *Liver* 1986; 6: 35–44.

17. Bar-Meir S et al. Effect of (+)-cyanidanol-3 on chronic active hepatitis: A double blind controlled trial. *Gut* 1985; 26: 975–79.

18. Magliulo E, Gagliardi B, Fiori GP. Results of a double blind study on the effect of silymarin in the treatment of acute viral hepatitis carried out at two medical centres. *Med Klin* 1978; 73: 1060–65 [in German].

19. Bode JC, Schmidt U, Durr HK. Silymarin for the treatment of acute viral hepatitis? Report of a controlled trial. *Med Klin* 1977; 72: 513–18 [in German].

20. Vailati A, Aristia L, Sozze E, et al. Randomized open study of the dose-affect relationship of a short course of IdB 1016 in patients with viral or alcoholic hepatitis. *Fitoterapia* 1993; 64: 219–27.

21. Buzzelli G, Moscarella S, Giusti A, et al. A pilot study on the liver protective effect of silybinphosphatidylcholine complex (IdB 1016) in chronic active hepatitis. *Int J Clin Pharmacol Ther Toxicol* 1993; 31: 456–60.

22. Lirussi F, Okolicsanyi L. Cytoprotection in the nineties: Experience with ursodeoxycholic acid and silymarin in chronic liver disease. *Acta Physiol Hung* 1992; 80: 363–67.

23. Ferenci P, Dragosics B, Dittrich H, et al. Randomized controlled trial of silymarin treatment in patients with cirrhosis of the liver. *J Hepat* 1989; 9: 105–13.

24. Velussi M, Cernigoi AM, Viezzoli L, et al. Silymarin reduces hyperinsulinemia, malondialdehyde levels, and daily insulin need in cirrhotic diabetic patients. *Curr Ther Res* 1993; 53: 533–45.

25. Salmi HA, Sarna S. Effect of silymarin on chemical, functional, and morphological alterations of the liver. A double-blind controlled study. *Scand J Gastroenterol* 1982; 17: 517–21.

26. Parés A, Planas R, Torres M, et al. Effects of silymarin in alcoholic patients with cirrhosis of the liver: Results of a controlled, double-blind, randomized and multicenter trial. *J Hepatol* 1998; 28: 615–21.

27. Doshi JC, Vaidya AB, Antarkar DS, et al. A two-stage clinical trial of *Phyllanthus amarus* in hepatitis B carriers: Failure to eradicate the surface antigen. *Ind J Gastroenterol* 1994; 13: 7–8.

28. Thyagarajan SP, Subramian S, Thirunalasundari T, et al. Effects of Phyllanthus amarus on chronic carriers of hepatitis B virus. *Lancet* 1988; 2: 764–66.

29. Leelarasamee A, Trakulsomboon S, Maunwongyathi P, et al. Failure of *Phyllanthus amarus* to eradicate hepatitis B surface antigen from symptomless carriers. *Lancet* 1990; 335: 1600–1601.

30. Meixa W, Cheng H, Li Y, et al. Herbs of the genus *Phyllanthus* in the treatment of chronic hepatitis B: Observations with three preparations from different geographical sites. *J Lab Clin Med* 1995; 126: 350–52.

31. Suzuki H, Ohta Y, Takino T, et al. Effects of glycyrrhizin on biochemical tests in patients with chronic hepatitis. Double blind trial. *Asian Med J* 1983; 26: 423–38.

32. Yasuda K, Hino K, Fujioka S, et al. Effects of high dose therapy with Stronger Neo-Minophagen C (SNMC) on hepatic histography in non-A, non-B chronic active hepatitis. In *Viral Hepatitis C, D, E,* eds. T Shikata, RH Purcell, T Uchida. Amsterdam: Excerpta Medica, 1991, 205–209.

33. Crance JM, L'eveque F, Biziagos E, et al. Studies on mechanism of action on glycyrrhizin against hepatitis A virus replication in vitro. *Antiviral Res* 1994; 23: 63–76.

34. Hobbs, C. *Medicinal Mushrooms.* Santa Cruz, CA: Botanica Press, 1995, 96–107.

35. Harada T, Kanetaka T, Suzuki H, Suzuki K. Therapeutic effect of LEM (extract of cultured *Lentinus edodes* mycelia) against HBeAg-positive chronic hepatitis B. *Gastroenterol Intl* 1988; 1(suppl 1): abstract 719.

36. Leung A, Foster S. *Encyclopedia of Common Natural Ingredients Used in Food, Drugs and Cosmetics* 2nd ed. New York: John Wiley & Sons, 1996, 469–72.

High Cholesterol (Hypercholesterolemia): Dietary and Lifestyle Changes

1. Kromhout D, Menotti A, Bloemberg B, et al. Dietary saturated and trans fatty acids and cholesterol and 25-year mortality from coronary heart disease: the Seven Countries Study. *Prev Med* 1995; 24: 308–15.

2. Tell GS, Evans GW, Folsom AR, et al. Dietary fat intake and carotid artery wall thickness: the atherosclerosis risk in communities (ARIC) study. *Am J Epidemiol* 1994; 139: 979–89.

3. Ornish D, Brown SE, Scherwitz LW, et al. Can lifestyle changes reverse coronary heart disease? The Lifestyle Heart Trial. *Lancet* 1990; 336: 129–33.

4. Denke MA, Grundy SM. Comparison of effects of lauric acid and palmitic acid on plasma lipids and lipoproteins. *Am J Clin Nutr* 1992; 56: 895–98.

5. Zock PL, de Vries JHM, Katan MB. Impact of myristic acid versus palmitic acid on serum lipid and lipoprotein levels in healthy women and men. *Arterioscler Thromb* 1994; 14: 567–75.

6. Kumar PD. The role of coconut and coconut oil in coronary heart disease in Kerala, south India. *Trop Doct* 1997; 27: 215–17.

7. Denke MA, Grundy SM. Comparison of effects of lauric acid and palmitic acid on plasma lipids and lipoproteins. *Am J Clin Nutr* 1992; 56: 895–98.

8. Mendis S, Kumarasunderam R. The effect of daily consumption of coconut fat and soya-bean fat on plasma lipids and lipoproteins of young normolipidaemic men. *Br J Nutr* 1990; 63: 547–52.

9. Dreon DM, Fernstrom HA, Williams PT, Krauss RM. A very-low-fat diet is not associated with improved lipoprotein profiles in men with a predominance of large, low-density lipoproteins. *Am J Clin Nutr* 1999; 69: 411–18.

10. Hepner G, Fried R, St Jeor S, et al. Hypocholesterolemic effect of yogurt and milk. *Am J Clin Nutr* 1979; 19–24.

11. de Roos NM, Schouten G, katan MB. Yoghurt enriched with *Lactobacillus acidophilus* does not lower blood lipids in healthy men and women with normal to borderline high serum cholesterol levels. *Eur J Clin Nutr* 1999; 53: 277–80.

12. Santos MJ, Lopez-Jurado M, Llopis J, et al. Influence of dietary supplementation with fish on plasma total cholesterol and lipoprotein cholesterol fractions in patients with coronary heart disease. *J Nutr Med* 1992; 3: 107–15.

13. Kromhout D, Bosschieter EB, Coulander CdL, The inverse relation between fish consumption and 20-year mortality from coronary heart disease. *N Engl J Med* 1985; 312: 1205–9.

14. Ascherio A, Rimm EG, Stampfer MJ, et al. Dietary intake of marine n-3 fatty acids, fish intake, and the risk of coronary disease among men. *N Engl J Med* 1995; 332: 977–82.

15. Albert CM, Manson JE, O'Donnoell C, et al. Fish consumption and the risk of sudden death in the Physicians' Health Study. *Circulation* 1996; 94 (suppl 1): I-578 [abstract #3382].

16. Thorogood M, Carter R, Benfield L, et al. Plasma lipids and lipoprotein cholesterol concentrations in people with different diets in Britain. *Br Med J* (Clin Res Ed) 1987; 295: 351–53.

17. Burr ML, Sweetnam PM. Vegetarianism, dietary fiber and mortality. *Am J Clin Nutr* 1982; 36: 873–77.

18. Resnicow K, Barone J, Engle A, et al. Diet and serum lipids in vegan vegetarians: a model for risk reduction. *J Am Dietet Assoc* 1991; 91: 447–53.

19. Ornish D, Brown SE, Scherwitz LW, et al. Can lifestyle changes reverse coronary heart disease? The Lifestyle Heart Trial. *Lancet* 1990; 336: 129–33.

20. Connor SL, Connor WE. The importance of dietary cholesterol in coronary heart disease. *Prev Med* 1983; 12: 115–23 [review].

21. Edington JD, Geekie M, Carter R, et al. Serum lipid response to dietary cholesterol in subjects fed a low-fat, high-fiber diet. *Am J Clin Nutr* 1989; 50: 58–62.

22. Raloff J. Oxidized lipids: a key to heart disease? *Sci News* 1985; 127: 278.

23. Levy Y, Maor I, Presser D, Aviram M. Consumption of eggs with meals increases the susceptibility of human plasma and low-density lipoprotein to lipid peroxidation. *Ann Nutr Metabol* 1996; 40: 243–51.

24. Shekelle RB, Stamler J. Dietary cholesterol and ischaemic heart disease. *Lancet* 1989; i: 1177–79.

25. Anderson JW, Chen WJL. Legumes and their soluble fiber: effect on cholesterol-rich lipoproteins. In *Unconventional Sources of Dietary Fiber*, ed. I Furda, Washington, DC: American Chemical Society, 1983.

26. Ripsin CM, Keenan JM, Jacobs DR, et al. Oat products and lipid lowering—a meta-analysis. *JAMA* 1992; 267: 3317–25.

27. Williams CL, Bollella M, Spark A, Puder D. Soluble fiber enhances the hypocholesterolemic effect of the Step I diet in childhood. *J Am Coll Nutr* 1995; 14: 251–57.

28. Miettinen TA, Tarpila S. Effect of pectin on serum cholesterol, fecal bile acids and biliary lipids in normolipidemic and hyperlipidemic individuals. *Clin Chim Acta* 1977; 79: 471–77.

29. Glore SR, Van Treeck D, Knehans AW, Guild M. Soluble fiber and serum lipids: a literature review. *J Am Dietet Assoc* 1994; 94: 425–36.

30. Rimm EB, Ascherio A, Giovannucci E, et al. Vegetable, fruit, and cereal fiber intake and risk of coronary heart disease among men. *JAMA* 1996; 275: 447–51.

31. Bierenbaum ML, Reichstein R, Watkins TR. Reducing atherogenic risk in hyperlipemic humans with flaxseed supplementation: a preliminary report. *J Am Coll Nutr* 1993; 12: 501–4.

32. Jenkins DJA, Kendall CWC, Vidgen E, et al. Health aspects of partially defatted flaxseed, including effects on serum lipids, oxidative measures, and ex vivo androgen and progestin activity: a controlled crossover trial. *Am J Clin Nutr* 1999; 69: 395–402.

33. Mantzioris E, James MJ, Bibson RA, Cleland LG. Dietary substitution with an alpha-linolenic acid-rich vegetable oil increases eicosapentaenoic acid concentrations in tissues. *Am J Clin Nutr* 1994; 59: 1304–9.

34. Harris WS. n-3 fatty acids and serum lipoproteins: human studies. *Am J Clin Nutr* 1997; 65(5 suppl): 1645S–54S [review].

35. Layne KS, Goh YK, Jumpsen JA, et al. Normal subjects consuming physiological levels of 18: 3(n-3) and 20: 5(n-3) from flaxseed or fish oils have characteristic differences in plasma lipid and lipoprotein fatty acid levels. *J Nutr* 1996; 126: 2130–40.

36. Nestel PJ, Pomeroy SE, Sasahara T, et al. Arterial compliance in obese subjects is improved with dietary plant n-3 fatty acid from flaxseed oil despite increased LDL oxidizability. *Arterioscler Thromb Vasc Biol* 1997; 17: 1163–70.

37. Anderson JW, Johnstone BM, Cook-Newell ME. Meta-analysis of the effects of soy protein intake on serum lipids. *N Engl J Med* 1995; 3333: 276–82.

38. Potter SM. Overview of proposed mechanisms for the hypocholes-

terolemic effect of soy. *J Nutr* 1995; 606S–11S [review].

39. Yudkin J, Kang SS, Bruckdorfer KR. Effects of high dietary sugar. *Br Med J* 1980; 281: 1396.

40. Reiser S. Effect of dietary sugars on metabolic risk factors associated with heart disease. *Nutr Health* 1985; 3: 203–16.

41. Liu K, Stamler J, Trevisan M, Moss D. Dietary lipids, sugar, fiber, and mortality from coronary heart disease. Bivariate analysis of international data. *Arteriosclerosis* 1982; 2: 221–27.

42. Urgert R, Schulz AGM, Katan MB. Effects of cafestol and kahweol from coffee grounds on serum lipids and serum liver enzymes in humans. *Am J Clin Nutr* 1995; 61: 149–54.

43. Superko HR, Bortz WM, Albers JJ, Wood PJ. Lipoprotein and apolipoprotein changes during a controlled trial of caffeinated and decaffeinated coffee drinking in men. *Circulation* 1989; 80: II-86.

44. Nygård O, Refsum H, Velanb PM, et al. Coffee consumption and plasma total homocysteine: The Hordaland Homocysteine Study. *Am J Clin Nutr* 1997; 65: 136–43.

45. Rosmarin PC, Applegate WB, Somes GW. Coffee consumption and serum lipids: a randomized, crossover clinical trial. *Am J Med* 1990; 88: 349–56.

46. Regular or decaf? Coffee consumption and serum lipoproteins. *Nutr Rev* 1992; 50: 175–78 [review].

47. Dai WS, Laporte RE, Hom DL, et al. Alcohol consumption and high density lipoprotein cholesterol concentration among alcoholics. *Am J Epidemiol* 1985; 122: 620–27.

48. Marques-Vidal P, Ducimetiere P, Evans A, et al. Alcohol consumption and myocardial infarction: a case-control study in France and northern Ireland. *Am J Epidemiol* 1996; 143: 1089–93.

49. Rimm EB, Klatsky A, Grobbee D, Stampfer MJ. Review of moderate alcohol consumption and reduced risk of coronary heart disease: is the effect due to beer, wine, or spirits? *BMJ* 1996; 312: 731–36 [review].

50. Hendriks HF, Veenstra J, Wierik EJMV, Schaafsma G, Kluft C. Effect of moderate dose of alcohol with evening meal on fibrinolytic factors. *BMJ* 1994; 304: 1003–6.

51. Doll R, Peto AR, Hall E, et al. Mortality in relation to consumption of alcohol: 13 years' observations on male British doctors. *BMJ* 1994; 309: 911–18.

52. Hein HO, Suadicani P, Gyntelberg F. Alcohol consumption, serum low density lipoprotein cholesterol concentration, and risk of ischaemic heart disease: six year follow up in the Copenhagen male study. *BMJ* 1996; 736–41.

53. Baggio G, Pagnan A, Muraca M, et al. Olive-oil-enriched diet: effect on serum lipoprotein levels and biliary cholesterol saturation. *Am J Clin Nutr* 1988; 47: 960–64.

54. Grundy SM. Monounsaturated fatty acids and cholesterol metabolism: implications for dietary recommendations. *J Nutr* 1989; 119: 529–33 [review].

55. Keys A, ed. Coronary heart disease in seven countries. *Circulation* 1970; 41(suppl q): I1–211.

56. Willett WC, Stampfer MJ, Manson JE, et al. Intake of *trans* fatty acids and risk of coronary heart disease among women. *Lancet* 1993; 341: 581–85.

57. Khosla P, Hayes KC. Dietary trans-monounsaturated fatty acids negatively impact plasma lipids in humans: critical review of the evidence. *J Am Coll Nutr* 1996; 15: 235–39.

58. Warshafsky S, Kamer RS, Sivak SL. Effect of garlic on total serum cholesterol—a meta-analysis. *Ann Intern Med* 1993; 119: 599–605.

59. McCrindle BW, Helden E, Conner WT. Garlic extract therapy in children with hypercholesterolemia. *Arch Pediatr Adolesc Med* 1998; 152: 1089–94.

60. Isaacsohn JL, Moser M, Stein EA, et al. Garlic powder and plasma lipids and lipoproteins. *Arch Intern Med* 1998; 158: 1189–94.

61. Berthold HK, Sudhop T, von Bergmann K. Effect of a garlic oil preparation on serum lipoproteins and cholesterol metabolism. *JAMA* 1998; 279: 1900–2.

62. Lawson L. Garlic oil for hypercholesterolemia–negative results. *Quart Rev Natural Med* Fall 1998; 185–86.

63. Lawson LD. Garlic powder for hyperlipidemia–analysis of recent negative results. *Quart Rev Natural Med* Fall, 1998; 187–89.

64. Lawson LD, Ransom DK, Hughes BG. Inhibition of whole blood platelet-aggregation by compounds in garlic clove extracts and commercial garlic products. *Thrombosis Res* 1992; 65: 141–56.

65. Mansell P, Reckless JPD. Garlic—effects on serum lipids, blood pressure, coagulation, platelet aggregation, and vasodilatation. *BMJ* 1991; 303: 379–80 [editorial].

66. Jenkins DJA, Khan A, Kenkins AL, et al. Effect of nibbling versus gorging on cardiovascular risk factors: serum uric acid and blood lipids. *Metabolism* 1995; 44: 549–55.

67. Edelstein SL, Barrett-Connor EL, Wingard DL, Cohn BA. Increased meal frequency associated with decreased cholesterol concentrations; Rancho Bernardo, CA, 1984–1987. *Am J Clin Nutr* 1992; 55: 664–69.

68. Reaven PD, McPhillips JB, Barrett-Connor EL, Criqui MH. Leisure time exercise and lipid and lipoprotein levels in an older population. *J Am Geriatr Soc* 1990; 38: 847–54.

69. Duncan JJ, Gordon NF, Scott CB. Women walking for health and fitness—how much is enough? *JAMA* 1991; 266: 3295–99.

70. Pekkanen J, Marti B, Nissinen A, Tuomilehto J. Reduction of premature mortality by high physical activity: a 20-year follow-up of middle-aged Finnish men. *Lancet* 1987; 1: 1473–77.

71. Willich SN, Lewis M, Lowel H, et al. Physical exertion as a trigger of acute myocardial infarction. *N Engl J Med* 1993; 329: 1684–90.

72. Hubert HB, Feinleib M, McNamara PM, Castelli WP. Obesity as an independent risk factor for cardiovascular disease: a 26-year follow-up of participants in the Framingham

Heart Study. *Circulation* 1983; 67: 968–77.

73. Glueck CJ, Taylor HL, Jacobs D, et al. Plasma high-density lipoprotein cholesterol: association with measurements of body mass: the Lipid Research Clinics Program Prevalence Study. *Circulation* 1980; 62(suppl IV): IV-62–69.

74. Wood PD, Stefanick ML, Dreon DM, et al. Changes in plasma lipids and lipoproteins in overweight men during weight loss through dieting as compared with exercise. *N Engl J Med* 1988; 319: 1173–79.

75. Dwyer JH, Rieger-Ndakorerwa GE, Semmer NK, et al. Low-level cigarette smoking and longitudinal change in serum cholesterol among adolescents. *JAMA* 1988; 2857–62.

76. Khosla S, Laddu A, Ehrenpreis S, Somberg JC. Cardiovascular effects of nicotine: relation to deleterious effects of cigarette smoking. *Am Heart J* 1994; 127: 1669–71 [editorial/review].

77. Nyboe J, Jensen G, Appleyard M, Schnohr P. Smoking and the risk of first acute myocardial infarction. *Am Heart J* 1991; 122: 438.

78. Kawachi I, Sparrow D, Spiro II A, et al. A prospective study of anger and coronary heart disease. *Circulation* 1996; 94: 2090–95.

79. Jiang W, Babyak M, Krantz DS, et al. Mental stress-induced myocardial ischemia and cardiac events. *JAMA* 1996; 275: 1651–56.

80. Bower B. Women take untype A behavior to heart. *Sci News* 1993; 144: 244.

81. A perspective on type A behavior and coronary disease. *N Engl J Med* 1988; 318: 110–12 [editorial/review].

82. McCann BS, Warnick R, Knopp RH. Changes in plasma lipids and dietary intake accompanying shifts in perceived workload and stress. *Psychosomatic Med* 1990; 52: 97–108.

83. Lundberg U, Hedman M, Melin B, Frankenhaeuser M. Type A Behavior in healthy males and females as related to physiological reactivity

and blood lipids. *Psychosomatic Med* 1989; 51: 113–22.

84. Friedman M, Theresen CE, Gill JJ, et al. Alteration of type A behavior and reduction in cardiac recurrences in postmyocardial infarction patients. *Am Heart J* 1984; 108: 237–48.

High Cholesterol (Hypercholesterolemia): Dietary Supplements and Herbs

1. Brown WV. Niacin for lipid disorders. *Postgrad Med* 1995; 98: 185–93.

2. Head KA. Inositol hexaniacinate: A safer alternative to niacin. *Alt Med Rev* 1996; 1: 176–84 [review].

3. Murray M. Lipid-lowering drugs vs. Inositol hexaniacinate. *Am J Natural Med* 1995; 2: 9–12 [review].

4. Dorner Von G, Fisher FW. Zur Beinflussung der Serumlipide und lipoproteine durch den Hexanicotinsaureester des m-Inositol. *Arzneimittel Forschung* 1961; 11: 110–13.

5. Cloarec MJ, Perdriset GM, Lamberdiere FA, et al., Alpha-tocopherol: effect on plasma lipoproteins in hypercholesterolemic patients. *Isr J Med Sci* 1987; 23: 869–72.

6. Kesaniemi YA, Grundy SM. Lack of effect of tocopherol on plasma lipids and lipoproteins in man. *Am J Clin Nutr* 1982; 36: 224–28.

7. Belcher JD, Balla J, Balla G, et al. Vitamin E, LDL, and endothelium: Brief oral vitamin supplementation prevents oxidized LDL-mediated vascular injury in vitro. *Arterioscler Thromb* 1993; 13: 1779–89.

8. Stampfer MJ, Hennekens CH, Manson JE, et al. Vitamin E consumption and the risk of coronary disease in women. *N Engl J Med* 1993; 328: 1444–49.

9. Rimm EB, Stampfer MJ, Ascherio A, et al. Vitamin E consumption and the risk of coronary heart disease in men. *N Engl J Med* 1993; 328: 1450–56.

10. Stephens NG, Parsons A, Schofield PM, et al. Randomised controlled trial of vitamin E in patients with coronary disease: Cambridge

Heart Antioxidant Study (CHAOS). *Lancet* 1996; 347: 781–86.

11. Frei B. Ascorbic acid protects lipids in human plasma and low-density lipoprotein against oxidative damage. *Am J Clin Nutr* 1991; 54: 1113S–8S.

12. Simon JA. Vitamin C and cardiovascular disease: a review. *J Am Coll Nutr* 1992; 11: 107–27.

13. Gatto LM, Hallen GK, Brown AJ, Samman S. Ascorbic acid induces a favorable lipoprotein profile in women. *J Am Coll Nutr* 1996; 15; 154–58.

14. Balz F. Antioxidant Vitamins and Heart Disease. Presented at the 60th Annual Biology Colloquium, Oregon State University, Corvallis, OR, February 25, 1999.

14. Galeone F, Scalabrino A, Giuntoli F, et al. The lipid-lowering effect of pantethine in hyperlipidemic patients: a clinical investigation. *Curr Ther Res* 1983; 34: 383–90.

15. Miccoli R, Marchetti P, Sampietro T, et al. Effects of pantethine on lipids and apolipoproteins in hypercholesterolemic diabetic and non diabetic patients. *Curr Ther Res* 1984; 36: 545–49.

16. Avogaro P, Bon B, Fusello M. Effect of pantethine on lipids, lipoproteins and apolipoproteins in man. *Curr Ther Res* 1983; 33; 488–93.

17. Ubbink JB, Hayward WJ, van der Merwe A, et al. Vitamin requirements for the treatment of hyperhomocysteinemia in humans. *J Nutr* 1994; 124: 1927–33.

18. Heinecke JW, Rosen H, Suzuki LA, Chait A. The role of sulfur-containing amino acids in superoxide production and modification of low density lipoprotein by arterial smooth muscle cells. *Biol Chem* 1987; 262: 10098–103.

19. Ronzio RA. Antioxidants, nutraceuticals and functional foods. *Townsend Letter for Doctors & Patients* 1996; Oct: 34–35 [review].

20. Hertog MGL, Feskens EJM, Hollman PCH, et al. Dietary antioxidant flavonoids and risk of coronary heart disease: the Zutphen Elderly Study. *Lancet* 1993; 342: 1007–11.

21. Hertog MGL, Kromhout D, Aravanis C, et al. Flavonoid intake and long-term risk of coronary heart disease and cancer in the Seven Countries Study. *Arch Intern Med* 1995; 155: 381–86.

22. Knekt P, Jarvinen R, Reunanen A, Maatela J. Flavonoid intake and coronary mortality in Finland: a cohort study. *BMJ* 1996; 312: 478–81.

23. Rimm EB, Katan MB, Aschario A, et al. Relation between intake of flavonoids and risk for coronary heart disease in male health professionals. *Ann Intern Med* 1996; 125: 384–89.

24. Riales R, Albrink MJ. Effect of chromium chloride supplementation on glucose tolerance and serum lipids including high-density lipoprotein of adult men. *Am J Clin Nutr* 1981; 34: 2670–78.

25. Press RI, Geller J, Evans GW. The effect of chromium picolinate on serum cholesterol and apolipoprotein fractions in human subjects. *West J Med* 1990; 152: 41–45.

26. Roeback JR, Hla KM, Chambless LE, Fletcher RH. Effects of chromium supplementation on serum high-density lipoprotein cholesterol levels in men taking beta-blockers. *Ann Intern Med* 1991; 115: 917–24.

27. Wang MM, Fox EA, Stoecker BJ, et al. Serum cholesterol of adults supplemented with brewer's yeast or chromium chloride. *Nutr Res* 1989; 9: 989–98.

28. Newman HAI, Leighton RF, Lanese RR, Freedland NA. Serum chromium and angiographically determined coronary artery disease. *Clin Chem* 1978; 541–44.

29. Yacowitz H, Fleischman AI, Bierenbaum ML. Effects of oral calcium upon serum lipids in man. *Br Med J* 1965; 1: 1352–54.

30. Bell L, Halstenson CE, Halstenson CJ, et al. Cholesterol-lowering effects of calcium carbonate in patients with mild to moderate hypercholesterolemia. *Arch Intern Med* 1992; 152: 2441–44.

31. Denke MA, Fox MM, Schulte MC. Short-term dietary calcium fortification increases fecal saturated fat content and reduces serum lipids in men. *J Nutr* 1993; 123: 1047–53.

32. Davis WH, Leary WP, Reyes AJ, Olhaberry JV. Monotherapy with magnesium increases abnormally low high density lipoprotein cholesterol: a clinical assay. *Curr Ther Res* 1984; 36: 341–46.

34. Nozue T, Kobayashi A, Uemasu F, et al. Magnesium status, serum HDL cholesterol, and apolipoprotein A-1 levels. *J Pediatr Gastroenterol Nutr* 1995; 20: 316–18.

35. Baxter GF, Sumeray MS, Walker JM. Infarct size and magnesium: insights into LIMIT-2 and ISIS-4 from experimental studies. *Lancet* 1996; 348: 1424–26.

36. Galloe A, Rasmussen HS, Jorgensen LN, et al. Influence of oral magnesium supplementation on cardiac events among survivors of an acute myocardial infarction. *BMJ* 1993; 307: 585–87.

37. Pola P, Savi L, Grilli M, et al. Carnitine in the therapy of dyslipidemic patients. *Curr Ther Res* 1980; 27: 208–16.

38. Maebashi M, Kawamura N, Sato M, et al. Lipid-lowering effect of carnitine in patients with type-IV hyperlipoproteinaemia. *Lancet* 1978; ii: 805–7.

39. Rossi CS, Siliprandi N. Effect of carnitine on serum HDL-cholesterol: report of two cases. *Johns Hopkins Med J* 1982; 150: 51–54.

40. Pola P, Savi L, Grilli M, et al. Carnitine in the therapy of dyslipidemic patients. *Curr Ther Res* 1980; 27: 208–16.

41. Davini P et al. Controlled study on L-carnitine therapeutic efficacy in post-infarction. *Drugs Exptl Clin Res* 1992; 18: 355–65.

42. Carrol KK, Kurowska EM. Soy consumption and cholesterol reduction: Review of animal and human studies. *J Nutr* 1995; 125: 594S–97.

43. Lees AM, Mok HYI, Lee RS, et al. Plant sterols as cholesterol-lowering agents: Clinical trials in patients with hypercholesterolemia and studies of sterol balance. *Atheroscler* 1977; 28: 325–38.

44. Pelletier X, Belbraouet S, Mirabel D, et al. A diet moderately enriched in phytosterols lowers plasma cholesterol concentrations in normocholesterolemic humans. *Ann Nutr Metab* 1995; 39: 291–95.

45. Grundy SM, Ahrens EH Jr, Davignon J. The interaction of cholesterol absorption and cholesterol synthesis in man. *J Lipid Res* 1969; 10: 304–15 [review].

46. Hendriks HFJ, Westrate JA, van Vliet T, Meijer GW. Spreads enriched with three different levels of vegetable oil sterols and the degree of cholesterol lowering in normocholesterolaemic and mildly hypercholesterolaemic subjects. *Eur J Clin Nutr* 1999; 53: 319–27.

47. Izuka K, Murata K, Nakazawa K, et al. Effects of chondroitin sulfates on serum lipids and hexosamines in atherosclerotic patients: With special reference to thrombus formation time. *Jpn Heart J* 1968; 9: 453–60.

48. Nakazawa K, Murata K. Comparative study of the effects of chondroitin sulfate isomers on atherosclerotic subjects. *ZFA* 1979; 34: 153–59.

49. Morrison LM, Enrick NL. Coronary heart disease: reduction of death rate by chondroitin sulfate A. *Angiology* 1973; 24: 269–87.

50. Pons P Rodríquez M, Más R, et al. One-year efficacy and safety of policosanol in patients with type II hypercholesterolemia. *Curr Ther Res* 1994; 55: 1084–92.

51. Aneiros E, Calderson B, Más R, et al. Effect of successive dose increases of policosanol on the lipid profile and tolerability of treatment. *Curr Ther Res* 1993; 54: 304–12.

52. Castano G, Canetti M, Moreira M, et al. Efficacy and tolerability of policosanol in elderly patients with type II hypercholesterolemia: A 12-month study. *Curr Ther Res* 1995; 56: 819–23.

53. Castano G, Tula L, Canetti M, et al. Effects of policosanol in hypertensive patients with type II hypercholesterolemia. *Curr Ther Res* 1996; 57: 691–95.

Part One: References

Part One: References

54. Menendez R, Arruzazabala L, Mas R, et al. Cholesterol-lowering effect of policosanol on rabbits with hypercholesterolaemia induced by a wheat starch-casein diet. *Br J Nutr* 1997; 77: 923–32.

55. Childs MT, Bowlin JA, Ogilvie JT, et al. The contrasting effects of a dietary soya lecithin product and corn oil on lipoprotein lipids in normolipidemic and familial hypercholesterolemic subjects. *Atherosclerosis* 1981; 38: 217–28.

56. Knuiman JT, Beynen AC, Katan MB. Lecithin intake and serum cholesterol. *Am J Clin Nutr* 1989; 49: 266–68.

57. Wilson TA, Meservey CM, Nicolosi RJ. Soy lecithin reduces plasma lipoprotein cholesterol and early atherogenesis in hypercholesterolemic monkeys and hamsters: beyond linoleate. *Atherosclerosis* 1998; 140: 147–53.

58. Koide SS. Chitin-chitosan: properties, benefits and risks. *Nutr Res* 1998; 18: 1091–101 [review].

59. Maezaki Y, Tsuji K, Nakagawa Y, et al. Hypocholesterolemic effect of chitosan in adult males. *Biosci Biotech Biochem* 1993; 57: 1439–44.

60. Abou-Hozaifa BM, Badr El-Din NK. Royal jelly, a possible agent to reduce the nicotine-induced atherogenic lipoprotein profile. *Saudi Med J* 1995; 16: 337–42.

61. Abou-Hozaifa BM, Roston AAH, El-Nokaly FA. Effects of royal jelly and honey on serum lipids and lipoprotein cholesterol in rats fed cholesterol-enriched diet. *J Biomed Sci Ther* 1993; 9: 35–44.

62. Cho YT. Studies on royal jelly and abnormal cholesterol and triglycerides. *Am Bee J* 1977; 117: 36–39.

63. Liusov VA, Zimin IU. Experimental rational and trial of therapeutic use of bee raising product in cardiovascular diseases. *Kardiologia* 1983; 23: 105–9 [in Russian].

64. Vittek J. Effect of royal jelly on serum lipids in experimental animals and humans with atherosclerosis. *Experientia* 1995; 51: 927–35.

65. Silagy C, Neil A. Garlic as a lipid-lowering agent—a meta-analysis. *J R Coll Physicians London* 1994; 28: 39–45.

66. Holzgartner J, Schmidt U, Kuhn U. Comparison of the efficacy of a garlic preparation vs. bezafibrate. *Arzneim-Forsch Drug Res* 1992; 42: 1473–77.

67. McCrindle BW, Helden E, Conner WT. Garlic extract therapy in children with hypercholesterolemia. *Arch Pediatr Adolesc Med* 1998; 152: 1089–94.

68. Isaacsohn JL, Moser M, Stein EA, et al. Garlic powder and plasma lipids and lipoproteins. *Arch Intern Med* 1998; 158: 1189–94.

69. Lawson L. Garlic oil for hypercholesterolemia—negative results. *Quart Rev Natural Med* Fall 1998; 185–86.

70. Garlic powder for hyperlipidemia—analysis of recent negative results. *Quart Rev Natural Med* Fall, 1998; 187–89.

71. Berthold HK, Sudhop T, von Bergmann K. Effect of a garlic oil preparation on serum lipoproteins and cholesterol metabolism. *JAMA* 1998; 279: 1900–2.

72. Silagy C, Neil A. Garlic as a lipid-lowering agent—a meta-analysis. *J R Coll Physicians London* 1994; 28: 39–45.

73. Silagy C, Neil A. Garlic as a lipid-lowering agent—a meta-analysis. *J R College Phys London* 1994; 28: 39–45.

74. Agarwal RC, Singh SP, Saran RK, et al. Clinical trial of gugulipid new hypolipidemic agent of plant origin in primary hyperlipidemia. *Indian J Med Res* 1986; 84: 626–34.

75. Nityanand S, Srivastava JS, Asthana OP. Clinical trials with Gugulipid—A new hypolipidemic agent. *J Assoc Phys India* 1989; 37: 323–28.

76. Foster S, Chongxi Y. *Herbal Emissaries*. Rochester, VT: Healing Arts Press, 1992, 79–85.

77. Foster S. *Herbal Renaissance*. Layton, Utah: Gibbs Smith, 1993, 40–41.

78. Araghiniknam M, Chung S, Nelson-White T, et al. Antioxidant activity of dioscorea and dehydroepiandrosterone (DHEA) in older humans. *Life Sci* 1996; 11: 147–57.

79. Olson BH, Anderson SM, Becker MP, et al. Psyllium-enriched cereals lower blood total cholesterol and LDL cholesterol, but not HDL cholesterol, in hypercholesterolemic adults: Results of a meta-analysis. *J Nutr* 1997; 127: 1973–80.

80. Fintelmann V. Antidyspeptic and lipid-lowering effect of artichoke leaf extract. *Zeitschirfit fur Allgemeinmed* 1996; 72: 1–19.

81. Heckers H, Dittmar K, Schmahl FW, Huth K. Inefficiency of cynarin as therapeutic regimen in familial type II hyperlipoproteinemia. *Atherosclerosis* 1977; 26: 249–53.

High Homocysteine

1. Stampfer MJ, Malinow R, Willett WC, et al. A prospective study of plasma homocysteine and risk of myocardial infarction in U.S. physicians. *JAMA* 1992; 268: 877–81.

2. Folsom AR, Nieto J, McGovern PG, et al. Prospective study of coronary heart disease incidence in relation to fasting total homocysteine, related genetic polymorphisms, and B vitamins. *Circulation* 1998; 98: 204–10.

3. Kuller LH, Evans RW. Homocysteine, vitamins, and cardiovascular disease. *Circulation* 1998; 98: 196–99 [editorial].

4. Perry IJ, Refsum H, Morris RW, et al. Prospective study of serum total homocysteine concentration and risk of stroke in middle-aged British men. *Lancet* 1995; 346: 1395–98.

5. Brattstrom LE, Hultberg BL, Hardebo JE. Folic acid responsive postmenopausal homocysteinemia. *Metabolism* 1985; 34: 1073–77.

6. Cattaneo M, Vecchi M, Zighetti ML, et al. High prevalence of hyperhomocysteinemia in patients with inflammatory bowel disease: a pathogenic link with thromboembolic complications? *Thromb Haemost* 1998; 80: 542–45.

7. Clarke R, Smith D, Jobst KA, et al. Folate, vitamin B_{12}, and serum total homocysteine levels in confirmed Alzheimer disease. *Arch Neruol* 1998; 55: 1449–55.

8. Nygård O, Refsum H, Ueland PM, Vollset SE. Major lifestyle determinants of plasma tota homocysteine distribution: the Hordaland Homocysteine Study. *Am J Clin Nutr* 1998; 67: 263–70.

9. Boers GHJ, Smals AGH, Trijbels FJM, et al. Heterozygosity for homocystinuria in premature peripheral and cerebral occlusive arterial disease. *N Engl J Med* 1985; 313: 709–15.

10. Glueck CJ, Shaw P, Land JE, et al. Evidence that homocysteine is an independent risk factor for atherosclerosis in hyperlipidemic patients. *Am J Cardiol* 1995; 75: 132–36.

11. Ubbink JB, Vermaak WJH, van der Merwe A, Becker PJ. Vitamin B$_{12}$, vitamin B$_6$, and folate nutritional status in men with hyperhomocysteinemia. *Am J Clin Nutr* 1993; 57: 47–53.

12. Ubbink JB, Vermaak WJH, ven der Merwe A, et al. Vitamin requirements for the treatment of hyperhomocysteinemia in humans. *J Nutr* 1994; 124: 1927–33.

13. Wilcken DEL, Wilcken B, Dudman NPB, Tyrrell PA. Homocystinuria—the effects of betaine in the treatment of patients not responsive to pyridoxine. *N Engl J Med* 1983; 309: 448–53.

14. Jancin B. Amino acid defect causes 20% of atherosclerosis in CHD. *Family Pract News* 1994; Oct 15: 7.

High Triglycerides (Hypertriglyceridemia)

1. Steinberg D, Pearson TA, Kuller LH. Alcohol and atherosclerosis. *Ann Intern Med* 1991; 114: 967–76.

2. Reiser S. Effect of dietary sugars on metabolic risk factors associated with heart disease. *Nutr Health* 1985; 3: 203–16.

3. Szanto S, Yudkin J. The effect of dietary sucrose on blood lipids serum insulin, platelet adhesiveness and body weight in human volunteers. *J Postgrad Med* 1969; 45: 602–7.

4. Anderson JW, Gustafson NJ. High-carbohydrate, high-fiber diet. *Postgrad Med* 1987; 82: 40–55 [review].

5. Glore SR, van Treeck D, Knehans AW, Guild M. Soluble fiber and serum lipids: a literature review. *J Am Dietet Assoc* 1994; 94: 425–36.

6. Cominacini L, Zocca I, Garbin U, et al. Long-term effect of a low-fat, high carbohydrate diet on plasma lipids of patients affected by familial endogenous hypertriglyceridemia. *Am J Clin Nutr* 1988; 48: 57–65.

7. West C, Sullivan DR, Katan MB, et al. Boys from populations with high-carbohydrate intake have higher fasting triglyceride levels than boys from populations with high-fat intake. *Am J Epidemiol* 1990; 131: 271–82.

8. Ullmann D, Connor WE, Hatcher LF, et al. Will a high-carbohydrate, low-fat diet lower plasma lipids and lipoproteins without producing hypertriglyceridemia? *Arterioscler Thromb* 1991; 11: 1059–67.

9. Consensus Development Panel. Treatment of hypertriglyceridemia. *JAMA* 1984; 251: 1196–200.

10. Burr ML, et al. Effects of changes in fat, fish, and fibre intakes on death and myocardial reinfarction: diet and reinfarction trial (DART). *Lancet* 1989; ii: 757–61.

11. Kromhout D et al. The inverse relation between fish consumption and 20-year mortality from coronary heart disease. *New Engl J Med* 1985; 312(19): 1205.

12. Ascherio A, Rimm EB, Stampfer MJ, et al. Dietary intake of marine n-3 fatty acids, fish intake, and the risk of coronary disease among men. *N Engl J Med* 1995; 332: 977–82.

13. Merril JR et al. Hyperlipemic response of young trained and untrained men after a high fat meal. *Arteriosclerosis* 1989; 9: 217–23.

14. Cowan LD, Wilcosky T, Criqui MH, et al. Demographic, behavioral, biochemical, and dietary correlates of plasma triglycerides. *Arteriosclerosis* 1985; 5: 466–80.

15. Despres J-P, Tremblay A, Leblanc C, Bouchard C. Effect of the amount of body fat on the age-associated increase in serum cholesterol. *Prev Med* 1988; 17: 423–31.

16. Prichard BN, Smith CCT, Ling KLE, Betteridge DJ. Fish oils and cardiovascular disease. *BMJ* 1995; 310: 819–20 [editorial/review].

17. Von Schacky C, Fischer S, Weber PC. Long-term effects of dietary marine omega-3 fatty acids upon plasma and cellular lipids, platelet function, and eicosanoid formation in humans. *J Clin Invest* 1985; 76(4): 626.

18. Leaf A, Weber PC. Cardiovascular effects of n-3 fatty acids. *N Engl J Med* 1988; 318(9): 549–57.

19. Adler AJ, Holub BJ. Effect of garlic and fish-oil supplementation on serum lipid and lipoprotein concentrations in hypercholesterolemic men. *Am J Clin Nutr* 1997; 65: 445–50.

20. Haglund O et al. The effects of fish oil on triglycerides, cholesterol, fibrinogen and malondialdehyde in humans supplemented with vitamin E. *J Nutr* 1991; 121: 165–69.

21. Pola P et al. Carnitine in the therapy of dyslipidemic patients. *Curr Ther Res* 1980; 27(2): 208.

22. Abdi-Aziz MT et al. Effect of carnitine on blood lipid pattern in diabetic patients. *Nutr Rep Int* 1984; 29(5): 1071.

23. Arsenio L et al. Effectiveness of long-term treatment with pantethine in patients with dyslipidemia. *Clin Ther* 1986; 8(5): 537–45.

24. Avogaro P et al. Effect of pantethine on lipids, lipoproteins and apolipoproteins in man. *Curr Ther Res* 1983; 33(3): 488–93.

25. Maggi GC et al. Pantethine: a physiological lipomodulating agent, in the treatment of hyperlipidemias. *Curr Ther Res* 1982; 32(3): 380–86.

26. Brown WV. Niacin for lipid disorders. *Postgrad Med* 1995; 98: 183–93 [review].

27. Head KA. Inositol hexaniacinate: a safer alternative to niacin. *Alt Med Rev* 1996; 1: 176–84 [review].

28. Murray M. Lipid-lowering drugs vs. Inositol hexaniacinate. *Am J Natural Med* 1995; 9–12 [review].

29. Silagy C, Neil A. Garlic as a lipid-lowering agent: A meta-analysis. *J Royal Coll Physicians London* 1994; 28: 39–45.

Part One: References

30. Holzgartner J, Schmidt U, Kuhn U. Comparison of the efficacy of a garlic preparation vs. bezafibrate. *Arzneim-Forsch Drug Res* 1992; 42: 1473–77.

31. Agarwal RC, Singh SP, Saran RK, et al. Clinical trial of gugulipid new hypolipidemic agent of plant origin in primary hyperlipidemia. *Indian J Med Res* 1986; 84: 626–34.

32. Araghiniknam M, Chung S, Nelson-White T, et al. Antioxidant activity of dioscorea and dehydroepiandrosterone (DHEA) in older humans. *Life Sci* 1996; 11: 147–57.

HIV Support

1. Ince S. Vitamin supplements may help delay onset of AIDS. *Med Tribune* 1993; November 9: 18.

2. Semba RD et al. Increased mortality associated with vitamin A deficiency during human immunodeficiency virus type 1 infection. *Arch Intern Med* 1993; 153: 2149–54.

3. Semba RD et al. Maternal vitamin A deficiency and mother-to-child transmission of HIV-1. *Lancet* 1994; 343: 1593–97.

4. Humphrey JH, Quinn T, Fine D, et al. Short-term effects of large-dose vitamin A supplementation on viral load and immune response in HIV-infected women. *J Acquired Immune Deficiency Syndromes Human Retrovirol* 1999; 20: 44–51.

5. Sappey C et al. Vitamin, trace element and peroxide status in HIV seropositive patients: asymptomatic patients present a severe beta-carotene deficiency. *Clin Chem Acta* 1994; 230: 35–42.

6. Coodley GO et al. Beta-carotene in HIV infection. *J Acquired Immune Deficiency Syndromes* 1993; 6: 272–76.

7. Coodley GO et al. Beta-carotene in HIV infection: an extended evaluation. *AIDS* 1996; 10: 967–73.

8. Butterworth RF et al. Thiamine deficiency in AIDS. *Lancet* 1991; 338: 1086.

9. Baum MK et al. Association of vitamin B$_6$ status with parameters of immune function in early HIV-1 infec-tion. *J Acquired Immunodeficiency Syndromes* 1991; 4: 1122–32.

10. Boudes P et al. Folate, vitamin B$_{12}$, and HIV infection. *Lancet* 1990; 335: 1401–2.

11. Harakeh S et al. Suppression of human immunodeficiency virus replication by ascorbate in chronically and acutely infected cells. *Proc Natl Acad Sci* 1990; 87: 7245–49.

12. Cathcart RF III. Vitamin C in the treatment of acquired immune deficiency syndrome (AIDS). *Med Hypotheses* 1984; 14: 423–33.

13. Gogu SR et al. Increased therapeutic efficacy of zidovudine in combination with vitamin E. *Biochem Biophys Res Commun* 1989; 165: 401–7.

14. Folkers K et al. Biochemical deficiencies of coenzyme Q$_{10}$ in HIV-infection and exploratory treatment. *Biochem Biophys Res Commun* 1988; 153: 888–96.

15. Fabris N et al. AIDS, zinc deficiency, and thymic hormone failure. *JAMA* 1988; 259: 839–40.

16. Dworkin BM. Selenium deficiency in HIV infection and the acquired immunodeficiency syndrome (AIDS). *Chem Biol Interact* 1994; 91: 181–86.

17. Castaldo A et al. Iron deficiency and intestinal malabsorption in HIV disease. *J Pediatr Gastroenterol Nutr* 1996; 22: 359–63.

18. Mocchegiani E et al. Benefit of oral zinc supplementation as an adjunct to zidovudine (AZT) therapy against opportunistic infections in AIDS. *Int J Immunopharmacol* 1995; 17: 719–27.

19. Schrauzer GN, Sacher J. Selenium in the maintenance and therapy of HIV-infected patients. *Chem Biol Interact* 1994; 91: 199–205.

20. Roederer M et al. Cytokine-stimulated human immunodeficiency virus replication is inhibited by N-acetyl-L-cysteine. *Proc Natl Acad Sci* 1990; 87: 4884–88.

21. Robinson MK et al. Glutathione deficiency and HIV infection. *Lancet* 1992; 339: 1603–4.

22. Blehaut H, Saint-Marc T, Touraine J. Double blind trial of *Saccharomyces boulardii* in AIDS-related diarrhea. International Conference on AIDS/Third STD World Congress, 1992, Abstract #2120, July 19–24.

23. Durant J, Chantre PH, Gonzalez G, et al. Efficacy and safety of Buxus sempervirens L. preparations (SPV30) in HIV-infected asymptomatic patients: a multicentre, randomized, double-blind, placebo-controlled trial. *Phytomedicine* 1998; 5(1): 1–10.

24. Abdullah TH et al. Enhancement of natural killer cell activity in AIDS with garlic. *Dtsch Zschr Onkol* 1989; 21: 52–53.

25. Ito M, Sato A, Hirabayashi K, et al. Mechanism of inhibitory effect of glycyrrhizin on replication of human immunodeficiency virus (HIV). *Antivir Res* 1988; 10: 289–98.

26. Hattori I, Ikematsu S, Koito A, et al. Preliminary evidence for inhibitory effect of glycyrrhizin on HIV replication in patients with AIDS. *Antivir Res* 1989; 11: 255–62.

27. Ikegami N et al. Prophylactic effect of long-term oral administration of glycyrrhizin on AIDS development of asymptomatic patients. *Int Conf AIDS* 1993; 9: 234 [abstract PO-A25-0596].

28. Yamada Y, Nanba H, Kuroda H. Antitumor effect of orally administered extracts from fruit body of *Grifola frondosa* (maitake). *Chemotherapy* 1990; 38: 790–96.

29. Nanba H. Immunostimulant activity in-vivo and anti-HIV activity in vitro of 3 branched b-1-6-glucans extracted from maitake mushrooms (*Grifola frondosa*). VIII International Conference on AIDS, 1992 [abstract].

30. Zhang QC. Preliminary report on the use of *Momordica charantia* extract by HIV patients. *J Naturopath Med* 1992; 3: 65–69.

31. Standish L, Guiltinan J, McMahon E, Lindstrom C. One year open trial of naturopathic treatment of HIV infection class IV-A men. *J Naturopathic Med* 1992; 3: 42–64.

High Blood Pressure (Hypertension)

1. P. LB, Damon A, Moellering RC Jr. Antecedents of cardiovascular disease in six Solomon Islands

Societies. *Circulation* 1974; 44: 1132–46.

2. Stamler J et al. Findings of the international cooperative INTER-SALT study. *Hypertension* 1991; 17(suppl I): I-9–15.

3. MacGregor GA et al. Double-blind study of three sodium intakes and long-term effects of sodium restriction in essential hypertension. *Lancet* 1989; ii: 1244–47.

4. Cutler JA, Follmann D, Allender PS. Randomized trials of sodium reduction: an overview. *Am J Clin Nutr* 1997; 65(suppl): 643S–51S.

5. Cutler JA, Follmann D, Allender PS. Randomized trials of sodium reduction: an overview. *Am J Clin Nutr* 1997; 65(suppl): 643S–51S.

6. Egan BM, Stepniakowski KT. Adverse effects of short-term, very-low-salt diets in subjects with risk-factor clustering. *Am J Clin Nutr* 1997; 65(suppl): 671S–77S.

7. Margetts BM et al. Vegetarian diet in mild hypertension: a randomised controlled trial. *BMJ* 1986; 293: 1468–71.

8. Cappuccio FP, MacGregor GA. Does potassium supplementation lower blood pressure? a meta-analysis of published trials. *J Hypertens* 1991; 9: 465–73.

9. Rossner S, Andersson I-L, Ryttig K. Effects of a dietary fibre-supplement to a weight reduction programme on blood pressure. *Acta Med Scand* 1988; 223: 353–57.

10. Appel LJ, Moore TJ, Boarzanek E, et al. A clinical trial of the effects of dietary patterns on blood pressure. *N Engl J Med* 1997; 336: 1117–24.

11. Svetkey LP, Simons-Morton D, Vollmer WM, et al. Effects of dietary patterns on blood pressure: a subgroup analysis of the Dietary Approaches to Stop Hypertension (DASH) randomized clinical trial. *Arch Intern Med* 1999; 159: 285–93.

12. Zein M, Areas JL, Breuss GH. Effects of excess sucrose ingestion on the lifespan of SHR. *J Am Coll Nutr* 1989; 8: 435 [abstr #42].

13. Rebello T, Hodges RE, Smith JL. Short-term effects of various sugars on antinatriuresis and blood pressure changes in normotensive young men. *Am J Clin Nutr* 1983; 38(1): 84–94.

14. Preuss HG, Fournier RD. Effects of sucrose ingestion on blood pressure. *Life Sci* 1982; 30: 879–86.

15. Rachima-Maoz C, Peleg E, Rosenthal T. The effect of caffeine on ambulatory blood pressure in hypertensive patients. *Am J Hypertens* 1998; 11: 1426–32.

16. Jee SH, He J, Whelton PK, et al. The effect of chronic coffee drinking on blood pressure. A meta-analysis of controlled clinical trials. *Hypertension* 1999; 33: 647–52.

17. Wakabayashi K, Kono S, Shinchi K, et al. Habitual coffee consumption and blood pressure: a study of self-defense officials in Japan. *Eur J Epidemiol* 1998; 14: 669–73.

18. Grant ECG. Food Allergies and migraine. *Lancet* 1979; i: 966–69.

19. Pirkle JL, Schwartz H, Landis JR, et al. The relationship between blood lead levels and blood pressure and its cardiovascular risk implications. *Am J Epidemiol* 1985; 121(2): 246–58.

20. Wu TN, Shen CY, Ko KN, et al. Occupational lead exposure and blood pressure. *Int J Epidemiol* 1996; 25: 791–96.

21. Narkiewicz K, Maraglino G, Biasion T, et al. Interactive effect of cigarettes and coffee on daytime systolic blood pressure in patients with mild essential hypertension. *J Hypertens* 1995; 13: 965–70.

22. Keil U, Liese A, Filipiak B, et al. Alcohol, blood pressure and hypertension. *Novartis Round Symp* 1998; 216: 125–44 [review].

23. Kukkonen K, Rauramaa R, Voutilainene E, Lansimies E. Physical training of middle-aged men with borderline hypertension. *Ann Clin Res* 1982; 14(suppl 34): 139–45.

24. Young DR, Appel LG, Jee SH, Miller ER III. The effect of aerobic exercise and T'ai Chi on blood pressure in older people: results of a randomized trial. *J Am Geriatr Soc* 1999; 47: 277–84.

25. Alderman MH. Nonpharmacologic approaches to the treatment of hypertension. *Lancet* 1994; 334: 307–11 [review].

26. Markovitz JH, Matthews KA, Kannel WB, et al. Psychological predictors of hypertension in the Framingham Study. Is there tension in hypertension? *JAMA* 1993; 270: 2439–43.

27. Schnall PL, Schwartz Landesbergis PA, et al. Relation between job strain, alcohol, and ambulatory blood pressure. *Hypertension* 1992; 19: 488–94.

28. Matthews KA, Cottington EM, Talbott E, et al. Stressful work conditions and diastolic blood pressure among blue collar factory workers. *Am J Epidemiol* 1987; 126: 280–91.

29. Pickering TG. Does psychological stress contribute to the development of hypertension and coronary heart disease? *Eur J Clin Pharmacol* 1990; 39(suppl 1): S1–S7.

30. Perini C, Müller FB, Bühler FR. Suppressed aggression accelerates early development of essential hypertension. *J Hypertens* 1991; 9: 499–503.

31. Eisenberg DM, Delbanco TL, Berkey CS, et al. Cognitive behavioral techniques for hypertension: are they effective? *Ann Intern Med* 1993; 118: 964–72.

32. Irvine MJ, Logan AG. Relaxation behavior therapy as sole treatment for mild hypertension. *Psychosomatic Med* 1991; 53: 587–97.

33. Johnston DW, Gold A, Kentish J, et al. Effect of stress management on blood pressure in mild primary hypertension. *BMJ* 1993; 306: 963–66.

34. Patel CH. Yoga and bio-feedback in the management of hypertension. *Lancet* 1973; ii: 1973–75.

35. Schneider RH, Staggers F, Alexander C, et al. A randomized controlled trial of stress reduction for hypertension in older African-Americans. *Hypertension* 1995; 26: 820–29.

36. Patel C, Marmot MG, Terry DJ, et al. Trial of relaxation in reducing coronary risk: four year follow up. *BMJ* 1985; 1104–6.

37. Griffith LE, Guyatt GH, Cook RJ, et al. The influence of dietary and nondietary calcium supplementation on blood pressure. An updated metaanalysis of randomized controlled trials. *Am J Hypertens* 1999; 12: 84–92.

38. Resnick LM. The role of dietary calcium in hypertension: a hierarchical review. *Am J Hypertens* 1999; 12: 99–112.

39. Motoyama T, Sano H, Fukuzaki H, et al. Oral magnesium supplementation in patients with essential hypertension. *Hypertension* 1989; 13: 227–32.

40. Patki PS, Singh J, Gokhale SV, et al. Efficacy of potassium and magnesium in essential hypertension: a double-blind, placebo controlled, crossover study. *BMJ* 1990; 301: 521–23.

41. Dyckner T, Wester PO. Effect of magnesium on blood pressure. *BMJ* 1983; 286: 1847–49.

42. Solzbach U, Hornig B, Jeserich M, Just H. Vitamin C improves endothelial dysfunction of epicardial coronary arteries in hypertensive patients. *Circulation* 1997; 96: 1513–19.

43. Ness AR, Chee D, Elliott P. Vitamin C and blood pressure—an overview. *J Human Hypertens* 1997; 11: 343–50.

44. Digiesi V, Cantini F, Bisi G, et al. Mechanism of action of coenzyme Q_{10} in essential hypertension. *Curr Ther Res* 1992; 51: 668–72.

45. Folkers K, Drzewoski J, Richardson PC, et al. Bioenergetics in clinical medicine. XVI. Reduction of hypertension in patients by therapy with coenzyme Q_{10}. *Res Commun Chem Pathol Pharmacol* 1981; 31: 129–40.

46. Langsjoen P, Langsjoen P, Willis R, Folkers K. Treatment of essential hypertension with coenzyme Q_{10}. *Mol Aspects Med* 1994; 15(suppl): S265–72.

47. Digiesi V, Cantini F, Oradei A, et al. Coenzyme Q_{10} in essential hypertension. *Molec Aspects Med* 1994; 15(suppl): S257–63.

48. Digiesi V, Cantini F, Brodbeck B. Effect of coenzyme Q_{10} on essential arterial hypertension. *Curr Ther Res* 1990; 47: 841–45.

49. Morris MC, Sacks F, Rosner B. Does fish oil lower blood pressure? A meta-analysis of controlled trials. *Circulation* 1993; 88: 523–33.

50. Kohashi N, Katori R. Decrease of urinary taurine in essential hypertension. *Jpn Heart J* 1983; 24: 91–102.

51. Abe M, Shibata K, Matsuda T, Furukawa T. Inhibition of hypertension and salt intake by oral taurine treatment in hypertensive rats. *Hypertension* 1987; 10: 383–89.

52. Fujita T, Ando K, Noda H, et al. Effects of increased adrenomedullary activity and taurine in young patients with borderline hypertension. *Circulation* 1987; 75: 525–32.

53. Kato H, Taguchi T, Okuda H, et al. Antihypertensive effect of chitosan in rats and humans. *J Trad Medicine* 1994; 11: 198–205.

54. Calver A, Collier J, Vallance P. Dilator actions of arginine in human peripheral vasculature. *Clin Sci* 1991; 81: 695–700.

55. Pezza V, Bernadini F, Pezza E, et al. Study of supplemental oral l-arginine in hypertensives treated with enalapril + hydrochlorothiazinde. *Am J Hypertens* 1998; 11: 1267–70 [letter].

56. Silagy C, Neil AW. A meta-analysis of the effect of garlic on blood pressure. *J Hypertension* 1994; 12: 463–68.

Hypoglycemia

1. Palardy J, Havrankova J, Lep. R, et al. Blood glucose measurements during symptomatic episodes in patients with suspected postprandial hypoglycemia. *N Engl J Med* 1989; 321: 1421–25.

2. Kwentus, JA, Achilles JT, Goyer PF. Hypoglycemia etiologic and psychosomatic aspects of diagnosis. *Postgrad Med* 1982; 71(6): 99–104.

3. Johnson DD, Dorr KE, Swenson WM, Service J. Reactive hypoglycemia. *JAMA* 1980; 243: 1151–55.

4. Yager J, Young RT. A non-editorial on non-hypoglycemia. *N Engl J Med* 1974; 291: 905–8.

5. Chalew, SA, McLaughlin JV, Mersey JH, et al. The use of the plasma epinephrine response in the diagnosis of idiopathic postprandial syndrome. *JAMA* 1984; 251(5): 612–15.

6. Sanders LR, Hofeldt FD, Kirk MC, Levin J. Refined carbohydrate as a contributing factor in reactive hypoglycemia. *Southern Med J* 1982; 75(9): 1072–75.

7. Permutt MA. Postprandial hypoglycemia. *Diabetes* 1976; 25: 719–33.

8. O'Keefe SJD, Marks V. Lunchtime gin and tonic as a cause of reactive hypoglycemia. *Lancet* 1977; i: 1286–88.

9. Hofeldt FD. Reactive hypoglycemia. *Metabol* 1975; 24(10): 1193–208.

10. Rippere V. A little something between meals: masked addiction not low blood blood-sugar. *Lancet* 1979; (June 23): 1349 [letter].

11. Anderson JW, Herman RH. Effects of carbohydrate restriction on glucose tolerance of normal men and reactive hypoglycemic patients. *Am J Clin Nutr* 1975; 28: 748.

12. Ullrich IH, Peters PJ, Albrink JA. Effect of low-carbohydrate diets high in either fat or protein on thyroid function, plasma insulin, glucose, and triglycerides in healthy young adults. *J Am Coll Nutr* 1985; 4: 451.

13. Anderson RA et al. Chromium supplementation of humans with hypoglycemia. *Fed Proc* 1984; 43: 471.

14. Stebbing JB et al. Reactive hypoglycemia and magnesium. *Mag Bull* 1982; 2: 131–34.

15. Shansky A. Vitamin B_3 in the alleviation of hypoglycemia. *Drug Cosm Ind* 1981; 129(4): 68–69, 104–5.

16. Gaby AR, Wright JV. Nutritional regulation of blood glucose. *J Advancement Med* 1991; 4(1): 57–71.

Hypothyroidism

1. Paynter OE, Burin GJ, Jaeger RB, Gregorio CA. Goitrogens and thyroid follicular cell neoplasia: evidence for a threshold process. *Regul Toxicol Pharmacol* 1988; 8: 102–19 [review].

2. McMillan M, Spinks EA, Fenwick GR. Preliminary observations on the effect of dietary Brussels sprouts on thyroid function. *Hum Toxicol* 1986; 5: 15–19.

3. Biassoni P, Ravera G, Bertocchi J, et al. Influence of dietary habits on thyroid status of a nomadic people, the Bororo shepherds, roaming a central African region affected by severe iodine deficiency. *Eur J Endocrinol* 1998; 138: 681–85.

4. Boyages SC. Iodine deficiency disorders. *J Clin Endocrinol Metab* 1993; 77: 587–91.

5. Galland L. Biochemical abnormalities in patients with multiple chemical sensitivities. *Occup Med* 1987; 2: 713–20 [review].

6. Robins JM, Cullen MR, Connors BB, Kayne RD. Depressed thyroid indexes associated with occupational exposure to inorganic lead. *Arch Intern Med* 1983; 143: 220–24.

7. Thilly CH, Swennen B, Bourdoux P, et al. The epidemiology of iodine-deficiency disorders in relation to goitrogenic factors and thyroid-stimulating-hormone regulation. *Am J Clin Nutr l* 1993; 57(2 suppl): 267S–70S.

8. Delange F. Risks and benefits of iodine supplementation. *Lancet* 1998; 351: 923–24.

9. Contempre B, Dumont JE, Ngo B, et al. Effect of selenium supplementation in hypothyroid subjects of an iodine and selenium deficient area: the possible danger of indiscriminate supplementation of iodine-deficient subjects with selenium. *J Clin Endocrinol Metab* 1991; 73: 213–15.

10. Chow CC, Phillips DIW, Lazarus JH, Parkes AB. Effect of low dose iodide supplementation on thyroid function in potentially susceptible subjects: are dietary iodide levels in Britain acceptable? *Clin Endocrinol* 1991; 34: 413–16.

11. Stewart JC, Vidor GI. Thyrotoxicosis induced by iodine contamination of food: a common unrecognized condition? *Br Med J* 1976; 1: 372–75.

12. Fujimoto S, Indo Y, Higashi A, et al. Conversion of thyroxine into tri-iodothyronine in zinc deficient rat liver. *J Pediatr Gastroenterol Nutr* 1986; 5: 799–805.

13. Hartoma TR, Sotaniemi EA, Maattanen J. Effect of zinc on some biochemical indices of metabolism. *Nutr Metab* 1979; 23: 294–300.

14. Weismann K, Roed-Petersen J, Hjorth N, Kopp H. Chronic zinc deficiency syndrome in a beer drinker with a Billroth II resection. *Int J Dermatol* 1976; 15: 757–61.

15. Wolf WR, Holden J, Greene FE. Daily intake of zinc and copper from self selected diets. *Fed Proc* 1977; 36: 1175.

16. Thilly CH, Swennen B, Bourdoux P, et al. The epidemiology of iodine-deficiency disorders in relation to goitrogenic factors and thyroid-stimulating-hormone regulation. *Am J Clin Nutr* 1993; 57(2 suppl): 267S–70S.

17. Contempre B, Dumont JE, Ngo B, et al. Effect of selenium supplementation in hypothyroid subjects of an iodine and selenium deficient area: the possible danger of indiscriminate supplementation of iodine-deficient subjects with selenium. *J Clin Endocrinol Metab* 1991; 73: 213–15.

18. Vanderpas JB, Contempre B, Duale NL, et al. Selenium deficiency mitigates hypothyroxinemia in iodine-deficient subjects. *Am J Clin Nutr* 1993; 57(2 suppl): 271S–5S [review].

19. Shakir KMM, Kroll S, Aprill BS, et al. Nicotinic acid decreases serum thyroid hormone levels while maintaining a euthyroid state. *Mayo Clin Proc* 1995; 70: 556–58.

20. O'Brien T, Silverberg JD, Nguyen TT. Nicotinic acid-induced toxicity associated with cytopenia and decreased levels of thyroxine-binding globulin. *Mayo Clin Proc* 1992; 67: 465–68.

21. Bunevicius R, Kazanavicius G, Zalinkevicius R, Prange AJ Jr. Effects of thyroxine as compared with thyroxine plus triiodothyronine in patients with hypothyroidism. *N Engl J Med* 1999; 340: 424–29.

22. Gaby AR. Treatment with thyroid hormone. *JAMA* 1989; 262: 1774 [letter].

23. Zha LL. Relation of hypothyroidism and deficiency of kidney yang. *Chung Kuo Chung His I Chieh Ho Tsa Chih* 1993; 13: 202–4 [in Chinese].

24. Zhang JQ, Zhao M. Effects of yin-tonics and yang-tonics on serum thyroid hormone levels and thyroid hormone receptors of hepatic cell nucleus in hyperthyroxinemic and hypothyroxinemic rats. *Chung His I Chieh Ho Tsa Chih* 1991; 11: 105–6,69–70 [in Chinese].

Immune Function

1. Chandra RK. Nutrition and the immune system: an introduction. *Am J Clin Nutr* 1997; 66: 460–63S [review].

2. Stallone DD. The influence of obesity and its treatment on the immune system. *Nutr Rev* 1994; 52: 37–50.

3. Nieman DC, Nehlsen-Cannarella SI, Henson DA, et al. Immune response to obesity and moderate weight loss. *Int J Obes Relat Metab Disord* 1996; 20: 353–60.

4. Nieman DC, Henson DA, Nehlsen-Cannarella SL. Influence of obesity on immune function. *J Am Diet Assoc* 1999; 99: 294–99.

5. Scanga CB, Verde TJ, Paolone AM, et al. Effects of weight loss and exercise training on natural killer cell activity in obese women. *Med Sci Sports Exerc* 1998; 30: 1666–71.

6. Sanchez A, et al. Role of sugars in human neutrophilic phagocytosis. *Am J Clin Nutr* 1973; 26: 1180.

7. Ringsdorf WM, et al. Sucrose, neutrophilic phagocytosis and resistance to disease. *Dental Survey* 1976; 52(12): 46.

8. Nutter RL, Gridley DS, Kettering JD, et al. Modification of a transplantable colon tumor and immune responses in mice fed different sources of protein, fat and carbohydrate. *Cancer Lett* 1983 Feb; 18(1): 49–62.

9. Kos WL, Kos KA, Kaplan AM. Impaired function of immune reactivity to Listeria monocytogenes in diet-fed mice. *Infect Immun* 1984; 43: 1094–96.

10. Ahmed FE. Toxicological effects of ethanol on human health. *Crit Rev Tox* 1995; 25(4): 347–67.

Part One: References

11. Szabo G. Monocytes, alcohol use, and altered immunity. *Alcohol Clin Exp Res* 1998; 22: 216–19S.

12. Seitz HK, Poschl G, Simanowski UA. Alcohol and cancer. *Recent Dev Alcohol* 1998; 14: 67–95 [review].

13. MacGregor RR, Louria DB. Alcohol and infection. *Curr Clin Top Infect Dis* 1997; 17: 291–315 [review].

14. Balla AK, Lischner HW, Pomerantz RJ, et al. Human studies on alcohol and susceptibility to HIV infection. *Alcohol* 1994; 11: 99–103 [review].

15. Engs RC, Aldo-Benson M. The association of alcohol consumption with self-reported illness in university students. *Psychol Rep* 1995; 76: 727–36.

16. Cohen S, Tyrrell DA, Russell MA, et al. Smoking, alcohol consumption, and susceptibility to the common cold. *Am J Public Health* 1993; 83: 1277–83.

17. Kelley DS, Daudu PA. Fat intake and immune response. *Prog Food Nutr Sci* 1993; 17: 41–63 [review].

18. Yaqoob P. Monounsaturated fats and immune function. *Proc Nutr Soc* 1998; 57: 511–20 [review].

19. Tashiro T, Yamamori H, Takagi K, et al. n-3 versus n-6 polyunsaturated fatty acids in critical illness. *Nutrition* 1998; 14: 551–3.

20. Gerster H. The use of n-3 PUFAs (fish oil) in enteral nutrition. *Int J Vitam Nutr Res* 1995; 65: 3–20 [review].

21. Meydani SN, Lichtenstein AH, Cornwall S, et al. Immunologic effects of national cholesterol education panel step-2 diets with and without fish-derived n-3 fatty acid enrichment. *J Clin Invest* 1993; 92: 105–13.

22. Wu D, Meydani SN. n-3 polyunsaturated fatty acids and immune function. *Proc Nutr Soc* 1998; 57: 503–9 [review].

23. Kelley DS, Dougherty RM, Branch LB, et al. Concentration of dietary N-6 polyunsaturated fatty acids and the human immune status. *Clin Immunol Immunopathol* 1992; 62: 240–44.

24. Rasmussen LB, Kiens B, Pedersen BK, et al. Effect of diet and plasma fatty acid composition on immune status in elderly men. *Am J Clin Nutr* 1994; 59: 572–77.

25. Wan JM, Teo TC, Babayan VK, et al. Invited comment: lipids and the development of immune dysfunction and infection. *JPEN J Parenter Enteral Nutr* 1988; 12: 43S–52S.

26. Horesh AJ. Allergy and infection VII. Support from the literature. *J Asthma Res* 1968; 6: 3–55 [review].

27. Pang LQ. The importance of allergy in otolaryngology. *Clin Ecology* 1982; 1(1): 53.

28. Nsouli TM, Nsouli SM, Linde RE, et al. Role of food allergy in serous otitis media. *Ann Allerg* 1994; 73: 215–19.

29. Horesh AJ. Allergy and recurrent urinary tract infections in childhood. II. *Ann Allergy* 1976; 36: 174–79.

30. Crandall, M. Allergic predisposition and recurrent vulvovaginal candidiasis. *J Advancement Med* 1991; 4: 21–38 [review].

31. Kudelco N. Allergy in chronic monilial vaginitis. *Ann Allerg* 1971; 29: 266–67.

32 Herbert TB, Cohen S. Stress and immunity in humans: a meta-analytic review. *Psychosom Med* 1993; 55: 364–79 [review].

33. Palmblad JE. Stress-related modulation of immunity: a review of human studies. *Cancer Detect Prev Suppl* 1987; 1: 57–64 [review].

34. Kemeny ME, Gruenewald TL. Psychoneuroimmunology update. *Semin Gastrointest Dis* 1999; 10: 20–29 [review].

35. Halley FM. Self-regulation of the immune system through biobehavioral strategies. *Biofeedback Self Regul* 1991; 16: 55–74 [review].

36. Whitehouse WG, Dinges DF, Orne EC, et al. Psychosocial and immune effects of self-hypnosis training for stress management throughout the first semester of medical school. *Psychosom Med* 1996; 58: 249–63.

37. Nieman DC. Exercise immunology: practical applications. *Int J Sports Med* 1997; 18: S91–100 [review].

38. Nieman DC. Exercise and resistance to infection. *Can J Physiol Pharmacol* 1998; 76: 573–80 [review].

39. Shephard RJ, Shek PN. Associations between physical activity and susceptibility to cancer: possible mechanisms. *Sports Med* 1998; 26: 293–315 [review].

40. Duchateau J, Delespesse G, Vereecke P. Influence of oral zinc supplementation on the lymphocyte response to mitogens of normal subjects. *Am J Clin Nutr* 1981; 34: 88–93.

41. Fraker PJ, Gershwin ME, Good RA, Prasad A. Interrelationships between zinc and immune function. *Fed Proc* 1986; 45: 1474–79.

42. Fortes C, Forastiere F, Agabiti N, et al. The effect of zinc and vitamin A supplementation on immune response in an older population. *J Am Geriatr Soc* 1998; 46: 19–26.

43. Girodon F, Lombard M, Galan P, et al. Effect of micronutrient supplementation on infection in institutionalized elderly subjects: a controlled trial. *Ann Nutr Metab* 1997; 41: 98–107.

44. Chandra RK. Excessive intake of zinc impairs immune responses. *JAMA* 1984; 252: 1443–46.

45. Macknin ML. Zinc lozenges for the common cold. *Cleveland Clin J Med* 1999; 66: 27–32 [review].

46. Semba RD. Vitamin A, immunity, and infection. *Clin Infect Dis* 1994; 19: 489–99 [review].

47. Glasziou PP, Mackerras DEM. Vitamin A supplementation in infectious diseases: a meta-analysis. *BMJ* 1993; 306: 366–70.

48. Stephensen CB, Franchi LM, Hernandez H, et al. Adverse effects of high-dose vitamin A supplements in children hospitalized with pneumonia. *Pediatrics* 1998; 101(5): E3 [abstract].

49. Bresee JS, Fischer M, Dowell SF, et al. Vitamin A therapy for children with respiratory syncytial virus infection: a multicenter trial in the United States. *Pediatr Infect Dis J* 1996; 15: 777–82.

50. Quinlan KP, Hayani KC. Vitamin A and respiratory syncytial virus infection. Serum levels and supplementation trial. *Arch Pediatr Adolesc Med* 1996; 150: 25–30.

51. Kjolhede CL, Chew FJ, Gadomski AM, et al. Clinical trial of vitamin A as adjuvant treatment for lower respiratory tract infections. *J Pediatr* 1995; 126: 807–12.

52. Pinnock CB, Douglas RM, Badcock NR. Vitamin A status in children who are prone to respiratory tract infections. *Aust Paediatr J* 1986; 22: 95–99.

53. Murphy S, West KP Jr, Greenough WB 3d, et al. Impact of vitamin A supplementation on the incidence of infection in elderly nursing-home residents: a randomized controlled trial. *Age Ageing* 1992; 21: 435–39.

54. Chew BP. Role of carotenoids in the immune response. *J Dairy Sci* 1993; 76: 2804–11.

55. Bendich A. Beta-carotene and the immune response. *Proc Nutr Soc* 1991; 50: 263–74.

56. Hughes DA, Wright AJ, Finglas PM, et al. The effect of beta-carotene supplementation on the immune function of blood monocytes from healthy male nonsmokers. *J Lab Clin Med* 1997; 129: 309–17.

57. Murata T, Tamai H, Morinobu T, et al. Effect of long-term administration of beta-carotene on lymphocyte subsets in humans. *Am J Clin Nutr* 1994; 60: 597–602.

58. Santos MS, Meydani SN, Leka L, et al. Natural killer cell activity in elderly men is enhanced by beta-carotene supplementation. *Am J Clin Nutr* 1996; 64: 772–77.

59. Santos MS, Leka LS, Ribaya-Mercado JD, et al. Short- and long-term beta-carotene supplementation do not influence T cell-mediated immunity in healthy elderly persons. *Am J Clin Nutr* 1997; 66: 917–24.

60. Kazi N, Radvany R, Oldham T, et al. Immunomodulatory effect of beta-carotene on T lymphocyte subsets in patients with resected colonic polyps and cancer. *Nutr Cancer* 1997; 28: 140–45.

61. Fuller CJ, Faulkner H, Bendich A, et al. Effect of beta-carotene supplementation on photo-suppression of delayed-type hypersensitivity in normal young men. *Am J Clin Nutr* 1992; 56: 684–90.

62. Coodley GO, Coodley MK, Lusk R, et al. Beta-carotene in HIV infection: an extended evaluation. *AIDS* 1996; 10: 967–73.

63. Fryburg DA, Mark RJ, Griffith BP, et al. The effect of supplemental beta-carotene on immunologic indices in patients with AIDS: a pilot study. *Yale J Biol Med* 1995; 68: 19–23.

64. Gerber WF, et al. Effect of ascorbic acid, sodium salicylate, and caffeine on the serum interferon level in response to viral infection. *Pharmacology* 1975; 13: 228.

65. Anderson R. The immunostimulatory, anti-inflammatory an anti-allergic properties of ascorbate. *Adv Nutr Res* 1984; 6: 19–45 [review].

66. Banic S. Immunostimulation by vitamin C. *Int J Vitam Nutr Res Suppl* 1982; 23: 49–52 [review].

67. Delafuente JC, Prendergast JM, Modigh A. Immunologic modulation by vitamin C in the elderly. *Int J Immunopharmacol* 1986; 8: 205–11.

68. Kennes B, Dumont I, Brohee D, et al. Effect of vitamin C supplements on cell-mediated immunity in old people. *Gerontology* 1983; 29: 305–10.

69. Murata A. Virucidal activity of vitamin C for prevention and treatment of viral diseases. In Proceedings of the First Intersectional Congress of IAMS, vol 3. Science Council Japan, 1975; 432.

70. Knodell RG, Tate MA, Akl BF, et al. Vitamin C prophylaxis for posttransfusion hepatitis: Lack of effect in a controlled trial. *Am J Clin Nutr* 1981; 34(1): 20–23.

71. Hemila H. Vitamin C and the common cold. *Br J Nutr* 1992; 67: 3–16.

72. Hemilá H. Vitamin C and common cold incidence: a review of studies with subjects under heavy physical stress. *Int J Sports Med* 1996; 17: 379–83.

73. Meydani SN, Barklund MP, Liu S, et al. Vitamin E supplementation enhances cell-mediated immunity in healthy elderly subjects. *Am J Clin Nutr* 1990; 52: 557–63.

74. Meydani SN, Meydani M, Blumberg JB, et al. Vitamin E supplementation and in vivo immune response in healthy elderly subjects: a randomized controlled trial. *JAMA* 1997; 277: 1380–86.

75. De Waart FG, Portengen L, Doekes G, et al. Effect of 3 months vitamin E supplementation on indices of the cellular and humoral immune response in elderly subjects. *Br J Nutr* 1997; 78: 761–74.

76. Penn ND, Purkins L, Kelleher J, et al. The effect of dietary supplementation with vitamins A, C and E on cell-mediated immune function in elderly long-stay patients: a randomized controlled trial. *Age Ageing* 1991; 20: 169–74.

77. de la Fuente M, Ferrandez MD, Burgos MS, et al. Immune function in aged women is improved by ingestion of vitamins C and E. *Can J Physiol Pharmacol* 1998; 76: 373–80.

78. Pike J, Chandra RK. Effect of vitamin and trace element supplementation on immune indices in healthy elderly. *Int J Vitam Nutr Res* 1995; 65: 117–21.

79. Chandra RK. Effect of vitamin and trace-element supplementation on immune responses and infection in elderly subjects. *Lancet* 1992; 340: 1124–27.

80. Chavance M, Herbeth B, Lemoine A, et al. Does multivitamin supplementation prevent infections in healthy elderly subjects? A controlled trial. *Int J Vitam Nutr Res* 1993; 63: 11–16.

81. Girodon F, Lombard M, Galan P, et al. Effect of micronutrient supplementation on infection in institutionalized elderly subjects: a controlled trial. *Ann Nutr Metab* 1997; 41: 98–107.

82. Berger MM, Spertini F, Shenkin A, et al. Trace element supplementation modulates pulmonary infection rates after major burns: a double-blind, placebo-controlled trial. *Am J Clin Nutr* 1998; 68: 365–71.

83. Caughey GE, Mantzioris E, Gibson RA, et al. The effect on human tumor necrosis factor alpha and interleukin 1 beta production of diets enriched in n-3 fatty acids from vegetable oil or fish oil. *Am J Clin Nutr* 1996; 63: 116–22.

84. Endres S, Meydani SN, Ghorbani R, et al. Dietary supplementation with n-3 fatty acids suppresses interleukin-2 production and mononuclear cell proliferation. *J Leukoc Biol* 1993; 54: 599–603.

85. Meydani SN, Endres S, Woods MM, et al. Oral (n-3) fatty acid supplementation suppresses cytokine production and lymphocyte proliferation: comparison between young and older women. *J Nutr* 1991; 121: 547–55.

86. Virella G, Fourspring K, Hyman B, et al. Immunosuppressive effects of fish oil in normal human volunteers: correlation with the in vitro effects of eicosapentanoic acid on human lymphocytes. *Clin Immunol Immunopathol* 1991; 61: 161–76.

87. Wu D, Meydani SN. n-3 polyunsaturated fatty acids and immune function. *Proc Nutr Soc* 1998; 57: 503–9 [review].

88. Jones C, Palmer TE, Griffiths RD. Randomized clinical outcome study of critically ill patients given glutamine-supplemented enteral nutrition. *Nutrition* 1999; 15: 108–15.

89. Griffiths RD. Outcome of critically ill patients after supplementation with glutamine. *Nutrition* 1997; 13: 752–54 [review].

90. Nieman DC. Exercise and resistance to infection. *Can J Physiol Pharmacol* 1998; 76: 573–80 [review].

91. Rohde T, MacLean DA, Pedersen BK. Effect of glutamine supplementation on changes in the immune system induced by repeated exercise. *Med Sci Sports Exerc* 1998; 30: 856–62.

92. Castell LM, Newsholme EA. Glutamine and the effects of exhaustive exercise upon the immune response. *Can J Physiol Pharmacol* 1998; 76: 524–32 [review].

93. Castell LM, Poortmans JR, Newsholme EA. Does glutamine have a role in reducing infections in athletes? *Eur J Appl Physiol* 1996; 73: 488–90.

94. Fernandes CF, Shahani KM, Amer MA. Therapeutic role of dietary lactobacilli and lactobacillic fermented dairy products. *FEMS Micro Rev* 1987; 46: 343–56.

95. Bengmark S. Immunonutrition: role of biosurfactants, fiber, and probiotic bacteria. *Nutrition* 1998; 14: 585–94 [review].

96. Rasic JL. Bifidobacteria and diarrhoea control in infants and young children. *Internat Clin Nutr Rev* 1992; 12: 27–30 [review].

97. Saavedra JM, Bauman NA, Oung I, et al. Feeding of Bifidobacterium bifidum and Streptococcus thermophilus to infants in hospital for prevention of diarrhoea and shedding of rotavirus. *Lancet* 1994; 344: 1046–49.

98. Kudsk KA, Minard G, Croce MA, et al. A randomized trial of isonitrogenous enteral diets after severe trauma. An immune-enhancing diet reduces septic complications. *Ann Surg* 1996; 224: 531–40.

99. Braga M, Gianotti L, Cestari A, et al. Gut function and immune and inflammatory responses in patients perioperatively fed with supplemented enteral formulas. *Arch Surg* 1996; 131: 1257–64.

100. Kemen M, Senkal M, Homann HH, et al. Early postoperative enteral nutrition with arginine-omega-3 fatty acids and ribonucleic acid-supplemented diet versus placebo in cancer patients: an immunologic evaluation of Impact. *Crit Care Med* 1995; 23: 652–59.

101. Alexander JW. Immunoenhancement via enteral nutrition. *Arch Surg* 1993; 128: 1242–45 [review].

102. Saffle JR, Wiebke G, Jennings K, et al. Randomized trial of immune-enhancing enteral nutrition in burn patients. *J Trauma* 1997; 42: 793–800.

103. Pichard C, Sudre P, Karsegard V, et al. A randomized double-blind controlled study of 6 months of oral nutritional supplementation with arginine and omega-3 fatty acids in HIV-infected patients. Swiss HIV Cohort Study. *AIDS* 1998; 12: 53–63.

104. See DM, Broumand N, Sahl L, Tilles JG. In vitro effects of echinacea and ginseng on natural killer and antibody-dependent cell cytotoxicity in healthy subjects and chronic fatigue syndrome or acquired immunodeficiency syndrome patients. *Immunopharmacology* 1997; 35: 229–35.

105. Melchart D, Linde K, Worku F, et al. Immunomodulation with echinacea—a systematic review of controlled clinical trials. *Phytomedicine* 1994; 1: 245–54.

106. Melchart D, Linde K, Worku F, et al. Results of five randomized studies on the immunomodulatory activity of preparations of echinacea. *J Alt Compl Med* 1995; 1: 145–60.

107. Scaglione F, Ferrara F, Dugnani S, et al. Immunomodulatory effects of two extracts of *Panax ginseng* CA Meyer. *Drugs Exptl Clin Res* 1990; 16: 537–42.

108. Baranov AI. Medicinal uses of ginseng and related plants in the Soviet Union: Recent trends in the Soviet literature. *J Ethnopharmacol* 1982; 6: 339–53 [review].

109. Bohn B, Nebe CT, Birr C. Flow-cytometric studies with *Eleutherococcus senticosus* extract as an immunomodulatory agent. *Arzneim Forsch* 1987; 37: 1193–96.

110. Bone K, Morgan M. *Clinical Applications of Ayurvedic and Chinese Herbs*. Warwick, Queensland, Australia: Phytotherapy Press, 1996, 13–20.

111. Nanba H. Antitumor activity of orally administered 'D-fraction' from maitake mushroom *(Grifola frondosa)*. *J Naturopathic Med* 1993; 4: 10–15.

112. Pengelly A. Medicinal fungi of the world. *Modern Phytotherapist* 1996; 2: 1,3–8 [review].

113. Keplinger H. Oxindole alkaloids having properties stimulating the immunologic system and preparation containing same. US Patent no. 5,302,611, April 12, 1994.

114. Stoner GD, Mukhtar H. Polyphenols as cancer chemopreven-

tive agents. *J Cell Bioch* 1995; 22: 169–80.

115. You SQ. Study on feasibility of Chinese green tea polyphenols (CTP) for preventing dental caries. *Chin J Stom* 1993; 28(4): 197–99.

116. Hamilton-Miller JM. Antimicrobial properties of tea (*Camellia sinensis* L.). *Antimicro Agents Chemo* 1995; 39(11): 2375–77.

117. Foster S, Chongxi Y. *Herbal Emissaries: Bringing Chinese Herbs to the West.* Rochester, VT: Healing Arts Press, 1992, 79–85.

118. Wagner H, Nörr H, Winterhoff H. Plant adaptogens. *Phytomed* 1994; 1: 63–76.

119. Bone K. *Clinical Applications of Ayurvedic and Chinese Herbs.* Queensland, Australia: Phytotherapy Press, 1996, 137–41.

120. Leung AY, Foster S. *Encyclopedia of Common Natural Ingredients Used in Foods, Drugs, and Cosmetics,* 2d ed. New York: John Wiley & Sons, 1996, 350–52.

Impotence

1. Aydin S, Ercan M, Çaskurlu T, et al. Acupuncture and hypnotic suggestions in the treatment of nonorganic male sexaul dysfunction. *Scand J Urol Nephrol* 1997; 31: 271–74.

2. Moody JA, Vernt D, Laidlaw S, et al. Effects of long-term oral administration of L-arginine on the rat erectile response. *J Urol* 1997; 158: 942–47.

3. Zorgniotti AW, Lizza EF. Effect of large doses of the nitric oxide precursor, L-arginine, on erectile dysfunction. *Int J Impot Res* 1994; 6: 33–36.

4. Reiter WJ, Pycha A, Schatzl G, et al. Dehydroepiandrosterone in the treatment of erectile dysfunction: a prospective, double-blind randomized, placebo-controlled study. *Urology* 1999; 53: 590–95.

5. Ernst E, Pittler MH. Yohimbine for erectile dysfunction: A systematic review and meta-analysis of randomized clinical trials. *J Urol* 1998; 159: 433–36.

6. Carey MP, Johnson BT. Effectiveness of yohimbine in the

treatment of erectile disorder: Four meta-analytic integrations. *Arch Sex Behav* 1996; 25: 341.

7. Kunelius P, Häkkinen J, Lukkarinen O. Is high-dose yohimbine hydrochloride effective in the treatment of mixed-type impotence? A prospective, randomized, controlled double-blind crossover study. *Urol* 1997; 49: 441–44.

8. Mann K, Klingler T, Noe S, et al. Effect of yohimbine on sexual experiences and nocturnal tumescence and rigidity in erectile dysfunction. *Arch Sex Behav* 1996; 25: 1–16.

9. Sohn M, Sikora R. *Ginkgo biloba* extract in the therapy of erectile dysfunction. *J Sec Educ Ther* 1991; 17: 53–61.

10. Cohen AJ, Bartlik B. *Ginkgo biloba* for antidepressant-induced sexual dysfunction. *J Sex Marital Ther* 1998; 24: 139–43.

Indigestion, Heartburn, and Low Stomach Acidity

1. Wright JV. *Dr. Wright's Guide to Healing with Nutrition.* New Canaan, CT: Keats Publishing, 1990, 155.

2. Murray MJ, Stein N. A gastric factor promoting iron absorption. *Lancet* 1968; 1: 614.

3. Ivanovich P et al. The absorption of calcium carbonate. *Ann Intern Med* 1967; 66: 917.

4. Recker RR. Calcium absorption and achlorhydria. *NEJM* 1985; 313: 70.

5. Sturniolo GC et al. Inhibition of gastric acid secretion reduces zinc absorption in man. *J Am Coll Nutr* 1991; 10: 372–75.

6. Allison JR. The relation of hydrochloric acid and vitamin B complex deficiency in certain skin conditions. *South Med J* 1945; 38: 235.

7. Russell RM et al. Correction of impaired folic acid (Pte Glu) absorption by orally administered HCl in subjects with gastric atrophy. *Am J Clin Nutr* 1984; 39: 656.

8. Mayron LW. Portals of entry: A review. *Ann Allergy* 1978; 40: 399.

9. Walker WA, Isselbacher KJ. Uptake and transport of macro-molecules by the intestine. Possible role in

clinical disorders. *Gastroenterology* 1974; 67: 531.

10. *Gastroenterology* 1969; 56(1): 71ff.

11. Giannella RA. Influence of gastric acidity on bacterial and parasitic enteric infections. A perspective. *Ann Int Med* 1973; 78: 271–76.

12. Wright, JV. *Dr. Wright's Guide to Healing with Nutrition.* New Canaan, CT: Keats Publishing, 1990, 33.

13. Rokkas T, Pursey C, Uzoechina E, et al. Non-ulcer dys-pepsia and short term De-Nol therapy: A placebo controlled trial with particular reference to the role of *Campylobacter pylori. Gut* 1988; 29: 1386–91.

14. Kang JY, Tay HH, Wee A, et al. Effect of colloidal bismuth subcitrate on symptoms and gastric histology in non-ulcer dyspepsia. A double blind placebo controlled study. *Gut* 1990; 31: 476–80.

15. *Matricaria flos.* ESCOP monograph, Oct 1990.

16. Mills SY. *Out of the Earth: The Essential Book of Herbal Medicine.* London: Viking Press, 1991, 448–51.

17. May B, Kuntz HD, Kieser M, Kohler S. Efficacy of a fixed peppermint/caraway oil combination in nonulcer dyspepsia. *Arzneim Forsch* 1996; 46: 1149–53.

18. Westphal J, Hörning M, Leonhardt K. Phytotherapy in functional upper abdominal complaints. Results of a clinical study with a preparation of several plants. *Phytomedicine* 1996; 2: 285–91.

19. Forster HB, Niklas H, Lutz S. Antispasmodic effects of some medicinal plants. *Planta Med* 1980; 40: 303–19.

20. Weiss RF. Herbal Medicine. Beaconsfield, UK: Beaconsfield Publishers Ltd, 1985.

21. Blumenthal M, Busse WR, Goldberg A, et al. (eds). *The Complete German Commission E Monographs: Therapeutic Guide to Herbal Medicines.* Austin: American Botanical Council and Boston: Integrative Medicine Communications, 1998, 425–26.

22. Blumenthal M, Busse WR, Goldberg A, et al. (eds). *The Complete German Commission E Monographs: Therapeutic Guide to Herbal Medicines*. Austin: American Botanical Council and Boston: Integrative Medicine Communications, 1998, 425–26.

23. Westphal J, Hörning M, Leonhardt K. Phytotherapy in functional upper abdominal complaints. Results of a clinical study with a preparation of several plants. *Phytomedicine* 1996; 2: 285–91.

24. Blumenthal M, Busse WR, Goldberg A, et al. (eds). *The Complete German Commission E Monographs: Therapeutic Guide to Herbal Medicines*. Austin: American Botanical Council and Boston: Integrative Medicine Communications, 1998, 425–26.

25. Schulz V, Hänsel R, Tyler VE. *Rational Phytotherapy: A Physician's Guide to Herbal Medicine*. 3rd ed, Berlin: Springer, 1998, 168–73.

26. Tewari JP, Srivastava MC, Bajpai JL. Pharmacologic studies of *Achillea millefolium* Linn. *Indian J Med Sci* 1994; 28(8): 331–36.

27. Leung AY, Foster S. *Encyclopedia of Common Natural Ingredients Used in Food, Drugs, and Cosmetics*, 2d ed. New York: John Wiley & Sons, 1996, 303.

28. Bradley PR. *British Herbal Compendium*, vol. 1. Great Britain: British Herbal Medicine Association, 1990, 218–19.

29. Kraft K. Artichoke leaf extract—recent findings reflecting effects on lipid metabolism, liver and gastrointestinal tracts. *Phytomedicine* 1997; 4: 370–78 [review].

30. Kirchhoff R, Beckers C, Kirchhoff GM, et al. Increase in choleresis by means of artichoke extract. *Phytomedicine* 1994; 1: 107–15.

31. Thamlikitkul V, Bunyapraphatsara N, Dechatiwongse T, et al. Randomized double blind study of *Curcuma domestica* Val for dyspepsia. *J Med Assoc Thai* 1989; 72: 613–20.

32. Goso Y, Ogata Y, Ishihara K, Hotta K. Effects of traditional herbal medicine on gastric acid. *Biochem Physiol* 1996; 113C: 17–21.

33. Reed PI, Davies WA. Controlled trial of a carbenoxolone/alginate antacid combination in reflux oesophagitis. *Curr Med Res Opin* 1978; 5: 637–44.

Infection

1. McIntosh WA, Kaplan HB, Kubena KS, et al. Life events, social support, and immune responses in elderly individuals. *Intl J Aging Hum Dev* 1993; 37: 23–36.

2. Nieman DC. Exercise, upper respiratory tract infection, and the immune system. *Med Sci Sports Med* 1994; 26(2): 128–39.

3. Sanchez A et al. Role of sugars in human neutrophilic phagocytosis. *Am J Clin Nutr* 1973; 26: 1180.

4. Ahmed FE. Toxicological effects of ethanol on human health. *Crit Rev Tox* 1995; 25(4): 347–67.

5. Kubena KS, McMurray DN. Nutrition and the immune system: A review of nutrient-nutrient interactions. *J Am Diet Assoc* 1996; 96(11): 1156–64.

6. Glaszious PP et al. Vitamin A supplementation in infectious diseases: A meta-analysis. *BMJ* 1993; 306: 366–70.

7. Duchateau J, Delespesse G, Vereecke P. Influence of oral zinc supplementation on the lymphocyte response to mitogens of normal subjects. *Am J Clin Nutr* 1981; 34: 88–93.

8. Fraker PJ, Gershwin ME, Good RA, Prasad A. Interrelationships between zinc and immune function. *Fed Proc* 1986; 45: 1474–79.

9. Gerber WF et al. Effect of ascorbic acid, sodium salicylate, and caffeine on the serum interferon level in response to viral infection. *Pharmacology* 1975; 13: 228.

10. Hemila H. Vitamin C and the common cold. *Br J Nutr* 1992; 67: 3–16.

11. Fernandes CF, Shahani KM, Amer MA. Therapeutic role of dietary lactobacilli and lactobacillic fermented dairy products. *FEMS Micro Rev* 1987; 343–56.

12. Brown DJ. *Herbal Prescriptions for Better Health*. Rocklin, CA: Prima Publishing, 1996, 213–14 [review].

13. Guiraud P, Steiman R, Campos-Takaki GM, et al. Comparison of antibacterial and antifungal activities of lapachol and beta-lapachone. *Planta Med* 1994; 60: 373–74.

14. Okazai K, Oshima S. Antibacterial activity of higher plants. XXIV. Antimicrobial effect of essential oils (5). *J Pharm Soc Japan* 1953; 73: 344–47.

Infertility (Female)

1. Grodstein F, Goldman MB, Ryan L, Cramer DW. Relation of female infertility to consumption of caffeinated beverages. *Am J Epidemiol* 1993; 137: 1353–60.

2. Hatch EE, Bracken MB. Association of delayed conception with caffeine consumption. *Am J Epidemiol* 1993; 138: 1082–92.

3. Wilcox A, Weinberg C, Baird D. Caffeinated beverages and decreased fertility. *Lancet* 1988; ii: 1453–56.

4. Williams MA, Monson RR, Goldman MG, et al. Coffee and delayed conception. *Lancet* 1990; 335: 1603 [letter].

5. Stanton CK, Gray RH. Effects of caffeine consumption on delayed conception. *Am J Epidemiol* 1995; 142: 1322–29.

6. Joesoef MR, Beral V, Rolfs RT, et al. Are caffeinated beverages risk factors for delayed conception? *Lancet* 1990; 335: 136–37.

7. Fenster L, Bubbard A, Windhan G, Hiatt R, et al. A prospective study of caffeine consumption and spontaneous abortion. *Am J Epidemiol* 1996; 143(11 suppl); 525 [abstract #99].

8. Cramer DW. Letter. *Lancet* 1990; 335: 792.

9. Howe G, Westhoff C, Vessey M, Yeates D. Effects of age, cigarette smoking, and other factors on fertility: findings in a large prospective study. *BMJ* 1985; 290: 1697–99.

10. Weinberg CR, Wilcox AJ, Baird DD. Reduced fecundability in

women with prenatal exposure to cigarette smoking. *Am J Epidemiol* 1989; 129: 1072–78.

11. Grodstein F, Goldman MB, Cramer DW. Infertility in women and moderate alcohol use. *Am J Public Health* 1994; 84: 1429–32.

12. Florack EIM, Zielhuis GA, Rolland R. Cigarette smoking, alcohol consumption, and caffeine intake and fecundability. *Prev Med* 1994; 23: 175–80.

13. Green BB et al. Risk of ovulatory infertility in relation to body weight. *Fertil Steril* 1988; 50: 621–26.

14. Werbach MR. Female Infertility. *Townsend Letter for Doctors and Patients* 1995; Aug: 34 [review].

15. Czeizel AE, Metneki J, Dudas I. The effect of preconceptional multivitamin supplementation on fertility. *Internat J Vit Nutr Res* 1996; 66: 55–58.

16. Thiessen DD et al. Vitamin E and sex behavior in mice. *Nutr Metabol* 1975; 18: 116–19.

17. Bayer R. Treatment of infertility with vitamin E. *Int J Fertil* 1960; 5: 70–78.

18. Rushton DH, Ramsay ID, Gilkes JJH, Norris MJ. Ferritin and fertility. *Lancet* 1991; 337: 1554 [letter].

19. Wiesel LL et al. The synergistic action of para-aminobenzoic acid and cortisone in the treatment of rheumatoid arthritis. *Am J Med Sci* 1951; 222: 243–48.

20. Sieve BF. The clinical effects of a new B-complex factor, para-aminobenzoic acid, on pigmentation and fertility. *South Med Surg* 1942(March); 104: 135–39.

21. Propping D, Katzorke T. Treatment of corpus luteum insufficiency. *Zeitschr Allgemeinmedizin* 1987; 63: 932–33.

Infertility (Male)

1. Fraga CG, Motchnik PA, Shigenaga MK, et al. Ascorbic acid protects against endogenous oxidative DNA damage in human sperm. *Proc Natl Acad Sci* 1991; 88: 11003–6.

2. Dawson EB, Harris WA, Teter MC, Powell LC. Effect of ascorbic acid supplementation on the sperm quality of smokers. *Fertil Steril* 1992; 58: 1034–39.

3. Dawson EB, Harris WA, McGanity WJ. Effect of ascorbic acid on sperm fertility. *Fed Proc* 1983; 42: 531 [abstr 31403].

4. Dawson EB, Harris WA, Powell LC. Relationship between ascorbic acid and male fertility. In: Aspects of Some Vitamins, Minerals and Enzymes in Health and Disease, ed. GH Bourne. *World Rev Nutr Diet* 1990; 62: 1–26 [review].

5. Hunt CD, Johnson PE, Herbel JoL, Mullen LK. Effects of dietary zinc depletion on seminal volume and zinc loss, serum testosterone concentrations, and sperm morphology in young men. *Am J Clin Nutr* 1992; 56: 148–57.

6. Netter A, Hartoma R, Nahoul K. Effect of zinc administration on plasma testosterone, dihydrotestosterone and sperm count. *Arch Androl* 1981; 7: 69–73.

7. Marmar JL et al. Semen zinc levels in infertile and postvasectomy patients and patients with prostatitis. *Fertil Steril* 1975: 26: 1057–63.

8. De Aloysio D, Mantuano R, Mauloni M, Nicoletti G. The clinical use of arginine aspartate in male infertility. *Acta Eur Fertil* 1982; 13: 133–67.

9. Tanimura J. Studies on arginine in human semen. Part II. The effects of medication with L-arginine-HCl on male infertility. *Bull Osaka Med School* 1967; 13: 84–89.

10. Schacter A, Goldman JA, Zukerman Z. Treatment of oligospermia with the amino acid arginine. *J Urol* 1973; 110: 311–13.

11. Schacter A et al. Treatment of oligospermia with the amino acid arginine. *Int J Gynaecol Obstet* 1973; 11: 206–9.

12. Mroueh A. Effect of arginine on oligospermia. *Fertil Steril* 1970: 21: 217–19.

13. Pryor JP, Blandy JP, Evans P, Chaput De Saintonge DM, Usherwood M. Controlled clinical trial of arginine for infertile men with oligozoospermia. *Brit J Urol* 1978; 50: 47–50.

14. Tanimura J. Studies on arginine in human semen. Part III. The influences of several drugs on male infertility. *Bull Osaka Med School* 1967; 13: 90–100.

15. Thiessen DD et al. Vitamin E and sex behavior in mice. *Nutr Metabol* 1975; 18: 116–19.

16. Bayer R. Treatment of infertility with vitamin E. *Int J Fertil* 1960; 5: 70–78.

17. Sandler B, Faragher B. Treatment of oligospermia with vitamin B$_{12}$. *Infertil* 1984; 7: 133–38.

18. Kumamoto Y, Maruta H, Ishigami J, et al. Clinical efficacy of mecobalamin in treatment of oligozoospermia. *Acta Urol Jpn* 1988; 34: 1109–32.

19. Costa M, Canale D, Filicori M, et al. L-carnitine in idiopathic asthenozoospermia: a multicenter study. *Andrologia* 1994; 26: 155–59.

20. Vitali G, Parente R, Melotti C. Carnitine supplementation in human idiopathic asthenospermia: clinical results. *Drugs Exptl Clin Res* 1995; 21: 157–59.

21. Piacentino R, Malara D, Zaccheo F, et al. Preliminary study of the use of s. adenosyl methionine in the management of male sterility. *Minerva Ginecologica* 1991; 43: 191–93 [in Italian].

Influenza

1. Clover RD, Abell T, Becker LA, et al. Family functioning and stress as predictors of influenza B infection. *J Fam Pract* 1989; 28: 535–39.

2. Renker K, Wegner S. Vitamin C-Prophylaxe in der Volkswertf Stralsund. *Deutsche Gesundheitswesen* 1954; 9: 702–6.

3. Klenner FR. The treatment of poliomyelitis and other virus diseases with vitamin C. *J Southern Med Surg* 1949; 111: 210–14.

4. Pauling L. *Vitamin C, the Common Cold and the Flu*. San Francisco: W. H. Freeman & Company, 1976 [review].

5. Braunig B, Dorn M, Limburg E, et al. *Echinacea purpurea* radix for strengthening the immune response in flu-like infections. *Z Phytother* 1992; 13: 7–13 [in German].

Part One: References

6. Zakay-Rones Z, Varsano N, Zlotnik M, et al. Inhibition of several strains of influenza virus in vitro and reduction of symptoms by an elderberry extract (*Sambucus nigra* L) during an outbreak of influenza B in Panama. *J Alt Comp Med* 1995; 1: 361–69.

7. Tsai Y, Cole LL, et al. Antiviral properties of garlic: In vitro effects of influenza B, herpes simplex and Coxsackie viruses. *Planta Med* 1985; (5): 460–61.

8. Woerdenbag HJ, Bos R, Hendriks H. *Eupatorium perfoliatum* L—the boneset. *Z Phytother* 1992; 13: 134–39.

9. Beuscher N, Kopanski L. Stimulation of immunity by the contents of *Baptisia tinctoria. Planta Med* 1985; 5: 381–84.

Insomnia

1. Weiss B, Laties VG. Enhancement of human performance by caffeine and the amphetamines. *Pharmacol Rev* 1962: 14: 1–36.

2. Hollingworth HL. The influence of caffeine on mental and motor efficiency. *Arch Psychol* 1912; 20: 1–66.

3. Blum I, Vered Y, Graff E, et al. The influence of meal composition on plasma serotonin and norepinephrine concentrations. *Metabolism* 1992; 41: 137–40.

4. Morin CM, Culbert JP, Schwartz SM. Nonpharmacological interventions for insomnia: a meta-analysis of treatment efficacy. *Am J Psychiatr* 1994; 151: 1172–80.

5. Fuerst ML. Insomniacs give up stress and medications. *JAMA* 1983; 249: 459–60.

6. Phillips BA, Danner FJ. Cigarette smoking and sleep disturbance. *Arch Intern Med* 1995; 155: 734–37.

7. Haimov I, Laudon M, Zisapel N, et al. Sleep disorders and melatonin rhythms in elderly people. *BMJ* 1994; 309: 167.

8. Singer C, McArthur A, Hughes R, et al. Melatonin and sleep in the elderly. *J Am Geriatr Soc* 1996; 44: 51 [abstr #A1].

9. Attenburrow MEJ, Dowling BA, Sharpley AL, Cowen PJ. Case-control study of evening melatonin concentration in primary insomnia. *BMJ* 1996; 312: 1263–64.

10. Zhadanova IV, Wurtman RJ, Lynch HJ, et al. Sleep-inducing effects of low doses of melatonin ingested in the evening. *Clin Pharmacol Ther* 1995; 57: 552–58.

11. Garfinkel D, Laudon M, Nof D, Zisapel N. Improvement of sleep quality in elderly people by controlled-release melatonin. *Lancet* 1995; 346: 541–44.

12. Schneider-Helmert D, Spinweber CL. Evaluation of L-tryptophan for treatment of insomnia: A review. *Psychopharmacology* (Berlin) 1986; 89: 1–7.

13. Leathwood PD, Chauffard F. Aqueous extract of valerian reduces latency to fall asleep in man. *Planta Medica* 1985; 51: 144–48.

14. Leathwood PD, Chauffard F, et al. Aqueous extract of valerian root (*Valeriana officinalis* L.) improves sleep quality in man. *Pharmacol Biochem Behav* 1982; 17: 65–71.

15. Dressing H, Riemann D, et al. Insomnia: Are valerian/balm combination of equal value to benzodiazepine? *Therapiewoche* 1992; 42: 726–36.

16. Brown DJ. *Herbal Prescriptions for Better Health.* Rocklin, CA: Prima Publishing, 1996, 279.

17. Blumenthal M, Busse WR, Goldberg A, et al. (eds). *The Complete German Commission E Monographs: Therapeutic Guide to Herbal Medicines.* Austin: American Botanical Council and Boston: Integrative Medicine Communications, 1998, 147, 160–61.

18. Buchbauer G, Jirovetz L, Jager W, et al. Aromatherapy: Evidence for sedative effects of the essential oil of lavender after inhalation. *Z Naturforsch [C]* 1991; 46: 1067–72.

19. Hardy M, Kirk-Smith MD, Stretch DD. Replacement of drug therapy for insomnia by ambient odour. *Lancet* 1995; 346: 701 [letter].

20. Blumenthal M, Busse WR, Goldberg A, et al. (eds). *The Complete German Commission E Monographs: Therapeutic Guide to Herbal Medicines.* Austin: American Botanical Council and Boston: Integrative Medicine Communications, 1998, 159–60.

Intermittent Claudication

1. Kiff RS, Wuick CRG. Does inositol nicotinate (Hexopal) influence intermittent claudication?—A controlled trial. *Brit J Clin Pract* 1988; 42: 141–45.

2. O'Hara J, Jolly PN, Nicol CG. The therapeutic efficacy of inositol nicotinate (Hexopal) in intermittent claudication: a controlled trial. *Brit J Clin Pract* 1988; 42: 377–83.

3. Haeger K. Long-time treatment of intermittent claudication with vitamin E. *Am J Clin Nutr* 1974; 27: 1179–81.

4. Williams HTG, Fenna D, Macbeth RA. Alpha tocopherol in the treatment of intermittent claudication. *Surg Gynecol Obstet* 1971; Apr: 662–66.

5. Donnan PT, Thomson M, Fowkes GR, et al. Diet as a risk factor for peripheral arterial disease in the general population: the Edinburgh Artery Study. *Am J Clin Nutr* 1993; 57: 917–21.

6. Livingstone PD, Jones C. Treatment of intermittent claudication with vitamin E. *Lancet* 1958; ii: 602–4 [reviews earlier studies].

7. Piesse JW. Vitamin E and peripheral vascular disease. *Internat Clin Nutr Rev* 1984; 4: 178–82 [review].

8. Neglen P et al. Peroral magnesium hydroxide therapy and intermittent claudication. *VASA* 1985; 14: 285–88.

9. Christie SBM, Conway N, Pearson HES. Observations on the performance of a standard exercise test by claudicants taking gamma-linolenic acid. *J Atheroscler Res* 1968; 8: 83–90.

10. Brevetti G, Chiariello M, Ferulano G, et al. Increases in walking distance in patients with peripheral vascular disease treated with L-carnitine: a double-blind, cross-over study. *Circulation* 1988; 77: 767–73.

11. Brevetti G, Perna S, Sabba C, et al. Effect of propionyl-L-carnitine

on quality of life in intermittent claudication. *Am J Cardiol* 1997; 79: 777–80.

12. Schneider B. *Ginkgo biloba* extract in peripheral arterial disease. Meta-analysis of controlled clinical trials. *Arzneim Forsch* 1992; 42: 428–36 [in German].

13. Bauer U. Six-month double-blind randomised clinical trial of *Ginkgo biloba* extract versus placebo in two parallel groups in patients suffering from peripheral arterial insufficiency. *Arzneim Forsch* 1984; 34: 716–20 [in German].

14. Blume, Kieser M, Ischer U. Placebo-controlled, double-blind study on the efficacy of *Ginkgo biloba* special extract EGb 761 in maximum-level trained patients with intermittent claudication. *VASA* 1996; 25: 265–74.

15. Kiesewetter H, Jung F, Jung EM, et al. Effects of garlic coated tablets in peripheral arterial occlusive disease. *Clin Invest* 1993; 71: 383–86.

Iron-Deficiency Anemia

1. Looker AC, Dallman PR, Carroll MD, et al. Prevalence of iron deficiency in the United States. *JAMA* 1997; 277: 973–76.

2. Sullivan JL. Stored iron and ischemic heart disease. *Circulation* 1992; 86: 1036 [editorial].

3. Morck TA, Lynch SR, Cook JD. Inhibition of food iron absorption by coffee. *Am J Clin Nutr* 1983; 37: 416–20

4. Mehta SW, Pritchard ME, Stegman C. Contribution of coffee and tea to anemia among NHANES II participants. *Nutr Res* 1992; 12: 209–22.

5. Kaltwasser JP, Werner E, Schalk K, et al. Clinical trial on the effect of regular tea drinking on iron accumulation in genetic haemochromatosis. *Gut* 1998; 43: 699–704.

6. Cook JD, Noble NL, Morck TA, et al. Effect of fiber on nonheme iron absorption. *Gastroenterology* 1983; 85: 1354–58.

7. Mejia LA, Chew F. Hematological effect of supplementing anemic children with vitamin A

alone and in combination with iron. *Am J Clin Nutr* 1988; 48: 595–600.

8. Ajayi OA, Nnaji UR. Effect of ascorbic acid supplementation on haematological response and ascorbic acid status of young female adults. *Ann Nutr Metab* 1990; 34: 32–36.

9. Hunt JR, Gallagher SK, Johnson LK. Effect of ascorbic acid on apparent iron absorption by women with low iron stores. *Am J Clin Nutr* 1994; 59: 1381–85.

Irritable Bowel Syndrome (IBS)

1. Bentley SJ, Pearson DJ, Rix KJ. Food hypersensitivity in irritable bowel syndrome. *Lancet* 1983; ii: 295–97.

2. McKee AM, Prior A, Whorwell PJ. Exclusion diets in irritable bowel syndrome: are they worthwhile? *J Clin Gastroenterol* 1987; 9: 526–28.

3. Farah DA, Calder I, Benson L, Mackenzie JF. Specific food intolerance: its place as a cause of gastrointestinal symptoms. *Gut* 1985; 26: 164–68.

4. King TS, Elia M, Hunter JO. Abnormal colonic fermentation in irritable bowel syndrome. *Lancet* 1998; 352: 1187–89.

5. Alun Jones V, McLaughlan P, Shorthouse M, et al. Food intolerance: A major factor in the pathogenesis of irritable bowel syndrome. *Lancet* 1982; ii: 1115–17.

6. Smith MA, Youngs GR, Finn R. Food intolerance, atopy, and irritable bowel syndrome. *Lancet* 1985; ii: 1064 [letter].

7. Parker TJ, Naylor SJ, Riordan AM, Hunter JO. Management of patients with food intolerance in irritable bowel syndrome: the development and use of an exclusion diet. *J Human Nutr Diet* 1995; 8: 159–66.

8. Alun Jones V, Shorthouse M, Workman E, Hunter JO. Food intolerance and the irritable bowel. *Lancet* 1983; ii: 633–34 [letter].

9. Birtwistle S. Letter. *Lancet* 1983; II: 634.

10. Fernandez-Banares F, Esteve-Pardo M, de Leon R, et al. Sugar malabsorption in functional bowel disease: clinical implications. *Am J Gastroenterol* 1993; 88: 2044–50.

11. Paganelli R, Fagiolo U, Cancian M, et al. Intestinal permeability in irritable bowel syndrome. Effect of diet and sodium cromoglycate administration. *Ann Allergy* 1990; 64: 377–80.

12. Alun Jones V, McLaughlan P, Shorthouse M, et al. Food intolerance: A major factor in the pathogenesis of irritable bowel syndrome. *Lancet* 1982; ii: 1115–17.

13. Manning AP, Heaton KW, Harvey RF, Uglow P. Wheat fibre and irritable bowel syndrome. *Lancet* 1977; ii: 417–18.

14. Hotz J, Plein K. Effectiveness of plantago seed husks in comparison with wheat bran no stool frequency and manifestations of irritable colon syndrome with constipation. *Med Klin* 1994; 89: 645–51.

15. Cann PA, Read NW, Holdsworth CD. What is the benefit of coarse wheat bran in patients with irritable bowel syndrome? *Gut* 1984; 25: 168–73.

16. Arffmann S, Andersen JR, Hegnhoj J, et al. The effect of coarse wheat bran in the irritable bowel syndrome. A double-blind cross-over study. *Scand J Gastroenterol* 1985; 20: 295–98.

17. Soloft J, Krag B, Gudmand-Hoyer E, et al. A double-blind trial of the effect of wheat bran on symptoms of irritable bowel syndrome. *Lancet* 1976; i: 270–73.

18. Lucey MR, Clark ML, Lowndes J, Dawson AM. Is bran efficacious in irritable bowel syndrome? A double blind placebo controlled crossover study. *Gut* 1987; 28: 221–25.

19. Francis CY, Whorwell PJ. Bran and irritable bowel syndrome: time for reappraisal. *Lancet* 1994; 344: 39–40.

20. Gaby AR. Commentary. *Nutrition and Healing* 1996; Feb: 1,10–11 [review].

21. Niec AM, Frankum B, Talley NJ. Are adverse food reactions linked to irritable bowel syndrome? *Am J Gastroenterol* 1998; 93: 2184–90 [review].

22. Whitehead WE, Palsson OS. Is rectal pain sensitivity a biological

marker for irritable bowel syndrome: psychological influences on pain perception. *Gastroenterology* 1998; 115: 1263–71.

23. Dancey CP, Taghavi M, Fox RJ. The relationship between daily stress and symptoms of irritable bowel: a time-series approach. *J Psychosom Res* 1998; 44: 537–45.

24. Guthrie E, Creed F, Dawson D, Tomenson BG. A controlled trial of psychological treatment for the irritable bowel syndrome. *Gastroenterology* 1991; 100: 450–57.

25. Harvey RF. Individual and group hypnotherapy in treatment of refractory irritable bowel syndrome. *Lancet* 1989; i: 424–26.

26. Waxman D. The irritable bowel: a pathological or a psychological syndrome? *J R Soc Med* 1988; 81: 718–20.

27. Houghton LA, Heyman DJ, Whorwell PJ. Symptomatology, quality of life and economic features of irritable bowel syndrome—the effect of hypnotherapy. *Aliment Pharmacol Ther* 1996; 10: 91–95.

28. Cotterell CJ, Lee AJ, Hunter JO. Double-blind cross-over trial of evening primrose oil in women with menstrually-related irritable bowel syndrome. In *Omega-6 Essential Fatty Acids: Pathophysiology and roles in clinical medicine.* New York: Alan R. Liss, 1990, 421–26.

29. Bohmer CJ, Tuynman HA. The clinical relevance of lactose malabsorption in irritable bowel syndrome. *Eur J Gastroenterol Hepatol* 1996; 8: 1013–16.

30. Rees WD, Evans BK, Rhodes J. Treating irritable bowel syndrome with peppermint oil. *Br Med J* 1979; 2(6194): 835–36.

31. Liu J-H, Chen G-H, Yeh H-Z, et al. Enteric-coated peppermint-oil capsules in the treatment of irritable bowel syndrome: a prospective, randomized trial. *J Gastroenterol* 1997; 32: 765–68.

32. Dew MJ, Evans BK, Rhodes J. Peppermint oil for the irritable bowel syndrome: A multi-center trial. *Br J Clin Pract* 1984; 38: 394–98.

33. May B, Kuntz HD, Kieser M, Kohler S. Efficacy of a fixed pepper-

mint/caraway oil combination in non-ulcer dyspepsia. *Arzneim Forsch Drug Res* 1996; 46: 1149–53.

34. Westphal J, Hörning M, Leonhardt K. Phytotherapy in functional abdominal complaints: Results of a clinical study with a preparation of several plants. *Phytomedicine* 1996; 2: 285–91.

35. Leicester RJ, Hunt RH. Peppermint oil to reduce colonic spasm during endoscopy. *Lancet* 1982; ii: 989 [letter].

36. Nash P, Gould SR, Barnardo DE. Peppermint oil does not relieve the pain of irritable bowel syndrome. *Br J Clin Pract* 1986; 40: 292–93.

37. Rogers J, Tay HH, Misiewicz JJ. Peppermint oil. *Lancet* 1988; ii: 98–99 [letter].

38. Achterrath-Tuckerman U, Kunde R, et al. Pharmacological investigations with compounds of chamomile. V. Investigations on the spasmolytic effect of compounds of chamomile and Kamillosan on isolated guinea pig ileum. *Planta Med* 1980; 39: 38–50.

39. Hotz J, Plein K. Effectiveness of plantago seed husks in comparison with wheat bran no stool frequency and manifestations of irritable colon syndrome with constipation. *Med Klin* 1994; 89: 645–51.

40. Jalihal A, Kurian G. Ispaghula therapy in irritable bowel syndrome: improvement in overall well-being is related to reduction in bowel dissatisfaction. *J Gastroenterol Hepatol* 1990; 5: 507–13.

41. Prior A, Whorwell PJ. Double blind study of ispaghula irritable bowel syndrome. *Gut* 1987; 11: 1510–13.

42. Mills SY. *Out of the Earth: The Essential Book of Herbal Medicine.* New York: Viking Arkana, 1991, 544–47.

43. Weiss RF. *Herbal Medicine.* Gothenburg, Sweden: Ab Arcanum and Beaconsfield, UK: Beaconsfield Publishers Ltd, 1988, 334–35.

Jet Lag

1. Petrie K, Dawson AG, Thompson L, et al. A double-blind trial of melatonin as a treatment for jet

lag in international cabin crew. *Bio Psych* 1993; 33(7): 526–30.

2. Suhner A, Schlagenhauf P, Johnson R, et al. Comparative study to determine the optimal melatonin dosage form for the alleviation of jet lag. *Chronobiol Int* 1998; 15: 655–66.

Kidney Stones

1. Blacklock N. Renal stone. In: *Western Diseases: Their Emergence and Prevention*, ed. DP Burkitt and HC Trowell. Cambridge, MA: Harvard Press, 1981, 60–70.

2. Massey LK, Roman-Smith H, Sutton RAL. Effect of dietary oxalate and calcium on urinary oxalate and risk of formation of calcium oxalate kidney stones. *J Am Dietet Assoc* 1993; 93: 901–6.

3. Massey LK, Roman-Smith H, Sutton RAL. Effect of dietary oxalate and calcium on urinary oxalate and risk of formation of calcium oxalate kidney stones. *J Am Dietet Assoc* 1993; 93: 901–6.

4. Brinkley L, McGuire J, Gregory J, Pak CYC, et al. Bioavailability of oxalate in foods. *Urology* 1981; 17: 534.

5. Curhan GC, Willett WC, Rimm EB, Stampfer MJ. A Prospective study of dietary calcium and other nutrients and the risk of symptomatic kidney stones. *N Engl J Med* 1993; 328: 833–38.

6. Hassapidou MN, Paraskevopoulos S Th, Karakoltsidis PA, et al. Dietary habits of patients with renal stone disease in Greece. *J Human Nutr Dietet* 1999; 12: 47–51.

7. Robertson WG, Peacock M, Marshall DH. Prevalence of urinary stone disease in vegetarians. *Eur Urol* 1982; 8: 334–39.

8. Hiatt RA, Ettinger B, Caan B, et al. Randomized controlled trial of a low animal protein, high fiber diet in the prevention of recurrent calcium oxalate kidney stones. *Am J Epidemiol* 1996; 144: 25–33.

9. Rao PN, Prendiville V, Buxton A, et al. Dietary management of urinary risk factors in renal stone formers. *Br J Urol* 1982; 54: 578–83.

10. Hughes J, Norman RW. Diet and calcium stones. *Can Med Assoc J* 1992; 146: 137–43 [review].

11. Hassapidou MN, Paraskevopoulos ST, Karakoltsidis PA, et al. Dietary habits of patients with renal stone disease in Greece. *J Human Nutr Dietet* 1999; 12: 47–51.

12. Muldowney FP, Freaney R, Moloney MF. Importance of dietary sodium in the hypercalciuria syndrome. *Kidney Int* 1982; 22: 292–96.

13. Sabto J, Powell MJ, Gurr B, Gurr FW. Influence of urinary sodium on calcium excretion in normal individuals. *Med J Austral* 1984; 140: 354–56.

14. Silver J, Rubinger D, Friedlaender MM, Popovitzer MM. Sodium-dependent idiopathic hypercalciuria in renal-stone formers. *Lancet* 1983; ii: 484–86.

15. Massey LK, Whiting SJ. Dietary salt, urinary calcium, and kidney stone risk. *Nutr Rev* 1995; 131–39 [review].

16. Hughes J, Norman RW. Diet and calcium stones. *Can Med Assoc J* 1992; 146: 137–43 [review].

17. Sakhaee K, Harvey JA, Padalino PK, et al. The potential role of salt abuse on the risk for kidney stone formation. *J Urol* 1993; 150(2 Pt. 1): 310–12.

18. Lehman J Jr, Pleuss JA, Gray RW, Hoffman RG. Potassium administration increases and potassium deprivation reduces urinary calcium excretion in healthy adults. *Kidney Int* 1991; 39: 973–83.

19. Curhan GC, Willett WC, Rimm EB, Stampfer MJ. A prospective study of dietary calcium and other nutrients and the risk of symptomatic kidney stones. *N Engl J Med* 1993; 328: 833–38.

20. Breslau NA, Padalino P, Kok DJ, et al. Physicochemical effects of a new slow-release potassium phosphate preparation (UroPhos-K) in absorptive hypercalciuria. *J Bone Miner Res* 1995; 10: 394–400.

21. Ettinger B, Pak CY, Citron JT, et al. Potassium-magnesium citrate is an effective prophylaxis against recurrent calcium oxalate nephrolithiasis. *J Urol* 1997; 158: 2069–73.

22. Pak CY. Medical prevention of renal stone disease. *Nephron* 1999; 81(suppl 1): 60–65 [review].

23. Pak CY. Nephrolithiasis from calcium supplementation. *J Urol* 1987; 137: 1212–13 [editorial].

24. Levine BS, Rodman JS, Wienerman S, et al. Effect of calcium citrate supplementation on urinary calcium oxalate saturation in female stone formers: implications for prevention of osteoporosis. *Am J Clin Nutr* 1994; 60: 592–96.

25. Seltzer MA, Low RK, McDonald M, et al. Dietary manipulation with lemonade to treat hypocitraturic calcium nephrolithiasis. *J Urol* 1996; 156: 907–9.

26. Curhan GC, Willett WC, Speizer FE, Stampfer MJ. Beverage use and risk for kidney stones in women. *Ann Intern Med* 1998; 128: 534–40.

27. Curhan GC, Willett WC, Rimm EB, et al. Prospective study of beverage use and the risk of kidney stones. *Am J Epidemiol* 1996; 143: 240–47.

28. Shah PJR. Unprocessed bran and its effect on urinary calcium excretion in idiopathic hypercalciuria. *Br Med J* 1980; 281: 426.

29. Ebisuno S, Morimoto S, Yoshida T, et al. Rice-bran treatment for calcium stone formers with idiopathic hypercalciuria. *Brit J Urol* 1986; 58: 592–95.

30. Rao PN, Gordon C, Davies D, Blacklock NJ. Are stone formers maladapted to refined carbohydrates? *Br J Urol* 1982; 54: 575–77.

31. Li MK, Kavanagh JP, Prendiville V, et al. Does sucrose damage kidneys? *Br J Urol* 1986; 58: 353–57.

32. Lemann J Jr, Piering WF, Lennon EJ. Possible role of carbohydrate-induced calciuria in calcium oxalate kidney-stone formation. *N Engl J Med* 1969; 280: 232–37.

33. Gaby AR. Commentary. *Nutr Healing* 1996; Jan: 1,10–11.

34. Piesse JW. Nutritional factors in calcium containing kidney stones with particular emphasis on vitamin C. *Int Clin Nutr Rev* 1985; 5: 110–29 [review].

35. Robertson WG, Peacock M, Heyburn PJ, Hanes FA. Epidemiological risk factors in calcium stone disease. *Scand J Urol Nephrol Supplement* 1980; 53: 15–30.

36. Hollingbery PW, Massey LK. Effect of dietary caffeine and sucrose on urinary calcium excretion in adolescents. *Fed Proc* 1986; 45: 375 [abstr #1280].

37. Kiel DP, Felson DT, Hannan MT, et al. Caffeine and the risk of hip fracture: the Framingham study. *Am J Epidemiol* 1990; 132: 675–84.

38. Curhan GC, Willett WC, Rimm EB, et al. Prospective study of beverage use and the risk of kidney stones. *Am J Epidemiol* 1996; 143: 240–47.

39. Shuster J, Finlayson B, Scheaffer RL, et al. Primary liquid intake and urinary stone disease. *J Chron Dis* 1985; 38: 907–14.

40. Curhan GC, Willett WC, Speizer FE, Stampfer MJ. Beverage use and risk for kidney stones in women. *Ann Intern Med* 1998; 128: 534–40.

41. Shuster J, Finlayson B, Scheaffer RL, et al. Primary liquid intake and urinary stone disease. *J Chron Dis* 1985; 38: 907–14.

42. Shuster J, Jenkins A, Logan C, et al. Soft drink consumption and urinary stone recurrence: a randomized prevention trial. *J Clin Epidemiol* 1992; 45: 911–16.

43. Curhan GC, Willett WC, Rimm EB, et al. Prospective study of beverage use and the risk of kidney stones. *Am J Epidemiol* 1996; 143: 240–47.

44. Marshall RW, Cochran M, Hodgkinson A. Relationship between calcium and oxalic acid intake in the diet and their excretion in the urine of normal and renal-stone forming subjects. *Clin Sci* 1972; 43: 91–99.

45. Lemann J Jr. Composition of the diet and calcium kidney stones. *N Engl J Med* 1993; 328: 880–82 [editorial].

46. Curhan GC, Willett WC, Rimm EB, Stampfer MJ. A prospective study of dietary calcium and other nutrients and the risk of symptomatic

kidney stones. *N Engl J Med* 1993; 328: 833–38.

47. Hassapidou MN, Paraskevopoulos S Th, Karakoltsidis PA, et al. Dietary habits of patients with renal stone disease in Greece. *J Human Nutr Dietet* 1999; 12: 47–51.

48. Sowers MFR, Hannausch M, Wood C, et al. Prevalence of renal stones in a population-based study with dietary calcium, oxalate, and medication exposures. *Am J Epidemiol* 1998; 147: 914–20.

49. Curhan GC, Willett WC, Speizer FE, et al. Comparison of dietary calcium with supplemental calcium and other nutrients as factors affecting the risk for kidney stones in women. *Ann Intern Med* 1997; 126: 497–504.

50. Curhan GC, Willett WC, Speizer FE, Stampfer MJ. A prospective study of dietary and supplemental calcium and the risk of kidney stones in women. *Am J Epidemiol* 1996; 143(11 suppl): S15 [abstr #57].

51. Pak CY. Nephrolithiasis from calcium supplementation. *J Urol* 1987; 137: 1212–13 [editorial].

52. Levine BS, Rodman JS, Wienerman S, et al. Effect of calcium citrate supplementation on urinary calcium oxalate saturation in female stone formers: implications for prevention of osteoporosis. *Am J Clin Nutr* 1994; 60: 592–96.

53. Pak CY, Sakhaee K, Hwang TIS, et al. Nephrolithiasis from calcium supplementation. *J Urol* 1987; 137: 1212–13 [editorial/review].

54. Bataille IP, Charransol G, Gregoire I, et al. Effect of calcium restriction on renal excretion of oxalate and the probability of stones in the various pathophsiological groups with calcium stones. *J Urol* 1983; 130: 218–23.

55. Bataille IP, Charransol G, Gregoire I, et al. Effect of calcium restriction on renal excretion of oxalate and the probability of stones in the various pathophysiological groups with calcium stones. *J Urol* 1983; 130: 218–23.

56. Broadus AE, Insogna KL, Lang R, et al. Evidence for disordered control of 1,25-dihydroxyvitamin D production in absorptive hypercalciuria. *N Engl J Med* 1984; 311: 73–80.

57. Netelenbos JC, Jongen MJM, van der Vijgh WJF, et al. Vitamin D status in urinary calcium stone formation. *Arch Intern Med* 1985; 145: 681–84.

58. Rao PN, Blacklock NJ. Hypercalciuria. *Lancet* 1983: ii: 747 [letter].

59. Nath R, Thind SK, Murthy MSR, et al. Role of pyridoxine in oxalate metabolism. *Ann NY Acad Sci* 1990; 585: 274–84 [review].

60. Watts RWE, Veall N, et al. The effect of pyridoxine on oxalate dynamics in three cases of primary hyperoxaluria (with glycollic aciduria). *Clin Sci* 1985; 69: 87–90.

61. Mitwalli A, Ayiomamitis W, Grass L, Oreopoulos DG. Control of hyperoxaluria with large doses of pyridoxine in patients with kidney stones. *Int Urol Nephrol* 1988; 20: 353–59.

62. Berkow R, Talbott JH, et al. *The Merck Manual of Diagnosis and Therapy*, 13th ed, Rahway, NJ: Merck Sharp & Dohme, 1977, 732.

63. Gershoff SN, Prien EL. Effect of daily MgO and vitamin B_6 administration to patients with recurring calcium oxalate kidney stones. *Am J Clin Nutr* 1967; 20(5)393–99.

64. Prien EL, Gershoff SF. Magnesium oxide-pyridoxine therapy for recurrent calcium oxalate calculi. *J Urol* 1974; 112: 509–12.

65. Johansson G, Backman U, Danielson BG, et al. Effects of magnesium hydroxide in renal stone disease. *J Am Coll Nutr* 1982; 1: 179–85.

66. Ettiniger B, Citron JT, Livermore B, Dolman LI. Chlorthalidone reduces calcium oxalate calculus recurrence but magnesium hydroxide does not. *J Urol* 1988; 139: 679–84.

67. Prien EL, Gershoff SF. Magnesium oxide-pyridoxine therapy for recurrent calcium oxalate calculi. *J Urol* 1974; 112: 509–12.

68. Will EJ, Bijvoet OL. Primary oxalosis: clinical and biochemical response to high-dose pyridoxine therapy. *Metabolism* 1979; 28: 542–48.

69. Lindberg J, Harvey J, Pak CY. Effect of magnesium citrate and mag-nesium oxide on the crystallization of calcium salts in urine: changes produced by food-magnesium interaction. *J Urol* 1990; 143: 248–51.

70. Piesse JW. Nutritional factors in calcium containing kidney stones with particular emphasis on vitamin C. *Int Clin Nutr Rev* 1985; 5(3): 110–29 [review].

71. Ringsdorf WM, Cheraskin WM. Medical complications from ascorbic acid: a review and interpretation (part one). *J Holistic Med* 1984; 6(1): 49–63.

72. Hoffer A. Ascorbic acid and kidney stones. *Can Med Assoc J* 1985; 32: 320 [letter].

73. Wandzilak TR, D'Andre SD, Davis PA, Williams HE. Effect of high dose vitamin C on urinary oxalate levels. *J Urol* 1994; 151: 834–37.

74. Levine M. Vitamin C and optimal health. Presented at the February 25, 1999 60th Annual Biology Colloquium, Oregon State University, Corvallis, Oregon.

75. Levine M, Conry-Cantilena C, Wang Y, et al. Vitamin C pharmacokinetics in healthy volunteers: evidence for a recommended dietary allowance. *Proc Natl Acad Sci U S A* 1996; 93: 3704–9.

76. Auer BL, Auer D, Rodgers AL. Relative hyperoxaluria, crystalluria and haematuria after megadose ingestion of vitamin C. *Eur J Clin Invest* 1998; 28: 695–700.

77. Baggio B, Gambaro G, Marchini F, et al. Correction of erythrocyte abnormalities in idiopathic calcium-oxalate nephrolithiasis and reduction of urinary oxalate by oral glycosaminoglycans. *Lancet* 1991; 338: 403–5.

78. Blumenthal M, Busse WR, Goldberg A, et al. (eds). *The Complete German Commission E Monographs: Therapeutic Guide to Herbal Medicines*. Austin: American Botanical Council and Boston: Integrative Medicine Communications, 1998, 428.

Lactose Intolerance

1. Gudmand-Hoyer E. The clinical significance of disaccharide

maldigestion. *Am J Clin Nutr* 1994; 59(3): 735S–41S.

2. Ledochowski M, Sperner-Unterweger S, Fuchs D. Lactose malabsorption is associated with early signs of mental depression in females: A preliminary report. *Digest Dis Sci* 1998; 43: 2513–17.

(Systemic Lupus Erythematosus [SLE])

1. Kardestuncer T, Frumkin H. Systemic lupus erythematosus in relation to environmental pollution: an investigation in an African-American community in North Georgia. *Arch Environ Health* 1997; 52: 85–90.

2. Fjellner B. Drug-induced lupus erythematosus aggravated by oral therapy. *Acta Derm Venereol* 1979; 59: 368–70.

3. Nagata C, Fuyita, Iwata H, et al. Systemic lupus erythematosus: a case-control epidemiologic study in Japan. *Int J Dermatol* 1995; 34: 333–37.

4. Minami Y, Sasaki Ti, Komatsu S, et al. Female systemic lupus erythematosus in Miyagi Prefecture, Japan: a case-control study of dietary and reproductive factors. *Tohoku J Exp Med* 1993; 169: 245–52.

5. Nagata C, Fuyita, Iwata H, et al. Systemic lupus erythematosus: a case-control epidemiologic study in Japan. *Int J Dermatol* 1995; 34: 333–37.

6. Kardestuncer T, Frumkin H. Systemic lupus erythematosus in relation to environmental pollution: an investigation in an African-American community in North Georgia. *Arch Environ Health* 1997; 52: 85–90.

7. Comstock GW, Burke AE, Hoffman SC, et al. Serum concentrations of alpha-tocopherol, beta-carotene, and retinol preceding the diagnosis of rheumatoid arthritis and systemic lupus erythematosus. *Ann Rheum Dis* 1997; 56: 323–35.

8. Nagata C, Fuyita, Iwata H, et al. Systemic lupus erythematosus: a case-control epidemiologic study in Japan. *Int J Dermatol* 1995; 34: 333–37.

9. Shigemasa C, Tanaka T, Mashiba H. Effect of vegetarian diet on systemic lupus erythematosus. *Lancet* 1992; 339: 1177 [letter].

10. Minami Y, Sasaki Ti, Komatsu S, et al. Female systemic lupus erythematosus in Miyagi Prefecture, Japan: a case-control study of dietary and reproductive factors. *Tohoku J Exp Med* 1993; 169: 245–52.

11. Corman LC. The role of diet in animal models of systemic lupus erythematosus: possible implications for human lupus. *Semin Arthritis Rheum* 1985; 15: 61–69 [review].

12. Clark WF, Parbtani A, Huff MW, et al. Flaxseed: a potential treatment for lupus nephritis. *Kidney Int* 1995; 48: 475–80.

13. Prasad K. Hydroxyl radical-scavenging property of secoisolariciresinol diglucoside (SDG) isolated from flax-seed. *Mol Cell Biochem* 1997; 168: 117–23.

14. Diumenjo MS, Lisanti M, Valles R, Rivero I. Allergic manifestations of systemic lupus erythematosus. *Allergol Immunopathol (Madr)* 1985; 13: 323–26 [in Spanish].

15. Nagata C, Fuyita, Iwata H, et al. Systemic lupus erythematosus: a case-control epidemiologic study in Japan. *Int J Dermatol* 1995; 34: 333–37.

16. Carr RI, Tilley D, Forsyth S, et al. Failure of oral tolerance in (NZB X NZW)F1 mice is antigen specific and appears to parallel antibody patterns in human systemic lupus erythematosus (SLE). *Clin Immunol Immunopathol* 1987; 42: 298–310.

17. Rutkowska-Sak L, Legatowicz-Koprowska M, Ryzko J, Socha J. Changes in the gastrointestinal system of children with inflammatory systemic connective tissue diseases. *Pediatr Pol* 1995; 70: 235–41 [in Polish].

18. Carr R, Forsyth S, Sadi D. Abnormal responses to ingested substances in murine systemic lupus erythematosus: apparent effect of a casein-free diet on the development of systemic lupus erythematosus in NZB/W mice. *J Rheumatol* 1987; 14 (suppl 13): 158–65.

19. Bardana EJ Jr, Malinow MR, Houghton DC, et al. Diet-induced systemic lupus erythematosus (SLE) in primates. *Am J Kidney Dis* 1982; 1: 345–52.

20. Roberts JL, Hayashi JA. Exacerbation of SLE associated with alfalfa ingestion. *N Engl J Med* 1983; 308(22): 1361 [letter].

21. Malinow MR, McLaughlin P, Bardana EJ Jr, Craig S. Elimination of toxicity from diets containing alfalfa seeds. *Food Chem Toxicol* 1984; 22: 583–87.

22. Hardy CJ, Palmer BP, Muir KR, et al. Smoking history, alcohol consumption, and systemic lupus erythematosus: a case-control study. *Ann Rheum Dis* 1998; 57: 451–55.

23. Kelley VE, Ferretti A, Izui S, Strom TB. A fish oil diet rich in eicosapentaenoic acid reduces cyclooxygenase metabolites, and suppresses lupus in MRL-1pr mice. *J Immunol* 1985; 134: 2914–19.

24. Walton AJE, Snaith ML, Locniskar M, et al. Dietary fish oil and the severity of symptoms in patients with systemic lupus erythematosus. *Ann Rheum Dis* 1991; 50: 463–66.

25. Westberg G, Tarkowski A. Effect of MaxEPA in patients with SLE. *Scand J Rheumatology* 1990; 19: 137–43.

26. Comstock GW, Burke AE, Hoffman SC, et al. Serum concentrations of alpha-tocopherol, beta-carotene, and retinol preceding the diagnosis of rheumatoid arthritis and systemic lupus erythematosus. *Ann Rheum Dis* 1997; 56: 323–35.

27. Weimann BJ, Weiser H. Effects of antioxidant vitamins C, E, and beta-carotene on immune functions in MRL/lpr mice and rats. *Ann N Y Acad Sci* 1992; 669: 390–92.

28. Ayres S Jr, Mihan R. Is vitamin E involved in the autoimmune mechanism? *Cutis* 1978; 21: 321–25.

29. Ayres S Jr, Mihan R. Lupus erythematosus and vitamin E: an effective and nontoxic therapy. *Cutis* 1979; 23: 49–54.

30. Yell JA, Burge S, Wojnarowska F. Vitamin E and discoid lupus erythematosus. *Lupus* 1992; 1: 303–5.

31. Newbold PC. Beta-carotene in the treatment of discoid lupus erythematosus. *Br J Dermatol* 1976; 95: 100–1.

Part One: References

32. Dubois EL, Patterson C. Ineffectiveness of beta-carotene in lupus erythematosus *JAMA* 1976; 236: 138–39 [letter].

33. Welsh AL. Lupus erythematosus: Treatment by combined use of massive amounts of pantothenic acid and vitamin E. *Arch Dermatol Syphilol* 1954; 70: 181–98.

34. Cochrane T, Leslie G. The treatment of lupus erythematosus with calcium pantothenate and panthenol. *J Invest Dermatol* 1952; 18: 365–67.

35. Van Vollenhoven RF, Engleman EG, McGuire JL. Dehydroepiandrosterone in systemic lupus erythematosus. Results of a double-blind, placebo-controlled, randomized clinical trial. *Arthritis Rheum* 1995; 38: 1826–31.

36. Van Vollenhoven RF, Morabito LM, Engleman EG, McGuire JL. Treatment of systemic lupus erythematosus with dehyroepiandrosterone: 50 patients treated up to 12 months. *J Rheumatol* 1998; 25: 285–89.

37. Van Vollenhoven RF, Engleman EG, McGuire JL. An open study of dehydroepiandrosterone in systemic lupus erythematosus. *Arthritis Rheum* 1994; 37: 1305–10.

38. Barry NN, McGuire JL, van Vollenhoven RF. Dehydroepiandrosterone in systemic lupus erythematosus: relationship between dosage, serum levels, and clinical response. *J Rheumatol* 1998; 25: 2352–56.

39. van Hollenhoven RF, Morabito LM, Engleman EG, McGuire JL. Treatment of systemic lupus erythematosus with dehydroepiandrosterone: 50 patients treated up to 12 months. *J Rheumatol* 1998; 25: 285–89.

40. Orner GA et al. Dehydroepiandrosterone is a complete hepatocarcinogen and potent tumor promoter in the absence of peroxisome proliferation in rainbow trout. *Carcinogenesis* 1995; 16: 2893–98.

41. Metzger C, Mayer D, et al. Sequential appearance and ultrastructure of amphophilic cell foci, adenomas, and carcinomas in the liver of male and female rats treated with dehydroepiandrosterone. *Taxicol Pathol* 1995; 23: 591–605.

42. Schwartz AG. Inhibition of spontaneous breast cancer formation in female C3H (A vy/a) mice by long-term treatment with dehydroepiandrosterone. *Cancer Res* 1979; 39: 1129–32.

43. McNeil C. Potential drug DHEA hits snags on way to clinic. *J Natl Cancer Inst* 1997; 89: 681–83.

44. Jones JA, Nguyen A, Strab M, et al. Use of DHEA in a patient with advanced prostate cancer: a case report and review. *Urology* 1997; 50: 784–88.

45. Zumoff B, Levin J, Rosenfeld RS, et al. Abnormal 24-hr mean plasma concentrations of dehydroisoandrosterone and dehydroisoandrosterone sulfate in women with primary operable breast cancer. *Cancer Res* 1981; 41: 3360–63.

46. Skolnick AA. Scientific verdict still out on DHEA. *JAMA* 1996; 276: 1365–67 [review].

47. Sahelian R. New supplements and unknown, long-term consequences. *Am J Natural Med* 1997; 4: 8 [editorial].

48. Casson PR, Santoro N, Elkind-Hirsch K, et al. Postmenopausal dehydroepiandrosterone administration increases free insulin-like growth factor-I and decreases high-density lipoprotein: a six-month trial. *Fertil Steril* 1998; 70: 107–10.

49. Wang ZY. Clinical and laboratory studies of the effect of an antilupus pill on systemic lupus erythematosus. *Chung His I Chieh Ho Tsa Chih* 1989; 9: 452,465–68 [in Chinese].

50. Ruan J, Ye RG. Lupus nephritis treated with impact therapy of cyclophosphamide and traditional Chinese medicine. *Chung Kuo Chung His I Chieh Ho Tsa Chih* 1994; 14: 260,276–78 [in Chinese].

51. Chen JR, Yen JH, Lin CC, et al. The effects of Chinese herbs on improving survival and inhibiting anti-ds DNA antibody production in lupus mice. *Am J Chin Med* 1993; 21: 257–62.

52. Werbach MR, Murray MT. *Botanical Influences on Illness*. Tarzana, CA: Third Line Press, 1994, 234–35 [review].

53. Werbach MR, Murray MT. *Botanical Influences on Illness*. Tarzana, CA: Third Line Press, 1994, 234–35 [review].

54. Roberts JL, Hayashi JA. Exacerbation of SLE associated with alfalfa ingestion. *N Engl J Med* 1995; 308(22): 1361 [letter].

55. Whittam J, Jensen C, Hudson T. Alfalfa, vitamin E, and autoimmune disorders. *Am J Clin Nut* 1995; 62: 1025–26.

Macular Degeneration

1. National Advisory Eye Council. Report of the Retinal and Choroidal Diseases Panel: Vision Research CA National Plan: 1983–1987. Bethesda, MD: U.S. Dept of Health and Human Services, 1984. National Institutes of Health publication 83-2471.

2. Young RW. Solar radiation and age-related macular degeneration. *Surv Ophthalmol* 1988: 32: 252–69.

3. Katz ML, Parker KR, Handelman GJ, et al. Effects of antioxidant nutrient deficiency on the retina and retinal pigment epithelium of albino rats: a light and electron microscopic study. *Exp Eye Res* 1982; 34: 339–69.

4. West S, Vitale S, Hallfrisch J, et al. Are anti-oxidants or supplements protective of age-related macular degeneration? *Arch Ophthalmol* 1994: 112: 222–27.

5. Eye Disease Case-Control Study Group. Antioxidant status and neovascular age-related macular degeneration. *Arch Ophthalmol* 1993: 111: 104–9.

6. Goldberg J, Flowerdew G, Smith E, et al. Factors associated with age-related macular degeneration. *Am J Epidemiol* 1988: 128: 700–10.

7. Bone RA. Landrum JT. Distribution of macular pigment components, zeaxanthin and lutein, in human retina. *Methods Enzymol* 1992: 213: 360–66.

8. Blumenkranz MS, Russell SR, Robey MG, et al. Risk factors in age-related maculopathy complicated by choroidal neovascularization. *Ophthalmol* 1986: 96: 552–58.

9. Mares-Perlman JA, Brady WE, Kleain R, et al. Serum antioxidants and age-related macular degeneration in a population-based case-control study. *Arch Ophthalmol* 1995; 113: 1518–23.

10. Seddon JM, Ajani UA, Sperduto RD, et al. Dietary carotenoids, vitamins A, C, and E, and advanced age-related macular degeneration. *JAMA* 1994: 272: 1413–20.

11. Newsome DA, Swartz M, Leone NC, et al. Oral zinc in macular degeneration. *Arch Ophthalmol* 1988: 106: 192–98.

12. Stur M, Tihl M, Reitner A, Meisinger V. Oral zinc and the second eye in age-related macular degeneration. *Invest Ophtholmol* 1966; 37: 1225–35.

13. Lebuisson DA, Leroy L, Reigal G. Treatment of senile macular degeneration with *Ginkgo biloba* extract: a preliminary double-blind study versus placebo. In *Rokan (Ginkgo biloba): Recent Results in Pharmacology and Clinic,* Fünfgeld FW, ed. Berlin: Springer-Verlag, 1988, 231–36.

14. Scharrer A, Ober M. Anthocyanosides in the treatment of retinopathies. *Klin Monatsbl Augenheikld Beih* 1981; 178: 386–89.

15. Mian E, Curri SB, et al. Anthocyanosides and the walls of microvessels: Further aspects of the mechanism of action of their protective in syndromes due to abnormal capillary fragility. *Minerva Med* 1977; 68: 3565–81.

Menopause

1. Baird DD, Umbach DM, Landsedell L, et al. Dietary intervention study to assess estrogenicity of dietary soy among postmenopausal women. *J Clin Endocrinol Metab* 1995; 80: 1685–90.

2. Cassidy A, Bingham S, Setchell KDR. Biological effects of a diet of soy protein rich in isoflavones on the men-strual cycle of premenopausal women. *Am J Clin Nutr* 1994; 60: 333–40.

3. Knight DC, Eden JA. A review of the clinical effects of phytoestrogens. *Obstet Gynecol* 1996; 87: 897–904 [review].

4. Albertazzi P, Pansini F, Bonaccorsi G, et al. The effect of dietary soy supplementation on hot flushes. *Obstet Gynecol* 1998; 91: 6–11.

5. Murkies AL, Lombard C, Strauss BJ, et al. Dietary flour supplementation decreases post-menopausal hot flushes: effect of soy and wheat. *Maturitas* 1995; 21: 189–95.

6. Brezinski A, Adlercreutz H, Shaoul R, et al. Short-term effects of phytoestrogen-rich diet on post-menopausal women. *Menopause* 1997; 4: 89–94.

7. Lee JR. *Natural Progesterone. The multiple roles of a remarkable hormone.* Sebastipol, CA: BLL Publishing, 1993, 31–37.

8. Gaby AR. Commentary. *Nutr Healing* 1996; June: 1,10–11.

9. Wright JV. Hormones for menopause. *Nutr Healing* 1996; June: 1–2,9.

10. Greendale GA, Reboussin BA, Hogan P, et al. Symptom relief and side effects of postmenopausal hormones: results from the Postmenopausal Estrogen/Progestin Interventions Trial. *Obstet Gynecol* 1998; 92: 982–88.

11. Bullock JL, Massey FM, Gambrell RD Jr. Use of medroxyprogesterone acetate to prevent menopausal symptoms. *Obstet Gynecol* 1975; 46: 165–68.

12. Morrison JC, Martin DC, Blair RA, et al. The use of medroxyprogesterone acetate for relief of climateric symptoms. *Am J Obstet Gynecol* 1980 138: 99–104.

13. Schiff I, Tulchinsky D, Cramer D, Ryan KJ. Oral medroxyprogesterone in the treatment of postmenopausal symptoms. *JAMA* 1980; 244: 1443–45.

14. Ivarsson T, Spetz AC, Hammar M. Physical exercise and vasomotor symptoms in postmenopausal women. *Mauritas* 1998; 29: 139–46.

15. Hammar M, Berg G, Lindgren R. Does physical exercise influence the frequency of postmenopausal hot flushes? *Acta Obstet Gynecol Scand* 1990; 69: 409–12.

16. Slaven L, Lee C. Mood and symptom reporting among middle-aged women: the relationship between menopausal status, hormone replacement therapy, and exercise participation. *Health Psychol* 1997; 16: 203–8.

17. Perloff WH. Treatment of the menopause. *Am J Obstet Gynecol* 1949; 58: 684–94.

18. Gozan HA. The use of vitamin E in treatment of the menopause. *NY State J Med* 1952; 52: 1289.

19. Christy CJ. Vitamin E in menopause: Preliminary report of experimental and clinical study. *Am J Obstet Gynecol* 1945: 50: 84.

20. Finkler RS. The effect of vitamin E in the menopause. *J Clin Endocrinol Metab* 1949; 9: 89–94.

21. Rubenstein BB. Vitamin E diminishes the vasomotor symptoms of menopause. *Fed Proc* 1948; 7: 106 [abstr].

22. Blatt MHG et al. Vitamin E and climacteric syndrome: failure of effective control as measured by menopausal index. *Arch Intern Med* 1953; 91: 792–99.

23. Barton DL, Loprinzi CL, Quella SK, et al. Prospective evaluation of vitamin E for hot flashes in breast cancer survivors. *J Clin Oncol* 1998; 16: 495–500.

24. CJ Smith. Non-hormonal control of vaso-motor flushing in menopausal patients. *Chicago Med* 1964; 67: 193–95.

25. Duker EM. Effects of extracts from *Cimicifuga racemosa* on gonadotropin release in menopausal women and ovariectomized rats. *Planta Med* 1991; 57: 420–24.

26. Lieberman S. A review of the effectiveness of *Cimicifuga racemosa* (black cohosh) for the symptoms of menopause. *J Womens Health* 1998; 7: 525–29.

27. Duke JA. *CRC Handbook of Medicinal Herbs.* Boca Raton, FL: CRC Press, 1985, 420–21[review].

28. Crawford AM. *The Herbal Menopause Book*. Freedom, CA: Crossing Press, 1996.

Menorrhagia (Heavy Menstruation)

1. Samuels, AJ. Studies in patients with functional menorrhagia: the antimenorrhagic effect of the adequate replication of iron stores. *Israel J Med Sci* 1965; 1: 851.

2. Taymor ML, Sturgis SH, Yahia C. The etiological role of chronic iron deficiency in production of menorrhagia. *JAMA* 1964; 187: 323–27.

3. Lithgow DM, Politzer WM. Vitamin A in the treatment of menorrhagia. *S Afr Med J* 1977; 51: 191–93.

4. Dasgupta PR, Dutta S, Banerjee P, Majumdar S. Vitamin E (alpha tocopherol) in the management of menorrhagia associated with the use of intrauterine contraceptive devices (IUCD). *Internat J Fertil* 1983; 28(1): 55–56.

5. Cohen JD, Rubin HW. Functional menorrhagia: treatment with bioflavonoids and vitamin C. *Curr Ther Res* 1960; 2: 539.

6. Leung AY, Foster S. *Encyclopedia of Common Natural Ingredients Used in Foods, Drugs, and Cosmetics,* 2d ed. New York: John Wiley & Sons, 1996, 168–70.

7. Ellingwood F. *American Materia Medica, Therapeutics and Pharmacognosy*. Sandy, OR: Eclectic Medical Publications, 1919, 1998, 354.

8. Mills SY. *Out of the Earth: The Essential Book of Herbal Medicine*. Middlesex, UK: Viking Arkana, 1991, 520–22.

Migraine Headaches

1. Grant EC. Food allergies and migraine. *Lancet* 1979; i: 966–69.

2. Monro J, Brostoff J, Carini C, Zilkha K. Food allergy in migraine. *Lancet* 1980; ii: 1–4.

3. Egger J, Carter CM, Wilson J, et al. Is migraine food allergy? A double-blind controlled trial of oligoantigenic diet treatment. *Lancet* 1983; ii: 865–69.

4. Hughs EC, Gott PS, Weinstein RC, Binggeli R. Migraine: a diagnostic test for etiology of food sensitivity by a nutritionally supported fast and confirmed by long-term report. *Ann Allergy* 1985; 55: 28–32.

5. Egger J, Carter CM, Soothill JF, Wilson J. Oligoantigenic diet treatment of children with epilepsy and migraine. *J Pediatr* 1989; 114: 51–58.

6. Brainard JB. Angiotensin and aldosterone elevation in salt-induced migraine. *Headache* 1981; 21: 222–26.

7. Ratner D, Shoshani E, Dubnov B. Milk protein-free diet for nonseasonal asthma and migraine in lactase-deficient patients. *Israel J Med Sci* 1983; 19(9): 806–9.

8. Hanington E. Preliminary report on tyramine headache. *BMJ* 1967; 2: 550–51.

9. Perkine JE, Hartje J. Diet and migraine: a review of the literature. *J Am Dietet Assoc* 1983; 83: 459–63.

10. Smith I, et al. A clinical and biochemical correlation between tyramine and migraine headache. *Headache* 1970; 10: 43–51.

11. Hasselmark L, Malmgren R, Hannerz J. Effect of a carbohydrate-rich diet, low in protein-tryptophan, in classic and common migraine. *Cephalalgia* 1987; 7: 87–92.

12. Unge G, Malmgren R, Olsson P, et al. Effects of dietary protein-tryptophan restriction upon 5-HT uptake by platelets and clinical symptoms in migraine-like headache. *Cephalalgia* 1983; 3: 213–18.

13. McCarren T, Hitzemann R, Allen C, et al. Amelioration of severe migraine by fish oil (omega-3) fatty acids. *Am J Clin Nutr* 1985; 41(4): 874 [abstract].

14. Glueck CJ, McCarren T, Hitzemann R, et al. Amelioration of severe migraine with omega-3 fatty acids: a double-blind placebo controlled clinical trial. *Am J Clin Nutr* 1986; 43(4): 710 [abstract].

15. Gallai V, Sarchielli P, Coata G, et al. Serum and salivary magnesium levels in migraine. Results in a group of juvenile patients. *Headache* 1992; 32: 132–35.

16. Weaver K. Magnesium and migraine. *Headache* 1990; 30: 168 [letter].

17. Mauskop A, Altura BT, Cracco RQ, Altura BM. Intravenous magnesium sulphate relieves migraine attacks in patients with low serum ionized magnesium levels: a pilot study. *Clin Sci* 1995; 89: 633–36.

18. Facchinetti F, Sances G, Borella P, et al. Magnesium prophylaxis of menstrual migraine: effects on intracellular magnesium. *Headache* 1991; 31: 298–301.

19. Thys-Jacobs S. Vitamin D and calcium in menstrual migraine. *Headache* 1994; 34: 544–46.

20. Thys-Jacobs S. Alleviation of migraines with therapeutic vitamin D and calcium. *Headache* 1994; 34: 590–92.

21. Schoenen J, Lenaerts M, Bastings E. High-dose riboflavin as a prophylactic treatment of migraine: results of an open pilot study. *Cephalalgia* 1994; 14: 328–29.

22. Gatto G et al. Analgesizing effect of a methyl donor (S-adenosyl-methionine) in migraine: an open clinical trial. *Int J Clin Pharmacol Res* 1986; 6: 15–17.

23. Kimball RW, Friedman AP, Vallejo E. Effect of serotonin in migraine patients. *Neurology* 1960; 10: 107–11.

24. Hepinstall S, White A, et al. Extracts of feverfew inhibit granule secretion in blood platelets and polymorphonuclear leukocytes. *Lancet* 1985; I: 1071–74.

25. Murphy JJ, Hepinstall S, Mitchell JRA. Randomized double-blind placebo controlled trial of feverfew in migraine prevention. *Lancet* 1988; ii: 189–92.

26. Johnson ES, Kadam NP, et al. Efficacy of feverfew as prophylactic treatment of migraine. *BMJ* 1985; 291: 569–73.

27. Palevitch D, Earon G, Carasso R. Feverfew *(Tanacetum parthenium)* as a prophylactic treatment for migraine: A double-blind placebo-controlled study. *Phytother Res* 1997; 11: 508–11.

28. Srivasta KC, Mustafa T. Ginger *(Zingiber officinale)* in migraine headache. *J Ethnopharmacol* 1992; 39: 267–73.

29. Lamant V, Mauco G, et al. Inhibition of the metabolism of platelet activating factor (PAF-acether) by three specific antagonist from *Ginkgo biloba*. *Biochem Pharmacol* 1987; 36: 2749–52.

30. Levy RL. Intranasal capsaicin for acute abortive treatment of migraine without aura. *Headache* 1995; 35(5): 277 [letter].

Minor Injuries—Sprains, Strains, and Skin Wounds

1. Souba WW, Wilmore D. Diet and nutrition in the care of the patient with surgery, trauma, and sepsis. In Shils ME, Olson JA, Shike M, et al. *Modern Nutrition in Health and Disease*, 9th ed. Baltimore, MD: Williams & Wilkins, 1999, 1589–618.

2. Bucci, L. *Nutrition Applied to Injury Rehabilitation and Sports Medicine*. Boca Raton, FL: CRC Press, 1995, 61–166.

3. Kanter M. Free radicals, exercise and antioxidant supplementation. *Proc Nutr Soc* 1998; 57: 9–13 [review].

4. Jakeman P, Maxwell S. Effect of antioxidant vitamin supplementation on muscle function after eccentric exercise. *Eur J Appl Physiol* 1993; 67: 426–30.

5. Kaminski M, Boal R. An effect of ascorbic acid on delayed-onset muscle soreness. *Pain* 1992; 50: 317–21.

6. McBride JM, Kraemer WJ, Triplett-McBride T, et al. Effect of resistance exercise on free radical production. *Med Sci Sports Exerc* 1998; 30: 67–72.

7. Rokitzki L, Logemann E, Huber G, et al. Alpha-Tocopherol supplementation in racing cyclists during extreme endurance training. *Int J Sport Nutr* 1994; 4: 253–64.

8. Meydani M, Evans WJ, Handelman, et al. Protective effect of vitamin E on exercise-induced oxidative damage in young and older adults. *Am J Physiol* 1993; 264(5 Pt. 2): R992–98.

9. Tiidus PM, Houston ME. Vitamin E status and response to exercise training. *Sports Med.* 1995; 20: 12–23 [review].

10. Kaikkonen J, Kosonen L, Nyyssonen K, et al. Effect of combined coenzyme Q$_{10}$ and d-alpha-tocopheryl acetate supplementation on exercise-induced lipid peroxidation and muscular damage: a placebo-controlled double-blind study in marathon runners. *Free Radic Res* 1998; 29: 85–92.

11. Fuchs J. Potentials and limitations of the natural antioxidants RRR-alpha-tocopherol, L-ascorbic acid and beta-carotene in cutaneous photoprotection. *Free Radic Biol Med* 1998; 25: 848–73.

12. Fuchs J, Kern H. Modulation of UV-light-induced skin inflammation by D-alpha-tocopherol and L-ascorbic acid: a clinical study using solar simulated radiation. *Free Radic Biol Med* 1998; 25: 1006–12.

13. Eberlein-Konig B, Placzek M, Przybilla B. Protective effect against sunburn of combined systemic ascorbic acid (vitamin C) and d-alpha-tocopherol (vitamin E). *J Am Acad Dermatol* 1998; 38: 45–48.

14. Werninghaus K, Meydani M, Bhawan J, et al. Evaluation of the photoprotective effect of oral vitamin E supplementation. *Arch Dermatol* 1994; 130: 1257–61.

15. Garmyn M, Ribaya-Mercado JD, Russel RM, et al. Effect of beta-carotene supplementation on the human sunburn reaction. *Exp Dermatol* 1995; 4: 104–11.

16. Ribaya-Mercado JD, Garmyn M, Gilchrest BA, et al. Skin lycopene is destroyed preferentially over beta-carotene during ultraviolet irradiation in humans. *J Nutr* 1995; 125: 1854–59.

17. Dreher F, Gabard B, Schwindt DA, et al. Topical melatonin in combination with vitamins E and C protects skin from ultraviolet-induced erythema: a human study in vivo. *Br J Dermatol* 1998; 139: 332–39.

18. Dreher F, Denig N, Gabard B, et al. Effect of topical antioxidants on UV-induced erythema formation when administered after exposure. *Dermatology* 1999; 198: 52–55.

19. Hunt TK. Vitamin A and wound healing. *J Am Acad Dermatol* 1986; 15: 817–21.

20. Hunt TK, Ehrlich HP, Garcia JA, et al. Effect of vitamin A on reversing the inhibitory effect of cortisone on healing of open wounds in animals and man. *Ann Surg* 1969; 170: 633–41.

21. Hunt TK. Vitamin A and wound healing. *J Am Acad Dermatol* 1986; 15: 817–21 [review].

22. Schwieger G, Karl H, Schonhaber E. Relapse prevention of painful vertebral syndromes in follow-up treatment with a combination of vitamins B$_1$, B$_6$, and B$_{12}$. *Ann NY Acad Sci* 1990; 585: 54–62.

23. Kuhlwein A, Meyer HJ, Koehler CO. Reduced diclofenac administration by B vitamins: results of a randomized double-blind study with reduced daily doses of diclofenac (75 mg diclofenac versus 75 mg diclofenac plus B vitamins) in acute lumbar vertebral syndromes. *Klin Wochenschr* 1990; 68: 107–15 [in German].

24. Bruggemann G, Koehler CO, Koch EM. Results of a double-blind study of diclofenac + vitamin B$_1$, B$_6$, B$_{12}$ versus diclofenac in patients with acute pain of the lumbar vertebrae. A multicenter study. *Klin Wochenschr* 1990; 68: 116–20 [in German].

25. Levine M. New concepts in the biology and biochemistry of ascorbic acid. *N Engl J Med* 1986; 314: 892–902 [review].

26. Mazzotta MY. Nutrition and wound healing. *J Am Podiatr Med Assoc* 1994; 84: 456–62 [review].

27. Ringsdorf WM Jr, Cheraskin E. Vitamin C and human wound healing. *Oral Surg Oral Med Oral Pathol* 1982; 53: 231–36 [review].

28. Greenwood J. Optimum vitamin C intake as a factor in the preservation of disc integrity. *Med Ann District of Columbia* 1964; 33: 274–76.

29. terRiet G, Kessels AG, Knipschild PG. Randomized clinical trial of ascorbic acid in the treatment of pressure ulcers. *J Clin Epidemiol* 1995; 48: 1453–60.

30. Gey GO, Cooper KH, Bottenberg RA. Effect of ascorbic acid on endurance performance and athletic injury. *JAMA* 1970; 211: 105.

Part One: References

31. Vaxman F, Olender S, Lambert A, et al. Can the wound healing process be improved by vitamin supplementation? Experimental study on humans. *Eur Surg Res* 1996; 28: 306–14.

32. Vaxman F, Olender S, Lambert A, et al. Effect of pantothenic acid and ascorbic acid supplementation on human skin wound healing process. A double-blind, prospective and randomized trial. *Eur Surg Res* 1995; 27: 158–66.

33. Gabor M. Pharmacologic effects of flavonoids on blood vessels. *Angiologica* 1972; 9: 355–74.

34. Hausteen B. Flavonoids, a class of natural products of high pharmacologic potency. *Biochem Pharm* 1983; 32: 1141–48 [review].

35. Miller MJ. Injuries to athletes. *Med Times* 1960; 88: 313–14.

36. Cragin RB. The use of bioflavonoids in the prevention and treatment of athletic injuries. *Med Times* 1962; 90: 529–32.

37. Jenkins M, Alexander JW, MacMillan BG, et al. Failure of topical steroids and vitamin E to reduce postoperative scar formation following reconstructive surgery. *J Burn Care Rehabil* 1986; 7: 309–12.

38. Bates B. Vitamin E gets an 'F' for wound healing, scarring. *Family Practice News* 1996; (Sep 1): 22.

39. Palmieri B, Gozzi G, Palmieri G. Vitamin E added silicone gel sheets for treatment of hypertrophic scars and keloids. *Int J Dermatol* 1995; 34: 506–9.

40. Sandstead HH. Understanding zinc: Recent observations and interpretations. *J Lab Clin Med* 1994; 124: 322–27.

41. Liszewski RF. The effect of zinc on wound healing: a collective review. *J Am Osteopath Assoc* 1981; 81: 104–6 [review].

42. Agren MS. Studies on zinc in wound healing. *Acta Derm Venereol Suppl* 1990; 154: 1–36 [review].

43. Liszewski RF. The effect of zinc on wound healing: a collective review. *J Am Osteopath Assoc* 1981; 81: 104–6 [review].

44. Tenaud I, Sainte-Marie I, Jumbou O, et al. In vitro modulation of keratinocyte wound healing integrins by zinc, copper and manganese. *Br J Dermatol* 1999; 140: 26–34.

45. Pereira CE, Felcman J. Correlation between five minerals and the healing effect of Brazilian medicinal plants. *Biol Trace Elem Res* 1998; 65: 251–59.

46. Carlisle EM. Silicon as an essential trace element in animal nutrition. *Ciba Found Symp* 1986; 121: 123–39.

47. Leach RM. Role of manganese in mucopolysaccharide metabolism. *Fed Proc* 1971; 30: 991.

48. Morrison LM, Murata K. Absorption, distribution, metabolism and excretion of acid mucopolysaccharides administered to animals and patients. In Morrison LM, Schjeide OA, Meyer K. *Coronary heart disease and the mucopolysaccharides (glycosaminoglycans)*. Springfield, IL: Charles C. Thomas, 1974: 109–27.

49. Denuziere A, Ferrier D, Damour O, et al. Chitosan-chondroitin sulfate and chitosan-hyaluronate polyelectrolyte complexes: biological properties. *Biomaterials* 1998; 19: 1275–85.

50. McCarty MF. Glucosamine for wound healing. *Med Hypotheses* 1996; 47: 273–75 [review].

51. Glade MJ. Polysulfated glycosaminoglycan accelerates net synthesis of collagen and glycosaminoglycans by arthritic equine cartilage tissues and chondrocytes. *Am J Vet Res* 1990; 51: 779–85.

52. Prudden JF, Wolarsky ER, Balassa L. The acceleration of healing. *Surg Gynecol Obstet* 1969; 128: 1321–26 [review].

53. Suyama T, Iga Y, Shirakawa H. The acceleration of wound healing with chondroitin sulfate A and its acidic hydrolysates. *Jpn J Exp Med* 1966; 36: 449–52.

54. Prudden JF, Allen J. The clinical acceleration of healing with a cartilage preparation; a controlled study. *JAMA* 1965; 192: 352–56.

55. Bucci L. Nutrition applied to injury rehabilitation and sports medicine. Boca Raton, FL: CRC Press, 1995, 193.

56. Sprengel H, Franke J, Sprengel A. Personal experiences in the conservative therapy of patellar chondropathy. *Beitr Orthop Traumatol* 1990; 37: 259–66 [in German].

57. Lysholm J. The relation between pain and torque in an isokinetic strength test of knee extension. *Arthroscopy* 1987; 3: 182–84.

58. Ziegler R, Rau R. Conservative or operative treatment for chondropathia patellae? *Beitr Orthop Traumatol* 1980; 27: 201–11 [in German].

59. Böhmer D, Ambrus P, Szögy A, et al. Treatment of chondropathia patellae in young athletes with glucosamine sulfate. In N Bachl, L Prokop, R Suckert, eds. *Current Topics in Sports Medicine*. Vienna: Urban & Schwarzenberg, 1984, 799.

60. Wilson RF, Tyburski JG. Metabolic responses and nutritional therapy in patients with severe head injuries. *J Head Trauma Rehabil* 1998; 13: 11–27.

61. Romito RA. Early administration of enteral nutrients in critically ill patients. *AACN Clin Issues* 1995; 6: 242–56.

62. Cynober L. Ornithine alpha-ketoglutarate in nutritional support. *Nutrition* 1991; 7: 313–22 [review].

63. Kirk SJ, Hurson M, Regan MC, et al. Arginine stimulates wound healing and immune function in elderly human beings. *Surgery* 1993; 114: 155–60.

64. Barbul A, Lazarou SA, Efron DT, et al. Arginine enhances wound healing and lymphocyte immune responses in humans. *Surgery* 1990; 108: 331–37.

65. Seligman B. Bromelain: An anti-inflammatory agent. *Angiology* 1962; 13: 508–10.

66. Castell JV, Friedrich G, Kuhn CS, et al. Intestinal absorption of undegraded proteins in men: presence of bromelain in plasma after oral intake. *Am J Physiol* 1997; 273: G139–46.

67. Miller JM. Absorption of orally introduced proteolytic enzymes. *Clin Med* 1968; 75: 35–42 [review].

68. Masson M. Bromelain in the treatment of blunt injuries to the musculoskeletal system. A case observation study by an orthopedic surgeon in private practice. *Fortschr Med* 1995; 113(19): 303–6.

69. Miller JN, Ginsberg M, McElfatrick GC, et al. The administration of bromelain orally in the treatment of inflammation and edema. *Exp Med Surg* 1964; 22: 293–99.

70. Cirelli MG. Five years experience with bromelains in therapy of edema and inflammation in postoperative tissue reaction, skin infections and trauma. *Clin Med* 1967; 74: 55–59.

71. Vallis C, Lund M. Effect of treatment with *Carica papaya* on resolution of edema and ecchymosis following rhinoplasty. *Curr Ther Res* 1969; 11: 356–59.

72. Trickett P. Proteolytic enzymes in treatment of athletic injuries. *Appl Ther* 1964; 6: 647–52.

73. Sweeny FJ. Treatment of athletic injuries with an oral proteolytic enzyme. *Med Times* 1963: 91: 765.

74. Boyne PS, Medhurst H. Oral anti-inflammatory enzyme therapy in injuries in professional footballers. *Practitioner* 1967; 198: 543–46.

75. Deitrick RE. Oral proteolytic enzymes in the treatment of athletic injuries: A double-blind study. *Pennsylvania Med J* 1965; Oct: 35–37.

76. Rathgeber WF. The use of proteolytic enzymes (Chymoral) in sporting injuries. *S Afr Med J* 1971; 45: 181–83.

77 Buck JE, Phillips N. Trial of Chymoral in professional footballers. *Br J Clin Pract* 1970; 24: 375–77.

78. Blonstein JL. Control of swelling in boxing injuries. *Practitioner* 1969; 203: 206.

79. Tsomides J, Goldberg RI. Controlled evaluation of oral chymotrypsin-trypsin treatment of injuries to the head and face. *Clin Med* 1969; 76: 40.

80. Holt HT. *Carica papaya* as ancillary therapy for athletic injuries. *Curr Ther Res* 1969; 11: 621–24.

81. Blonstein JL. Oral enzyme tablets in the treatment of boxing injuries. *Practitioner* 1967; 198: 547.

82. Baumüller M. Therapy of ankle joint distortions with hydrolytic enzymes—results from a double blind clinical trial. In GPH Hermans, WL Mosterd, eds. *Sports, Medicine and Health*. Amsterdam: Excerpta Medica, 1990, 1137.

83. Craig RP. The quantitative evaluation of the use of oral proteolytic enzymes in the treatment of sprained ankles. *Injury* 1975; 6: 313–16.

84. Swanson BN. Medical use of dimethyl sulfoxide (DMSO). *Rev Clin Basic Pharmacol* 1985; 5: 1–33 [review].

85. American Medical Association. Dimethyl sulfoxide. Controversy and Current Status—1981. *JAMA* 1982; 248: 1369–71 [review].

86. Jacob SW, Wood DC. Dimethyl sulfoxide (DMSO). Toxicology, pharmacology, and clinical experience. *Am J Surg* 1967; 114: 414–26 [review].

87. Kneer W, Kuhnau S, Bias P, et al. Dimethylsulfoxide (DMSO) gel in treatment of acute tendopathies. A multicenter, placebo-controlled, randomized study. *Fortschritte Med* 1994; 112: 142–46 [in German].

88. Carson JD, Percy EC. The use of DMSO in tennis elbow and rotator cuff tendinitis: a double-blind study. *Med Sci Sports Exer* 1981; 13: 215–19.

89. Giamberardino MA et al. Effects of prolonged L-carnitine administration on delayed muscle pain and CK release after eccentric effort. *Int J Sports Med* 1996; 17: 320–24.

90. Pennies NS. Inhibition of arachidonic acid oxidation in vitro by vehicle components. *Acta Derm Venerol Stockh* 1981; 62: 59–61.

91. Fulton JE Jr. The stimulation of postdermabrasion wound healing with stabilized aloe vera gel-polyethylene oxide dressing. *J Dermatol Surg Oncol* 1990; 16: 460–67.

92. Schmidt JM, Greenspoon JS. Aloe vera dermal wound gel is associated with a delay in wound healing. *Obstet Gynecol* 1991; 78: 115–17.

93. Carson CF, Riley TV. Antimicrobial activity of the essential oil of Melaleuca alternifolia: A review. *Lett Appl Microbiol* 1993; 16: 49–55.

94. Faoagali J, George N, Leditschke JF. Does tea tree oil have a place in the topical treatment of burns? *Burns* 1997; 23: 349–51.

95. Hobbs C. Echinacea: A literature review. *HerbalGram* 1994; 30: 33–48 [review].

96. Blumenthal M, Busse WR, Goldberg A, et al. (eds). *The Complete German Commission E Monographs: Therapeutic Guide to Herbal Medicines*. Austin: American Botanical Council and Boston: Integrative Medicine Communications, 1998, 122–23.

97. Leung A, Foster S. *Encyclopedia of Common Natural Ingredients Used in Food, Drugs and Cosmetics*, 2d ed. New York: John Wiley & Sons, 1996, 113–14.

98. Blumenthal M, Busse WR, Goldberg A, et al. (eds). *The Complete German Commission E Monographs: Therapeutic Guide to Herbal Medicines*. Austin: American Botanical Council and Boston: Integrative Medicine Communications, 1998, 100.

99. Weiss R. *Herbal Medicine*. Gothenburg, Sweden: Ab Arcanum and Beaconsfield, UK: Beaconsfield Publishers Ltd, 1988, 342.

100. Blumenthal M, Busse WR, Goldberg A, et al. (eds). *The Complete German Commission E Monographs: Therapeutic Guide to Herbal Medicines*. Austin: American Botanical Council and Boston: Integrative Medicine Communications, 1998, 83.

101. Weiss R. *Herbal Medicine*. Gothenburg, Sweden: Ab Arcanum and Beaconsfield, UK: Beaconsfield Publishers Ltd, 1988, 342.

102. Duke JA. *CRC Handbook of Medicinal Herbs*. Boca Raton, FL: CRC Press, 1985, 221.

103. Rask MR. Colchicine use in five hundred patients with disk disease. *J Neurol Orth Surg* 1980; 1(5): 1–19.

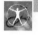

104. Simmons JW, Harris WP, Koulisis CW, et al. Intravenous colchicine for low back pain: A double blind study. *Spine* 1990; 15: 716–17.

105. Kiriluk JE. Experimental basis for the applications of St. John's wort and Kolanch preparations in the treatment of infected wounds. *Vestnik Khirurgii* 1978; 123: 126–30.

106. Guillaume M, Padioleau F. Veinotonic effect, vascular protection, anti-inflammatory and free radical scavenging properties of horse chestnut extract. *Arzneim-Forsch Drug Res* 1994; 44: 25–35.

107. Morisset R, Cote NG, Panisset JC, et al. Evaluation of the healing activity of hydrocotyle tincture in the treatment of wounds. *Phytother Res* 1987; 1: 117–21.

108. Zeylstra H. *Filipendila ulmaria. Br J Phytotherapy* 1998; 5: 8–12.

Mitral Valve Prolapse

1. Frederickson L. *Confronting Mitral Valve Prolapse Syndrome.* New York: Warner Books, 1992.

2. Galland LD, Baker SM, McLellan RK. Magnesium deficiency in the pathogenesis of mitral valve prolapse. *Magnesium* 1986; 5: 165–74.

3. Lichodziejewska B, Klos J, Rezler J, et al. Clinical symptoms of mitral valve prolapse are related to hypomagnesemia and attenuated by magnesium supplementation. *Am J Cardiol* 1997; 79: 768–72.

4. Oda T, Hamamoto K. Effect of coenzyme Q_{10} on the stress-induced decrease of cardiac performance in pediatric patients with mitral valve prolapse. *Jpn Circ J* 1984; 48: 1387.

5. Langsjoen PH, Langsjoen PH, Folkers K. Isolated diastolic dysfunction of the myocardium and its response to coQ_{10} treatment. *Clin Invest* 1993; 71(suppl): S140–44.

Morning Sickness

1. Signorello LB, Harlow BL, Wang SP, Erick MA. Saturated fat intake and the risk of severe hyperemesis gravidarum. *Am J Epidemiol* 1996; 143 (11 suppl): S25 [abstr# 97].

2. Merkel RL. The use of menadione bisulfite and ascorbic acid in the treatment of nausea and vomiting of pregnancy. *Am J Obstet Gynecol* 1952; 64: 416–18.

3. Sahakian V, Rouse D, Sipes S, et al. Vitamin B_6 is effective therapy for nausea and vomiting of pregnancy: a randomized, double-blind placebo-controlled study. *Obstet Gynecol* 1991; 78: 33–36.

4. Vutyavanich T, Wongtra-ngan S, Ruangsri R. Pyridoxine for nausea and vomiting of pregnancy: a randomized, double blind, placebo-controlled trial. *Am J Obstet Gynecol* 1995; 173: 881–84.

5. Fischer-Rasmussen W, Kjaer SK, et al. Ginger treatment of hyperemesis gravidarum. *Eur J Obstet Gynecol Reprod Biol* 1990; 38: 19–24.

6. Fischer-Rasmussen W, Kjaer SK, Dahl C, Asping U. Ginger treatment of hyperemesis gravidarum. *Eur J Obstet Gynecol Reproductive Biol* 1990; 38: 19–24.

Motion Sickness

1. Mowrey DB, Clayson DE. Motion sickness, ginger, and psychophysics. *Lancet* 1982; i: 655–57.

2. Grontved A, Brask T, Kambskard J, et al. Ginger root against seasickness. *Acta Otolaryngol* 1988; 105: 45–49.

3. Holtmann S, Clarke AH, Scherer H, et al. The anti-motion sickness mechanism of ginger. *Acta Otolaryngol* 1989; 108: 168–74.

4. Grontved A, Hentzer E. Vertigo-reducing effect of ginger root. *ORL* 1986; 48: 282.

Multiple Sclerosis

1. Landtblom AM, Flodin U, Karlsson M, et al. Multiple sclerosis and exposure to solvents, ionizing radiation and animals. *Scand J Work Environ Health* 1993; 19: 399–404.

2. Haahr S, Koch-Henriksen N, Moller-Larsen A, et al. Increased risk of multiple sclerosis after late Epstein-Barr virus infection: a historical prospective study. *Mult Scler* 1995; 1: 73–77.

3. Swank RL. Multiple sclerosis: fat-oil relationship. *Nutrition* 1991; 7: 368–76.

4. Esparza ML, Saski S, Kesteloot H. Nutrition, latitude, and multiple sclerosis mortality: an ecologic study. *Am J Epidemiol* 1995; 142: 733–37.

5. Esparza ML, Saski S, Kesteloot H. Nutrition, latitude, and multiple sclerosis mortality: an ecologic study. *Am J Epidemiol* 1995; 142: 733–37.

6. Ghadirian P, Jain M, Ducic S, et al. Nutritional factors in the aetiology of multiple sclerosis: a case-control study in Montreal, Canada. *Int J Epidemiol* 1998; (5): 845–52.

7. Malosse D, Perron H, Sasco A, Seigneurin JM. Correlation between milk and dairy product consumption and multiple sclerosis prevalence: a worldwide study. *Neuroepidemiology* 1992; 11: 304–12.

8. Tola MR, Granieri E, Malagu S, et al. Dietary habits and multiple sclerosis. A retrospective study in Ferrara, Italy. *Acta Neurol (Napoli)* 1994; 16: 189–97.

9. Esparza ML, Saski S, Kesteloot H. Nutrition, latitude, and multiple sclerosis mortality: an ecologic study. *Am J Epidemiol* 1995; 142: 733–37.

10. Ghadirian P, Jain M, Ducic S, et al. Nutritional factors in the aetiology of multiple sclerosis: a case-control study in Montreal, Canada. *Int J Epidemiol* 1998; 27: 845–52.

11. Hadjivassiliou M, Gibson A, Davies-Jones GA, et al. Does cryptic gluten sensitivity play a part in neurological illness? *Lancet* 1996; 347: 369–71.

12. Mortensen JT, Bronnum-Hansen H, Rasmussen K. Multiple sclerosis and organic solvents. *Epidemiology* 1998; 9: 168–71.

13. Juntunen J, Kinnunen E, Antti-Poika M, Koskenvuo M. Multiple sclerosis and occupational exposure to chemicals: a co-twin control study of a nationwide series of twins. *Br J Ind Med* 1989; 46: 417–19.

14. Landtblom AM, Flodin U, Soderfeldt B, et al. Organic solvents and multiple sclerosis: a synthesis of the current evidence. *Epidemiology* 1996; 7: 429–33 [review].

15. Blisard KS, Kornfeld M, McFeeley PJ, Smialek JE. The investigation of alleged insecticide toxicity: a case involving chlordane exposure, multiple sclerosis, and peripheral neuropathy. *J Forensic Sci* 1986; 31: 1499–504.

16. Landtblom AM, Flodine U, Karlsson M, et al. Multiple sclerosis and exposure to solvents, ionizing radiation and animals. *Scand J Work Environ Health* 1993; 19: 399–404.

17. Krebs JM, Park RM, Boal WL. A neurological disease cluster at a manufacturing plant. *Arch Environ Health* 1995; 50: 190–95.

18. Emre M, de Decker C. Effects of cigarette smoking on motor functions in patients with multiple sclerosis. *Arch Neurol* 1992; 49: 1243–47.

19. Fung YK, Meade AG, Rack EP, Blotcky AJ. Brain mercury in neurodegenerative disorders. *J Toxicol Clin Toxicol* 1997; 35: 49–54.

20. Siblerud RL, Kienholz E. Evidence that mercury from silver dental fillings may be an etiological factor in multiple sclerosis. *Sci Total Environ* 1994; 142: 191–205.

21. Bangsi D, Ghadirian P, Ducic S, et al. Dental amalgam and multiple sclerosis: a case-control study in Montreal, Canada. *Int J Epidemiol* 1998; 27: 667–71.

22. Craelius W. Comparative epidemiology of multiple sclerosis and dental caries. *J Epidemiol Community Health* 1978; 32: 155–65.

23. Cendrowski W. Multiple sclerosis and MaxEPA. *Br J Clin Pract* 1986; 40: 365–67.

24. Bates D, Cartlidge NE, French JM, et al. A double-blind controlled trial of long chain n-3 polyunsaturated fatty acids in the treatment of multiple sclerosis. *J Neurol Neurosurg Psychiatry* 1989; 52: 18–22.

25. Goldberg P, Fleming MC, Picard EH. Multiple sclerosis: decreased relapse rate through dietary supplementation with calcium, magnesium and vitamin D. *Med Hypothesis* 1986; 21: 193–200.

26. DeLuca HF, Zierold C. Mechanisms and functions of vitamin D. *Nutr Rev* 1998; 56(two Pt. 2): S4–10 [review].

27. Yasui M, Yase Y, Ando K, et al. Magnesium concentration in brains from multiple sclerosis patients. *Acta Neurol Scand* 1990; 81: 197–200.

28. Yasui M, Ota K. Experimental and clinical studies on dysregulation of magnesium metabolism and the aetiopathogenesis of multiple sclerosis. *Magnes Res* 1992; 5: 295–302.

29. Werbach M. *Nutritional Influences on Illness.* Tarzana, CA: Third Line Press, 1996, 434 [review].

30. Dworkin RH, Bates D, Millar JHD, Paty DW. Linoleic acid and multiple sclerosis: a reanalysis of three double-blind trials. *Neurology* 1984; 34: 1441–45 [review].

31. Dines KC, Powell HC. Mast cell interactions with the nervous system: relationship to mechanisms of disease. *J Neuropathol Exp Neurol* 1997; 56: 627–40.

32. Stern EI. The intraspinal injection of vitamin B$_1$ for the relief of intractable pain, and for inflammatory and degenerative diseases of the central nervous system. *Am J Surg* 1938; 34: 495.

33. Moore MT. Treatment of multiple sclerosis with nicotinic acid and vitamin B$_1$. *Arch Int Med* 1940; 65: 18.

34. Werbach MR, Murray MT. *Botanical Influences on Illness.* Tarzana, CA: Third Line Press, 1994, 239 [review].

35. Werbach MR, Murray MT. *Botanical Influences on Illness.* Tarzana, CA: Third Line Press, 1994, 239 [review].

MSG Sensitivity (Chinese Restaurant Syndrome)

1. Wen C-P, Gershoff SN. Effects of dietary vitamin B$_6$ on the utilization of monosodium glutamate by rats. *J Nutr* 1972; 102: 835–40.

2. Folkers K, Shizukuishi S, Scudder SL, et al. Biochemical evidence for a deficiency of vitamin B$_6$ in subjects reacting to monosodium-L-glutamate by the Chinese restaurant syndrome. *Biochem Biophys Res Comm* 1981; 100: 972–77.

Night Blindness

1. Anonymous. Zinc-responsive night blindness in sickle cell anemia. *Nutr Rev* 1982; 40: 175–77.

2. Alfieri R, Sole P. Influencedes anthocyanosides admintres parvoie parenterale su l'adaptoelectroretinogramme du lapin. *CR Soc Biol* 1964; 15: 2338.

3. Sala D, Rolando M, et al. Effect of anthocyanosides on visual performance at low illumination. *Minerva Oftalmol* 1979; 21: 283–85.

Osgood-Schlatter Disease

1. Riech, CJ. Vitamin E, selenium, and knee problems. *Lancet* 1976; i: 257 [letter].

2. Jonathan V Wright, MD, personal correspondence with author, Apr 1997.

Osteoarthritis

1. Warmbrand M. *How Thousands of My Arthritis Patients Regained Their Health.* New York: Arco Publishing, 1974.

2. Childers NF. A relationship of arthritis to the solanaceae (nightshades). *J Internat Acad Pre Med* 1982; Nov: 31–37.

3. Childers NF, Margoles MS. An apparent relation of nightshades (Solanaceae) to arthritis. *J Neurol Orthop Med Surg* 1993; 14: 227–31.

4. Taylor MR. Food allergy as an etiological factor in arthropathies: a survey. *J Internat Acad Prev Med* 1983; 8: 28–38 [review].

5. Altman RD, Lozada CJ. Practice guidelines in the management of osteoarthritis. *Osteoarthritis Cartilage* 1998; 6(suppl A): 22–24 [review].

6. Tapadinhas MJ, Rivera IC, Bignamini AA. Oral glucosamine sulphate in the management of arthrosis: report on a multi-centre open investigation in Portugal. *Pharmtherapeutica* 1982; 3: 157–68.

7. Giordano N, Nardi P, Senesi M, et al. The efficacy and safety of glucosamine sulfate in the treatment of gonarthritis. *Clin Ter* 1996; 147: 99–105.

8. D'Ambrosio E, Casa B, Bompani G, et al. Glucosamine sulphate: a controlled clinical investigation in arthrosis. *Pharmatherapeutica* 1981; 2(8): 504–8.

9. Crolle G, DiEste E. Glucosamine sulfate for the management of arthrosis. *Curr Ther Res* 1980; 7: 104–9.

10. Qiu GX, Gao SN, Giacovelli G, et al. Efficacy and safety of glucosamine sulfate versus ibuprofen in patients with knee osteoarthritis. *Arzneimforsch Drug Res* 1998; 48: 469–74.

11. Reichelt A, Förster KK, Fischer M, et al. Efficacy and safety of intramuscular glucosamine sulfate in osteoarthritis of the knee. *Arzneimforsch Drug Res* 1994; 44: 75–80.

12. Drovanti A, Bignamini AA, Rovati AL. Therapeutic activity of oral glucosamine sulfate in osteoarthritis: a placebo-controlled double-blind investigation. *Clin Ther* 1980; 3(4): 260–72.

13. Vaz AL. Double-blind clinical evaluation of the relative efficacy of ibuprofen and glucosamine sulphate in the management of osteoarthritis of the knee in out-patients. *Curr Med Res Opin* 1982; 8(3): 145–49.

14. Pujalte JM, Llavore EP, Ylescupidez FR. Double-blind clinical evaluation of oral glucosamine sulphate in the basic treatment of osteoarthrosis. *Curr Med Res Opin* 1980; 7(2): 110–14.

15. da Camara CC, Dowless GV. Glucosamine sulfate for osteoarthritis. *Ann Pharmacother* 1998; 32: 580–87.

16. Barclay TS, Tsourounis C, McCarthy GM. Glucosamine. *Ann Pharmacother* 1998; 32(5): 574–79.

17. Kerzberg EM, Roldan EJA, Castelli G, Huberman ED. Combination of glycosaminoglycans and acetylsalicylic acid in knee osteoarthritis. *Scand J Rheum* 1987; 16: 377.

18. Baici A, Hörler D, Moser B, et al. Analysis of glycosaminoglycans in human serum after oral administration of chondroitin sulfate. *Rheumatol Int* 1992; 12: 81–88.

19. Kerzberg EM, Roldán EJA, Castelli G, Huberman ED. Combination of glycosaminoglycans and acetylsalicylic acid in knee osteoarthrosis. *Scand J Pheumatol* 1987; 16: 377–80.

20. Rovetta G. Galactosaminoglycuronoglycan sulfate (Matrix) in therapy of tibiofibular osteoarhtirits of the knee. *Drugs Exptl Clin Res* 1991; 17: 53–57.

21. Conte A, Volpi N, Palmieri L, et al. Biochemical and pharmacokinetic aspects of oral treatment with chondroitin sulfate. *Arzneim-Forsch* 1995; 45: 918–25.

22. Ronca F, Palmieri L, Panicucci P, Ronca G. Anti-inflammatory active of chondroitin sulfate. *Osteoarthritis Cartilage* 1998; 6(Suppl A): 14–21.

23. Uebelhart D, Thonar EJ-M, Delmas PD, et al. Effects of oral chondroitin sulfate on the progression of knee osteoarthritis: a pilot study. *Osteoarthritis Cartilage* 1998; 6(suppl A): 39–46.

24. Verbruggen G, Goemaere S, Veys EM. Chondroitin sulfate: S/DMOAD (structure/disease modifying anti-osteoarthritis drug) in the treatment of finger joint OA. *Osteoarthritis Cartilage* 1998; 6(suppl A): 37–38.

25. Bucsi L, Poór G. Efficacy and tolerability of oral chondroitin sulfate as a symptomatic slow-acting drug for osteoarthritis (SYSADOA) in the treatment of knee osteoarthritis. *Osteoarthritis Cartilage* 1998; 6(suppl A): 31–36.

26. Bourgeois P, Chales G, Dehais J, et al. Efficacy and tolerability of chondroitin sulfate 1200 mg/day vs chondroitin sulfate 3 × 400 mg/day vs placebo. *Osteoarthritis Cartilage* 1998; 6(suppl A): 25–30.

27. Pipitone V, Ambanelli U, Cervini C, et al. A multicenter, triple-blind study to evaluate galactosaminoglucuronoglycan sulfate versus placebo in patients with femorotibial gonarthritis. *Curr Ther Res* 1992; 52: 608–38.

28. Bazières B, Loyau G, Menkès CJ, et al. Le chondroïtine sulfate dans le traitement de la gonarthrose et de la coxarthrose. *Rev Rhum Mal Ostéoartic* 1992; 59: 466–72.

29. Conrozier T, Vignon E. Die Wirkung von Chondroitinsulfat bei der Behandlung der Hüft Gelenksarthrose. Eine Doppelblindstudie gegen Placebo. *Litera Rheumatologica* 1992; 14: 69–75.

30. L'Hirondel JLL. Klinische Doppelblind-Studie mit oral verabreichtem Chondroitinsulfat gegen Placebo bei der tibiofermoralen Gonarthrose (125 Patienten). *Litera Rheumatologica* 1992; 14: 77–82.

31. Morreale P, Manopulo R, Galati M, et al. Comparison of the antiinflammatory efficacy of chondroitin sulfate and diclofenac sodium in patients with knee osteoarthritis. *J Rheumatol* 1996; 23: 1385–91.

32. Leeb BF, Petera P, Neumann K. Results of a multicenter study of chondroitin sulfate (Condrosulf) use in arthroses of the finger, knee and hip joints. *Wien Med Wochenschr* 1996; 146: 609–14.

33. Bourgeois P, Chales G, Dehais J, et al. Efficacy and tolerability of chondroitin sulfate 1200 mg/day vs chondroitin sulfate 3 × 400 mg/day vs placebo. *Osteoarthritis Cartilage* 1998; 6(suppl A): 25–30.

34. Murray MT. Which is better: aged versus fresh garlic; glucosamine sulfate versus chondroitin sulfate. *Am J Natural Med* 1997; 4: 5–8.

35. Theodosakis J, Adderly B, Fox B. *The Arthritis Cure*. St. New York: Martin's Press, 1997.

36. Schumacher HR. Osteoarthritis: The clinical picture, pathogenesis, and management with studies on a new therapeutic agent, S-adenosylmethionine. *Am J Med* 1987; 83(suppl 5A): 1–4 [review].

37. Harmand MF, Vilamitjana J, Maloche E, et al. Effects of S-adenosylmethionine on human articular chondrocyte differentiation: An in vitro study. *Am J Med* 1987; 83(suppl 5A): 48–54.

38. Konig H et al. Magnetic resonance tomography of finger polyarthritis: Morphology and cartilage signals after ademetionine therapy. *Aktuelle Radiol* 1995; 5: 36–40.

39. Domljan Z et al. A double-blind trial of ademetionine vs naproxen in activated gonarthrosis. *Int J Clin Pharmacol Ther Toxicol* 1989; 27: 329–33.

Part One: References

40. Müller-Fassbender H. Double-blind clinical trial of S-adenosylmethionine in versus ibuprofen in the treatment of osteoarthritis. *Am J Med* 1987; 83(suppl 5A): 81–83.

41. Vetter G. Double-blind comparative clinical trial with S-adenosyl-methionine and indomethacin in the treatment of osteoarthritis. *Am J Med* 1987; 83(suppl 5A): 78–80.

42. Maccagno A. Double-blind controlled clinical trial of oral S-adenosylmethionine versus piroxicam in knee osteoarthritis. *Am J Med* 1987; 83(suppl 5A): 72–77.

43. Caruso I, Pietrogrande V. Italian double-blind multicenter study comparing S-adenosylmethionine, naproxen, and placebo in the treatment of degenerative joint disease. *Am J Med* 1987; 83(suppl 5A): 66–71.

44. Marcolongo R, Giordano N, Colombo B, et al. Double-blind multicentre study of the activity of s-adenosyl-methionine in hip and knee osteoarthritis. *Curr Ther Res* 1985; 37: 82–94.

45. Glorioso S, Todesco S, Mazzi A, et al. Double-blind multicentre study of the activity of S-adenosylmethionine in hip and knee osteoarthritis. *Int J Clin Pharmacol Res* 1985; 5: 39–49.

46. Montrone F, Fumagalli M, Sarzi Puttini P, et al. Double-blind study of S-adenosyl-methionine versus placebo in hip and knee arthrosis. *Clin Rheumatol* 1985; 4: 484–85.

47. Kaufman W. The use of vitamin therapy for joint mobility. Therapeutic reversal of a common clinical manifestation of the 'normal' aging process. *Conn State Med J* 1953; 17(7): 584–89.

48. Kaufman W. The use of vitamin therapy to reverse certain concomitants of aging. *J Am Geriatr Soc* 1955; 11: 927.

49. Hoffer A. Treatment of arthritis by nicotinic acid and nicotinamide. *Can Med Assoc J* 1959; 81: 235–38.

50. Jonas WB, Rapoza CP, Blair WF. The effect of niacinamide on osteoarthritis: A pilot study. *Inflamm Res* 1996; 45: 330–34.

51. McAlindon TE, Jacques P, Azang Y. Do antioxidant micronutrients protect against the development and progression of knee osteoarthritis? *Arthrit Rheum* 1996; 39: 648–56.

52. Machtey I, Ouaknine L. Tocopherol in osteoarthritis: a controlled pilot study. *J Am Geriatr Soc* 1978; 25(7): 328–30.

53. Blankenhorn G. Klinische Wirtsamkeit von Spondyvit (vitamin E) bei aktiverten arthronsen. *Z Orthop* 1986; 124: 340–43.

54. Scherak O, Kolarz G, Schödl Ch, Blankenhorn G. Hochdosierte Vitamin-E-Therapie bei Patienten mit aktivierter Arthrose. *Z Rheumatol* 1990; 49: 369–73.

55. Newnham RE. The role of boron in human nutrition. *J Applied Nutr* 1994; 46: 81–5.

56. Helliwell TR, Kelly SA, Walsh HP, et al. Elemental analysis of femoral bone from patients with fractured neck of femur or osteoarthrosis. *Bone* 1996; 18: 151–57.

57. Travers RL, Rennie GC, Newnham RE. Boron and arthritis: the results of a double-blind pilot study. *J Nutr Med* 1990; 1: 127–32.

58. Altman R, Gray R. Inflammation in osteoarthritis. *Clin Rheum Dis* 1985; 11: 353.

59 Stammers T, Sibbald B, Freeling P. Fish oil in osteoarthritis. *Lancet* 1989; ii: 503 [letter].

60. Balagot RC, Ehrenpreis S, Kubota K, Greenberg J. Analgesia in mice and humans by D-phenylalanine: Relation to inhibition of enkephalin degradation and enkephalin levels. In *Advances in Pain Research and Therapy*, vol. 5, eds. JJ Bonica, JC Liebeskind, DG Albe-Fessard. New York: Raven Press, 1983, 289–93.

61. Budd K. Use of D-phenylalanine, an enkephalinase inhibitor, in the treatment of intractable pain. In *Advances in Pain Research and Therapy*, vol 5, eds. JJ Bonica, JC Liebeskind, DG Albe-Fessard. New York: Raven Press, 1983, 305–8.

62. Seltzer S, Marcus R, Stoch R. Perspectives in the control of chronic pain by nutritional manipulation. *Pain* 1981; 11: 141–48 [review].

63. Prudden JF, Balassa LL. The biological activity of bovine cartilage preparations. *Semin Arthritis Rheum* 1974; 3: 287–320.

64. Reijholec V. Long term studies of antiosteoarthritic drugs: an assessment. *Semin Arthritis Rheum* 1987; 17(2 suppl 1): 35–53.

65. American Medical Association. Dimethyl sulfoxide. Controversy and Current Status—1981. *JAMA* 1982; 248: 1369–71.

66. Jimenez RAH, Willkens RF. Dimethyl sulfoxide: A perspective of its use in rheumatic diseases. *J Lab Clin Med* 1982; 100: 489–500.

67. Jacob SW, Wood DC. Dimethyl sulfoxide (DMSO). Toxicology, pharmacology, and clinical experience. *Am J Surg* 114: 414–26.

68. Safayhi H, Mack T, Saieraj J, et al. Boswellic acids: Novel, specific, nonredox inhibitors of 5-lipoxygenase. *J Pharmacol Exp Ther* 1992; 261: 1143–46.

69. Mills SY, Jacoby RK, Chacksfield M, Willoughby M. Effect of a proprietary herbal medicine on the relief of chronic arthritic pain: A double-blind study *Br J Rheum* 1996; 35: 874–88.

70. McCarthy GM, McCarty DJ. Effect of topical capsaicin in the therapy of painful osteoarthritis of the hands *J Rheumatol* 1992; 19: 604–7.

71. Bingham R, Bellow BA, Bellow JG. Yucca plant saponin in the management of arthritis. *J Appl Nutr* 1975; 27: 45–51.

Osteoporosis

1. Feskanich D, Willett WC, Stampfer MJ, Colditz GA. Protein consumption and bone fractures in women. *Am J Epidemiol* 1996; 143: 472–79.

2. Abelow BJ, Holford TR, Insogna KL. Cross-cultural associations between dietary animal protein and hip fracture: a hypothesis. *Calcif Tissue Int* 1992; 50: 14–18.

3. Heaney RP. Nutrient interactions and the calcium requirement. *J Lab Clin Med* 1994; 124: 15–16 [editorial/review].

4. Kerstetter JE, Allen LH. Dietary protein increases urinary calcium. *J Nutr* 1990; 120: 134–36.

5. Draper HH, Piché LA, Gibson RS. Effects of a high protein intake

from common foods on calcium metabolism in a cohort of post-menopausal women. *Nutr Res* 1991; 11: 273–81.

6. Tkatch L, Rapin C-H, Rizzoli R, et al. Benefits of oral protein supplementation in elderly patients with fracture of the proximal femur. *J Am Coll Nutr* 1992; 11: 519–25.

7. Munger RG, Cerhan JR, Chiu BC-H. Prospective study of dietary protein intake and risk of hip fracture in postmenopausal women. *Am J Clin Nutr* 1999; 69: 147–52.

8. Schürch M-A, Rizzoli R, Slosman D, et al. Protein supplements increase serum insulin-like growth factor-I levels and attenuate proximal femur bone loss in patients with recent hip fracture. A randomized, double blind, placebo-controlled trial. *Ann Intern Med* 1998; 128: 801–9.

9. Zarkadas M, Geougeon-Reyburn R, Marliss EB, et al. Sodium chloride supplementation and urinary calcium excretion in postmenopausal women. *Am J Clin Nutr* 1989; 50: 1088–94.

10. Evans CEL, Chughtai AY, Blumsohn A, et al. The effect of dietary sodium on calcium metabolism in premenopausal and postmenopausal women. *Eur J Clin Nutr* 1997; 51: 394–99.

11. McParland BE, Boulding A, Campbell AJ. Dietary salt affects biochemical markers of resorption and formation of bone in elderly women. *Br Med J* 1989; 299: 834–35.

12. Devine A, Criddle RA, Dick IM, et al. A longitudinal study of the effect of sodium and calcium intakes on regional bone density in postmenopausal women. *Am J Clin Nutr* 1995; 62: 740–45.

13. Hernandez-Avila M, Colditz GA, Stampfer MJ, et al. Caffeine, moderate alcohol intake, and risk of fractures of the hip and forearm in middle-aged women. *Am J Clin Nutr* 1991; 54: 157–63.

14. Kynast-Gales SA, Massey LK. Effect of caffeine on circadian excretion of urinary calcium and magnesium. *J Am Coll Nutr* 1994; 13: 467–72.

15. Harris SS, Dawson-Hughes B. Caffeine and bone loss in healthy postmenopausal women. *Am J Clin Nutr* 1994; 60: 573–78.

16. Wyshak G, Frisch RE. Carbonated beverages, dietary calcium, the dietary calcium/phosphorus ratio, and bone fractures in girls and boys. *J Adolescent Health* 1994; 15: 210–15.

17. Smith S, Swain J, Brown EM, et al. A preliminary report of the short-term effect of carbonated beverage consumption on calcium metabolism in normal women. *Arch Intern Med* 1989; 149: 2517–19.

18. Mazariegos-Ramos E, Guerrero-Romero F, Rodríquez-Morán F, et al. Consumption of soft drinks with phosphoric acid as a risk factor for the development of hypocalcemia in children: a case-control study. *J Pediatr* 1995; 126: 940–42.

19. Shuster J, Jenkins A, Logan C, et al. Soft drink consumption and urinary stone recurrence: a randomized prevention trial. *J Clin Epidemiol* 1992; 45: 911–16.

20. Kim SH, Morton DJ, Barrett-Connor EL. Carbonated beverage consumption and bone mineral density among older women: The Rancho Bernardo Study. *Am J Public Health* 1997; 87: 276–79.

21. Anderson JJB, Ambrose WW, Garner SC. Biphasic effects of genistein on bone tissue in the ovariectomized, lactating rat model (44243). *Proc Soc Exp Biol Med* 1998; 217: 345–50.

22. Potter SM, Baum JA, Teng H, et al. Soy protein and isoflavones: Their effects on blood lipids and bone density in postmenopausal women. *Am J Clin Nutr* 1998; 68(suppl): 1375S–79S.

23. Head KA. Ipriflavone: an important bone-building isoflavone. *Altern Med Rev* 1999; 4: 10–22 [review].

24. Prior JC. Progesterone as a bone-trophic hormone. *Endocr Rev* 1990; 11: 386–98.

25. Lee JR. Osteoporosis reversal: the role of progesterone. Int C*lin Nutr Rev* 1990; 10: 384–91.

26. Riis BJ, Thomsen K, Strom V, Christiansen C. The effect of percutaneous estradiol and natural progesterone on postmenopausal bone loss. *Am J Obstet Gynecol* 1987; 156: 61–65.

27. Hopper JL, Seeman E. The bone density of female twins discordant for tobacco use. *N Engl J Med* 1994; 330: 387–92.

28. Chow R, Harrison JE, Notarius C. Effect of two randomised exercise programmes on bone mass of healthy postmenopausal women. *Br Med J* 1987; 295: 1441–44.

29. Lloyd T, Triantafyllou SJ, Baker ER, et al. Women athletes with menstrual irregularity have increased musculoskeletal injuries. *Med Sci Sports Exercise* 1986; 18(4): 374–79.

30. Reid IR, Ames RW, Evans MC, et al. Long-term effects of calcium supplementation on bone loss and fractures in postmenopausal women: a randomized controlled trial. *Am J Med* 1995; 98: 331–35.

31. Owusu W, Willett WC, Feskanich D, et al. Calcium intake and the incidence of forearm and hip fractures among men. *J Nutr* 1997; 127: 1782–87.

32. Hosking DJ, Ross PD, Thompson DE, et al. Evidence that increased calcium intake does not prevent early postmenopausal bone loss. *Clin Ther* 1998; 20: 933–44.

33. Nieves JW, Komar L, Cosman F, Lindsay R. Calcium potentiates the effect of estrogen and calcitonin on bone mass: review and analysis. *Am J Clin Nutr* 1998; 67: 18–24.

34. Bonjour J-P, Carrie A-L, Ferrari S, et al. Calcium-enriched foods and bone mass growth in prepubertal girls: a randomized, double-blind, placebo-controlled trial. *J Clin Invest* 1997; 99: 1287–94.

35. Welten DC, Kemper HCG, Post GB, van Stavberen WA. A meta-analysis of the effect of calcium intake on bone mass in young and middle aged females and males. *J Nutr* 1995; 125: 2802–13.

36. Nordin BEC, Baker MR, Horsman A, Peacock M. A prospective trial of the effect of vitamin D supplementation on metacarpal bone loss

in elderly women. *Am J Clin Nutr* 1985; 42(3): 470–74.

37. Lips P, Graafmans WC, Ooms ME, et al. Vitamin D supplementation and fracture incidence in elderly persons. *Ann Intern Med* 1996; 124: 400–6.

38. Komulainen M, Tupperainen MT, Kröger H, et al. Vitamin D and HRT: No benefit additional to that of HRT alone in prevention of bone loss in early postmenopausal women. A 2.5-year randomized placebo-controlled study. *Osteoporos Int* 1997; 7: 126–32.

39. Chapuy MC, Arlot ME, Duboeuf F, et al. Vitamin D3 and calcium to prevent hip fractures in elderly women. *N Engl J Med* 1992; 327: 1637–42.

40. Dawson-Hughes B, Dallal GE, Krall EA, et al. Effect of vitamin D supplementation on wintertime and overall bone loss in healthy postmenopausal women. *Ann Intern Med* 1991; 115: 505–12.

41. Dawson-Hughes B, Harris SS, Krall EA, et al. Rates of bone loss in postmenopausal women randomly assigned to one of two dosages of vitamin D. *Am J Clin Nutr* 1995; 61: 1140–45.

42. Cohen L, Laor A, Kitzes R. Magnesium malabsorption in postmenopausal osteoporosis. *Magnesium* 1983; 2: 139–43.

43. Cohen L, Kitzes R. Infrared spectroscopy and magnesium content of bone mineral in osteoporotic women. *Isr J Med Sci* 1981; 17: 1123–25.

44. Geinster JY, Strauss L, Deroisy R, et al. Preliminary report of decreased serum magnesium in postmenopausal osteoporosis. *Magnesium* 1989; 8: 106–9.

45. Dimai H-P, Porta S, Wirnsberger G, et al. Daily oral magnesium supplementation suppresses bone turnover in young adult males. *J Clin Endocrinol Metab* 1998; 83: 2742–48.

46. Stendig-Lindberg G, Tepper R, Leichter I. Trabecular bone density in a two year controlled trial of peroral magnesium in osteoporosis. *Magnesium Res* 1993; 6: 155–63.

47. Abraham GE, Grewal H. A total dietary program emphasizing magnesium instead of calcium. *J Reprod Med* 1990; 35: 503–7.

48. Sahap Atik O. Zinc and senile osteoporosis. *J Am Geriatr Soc* 1983; 31: 790–91.

49. Relea P, Revilla M, Ripoll E, et al. Zinc, biochemical markers of nutrition, and type I osteoporosis. *Age Ageing* 1995; 24: 303–7.

50. Elmståhl S, Gullberg B, Janzon L, et al. Increased incidence of fractures in middle-aged and elderly men with low intakes of phosphorus and zinc. *Osteoporos Int* 1998; 8: 333–40.

51. Strause L, Saltman P, Smith KT, et al. Spinal bone loss in postmenopausal women supplemented with calcium and trace minerals. *J Nutr* 1994; 124: 1060–64.

52. Eaton-Evans J, McIlrath EM, Jackson WE, et al. Copper supplementation and bone-mineral density in middle-aged women. *Proc Nutr Soc* 1995; 54: 191A.

53. Nielson FH, Hunt CD, Mullen LM, Hunt JR. Effect of dietary boron on mineral, estrogen, and testosterone metabolism in postmenopausal women. *FASEB J* 1987; 1: 394–97.

54. Meacham SL, Taper LJ, Volpe SL. Effect of boron supplementation on blood and urinary calcium, magnesium, and phosphorus, and urinary boron in athletic and sedentary women. *Am J Clin Nutr* 1995; 61: 341–45.

55. Hunt CD, Herbel JL, Nielsen FH. Metabolic responses of postmenopausal women to supplemental dietary boron and aluminum during usual and low magnesium intake: boron, calcium, and magnesium absorption and retention and blood mineral concentrations. *Am J Clin Nutr* 1997; 65: 803–13.

56. Nielson FH, Hunt CD, Mullen LM, Hunt JR. Effect of dietary boron on mineral, estrogen, and testosterone metabolism in postmenopausal women. *FASEB J* 1987; 1: 394–97.

57. Gold M. Basketball bones. *Science* 1980; 80: 101–2.

58. Raloff J. Reasons for boning up on manganese. *Science News 1986;* (Sep 27): 199 [review].

59. Strause L, Saltman P, Smith KT, et al. Spinal bone loss in postmenopausal women supplemented with calcium and trace minerals. *J Nutr* 1994; 124: 1060–64.

60. Carlisle EM. Silicon localization and calcification in developing bone. *Fed Proc* 1969; 28: 374.

61. Hott M, de Pollak C, Modrowski D, Marie PJ. Short-term effects of organic silicon on trabecular bone in mature ovariectamized rats. *Calcif Tissue Int* 1993; 53: 174–79.

62. Eisinger J, Clairet D. Effects of silicon, fluoride, etidronate and magnesium on bone mineral density: a retrospective study. *Magnes Res* 1993; 6: 247–49.

63. Ferrari S, Zolezzi C, Savarino L, et al. The oral strontium load test in the assessment of intestinal calcium absorption. *Minerva Med* 1993; 84: 527–31.

64. McCaslin FE, Janes JM. The effect of strontium lactate in the treatment of osteoporosis. *Proc Staff Meetings Mayo Clinic* 1959; 34(13): 329–34.

65. Gaby AR. *Preventing and Reversing Osteoporosis.* Rocklin, CA: Prima Publishing, 1994, 88–89 [review].

66. Gaby AR. *Preventing and Reversing Osteoporosis.* Rocklin, CA Prima Publishing, 1994 [review].

67. Hart JP. Circulating vitamin K$_1$ levels in fractured neck of femur. *Lancet* 1984; ii: 283 [letter].

68. Tamatani M, Morimoto S, Nakajima M, et al. Decreased circulating levels of vitamin K and 25-hydroxyvitamin D in osteopenic elderly men. *Metabolism* 1998; 47: 195–99.

69. Feskanich D, Weber P, Willett WC, et al. Vitamin K intake and hip fractures in women: a prospective study. *Am J Clin Nutr* 1999; 69: 74–79.

70. Knapen MHJ, Hamulyak K, Vermeer C. The effect o f vitamin K supplementation on circulating osteocalcin (Bone Gla protein) and urinary calcium excretion. *Ann Intern Med* 1989; 111: 1001–5.

71. Orimo H, Shiraki M, Fujita T, et al. Clinical evaluation of Menatetrenone in the treatment of involutional osteoporosis—a double-blind multicenter comparative study with 1–alpha-hydroxyvitamin D$_3$. *J Bone Mineral Res* 1992; 7(suppl 1): S122.

72. Iwamoto I, Kosha S, Noguchi S, et al. A longitudinal study of the effect of vitamin K$_2$ on bone mineral density in postmenopausal women: a comparative study with vitamin D$_3$ and estrogen–progestin therapy. *Maturitas* 1999; 31: 161–64.

73. Cracium AM, Wolf J, Knapen MJH, et al. Improved bone metabolism in female elite athletes after vitamin K supplementation. *Int J Sports Med* 1998; 19: 479–84.

74. Kadota S, Li JX, Li HY, et al. Effects of cimicifugae rhizome on serum calcium and phosphate levels in low calcium dietary rats and on bone mineral density in ovariectomized rats. *Phytomed* 1996/97; 3(4): 379–85.

75. Gaby AR. Literature review & commentary. *Townsend Letter for Doctors and Patients.* Jun 1990: 338–39.

76. Parry G, Bredesen DE. Sensory neuropath with low-dose pyridoxine. *Neurology* 1985; 35: 1466–68.

77. Schaumburg H, Kaplan J, Windebank A, et al. Sensory neuropathy from pyridoxine abuse. *N Engl J Med* 1983; 309(8): 445–48.

Pap Smear (Abnormal)

1. Palan PR et al. Plasma levels of antioxidant β-carotene and alpha-tocopherol in uterine cervix dysplasias and cancer. *Nutr Cancer* 1991; 15: 13–20.

2. Dawson EB et al. Serum vitamin and selenium changes in cervical dysplasia. *Fed Proc* 1984; 43: 612.

3. Wassertheil-Smoller S et al. Dietary vitamin C and uterine cervical dysplasia. *Am J Epidemiol* 1981; 114: 714–724.

4. Romney SL et al. Retinoids and the prevention of cervical dysplasias. *Am J Obstet Gynecol* 1981; 141: 890–894.

5. Mackerras D, Irwig L, Simpson JM, et al. Randomized double-blind trial of beta-carotene and vitamin C in women with minor cervical abnormalities. *Br J Cancer* 1999; 79: 1448–53.

6. Butterworth CE et al. Improvement in cervical dysplasia associated with folic acid therapy in users of oral contraceptives. *Am J Clin Nutr* 1982; 35: 73–82.

7. Zarcone R, Bellini P, Carfora E, et al. Folic acid and cervix dysplasia. *Minerva Ginecol* 1996; 48: 397–400.

8. Butterworth CE, Hatch KD, Soong S-J, et al. Oral folic acid supplementation for cervical dysplasia: A clinical intervention trial. *Am J Obstet Gynecol* 1992; 166: 803–809.

9. Butterworth CE Jr. et al. Folate deficiency and cervical dysplasia. *JAMA* 1992; 267: 528–33.

10. Hudson T. *Gynecology and Naturopathic Medicine: A Treatment Manual* 3rd ed. Aloha, OR: TK Publications, 1994, 2–4.

Parasites

1. Mirelman D, Monheit D, Varon S. Inhibition of growth of *Entamoeba histolytica* by allicin, the active principle of garlic extract (*Allium sativum*). *J Infect Dis* 1987; 156: 243–44.

2. Bastidas CJ. Effect of ingested garlic on *Necator americanus* and *Ancylostoma caninum*. *Am J Trop Med Hyg* 1969; 13: 920–23.

3. Koch HP, Lawson LD, eds. *Garlic: The Science and Therapeutic Application of Allium sativum L. and Related Species.* Baltimore: Williams & Wilkins, 1996, 173–74.

4. Gupte S. Use of berberine in treatment of giardiasis. *Am J Dis Child* 1975; 129: 866.

5. Choudhry VP, Sabir M, Bhide VN. Berberine in giardiasis. *Indian Pediatr* 1972; 9: 143–46.

6. Kaneda Y, Torii M, Tanaka T, Aikawa M. In vitro effects of berberine sulphate on the growth and structure of *Entamoeba histolytica, Giardia lamblia* and *Trichomonas vaginalis*. *Ann Trop Med Parasitol* 1991; 85: 417–25.

7. Kliks MM. Studies on the traditional herbal anthelmintic *Chenopodium ambrosioides* L.: Ethnopharmacological evaluation and clinical field trials. *Soc Sci Med* 1985; 21: 879–86.

8. Weiss RF. *Herbal Medicine.* Beaconsfield, UK: Beaconsfield Publishers Ltd., 1985, 119–20.

9. Mendiola J, Bosa M, Perez N, et al. Extracts of *Artemisia abrotanum* and *Artemisia absinthium* inhibit growth of *Naegleria fowleri* in vitro. *Trans R Soc Trop Med Hyg* 1991; 85: 78–79.

Peptic Ulcer

1. Katchinski BD, Logan RFA, Edmond M, Langman MJS. Duodenal ulcer and refined carbohydrate intake: a case-control study assessing dietary fiber and refined sugar intake. *Gut* 1990; 31: 993–96.

2. Suadicani P, Hein HO, Gyntelberg F. Genetic and life-style determinants of peptic ulcer. A study of 3387 men aged 54 to 74 years: The Copenhagen Male Study. *Scand J Gastroenterol* 1999; 34: 12–17.

3. Yudkin J. Eating and ulcers. *BMJ* 1980; (Feb 16): 483 [letter].

4. Sonnenberg A. Dietary salt and gastric ulcer. *Gut* 1986; 27: 1138–42.

5. Cheney G. Rapid healing of peptic ulcers in patients receiving fresh cabbage juice. *Cal Med* 1949; 70: 10.

6. Doll R, Pygott F. Clinical trial of Robaden and of cabbage juice in the treatment of gastric ulcer. *Lancet* 1954; ii: 1200.

7. Thaly H. A new therapy of peptic ulcer: The anti-ulcer factor of cabbage. *Gaz Med Fr* 1965; 72: 1992–93.

8. Dunaevskii GA, Migonova DK, Rozka IM, Chibisova SM. Value of preserved juice of white cabbage in the complex therapy of peptic ulcer. *Vopr Pitan* 1970; 29: 29–33.

9. Noess K. Ulcer-fiber-cabbage and vitamin U. *Tidsskr Nor Laegeforen* 1986; 106: 693–94.

10. Grimes DS, Goddard J. Gastric emptying of wholemeal and white bread. *Gut* 1977; 18: 725–29.

11. Rydning A, Berstad A, Aadland E, Odegaard B. Prophylactic

effect of dietary fiber in duodenal ulcer disease. *Lancet* 1982; ii: 736–39.

12. Ryndning A, Berstad A. Fiber diet and antacids in the short-term treatment of duodenal ulcer. *Scand J Gastroenterol* 1985; 20: 1078–82.

13. Hills BA, Kirwood CA. Surfactant approach to the gastric mucosal barrier: Protection of rats by banana even when acidified. *Gastroenterology* 1989; 97: 294–303.

14. Sikka KK, Singhai CM, Vajpcyi GN. Efficacy of dried raw banana powder in the healing of peptic ulcer. *J Assoc Phys India* 1988; 36(1): 65 [abstract].

15. Kern RA, Stewart G. Allergy in duodenal ulcer: incidence and significance of food hypersensitivities as observed in 32 patients. *J Allergy* 1931; 3: 51.

16. Reimann HJ, Lewin J. Gastric mucosal reactions in patients with food allergy. *Am J Gastroenterol* 1988; 83: 1212–19.

17. Allison MC, Howatson AG, Caroline MG, et al. Gastrointestinal damage associated with the use of nonsteroidal antiinflammatory drugs. *N Engl J Med* 1992; 327: 749–54.

18. Lenz HJ, Ferrari-Taylor J, Isenberg JI. Wine and five percent ethanol are potent stimulants of gastric acid secretion in humans. *Gastroenterology* 1983; 85: 1082–87.

19. Cohen S, Booth GH Jr. Gastric acid secretion and lower-esophageal-sphincter pressure in response to coffee and caffeine. *N Engl J Med* 1975; 293: 897–99.

20. Feldman EJ, Isenberg JI, Grossman MI. Gastric acid and gastrin response to decaffeinated coffee and a peptone meal. *JAMA* 1981; 246: 248–50.

21. Dubey P, Sundram KR, Nundy S. Effect of tea on gastric acid secretion. *Dig Dis Sci* 1984; 29: 202–6.

22. Korman MG, Hansky J, Eaves ER, Schmidt GT. Influence of cigarette smoking on healing and relapse in duodenal ulcer disease. *Gastroenterology* 1983; 85: 871–74.

23. Patty I, Benedek S, Deak G, et al. Controlled trial of vitamin A therapy in gastric ulcer. *Lancet* 1982; ii: 876 [letter].

24. Patty I, Tarnok F, Simon L, et al. A comparative dynamic study of the effectiveness of gastric cytoprotection by vitamin A, De-Nol, sucralfate and ulcer healing by pirenzepine in patients with chronic gastric ulcer (a multiclinical and randomized study). *Acta Physiol Hung* 1984; 64: 379–84.

25. Pfeiffer CJ, Cho CH, Cheema A, Saltman D. Reserpine-induced gastric ulcers: protection by lysosomal stabilization due to zinc. *Eur J Pharmacol* 1980; 61: 347–53.

26. Jimenez E, Bosch F, Galmes JL, Banos JE. Meta-analysis of efficacy of zinc acexamate in peptic ulcer. *Digestion* 1992; 51: 18–26.

27. Frommer DJ. The healing of gastric ulcers by zinc sulphate. *Med J Aust* 1975; 2: 793.

28. Shive W, Snider RN, DuBilier B, et al. Glutamine in treatment of peptic ulcer. *Texas State J Med* 1957; Nov: 840.

29. Yan R, Sun Y, Sun R. Early enteral feeding and supplement of glutamine prevent occurrence of stress ulcer following severe thermal injury. *Chung Hwa Cheng Hsing Shao Shang Wai Ko Tsa Chih* 1995; 11: 189–92.

30. Beil W, Birkholz C, Sewing KF. Effects of flavonoids on parietal cell acid secretion, gastric mucosal prostaglandin production and *Helicobacter pylori* growth. *Arzneim-Forsch Drug Res* 1995; 45: 697–700.

31. Wendt P, Reiman H, et al. The use of flavonoids as inhibitors of histidine decarboxylase in gastric diseases: Experimental and clinical studies. *Naunyn-Schmeidbergs Arch Pharmakol* 1980; 313(suppl): 238.

32. Salim AS. The relationship between *Helicobacter pylori* and oxygen-derived free radicals in the mechanism of duodenal ulceration. *Internal Med* 1993; 32: 359–64.

33. Salim AS. Allopurinol and dimethyl sulfoxide improve treatment outcomes in smokers with peptic ulcer disease. *J Lab Clin Med* 1992; 119: 702–9.

34. Goso Y, Ogata Y, Ishihara K, Hotta K. Effects of traditional herbal medicine on gastric mucin against ethanol-induced gastric injury in rats. *Comp Biochem Physiol* 1996; 113C: 17–21.

35. Beil W, Birkholz W, Sewing KF. Effects of flavonoids on parietal cell acid secretion, gastric mucosal prostaglandin production and *Helicobacter pylori* growth. *Arzneim Forsch* 1995; 45: 697–700.

36. Brogden RN, Speight TM, Avery GS. Deglycyrrhizinated licorice: A report of its pharmacological properties and therapeutic efficacy. *Drugs* 1974; 8: 330–39.

37. D'imperio N, Piccari GG, Sarti F, et al. Double blind trial in duodenal and gastric ulcers. Cimetidine and deglycyrrhizinized liquorice. *Acta Gastro-Enterologica Belgica* 1978; 41: 427–34.

38. Morgan AG, Pacsoo C, McAdam WAF. Maintenance therapy: a two year comparison between Caved-S and cimetidine treatment in the prevention of symptomatic gastric ulcer recurrence. *Gut* 1985; 26: 599–602.

39. Bardhan KD, Cumberland DC, Dixon RA, Holdsworth CD. Clinical trial of deglycyrrhizinised liquorice in gastric ulcer. *Gut* 1978; 19: 779–82.

40. Gaby AR. Deglycyrrhizinated licorice treatment of peptic ulcer. *Townsend Letter for Doctors* 1988; July: 306 [editorial/review].

41. Al-Said MS, Ageel AM, Parmar NS, Tariq M. Evaluation of mastic, a crude drug obtained from Pistacia lentiscus for gastric and duodenal anti-ulcer activity. *J Ethnopharmacol* 1986; 15: 271–78.

42. Huwez FU, Al-Habbal MJ. Mastic in treatment of benign gastric ulcers. *Gastroenterol Japon* 1986; 21: 273–74.

43. Huwez FU, Thirlwell D, Cockayne A, Ala'Aldeen DA. Mastic gum kills *Helicobacter pylori*. *New Engl J Med* 1998; 339: 1946 [letter].

44. Sivam GP, Lampe JW, Ulness B, et al. *Helicobacter pylori*—in vitro susceptibility to garlic (*Allium sativum*) extract. *Nutr Cancer* 1997; 27: 118–21.

45. Tabak M, Armon R, Potasman I, Neeman I. In vitro inhibi-

tion of *Helicobacter pylori* by extracts of thyme. *J Appl Bacteriol* 1996; 80(6): 667–72.

46. Mills SY. *Out of the Earth: The Essential Book of Herbal Medicine.* New York: Viking Arkana, 1991, 544–47.

47. Weiss RF. *Herbal Medicine.* Gothenburg, Sweden: Ab Arcanum and Beaconsfield, UK: Beaconsfield Publishers Ltd, 1988, pp 334–35.

Photosensitivity

1. Cripps DJ. Diet and alcohol effects on the manifestation of hepatic porphyrias. *Fed Proc* 1987; 46: 1894–1900.

2. Mathews-Roth MM, Pathak MA, Fitzpatrick TB, et al. Beta-carotene as an oral photoprotective agent in erythropoietic protoporphyria. *JAMA* 1974; 228: 1004–1008.

3. Nordlund JJ, Klaus SN, Mathews-Roth MM, Pathak MA. New therapy for polymorphous light eruption. *Arch Dermatol* 1973; 108: 710–12.

4. Mathews-Roth MM, Pathak MA, Fitzpatrick TB, et al. Beta-carotene as a photoprotective agent in erythropoietic protoporphyria. *N Engl J Med* 1970; 282: 1231–34.

5. Mathews-Roth MM. Photoprotection by carotenoids. *Fed Proc* 1987; 46: 1890–93 [review].

6. Ayres S Jr, Mihan R. Porphyrea cutanea tarda: response to vitamin E. *Cutis* 1978; 22: 50.

7. Werninghaus K, Meydani M, Bhawan J, et al. Evaluation of the photoprotective effect of oral vitamin E supplementation. *Arch Dermatol* 1994; 130: 1257–61.

8. Kaufman G. Pyridoxine against amiodarone-induced photosensitivity. *Lancet* 1984; I: 51–52 [letter].

9. Ross JB, Moss MA. Relief of the photosensitivity of erythropoietic protoporphyria by pyridoxine. *J Am Acad Dermatol* 1990; 22: 340–42.

10. Neuman R et al. Treatment of polymorphous light eruption with nicotinamide: a pilot study. *Brit J Dermatol* 1986; 115: 77–80.

11. Gajdos A. AMP in porphyria cutanea tarda. *Lancet* 1974; I: 163 [letter].

PMS (Premenstrual Syndrome)

1. Rossignol AM, Bonnlander H. Prevalence and severity of the premenstrual syndrome. Effects of foods and beverages that are sweet or high in sugar content. *J Reprod Med* 1991; 36: 131–36.

2. Halliday A, Bush B, Cleary P, et al. Alcohol abuse in women seeking gynecologic care. *Obstet Gynecol* 1986; 68; 322–26.

3. Rossignol AM, Zhang J, Chen Y, Xiang Z. Tea and premenstrual syndrome in the People's Republic of China. *Am J Public Health* 1989; 79: 67–6.

4. Rossignol AM. Caffeine-containing beverages and premenstrual syndrome in young women. *Am J Public Health* 1985; 75(11): 1335–37.

5. Rossignol AM, Bonnlander H. Caffeine-containing beverages, total fluid consumption, and premenstrual syndrome. *Am J Public Health* 1990; 80: 1106–10.

6. Werbach MR. *Nutritional Influences on Illness, 2d ed.* Tarzana, CA: Third Line Press, 1993, 540–41 [review].

7. Freeman E et al. Ineffectiveness of progesterone suppository treatment for premenstrual syndrome. *JAMA* 1990; 264: 349–53.

8. Martorano JT, Ahlgrimm M, Colbert T. Differentiating between natural progesterone and synthetic progestins: clinical implications for premenstrual syndrome and perimenopause management. *Comp Ther* 1998; 24: 336–39.

9. Prior JC, Vigna Y, Sciarretta D, et al. Conditioning exercise decreases premenstrual symptoms: a prospective, controlled 6-month trial. *Fertil Steril* 1987; 47(3): 402–408.

10. Barr W. Pyridoxine supplements in the premenstrual syndrome. *Practitioner* 1984; 228: 425–27.

11. Gunn ADG. Vitamin B₆ and the premenstrual syndrome. *Int J Vitam Nutr Res* 1985; (suppl 27: 213–24 [review].

12. Kleijnen J, Riet GT, Knipschild P. Vitamin B₆ in the treatment of the premenstrual syndrome—a review. *Br J Obstet Gynaecol* 1990; 97: 847–52 [review].

13. Williams MJ, Harris RI, Deand BC. Controlled trial of pyridoxine in the treatment of premenstrual syndrome. *J Int Med Res* 1985; 13: 174–79.

14. Brush MG, Perry M. Pyridoxine and the premenstrual syndrome. *Lancet* 1985; i: 1399 [letter].

15. Hagen I, Nesheim B-I, Tuntland T. No effect of vitamin B₆ against premenstrual tension. *Acta Obstet Gynecol Scand* 1985; 64: 667–70.

16. Biskind MS. Nutritional deficiency in the etiology of menorrhagia, metrorrhagia, cystic mastitis and premenstrual tension: treatment with vitamin B-complex. *J Clin Endocrinol Metabol* 1943; 3: 227–34.

17. Biskind MS, Biskind GR, Biskind LH. Nutritional deficiency in the etiology of menorrhagia, metrorrhagia, cystic mastitis and premenstrual tension. *Surg Gynecol Obstet* 1944; 78: 49–57.

18. Piesse JW. Nutritional factors in the premenstrual syndrome. *Int Clin Nutr Rev* 1984; 4(2): 54–80 [review].

19. Horrobin DF, Manku MS, Brush M, et al. Abnormalities in plasma essential fatty acid levels in women with premenstrual syndrome and with nonmalignant breast disease. *J Nutr Med* 1991; 2: 259–64.

20. Puolakka J, Makarainen L, Viinikka L, Ylikorkola O. Biochemical and clinical effects of treating the premenstrual syndrome with prostaglandin synthesis precursors. *J Reprod Med* 1985; 30: 149–53.

21. Ockerman PA, Bachrack I, Glans S, Rassner S. Evening primrose oil as a treatment of the premenstrual syndrome. *Rec Adv Clin Nutr* 1986; 2: 404–405.

22. Massil H, O'Brien PMS, Brush MG. A double blind trial of Efamol evening primrose oil in premenstrual syndrome. *2nd International Symposium on PMS*, Kiawah Island, Sep 1987.

23. Casper R. A double blind trial of evening primrose oil in premenstrual syndrome. *2nd International Symposium on PMS*, Kiawah Island, Sep 1987.

24. Khoo SK, Munro C, Battisutta D. Evening primrose oil and treatment of premenstrual syndrome. *Med J Aust* 1990; 153: 189–92.

25. Collins A, Cerin A, Coleman G, Landgren B-M. Essential fatty acids in the treatment of premenstrual syndrome. *Obstet Gynecol* 1993; 81: 93–98.

26. McFayden IJ, Forest AP, et al. Cyclical breast pain—some observations and the difficulties in treatment. *Br J Clin Pract* 1992; 46: 161–64.

27. Abraham GE, Lubran MM. Serum and red cell magnesium levels in patients with premenstrual tension. *Am J Clin Nutr* 1981; 34: 2364–66.

28. Sherwood RA, Rocks BF, Stewart A, Saxton RS. Magnesium and the premenstrual syndrome. *Ann Clin Biochem* 1986; 23: 667–70.

29. Nicholas A. Traitement du syndrome pre-menstruel et de la dysmenorrhee par l'ion magnesium. In *First International Symposium on Magnesium Deficit in Human Pathology*, ed. J Durlach. Paris: Springer-Verlag, 1973, 261–63.

30. Facchinetti F, Borella P, Sances G, et al. Oral magnesium successfully relieves premenstrual mood changes. *Obstet Gynecol* 1991; 78: 177–81.

31. Werbach MR. Premenstrual syndrome: magnesium. *Int J Alternative Complementary Med* 1994; Feb: 29 [review].

32. Rossignol AM, Bonnlander H. Premenstrual symptoms and beverage consumption. *Am J Obstet Gynecol* 1993; 168: 1640 [letter].

33. Thys-Jacobs S, Ceccarelli S, Bierman A, et al. Calcium supplementation in premenstrual syndrome. *J Gen Intern Med* 1989; 4: 183–89.

34. Penland JG, Johnson PE. Dietary calcium and manganese effects on menstrual cycle symptoms. *Am J Obstet Gynecol* 1993; 168: 1417–23.

35. Panth M, Raman L, Ravinder P, Sivakumar B. Effect of vitamin A supplementation on plasma progesterone and estradiol levels during pregnancy. *Int J Vitam Nutr Res* 1991; 61: 17–19.

36. Block E. The use of vitamin A in premenstrual tension. *Acta Obstet Gynecol Scand* 1960; 39: 586–92.

37. Argonz J, Abinzano C. Premenstrual tension treated with vitamin A. *J Clin Endocrinol* 1950; 10: 1579–89.

38. Chuong CJ, Dawson EB, Smith ER. Vitamin E levels in premenstrual syndrome. *Am J Obstet Gynecol* 1990; 163: 1591–95.

39. London RS, Sundaram GS, Murphy L, Goldstein PJ. The effect of alpha-tocopherol on premenstrual symptomatology: a double blind study. *J Am Coll Nutr* 1983; 2(2): 115–22.

40. London RS, Bradley L, Chiamori NY. Effect of a nutritional supplement on premenstrual symptomatology in women with premenstrual syndrome: a double-blind longitudinal study. *J Am Coll Nutr* 1991; 10: 494–99.

41. Stewart A. Clinical and biochemical effects of nutritional supplementation on the premenstrual syndrome. *J Reprod Med* 1987; 32: 435–41.

42. Böhnert KJ, Hahn G. Phytotherapy in gynecology and obstetrics—Vitex agnus castus. *Erfahrungsheilkunde* 1990; 39: 494–502.

43. Dittmar FW, Böhnert KJ, et al. Premenstrual syndrome: Treatment with a phytopharmaceutical. *Therapiwoche Gynäkol* 1992; 5: 60–68.

44. Lauritzen C, Reuter HD, Repges R, et al. Treatment of premenstrual tension syndrome with Vitex agnus castus. Controlled, double-blind study versus pyridoxine. *Phytomedicine* 1997; 4: 183–89.

45. Qi-bing M, Jing-yi T, Bo C. Advance in the pharmacological studies of radix *Angelica sinensis* (oliv) diels (Chinese danggui). *Chin Med J* 1991; 104: 776–81.

46. Mills SY. *Out of the Earth: The Essential Book of Herbal Medicine*. Middlesex, UK: Viking Arkana, 1991, 520–22.

47. Blumenthal M, Busse WR, Goldberg A, et al. (eds). *The Complete German Commission E Monographs: Therapeutic Guide to Herbal Medicines*. Austin: American Botanical Council and Boston: Integrative Medicine Communications, 1998, 90.

48. Weiss RF. *Herbal Medicine*. Gothenburg, Sweden: Ab Arcanum and Beaconsfield, UK: Beaconsfield Publishers Ltd, 1988, 315.

Pregnancy and Postpartum Support

1. Barnes B, Bradley SG. *Planning for a Healthy Baby*. London: Ebury Press, 1990.

2. Price WA. *Nutrition and Physical Degeneration*, 50th anniv. Ed. New Canaan, CT: Keats Pulishing, Inc., 1989.

3. Gold S, Sherry L. Hyperactivity, learning disabilities, and alcohol. *J Learn Disabil* 1984; 17: 3–6.

4. Northrup C. *Women's Bodies, Women's Wisdom*. New York: Bantam, 1994, 613.

5. Haglund B et al. Cigarette smoking as a risk factor for sudden infant death syndrome. *Am J Public Health* 1990; 80: 29–32.

6. Fenster I et al. Caffeine consumption during pregnancy and fetal growth. *Am J Public Health* 1991; 81: 458–61.

7. Truswell AS. ABC of nutrition. Nutrition for pregnancy. *Br Med J* 1985; 291: 263–66.

8. MRC Vitamin Study Research Group. Prevention of neural tube defects: Results of the Medical Research Council Vitamin Study. *Lancet* 1991; 338: 131–37.

9. Tamura T, Goldenberg R, Freeberg L, et al. Maternal serum folate and zinc concentrations and their relationships to pregnancy outcome. *Am J Clin Nutr* 1992: 56; 365–370.

10. Romslo I, Haram K, Sagen N, Augensen K. Iron requirement in normal pregnancy as assessed by serum ferritin, serum transferrin saturation and erythrocyte protoporphyrin determinations. *Br J Obstet Gynaecol* 1983; 90: 101–107.

11. Bloxam DL, Williams NR, Waskett RJD, et al. Maternal zinc during oral iron supplementation in pregnancy: a preliminary study. *Clin Sci* 1989; 76: 59–65.

Part One: References

12. Mukherjee MD, Sandstead HH, Ratnaparkhi MV, et al. Maternal zinc, iron, folic acid, and protein nutriture and outcome of human pregnancy. *Am J Clin Nutr* 1984; 40: 496–507.

13. Nelson MM, Forfar JO. Associations between drugs administered during pregnancy and congenital abnormalities of the fetus. *Br Med J* 1971; 1: 523–527.

14. Doyle W et al. The association between maternal diet and birth dimensions. *J Nutr Med* 1990; 1: 9–17.

15. Truswell AS. ABC of nutrition: Nutrition for pregnancy. *Br Med J* 1985; 291: 263–66.

16. Villar J, Repke JT. Calcium supplementation during pregnancy may reduce preterm delivery in high-risk populations. *Am J Obstet Gynecol* 1990; 163: 1124–31.

17. Rothman KJ, Moore LL, Singer MR, et al. Teratogenicity of high vitamin A intake. *N Engl J Med* 1995; 333: 1369–73.

18. Mastroiacovo P, Mazzone T, Addis A, et al. High vitamin A intake in early pregnancy and major malformations: a multicenter prospective controlled study. *Teratology* 1999; 59: 7–11.

19. Gladstar R. *Herbal Healing for Women.* New York: Simon and Schuster, 1993, 176.

20. Gladstar R. *Herbal Healing for Women.* New York: Simon and Schuster, 1993, 177.

21. Gladstar R. *Herbal Healing for Women.* New York: Simon and Schuster, 1993, 177.

22. Dale A, Cornwell S. The role of lavender oil in relieving perineal discomfort following childbirth: A blind randomized trial. *J Adv Nursing* 1994; 19: 89–96.

23. Bingel AS, Farnsworth NR. Higher plants as potential sources of galactagogues. *Econ Med Plant Res* 1994; 6: 1–54 [review].

24. Mohr H (1954) [Clinical investigations of means to increase lactation.] *Dtsch Med Wschr* 79: 1513–16 [in German].

25. Weiss RF. *Herbal Medicine.* Gothenburg, Sweden: Ab Arcanum and Beaconsfield, UK: Beaconsfield Publishers Ltd., 1988, 318.

26. Weiss RF. *Herbal Medicine.* Gothenburg, Sweden: Ab Arcanum and Beaconsfield, UK: Beaconsfield Publishers Ltd., 1988, 229–30.

Prostatic Hyperplasia, Benign (BPH)

1. Hart JP, Cooper WL. Vitamin F in the treatment of prostatic hypertrophy. Report Number 1, Lee Foundation for Nutritional Research, Milwaukee, Wisconsin, 1941.

2. Bush IM, Berman E, Nourkayhan S, et al. Zinc and the prostate. Presented at the annual meeting of the American Medical Association Chicago, 1974.

3. Fahim MS, Fahim Z, Der R, Harman J. Zinc treatment for reduction of hyperplasia of prostate. *Fed Proc* 1976; 35(3): 361.

4. Damrau F. Benign prostatic hypertrophy: amino acid therapy for symptomatic relief. *J Am Geriatr Soc* 1962; 10: 426–30.

5. Berges RR, Windeler J, Trampisch HJ, et al. Randomized, placebo-controlled, double-blind clinical trial of beta-sitosterol in patients with benign prostatic hyperplasia. *Lancet* 1995; 345: 1529–32.

6. Horii A, Iwai S, Maekawa M, Tsujita M. Clinical evaluation of Cernilton in the treatment of the benign prostatic hypertrophy. *Hinyokika Kiyo* 1985; 31: 739–45 (in Japanese).

7. Schneider HJ, Honold E, Mashur T. Treatment of benign prostatic hyperplasia. Results of a surveillance study in the practices of urological specialists using a combined plant-base preparation. *Fortschr Med* 1995; 113: 37–40.

8. Koch E, Biber A. Pharmacological effects of sabal and urtica extracts as a basis for a rational medication of benign prostatic hyperplasia. *Urologe* 1994; 334: 90–95.

9. Bach D, Ebeling L. Long-term drug treatment of benign prostatic hyperplasia—results of a prospective 3-year multicenter study using Sabal extract IDS 89. *Phytomedicine* 1996; 3: 105–11 (originally published in *Urologe [B]* 1995; 35: 178–83).

10. Carraro JC, Raynaud JP, Koch G, et al. Comparison of phytotherapy (Permixon) with finasteride in the treatment of benign prostate hyperplasia: A randomized international study of 1,098 patients. *Prostate* 1996; 29: 231–40.

11. Braeckman J, Bruhwyler J, Vandekerckhove K, Géczy J. Efficacy and safety of the extract of *Serenoa repens* in the treatment of benign prostatic hyperplasia: Therapeutic equivalence between twice and once daily dosage forms. *Phytotherapy Res* 1997; 11: 558–63.

12. Wilt TJ, Ishani A, Stark G, et al. Saw palmetto extracts for treatment of benign prostatic hyperplasia. A systematic review. *JAMA* 1998; 280: 1604–1609.

13. Andro MC, Riffaud JP. *Pygeum africanum* extract for the treatment of patients with benign prostatic hyperplasia: a review of 25 years of published experience. *Curr Ther Res* 1995; 56: 796–817.

14. Koch E, Biber A. Pharmacological effects of sabal and urtica extracts as a basis for a rational medication of benign prostatic hyperplasia. *Urologe* 1994; 334: 90–95.

15. Metzker H, Kieser M, Hölscher U. Efficacy of a combined Sabal-Urtica preparation in the treatment of benign prostatic hyperplasia (BPH). *Urologe [B]* 1996; 36: 292–300.

16. Blumenthal M, Busse WR, Goldberg A, et al. (eds). *The Complete German Commission E Monographs: Therapeutic Guide to Herbal Medicines.* Austin: American Botanical Council and Boston: Integrative Medicine Communications, 1998, 193.

Psoriasis

1. Poikolainen K, Reunala T, Karvonen J, et al. Alcohol intake: a risk factor for psoriasis in young and middle aged men? *BMJ* 1990; 300: 780–83.

2. Monk BE, Neill SM. Alcohol consumption and psoriasis. *Dermatologica* 1986; 173: 57–60.

3. Douglas JM. Psoriasis and diet. *West J Med* 1980; 133: 450 [letter].

4. Michaelsson G, Gerden B. How common is gluten intolerance among patients with psoriasis? *Acta Derm Venereol* 1991; 71: 90.

5. Bittiner SB, Tucker WFG, Cartwright I, Bleehen SS. A double-blind, randomised, placebo-controlled trial of fish oil in psoriasis. *Lancet* 1988; i: 378–80.

6. Kojima T, Terano T, Tanabe E, et al. Long-term administration of highly purified eicosapentaenoic acid provides improvement of psoriasis. *Dermatologica* 1991; 182: 225–30.

7. Kojima T, Ternao T, Tanabe E, et al. Effect of highly purified eicosapentaenoic acid on psoriasis. *J Am Acad Dermatol* 1989; 21: 150–51.

8. Soyland E, Funk J, Rajka G, et al. Effect of dietary supplementation with very-long-chain n-3 fatty acids in patients with psoriasis. *N Engl J Med* 1993; 328: 1812–16.

9. Dewsbury CE, Graham P, Darley CR. Topical eicosapentaenoic acid (EPA) in the treatment of psoriasis. *Br J Dermatol* 1989; 120: 581–84.

10. Ashley JM, Lowe NJ, Borok ME, Alfin-Slater RB. Fish oil supplementation results in decreased hypertriglyceridemia in patients with psoriasis undergoing etretinate or acitretin therapy. *J Am Acad Dermatol* 1988; 19: 76–82.

11. Morimoto S, Yoshikawa K, Kozuka T, et al. An open study of vitamin D_3 treatment in psoriasis vulgaris. *Br J Dermatol* 1986; 115: 421–29.

12. Morimoto S, Yoshikawa K. Psoriasis and vitamin D_3. *Arch Dermatol* 1989; 125: 231–34.

13. Kragballe K. Treatment of psoriasis by the topical application of the novel cholecalciferol analogue calcipotriol. *Arch Dermatol* 1989; 125: 1647–52.

14. Smith EL, Pincus SH, Donovan L, Holick MF. A novel approach for the evaluation and treatment of psoriasis. *J Am Acad Dermatol* 1988; 19: 516–28.

15. Kragballe K, Beck HI, Sogaard H. Improvement of psoriasis by a topical vitamin D_3 analogue (MC

903) in a double-blind study. *Br J Dermatol* 1988; 119: 223–30.

16. Henderson CA, Papworth-Smith J, Cunliffe WJ, et al. A double-blind, placebo-controlled trial of topical 1,25-dihydroxycholecalciferol in psoriasis. *Br J Dermatol* 1989; 121: 493–96.

17. Van de Kerkhof PCM, Van Bokhoven M, Zultak M, Czarnetzki BM. A double-blind study of topical 1 alpha,25-dihydroxyvitamin D_3 in psoriasis. *Br J Dermatol* 1989; 120: 661–64.

18. Kolbach DN, Nieboer C. Fumaric acid therapy in psoriasis: results and side effects of 2 years of treatment. *J Am Acad Dermatol* 1992; 27: 769–71.

19. Altmeyer PJ, Matthes U, Pawlak F, et al. Antipsoriatic effect of fumaric acid derivatives. *J Am Acad Dermatol* 1994; 30: 977–81.

20. Ellis CN, Berberian B, Sulica VI, et al. A double-blind evaluation of topical capsaicin in pruritic psoriasis. *J Am Acad Dermatol* 1993; 29: 438–42.

21. Hoffman D. *The Herbal Handbook: A User's Guide to Medical Herbalism.* Rochester, VT: Healing Arts Press, 1988, 23–24 [review].

22. Wiesenauer M, Lüdtke R. *Mahonia aquifolium* in patients with psoriasis vulgaris—an intraindividual study. *Phytomedicine* 1996; 3: 231–35.

23. Galle K, Müller-Jakic B, Proebstle A, et al. Analytical and pharmacological studies on *Mahonia aquifolium*. *Phytomedicine* 1994; 1: 59–62.

Raynaud's Disease

1. Aylward M. Hexopal in Raynaud's disease. *J Int Med Res* 1979; 7: 484–91.

2. Holti G. An experimentally controlled evaluation of the effect of inositol nicotinate upon the digital blood flow in patients with Raynaud's phenomenon. *J Int Med Res* 1979; 7: 473–83.

3. Ring EFJ et al. Quantitative thermographic assessment of inositol nicotinate therapy in Raynaud's phe-

nomenon. *J Int Med Res* 1977; 5: 217–22.

4. Belch JJF, Shaw B, O'Dowd A, et al. Evening primrose oil (Efamol) in the treatment of Raynaud's phenomenon: A double-blind study. *Throm Haemost* 1985; 54(2): 490–94.

5. Leppert J, Aberg H, Levin K, et al. The concentration of magnesium in erythrocytes in female patients with primary Raynaud's phenomenon; fluctuation with the time of year. *Angiology* 1994; 45: 283–88.

6. Smith WO, Hammarsten JF, Eliel LP. The clinical expression of magnesium deficiency. *JAMA* 1960; 174: 77–78.

7. Turlapaty P, Altura BM. Magnesium deficiency produces spasms of coronary arteries; relationship to etiology of sudden death ischemic heart disease. *Science* 1980; 208: 198–200.

8. Gasser P, Martina B, Dubler B. Reaction of capillary blood cell velocity in nailfold capillaries to L-carnitine in patients with vasospastic disease. *Drugs Exptl Clin Res* 1997; 23: 39–43.

9. Digiacomo RA, Kremer JM, Shah DM. Fish-oil dietary supplementation in patients with Raynaud's phenomenon: a double-blind, controlled, prospective study. *Am J Med* 1989; 86: 158–64.

10. Kleijnen J, Knipschild P. *Ginkgo biloba. Lancet* 1992; 340: 1136–39 [review].

Restless Legs Syndrome

1. Kanter AH. The effect of sclerotherapy on restless legs syndrome. *Dermatol Surg* 1995; 21: 328–32.

2. Mountifield JA. Restless leg syndrome relieved by cessation of cigarette smoking. *Can Med Assoc J* 1985; 133: 426.

3. Roberts HJ. Spontaneous leg cramps and "restless legs" due to diabetogenic hyperinsulinism: observations on 131 patients. *J Am Geriatr Soc* 1965; 13: 602–608.

4. Lutz EG. Restless legs, anxiety and caffeinism. *J Clin Psychiatry* 1978; 39: 693–98.

5. O'Keeffe ST, Gavin K, Lavan JN. Iron status and restless legs syn-

drome in the elderly. *Age Ageing* 1994; 23: 200–203.

6. Botez MI. Folate deficiency and neurological disorders in adults. *Med Hypotheses* 1976; 2: 135–40.

7. Ayres S Jr, Mihan R. "Restless legs" syndrome: Response to vitamin E. *J Appl Nutr* 1973; 25: 8–15.

Retinopathy

1. Paetkau ME, Boyd TAS, Winship B, Grace M. Cigarette smoking and diabetic retinopathy. *Diabetes* 1977; 26: 46–49.

2. McCance DR, Hadden DR, Atkinson AB, et al. Long-term glycaemic control and diabetic retinopathy. *Lancet* 1989; 2: 824–28.

3. Anonymous. Retinopathic effect of sucrose-rich diets due to fructose. *Nutr Rev* 1982; 40: 117–18,128.

4. Gaby AR. Fructose, glycosylation, and aging. *Townsend Letter for Doctors and Patients* 1999; Apr: 107–108.

5. Alieva ZA, Gadzhiev RV, Sultanov M. Possible role of the antioxidant system of the vitreous body in delaying the development of diabetic retinopathy. *Oftalmol Zh* 1985; (3): 142–45 [in Russian].

6. Johnson L, Quinn GE, Abbasi S, et al. Effect of sustained pharmacological vitamin E levels on incidence and severity of retinopathy of prematurity: A controlled clinical trial. *J Pediatr* 1989; 114: 827–38.

7. Runge P, Muller DP, McAllister J, et al. Oral vitamin E supplements can prevent the retinopathy of abetalipoproteinaemia. *Br J Ophthalmol* 1986; 70: 166–73.

8. De Hoff JB, Ozazewski J. Alpha tocopherol to treat diabetic retinopathy. *Am J Ophthalmol* 1954; 37: 581–82.

9. Crary EJ, McCarty MF. Potential clinical applications for high-dose nutritional antioxidants. *Med Hypotheses* 1984; 13: 77–98.

10. Jialal I, Joubert SM. The biochemical profile in Indian patients with non-insulin-dependent diabetes in the young with retinopathy. *Diabetes Metabol* 1985; 11: 262–65.

11. McNair P, Christiansen C, Madsbad S, et al. Hypomagnesemia, a risk factor in diabetic retinopathy. *Diabetes* 1978; 27: 1075–78.

12. Erasmus RT, Olukoga AO, Alanamu RA, et al. Plasma magnesium and retinopathy in black African diabetics. *Trop Geogr Med* 1989; 41: 234–37.

13. Ellis JM, Folkers K, Minadeo M, et al. A deficiency of vitamin B_6 is a plausible molecular basis of the retinopathy of patients with diabetes mellitus. *Biochem Biophys Res Commun* 1991; 179: 615–19.

14. Kornerup T, Strom L. Vitamin B_{12} and retinopathy in juvenile diabetics. *Acta Paediatr* 1958: 47: 646–51.

15. Varma D. Inhibition of aldose reductase by flavonoids: Possible attenuation of diabetic complications. *Progr Clin Biol Res* 1986; 213: 343–58.

16. Scharrer A, Ober M. Anthocyanosides in the treatment of retinopathies. *Klin Monatsblatt Augenheilk* 1981; 178: 386–89.

17. Lanthony P, Cosson JP. The course of color vision in early diabetic retinopathy treated with *Ginkgo biloba* extract. A preliminary double-blind versus placebo study. *J Fr Ophtalmol* 1988; 11: 671–74 [in French].

Rheumatoid Arthritis (RA)

1. Levy JA, Ibrahim AB, Shirai T, et al. Dietary fat affects immune response, production of antiviral factors, and immune complex disease in NZP/NZW mice. *Proc Natl Acad Sci* 1982; 79: 1974–78.

2. Jacobson I et al. Correlation of fatty acid composition of adipose tissue lipids and serum phosphatidylcholine and serum concentrations of micronutrients with disease duration in rheumatoid arthritis. *Ann Rheum Dis* 1990; 49: 901–905.

3. Lucas CP, Power L. Dietary fat aggravates active rheumatoid arthritis. *Clin Res* 1981; 29: 754A [abstract].

4. Skoldstram L. Fasting and vegan diet in rheumatoid arthritis. *Scand J Rheumatol* 1987; 15: 219–21.

5. Nenonen M, Helve T, Hanninen O. Effects of uncooked vegan food—"living food"—on rheumatoid arthritis, a three month controlled and randomised study. *Am J Clin Nutr* 1992; 56: 762 [abstr #48].

6. Kjeldsen-Kragh J, Haugen M, Borchgrevink CF, et al. Controlled

trial of fasting and one-year vegetarian diet in rheumatoid arthritis. *Lancet* 1991; 338: 899–902.

7. Warmbrand M. *How Thousands of My Arthritis Patients Regained Their Health*. New York: Arco Publishing, 1974.

8. Panush RS, Carter RL, Katz P, et al. Diet therapy for rheumatoid arthritis. *Arthrit Rheum* 1983; 26: 462–71.

9. Childers NF. A relationship of arthritis to the solanaceae (nightshades). *J Internat Acad Pre Med* 1982; Nov: 31–37.

10. Zeller M. Rheumatoid arthritis—food allergy as a factor. *Ann Allerg* 1949; 7: 200–5,239.

11. Darlington LG, Ramsey NW, Mansfield JR. Placebo-controlled, blind study of dietary manipulation therapy in rheumatoid arthritis. *Lancet* 1986; i: 236–38.

12. Beri D et al. Effect of dietary restrictions on disease activity in rheumatoid arthritis. *Ann Rheum Dis* 1988; 47: 69–72.

13. Panush RS. Possible role of food sensitivity in arthritis. *Ann Allerg* 1988; 61(part 2): 31–35.

14. Taylor MR. Food allergy as an etiological factor in arthropathies: a survey. *J Internat Acad Prev Med* 1983; 8: 28–38 [review].

15. Darlington LG, Ramsey NW. Diets for rheumatoid arthritis. *Lancet* 1991; 338: 1209 [letter].

16. Kay DR, Webel RB, Drisinger TE, et al. Aerobic exercise improves performance in arthritis patients. *Clin Res* 1985; 33: 919A [abstract].

17. Harkcom TM, Lampman RM, Banwell BF, Castor CW. Therapeutic value of graded aerobic exercise training in rheumatoid arthritis. *Arthrit Rheum* 1985; 28: 32–38.

18. Fairburn K, Grootveld M, Ward RJ, et al. Alpha-tocopherol, lipids and lipoproteins in knee-joint synovial fluid and serum from patients with inflammatory joint disease. *Clin Sci* 1992; 83: 657–64.

19. Scherak O, Kolarz G. Vitamin E and rheumatoid arthritis. *Arthrit Rheum* 1991; 34: 1205–1206 [letter].

20. Barton-Wright EC, Elliott WA. The pantothenic acid metabolism of rheumatoid arthritis. *Lancet* 1963; ii: 862–63.

21. General Practitioner Research Group. Calcium pantothenate in arthritic conditions. *Practitioner* 1980; 224: 208–211.

22. Simkin PA. Oral zinc sulphate in rheumatoid arthritis. *Lancet* 1976; ii: 539–42.

23. Peretz A, Neve J, Jeghers O, Pelen F. Zinc distribution in blood components, inflammatory status, and clinical indexes of disease activity during zinc supplementation in inflammatory rheumatic diseases. *Am J Clin Nutr* 1993; 57: 690–94.

24. Job C, Menkes CJ, de Gery A, et al. Zinc sulphate in the treatment of rheumatoid arthritis. *Arthrit Rheum* 1980; 23: 1408.

25. Simkin PA. Treatment of rheumatoid arthritis with oral zinc sulfate. *Agents Actions* 1981; 8(suppl): 587–96.

26. DiSilvestro RA, Marten J, Skehan M. Effects of copper supplementation on ceruloplasmin and copper-zinc superoxide dismutase in free-living rheumatoid arthritis patients. *J Am Coll Nutr* 1992; 11: 177–80.

27. Medical News. Copper boosts activity of anti-inflammatory drugs. *JAMA* 1974; 229: 1268–69.

28. Sorenson JRJ. Copper complexes—a unique class of anti-arthritic drugs. *Progress Med Chem* 1978; 15: 211–60 [review].

29. Walker WR, Keats DM. An investigation of the therapeutic value of the 'copper bracelet'—dermal assimilation of copper in arthritic/rheumatoid conditions. *Agents Actions* 1976; 6: 454–59.

30. Blake DR, Lunec J. Copper, iron, free radicals and arthritis. *Brit J Rheumatol* 1985; 24: 123–27 [editorial].

31. Kremer JM, Jubiz W, Michalek A, et al. Fish-oil fatty acid supplementation in active rheumatoid arthritis. *Ann Int Med* 1987; 106(4): 497–503.

32. Kremer JM, Lawrence DA, Jubiz W, et al. Dietary fish oil and olive oil supplementation in patients with rheumatoid arthritis. *Arthrit Rheum* 1990; 33(6): 810–20.

33. Geusens P, Wouters C, Nijs J, et al. Long-term effect of omega-3 fatty acid supplementation in active rheumatoid arthritis. *Arthrit Rheum* 1994; 37: 824–29.

34. van der Tempel H, Tulleken JE, Limburg PC, et al. Effects of fish oil supplementation in rheumatoid arthritis. *Ann Rheum Dis* 1990; 49: 76–80.

35. Cleland LG, French JK, Betts WH, et al. Clinical and biochemical effects of dietary fish oil supplements in rheumatoid arthritis. *J Rheumatol* 1988; 151471–75.

36. Kremer JM, Lawrence DA, Petrillow GF, et al. Effects of high-dose fish oil on rheumatoid arthritis after stopping nonsteroidal antiinflammatory drugs. *Arthrit Rheum* 1995; 38: 1107–14.

37. Lee TH, Hoover RL, Williams JD, et al. Effect of dietary enrichment with eicosapentaenoic and docosahexaenoic acids on in vitro neutrophil and monocyte leukotriene generation and neutrophil function. *N Engl J Med* 1985; 312(19): 1217–24.

38. Leventhal LJ, Boyce EG, Zurier RB. Treatment of rheumatoid arthritis with gammalinolenic acid. *Ann Intern Med* 1993; 119: 867–73.

39. Zurier RB, Rossetti RG, Jacobson EW, et al. Gamma-liolenic acid treatment of rheumatoid arthritis. A randomized, placebo-controlled trial. *Arthritis Rheum* 1996; 39: 1808–17.

40. Leventahn LJ, Boyce EG, Zuerier RB. Treatment of rheumatoid arthritis with black currant seed oil. *Brit J Rheumatol* 1994; 33: 847–52.

41. Brzeski M, Madhok R, Capell HA. Evening primrose oil in patients with rheumatoid arthritis and side-effects of non-steroidal anti-inflammatory drugs. *Brit J Rheumatol* 1991; 30: 370–72.

42. Jantti J, Seppala E, Vapaatalo H, Isomaki H. Evening primrose oil and olive oil in treatment of rheumatoid arthritis. *Clin Rheumatol* 1989; 8: 238–44.

43. Belch JJF, Ansell D, Madhok R, et al. Effects of altering dietary essential fatty acids on requirements for non-steroidal anti-inflammatory drugs in patients with rheumatoid arthritis: a double blind placebo controlled study. *Ann Rheum Dis* 1988; 47: 96–104.

44. Newnham RE. Arthritis or skeletal fluorosis and boron. *Int Clin Nutr Rev* 1991; 11: 68–70 [letter].

45. Balagot RC, Ehrenpreis S, Kubota K, et al. Analgesia in mice and humans by D-phenylalanine: Relation to inhibition of enkephalin degradation and enkephalin levels. *Adv Pain Res Ther* 1983; 5: 289–93.

46. American Medical Association. Dimethyl sulfoxide. Controversy and Current Status—1981. *JAMA* 1982; 248: 1369–71.

47. Jimenez RAH, Willkens RF. Dimethyl sulfoxide: A perspective of its use in rheumatic diseases. *J Lab Clin Med* 1982; 100: 489–500.

48. Jacob SW, Wood DC. Dimethyl sulfoxide (DMSO). Toxicology, pharmacology, and clinical experience. *Am J Surg* 1967; 114: 414–26.

49. Hartung EF, Steinbroker O. Gastric acidity in chronic arthritis. *Ann Intern Med* 1935; 9: 252.

50. Cohen A, Goldman J. Bromelains therapy in rheumatoid arthritis. *Pennsyl Med J* 1964; 67: 27–30.

51. Singh GB, Singh S, Bani S. New phytotherapeutic agent for the treatment of arthritis and allied disorders with novel mode of action. *4th International Congress on Phytotherapy*, Munich, Germany, Sep 10–13, 1992.

52. Kulkarni RR, Patki VP, et al. Treatment of osteoarthritis with a herbomineral formulation: A double-blind, placebo-controlled, cross-over study. *J Ethnopharm* 1991; 33: 91–95.

53. Deodhar SD, Sethi R, Srimal RC Preliminary studies on antirheumatic activity of curcumin (diferuloyl methane). *Ind J Med Res* 1980; 71: 632–34.

54. Srivastava KC, Mustafa T. Ginger (*Zingiber officinale*) in rheumatism and musculoskeletal disorders. *Med Hypoth* 1992; 39: 342–48.

55. Deal CL, Schnitzer TJ, Lipstein E, et al. Treatment of arthritis with topical capsaicin: A double-blind trial. *Clin Ther* 1991; 13: 383–95.

56. Bone K. The story of devil's claw: Is it an herbal antirheumatic? *Nutrition and Healing* 1998; October: 3,4,8 [review].

Part One: References

57 Blumenthal M, Busse WR, Goldberg A, et al. (eds). *The Complete German Commission E Monographs: Therapeutic Guide to Herbal Medicines*. Austin: American Botanical Council and Boston: Integrative Medicine Communications, 1998, 230.

58. Blumenthal M, Busse WR, Goldberg A, et al. (eds). *The Complete German Commission E Monographs: Therapeutic Guide to Herbal Medicines*. Austin: American Botanical Council and Boston: Integrative Medicine Communications, 1998, 430–31.

Shingles (Herpes Zoster) and Postherpetic Neuralgia

1. Schiller F. Herpes zoster: review, with preliminary report on new method for treatment of postherpetic neuralgia. *J Am Geriatr Soc* 1954; 2: 726–35.

2. Heyblon R. Vitamin B_{12} in herpes zoster. *JAMA* 1951; 146: 1338 [abstract].

3. Ayres S Jr, Mihan R. Post-herpes zoster neuralgia: response to vitamin E therapy. *Arch Dermatol* 1973; 108: 855–66.

4. Ayres S Jr, Mihan R. Post-herpes zoster neuralgia: response to vitamin E therapy. *Arch Dermatol* 1975; 111: 396.

5. Cochrane T. Post-herpes zoster neuralgia: response to vitamin E therapy. *Arch Dermatol* 1975; 111: 396.

6. Bernstein JE, Korman NJ, Bickers DR, et al. Topical capsaicin treatment of chronic postherpetic neuralgia. *J Am Acad Dermatol* 1989; 21: 265–70.

7. Sklar SH, Blue WT, Alexander EJ, et al. Herpes zoster. The treatment and prevention of neuralgia with adenosine monophosphate. *JAMA* 1985; 253: 1427–30.

8. Sklar SH, Wigand JS. Herpes zoster. *Br J Dermatol* 1981; 104: 351–52.

9. Bernstein JE, Korman NJ, Bickers DR, et al. Topical capsaicin treatment of chronic postherpetic neuralgia. *J Am Acad Dermatol* 1989; 21: 265–70.

10. Bernstein JE, Bickers DR, Dahl MV, Roshal JY. Treatment of chronic postherpetic neuralgia with topical capsaicin. *J Am Acad Dermatol* 1987; 17: 93–96.

11. Baba M, Shigeta S. Antiviral activity of glycyrrhizin against varicella-zoster virus in vitro. *Antivir Res* 1987; 7: 99–107.

Sinusitis

1. Bullock C. Chronic infectious sinusitis linked to allergies. *Med Trib* 1995; Dec 7: 1.

2. Derebery MJ. Otoplaryngic allergy. *Otolaryngol Clin North Am* 1993; 26: 593–611 [review].

3. Host A. Mechanisms in adverse reactions to food. *Allergy* 1995; 50(20 suppl): 60–63 [review].

4. Martin W. On treating allergic disorders! *Townsend Letter for Doctors* 1991; Aug/Sept: 670–71 [letter].

5. Clemetson, CA. Histamine and ascorbic acid in human blood. *J Nutr* 1980; 110: 662–68.

6. Bucca C, Rolla G, Oliva A, Farina JC. Effect of vitamin C on histamine bronchial responsiveness of patients with allergic rhinitis. *Ann Allergy* 1990; 65: 311–14.

7. Bellioni P et al. La provocazione istaminica in soggetti allergici. Il ruolo dell'acido ascorbico. *Eur Rev Med Pharm Sci* 1987; 9: 419–22.

8. Nikolaev MP, Longunov AI, Tsyrulnikova LG, Dzhalilov DS. Clinical and biochemical aspects in the treatment of acute maxillary sinusitis with antioxidants. *Vestn Otorinolaringol* 1994; Jan/Feb: 22–26.

9. Ryan R. A double blind clinical evaluation of bromelains in the treatment of acute sinusitis. *Headache* 1967; 7: 13–17.

10. Taub SJ. The use of bromelains in sinusitis: a double-blind evaluation. *EENT Monthly* 1967; 46(3): 361–65.

11. Seltzer AP. Adjunctive use of bromelains in sinusitis: a controlled study. *EENT Monthly* 1967; 46(10): 1281–88.

12. Gaby AR. The story of bromelain! *Nutr Healing* 1995; May: 3,4,11.

13. Mittman P. Randomized, double blind study of freeze dried *Urtica dioica* in the treatment of allergic rhinitis. *Planta Med* 1990; 56: 44–47.

14. Schulz V, Hansel R, Tyler VE. *Rational Phytotherapy*, 3rd ed. Berlin, Germany: Springer Verlag, 1998, 146–47.

Tardive Dyskinesia

1. Tkacz C. A preventive measure for tardive dyskinesia. *J Int Acad Prev Med* 1984; 8: (5)5–8.

2. Toll N. To the editor. *J Orthomolec Psychiatry* 1982; 11: 42.

3. Adler LA, Peselow E, Rotrosen J, et al. Vitamin E treatment of tardive dyskinesia. *Am J Psychiatry* 1993; 150: 1405–7.

4. Sajjad SHA. Vitamin E in the treatment of tardive dyskinesia: a preliminary study over 7 months a tdifferent doses. *Int Clin Psychopahrmacol* 1998; 13: 147–55.

5. Elkashef AM, Ruskin PE, Bacher N, Barrett D. Vitamin E in the treatment of tardive dyskinesia. *Am J Psychiatry* 990; 147: 505–6.

6. Lohrr JB, Cadet JL, Lohr MA. Alpha-tocopherol in trdive dyskinesia. *Lancet* 1987; 1: 913–14.

7. Shriqui CL, Bradwejn J, Annable L, Jones BD. Vitamin E in the treatment of tardive dyskinesia: a double-blind placebo-controlled study. *Am J Psychiatry* 1992; 149: 391–93.

8. Dorevitch A, Kalian M, Shlafman M, Lerner V. Treatment of long-term tardive dyskinesia with vitamin E. *Biol Psychiatry* 1997; 41: 114–16.

9. Egan MF, Hyde TH, Albers GW, et al. Treatment of tardive dyskinesia with vitamin E. *Am J Psychiatry* 1992; 149: 773–77.

10. Lohr JB, Caligiuri MP. A double-blind placebo-controlled study of vitamin E treatment of tardive dyskinesia. *J Clin Psychiatry* 1996; 57: 167–73.

11. Kunin RA. Manganese in dyskinesias. *Am J Psychiatry* 1976; 133: 105.

12. Norris JP, Sams RE. More on the use of manganese in dyskinesia. *Am J Psychiatry* 1997; 134: 1448.

13. Vaddadi KS. Essential fatty acids and neuroleptic drug-associated tardive dyskinesia: preliminary clinical

observations. *IRCS Med Sci* 1984; 12: 678.

14. Vaddadi KS, Courtney P, Gilleard CJ, et al. A double-blind trial of essential fatty acid supplementation in patients with tardive dyskinesia. *Psychiatr Res* 1989; 27: 313–23.

15. Davis KL, Hollister LE, Barchas JD, Berger PA. Choline in tardive dyskinesia and Huntington's disease: preliminary results from a pilot study. *Am J Psychiatry* 1979; 136: 772–76.

17. Anderson BG, Reker D, Ristich M, et al. Lecithin treatment of tardive dyskinesia—a progress report. *Psychopharmacol Bull* 1982; 18: 87–88.

Tinnitus (Ringing in the Ears)

1. Spencer JT Jr. Hyperlipoproteinemia, hyperinsulinism, and Ménière's disease. *South Med J* 1981; 74: 1194–97.

2. Shemesh Z et al. Vitamin B_{12} deficiency in patients with chronic tinnitus and noise-induced hearing loss. *Am J Otolaryngol* 1993; 14: 94–99.

3. Shambaugh GE. Zinc and presbycusis. *Am J Otol* 1985; 6: 116–17.

4. Paaske PB, Kjems G, Pedersen CB, Sam ILK. Zinc in the management of tinnitus. Placebo-controlled trial. *Ann Otol Rhinol Laryngol* 1991; 100: 647–49.

5. Rosenberg SI, Silverstein H, Rowan PT, Olds MJ. Effect of melatonin on tinnitus. *Laryngoscope* 1998; 108: 305–10.

6. Meyer B. A multicenter, double-blind, drug versus placebo study of *Ginkgo biloba* extract in the treatment of tinnitus. *Presse Med* 1986; 5: 1562–64 [in French].

7. Meyer B. A multicenter randomized double-blind study of *Ginkgo biloba* extract versus placebo in the treatment of tinnitus. In *Rokan (Ginkgo biloba): Recent Results in Pharmacology and Clinic,* ed. EW Funfgeld. New York: Springer-Verlag, 1988, 245–50.

8. Holgers K, Axelsson A, Pringle I. *Ginkgo biloba* extract from the treatment of tinnitus. *Audiol* 1994; 33: 85–92.

9. Weiss RF. *Herbal Medicine.* Gothenburg, Sweden: Ab Arcanum and Beaconsfield, UK: Beaconsfield Publishers Ltd, 1988, 181.

Ulcerative Colitis

1. Pullan RD, Rhodes J, Ganesh S, et al. Transdermal nicotine for active ulcerative colitis. *N Engl J Med* 1994; 330: 811–15.

2. Thomas GA, Rhodes J, Mani V, et al. Transdermal nicotine as maintenance therapy for ulcerative colitis. *N Engl J Med* 1995; 332: 988–92.

3. Rhodes J, Thomas GA. Smoking: good or bad for inflammatory bowel disease? *Gastroenterol* 1994; 106: 907–10[editorial].

4. Reif S, Klein I, Lubin F, et al. Pre-illness dietary factors in inflammatory bowel disease. *Gut* 1997; 40: 754–60.

5. Thornton JR, Emmett PM, Heaton KW. Diet and ulcerative colitis. *BMJ* 1980; 1: 293–94.

6. Jarmerot G, Jammark I, Nilsson K. Consumption of refined sugar by patients with Crohn's disease, ulcerative colitis or irritable bowel syndrome. *Scand J Gastroenterol* 1983; 18: 999–1002.

7. Reif S, Klein I, Lubin F, et al. Pre-illness dietary factors in inflammatory bowel disease. *Gut* 1997; 40: 754–60.

8. Kono S. Dietary and other risk factors of ulcerative colitis. A case-control study in Japan. *J Clin Gastroenterol* 1994; 19: 166–71.

9. Rowe AH. Chronic ulcerative colitis—allergy in its etiology. *Ann Intern Med* 1942; 17: 83–100.

10. Andresen AFR. Ulcerative colitis—an allergic phenomenon. *Am J Dig Dis* 1942; 9: 91–98.

11. Candy S, Borok G, Wright JP, et al. The value of an elimination diet in the management of patients with ulcerative colitis. *S Afr Med J* 1995; 85: 1176–79.

12. Lashner BA, Heidnreich PA, Su GL, et al. Effect of folate supplementation on the incidence of dysplasia and cancer in chronic ulcerative colitis. *Gastroenterol* 1989; 97: 255–59.

13. Lashner BA. Red blood cell folate is associated with the development of dysplasia and cancer in ulcer-ative colitis. *J Cancer Res Clin Oncol* 1993; 119: 549–54.

14. Lashner BA, Provencher KS, Seidner DL, et al. The effect of folic acid supplementation on the risk for cancer or dysplasia in ulcerative colitis. *Gastroenterol* 1997; 112: 29–32.

15. Kim YI, Salomon RN, Graeme-Cooke F, et al. Dietary folate protects against the development of macroscopic colonic neoplasia in a does responsive manner in rats. *Gut* 1996; 39: 732–40.

16. Elsbord L, Larsen L. Folate deficiency in chronic inflammatory bowel disease. *Scand J Gastroenterol* 1979; 14: 1019–24.

17. Halsted CH, Gandhi G, Tamura T. Sulfasalazine inhibits the absorption of folates in ulcerative colitis. *N Engl J Med* 1981; 317: 1513–17.

18. Kaltsky AL, Armstrong MA, Friedman GD, Hiatt RA. The relations of alcoholic beverage use to colon and rectal cancer. *Am J Epidemiol* 1988; 128: 1007–15.

19. Stenson WF, Cort D, Rodgers J, et al. Dietary supplementation with fish oil in ulcerative colitis. *Ann Intern Med* 1992; 116: 609–14.

20. Hawthorne AB, Daneshmend TK, Hawkey CJ, et al. Treatment of ulcerative colitis with fish oil supplementation: a prospective 12 month randomised controlled trial. *Gut* 1992; 33: 922–28.

21. Aslan A, Triadafílopoulos G. Fish oil fatty acid supplementation in active ulcerative colitis: a double-blind, placebo-controlled, crossover study. *Am J Gastroenterol* 1992; 87: 432–37.

22. Salomon P, Kornbluth AA, Janowitz HD. Treatment of ulcerative colitis with fish oil n-3-omega-fatty acid: an open trial. *J Clin Gastroenterol* 1990; 12: 157–61.

23. Scheppach W, Sommer H, Kirchner T, et al. Effect of butyrate enemas on the colonic mucosa in distal ulcerative colitis. *Gastroenterol* 1992; 103: 51–56.

24. Gupta I, Parihar A, Malhotra P, et al. Effects of *Boswellia serrata* gum resin in patients with ulcerative colitis. *Eur J Med Res* 1997; 2: 37–43.

25. Weiss RF. *Herbal Medicine.* Beaconsfield, UK: Beaconsfield Publishers Ltd, 1989: 114–15.

26. Weiss RF. *Herbal Medicine.* Beaconsfield, UK: Beaconsfield Publishers Ltd, 1989: 26.

27. Weiss RF. *Herbal Medicine.* Beaconsfield, UK: Beaconsfield Publishers Ltd, 1989: 114–15.

Urinary Tract Infection (UTI)

1. Sanchez A, Reeser JL, Lau HS, et al. Role of sugars in human neutrophilic phagocytosis. *Am J Clin Nutr* 1973; 26: 1180–84.

2. MacGregor RR. Alcohol and immune defense. *JAMA* 1986; 256: 1474.

3. Barone J, Herbert JR, Reddy MM. Dietary fat and natural-killer-cell activity. *Am J Clin Nutr* 1989; 50: 861–67.

4. Horesh AJ. Allergy and infection. Proof of infectious etiology. *J Asthma Res* 1967; 4: 269–82.

5. Rudolph JA. Allergy as a cause of frequent recurring colds and coughs in children. *Dis Chest* 1940; 6: 138.

6. Berman BA. Pseudomononucleosis of allergic origin: a new clinical entity. *Ann Allerg* 1964; 22: 403–409.

7. Randolph TG, Hettig RA. The coincidence of allergic disease, unexplained fatigue, and lymphadenopathy; possible diagnostic confusion with infectious mononucleosis. *Am J Med Sci* 1945; 209: 306–14.

8. Sirsi M. Antimicrobial action of vitamin C on M. tuberculosis and some other pathogenic organisms. *Indian J Med Sci* 1952; 6: 252–55.

9. Axelrod DR. Ascorbic acid and urinary pH. *JAMA* 1985; 254: 1310–11.

10. Hussey GD, Klein M. A randomized, controlled trial of vitamin A in children with severe measles. *N Engl J Med* 1990; 323: 160–64.

11. Mori S, Ojima Y, Hirose T, et al. The clinical effect of proteolytic enzyme containing bromelain and trypsin on urinary tract infection evaluated by double blind method. *Acta Obstet Gynaecol Jpn* 1972; 19: 147–53.

12. Chandra RK. Effect of vitamin and trace-element supplementation on immune responses and infection in elderly subjects. *Lancet* 1992; 340: 1124–27.

13. Avorn J, Monane M, Gurwitz JH, et al. Reduction of bacteriuria and pyuria after ingestion of cranberry juice. *JAMA* 1994; 271: 751–54.

14. Dignam R, Ahmed M, Denman S, et al. The effect of cranberry juice on UTI rates in a long term care facility. *J Am Geriatr Soc* 1997; 45: S53.

15. Sobota AE. Inhibition of bacterial adherence by cranberry juice: Potential use for the treatment of urinary tract infections. *J Urol* 1984; 131: 1013–16.

16. Bodel PT, Cotran R, Kass EH. Cranberry juice and the antibacterial action of hippuric acid. *J Lab Clin Med* 1959; 54: 881–88.

17. Sun DX, Abraham SN, Beachey EH. Influence of berberine sulfate on synthesis and expression of pap fimbrial adhesin in uropathogenic *Escherichia coli. Antimicr Agents Chemother* 1988; 32: 1274–77.

18. European Scientific Cooperative for Phytotherapy. *Proposal for European Monographs*, Vol. 3. Bevrijdingslaan, Netherlands: ESCOP Secretariat, 1992.

19. Blumenthal M, Busse WR, Goldberg A, et al. (eds). *The Complete German Commission E Monographs: Therapeutic Guide to Herbal Medicines.* Austin: American Botanical Council and Boston: Integrative Medicine Communications, 1998, 224–25.

20. Blumenthal M, Busse WR, Goldberg A, et al. (eds). *The Complete German Commission E Monographs: Therapeutic Guide to Herbal Medicines.* Austin: American Botanical Council and Boston: Integrative Medicine Communications, 1998, 428.

21. Leung AY, Foster S. *Encyclopedia of Common Natural Ingredients Used in Food, Drugs and Cosmetics.* New York: John Wiley & Sons, 1996, 104–105.

22. Blumenthal M, Busse WR, Goldberg A, et al. (eds). *The Complete German Commission E Monographs:*

Therapeutic Guide to Herbal Medicines. Austin: American Botanical Council and Boston: Integrative Medicine Communications, 1998, 317.

23. Kienholz VM, Kemkes B. The anti-bacterial action of ethereal oils obtained from horse radish root (*Cochlearia armoracia* L.). *Arzneimittelforschung* 1961; 10: 917–18 [in German].

24. Schindler VE, Zipp H, Marth I. Comparative clinical investigations of an enzyme glycoside mixture obtained from horse radish roots (*Cochlearia armoracia* L.). *Arzneimittelforschung* 1961; 10: 919–21 [in German].

25. Mills SY. *Out of the Earth: The Essential Book of Herbal Medicine.* London: Viking Arkana, 1991, 493–94.

Vaginitis

1. Heidrich F, Berg A, Bergman J. Clothing factors and vaginitis. *J Fam Prac* 1984; 19: 491–94.

2. Kudelco N. Allergy in chronic monilial vaginitis. *Ann Allergy* 1971; 29: 266–67.

3. Horowitz BJ, Edelstein SW, Lippman L. Sugar chromatography studies in recurrent candida vulvovaginitis. *J Reprod Med* 1984; 29: 441–43.

4. Hilton E, Isenberg H, Alperstein P, et al. Ingestion of yogurt containing *Lactobacillus acidophilus* as prophylaxis for candidal vaginitis. *Ann Intern Med* 1992; 116: 353–57.

5. Wilcox G, Wahlqvist M, Burger H, et al. Oestrogenic effects of plant foods in postmenopausal women. *Br Med J* 1990; 301: 905–906.

6. Jovanovic R, Congema E, Nguyen H. Antifungal agents vs. boric acid for treating chronic mycotic vulvovaginitis. *J Reprod Med* 1991; 36: 593–97.

7. Pena E. *Melaleuca alternifolia* oil: Its use for trichomonal vaginitis and other vaginal infections. *Obstet Gynecol* 1962; 19: 793–95.

8. Hughes BG, Lawson LD. Antimicrobial effects of *Allium sativum* (garlic), *Allium ampelopra-*

sum L (elephant garlic), and *Allium cepa* (onion), garlic compounds and commercial garlic supplement products. *Phytother Res* 1991; 5: 154–58.

9. Melchart D, Linde K, Worku F, et al. Immunomodulation with *Echinacea*—a systematic review of controlled clinical trials. *Phytomedicine* 1994; 1: 245–54.

Varicose Veins

1. European Scientific Cooperative on Phytotherapy. *Hamamelidis folium* (Hamamelis leaf). *ESCOP Monographs on the Medicinal Uses of Plant Drugs.* Exeter, UK: ESCOP, 1997.

2. Blumenthal M, Busse WR, Goldberg A, et al. (eds). *The Complete German Commission E Monographs: Therapeutic Guide to Herbal Medicines.* Austin, TX: American Botanical Council and Boston: Integrative Medicine Communications, 1998, 231.

3. Blumenthal M, Busse WR, Goldberg A, et al. (eds). *The Complete German Commission E Monographs: Therapeutic Guide to Herbal Medicines.* Austin, TX: American Botanical Council and Boston: Integrative Medicine Communications, 1998, 149.

4. Kreysel HW, Nissen HP, Enghofer E. A possible role of lysosomal enzymes in the pathogenesis of varicosis and the reduction in their serum activity by Venostasin. *Vasa* 1983; 12: 377–82.

Vitiligo

1. Ortonne JP, Bose SK. Vitiligo: where do we stand? *Pigment Cell Res* 1993; 6: 61–72.

2. Montes LF, Diaz ML, Lajous J, Garcia NJ. Folic acid and vitamin B_{12} in vitiligo: a nutritional approach. *Cutis* 1992; 50: 39–42.

3. Juhlin L, Olsson MJ. Improvement of vitiligo after oral treatment with vitamin B_{12} and folic acid and the importance of sun exposure. *Acta Derm Venereol* 1997; 77: 460–62.

4. Siddiqui AH, Stolk LM, Bhaggoe R, et al. L-phenylalanine and UVA irradiation in the treatment of vitiligo. *Dermatology* 1994; 188: 215–18.

5. Schulpis CH, Antoniou C, Michas T, Strarigos J. Phenylalanine plus ultraviolet light: preliminary report of a promising treatment for childhood vitiligo. *Pediatr Dermatol* 1989; 6: 332–35.

6. Camacho F, Mazuecos J. Treatment of vitiligo with oral and topical phenylalanine: 6 years of experience. *Arch Dermatol* 1999; 135: 216–17.

7. Francis HW. Achlorhydria as an etiological factor in vitiligo, with report of four cases. *Nebraska State Med J* 1931; 16(1): 25–26.

8. Sieve BF. Further investigations in the treatment of vitiligo. *Virginia Med Monthly* 1945; Jan: 6–17.

9. Abdel-Fattah, Aboul-Enein MN, Wassel GM, El-Menshawi BS. An approach to the treatment of vitiligo by khellin. *Dermatologica* 1982; 165: 136–40.

10. Brown DJ. *Herbal Prescriptions for Better Health.* Rocklin, CA: Prima Publishing, 1996, 294–95.

Weight Loss and Obesity

1. Duncan KH, Bacon JA, Weinsier RL. The effects of high and low energy density diets on satiety, energy intake, and eating time of obese and nonobese subjects. *Am J Clin Nutr* 1983; 37: 763–67.

2. Marquette CJ Jr. Effects of bulk producing tablets on hunger intensity in dieting patients. *Obes Bariatr Med* 1976; 5(3): 84–88.

3. Rossner S, von Zweigbergk D, Ohlin A, Ryttig K. Weight reduction with dietary fibre supplements. *Acta Med Scand* 1987; 222: 83–88.

4. Biancardi G, Palmiero L, Ghirardi PE. Glucomannan in the treatment of overweight patients with osteoarthritis. *Curr Ther Res* 1989; 46: 908–12.

5. Hylander B, Rössner S. Effects of dietary fiber intake before meals on weight loss and hunger in a weight-reducing club. *Acta Med Scand* 1983; 213: 217–20.

6. Randolph TG. Masked food allergy as a factor in the development

and persistence of obesity. *J Lab Clin Med* 1947; 32: 1547.

7. Muls E, Kempen K, Vansant G, et al. Is weight cycling detrimental to health? A review of the literature in humans. *Int J Obes* 1995; 19(3): S46–S50.

8. Anonymous. Effect of exercise alone on obesity. *Br Med J* 1976; 1: 417–18.

9. Racette SB, Schoeller DA, Kushner RF, Neil KM. Exercise enhances dietary compliance during moderate energy restriction in obese women. *Am J Clin Nutr* 1995; 62: 345–49.

10. P. TG, Southern LL, Ward TL, Thompson DL Jr. Effect of chromium picolinate on growth and serum and carcass traits of growing-finishing pigs. *J Anim Sci* 1993; 71: 656–62.

11. Lefavi R, Anderson R, Keith R, et al. Efficacy of chromium supplementation in athletes: Emphasis on anabolism. *Int J Sport Nutr* 1992; 2: 111–22.

12. McCarty MF. The case for supplemental chromium and a survey of clinical studies with chromium picolinate. *J Appl Nutr* 1991; 43: 59–66.

13. Hallmark MA, Reynolds TH, DeSouza CA, et al. Effects of chromium and resistive training on muscle strength and body composition. *Med Sci Sports Exerc* 1996; 28: 139–44.

14. Lowenstein JM. Effect of (-)-hydroxycitrate on fatty acid synthesis by rat liver in vivo. *J Biol Chem* 1971; 246: 629–32.

15. Triscari J, Sullivan AC. Comparative effects of (-)-hydroxycitrate and (+)-allo-hydroxycitrate on acetyl CoA carboxylase and fatty acid and cholesterol synthesis in vivo. *Lipids* 1977; 12: 357–63.

16. Cheema-Dhadli S, Harlperin ML, Leznoff CC. Inhibition of enzymes which interact with citrate by (-)-hydroxycitrate and 1,2,3,-tricarboxybenzene. *Eur J Biochem* 1973; 38: 98–102.

17. Sullivan AC, Hamilton JG, Miller ON, et al. Inhibition of lipogenesis in rat liver by (-)-hydroxycitrate.

Arch Biochem Biophys 1972; 150: 183–90.

18. Greenwood MRC, Cleary MP, Gruen R, et al. Effect of (-)-hydroxycitrate on development of obesity in the Zucker obese rat. *Am J Physiol* 1981; 240: E72–78.

19. Sullivan AC, Triscari J. Metabolic regulation as a control for lipid disorders. *Am J Clin Nutr* 1977; 30: 767–76.

20. Sullivan AC, Triscari J, Hamilton JG, et al. Effect of (-)-hydroxycitrate upon the accumulation of lipid in the rat: I. Lipogenesis. *Lipids* 1974; 9: 121–28.

21. Sullivan AC, Triscari J, Hamilton JG, et al. Effect of (-)-hydroxycitrate upon the accumulation of lipid in the rat: II. Appetite. *Lipids* 1974; 9: 129–34.

22. Sergio W. A natural food, the Malabar Tamarind, may be effective in the treatment of obesity. *Med Hypotheses* 1988; 27: 39–40.

23. Stanko RT, Tietze DL, and Arch JE. Body composition, energy utilization, and nitrogen metabolism with a 4.25-MJ/d low-energy diet supplemented with pyruvate. *Am J Clin Nutr* 1992; 56: 630–35.

24. Stanko RT, Reynolds HR, Hoyson R, et al. Pyruvate supplementation of a low-cholesterol, low-fat diet: Effects on plasma lipid concentration and body composition in hyperlipidemic patients. *Am J Clin Nutr* 1994; 59: 423–27.

29. Ivy JL, Cortez MY, Chandler RM, et al. Effects of pyruvate on the metabolism and insulin resistance of obese Zucker rats. *Am J Clin Nutr* 1994; 59: 331–37.

26. Becher EW, Jakober B, Luft D, et al. Clinical and biochemical evaluations of the alga spirulina with regard to its application in the treatment of obesity. A double-blind crossover study. *Nutr Rep Intl* 1986; 33: 565–73.

27. Ceci F, Cangiano C, Cairella M, et al. The effects of oral 5-hydroxytryptophan administration on feeding behavior in obese adult female subjects. *J Neural Transm* 1989; 76: 109–17.

28. Cangiano C, Ceci F, Cascino A, et al. Eating behavior and adherence to dietary prescriptions in obese adult subjects treated with 5-hydroxytryptophan. *Am J Clin Nutr.* 1992; 56: 863–67.

29. Leung A, Foster S. *Encyclopedia of Common Natural Ingredients Used in Food, Drugs, and Cosmetics*, 2d ed. New York: John Wiley & Sons, 1996, 293–94.

30. Breum L, Pedersen JK, Ahlstrom F, et al. Comparison of an ephedrine/caffeine combination and dexfenfluramine in the treatment of obesity. A double-blind multi-centre trial in general practice. *Int J Obes Relat Metab Disord* 1994; 18: 99–103.

31. Toubro S, Astrup A, Breum L, et al. The acute and chronic effects of ephedrine/caffeine mixtures on energy expenditure and glucose metabolism in humans. *Int J Obes Relat Metab Disord* 1993; 17(suppl 3): 73–77.

Wilson's Disease

1. Hoogenraad TU, Van den Hammer CJA, Van Hattum J. Effective treatment of Wilson's disease with oral zinc sulphate: two case reports. *Br Med J* 1984; 289: 273–76.

2. Cossack ZT. The efficacy of oral zinc therapy as an alternative to penicillamine for Wilson's disease. *N Engl J Med* 1988; 318: 322–23 [letter/review].

3. Brewer GJ, Yuzbasiyan-Gurkan V. The use of zinc-copper metabolic interactions in the treatment of Wilson's disease. *J Am Coll Nutr* 1989; 8: 452 [abstr# 103].

4. Brewer GJ, Hill GM, Dick RD, et al. Treatment of Wilson's disease with zinc. III. Prevention of reaccumulation of hepatic copper. *J Lab Clin Med* 1987; 109: 526–31.

5. Brewer GJ, Yuzbasiyan-Gurkan V. Use of zinc-copper metabolic interactions in the treatment of Wilson's disease. *J Am Coll Nutr* 1990; 9: 487–91.

6. Brewer JG, Yuzbasiyan-Gurkan V, Lee D-Y, Appelman H. Treatment of Wilson's disease with zinc. VI. Initial treatment studies. *J Lab Clin Med* 1989; 114: 633–38.

7. Van den Hamer CJA, Hoogenraad TU. Copper deficiency in Wilson's disease. *Lancet* 1989; ii: 442 [letter].

8. van Caillie-Bertrand M, Degenhart HJ, Visser HKA, et al. Oral zinc sulphates for Wilson's disease. *Arch Dis Child* 1985; 60: 656–59.

9. Brewer JG, Yuzbasiyan-Gurkan V, Lee D-Y, Appelman H. Treatment of Wilson's disease with zinc. VI. Initial treatment studies. *J Lab Clin Med* 1989; 114: 633–38.

Wound Healing

1. Declair V. The usefulness of topical application of essential fatty acids (EFA) to prevent pressure ulcers. *Ostomy Wound Manage* 1997; 43(5): 48–52,54.

2. Breslow RA, Hallfrisch J, Guy DG, et al. The importance of dietary protein in healing pressure ulcers. *J Am Geriatr Soc* 1993; 41(4): 357–362.

3. Ringsdorf WM, Cheraskin E. Vitamin C and human wound healing. *Oral Surg Oral Med Oral Pathol* 1982; 53(3): 231–36.

4. Taylor TV, Rimmer S, Day B, Butcher J, Dymock IW. Ascorbic acid supplementation in the treatment of pressure-sores. *Lancet* 1974; 2: 544–46.

5. Weismann K. What is the use of zinc for wound healing? *Int J Dermatol* 1978; 17: 568–70.

6. Pories WJ, Henzel JH, Rob CG, Strain WH. Acceleration of healing with zinc sulfate. *Ann Surg* 1967; 165: 432–36.

7. Carruthers R. Oral zinc sulphate in leg ulcers. *Lancet* 1969; 1: 1264.

8. Cohen C. Zinc sulphate and bedsores. *Br Med J* 1968; 2: 561.

9. Faure H, Peyrin J-C, Richard M-J, Favier A. Parenteral supplementation with zinc in surgical patients corrects postoperative serum-zinc drop. *Biol Trace Elem Res* 1991; 30: 37–45.

10. Agren MS. Studies on zinc in wound healing. *Acta Derm Venereol Supll* (Stockh) 1990; 154: 1–36.

11. Stromberg HE, Agren MS. Topical zinc oxide treatment improves arterial and venous leg ulcers. *Br J Dermatol* 1984; 111(4): 461–68.

12. Seifter E, Crowley LV, Rettura G, et al. Influence of vitamin A on wound healing in rats with femoral fracture. *Ann Surg* 1975; 181(6): 836–41.

13. Demetriou AA, Levenson SM, Rettura G, Seifter E. Vitamin A and retinoic acid: induced fibroblast differentiation in vitro. *Surgery* 1985 Nov; 98: 931–34.

14. Bartolomucci E. Action of vitamin E on healing of experimental wounds on parenchymatous organs. *JAMA* 1939; 113: 1079 [abstract].

15. Ehrlich HP, Tarver H, Hunt TK. Inhibitory effects of vitamin E on collagen synthesis and wound repair. *Ann Surg* 1972; 175: 235–40.

16. Rucker RB, Kosonen T, Clegg MS, et al. Copper lysyl oxidase, and extracellular matrix protein cross-linking. *Am J Clin Nutr* 1998; 67(5 suppl): 996s–1002s.

17. Alvarez OM, Gilbreath RL. Effect of dietary thiamine on intermolecular collagen cross-linking during wound repair: a mechanical and biochemical assessment. *J Trauma* 1982 Jan; 22(1): 20–24.

18. Aprahamian M, Dentinger A, Stock-Damge C, et al. Effects of supplemental pantothenic acid on wound healing: experimental study in rabbit. *Am J Clin Nutr* 1985; 41(3): 578–89.

19. Bosse MD, Axelrod AE. Wound healing in rats with biotin, pyridoxin, or riboflavin deficiencies. *Proc Soc Exp Biol Med* 1948; 67: 418–21.

20. Tassman G, Zafran J, Zayon G. A double-blind crossover study of a plant proteolytic enzyme in oral surgery. *J Dent Med* 1965; 20: 51–54.

21. Blonstein J. Control of swelling in boxing injuries. *Practitioner* 1960; 203: 206.

22. Della Loggia R, Tubaro A, Sosa S, et al. The role of triterpenoids in the topical anti-inflammatory activity of *Calendula officinalis* flowers. *Planta Med* 1994; 60(6): 516–20.

23. Zitterl-Eglseer K, Sosa S, Jurenitsch J, et al. Anti-oedematous activities of the main triterpendiol esters of marigold (*Calendula officinalis* L.). *J Ethnopharmacol* 1997; 57(2): 139–44.

24. Shipochliev T, Dimitrov A, Aleksandrova E. Anti-inflammatory action of a group of plant extracts. *Vet Med Nauki* 1981; 18(6): 87–94 [in Bulgarian].

25. Blumenthal M, Busse WR, Goldberg A, et al. *The Complete German Commission E Monographs. Therapeutic Guide to Herbal Medicines.* Austin, Texas: American Botanical Council, 1998, 186–87.

26. Blumenthal M, Busse WR, Goldberg A, et al. *The Complete German Commission E Monographs. Therapeutic Guide to Herbal Medicines.* Austin, Texas: American Botanical Council, 1998, 214–15.

27. Blumenthal M, Busse WR, Goldberg A, et al. *The Complete German Commission E Monographs. Therapeutic Guide to Herbal Medicines.* Austin, Texas: American Botanical Council, 1998, 115–16.

28. Blumenthal M, Busse WR, Goldberg A, et al. *The Complete German Commission E Monographs. Therapeutic Guide to Herbal Medicines.* Austin, Texas: American Botanical Council, 1998, 231.

29. Blumenthal M, Busse WR, Goldberg A, et al. *The Complete German Commission E Monographs. Therapeutic Guide to Herbal Medicines.* Austin, Texas: American Botanical Council, 1998, 150–51.

30. Davis RH, Stewart GH, Bregman PJ. Aloe vera and the inflamed synovial pouch model. *J Am Podiatr Med Assoc* 1992; 82(3): 140–48.

31. Davis RH, Leitner MG, Russo JM, Byrne ME. Wound healing. Oral and topical activity of Aloe vera. *J Am Podiatr Med Assoc* 1989: 79(11): 559–62.

Yeast Infection

1. Horowitz BJ, Edelstein SW, Lippman L. Sugar chromatography studies in recurrent candida vulvovaginitis. *J Reproduc Med* 1984; 29: 441–43.

2. Heidrich F, Berg A, Gergman R, et al. Clotting factors and vaginitis. *J Family Pract* 1984; 19: 491–94.

3. Kudelco N. Allergy in chronic monilial vaginitis. *Ann Allergy* 1971; 29: 266–67.

4. Hilton E, Isenberg HD, Alperstein P, et al. Ingestion of yogurt containing *Lactobacillus acidophilus* as prophylaxis for candidal vaginitis. *Ann Intern Med* 1992; 116: 353–57.

5. Neri A, Sabah G, Samra Z. Bacterial vaginosis in pregnancy treated with yogurt. *Acta Obstet Gynecol Scand* 1993; 72: 17–19.

6. Eschenback H. Vaginal infection. *Clin Obstet Gynecol* 1983; 26: 186–202.

7. Vincent J, Voomett R, and Riley R. Antibacterial activity associated with *Lactobaccillus acidophilus*. *J Bacteriol* 1959; A78: 477–84.

8. Jovanovic R, Congema E, Nguyen HT. Antifungal agents vs. boric acid for treating chronic mycotic vulvovaginitis. *J Reprod Med* 1977; 36: 593–97.

9. Pena EO. *Melaleuca alternifolia* oil. Uses for trichomonal vaginitis and other vaginal infections. *Obstet Gynecol* 1962; 19: 793–95.

12. Hughes BG, Lawson LD. Antimicrobial effects of *Allium sativum* L. (garlic), *Allium ampeloprasum* L. (elephant garlic) and *Allium cepa* L. (onion), garlic compounds and commercial garlic supplement products. *Phytother Res* 1991; 5: 154–58.

11. Guiraud P, Steiman R, Campos-Takaki GM, et al. Comparison of the antibacterial and antifungal activities of lapachol and beta-lapachone. *Planta Med* 1994; 60: 373–74.

12. Coeugniet E, Kuhnast R. Recurrent candidiasis: Adjuvant immunotherapy with different formulations of Echinacin. *Therapiewoche* 1986; 36: 3352–58.

13. Singh HB, Srivastava M, Singh AB, Srivastava AK. Cinnamon bark oil, a potent fungitoxicant against fungi causing respiratory tract mycoses. *Allergy* 1995; 50: 995–99.

14. Quale JM, Landman D, Zaman MM, et al. In vitro activity of *Cinnamomum zeylanicum* against azole resistant and sensitive candida species and a pilot study of cinnamon for oral candidiasis. *Am J Chin Med* 1996; 24: 103–9.

Yellow Nail Syndrome

1. Norton L. Further observations on the yellow nail syndrome with therapeutic effects of oral alpha-tocopherol. *Cutis* 1985; 36: 457–62.

2. Ayres S Jr, Hihan R. Yellow nail syndrome: response to vitamin E. *Arch Dermatol* 1973; 108: 267–68.

3. Ayres S Jr. Yellow nail syndrome controlled by vitamin E therapy. J *Am Acad Dermatol* 1986; 15: 714–16 [letter].

4. Williams HC, Buffham R, du Vivier A. Successful use of topical vitamin E solution in the treatment of nail changes in yellow nail syndrome. *Arch Dermatol* 1991; 127: 1023–28.

Part Two

Nutritional
Supplements

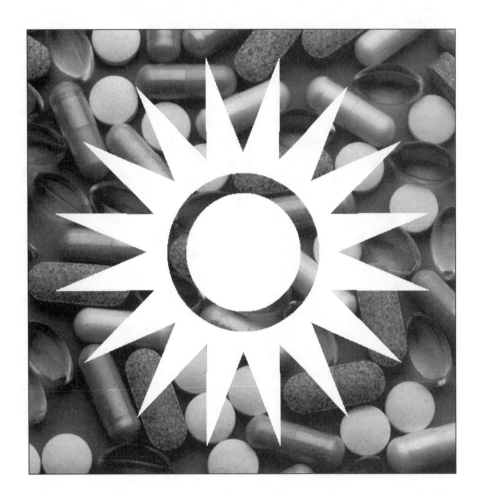

Acetyl-L-Carnitine

Acetyl-L-carnitine is similar in form to the amino acid **carnitine** (p. 279) and also has some similar functions, such as being involved in the metabolism of food into energy.

The acetyl group that is part of acetyl-L-carnitine contributes to the production of the neurotransmitter acetylcholine. Several double-blind clinical trials suggest that acetyl-L-carnitine delays the progression of **Alzheimer's disease** (p. 11)[1,2] and enhances overall performance in some individuals with Alzheimer's disease.[3] Alzheimer's research has been done with the acetyl-L-carnitine form, rather than the L-carnitine form, of this nutrient.

Where Is It Found?

Acetyl-L-carnitine is a molecule that occurs naturally in the brain and other tissues. It is also available as a supplement.

Acetyl-L-Carnitine Has Been Used in Connection with the Following Condition*

Ranking	Health Concern
Primary	Alzheimer's disease (p. 11)

*Refer to the Individual Health Concern for Complete Information

Who Is Likely to Be Deficient?

Acetyl-L-carnitine levels may decrease with advancing age; however, because it is not an essential nutrient, deficiencies do not occur.

How Much Is Usually Taken?

Most research involving acetyl-L-carnitine uses 500 mg 3 times per day, though some research uses double this amount.

Are There Any Side Effects or Interactions? Acetyl-L-carnitine is safe, although skin rash, increased appetite, nausea, vomiting, agitation, and body odor have been reported in individuals taking acetyl-L-carnitine.[4,5]

Adenosine Monophosphate (AMP)

Adenosine monophosphate (AMP) is an intermediary substance formed during the body's process of creating energy in the form of adenosine triphosphate (ATP) from food. AMP may play a role in limiting postherpetic neuralgia, which is the pain that sometimes lingers after a bout of **shingles** *(herpes zoster)* (p. 155). One double-blind study involving 32 adults with shingles found that injections of AMP given 3 times per week for a month following a flare-up of shingles relieved the pain more quickly than placebo.[1] Whether oral supplementation would have the same effect remains unclear. AMP also helps heal the lesions and prevents recurrence of pain or lesions.

Nineteen out of twenty-one people with porphyria cutanea tarda (a disease that develops in adulthood and causes **photosensitivity** (p. 140), among other symptoms, responded well to 160–200 mg of AMP per day taken for at least 1 month, according to one group of researchers.[2] Partial and even complete alleviation of photosensitivity associated with this condition occurred in several people.

Where Is It Found?

The body creates AMP within cells during normal metabolic processes. AMP is also found as a supplement, although it is not widely available.

Adenosine Monophosphate (AMP) Has Been Used in Connection with the Following Conditions*

Ranking	Health Concerns
Other	Photosensitivity (p. 140) Shingles (herpes zoster)/postherpetic neuralgia (p. 155)

*Refer to the Individual Health Concern for Complete Information

Who Is Likely to Be Deficient?

Preliminary research suggests that individuals with herpes simplex or herpes zoster (shingles) infections may have low levels of AMP; however, the clinical significance of this finding is unclear.[3]

How Much Is Usually Taken?

The trials using AMP for photosensitivity have used 160–200 mg of AMP per day; however, the ideal intake of this supplement has not been determined. Research with shingles has used a special gel form of AMP injected into muscle; a doctor of natural medicine should be consulted for this form of AMP.

Are There Any Side Effects or Interactions? The limited number of human studies involving oral AMP have not indicated any side effects. However, some researchers have expressed concern that supplemental intake of AMP is hypothetically associated with increased levels of adenosine, a substance related to AMP that may interfere with immune function.[4] Doctors using intramuscular AMP shots report that too-rapid administration can cause life-threatening arrythmias of the heart.[5]

Alanine

Alanine is a nonessential **amino acid** (p. 265) used by the body to build proteins. Alanine is present in prostate fluid, and it may play a role in supporting prostate health. One study, involving forty-five men with **benign prostatic hyperplasia** (p. 145), found that 780 mg of alanine per day for 2 weeks and then 390 mg for the next 2½ months, taken in combination with equal amounts of the amino acids **glycine** (p. 300) and **glutamic acid** (p. 299), reduced symptoms of benign prostatic hyperplasia;[1] this work has been independently confirmed.[2]

Where Is It Found?

As with the other amino acids, excellent sources of alanine include meat, poultry, fish, eggs, and dairy products. Some protein-rich plant foods also supply alanine.

Alanine Has Been Used in Connection with the Following Condition*

Ranking	Health Concern
Secondary	Benign prostatic hyperplasia (p. 145)
*Refer to the Individual Health Concern for Complete Information	

Who Is Likely to Be Deficient?

Since most food sources of protein supply alanine, only an individual deficient in protein would become deficient in alanine.[3]

How Much Is Usually Taken?

Most people do not need to supplement with alanine; for those who do use this amino acid as a supplement, appropriate amounts should be determined with the consultation of a nutritionally oriented physician.

Are There Any Side Effects or Interactions?

Alanine is free of side effects for the vast majority of people who take it; however, individuals with kidney

or liver disease should not consume high intakes of amino acids without consulting a healthcare professional.

Alpha Lipoic Acid

Alpha lipoic acid (also known as thioctic acid) is a vitamin-like **antioxidant** (p. 267). Alpha lipoic acid is sometimes referred to as the "universal antioxidant," because it is soluble in both fat and water.[1]

Alpha lipoic acid has several potential benefits for **diabetics** (p. 53). It enhances glucose uptake in non-insulin-dependent diabetes (NIDDM), inhibits glycosylation (the abnormal attachment of sugar to protein), and has been used to improve diabetic nerve damage and reduce pain associated with that nerve damage.[2] Most studies have used intravenous alpha lipoic acid, but oral supplementation has nonetheless proved partially helpful in treating at least one form of diabetic neuropathy, using 800 mg per day.[3]

Preliminary evidence indicates that 150 mg of alpha lipoic acid, taken daily for one month, improves visual function in people with **glaucoma** (p. 74).[4]

Alpha lipoic acid has been shown to inhibit the replication of the **HIV** (p. 87) virus in the test tube. However, it is not known whether supplementing with alpha lipoic acid would benefit HIV-positive people.[5]

Alpha lipoic acid has significantly increased the survival rate of people who have eaten poison mushrooms.[6] Such a treatment should be prescribed by a nutritionally oriented doctor and should not be attempted on one's own.

Where Is It Found?

The body makes small amounts of alpha lipoic acid. There is only limited knowledge about the food sources of this nutrient; however, foods that contain mitochondria (a specialized component of cells), such as red meats, are believed to provide the most alpha lipoic acid. Supplements are also available.

Alpha Lipoic Acid Has Been Used in Connection with the Following Conditions*

Ranking	Health Concerns
Primary	Diabetes (p. 53)
Other	Glaucoma (p. 74)
*Refer to the Individual Health Concern for Complete Information	

Who Is Likely to Be Deficient?

Although alpha lipoic acid was thought to be a vitamin when it was first discovered, subsequent research determined that it is created in the human body—and thus is not an essential nutrient. For this reason, humans are not known to be deficient in alpha lipoic acid.

How Much Is Usually Taken?

The amount of alpha lipoic acid used in research to improve diabetic neuropathies is 800 mg per day and 150 mg per day for glaucoma. However, much lower amounts, such as 20–50 mg per day, are recommended by some doctors of natural medicine for general antioxidant protection, although there remains no clear evidence that such general use has any benefit.

Are There Any Side Effects or Interactions? Side effects with alpha lipoic acid are rare but can include skin rash and the potential of hypoglycemia in diabetic patients. Individuals who may be deficient in **vitamin B₁** (p. 237), such as alcoholics, should take vitamin B₁ along with alpha lipoic acid supplements. Chronic administration of alpha lipoic acid in animals has interfered with the actions of the vitamin **biotin** (p. 272). Whether this has significance for humans remains unknown.[7]

Amino Acids (Overview)

Amino acids are the building blocks of protein. Twenty amino acids are needed to build the various proteins used in the growth, repair, and maintenance of body tissues. Eleven of these amino acids can be made by the body itself, while the other nine (called essential amino acids) must come from the diet. The classification of an amino acid as essential or nonessential does not reflect its importance because all twenty amino acids are necessary for health. Instead, this classification system simply reflects whether or not the body is capable of manufacturing a particular amino acid.

The essential amino acids are **isoleucine** (p. 274), **leucine** (p. 274), **lysine** (p. 309), **methionine** (p. 313), **phenylalanine** (p. 320), threonine, **tryptophan** (p. 295), and **valine** (p. 274). Another amino acid, **histidine** (p. 301), is considered semiessential because the body does not always require dietary sources for it. The nonessential amino acids are **arginine** (p. 268), **alanine** (p. 264), asparagine, aspartic acid, **cysteine** (p. 286), **glutamine** (p. 300), **glutamic acid** (p. 299), **glycine** (p. 300), proline, serine, and **tyrosine** (p. 335). Other amino acids, such as **carnitine** (p. 279), are made from the combination of other amino acids, in this case lysine and methionine.

Where Are They Found?

Foods of animal origin, such as meat, fish, poultry, eggs, and dairy products, are the richest dietary sources of the essential amino acids. However, the outdated belief that vegetarians need to be concerned about combining certain foods to obtain enough essential amino acids has now been disproved by research[1] and is almost universally rejected by scientists. Part of the reason that vegetarians do not need to "balance" amino acids is that the body's requirement for essential amino acids now appears to be much less important than researchers once believed, especially in adults. In fact, research indicates that protein deficiencies rarely occur in people who simply eat enough calories. As a result, the old scientific term for protein deficiency, "kwashiorkor," has been dropped from use and replaced by the term "protein-calorie malnutrition."

Who Is Likely to Be Deficient?

The vast majority of Americans eat more than enough protein and also more than enough of each essential amino acid for normal purposes. Anyone not consuming an adequate number of calories, dieters, and some strict vegetarian bodybuilders may not consume adequate amino acids. In these cases, the body will either break down the protein in muscle tissue and use those amino acids to meet the needs of more important organs or simply not build more muscle mass despite increasing exercise.

How Much Is Usually Taken?

Nutrition experts recommend that protein, as a source of amino acids, account for 10–12% of the calories in a balanced diet. However, requirements for protein are affected by age, weight, state of health, and other factors. On average, a normal adult requires approximately 0.36 grams of protein per pound of body weight. Using this formula, a 140-pound person would need 50 grams (or less than 2 ounces) of protein per day. An appropriate range of protein intake for healthy adults may be as low as 45–65 grams daily. Some athletes have higher amino acid requirements.[2] Most American adults eat about

Androstenedione (Andro)

Amino Acids Have Been Used in Connection with the Following Conditions*

Ranking	Health Concerns
Primary	Alzheimer's disease (p. 11) (acetyl-L-carnitine [p. 263]) Angina (p. 13) (carnitine [p. 279]) Bronchitis (N-acetyl cysteine [p. 317]) Chronic obstructive pulmonary disease (p. 45) (N-acetyl cysteine [p. 317]) Congestive heart failure (p. 43) (taurine [p. 334])
Secondary	Angina (p. 13) (arginine [p. 268]) Athletic performance (p. 515) (creatine [p. 285]) Benign prostatic hyperplasia (p. 145) (alanine [p. 264], glutamic acid [p. 299], glycine [p. 300]) Cancer risk reduction (soy protein [p. 332]) Chronic fatigue syndrome (p. 36) (carnitine [p. 279]) Cold sores (p. 39) (lysine [p. 309]) Congestive heart failure (p. 43) (arginine [p. 268], carnitine [p. 279]) Depression (p. 532) (5-HTP [p. 295], DLPA [p. 320], L-phenylalanine [p. 320], tyrosine [p. 335]) Diabetes (p. 53) (carnitine [p. 279]) Emphysema (N-acetyl cysteine [p. 317]) Fibromyalgia (p. 68) (5-HTP [p. 295]) High triglycerides (p. 85) (carnitine [p. 279]) HIV support (p. 87) (N-acetyl cysteine [p. 317]) Infertility (male) (p. 103) (arginine [p. 268], carnitine [p. 279]) Intermittent claudication (p. 106) (carnitine [p. 279]) Liver support (taurine [p. 34])
Other	Alcohol withdrawal (p. 6) (DLPA [p. 320], glutamine [p. 300], tyrosine [p. 335]) Athletic performance (p. 20) (carnitine [p. 279], isoleucine [p. 274], leucine [p. 274], ornithine [p. 318], ornithine alpha-ketoglutarate [p. 319], valine [p. 274], whey protein [p. 346]) Diabetes (p. 53) (taurine [p. 334]) Epilepsy (taurine [p. 334]) High blood pressure (p. 89) (arginine [p. 268], taurine [p. 334]) HIV support (p. 87) (glutamine [p. 300], methionine [p. 313]) Insomnia (p. 105) (5-HTP [p. 295]) Liver support (methionine [p. 313]) Migraine headaches (p. 121) (5-HTP [p. 295]) Osteoarthritis (p. 130) (DLPA [p. 320]) Pain (DLPA [p. 320]) Peptic ulcer (p. 138) (glutamine [p. 300]) Phenylketonuria (leucine [p. 274], tyrosine [p. 335]) Postsurgery recovery (creatine [p. 285]) Rheumatoid arthritis (p. 151) (DLPA [p. 320], histidine [p. 301]) Ulcerative colitis (p. 158) (glutamine [p. 300]) Vitiligo (p. 164) (L-phenylalanine [p. 320]) Weight loss and obesity (p. 165) (5-HTP [p. 295])

*Refer to the Individual Health Concern for Complete Information

100 grams of protein per day, or about twice what their bodies need and at least as much as any athlete requires.

Supplements of individual amino acids are recommended by nutritionally oriented doctors for specific purposes, such as lysine for herpes or phenylalanine for pain. **Are There Any Side Effects or Interactions?** Most diets provide more protein than the body needs, causing excess nitrogen to be excreted as urea in urine. The excess nitrogen has been linked in some studies with reduced kidney function in old age. Moreover, several studies have found that when people have impaired kidney function, restricting dietary intake of protein improves their health status.[3]

Excessive protein intake also can increase excretion of **calcium** (p. 277), and some evidence has linked high-protein diets with **osteoporosis** (p. 133),[4] particularly regarding animal protein.[5] On the other hand, some protein is needed for bone formation. Double-blind evidence indicates that elderly individuals who eat barely below the recommended amount suffer less bone loss when supplemented with an additional 20 grams of protein per day.[6] A nutritionally oriented doctor can help people assess their protein intake.

Androstenedione (Andro)

Androstenedione is an androgen hormone. It is produced in the adrenal glands and gonads from dehydroepiandrosterone (**DHEA** [p. 288]) or 17 alpha-hydroxyprogesterone and is converted to testosterone by several tissues, including muscle and bone. One study reported that 100 mg of androstenedione raised testosterone levels in women to six times the normal range and was significantly more effective in this than a similar amount of DHEA.[1] A German patent claims that oral androstenedione briefly raises blood levels of testosterone in men[2] but no formally published studies are available to corroborate this. No studies have investigated the effects of androstenedione on body composition or **athletic performance** (p. 20).

Animal studies have demonstrated a protective effect of androstenedione against bone loss when normal hormone production is reduced.[3]

Where Is It Found?

Androstenedione is made in the human adrenal glands and gonads. It also occurs naturally in animal foods and in the pollen of Scotch pine trees.[4]

Who Is Likely to Be Deficient?

The concentration of androgens such as androstenedione peaks in early adulthood. Androstenedione probably declines steadily thereafter in men, but levels in women decline abruptly at menopause,[5] after which they actually rise.[6] It remains unclear whether or not these normal declines with age should be considered a "deficiency." Lower androstenedione levels have been found in postmenopausal women who were either underweight[7] or had lower bone mineral density.[8] Men with **systemic lupus erythematosus** (p. 115) also show reduced production of androstenedione.[9]

How Much Is Usually Taken?

One human trial used 100 mg per day in an attempt to increase testosterone levels. However, ideal intake remains unknown.

Are There Any Side Effects or Interactions? Androstenedione has been banned by the International Olympic Committee, the National Football League, and the National Collegiate Athletic Association. No reports of side effects from use of androstenedione have been published. However, common side effects of elevated testosterone include enlargement of breasts, prostate, and other glandular tissues, as well as increased risk of glandular cancers, hair loss, water retention, lower LDL levels, **impotence** (p. 98), **acne** (p. 5), oily skin, and increased sex drive. Women should avoid elevated testosterone levels because they could lead to permanent changes, such as deep voice, beard, enlargement of genitals, and other masculine characteristics. Androgen steroid hormones may aggravate certain diseases, including **diabetes** (p. 53), heart disease, psychological disorders, **benign prostatic hyperplasia (BPH)** (p. 145), and hormonal abnormalities. It should also not be used by growing children and pregnant or lactating women.

Antioxidants and Free Radicals

Free radicals are highly reactive compounds that are created in the body during normal metabolic functions or introduced from the environment.

Free radicals are inherently unstable, since they contain "extra" energy. To reduce their energy load, free radicals react with certain cells in the body, interfering with the cells' ability to function normally. In fact, free radicals are believed to play a role in more than sixty different health conditions, including the aging process, cancer, and **atherosclerosis** (p. 17).[1] Reducing exposure to free radicals and increasing intake of antioxidant nutrients can reduce the risk of free radical-related health problems.

Oxygen, although essential to life, is the source of potentially damaging compounds called free radicals. Free radicals are also found in the environment. Environmental sources of free radicals include exposure to ionizing radiation (from industry, sun exposure, cosmic rays, and medical X-rays), ozone and nitrous oxide (primarily from automobile exhaust), heavy metals (such as mercury, cadmium, and lead), cigarette smoke (both active and passive), alcohol, unsaturated fat, and other chemicals and compounds from food, water, and air.

Antioxidants work in several ways: they may reduce the energy of the free radical, stop the free radical from forming in the first place, or interrupt an oxidizing chain reaction to minimize the damage of free radicals.

The body produces several enzymes, including superoxide dismutase (SOD), catalase, and glutathione peroxidase, that neutralize many types of free radicals. Supplements of these compounds are available to augment the body's supply; however, these antioxidant enzymes may not absorb well. Supplementing with the "building blocks" the body requires to make SOD, catalase, and glutathione peroxidase may be more effective. These building block nutrients include the minerals **manganese** (p. 311), **zinc** (p. 346), and **copper** (p. 285) for SOD, and **selenium** (p. 331) for glutathione peroxidase.

In addition to enzymes, many vitamins and minerals act as antioxidants in their own right, such as **vitamin C** (p. 341), **vitamin E** (p. 344), **beta-carotene** (p. 268), **lutein** (p. 308), **lycopene** (p. 308), **vitamin B$_3$** (p. 339) in the form of niacin, **vitamin B$_2$** (p. 338), **vitamin B$_6$** (p. 340), **coenzyme Q$_{10}$** (p. 283), and **cysteine** (p. 286), an amino acid. Herbs, such as **bilberry** (p. 396), **turmeric** (p. 465) (curcumin), **grape seed or pine bark** (p. 324) extracts, and **ginkgo** (p. 427) can also provide powerful antioxidant protection for the body.

A wide variety of antioxidant enzymes, vitamins, minerals, and herbs may be the best way to provide the body with the most complete protection against free radical damage.

Antioxidants and Free Radicals

Arginine

The **amino acid** (p. 265) arginine has several roles in the body, such as assisting in **wound healing** (p. 167), helping remove excess ammonia from the body, stimulating **immune function** (p. 94), and promoting secretion of several hormones, including glucagon, insulin, and growth hormone.

The effect on growth hormone levels[1] has interested bodybuilders. In a controlled trial, when arginine was combined with weight training and **ornithine** (p. 318) (taken as 500 mg of each, twice per day, 5 times per week), a greater decrease in body fat was obtained after only 5 weeks than when the same exercise was combined with placebo.[2]

Arginine is also needed to increase protein synthesis, which can in turn increase cellular replication. Therefore, arginine may help people with inadequate numbers of certain cells. For example, some[3] (though not all[4]) studies have found that men with low sperm counts experienced an increase in the number of sperm when supplemented with arginine.

Arginine's effect on increasing protein synthesis improves wound healing. This effect has been shown in both animals[5] and, at 17 grams per day, in people as well.[6]

Arginine is also a precursor to nitric oxide, which the body uses to keep blood vessels dilated, allowing the heart to receive adequate oxygen. Preliminary evidence suggests that arginine may help regulate **cholesterol levels** (p. 79).[7] Arginine also appears to act as a natural blood thinner by reducing platelet aggregation.[8]

According to researchers, the effect arginine has on increasing nitric oxide might help people with interstitial cystitis. In a preliminary trial using 1.5 grams of arginine per day, symptoms of this condition were significantly reduced.[9]

Where Is It Found?

Dairy, meat, poultry, and fish are good sources of arginine. Nuts and chocolate also contain significant amounts of this amino acid.

Who Is Likely to Be Deficient?

Normally, the body makes enough arginine, even when it is lacking in the diet. However, during times of unusual stress (including infection, burns, and injury), the body may not be able to keep up with increased requirements.

How Much Is Usually Taken?

Most people do not need to take extra arginine. While some people with serious infections, burns, or other

Arginine Has Been Used in Connection with the Following Conditions*

Ranking	Health Concerns
Secondary	Angina (p. 13) Congestive heart failure (p. 43) Infertility (male) (p. 103) Minor injuries (p. 122)
Other	Athletic performance (p. 20) (for body composition and strength) Gastritis (p. 71) High blood pressure (p. 89) Impotence (p. 98) Wound healing (p. 167)

*Refer to the Individual Health Concern for Complete Information

trauma should take arginine, appropriate doses must be determined by a doctor. Levels used in research vary considerably (2–30 grams per day). Optimal intakes remain unknown and are likely to vary depending upon the individual.

Are There Any Side Effects or Interactions? Arginine has so far appeared to be free of obvious side effects, although some doctors are concerned that increases in growth hormone triggered by arginine could overwork the pancreas.

Individuals with kidney or liver disease should consult their nutritionally oriented doctor before supplementing with arginine. Individuals with **herpes** (p. 155), either cold sores or genital herpes, should not take arginine supplements because arginine can stimulate replication of the virus.

Large amounts of arginine in animals can both promote[10] and interfere with cancer growth.[11] In preliminary research, high intake (30 grams per day) of arginine has increased cancer cell growth in humans.[12] On the other hand, in people with cancer, arginine has been found to stimulate the immune system.[13] At this time it remains unclear whether arginine is dangerous or helpful for people with cancer.

Arginine works with **ornithine** (p. 318) in the synthesis of growth hormone.

Beta-Carotene

Beta-carotene, a substance from plants that the body can convert into **vitamin A** (p. 336), also acts as an **antioxidant** (p. 267) and **immune system** (p. 94) booster. Other members of the antioxidant carotene family include cryptoxanthin, alpha-carotene, zeaxanthin, **lutein** (p. 308), and **lycopene** (p. 308); however, unlike beta-carotene, most of these nutrients do not convert to significant amounts of vitamin A.

How Do Natural and Synthetic Beta-Carotene Differ?

Most, but not all, beta-carotene in supplements is synthetic, consisting of only one molecule called all trans beta-carotene. Natural beta-carotene found in food is made of two molecules—all trans beta-carotene plus 9-cis beta-carotene.

Researchers originally saw no meaningful difference between natural and synthetic beta-carotene. This view was questioned when the link between beta-carotene-containing foods (all natural) and lung cancer prevention[1] was not duplicated in studies using synthetic pills.[2] In smokers, synthetic beta-carotene has apparently caused an increased risk of lung cancer in double-blind research.[3,4] Animal research has begun to identify the ways in which synthetic beta-carotene causes damage to lungs, particularly when animals are exposed to cigarette smoke. [5]

Much of natural beta-carotene is in the all trans molecule form—the same as synthetic beta-carotene. Moreover, much of the 9-cis molecule found only in natural beta-carotene converts to the synthetic molecule before it reaches the bloodstream.[6] Also, absorption of 9-cis beta-carotene appears to be poor,[7] though some researchers question this finding.[8]

Despite the overlap between natural and synthetic forms, natural beta-carotene may possibly have activity that is distinct from the synthetic form. For example, the natural form has antioxidant activity that the synthetic form has been reported to lack in both animals[9] and in people.[10] Also, in one trial, precancerous changes in people reverted to normal tissue with natural beta-carotene supplements, but not with synthetic supplements.[11] Increasingly, nutritionally oriented doctors recommend that people supplement only natural beta-carotene. However, no animal research has yet explored whether the precancerous effects caused by synthetic beta-carotene might result from a combination of cigarette smoke plus *natural* beta-carotene supplementation. Until more is known, smokers should avoid all beta-carotene supplements and others should avoid synthetic beta-carotene.

In supplements, the natural form can be identified by the phrases "from *D. salina*," "from an algal source," "from a palm source," or as "natural beta-carotene" on the label. The synthetic form is identified as "beta-carotene."

Where Is It Found?

Dark green and orange-yellow vegetables are good sources of beta-carotene, which is also available in supplements.

Beta-Carotene Has Been Used in Connection with the Following Conditions*

Ranking	Health Concerns
Primary	Immune function (for elderly people) (p. 94) Night blindness (p. 129) Photosensitivity (p. 140)
Secondary	Immune function (p. 94)
Other	Alcohol withdrawal support (p. 6) Cataracts (p. 34) Gastritis (p. 71) HIV support (p. 87) Macular degeneration (p. 118)

*Refer to the Individual Health Concern for Complete Information

Who Is Likely to Be Deficient?

Individuals who limit their consumption of beta-carotene-containing vegetables could be at higher risk of developing a vitamin A deficiency; however, because beta-carotene is not an essential nutrient, deficiencies do not occur.

How Much Is Usually Taken?

The most common beta-carotene supplement intake is probably 25,000 IU (15 mg) per day, though some people take as much as 100,000 IU (60 mg) per day. Whether the average person would benefit from supplementation with beta-carotene remains unclear.

Are There Any Side Effects or Interactions? Beta-carotene does not cause any side effects; however, excessive intake (more than 100,000 IU, or 60 mg per day) sometimes gives the skin a yellow-orange hue. Individuals taking beta-carotene for long periods of time should also supplement with **vitamin E** (p. 344), as beta-carotene may reduce vitamin E levels.[12] As noted above, synthetic beta-carotene has now been linked to increased risk of lung cancer in smokers. Precancerous changes to lungs have appeared in animals given synthetic beta-carotene supplements, particularly those exposed to tobacco smoke. Though some research suggests that differences between synthetic and natural supplements may exist, conclusive proof of such a difference has not yet been shown.

Betaine Hydrochloride
(Hydrochloric Acid)

The digestive process takes place as food passes through the mouth, stomach, small intestine, and large intestine. One of the most important parts of digestion occurs in the stomach, where gastric (stomach) acid helps break down proteins for further digestion in the small intestine.

A low level of gastric acid increases the likelihood and severity of certain bacterial and parasitic intestinal infections. A normal stomach's level of gastric acid is sufficient to destroy bacteria.[1] In one study, most fasting people who had normal gastric acid in the stomach had virtually no bacteria in the small intestine. Some bacterial colonization of the stomach occurred in individuals who had low levels of hydrochloric acid.[2]

Where Is It Found?

Gastric acid is produced by the parietal cells of the stomach. The acidity is quite strong in a normal stomach. In fact, the stomach can be between 100,000 and almost 1,000,000 times more acidic than water.

Who Is Likely to Be Deficient?

Some research suggests that people with a wide variety of chronic disorders, such as **allergies** (p. 8),[3] **asthma** (p. 15),[4] and **gallstones** (p. 69),[5] do not produce adequate amounts of stomach acid.

How Much Is Usually Taken?

Betaine hydrochloride (HCl) is the most common hydrochloric acid-containing supplement. Normally it comes in tablets or capsules measured in grains or milligrams. Only people who have reduced levels of stomach acid ("hypochlorhydria") should take betaine HCl; this condition can be diagnosed by a nutritionally oriented doctor. When appropriate, some nutritionally oriented doctors recommend taking one or more tablets or capsules, each 5–10 grains (325 – 650 mg), with a meal that contains protein. Occasionally, betaine is recommended to reduce blood levels of a substance called **homocysteine** (p. 84), which is associated with heart disease. This form of betaine is different from betaine HCl.

Are There Any Side Effects or Interactions? Large amounts of betaine HCl can burn the lining of the stomach. If a burning sensation is experienced, betaine HCl should be immediately discontinued. People should not take more than 10 grains (650 mg) of betaine HCl without the recommendation of a nutritionally oriented physician. All people with a history of **ulcers** (p. 138), **gastritis** (p. 71), or gastrointestinal symptoms—particularly **heartburn** (p. 99)—should see a nutritionally oriented doctor before taking betaine HCl. People taking nonsteroidal anti-inflammatory drugs (NSAIDs), cortisone-like drugs, or other medications that might cause a **peptic ulcer** (p. 138) should not take betaine HCl. Betaine HCl helps make some minerals and other nutrients more absorbable.[6,7]

Betaine Hydrochloride Has Been Used in Connection with the Following Conditions*

Ranking	Health Concerns
Secondary	High homocysteine (p. 84)
Other	Anemia (p. 107) Asthma (p. 15) Gallstones (p. 69) Indigestion and heartburn (p. 99) Rheumatoid arthritis (p. 151) Thyroid conditions Tic douloureux Vitiligo (p. 164)

*Refer to the Individual Health Concern for Complete Information

Beta-Sitosterol

Beta-sitosterol—alone and in combination with similar plant sterols—reduces blood levels of **cholesterol** (p. 79).[1,2] This appears to be because beta-sitosterol blocks absorption of cholesterol.[3] It has also been effective in reducing symptoms of **benign prostatic hyperplasia** (p. 145).[4]

Although molecules quite similar to beta-sitosterol inhibit cancer cells in test tubes, the relevance of this information for people remains unknown.[5]

Where Is It Found?

Beta-sitosterol is one of several plant sterols (cholesterol is the main animal sterol) found in almost all plants; high levels are found in rice bran, wheat germ, corn oils, and **soybeans** (p. 332).

Beta-Sitosterol Has Been Used in Connection with the Following Conditions*

Ranking	Health Concerns
Primary	Benign prostatic hyperplasia (p. 145)
Secondary	High cholesterol (p. 79)

*Refer to the Individual Health Concern for Complete Information

Who Is Likely to Be Deficient?

Because beta-sitosterol is not an essential nutrient, deficiencies do not occur.

How Much Is Usually Taken?

From 500 mg up to 10 grams of beta-sitosterol have been used each day for reduction of elevated blood cholesterol in clinical research. Between 60 (20 mg 3 times per day) and 130 mg per day have been used in trials successfully reporting a reduction in prostatic hyperplasia-related symptoms.[6,7]

Are There Any Side Effects or Interactions? No significant side effects or interactions have yet been reported in studies on beta-sitosterol.

Bioflavonoids

Bioflavonoids are a class of water-soluble plant pigments. Bioflavonoids are broken down into categories, though the issue of how to divide them is not universally agreed upon. One system breaks bioflavonoids into isoflavones, anthocyanins, flavans, flavonols, flavones, and flavanones.[1] Some of the best-known bioflavonoids, such as genistein in **soy** (p. 332) and **quercetin** (p. 328) in onions, can be considered subcategories of the categories. Although they are all structurally related, their functions are different.

While they are not considered essential, some bioflavonoids do support health as anti-inflammatory, antihistaminic, and antiviral agents. Quercetin has been reported to block the "sorbitol pathway" that is linked to many problems associated with **diabetes** (p. 53). Rutin and several other bioflavonoids may also protect blood vessels.

As antioxidants, some bioflavonoids, such as quercetin, protect LDL-cholesterol from oxidative damage. Others, such as the anthocyanidins from **bilberry** (p. 396), may help protect the lens of the eye from **cataracts** (p. 34). Animal research suggests that naringenin may have anticancer activity.[2] Soy isoflavones are also currently being studied to see if they help fight cancer.

Where Are They Found?

Bioflavonoids are found in a wide range of foods. For example, flavanones are in citrus, isoflavones in soy products, anthocyanins in wine and bilberry, flavans in apples and tea, etc.

Who Is Likely to Be Deficient?

Bioflavonoid deficiencies have not been reported.

How Much Is Usually Taken?

Bioflavonoid supplements are not required to prevent deficiencies in individuals eating a healthy diet. When doctors of natural medicine recommend supplementation (typically to people with one of the conditions listed above), the most common amounts suggested are 1,000 mg of citrus bioflavonoids or 400 mg of quercetin, each taken 3 times per day.

Are There Any Side Effects or Interactions? No consistent toxicity has been linked to the bio-

Bioflavonoids Have Been Used in Connection with the Following Conditions*

Ranking	Health Concerns
Primary	Capillary fragility (p. 32) (hesperidin, quercetin [p. 328], rutin) Chronic venous insufficiency (p. 38) (rutin) Injury (minor) (p. 122) (for prevention only)
Secondary	Bruising (p. 28) Chronic venous insufficiency (p. 38) (hesperidin) Diabetes (p. 53) (bilberry [p. 396]) Hepatitis (p. 77) (catechin)
Other	Atherosclerosis (p. 17) (quercetin [p. 328], bilberry [p. 396]) Cataracts (p. 34) (quercetin [p. 328], bilberry [p. 396]) Diabetes (p. 53) (quercetin [p. 328]) Edema (water retention) (p. 65) (quercetin [p. 328], rutin) Gingivitis (periodontal disease) (p. 73) Glaucoma (p. 74) (rutin) Hay fever (p. 76) (quercetin [p. 328], hesperidin, rutin) High cholesterol (p. 79) (quercetin) (p. 328) Macular degeneration (p. 118) (bilberry [p. 396]) Menopause (p. 118) (hesperidin) Menorrhagia (heavy menstruation) (p. 120) Night blindness (p. 129) (bilberry [p. 396]) Peptic ulcer (p. 138) (quercetin [p. 328]) Retinopathy (p. 150) (quercetin [p. 328]) Varicose veins (p. 163) (bilberry [p. 396])

*Refer to the Individual Health Concern for Complete Information

flavonoids. The exception is for a bioflavonoid called cianidanol, which is not found in supplements.

Years ago, **quercetin** (p. 328) was reported to induce cancer in animals.[3] Most further research did not find this to be true, however.[4,5] While quercetin is mutagenic in test tube studies, it does not appear to be mutagenic in real animals.[6] In fact, quercetin has been found to inhibit both tumor promoters[7] and human cancer cells.[8] People who eat high levels of bioflavonoids have been found to have an overall *lower* risk of getting a wide variety of cancers,[9] though preliminary human research studying only foods high in quercetin has found no relation to cancer risk one way or the other.[10]

Despite the confusion, in recent years, experts have shifted their view of quercetin from concerns that it might cause cancer in test tube studies to guarded hope that quercetin has *anti*cancer effects in humans.[11]

The bioflavonoids help protect **vitamin C** (p. 341); the citrus bioflavonoids, in particular, improve the absorption of vitamin C.[12,13]

Bioflavonoids

Biotin

Biotin, a water-soluble B vitamin, acts as a coenzyme during the metabolism of protein, fats, and carbohydrates.

Where Is It Found?

Good dietary sources of biotin include organ meats, oatmeal, egg yolk, **soy** (p. 332), mushrooms, bananas, peanuts, and **brewer's yeast** (p. 275). Bacteria in the intestine produce significant amounts of biotin, which is probably available for absorption and use by the body.

Biotin Has Been Used in Connection with the Following Conditions*

Ranking	Health Concerns
Secondary	Brittle nails (p. 28)
	Diabetes (p. 53)
Other	Cradle cap
*Refer to the Individual Health Concern for Complete Information	

Who Is Likely to Be Deficient?

Certain rare inborn diseases can leave people with depletion of biotin due to the inability to metabolize the vitamin normally. A dietary deficiency of biotin, however, is quite uncommon, even in those consuming a diet low in this B vitamin. Nonetheless, if someone eats large quantities of raw egg whites, a biotin deficiency can develop, because a protein in the raw egg white inhibits the absorption of biotin. Cooked eggs do not present this problem. Long-term antibiotic use can interfere with biotin production in the intestine and increase the risk of deficiency symptoms, such as **dermatitis** (p. 64), **depression** (p. 50), hair loss, anemia, and nausea. Long-term use of anti-seizure medications may also lead to biotin deficiency.[1] Alcoholics, people with inflammatory bowel disease, and those with diseases of the stomach have been reported to show evidence of poor biotin status; however, the usefulness of biotin supplementation for these individuals remains unclear.[2] In animals, biotin deficiency can cause birth defects.

How Much Is Usually Taken?

The ideal intake of biotin is unknown; however, the amount of biotin found in most diets, combined with intestinal production, appears to be adequate for preventing deficiency symptoms. Researchers have estimated that 30 mcg per day appears to be an adequate intake for adults.[3] Typically, consumption from a Western diet has been estimated to be 30–70 mcg per day. Larger amounts of biotin (8–16 mg per day) may be supportive for **diabetics** (p. 53) by lowering blood glucose levels and preventing diabetic neuropathy.[4,5] Biotin in the amount of 2.5 mg per day strengthened the fingernails of two-thirds of the individuals with **brittle nails** (p. 28), according to one clinical trial.[6]

Are There Any Side Effects or Interactions? Excess intake of biotin is excreted in the urine; no toxicity symptoms have been reported.

Biotin works with some other B vitamins, such as **folic acid** (p. 297), **pantothenic acid** (p. 340) (also known as vitamin B$_5$), and **vitamin B$_{12}$** (p. 340); however, no solid evidence indicates that people supplementing with biotin need to also take these other vitamins. Symptoms of pantothenic acid or **zinc** (p. 346) deficiency have been reported to be lessened with biotin,[7] though people with these deficiencies should supplement with the nutrients they are deficient in. Researchers have speculated that biotin and **alpha lipoic acid** (p. 264) may compete with each other for absorption or uptake into cells; but little is known about the importance of these interactions in humans.[8]

Boric Acid

Boric acid is a chemical substance with mild antiseptic properties.[1] Dilute boric acid is commonly used as a suppository inserted in the vagina to treat **yeast infection** (p. 169).

In one study of 100 women with chronic yeast vaginitis who were not successfully treated with any over-the-counter or prescription antifungal medicines, 98% of the women successfully treated their infections with boric acid capsules inserted into the vagina twice per day for two to four weeks.[2] Several commercial douching products contain boric acid.

The antiseptic activity of boric acid is also used in commercial "artificial tears" and eyewash products.

Boric acid also has antiviral activity. Topical dilute boric acid ointment in the form of sodium borate has been used to shorten the outbreak of **cold sores** (p. 39) in a double-blind trial.[3] Duration of cold sores was approximately 4 days with boric acid but 6 days with placebo.

Where Is It Found?

Boric acid is a white, odorless powder or crystalline substance that is used in some cosmetics, many over-the-counter pharmaceutical products for topical use, alone as a topical antiseptic, and in some manufacturing materials.

Boric Acid Has Been Used in Connection with the Following Conditions*

Ranking	Health Concerns
Secondary	Yeast infection (p. 169)
Other	Cold sores (p. 39) Vaginitis (p. 162)

*Refer to the Individual Health Concern for Complete Information

Who Is Likely to Be Deficient?

Boric acid is not taken internally and is not a nutrient; no deficiency exists.

How Much Is Usually Taken?

Boric acid is available in powder form from a pharmacy without a prescription. This powder is packed tightly into empty gelatin capsules and used as a suppository. For women with **vaginitis** (p. 162), some doctors of natural medicine recommend one such capsule to be inserted into the vagina each night for 2 weeks. Products designed for vaginitis are typically diluted to between 1–4% boric acid. Some health-food stores have prepared suppositories of a combination of boric acid and herbs.

In the trial studying cold sores, an ointment diluted to 4% boric acid was applied 4 times per day. Because of the potential toxicity, people should consult their doctors before using boric acid.

Are There Any Side Effects or Interactions? Suppository boric acid capsules should not be used during pregnancy. Boric acid is very toxic when taken internally and should also never be used on open wounds. When boric acid enters the body, it can cause nausea, vomiting, diarrhea, dermatitis, kidney damage, acute failure of the circulatory system, and even death. Boric acid used to be applied to infants with diaper rash, but even in dilute (3%) topical form caused significant toxicity and two deaths.[4] Therefore, boric acid should not be applied to infants and small children. In fact, experts in the field have stated, "The minor therapeutic value of this compound, in comparison with its potential as a poison, has led to the general recommendation that it no longer be used as a therapeutic agent."[5]

Boron

Whether boron is an essential nutrient remains in debate. Boron appears to affect the metabolism of **calcium** (p. 277), **magnesium** (p. 310), **copper** (p. 285), and phosphorus, as well as **vitamin D** (p. 343).

Preliminary research suggests that boron might affect bone and joint health, but very little is known regarding specifics. The most promising research with boron has linked supplementation to reduced loss of calcium in urine. This effect might help prevent **osteoporosis** (p. 133), but so far decreased loss of calcium from boron supplementation occurs mostly when people are not getting enough magnesium in their diets.[1]

The ability to use energy and to think clearly may also depend somewhat on boron, but details are poorly understood.

Where Is It Found?

Raisins, prunes, and nuts are generally excellent sources. Fruit (other than citrus), vegetables, and legumes also typically contain significant amounts. Actual amounts vary widely, however, depending upon boron levels in soil where the food is grown.

Boron Has Been Used in Connection with the Following Conditions*

Ranking	Health Concerns
Other	Osteoarthritis (p. 130) Osteoporosis (p. 133) Rheumatoid arthritis (p. 151)

*Refer to the Individual Health Concern for Complete Information

Who Is Likely to Be Deficient?

This is unknown; however, people who eat little fruit and few vegetables will consume less boron than do others.

How Much Is Usually Taken?

A leading boron expert has suggested 1 mg per day of boron is a reasonable amount to consume per day.[2] People who eat adequate amounts of produce, nuts, and legumes are likely to already be eating two to six times this amount.[3] Therefore, whether the average person would benefit by supplementing this mineral remains unclear.

Are There Any Side Effects or Interactions?

Accidental acute exposure to high levels of boron can cause nausea, vomiting, abdominal pain, rash, convulsions, and other symptoms.[4] Although chronic exposures can cause related problems, the small (usually 1–3 mg per day) amounts found in supplements have not been linked with toxicity. Supplemental levels do not lead to accumulations within the body.[5] This probably accounts for the lack of toxicity.

However, one study found that 3 mg per day resulted in an increase of estrogen and testosterone levels.[6] In particular, the increase in estrogen is a concern because it may increase the risk of several cancers.

Boron

Until more is known, some doctors of natural medicine recommend that supplemental boron intake should be limited to a maximum of 1 mg per day.

The relationship between boron and other minerals is complex and remains poorly understood. Boron may conserve the body's use of **calcium** (p. 277), **magnesium** (p. 310), and **vitamin D** (p. 343). In one study, the ability of boron to reduce urinary loss of calcium disappeared when subjects were also given magnesium.[7] Therefore, boron may provide no special benefit in maintaining bone mass in the presence of adequate amounts of dietary magnesium.

Branched-Chain Amino Acids (BCAAs)

Branched-chain **amino acids** (BCAAs) (p. 265) include leucine, isoleucine, and valine. BCAAs are essential to the human body. They are needed for the maintenance of muscle tissue and appear to preserve muscle glycogen stores[1] and help prevent muscle protein breakdown during **exercise** (p. 20).[2]

Some research has shown that BCAA supplementation (typically 10–20 grams per day) does not result in meaningful changes in body composition,[3] nor does it improve exercise performance [4,5,6,7] or enhance the effects of physical training.[8,9] However, BCAA supplementation may be useful in special situations, such as preventing muscle loss at high altitudes[10] and prolonging endurance performance in the heat.[11] Studies by one group of researchers suggest that BCAA supplementation may also improve exercise-induced declines in some aspects of mental functioning.[12,13,14]

BCAAs can activate glutamate dehydrogenase—an enzyme that is deficient in amyotrophic lateral sclerosis (ALS), also called Lou Gehrig's disease. In one double-blind trial, 26 grams per day of BCAA supplements helped those with ALS maintain muscle strength.[15] However, a larger study was ended early when people using BCAA not only failed to improve, but experienced higher death rates than the placebo group.[16] Other studies have shown no benefit of BCAA supplementation for ALS or other neuromuscular diseases.[17,18]

One study investigating the advantages of BCAA supplementation for **diabetics** (p. 53) undergoing an intense exercise program found no additional benefit of BCAA on reducing abdominal fat or improving glucose metabolism.[19]

Patients with liver diseases that lead to coma—called hepatic encephalopathy—have low concentrations of BCAAs and excess levels of certain other amino acids. Preliminary research suggested that individuals with this condition might be helped by BCAAs. Double-blind studies have produced somewhat inconsistent results,[20,21,22] but a reanalysis of these studies found an overall benefit for the symptoms of encephalopathy.[23] Therapeutic effects of BCAAs have also been shown in children with liver failure[24] and adults with cirrhosis of the liver.[25] Any treatment of people with liver failure requires the direction of a physician.

People with chronic renal failure may also benefit from BCAA supplementation. A preliminary study found improved breathing and sleep quality in people given intravenous BCAAs during kidney dialysis.[26]

Phenylketonuria (PKU) is a genetic disease that allows abnormally high amounts of phenylalanine and its end products to accumulate in the blood, causing damage to the nervous system. A controlled trial demonstrated that regular use of BCAAs by adolescents and young adults with PKU improved performance on some tests of mental functioning.[27]

Where Are They Found?

Dairy products and red meat contain the greatest amounts of BCAAs, although they are present in all protein-containing foods. **Whey** (p. 346) protein and egg protein supplements are other sources of BCAAs. BCAA supplements provide the amino acids leucine, isoleucine, and valine.

BCAAs Have Been Used in Connection with the Following Conditions*

Ranking	Health Concerns
Secondary	Chronic renal failure (intravenous BCAA) Phenylketonuria
Other	Athletic performance (p. 20) (for high altitude and extreme temperature only) Hepatic encephalopathy

*Refer to the Individual Health Concern for Complete Information

Who Is Likely to Be Deficient?

Only an individual deficient in protein would become deficient in BCAAs because most food sources of protein supply BCAAs. Few people in Western societies are protein deficient.

How Much Is Usually Taken?

Most diets provide an adequate amount of BCAAs for most people, which is about 25–65 mg per pound of body weight.[28,29] Athletes involved in intense training often take 5 grams of leucine, 4 grams of valine, and

2 grams of isoleucine per day to prevent muscle loss and increase muscle gain, though most research does not support this use of BCAAs.

Are There Any Side Effects or Interactions? Side effects have not been reported with the use of BCAAs, except in the one study of ALS described above. At high intakes, BCAAs are simply converted into other amino acids, used as energy, or converted to fat for storage. However, individuals with kidney or liver disease should not consume high intakes of amino acids without consulting their doctor.

Brewer's Yeast

Brewer's yeast is the dried, pulverized cells of Saccharomyces cerevisiae, a type of fungus.

It is a rich source of the **B-complex** (p. 341) vitamins, protein (providing all the essential **amino acids** [p. 265]), and minerals, particularly **chromium** (p. 282). Brewer's yeast should not be confused with baker's yeast, nutritional yeast, or torula yeast, which are low in chromium.

Brewer's yeast, perhaps by changing bacterial flora in the large intestine, might be helpful in treating of some cases of infectious **diarrhea** (p. 58).

Where Is It Found?

Brewer's yeast, which has a very bitter taste, is recovered after being used in the beer-brewing process. Brewer's yeast can also be grown specifically for harvest as a nutritional supplement. "De-bittered" yeast is also available, though most yeast sold in health-food stores not tasting bitter is not real brewer's yeast—particularly if found in bulk.

Who Is Likely to Be Deficient?

Brewer's yeast is not an essential nutrient, but it can be used as a source of **B-complex vitamins** (p. 341) and protein. It is by far the best source of **chromium** (p. 282), both in terms of quantity and bioavailability.

How Much Is Usually Taken?

Brewer's yeast is often taken as a powder, tablets, or capsules. High-quality brewer's yeast powder or flakes contain as much as 60 mcg of chromium per tablespoon. When doctors recommend brewer's yeast, they will often suggest 1–2 tablespoons of this high-potency bulk product, usually as an optimal way to supply chromium. Remember: if it is not bitter, it is not likely to be real brewer's yeast and therefore will not contain chromium.

Are There Any Side Effects or Interactions? Side effects have not been reported from the use of

Brewer's Yeast Has Been Used in Connection with the Following Conditions*

Ranking	Health Concerns
Primary	Diabetes (p. 53) High cholesterol (p. 79)
Secondary	Diarrhea (p. 58) (infectious)
*Refer to the Individual Health Concern for Complete Information	

brewer's yeast, although allergies to it exist in some people. It is not related to *Candida albicans* fungus, which causes **yeast infection** (p. 169).

Bromelain

Bromelain is a group of **proteolytic enzymes** (p. 289), which means that it is capable of digesting protein. Although most enzymes are widely believed to absorb poorly, significant amounts of bromelain do absorb.[1] Proteolytic enzymes other than bromelain are often used with people who suffer from malabsorption. Although bromelain in combination with other enzymes and ox bile has been reported to help digest food,[2] it is generally not used for this purpose. Although many doctors of natural medicine assume that other proteolytic enzymes, such as those found in pancreatin, are more effective than bromelain in helping digestion and absorption, almost no research compares the relative effects of these enzymes.

Bromelain is an anti-inflammatory agent, and for this reason is helpful in healing **minor injuries** (p. 122), particularly sprains and strains, muscle injuries, and the pain, swelling, and tenderness that accompany sports injuries.[3,4,5]

Also as a result of its anti-inflammatory effect, bromelain has been found to dramatically reduce postoperative swelling in controlled human research.[6] Double-blind research has found bromelain effective in reducing swelling, bruising,[7] and pain for women having minor surgery after giving birth (episiotomy).[8]

The anti-inflammatory effect of bromelain is the probable reason this enzyme has been found effective for people suffering from **sinusitis** (p. 156).[9] Some of the evidence supporting bromelain in the treatment of sinusitis comes from double-blind research.[10]

Bromelain, in combination with trypsin, another enzyme, may alleviate symptoms of **urinary tract infection** (p. 160) due to its anti-inflammatory action. One double-blind study comparing the two enzymes in combination with antibiotics to placebo plus antibiotics reported that reduction of symptoms was good to excellent in all of the subjects given the

Calcium

enzymes and antibiotics, but less than half of those given antibiotics only.[11]

Bromelain has been reported to increase absorption of amoxicillin when it is taken with this antibiotic.

Again, probably due to its anti-inflammatory action, bromelain was reported to help patients with **rheumatoid arthritis** (p. 151) in preliminary research.[12] In that trial, in which bromelain was given for varying (3-week to 13-month) periods, 73% had good to excellent results.

Bromelain is a natural blood thinner because it prevents excessive blood platelet stickiness.[13] This may explain, in part, the positive reports in a few clinical trials of bromelain to decrease symptoms of **angina** (p. 13) and thrombophlebitis.[14,15] In addition, bromelain reduces the thickness of mucus, which may benefit patients with **asthma** (p. 15) or chronic bronchitis.[16]

Preliminary evidence in both animals and people suggests that bromelain may possess antitumor activity, though the true importance of this effect is poorly understood.[17]

Where Is It Found?

Bromelain is found mostly in the stems of pineapples and is available as a dietary supplement.

Bromelain Has Been Used in Connection with the Following Conditions*

Ranking	Health Concerns
Primary	Minor injuries (p. 122) Sinusitis (p. 156) Wound healing (p. 167)
Secondary	Postsurgical healing Urinary tract infection (p. 160)
Other	Angina (p. 13) Asthma (p. 15) Rheumatoid arthritis (p. 151) Thrombophlebitis
*Refer to the Individual Health Concern for Complete Information	

Who Is Likely to Be Deficient?

Since bromelain is not essential, deficiencies of this plant-based enzyme do not exist.

How Much Is Usually Taken?

Assessing the right dose of bromelain is complicated. Most bromelain research was conducted years ago, when amounts used were listed in units of activity that no longer exist; these old units do not precisely convert to new ones. Today, bromelain is measured in MCUs (milk clotting units) or GDUs (gelatin dissolv-

ing units). One GDU equals approximately 1.5 MCU. Strong products contain at least 2,000 MCU (1,200–1,333 GDU) per gram (1,000 mg). A supplement containing 500 mg labeled "2,000 MCU per gram" would have 1,000 MCU of activity. Some doctors of natural medicine recommend as much as 3,000 MCU taken 3 times per day for several days, followed by 2,000 MCU 3 times per day.[18] Much of the research, however, uses smaller amounts, more like the equivalent of approximately 2,000 MCU in divided amounts in the course of a day (500 MCU taken 4 times per day).

Are There Any Side Effects or Interactions?
Bromelain is generally safe and free of side effects when taken in moderate amounts; however, one preliminary report indicates increased heart rate with the use of bromelain.[19] In addition, some people are allergic to bromelain. Because bromelain acts as a blood thinner and little is known about how bromelain interacts with blood-thinning drugs, individuals should avoid combining such drugs with bromelain, in order to reduce the theoretical risk of excessive bleeding.

Calcium

Calcium is the most abundant mineral in the human body. Of the 2 to 3 pounds of calcium contained in the average body, 99% is located in the bones and teeth. Calcium is needed to form bones and teeth and is also required for blood clotting, transmission of signals in nerve cells, and muscle contraction. The importance of calcium for preventing **osteoporosis** (p. 133) is probably its most well-known role.

Although calcium plays at least some minor role in lowering **blood pressure** (p. 89), the mechanisms involved appear complex and remain somewhat unclear.[1]

By reducing absorption of oxalate,[2] a substance found in many foods, calcium may be able to indirectly reduce the risk of **kidney stones** (p. 111).[3] However, people with a history of kidney stones must talk with a doctor before supplementing calcium because such supplementation might actually increase the risk of forming stones for the small number of people who absorb too much calcium.

Calcium also appears to partially bind some fats and cholesterol in the gastrointestinal tract. Perhaps as a result, some older research suggests that calcium supplementation may help lower **cholesterol** (p. 79) levels.[4]

Where Is It Found?

Most dietary calcium comes from dairy products. The myth that calcium from dairy products "doesn't absorb" is not supported by scientific research.[5,6] Other good sources include sardines, canned salmon, green leafy vegetables, and tofu.

Choosing a form of calcium supplement can be confusing. While fewer pills of the calcium carbonate form are needed, this form doesn't absorb as well as some other forms of calcium. Most,[7,8] but not all,[9] studies suggest that calcium citrate is better absorbed than calcium carbonate. Virtually all comparative studies find that calcium citrate/malate (CCM) absorbs somewhat better than calcium carbonate. CCM is increasingly the form of calcium recommended by nutritionally oriented doctors. The microcrystalline hydroxyapatite (MCHC), a variation on the bonemeal form of calcium, has been shown to improve bone mass,[10] but the absorption of MCHC appears to be poor.[11,12] Only preliminary research exists regarding the amino acid chelates of calcium, and conclusions cannot be drawn at this time. Please refer to **Calcium: Which Form is Best?** (p. 278) for more information about choosing a calcium supplement.

Calcium Has Been Used in Connection with the Following Conditions*

Ranking	Health Concerns
Primary	Celiac disease (p. 35) (if deficient) Osteoporosis (p. 133) Rickets (p. 154)
Secondary	High blood pressure (p. 89) High cholesterol (p. 79) Premenstrual syndrome (p. 141)
Other	Gingivitis (periodontal disease) (p. 73) Kidney stones (p. 111) Menstruation painful (dysmenorrhea) (p. 61) Migraine headaches (p. 121) Multiple sclerosis (p. 127) Pregnancy and postpartum support (p. 143)
*Refer to the Individual Health Concern for Complete Information	

Who Is Likely to Be Deficient?

Severe deficiency of both calcium and **vitamin D** (p. 343) is called **rickets** (p. 154) in children and **osteomalacia** (p. 154) in adults. Vegans (pure vegetarians), people with dark skin, those who live in northern climates, and people who stay indoors almost all the time are more likely to be vitamin D deficient than are other people. Vegans often eat less calcium and vitamin D than do other people. Most people eat well below the recommended amount of calcium. This lack of dietary

calcium is thought to contribute to the risk of osteoporosis, particularly in white and Asian women.

How Much Is Usually Taken?

The National Academy of Sciences has established guidelines for calcium that are 25–50% higher than previous recommendations. For ages 19 to 51, calcium intake is recommended to be 1,000 mg daily; for adults over age 51, the recommendation is 1,200 mg daily. The most common supplemental amount for adults is 800–1,000 mg per day.[13] General recommendations for higher intakes (1,200–1,500 mg) usually include the several hundred milligrams of calcium most people consume from their diets.

Are There Any Side Effects or Interactions? Constipation, bloating, and gas are sometimes reported with the use of calcium supplements.[14] A very high intake of calcium from dairy taken with calcium carbonate used to cause a condition called "milk alkali syndrome." This toxicity is rarely reported today because most medical doctors no longer tell people with ulcers to take this combination.

People with hyperparathyroidism, or chronic kidney disease should not supplement with calcium without consulting a nutritionally oriented physician. People who have had kidney stones should read the section on **kidney stones** (p. 111) before considering supplementation. For other adults, the highest amount typically suggested by nutritionally oriented doctors (1,200 mg per day) is considered quite safe.

In some cases, calcium supplements in the forms of bonemeal (including MCHC), dolomite, and oyster shell have higher lead levels than permitted by California regulations, though generally less than the levels set by the federal government.[15] "Refined" forms (which would include CCM, calcium citrate, and most calcium carbonate) had low levels.[16] In that report, only bonemeal exceeded federal levels. People who decide to take bonemeal, dolomite, or oyster shell for long periods of time should contact the supplying supplement company to request independent laboratory analysis showing minimal lead levels.

Vitamin D (p. 343) is needed for calcium to absorb. Therefore, many nutritionally oriented doctors recommend that those supplementing with calcium also supplement with 400 IU of vitamin D per day.

Calcium competes for absorption with a number of other minerals. Therefore, individuals taking calcium for more than a few weeks should also take a multimineral supplement.

Lysine (p. 309) supplementation increases the absorption of calcium and may reduce its excretion.[17] As a result some researchers believe that lysine may

Calcium

eventually be shown to have a role in the prevention and treatment of **osteoporosis** (p. 133).[18]

Calcium: Which Form Is Best?

Dietary supplements may contain one of several different forms of **calcium** (p. 277). One difference between the various calcium compounds is the percentage of elemental calcium present. A greater percentage of elemental calcium means that fewer tablets will be needed to achieve the desired calcium intake. For instance, in the calcium carbonate form, calcium accounts for 40% of the compound, while the calcium citrate form provides 24% elemental calcium.

Many medical doctors recommend calcium carbonate because it requires the fewest pills to reach a given level of calcium and also because it is readily available and inexpensive. For people concerned about cost and only willing to swallow two to three calcium pills per day, calcium carbonate is a sensible choice. Even for these people, however, low-quality calcium carbonate supplements are less than ideal. Depending on how the tablet is manufactured, some calcium carbonate pills have been found to disintegrate and dissolve improperly, which could interfere with absorption.[19] The disintegration of calcium carbonate pills can be easily evaluated by putting a tablet in a half cup of vinegar and stirring occasionally. After half an hour, no undissolved chunks of tablet should remain at the bottom.[20]

Calcium carbonate may not always show optimal absorption, but it clearly has positive effects. For example, calcium carbonate appears to be as bioavailable as the calcium found in milk.[21] In fact, some studies indicate that calcium carbonate absorbs as well as most other forms besides calcium citrate/malate (CCM).[22,23] For example, a recent study found absorption of calcium from calcium carbonate to be virtually identical to absorption of calcium from calcium citrate.[24]

For people willing to take more pills to achieve a given amount of calcium (typically 800–1,000 mg), calcium carbonate does not appear to be the optimal choice, because other forms have been reported to absorb better (however, they do require more pills per day because each pill contains less calcium). For this reason, some nutritionally oriented doctors recommend other forms of calcium—CCM. Research shows that CCM absorbs better than most other forms.[25,26,27] CCM may also be more effective in maintaining bone mass than some other forms of calcium supplements.[28] Because of their similarity in both name and structure, CCM can be confused with calcium citrate, but they are not the same.

CCM is not the only form of calcium that might absorb better than carbonate. For example, most,[29,30]

though not all,[31] studies suggest that calcium citrate might have some absorption advantage over calcium carbonate. However, no evidence suggests that calcium citrate absorption equals the absorption from CCM.

Microcrystalline hydroxyapatite (MCHC), a variation on bonemeal, has attracted attention because of studies reporting increases in bone mass[32] and better effects on bone mass than calcium carbonate.[33] Similar positive studies exist using CCM.[34] However, unlike CCM, MCHC has only occasionally been compared with other forms of calcium. In limited research that does make comparisons, MCHC fared poorly in terms of solubility, absorption, and effect on calcium metabolism.[35,36]

Remarkably little is known about the relative efficacy of amino acid chelates (pronounced "kee-lates") of calcium. In the only commonly cited trial, absorption was measured for an amino acid chelate called calcium bisglycinate and compared with absorption from citrate, carbonate, and MCHC.[37] In that trial, the amino acid chelate showed the best absorption, and MCHC the worst. Although CCM was studied in that trial, it was taken under different circumstances than the chelate (with meals), so it is difficult to draw conclusions.

Whatever the form, calcium supplements typically absorb better when eaten with meals.[38] Moreover, research indicates that taking calcium with meals may reduce the risk of **kidney stones** (p. 111) and supplementing calcium between meals might actually increase the risk.[39]

Besides *how* to take calcium supplements, scientists have also been studying *when* to take them. Supplementing calcium in the evening appears better for **osteoporosis** (p. 133) prevention than taking calcium in the morning, based on the circadian rhythm of bone loss.[40]

What Is the Relationship Between Calcium Supplements and Stomach Acid?

Years ago, researchers reported that people who do not make **hydrochloric acid** (p. 269) in their stomachs cannot absorb calcium adequately when the calcium is taken alone.[41] In that report, adding hydrochloric acid restored normal calcium absorption. Although researchers have subsequently confirmed these findings, they have also discovered that these same people absorb calcium normally if they take it with meals. In addition, researchers have noted that giving these people hydrochloric acid does not further improve absorption during meals.[42] Many others have confirmed that hydrochloric acid, either from pills or from the stomach, is unnecessary for the absorption

Calcium

of calcium, as long as the calcium supplement is taken with meals.[43,44,45,46]

L-Carnitine

L-carnitine is made in the body from the **amino acids** (p. 265) **lysine** (p. 309) and **methionine** (p. 313). It is needed to release energy from fat. Its actions appear to be particularly important in the heart. For congestive heart failure, much of the research has used a modified form of carnitine called propionyl-L-carnitine (PC). In one double-blind trial, using 500 mg PC per day led to a 26% increase in exercise capacity after 6 months.[1]

Research shows that individuals who supplement with carnitine while engaging in an exercise regimen are less likely to experience muscle soreness.[2] However, the belief that carnitine's effect on energy release will help build muscle or improve **athletic performance** (p. 20) has, so far, not been supported by most research.[3,4]

However, carnitine has been given to people with chronic lung disease in trials investigating how the body responds to exercise.[5,6] In these double-blind reports, 2 grams of carnitine taken twice per day for 2 to 4 weeks led to positive changes in breathing response to exercise.

Where Is It Found?

Dairy and red meat contain the greatest amounts of carnitine. Therefore, people who have a limited intake of meat and dairy products tend to have lower carnitine intakes.

Who Is Likely to Be Deficient?

Carnitine deficiencies are rare, even in strict vegetarians, because the body produces carnitine relatively easily.

Rare genetic diseases can cause a carnitine deficiency. Also, deficiencies are occasionally associated with other diseases, such as **diabetes** (p. 53) and cirrhosis.[7,8] A carnitine deficiency can also result from oxygen deprivation, which can occur in some heart conditions. In Italy, carnitine is prescribed for heart failure, heart arrhythmias, **angina** (p. 13) pectoris, and lack of oxygen to the heart.[9]

How Much Is Usually Taken?

Most people do not need carnitine supplements. For therapeutic use, typical amounts are 1–3 grams per day.

It remains unclear whether the propionyl-L-carnitine form of carnitine used in congestive heart failure

L-Carnitine Has Been Used in Connection with the Following Conditions*

Ranking	Health Concerns
Primary	Angina (p. 13) Congestive heart failure (p. 43) (propionyl-L-carnitine)
Secondary	Chronic fatigue syndrome (p. 36) Chronic obstructive pulmonary disease (COPD) (p. 45) Diabetes (p. 53) High triglycerides (p. 85) Infertility (male) (p. 103) Intermittent claudication (p. 106) Minor injuries (p. 122) (for exercise-related muscle injury)
Other	Athletic performance (p. 20) (for ultra-endurance only) High cholesterol (p. 79) Raynaud's disease (p. 148)

*Refer to the Individual Health Concern for Complete Information

research has greater benefits than the L-carnitine form, since limited research in both animals and humans with the more common L-carnitine has also shown very promising effects.[10]

Are There Any Side Effects or Interactions? L-carnitine has not been consistently linked with any toxicity.

The body needs **lysine** (p. 309), **methionine** (p. 313), **vitamin C** (p. 341), **iron** (p. 304), **niacin** (p. 339), and **vitamin B$_6$** (p. 340) to produce carnitine.

Cartilage (Bovine and Shark)

Cartilage, derived from shark and bovine (cow) sources, is a type of connective tissue comprised of mucopolysaccharides, protein substances, **calcium** (p. 277), **sulfur** (p. 334), and collagen. Early research in the 1950s and 1960s, using chips of bovine cartilage inserted into wounds, demonstrated that cartilage enhances **wound healing** (p. 167).[1,2] Since then, cartilage has been investigated for its potential role in regulating **immune function** (p. 94) and stopping the growth of tumors.[3] The role of shark cartilage in inhibiting angiogenesis (the growth of new blood vessels) is hypothesized to be beneficial in halting the growth and spread of cancer.[4] A few studies suggest that individuals with cancer may benefit from cartilage supplements;[5,6] however, well-designed research is lacking, and many experts question the use of

Chitosan

cartilage in this regard. A similar situation is seen with the use of cartilage in individuals with **arthritis** (p. 130, 562).

Where Is It Found?

Cartilage is derived from either sharks or cows.

Cartilage Has Been Used in Connection with the Following Conditions*

Ranking	Health Concerns
Other	Osteoarthritis (p. 130) Rheumatoid arthritis (p. 151, 571)

*Refer to the Individual Health Concern for Complete Information

Who Is Likely to Be Deficient?

Since it is not an essential nutrient, cartilage is not associated with deficiency states.

How Much Is Usually Taken?

Anyone who is interested in taking bovine or shark cartilage supplements should consult a nutritionally oriented doctor for advice.

Are There Any Side Effects or Interactions?

Reports have suggested that some people should not use a cartilage supplement—this concern is based only on theory, not clinical evidence. This would include those people with cardiovascular disease, women who are planning to be or are pregnant, nursing mothers, anyone having or having had surgery within 30 days, and athletes training intensely. None of these contraindications has been proven, however. The calcium in the huge amount of shark cartilage taken by some people with cancer (greater than 50 grams per day) could lead to toxicity. However, remarkably few instances of actual calcium toxicity have been reported.

Chitosan

Like dietary fiber, chitosan is not digestible but may have beneficial effects on the gastrointestinal tract. Chitosan may reduce the absorption of bile acids or cholesterol, either of which may cause a lowering of blood **cholesterol** (p. 79).[1] This effect has been repeatedly demonstrated in animals, and a preliminary human study showed that 3–6 grams per day of chitosan taken for 2 weeks resulted in a 6% drop in cholesterol and a 10% increase in HDL (the "good") cholesterol.[2] Another preliminary study showed a 43% lowering of total cholesterol in people being treated

for kidney failure with dialysis who took 4 grams per day of chitosan for 12 weeks. This group also appeared to have improved kidney function and less severe anemia after chitosan treatment.[3]

Chitosan in large amounts given with **vitamin C** (p. 341) has been shown to reduce dietary fat absorption in animals fed a high-fat diet.[4,5,6] Unfortunately, mineral and fat-soluble vitamin absorption is also reduced by feeding animals large amounts of chitosan.[7] No studies have been done on the effects of chitosan on dietary fat absorption in humans.

Animal and preliminary human research suggests that chitosan may prevent the **blood pressure** (p. 89) elevating effects of a high-salt meal, possibly by reducing the absorption of chloride. A small study showed that men taking 5 grams of chitosan with a meal high in salt resulted in no elevation in blood pressure, while the same meal without chitosan significantly elevated systolic blood pressure.[8]

Chitosan may also have an effect on bacteria in the intestines. A small human study found that taking 3–6 grams per day of chitosan for 2 weeks reduced indicators of putrefaction in the intestines,[9] a change that might help prevent diseases, such as colon cancer.[10]

Where Is It Found?

Chitosan is a supplement commonly extracted from the shells of crustaceans, such as shrimp and crab.

Chitosan Has Been Used in Connection with the Following Conditions*

Ranking	Health Concerns
Other	High blood pressure (p. 89) High cholesterol (p. 79) Kidney failure

*Refer to the Individual Health Concern for Complete Information

Who Is Likely to Be Deficient?

Chitosan is not an essential nutrient, so deficiencies do not occur.

How Much Is Usually Taken?

Most human research has used 3–6 grams per day with meals.

Are There Any Side Effects or Interactions?

While no long-term studies of the effects of chitosan on human health have been done, animal studies suggest that harmful effects on mineral and fat-soluble vitamin absorption, on maintenance of normal intestinal flora, and on normal growth in children and during pregnancy are possible.[11] People with intestinal malabsorption syndromes should not use chitosan.

Chlorophyll

Chlorophyll, the substance responsible for the green color in plants, has been used traditionally to ameliorate bad breath, as well as to reduce the odors of urine, feces, and infected **wounds** (p. 167). Chlorophyll has anti-inflammatory, **antioxidant** (p. 267), and wound-healing properties.[1,2]

Historically, chlorophyll was used for gastrointestinal problems, such as **constipation** (p. 44), and to stimulate blood cell formation in anemia. Some preliminary evidence suggests that chlorophyll might help detoxify cancer-promoting substances.[3,4]

Where Is It Found?

Good dietary sources of chlorophyll include dark green leafy vegetables, algae, **spirulina** (p. 333), chlorella, wheat grass, and barley grass. Supplements of chlorophyll as powder, capsule, tablet, and drinks are also available.

Chlorophyll Has Been Used in Connection with the Following Conditions*

Ranking	Health Concerns
Other	Constipation (p. 44) Halitosis (bad breath)
*Refer to the Individual Health Concern for Complete Information	

Who Is Likely to Be Deficient?

Because chlorophyll is not known to be an essential nutrient, a deficiency does not exist. Individuals who do not eat plenty of green foods lack chlorophyll in their diets.

How Much Is Usually Taken?

Optimal levels remain unknown. Chlorophyll in the amount of 100 mg 2 or 3 times per day can be used for deodorization.

Are There Any Side Effects or Interactions? No side effects have been reported with the use of chlorophyll.

Chondroitin Sulfate

Chondroitin sulfate consists of repeating chains of molecules called mucopolysaccharides. Chondroitin sulfate is a major constituent of cartilage, providing structure, holding water and nutrients, and allowing other molecules to move through cartilage—an important property, as there is no blood supply to cartilage.

Animal studies indicate that chondroitin sulfate may promote healing of bone, which is consistent with the fact that the majority of glycosaminoglycans found in bone consist of chondroitin sulfate.[1] Chondroitin sulfate also appears to help restore joint function in people with **osteoarthritis** (p. 130),[2] a finding confirmed in double-blind research.[3,4]

Chondroitin and similar compounds are present in the lining of blood vessels and the urinary bladder. They help prevent abnormal movement of blood, urine, or components across the barrier of the vessel or bladder wall. Part of chondroitin's role in blood vessels is to prevent excessive blood clotting. However, whether supplements of chondroitin are able to favorably affect blood clotting remains unclear. In addition, chondroitin sulfate may lower blood **cholesterol levels** (p. 53).[5] Older preliminary research showed that chondroitin sulfate may prevent **atherosclerosis** (p. 17) in animals and humans and may also prevent heart attacks in people who already have atherosclerosis.[6,7,8]

Chondroitin sulfate can help form a coating on nasal passages. Perhaps as a result, researchers found that when chondroitin sulfate was sprayed onto nasal passages in a small group of snorers, the amount of time people spent snoring was reduced about one-third in a double-blind trial.[9] No further studies have investigated the effects of oral chondroitin sulfate on snoring.

Chondroitin sulfate is classified as a type of glycosaminoglycan; it is rich in **sulfur** (p. 334) and is related to **glucosamine** (p. 299). Glycosaminoglycans affect how the body processes oxalate, a substance linked to kidney stones. In one study of forty people with a history of **kidney stones** (p. 111), 30 mg twice a day of mixed glycosaminoglycans reduced urinary oxalate excretion in 15 days—a change that could drop the risk of stone formation.[10] However, while experts believe that glycosaminoglycans effectively prevent formation of kidney stones in test tube studies, effects in humans have been inconsistent.[11]

Where Is It Found?

The only significant food source of chondroitin sulfate is animal cartilage.

Who Is Likely to Be Deficient?

Because the body makes chondroitin, the possibility of a dietary deficiency remains uncertain. Nevertheless, chondroitin sulfate may be reduced in joint cartilage affected by osteoarthritis and possibly other forms of arthritis.

Chondroitin Sulfate

How Much Is Usually Taken?

For atherosclerosis, researchers have sometimes started therapy using very high amounts, such as 5 grams twice per day with meals, lowering the amount to 500 mg 3 times per day after a few months. Before taking such high amounts, people should consult a nutritionally oriented doctor. For osteoarthritis, a typical level is 400 mg 3 times per day. The ability for chondroitin to be absorbed orally is still under question.

Are There Any Side Effects or Interactions?

Nausea may occur at intakes greater than 10 grams per day. No other adverse effects have been reported.

The hypothesis that **glucosamine sulfate** (p. 111) and chondroitin sulfate work synergistically in the support of osteoarthritis remains unproven. The fact that they are structurally similar suggests that they may act in similar ways.

Chondroitin Sulfate Has Been Used in Connection with the Following Conditions*

Ranking	Health Concerns
Primary	Osteoarthritis (p. 130)
Other	Atherosclerosis (p. 17) High cholesterol (p. 79) Kidney stones (p. 111) Minor injuries (p. 122)

*Refer to the Individual Health Concern for Complete Information

Chromium

Chromium is an essential trace mineral that helps the body maintain normal blood sugar levels. In addition to its well-studied effects in **diabetes** (p. 53), preliminary research has found that chromium supplementation also improves glucose tolerance in people with Turner's syndrome—a disease linked with glucose intolerance.[1]

Chromium may also play a role in increasing HDL (the "good" cholesterol),[2] yet lowering overall **cholesterol levels** (p. 79).[3]

Chromium, in a form called chromium picolinate, has been studied for its potential role in altering body composition. Preliminary research in animals[4] and humans[5,6] suggested that chromium picolinate increases fat loss and lean muscle tissue gain. Though some follow-up research in people has not confirmed chromium picolinate to have a significant effect in altering body composition,[7] double-blind research has reported reduction in body fat[8] and body weight[9] in

people given 400 mcg of chromium picolinate per day for 3 months.

Where Is It Found?

The best source of chromium is true **brewer's yeast** (p. 275). Nutritional yeast and torula yeast do not contain significant amounts and are not substitutes. Chromium is also found in grains and cereals, although it is lacking when these foods are refined. Stainless steel scrapings from pots and pans provide much of the chromium in many people's diets. Some brands of beer contain significant amounts.

Chromium Has Been Used in Connection with the Following Conditions*

Ranking	Health Concerns
Primary	Diabetes (p. 53) High cholesterol (p. 79) Hypoglycemia (p. 92)
Other	Athletic performance (p. 20) Weight loss and obesity (p. 165)

*Refer to the Individual Health Concern for Complete Information

Who Is Likely to Be Deficient?

Most people eat less than the U.S. National Academy of Science's recommended range of 50–200 mcg per day. The high incidence of adult-onset diabetes suggests to many doctors of nutritional medicine that most people should be supplementing small amounts of chromium.

How Much Is Usually Taken?

A daily intake of 200 mcg is recommended by many doctors of nutritional medicine.

Are There Any Side Effects or Interactions? In

supplemental doses (typically 50–300 mcg per day), chromium has not been linked consistently with human toxicity. One study suggested that chromium in very high concentrations in a test tube could cause chromosomal mutations in ovarian cells of hamsters.[10,11] This risk, however, has not been demonstrated in humans.[12] There is one report of severe illness (including liver and kidney damage) occurring in an individual who was taking 1,000 mcg of chromium per day.[13] However, chromium supplementation was not proven to be the cause of these problems.

Two single, unrelated cases of toxicity have been reported. A case of kidney failure appeared after taking 600 mcg per day for 6 weeks;[14] and a case of anemia, liver dysfunction, and other problems appeared after 4 to 5 months of 1,200–24,000 mcg chromium picolinate per day.[15] Whether these problems were caused by chromium picolinate or, if so, whether other forms of chromium might have the same effects at these high amounts remains unclear. No one should take more than 300 mcg per day of chromium without the supervision of a nutritionally oriented doctor.

Preliminary research has found that **vitamin C** (p. 341) increases the absorption of chromium.[16]

Coenzyme Q$_{10}$

Coenzyme Q$_{10}$ is a powerful **antioxidant** (p. 267) that protects the body from free radicals.[1] Coenzyme Q$_{10}$ is also called ubiquinone, a name that signifies its ubiquitous (widespread) distribution in the human body. As a coenzyme, this nutrient aids metabolic reactions, such as the complex process of transforming food into ATP, the energy on which the body runs.

Coenzyme Q$_{10}$ supplementation has been investigated as a way to improve physical endurance because of its effect on energy production. However, most research shows that coenzyme Q$_{10}$ does not improve **athletic performance** (p. 20).[2]

Synthesis of sperm requires considerable energy. Due to its role in energy production, coenzyme Q$_{10}$ has been studied in **infertile men** (p. 103). Preliminary research reports that supplementation of coenzyme Q$_7$, a related molecule, increased sperm counts in a group of infertile men.[3]

Healing of periodontal tissue (the gums of the mouth) may require increased energy production; therefore, researchers have explored the effects of coenzyme Q$_{10}$ supplementation in people with **periodontal disease** (p. 73), which has been linked to coenzyme Q$_{10}$ deficiency. Double-blind research shows that people with gum disease given coenzyme Q$_{10}$ achieve better results than do those given placebo.[4]

The role of coenzyme Q$_{10}$ in energy formation also relates to how the body uses carbohydrates. Preliminary research suggests that a close relative of this nutrient lowered blood sugar levels in a group of **diabetics** (p. 53).[5]

Virtually every cell of the human body contains coenzyme Q$_{10}$. The mitochondria, the area of cells where energy is produced, contain the most coenzyme Q$_{10}$. The heart and liver, because they contain the most mitochondria per cell, have the greatest amount of coenzyme Q$_{10}$. Coenzyme Q$_{10}$ helps people with **congestive heart failure**[6] (p. 43)—an effect proven in double-blind research.[7] Coenzyme Q$_{10}$ may take several

months to show beneficial results. People with congestive heart failure taking coenzyme Q$_{10}$ should not stop taking it suddenly because sudden withdrawal may exacerbate the symptoms of congestive heart failure.[8]

Similar improvements have been reported in people with cardiomyopathies—a group of diseases affecting heart muscle. Research (including double-blind studies) in this area has been consistently positive.[9]

Also, due to its effect on heart muscle, researchers have studied coenzyme Q$_{10}$ in people with heart arrhythmias. Preliminary research in this area reported improvement after approximately 1 month in people with premature ventricular beats (a form of arrhythmia) who also suffer from diabetes.[10]

Angina (p. 13) patients taking 150 mg per day of coenzyme Q$_{10}$ report a greater ability to exercise without problems.[11] This has been confirmed in independent investigations.[12]

Coenzyme Q$_{10}$ appears to increase the heart's tolerance to a lack of oxygen. Perhaps as a result, preliminary research has shown that problems resulting from heart surgery occurred less frequently in people given coenzyme Q$_{10}$ compared with the control group.[13]

Muscle mitochondria lack adequate coenzyme Q$_{10}$ in people with muscular dystrophy, a problem that could affect muscle function. In a preliminary double-blind 3-month trial, four of eight people with muscular dystrophy had improvements in heart function and sense of well-being when supplementing coenzyme Q$_{10}$.[14]

Mitochondrial function also appears to be impaired in people with **Alzheimer's disease** (p. 11). Due to coenzyme Q$_{10}$'s effects on mitochondrial functioning, one group of researchers has given coenzyme Q10 (along with **iron** [p. 304] and **vitamin B$_6$** [p. 340]) to several people with Alzheimer's disease and reported that the progression of the disease appeared to have been prevented for 1½ to 2 years.[15]

Coenzyme Q$_{10}$ also modulates **immunity** (p. 94).[16] Perhaps as a result, preliminary research suggests that women with a high risk of breast cancer recurrence show evidence of protection when given very high (390 mg per day) levels of coenzyme Q10 for up to 5 years.[17]

Coenzyme Q$_{10}$ appears to modulate **blood pressure** (p. 89) by reducing resistance to blood flow.[18] Several trials have reported that supplementation with coenzyme Q$_{10}$ for at least several months significantly reduces blood pressure in people with **hypertension** (p. 89).[19]

Where Is It Found?

Coenzyme Q_{10} is primarily found in fish and meat.

Coenzyme Q_{10} Has Been Used in Connection with the Following Conditions*

Ranking	Health Concerns
Primary	Angina (p. 13) Congestive heart failure (p. 43)
Secondary	Diabetes (p. 53) Gingivitis (periodontal disease) (p. 73) High blood pressure (p. 89) Mitral valve prolapse (p. 125)
Other	Alzheimer's disease (p. 11) Athletic performance (p. 20) Chronic obstructive pulmonary disease (COPD) (p. 45) HIV support (p. 87) Infertility (male) (p. 103)

*Refer to the Individual Health Concern for Complete Information

Who Is Likely to Be Deficient?

Deficiency is poorly understood, but it may be caused by synthesis problems in the body rather than an insufficiency in the diet. Low blood levels have been reported in people with heart failure, cardiomyopathies, gingivitis (inflammation of the gums), morbid obesity, hypertension, muscular dystrophy, AIDS, and in some people on kidney dialysis. Coenzyme Q_{10} levels are also generally lower in older individuals. The test used to assess coenzyme Q_{10} status is not routinely available from medical laboratories.

How Much Is Usually Taken?

Adult levels of supplementation are usually 30–90 mg per day, although individuals with specific health conditions may supplement with higher levels (with the involvement of a nutritionally oriented physician). Most of the research on heart conditions has used 90–150 mg of coenzyme Q_{10} per day. People with cancer who consider taking much higher amounts should discuss this issue with a nutritionally oriented doctor before supplementing. Most nutritionally oriented doctors recommend that coenzyme Q_{10} be taken with meals to improve absorption.

Which Form of Coenzyme Q_{10} Is Best?

Some,[20] but not all,[21] research supports the idea that oil-based suspension of coenzyme Q_{10} absorbs better than forms that lack oil. Of the oil-based products, solubilized coenzyme Q_{10} absorbed the best, according to one group of researchers.[22]

Are There Any Side Effects or Interactions?

Congestive heart failure patients who are taking coenzyme Q_{10} should not discontinue taking coenzyme Q_{10} supplements without first consulting a doctor.

An isolated test tube study reported that the anticancer effect of a certain cholesterol-lowering drug was blocked by addition of coenzyme Q_{10}.[23] So far, experts in the field have put little stock in this report because its results have not yet been confirmed in animal, human, or even other test tube studies; the drug used in the test tube is not used to treat cancer; and preliminary information regarding the use of high amounts of coenzyme Q_{10} in humans suggests the possibility of *anti*cancer activity.[24,25,26]

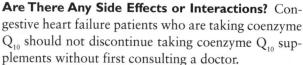

Conjugated Linoleic Acid (CLA)

Conjugated linoleic acid (CLA) is a slightly altered form of the essential fatty acid linoleic acid. Preliminary animal and test tube research suggests that CLA might reduce the risk of cancers at several sites, including breast, prostate, colorectal, lung, skin, and stomach.[1,2,3,4] Whether CLA will have a similar protective effect for people has yet to be demonstrated in human research.

Animal research also suggests an effect of CLA supplementation on reducing **body fat** (p. 165),[5,6] limiting food allergy reactions,[7] preventing **atherosclerosis** (p. 17),[8,9] and improving **glucose tolerance** (p. 53).[10] As with the cancer research, the effects of CLA on these conditions in humans remain unclear.

Where Is It Found?

CLA is found mainly in dairy products and also in beef, poultry, eggs, and corn oil. Bacteria that live in the intestine of humans can produce CLA from linoleic acid, but supplementation of a rich source of linoleic acid did not produce increases in blood levels of CLA in one human study.[11] CLA is available as a supplement.

Who Is Likely to Be Deficient?

No deficiencies of CLA are reported or believed to occur, since it is not an essential nutrient.

How Much Is Usually Taken?

Animal research uses very large amounts, equivalent to several grams per day for humans. Until human research is conducted with CLA, the appropriate amount to take of this nutrient remains unclear.

Are There Any Side Effects or Interactions? The side effects of CLA are unknown, due to the limited research in humans. However, one unpublished human trial reported isolated cases of gastrointestinal upset.[12]

Copper

Copper is needed to absorb and utilize **iron** (p. 304). It is also part of the antioxidant enzyme superoxide dismutase (SOD). Copper is needed to make adenosine triphosphate (ATP), the energy the body runs on. Synthesis of some hormones requires copper, as does collagen (the "glue" that holds muscle tissue together) and tyrosinase (the enzyme that puts pigment into the skin).

Where Is It Found?

The best source of copper is oysters. Nuts, dried legumes, cereals, potatoes, vegetables, and meat also contain copper.

Who Is Likely to Be Deficient?

Copper deficiency is uncommon. Children with Menke's syndrome are unable to absorb copper normally and become severely deficient unless medically treated early in life. Deficiency can also occur in people who supplement with zinc without also increasing copper intake. **Zinc** (p. 346) interferes with copper absorption.[1] Health consequences of zinc-induced copper deficiency can be quite serious.[2] In the absence of copper supplementation, **vitamin C** (p. 341) supplementation has also been reported to mildly impair copper metabolism.[3] Copper deficiency can cause anemia, a drop in HDL cholesterol (the "good" cholesterol), and several other health problems.

How Much Is Usually Taken?

Most people consume less than the recommended amount of this mineral. Nonetheless, supplementing with 1–3 mg per day is important only for people who take zinc supplements, including the zinc found in **multiple-vitamin/mineral supplements** (p. 314).

Are There Any Side Effects or Interactions? The

level at which copper causes problems is unclear. But in combination with zinc, up to 3 mg per day is considered safe. People drinking tap water from new copper pipes should consult their nutritionally oriented doctor before supplementing, since they might be getting enough (or even too much) copper from their water. People with **Wilson's disease** (p. 166) should never take copper.

Copper Has Been Used in Connection with the Following Conditions*

Ranking	Health Concerns
Secondary	Wound healing (p. 167)
Other	Benign prostatic hyperplasia (p. 145) Hypoglycemia (p. 92) Minor injuries (p. 122) Rheumatoid arthritis (p. 151)
*Refer to the Individual Health Concern for Complete Information	

Zinc interferes with copper absorption. People taking zinc supplements for more than a few weeks should also take copper (unless they have Wilson's disease). In the absence of copper supplementation, vitamin C may interfere with copper metabolism. Copper improves absorption and utilization of iron.

Creatine Monohydrate

Creatine (creatine monohydrate) is used in muscle tissue for the production of phosphocreatine, an important factor in the formation of ATP, the source of energy for muscle contraction and many other functions in the body.[1,2] Creatine monohydrate supplementation increases phosphocreatine levels in muscle, especially when accompanied by exercise or carbohydrate intake.[3,4] It may also increase **exercise** (p. 20) -related gains in lean body mass, though whether this represents more muscle or simply water retention is unclear.[5]

Most, though not all, controlled studies have shown that 20 grams per day of creatine monohydrate for 5 to 6 days in sedentary or moderately active people improves performance and delays muscle fatigue during short-duration, high-intensity exercise such as sprinting and weight lifting.[6,7] However, outcomes for trained athletes in competitive situations have not been consistent.[8,9,10] Creatine supplementation does not appear to increase endurance performance and may impair it by contributing to weight gain.[11] Only one controlled study has been done to evaluate the long-term (over 1 month) effects of creatine monohydrate supplementation;[12] more research is needed.

Creatine supplementation has been reported to improve strength in rare diseases of muscle and energy metabolism.[13,14,15] For people with **congestive heart failure** (p. 43), intravenous creatine has been found to improve heart function, but oral supplementation has not been effective, though skeletal muscle function does improve.[16,17]

A recent double-blind placebo-controlled study found that a supplement of 5 grams of creatine plus 1 gram of glucose taken 4 times per day for 5 days followed by twice a day for 51 days significantly lowered serum total **cholesterol** (p. 79) and **triglycerides** (p. 85), but did not change either LDL or HDL cholesterol, in both men and women.[18]

Where Is It Found?

Creatine is produced naturally in the human liver, pancreas, and kidneys. It is concentrated primarily in muscle tissues, including the heart. Animal proteins, including fish, are the main source of the 1–2 grams per day of dietary creatine most people consume. Supplements in the form of creatine monohydrate are well absorbed and tolerated by the stomach.

Who Is Likely to Be Deficient?

Individuals involved in intense physical activity, especially those limiting their intake of red meat, may have low muscle stores of creatine.

How Much Is Usually Taken?

Two methods are used for supplementing with creatine. In the loading method, 20 grams of creatine per day (in 4 divided doses mixed well in warm liquid) are taken for 5 to 6 days.[19] Muscle creatine levels increase rapidly, which is beneficial if a short-term rise in force is needed, such as during a weight-lifting competition, football game, or sprinting.

In the other method, 3 grams of creatine monohydrate per day can be taken over an extended training period of at least 4 weeks, during which muscle creatine rises more slowly, yet eventually reaches levels similar to those achieved with the loading method.[20] Smaller daily doses of 2–5 grams may be adequate for maintaining elevated muscle creatine concentrations. Taking creatine with sugar appears to maximize muscle uptake.[21,22]

Caffeine intake should not be excessive, as large amounts may counteract the benefits of creatine supplementation.[23]

Are There Any Side Effects or Interactions? Little

is known about long-term side effects of creatine, but no consistent toxicity appears in most reports of creatine supplementation. Kidney, liver, and blood functions have been reported by some to not be affected by short-term higher dose[24,25] or long-term lower dose (10 grams/day for up to 51 days)[26,27] creatine supplementation in healthy young adults. However, interstitial nephritis, a serious kidney condition, developed in an otherwise healthy young man supplementing with 20 grams of creatine per day.[28] Improvement in kidney function followed avoidance of creatine. Details of this case strongly suggest that creatine supplementa-

tion triggered this case of kidney disease. Creatine supplementation may also be dangerous for people with existing kidney disease; a patient with nephrotic syndrome developed glomerulosclerosis, another serious kidney condition, while taking creatine, which reversed when the supplement was discontinued.[29]

Creatine Monohydrate Has Been Used in Connection with the Following Conditions*

Ranking	Health Concerns
Secondary	Athletic performance (p. 20)
Other	Congestive heart failure (p. 43) High cholesterol (p. 79) High triglycerides (p. 85)
*Refer to the Individual Health Concern for Complete Information	

Cysteine

Cysteine is a nonessential **amino acid** (p. 265) (protein building block) and is one of the few that contains **sulfur** (p. 334). This allows cysteine to bond in a special way and maintain the structure of proteins in the body. Cysteine is a component of the **antioxidant** (p. 267) glutathione. The body also uses cysteine to produce **taurine** (p. 334), another amino acid.

Cysteine is occasionally converted into glucose and used as a source of energy. Cysteine strengthens the protective lining of the stomach and intestines, which may help prevent damage caused by aspirin and similar drugs.[1] In addition, cysteine may play an important role in the communication between **immune system** (p. 94) cells.[2] Cysteine is rarely used as a dietary supplement. **N-acetyl cysteine (NAC)** (p. 317), which contains cysteine, is more commonly used as a supplement.

Where Is It Found?

The body can synthesize cysteine from **methionine** (p. 313) and other building blocks. Cysteine, the amino acid from which NAC is derived, is found in most high-protein foods.

Refer to N-acetyl cysteine (p. 317) **for corresponding health concerns.**

Who Is Likely to Be Deficient?

According to several studies, blood levels of cysteine and glutathione are low in individuals infected with **HIV** (p. 87).[3,4,5] Cysteine has a role in the proper function of the immune system, so a deficiency of this amino acid may either contribute to or result from immune suppression associated with HIV.

How Much Is Usually Taken?

Most people do not need to supplement cysteine. Almost nothing is known about appropriate supplemental levels, in part because almost all clinical research has been done with N-acetyl cysteine and not cysteine itself. Refer to the section on **N-acetyl cysteine (NAC)** (p. 317) for information about that variation of the cysteine molecule.

Are There Any Side Effects or Interactions? No consistent adverse effects of NAC have been reported in humans. One small study found that daily amounts of 1.2 grams or more could lead to oxidative damage.[6] Extremely large amounts of cysteine, the amino acid NAC is derived from, may be toxic to nerve cells in rats.[7]

Adequate amounts of **methionine** (p. 313) are needed in the diet, as the precursor to cysteine, to prevent cysteine deficiency.

DHA (Docosahexaenoic Acid)

Omega-3 oil, such as docosahexaenoic acid (DHA), belongs to the class of nutrients called essential fatty acids. DHA has been shown to reduce levels of blood triglycerides. **High triglycerides** (p. 85) are linked with **heart disease** (p. 32) in most, but not all, research. DHA alone appears to be just as effective as **fish oils** (p. 294) (which contain both DHA and EPA) in beneficially lowering triglyceride levels in individuals at risk for heart disease.[1] In part, this may be because some DHA converts to EPA in the body.[2] Unlike EPA, however, DHA may not reduce excessive blood clotting. [3]

DHA is essential for normal visual and neurological (nervous system) development in infants.[4,5] Double-blind evidence links DHA supplementation in premature infants to better brain functioning.[6] The effects of DHA on the nervous system may well extend beyond infancy. Young adults given 1.5–1.8 grams DHA per day showed less evidence of aggression in response to mental stress compared with people in the control group in a double-blind trial. [7]

Where Is It Found?

Cold-water fish, such as mackerel, salmon, herring, sardines, black cod, anchovies, and albacore tuna, are rich sources of DHA and EPA. Similarly, cod liver oil contains large amounts of DHA and EPA. However, due to its very high levels of **vitamin A** (p. 336) and

vitamin D (p. 343), cod liver oil should not be taken by women who are or who could become pregnant before consulting a nutritionally oriented doctor. Other adults should make sure the cod liver oil taken (plus other supplements) does not contain more than 25,000 IU (7,500 mcg) per day of vitamin A or 800 IU of vitamin D per day without consulting a nutritionally oriented doctor. Certain microalgae contain DHA and are used as a vegetarian source of this nutrient in some supplements. Most fish oil supplements contain 12% DHA.

Since DHA is a component of fish oil, see the fish oil (p. 294) entry for corresponding health concerns.

Who Is Likely to Be Deficient?

Premature infants who are not breast-fed are often DHA deficient.[8] A link has appeared between DHA deficiency and **Alzheimer's disease** (p. 11); however, no evidence at this time indicates that supplementation with DHA will help Alzheimer's patients.[9] Similarly, preliminary evidence shows that children with **attention deficit disorder** (ADD) (p. 26) have low DHA levels; however, no evidence demonstrates that DHA supplementation improves ADD.[10] Many nutritionally oriented doctors believe that the diets of most people eating a Western diet do not provide optimal amounts of omega-3 oil.

How Much Is Usually Taken?

Most healthy people do not supplement fish oil containing DHA or vegetarian sources of DHA. The level of DHA given premature infants who are not breast-fed should be determined by a pediatrician. Much of the research in adults has been based on 1–3 grams per day of DHA from fish oil, although higher levels have been taken when isolated DHA from microalgae sources is used.

Are There Any Side Effects or Interactions? While those with **heart disease** (p. 32) and **diabetes** (p. 53) often benefit from fish oil (the primary source of DHA in the diet),[11,12] such individuals should check with their nutritionally oriented doctor before taking more than 3 or 4 grams of fish oil for several months. Elevations in blood sugar have sometimes been reported,[13] though this may simply be due to small increases in weight resulting from high dietary fish oil.[14] While DHA combined with EPA from fish oil consistently lowers triglycerides, it occasionally increases LDL cholesterol.[15]

Fish oil is easily damaged by oxygen, so small amounts of **vitamin E** (p. 344) are often included in fish oil supplements.[16] Nutritionally oriented doctors often recommend that people who supplement with fish oil or DHA take vitamin E supplements to protect

DHA (Docosahexaenoic Acid)

EPA and DHA within the body from oxidative damage. Some evidence indicates that vitamin E may be protective against oxidative damage caused by fish oil.[17] However, animal researchers have reported that the oxidative damage caused by DHA alone was not prevented with vitamin E supplementation.[18] The level of oxidative damage caused by DHA has not been shown to result in significant health problems.

Some evidence suggests that adding vitamin E to EPA/DHA may prevent this fish oil–induced increase in serum glucose.[19] Similarly, the impairment of glucose tolerance sometimes caused by the omega-3 oil has been prevented by the addition of half an hour of moderate exercise 3 times a week.[20] The effect of DHA by itself on glucose levels has not been adequately studied.

People who take fish oil containing EPA and DHA and who also take 15 grams of pectin per day have been reported to have reductions in LDL cholesterol.[21] This suggests that pectin may overcome the occasional problem of increased LDL cholesterol from fish oil supplementation. The LDL cholesterol-raising effect of EPA and DHA may also be successfully prevented by taking **garlic** (p. 425) supplements (or presumably adding garlic to the diet) along with EPA and DHA.[22] Adding pectin or garlic when people supplement DHA by itself has yet to be studied.

DHEA (Dehydroepiandrosterone)

Little is known about how dehydroepiandrosterone (DHEA) works in the body.[1] Confusing the picture is the fact that DHEA has very different effects in men, premenopausal women, and postmenopausal women.[2]

DHEA is the most prevalent of the hormones produced by the adrenal glands. After being secreted by the adrenals, it circulates in the bloodstream as DHEA-sulfate (DHEAS) and is converted as needed into other hormones.

DHEA converts, in part, to testosterone,[3] which may account for the fact that low blood levels of DHEA have been reported in some men with erectile dysfunction. Double-blind research reported that 50 mg supplements of DHEA taken daily for 6 months significantly improved erectile function. [4]

Some,[5,6] but not all[7,8] studies find that DHEA supplementation lowers fat mass without reducing total **body weight** (p. 165).[9] In one trial, the reduction in fat mass occurred in men, but not in women.[10]

DHEA is believed to indirectly affect blood sugar levels, but information remains incomplete and contradictory. Attempts to affect blood sugar levels in humans have led to improvements,[11] no effect,[12] and, at very high amounts (1,600 mg DHEA per day), a worsening of tolerance to sugar.[13]

DHEA modulates **immunity** (p. 94). A group of elderly men with low DHEA levels who were given a high level of DHEA (50 mg per day) for 20 weeks, experienced a significant activation of immune function.[14] Postmenopausal women have also shown increased immune functioning in just 3 weeks when given DHEA in double-blind research.[15]

Reports have suggested that DHEA might reduce the risk of **heart disease** (p. 32), perhaps by lowering **cholesterol levels** (p. 79). Most research supports this idea weakly for men, but not at all for women.[16,17] DHEA has also been reported to act as a blood thinner.[18] Unfortunately, DHEA has also been reported to lower HDL (the "good" cholesterol).[19]

Claims have appeared that DHEA is an anti-aging hormone; but to date, no human research supports this claim. The fact that young people have higher levels of DHEA than older people does not necessarily mean that supplementing DHEA will make people younger. In double-blind research, DHEA has improved a sense of well-being in some,[20] but not all,[21] studies.

Systemic lupus erythematosus (SLE) (p. 115), an autoimmune disease, has been linked to abnormalities in sex hormone metabolism.[22] Using very high levels of DHEA (200 mg per day) in a double-blind study, researchers have shown that people with SLE are less likely to suffer exacerbations of their disease than people given placebo.[23] An uncontrolled study confirmed the benefit of 50–200 mg per day of DHEA for people with SLE.[24]

Where Is It Found?

DHEA is produced by the adrenal glands. A synthetic form of this hormone is also available as a supplement in tablet, capsule, liquid, and sublingual form. Some products claim to contain "natural" DHEA precursors from **wild yam** (p. 469); however, the body cannot convert any compounds in the yam into DHEA[25] (although a series of reactions in a laboratory can make the conversion).

Who Is Likely to Be Deficient?

Meaningful levels of DHEA do not appear in food, and therefore "dietary deficiency" does not exist. Some people, however, may not synthesize enough DHEA. DHEA levels peak in early adulthood and then start a lifelong descent. By the time people reach the age of 60, DHEA levels are only about 5–15% of what they were at their peak at younger ages.[26]

Dehydroepiandrosterone (DHEA) Has Been Used in Connection with the Following Conditions*

Ranking	Health Concerns
Secondary	Impotence (p. 98) Lupus (SLE) (p. 115)

*Refer to the Individual Health Concern for Complete Information

Whether the lower level associated with age represents a deficiency remains unclear. Women with **asthma** (p. 15) have been reported to have depressed levels of DHEA.[27]

Researchers from the University of California, San Francisco, report that DHEA and DHEAS levels may be lower in **depressed** (p. 50) patients, and DHEA supplements of 30–90 mg per day for 4 weeks significantly improved depression in six depressed patients.[28] However, experts maintain that DHEA may only be effective for a minority of people with depression.[29]

People with **diabetes** (p. 53) who use insulin have been reported to have low levels of DHEA.[30] People infected with **HIV** (p. 87) (AIDS virus) and those with asthma, **osteoporosis** (p. 133), and a host of other conditions have been reported to have low levels of DHEA.[31] In most cases, the meaning of this apparent deficiency is not well understood.

How Much Is Usually Taken?

Most people do not need to supplement DHEA. The question of who should take this hormone remains controversial. Some experts believe that 5–15 mg of DHEA for women and 10–30 mg for men are appropriate amounts, depending in part on blood levels of DHEA or DHEAS.[32] Due to problems with absorption, a few experts have suggested levels as high as 50 mg per day in postmenopausal women.[33] People should consult a nutritionally oriented doctor to have DHEA levels monitored before and during supplementation. Only people with low blood levels of DHEA or DHEAS should take this hormone until more is known about its effects.

People with SLE appear to require high levels (100–200 mg per day) of DHEA. Such levels should never be taken without medical supervision.

Are There Any Side Effects or Interactions?

Experts have concerns about the use of DHEA, particularly because long-term safety data do not exist.

Side effects at high intakes (50–200 mg per day) appear to be acne (in over 50% of people), increased facial hair (18%), and increased perspiration (8%). Less common problems reportedly caused by DHEA include breast tenderness, weight gain, mood alter-ation, headache, oily skin, and menstrual irregularity.[34] Because this trial was not controlled, some of the less common "side effects" were possibly unrelated to DHEA and might have occurred even with placebo.

High amounts of DHEA have caused cancer in animals.[35,36] Although *anti*cancer effects of DHEA have also been reported,[37] they involve trials using animals that do not process DHEA the way humans do; therefore, these positive effects may have no relevance for people.

Links have begun to appear between higher DHEA levels and risks of prostate cancer in humans.[38] At least one person with prostate cancer has been reported to have had a worsening of his cancer, despite feeling better, while taking very high amounts (up to 700 mg per day) of DHEA.[39] While younger women with breast cancer may have low levels of DHEA, postmenopausal women with breast cancer appear to have high levels of DHEA, which has researchers concerned.[40] These cancer concerns make sense because DHEA is a precursor to testosterone (linked to prostate cancer) and estrogen (linked to breast cancer). Until more is known, individuals with breast or prostate cancer or a family history of these conditions should avoid supplementing with DHEA. Preliminary evidence has also linked higher DHEA levels to ovarian cancer in women.[41]

Some doctors recommend that people taking DHEA have liver enzymes measured routinely. Anecdotes of DHEA supplementation (of at least 25 mg per day) leading to heart arrhythmias have appeared.[42]

At only 25 mg per day, DHEA has lowered HDL cholesterol while increasing insulin-like growth factor (IGF).[43] Decreasing HDL could increase the risk of heart disease. Increasing IGF might increase the risk of breast cancer.

Digestive Enzymes
(see also **Bromelain**, p. 276)

Digestive enzymes—also called pancreatic enzymes—include three classes: proteolytic enzymes needed to digest protein, **lipases** (p. 307) needed to digest fat, and amylases needed to digest carbohydrates. In several conditions that cause malabsorption, such as pancreatic insufficiency and cystic fibrosis, doctors sometimes prescribe digestive enzymes to improve absorption of food.

Nutritionally oriented doctors often tell people to try using pancreatic enzymes with meals when they

Digestive Enzymes

have symptoms of **indigestion** (p. 99) that cannot be attributed to a specific cause. Research has not explored whether this use of enzymes is helpful.

According to one theory, **allergies** (p. 8) are triggered by partially undigested protein, while proteolytic enzymes reduce allergy symptoms.[1] Limited scientific evidence supports this theory.[2] Proteolytic enzymes such as trypsin, chymotrypsin, and **bromelain** (p. 276) are partially absorbed by the body.[3,4,5] Once absorbed, they have anti-inflammatory activity and may even demonstrate anti-tumor effects.[6,7,8,9] Proteolytic enzymes may also improve immune system function, for example, in people with **shingles** (herpes zoster) (p. 155), though this area of research has been poorly explored.[10]

Where Are They Found?

Only small amounts of the animal-based proteolytic enzymes trypsin and chymotrypsin are found in the diet; however, the pancreas can synthesize these enzymes. The plant-based proteolytic enzyme **bromelain** (p. 276) comes from pineapples and is useful in many conditions; papain comes from unripe papayas. All of these enzymes are available as supplements.

Digestive Enzymes Have Been Used in Connection with the Following Conditions*

Ranking	Health Concerns
Primary	Pancreatic insufficiency (including pancreatitis)
Secondary	Cystic fibrosis
Other	Indigestion and heartburn (p. 99)
*Refer to the Individual Health Concern for Complete Information	

Who Is Likely to Be Deficient?

People with pancreatic insufficiency and cystic fibrosis frequently require supplemental pancreatic enzymes, which include proteolytic enzymes, **lipases** (p. 307), and amylases. In addition, those with celiac disease, **Crohn's disease** (p. 48), and perhaps **indigestion** (p. 99) may be deficient in pancreatic enzymes.[11] As bromelain and papain are not essential, deficiencies do not exist.

How Much Is Usually Taken?

The digestive enzymes—proteolytic enzymes, lipases, and amylases—are generally taken together. Pancreatin, which contains all three digestive enzymes, is rated against a standard established by the United States Pharmacopeia (USP). For example, "4X pancreatin" is four times stronger than the USP stan-

dard. Each "X" contains 25 USP units of amylase, 2 USP units of lipase, and 25 USP units of protease (or proteolytic enzymes). A dose of 3–4 grams of 4X pancreatin (or a lower amount at higher potency) with each meal is likely to help digest food in some people with pancreatic insufficiency.

Those with chronic pancreatitis need to discuss enzyme intakes with their physician. Under medical supervision, seriously ill people with pancreatic insufficiency caused by pancreatitis are given very high levels of enzymes to improve fat digestion. In one successful trial, enough pancreatin was used with each meal to supply slightly over 1,000,000 USP units of lipase.[12]

Supplemental enzymes that state only product weight but not activity units may lack potency.

Are There Any Side Effects or Interactions? The most important digestive enzymes in malabsorption diseases are usually fat-digesting enzymes called lipases. Proteolytic enzymes can digest lipases; therefore, people with enzyme deficiencies may want to avoid proteolytic enzymes in order to spare lipases.[13] If this is not possible (as most enzyme products contain both), people with malabsorption syndromes should talk with their doctor to see if their condition warrants finding products that contain the most lipase and the least protease.

In theory, too much enzyme activity could be irritating because it could start to "digest" parts of the body as the enzymes traveled through the digestive system. Fortunately, that does not happen with supplemental amounts. Research has not determined the level at which such problems might arise.

Digestive enzymes should not be taken with **betaine HCl** (p. 269), or hydrochloric acid, which breaks down enzymes, reducing their activity.

DMAE (2-Dimethylaminoethanol)

DMAE (2-dimethylaminoethanol), like **choline** (p. 290), may increase levels of the brain neurotransmitter acetylcholine; however, not all studies confirm that DMAE serves as a precursor to acetylcholine.[1] Early research with DMAE focused on the possible benefits of this substance for relieving **tardive dyskinesia** (p. 157), a trembling disorder caused by long-term antipsychotic medication);[2] but several controlled studies did not find the effects of DMAE better than placebo.[3]

One uncontrolled 4-week trial of fourteen senile patients given DMAE supplements of 600 mg 3 times per day failed to show any changes in memory but did produce positive behavior changes in some of the patients.[4] However, subsequent double-blind research did not find a significant benefit from the use of DMAE in people with **Alzheimer's disease** (p. 71).[5]

Where Is It Found?

DMAE is found as a supplement, although it is not widely available.

Who Is Likely to Be Deficient?

No deficiencies of DMAE are reported or believed to occur.

How Much Is Usually Taken?

DMAE supplementation is not recommended at this time.

Are There Any Side Effects or Interactions?

Clinical studies of DMAE have used up to 1,600 mg per day with no reports of side effects,[6] and for this reason DMAE is believed to be relatively nontoxic. However, one study using higher intakes for Alzheimer's disease patients did report symptoms of drowsiness and confusion with the use of DMAE.[7] A possible side effect of lucid dreaming (in which the dreamer is conscious and in control of a dream) is suggested with DMAE use.[8]

DMAE Has Been Used in Connection with the Following Condition*

Ranking	Health Concern
Other	Alzheimer's disease (p. 11)
*Refer to the Individual Health Concern for Complete Information	

DMSO
(Dimethyl Sulfoxide)

DMSO (dimethyl sulfoxide) is a colorless, slightly oily liquid that is primarily used as an industrial solvent. The use of DMSO for therapeutic applications is controversial, but some evidence indicates that DMSO has anti-inflammatory properties and alleviates pain when applied to the skin. These effects have been reported particularly with connective tissue diseases, such as scleroderma, **osteoarthritis** (p. 130), and **rheumatoid arthritis** (p. 151), and with **muscle injuries** (p. 122).[1,2,3] DMSO appears to reduce pain by

inhibiting transmission of pain messages by nerves and may also soften the abnormal connective tissue associated with disorders such as **Dupuytren's contracture** (p. 61), keloids, Peyronie's disease, and scleroderma. [4]

Double-blind and other placebo-controlled studies have found a 25% DMSO gel effective for pain relief in osteoarthritis of the knee[5] and a 50% DMSO cream helpful for symptoms of acute reflex sympathetic dystrophy.[6] A similarly controlled study successfully used a 10% DMSO gel to reduce pain and improve movement in people with acute tendinitis of the shoulder or elbow,[7] confirming the findings of an older study.[8]

Uncontrolled research has suggested that DMSO may help relieve symptoms of amyloidosis of the skin.[9]

Some medical doctors have instilled DMSO into the bladder to treat interstitial cystitis.[10] A study from Malaysia reports that oral DMSO reduced relapse rates for **peptic ulcer** (p. 138) significantly better than placebo or the ulcer drug cimetidine.[11] DMSO is sometimes used by physicians as a vehicle to help absorb other therapeutic agents through the skin.

Where Is It Found?

DMSO is derived from trees as a manufacturing byproduct from the processing of paper. Metabolites of DMSO, such as the sulfide and sulfone form, are naturally present in the human body; however, the role of these in the body is not clear.

DMSO Has Been Used in Connection with the Following Conditions*

Ranking	Health Concerns
Primary	Minor injuries (p. 122) (topical) Tendinitis
Secondary	Osteoarthritis (p. 130) Rheumatoid arthritis (p. 151)
Other	Amyloidosis Dupuytren's contracture (p. 61) Keloid scars Peptic ulcer (p. 138) Peyronie's disease Reflex sympathetic dystrophy Scleroderma
*Refer to the Individual Health Concern for Complete Information	

Who Is Likely to Be Deficient?

DMSO is not an essential nutrient and is not needed in the functions of a healthy body; therefore, deficiencies do not exist.

How Much Is Usually Taken?

DMSO is not indicated for healthy people; those who do use this substance should consult a doctor familiar with its use. Some physicians do not recommend the use of DMSO, due to concerns about safety and questions about efficacy. The potential for contamination exists in some DMSO products designed for industrial uses. DMSO used topically is rapidly absorbed through intact skin; therefore, the area of skin (and the hands applying DMSO) must be clean, because anything on the skin will also be absorbed along with the DMSO.

Are There Any Side Effects or Interactions?

DMSO frequently causes a garlic-like body odor and taste in the mouth. Other reported side effects include stomach upset, sensitivity to light, visual disturbances, and headache. Skin irritation can develop at the site where DMSO is applied. Only highly purified DMSO should be used and the skin site and applying hand should be thoroughly cleaned before application because the solvent properties of DMSO allow any contaminants to be absorbed through the skin and transported into the bloodstream.

Evening Primrose Oil

Evening primrose oil (EPO), black currant seed oil, and borage oil contain gamma linolenic acid (GLA), a fatty acid that the body converts to a hormone-like substance called prostaglandin E1 (PGE1). PGE1 has anti-inflammatory properties and may also act as a blood thinner and blood vessel dilator.

The anti-inflammatory properties of EPO have been studied in double-blind research with people suffering from **rheumatoid arthritis** (p. 151). Some, but not all, studies have reported that EPO supplementation provides significant benefit to these people.[1]

GLA, the primary active ingredient in EPO, has anti-cancer activity in test tube studies[2] and in some,[3] but not all,[4] animal studies. Injecting GLA into tumors has caused regression of cancer in people in preliminary research.[5] Very preliminary evidence in people with cancer suggested "marked subjective improvement,"[6] though not all studies find GLA helpful.[7]

EPO has been reported to lower **cholesterol levels** (p. 79) in people in some,[8] but not all,[9] research.

Linoleic acid, a common fatty acid found in nuts, seeds, and most vegetable oils (including EPO), should theoretically convert to PGE1. But many things can interfere with this conversion, including disease, the aging process, saturated fat, hydrogenated

oils, blood sugar problems, and inadequate **vitamin C** (p. 341), **magnesium** (p. 310), **zinc** (p. 346), and **B vitamins** (p. 341). Supplements that provide GLA circumvent these conversion problems, leading to more predictable formation of PGE1.[10]

Where Is It Found?

EPO is found primarily in supplements. The active ingredient, GLA, can also be found in black currant seed oil and borage oil supplements.

Who Is Likely to Be Deficient?

Those with **premenstrual syndrome** (p. 141),[11] **diabetes** (p. 53),[12] scleroderma,[13] Sjogren's syndrome,[14] **tardive dyskinesia** (p. 157),[15] and **eczema** (p. 64),[16] and other skin conditions[17] can have a metabolic block that interferes with the body's ability to make GLA. In preliminary research, supplementation with EPO has helped people with these conditions.[18,19,20,21,22]

Evening Primrose Oil Has Been Used in Connection with the Following Conditions*

Ranking	Health Concerns
Primary	Diabetes (p. 53) Eczema (p. 64) Rheumatoid arthritis (p. 151)
Secondary	Alcohol withdrawal (p. 6) Fibrocystic breast disease (p. 66) Premenstrual syndrome (PMS) (p. 141)
Other	Atherosclerosis (p. 17) Attention deficit disorder (p. 26) Intermittent claudication (p. 106) Irritable bowel syndrome (IBS) (p. 109) Multiple sclerosis (p. 127) Raynaud's disease (p. 148) Scleroderma Sjögren's syndrome Tardive dyskinesia (p. 157)
*Refer to the Individual Health Concern for Complete Information

Though preliminary, double-blind evidence suggests that alcoholics may be deficient in GLA and that **alcohol withdrawal** (p. 6) may be facilitated with EPO supplementation,[23] many people in Western societies may be at least partially GLA deficient as a result of aging, glucose intolerance, dietary fat intake, and other problems. Individuals with deficiencies benefit from supplemental GLA intake from EPO, black currant seed oil, or **borage** (p. 402) oil.

How Much Is Usually Taken?

Although many people may have inadequate levels of GLA, the optimal intake for this nutrient remains unknown. Researchers often use 3,000–6,000 mg of

EPO per day, which provides approximately 270–540 mg of GLA.

Are There Any Side Effects or Interactions? Consistent, reproducible problems from taking EPO have not been reported.

Other nutrients are needed by the body, along with EPO, to make PGE1. Consequently, some experts suggest that **magnesium** (p. 310), **zinc** (p. 346), **vitamin C** (p. 341), **niacin** (p. 339), and **vitamin B$_6$** (p. 340) should be taken along with EPO.

Fiber

Fiber is divided into two general categories—water soluble and water insoluble. Soluble fiber **lowers cholesterol** (p. 79).[1] For unknown reasons, however, diets higher in insoluble fiber appear to correlate better with protection against **heart disease** (p. 37).[2]

Soluble fibers can also lower blood sugar levels in people with **diabetes** (p. 53), and some researchers find that increasing fiber decreases the body's need for insulin—a good sign for diabetics.[3] However, a research review reveals that just how much moderate amounts of soluble fiber really help people with diabetes remains unclear.[4] As with heart disease, a clear mechanism to explain how insoluble fiber helps diabetics has not been identified. Nonetheless, diets high in insoluble fiber (from whole grains) associate with protection from adult-onset diabetes.[5]

Insoluble fiber softens stool, which helps move it through the body in less time. For this reason, insoluble fiber is partially effective as a treatment for **constipation** (p. 44).[6] The reduction in "transit time" is thought to also explain why fiber is associated with protection from colon and other gastrointestinal (GI) cancers. However, the true relationship between fiber and colon cancer risk appears more complicated than first believed. For example, wheat bran has been reported in animal research to be significantly more protective than diets not containing wheat bran, but equally high in insoluble fibers.[7] Fiber may have other anticancer effects unrelated to "transit time" or even to the GI tract.[8] Some researchers believe that changes in bile acid metabolism in the GI tract may partially explain the special link between wheat bran and prevention of colon cancer,[9] a protective link sometimes not found when scientists study total fiber or even total grain fiber intake and colon cancer incidence.[10]

Fiber also fills the stomach, reducing appetite. In theory, fiber should therefore reduce eating, leading to **weight loss** (p. 165). However, at least some research has found increased fiber to have no effect on body weight despite decreasing appetite.[11]

Lignan, a fiber-like substance, has mild antiestrogenic activity. Probably for this reason, high lignan levels in urine (and therefore dietary intake) have been linked to protection from breast cancer in humans.[12]

Where Is It Found?

Whole grains are particularly high in insoluble fiber. **Oats** (p. 448), barley, beans, fruit (but not fruit juice), **psyllium** (p. 452), and some vegetables contain significant amounts of both soluble and insoluble fiber. The best source of lignan, by far, is flaxseed (not flaxseed oil, regardless of packaging claims to the contrary).

Fiber Has Been Used in Connection with the Following Conditions*

Ranking	Health Concerns
Primary	Constipation (p. 44) Diabetes (p. 53) High cholesterol (p. 79) Weight loss and obesity (p. 165)
Secondary	Diarrhea (p. 58) Hemorrhoids (p. 77) High blood pressure (p. 89)
Other	High triglycerides (p. 85) Irritable bowel syndrome (p. 109) (fiber other than wheat) Kidney stones (p. 111) Peptic ulcer (p. 138) Premenstrual syndrome (p. 141)
*Refer to the Individual Health Concern for Complete Information	

Who Is Likely to Be Deficient?

Most people are fiber deficient. Eating white flour, white rice, and fruit juice (as opposed to whole fruit) all contribute to this problem. Many so-called whole wheat products contain mostly white flour. Read labels and avoid "flour" and "unbleached flour," both of which are simply white flour. Junk food is also fiber depleted. The diseases listed above (plus colon and breast cancers) are much more likely to occur with low-fiber diets.

How Much Is Usually Taken?

Western diets generally provide approximately 10 grams of fiber per day. So-called primitive societies consume 40–60 grams per day. Increasing fiber intake similar to the "primitive" diets is desirable.

Are There Any Side Effects or Interactions? While individuals can be allergic to certain high-fiber foods (most commonly wheat), high-fiber diets are more

Fiber

likely to improve health than cause any health problems. Beans, a good source of soluble fiber, also contain special sugars that are often poorly digested, leading to gas. Special enzyme products are now available in supermarkets to reduce this problem by improving digestion of these sugars.

Fiber reduces the absorption of most minerals. To minimize this effect, **multimineral supplements** (p. 314) should not be taken at the same time as a high-fiber meal.

Bran, an insoluble fiber, reduces the absorption of **calcium** (p. 277) enough to cause urinary calcium to fall.[13] As a result of this interaction, **kidney stones** (p. 111) can sometimes be prevented simply by incorporating ½ ounce of bran per day into the diet.[14] Before supplementing with bran, people should check with a nutritionally oriented doctor, because some people—even a few with kidney stones—don't absorb enough calcium. For those people, supplementing with bran might deprive them of much-needed calcium.

Fish Oil (EPA and DHA) and Cod Liver Oil

Fish oil contains EPA (eicosapentaenoic acid) and **DHA** (p. 287) (docosahexaenoic acid); both are omega-3 oils. Most fish oil supplements are 18% EPA and 12% DHA, or a total of 30% omega-3. These special omega-3 oils, unlike other omega-3 oils, keep blood triglycerides in check. **High triglycerides** (p. 85) are generally linked with increased risk of **heart disease** (p. 32). EPA and DHA keep blood from clotting too quickly. They also have anti-inflammatory activity. As a result, fish oil is used to help people with various inflammatory conditions, including **Crohn's disease** (p. 48).[1] Fish oil may help people with a wide variety of disorders, including chronic kidney diseases.[2,3] **Chronic obstructive pulmonary disease** (p. 45) may be less likely to develop in those with a greater intake of omega-3 fatty acids.[4]

Due to its effects on prostaglandin metabolism, fish oil has helped some people with **Raynaud's disease** (p. 148) in double-blind research.[5] Schizophrenia is linked with abnormalities in fatty acid metabolism, and preliminary research has found fish oil helpful in people with schizophrenia.[6]

DHA is essential for vision in infants. Fish oil may also help prevent some types of cancer in animals[7,8,9] and humans,[10] but this evidence remains preliminary. Preliminary evidence shows that fish oil may help pre-

vent **cardiac arrhythmias** (p. 32).[11] Finally, fish oil modulates **immune function** (p. 94),[12] though details remain unclear.

Where Is It Found?

EPA and DHA are found in mackerel, salmon, herring, sardines, sable fish (black cod), anchovies, albacore tuna, and wild game. Cod liver oil contains large amounts of EPA and DHA.

Who Is Likely to Be Deficient?

To a very limited extent, omega-3 oil from vegetable sources, such as **flaxseed oil** (p. 296), can convert to EPA. Most nutritionally oriented doctors believe most people do not eat enough EPA and DHA. So-called primitive diets have much higher levels than modern diets.

Fish Oil Has Been Used in Connection with the Following Conditions*

Ranking	Health Concerns
Primary	Crohn's disease (p. 48) (enteric-coated free fatty acid form of fish oil) High blood pressure (p. 89) High triglycerides (p. 85) Rheumatoid arthritis (p. 151) Ulcerative colitis (p. 158)
Secondary	Chronic kidney disease Eczema (p. 64) Lupus (SLE) (p. 115) Psoriasis (p. 147) Raynaud's disease (p. 145)
Other	Angina (p. 13) Asthma (p. 15) Chronic obstructive pulmonary disease (p. 45) Depression (p. 50) Diabetes (p. 53) Menstruation painful (dysmenorrhea) (p. 61) Migraine headaches (p. 121) Multiple sclerosis (p. 127) Osteoarthritis (p. 133) Schizophrenia

*Refer to the Individual Health Concern for Complete Information

How Much Is Usually Taken?

Most of the research with fish oil has given people with a variety of health conditions at least 3 grams of EPA plus DHA—an amount that may require 10 grams of fish oil, because most fish oil contains only 18% EPA and 12% DHA. A lesser, ideal amount for healthy people has not been determined.

The health benefits for individuals with Crohn's disease have been reported with a special enteric-coated, "free fatty acid" form of EPA/DHA taken from fish oil. The enteric-coated free fatty acid form has also been reported to not cause the gastrointestinal symptoms often resulting from taking regular fish oil supplements, again suggesting unique benefit.[13]

Are There Any Side Effects or Interactions? While those with heart disease and **diabetes** (p. 53) often benefit from fish oil,[14,15] both groups should check with their nutritionally oriented doctor before taking more than 3 or 4 grams of fish oil for several months. Elevations in blood sugar and **cholesterol** (p. 79) levels may occur in some individuals who take fish oil.[16] The increase in blood sugar appears to be related in part to the amount of fish oil used.[17] While supplementation with fish oil consistently lowers **triglycerides** (p. 85), the effect of fish oil on LDL cholesterol varies, and sometimes the levels actually increase.[18] Also, because EPA and DHA reduce blood clotting, people taking them sometimes get nose bleeds.[19] Some people who supplement several grams of fish oil will experience gastrointestinal upset and burp up a "fishy" smell.

Due to its very high levels of **vitamin A** (p. 336) and **vitamin D** (p. 343), cod liver oil should not be taken by women who are or who could become pregnant before consulting a nutritionally oriented doctor. Other adults should consult with a nutritionally oriented doctor before taking cod liver oil (or other supplements) containing more than 25,000 (7,500 mcg) of vitamin A per day or 800 IU of vitamin D per day.

Fish oil is easily damaged by oxygen, so a few milligrams or IUs of **vitamin E** (p. 344) should be included in all fish oil supplements.[20] In addition, people who supplement with fish oil should take additional vitamin E supplements (several hundred IUs) to protect EPA and DHA within the body from oxidative damage.[21]

Some evidence suggests that adding vitamin E to EPA/DHA may prevent the fish oil-induced increase in serum glucose.[22] Similarly, the impairment of glucose tolerance sometimes caused by the omega-3 oil has been prevented by the addition of half an hour of moderate exercise 3 times a week.[23]

People who take fish oil containing EPA and DHA and who also take 15 grams of pectin per day have been reported to have reductions in LDL cholesterol.[24] This suggests that pectin may overcome the occasional problem of increased LDL cholesterol from fish oil supplementation. The LDL-C raising effect of EPA and DHA may also be successfully prevented by taking **garlic** (p. 425) supplements (or presumably including garlic in the diet) along with EPA and DHA.[25]

5-Hydroxytryptophan (5-HTP)

5-HTP is used by the human body to make serotonin, an important substance for normal nerve and brain function. Serotonin appears to play significant roles in sleep, emotional moods, pain control, inflammation, intestinal peristalsis, and other body functions.[1]

Where Is It Found?

5-HTP is not present in significant amounts in a typical diet. The human body manufactures 5-HTP from L-tryptophan, a natural **amino acid** (p. 265) found in many dietary proteins. However, eating food that contains tryptophan does not significantly increase 5-HTP levels. Supplemental 5-HTP is naturally derived from the seeds of the *Griffonia simplicifolia,* a West African medicinal plant.

5-HTP Has Been Used in Connection with the Following Conditions*

Ranking	Health Concerns
Secondary	Depression (p. 50) Fibromyalgia (p. 68)
Other	Insomnia (p. 105) Migraine headaches (p. 121) Weight loss and obesity (p. 165)

*Refer to the Individual Health Concern for Complete Information

Who Is Likely to Be Deficient?

Disruptions in emotional well-being, including **depression** (p. 50) and **anxiety** (p. 14), have been linked to serotonin imbalances in the brain.[2] Individuals with **fibromyalgia** (p. 68) often have low serotonin levels in their blood.[3,4,5] Supplements of 5-HTP may increase serotonin synthesis in these cases. The cause of **migraine** (p. 121) headaches is related to abnormal serotonin function in blood vessels,[6] and 5-HTP may help correct this abnormality. **Insomnia** (p. 105) has been associated with tryptophan deficiency in the tissues of the brain;[7] therefore, 5-HTP may provide a remedy for this condition.

How Much Is Usually Taken?

In a controlled trial, 5-HTP (300 mg per day) was shown to be effective in reducing many symptoms of fibromyalgia, including pain, morning stiffness, sleep disturbances, and anxiety.[8] Migraine attacks were reduced in frequency, severity, and duration in 90% of those taking 400 mg per day of 5-HTP in a well-controlled trial.[9] Larger doses of 5-HTP (600 mg per day) were found to be as effective as medications for reducing migraine headache attacks in adults in two double-blind studies,[10,11] though another trial found no benefit of 5-HTP.[12] Children who suffered from migraines and had problems sleeping responded well to a daily dose of 5-HTP equal to 20 mg for every 10 pounds of body weight in a controlled study.[13] For depression, 300 mg per day is often effective, though much of the research used 5-HTP in combination with drugs or was uncontrolled.[14,15,16] A single 100 mg nighttime dose of 5-HTP was sufficient to improve the duration and depth of sleep in one placebo-controlled study.[17] Appetite reduction and **weight loss** (p. 165) (averaging 11 pounds in 12 weeks) have occurred with doses of 600–900 milligrams daily.[18,19]

Are There Any Side Effects or Interactions?

During the research studies described above, some people taking large amounts of 5-HTP experienced gastrointestinal upset or, less often, headache, sleepiness, muscle pain, or anxiety. Rarely, some 5-HTP supplements have been reported to cause symptoms resembling a disorder known as eosinophilia-myalgia syndrome (EMS).[20] This syndrome appears to be related to contaminants that may be present in many 5-HTP products.[21] It is not known if very small amounts of contaminant are safe. It is impossible for most people to determine if such contaminants exist in any given 5-HTP product, though some reputable manufacturers routinely test for contamination.

5-HTP should not be taken with antidepressants, weight-control drugs, other serotonin-modifying agents, or substances known to cause liver damage, because in these cases 5-HTP may have excessive effects. Individuals with liver disease may not be able to regulate 5-HTP adequately, and those suffering from autoimmune diseases such as scleroderma may be more sensitive to 5-HTP.[22] These people should not take 5-HTP without consulting a knowledgeable health-care professional. The safety of 5-HTP therapy during pregnancy or lactation is not known at this time.

Flaxseed Oil

Like most vegetable oils, flaxseed oil contains linoleic acid, an essential fatty acid needed for survival. But unlike most oils, it also contains significant amounts of another essential fatty acid, alpha linolenic acid (ALA) (p. 264).

ALA is an omega-3 oil. To a limited extent, the body turns ALA into **EPA** (p. 294)—an omega-3 oil found in **fish oil** (p. 294). EPA in turn converts to 3-series prostaglandins. (Prostaglandins are hormone-like substances made in many parts of the body rather than coming from one organ, as most hormones do.) Indirectly, the 3-series prostaglandins have anti-inflammatory activity. Because the conversion from ALA to EPA is quite limited, some of the effects of fish oil (like controlling triglycerides) do not result when people supplement flaxseed oil.

In theory, flaxseed should be useful in the same conditions for which **fish oil** (p. 294) is used. However, it does not **lower triglycerides** (p. 85) and may not protect against **heart disease** (p. 32). Its anti-inflammatory activity also has yet to be proven, though researchers remain hopeful.

In 1994, a diet purportedly high in ALA was successful in preventing heart disease.[1] But this study altered many dietary factors, so ALA may not have been solely responsible for the outcome.[2] In general, flaxseed oil does not appear to be a good replacement for fish oil for people with elevated triglycerides,[3,4] though it may help **lower cholesterol** (p. 79).[5] Even outside the realm of heart disease, most omega-3 oil research has been done with fish oil and not flaxseed oil.

However, research specific to flaxseed oil indicates that it may **lower blood pressure** (p. 89).[6] Flaxseed oil will not cause a fishy-smelling burp (a possible side effect of fish oil). Although it is not suitable for cooking, flaxseed oil (unlike fish oil) can be used in salads. Some conversion to EPA does occur,[7] and this conversion can be increased by restricting the intake of other vegetable oils.[8]

Where Is It Found?

In addition to its presence in flaxseed oil, small amounts of ALA are found in canola, **soy** (p. 332), black currant, and walnut oils.

Flaxseed Oil Has Been Used in Connection with the Following Conditions*

Ranking	Health Concerns
Primary	Constipation (p. 44) (flaxseed)
Other	Benign prostatic hyperplasia (BPH) (p. 145) (flaxseed oil) Constipation (p. 44) (flaxseed oil) Ulcerative colitis (p. 158) (flaxseed) Vaginitis (p. 162) (flaxseed)
*Refer to the Individual Health Concern for Complete Information	

Who Is Likely to Be Deficient?

ALA deficiencies are possible but believed to be rare, except in infants who are fed formula that is omega-3 deficient.

How Much Is Usually Taken?

Some nutritionally oriented doctors recommend that people use 1 tablespoon per day as a supplement in salads or on vegetables to ensure a supply of essential fatty acids.

For those who wish to replace fish oil with flaxseed oil, research suggests taking up to ten times as much ALA as EPA.[9] Typically, this means that 7.2 grams of flaxseed oil should equal 1 gram of fish oil.

Are There Any Side Effects or Interactions? Flaxseed oil toxicity has not been reported. However, metabolites, blood levels, or dietary levels of ALA have been reported to increase mammary tumors in animals[10] and to correlate with increased risk of prostate cancer in men[11] and breast cancer risk in women.[12] Also, ALA becomes mutagenic when heated.[13] Therefore, the previous belief held by some nutritionally oriented doctors that flaxseed oil may have anticancer effects, based on very preliminary research,[14] appears to be unfounded. In addition, the possibility exists that flaxseed oil may eventually be shown to increase cancer risks, though to date studies supporting such a link are far from conclusive.

Folic Acid

Folic acid is needed for DNA synthesis. DNA allows cells—including cells in the fetus when a woman is **pregnant** (p. 143)— to replicate normally. Adequate intake of folic acid early in pregnancy is important for preventing most neural tube birth defects[1] and may also protect against some birth defects of the arms, legs, and heart.[2] It also appears to protect against cleft palate and cleft lip formation in most,[3,4] though not all,[5] studies.

Folic acid is needed to make **SAMe** (S-adenosyl-L-methionine) (p. 330), which affects (and may improve) mood. Folic acid is also needed to keep **homocysteine** (p. 84) (an amino acid) levels in blood from rising. Excess homocysteine has been linked to an increased risk of **heart disease** (p. 32) in most studies and may also be linked to **osteoporosis** (p. 133, 563), strokes, and **Alzheimer's disease** (p. 11).

Where Is It Found?

Beans, leafy green vegetables, citrus fruits, beets, wheat germ, and meat are good sources of folic acid.

Who Is Likely to Be Deficient?

Most people do not consume the recommended amount of folic acid. Recently, scientists have found that many people with heart disease have elevated blood levels of homocysteine, which is often controllable with folic acid. This suggests that many people in Western societies have a mild folic acid deficiency. In fact, increasing folic acid intake could potentially prevent an estimated 13,500 deaths from cardiovascular diseases each year.[6] Folic acid deficiency is also common in alcoholics, people living at poverty level, those with malabsorption disorders, and women taking the birth control pill. Recently, elderly people with hearing loss have been reported to be much more likely to be folic acid deficient than healthy elderly individuals.[7]

Folic Acid Has Been Used in Connection with the Following Conditions*

Ranking	Health Concerns
Primary	Celiac disease (p. 35) (if deficient) Crohn's disease (p. 48) Depression (p. 50) Gingivitis (periodontal disease) (p. 73) (rinse only) High homocysteine (p. 84) Pap smear (abnormal) (p. 136) Pregnancy and postpartum support (p. 143)
Secondary	Atherosclerosis (p. 17) Ulcerative colitis (p. 158)
Other	Alzheimer's disease (p. 11) Diarrhea (p. 58) Gout (p. 75) High cholesterol (p. 79) (protection of LDL cholesterol) HIV support (p. 87) Osteoporosis (p. 133) Restless legs syndrome (p. 149) Vitiligo (p. 164)

*Refer to the Individual Health Concern for Complete Information

How Much Is Usually Taken?

All women who are or who could become pregnant should take 400–800 mcg per day in order to reduce the risk of birth defects. Many nutritionally oriented doctors recommend 400 mcg to others. Dietary folate is much less available to the body compared with synthetic folic acid found in most supplements. Therefore adding supplemental folic acid from a vitamin pill is probably important.

Are There Any Side Effects or Interactions? Folic acid is not generally associated with side effects.[8] However, folic acid supplementation can interfere with the laboratory diagnosis of **vitamin B$_{12}$** (p. 337) deficiency, possibly allowing the deficiency to progress undetected to the point of irreversible nerve damage.[9] Although vitamin B$_{12}$ deficiency is uncommon, no one should supplement with 1,000 mcg or more of folic acid without consulting a nutritionally oriented doctor.

Vitamin B$_{12}$ deficiencies often occur without anemia (even in people who don't take folic acid supplements). Some doctors do not know that the absence of anemia does not rule out a B$_{12}$ deficiency. If this confusion delays diagnosis of a vitamin B$_{12}$ deficiency, the patient could be injured, sometimes permanently. This problem is rare and should not happen with doctors knowledgeable in this area using correct testing procedures.

Folic acid is needed by the body to utilize vitamin B$_{12}$. **Proteolytic enzymes** (p. 289) and antacids[10] inhibit folic acid absorption.[11] People taking either of these are advised to supplement with folic acid.

Folic acid-containing supplements may interfere with methotrexate therapy in people with cancer. People using methotrexate for cancer treatment should ask their prescribing doctor before using any folic acid-containing supplements. Until recently, methotrexate was believed to help people with **rheumatoid arthritis** (p. 151) also by interfering with folic acid metabolism. However, recent research has shown that this is not so. In fact, people with rheumatoid arthritis taking methotrexate should supplement large amounts of folic acid. The same now appears to be true for people with severe psoriatic arthritis who are taking methotrexate. However, high levels of folic acid should not be taken without clinical supervision.

Fumaric Acid

Fumaric acid is related to **malic acid** (p. 311), and like malic acid, it is involved in the production of energy (in the form of ATP) from food. Fumaric acid has been used with some success to alleviate **psoriasis** (p. 147) symptoms.[1,2,3,4,5]

Typically, the amount used in these trials begins with 60–105 mg per day of fumaric acid esters, gradually increasing to as much as 1,290 mg per day.

Where Is It Found?

Fumaric acid is formed in the skin during exposure to sunlight, as well as being available as an oral supplement and as a preparation for topical use.

Fumaric Acid Has Been Used in Connection with the Following Condition*

Ranking	Health Concern
Other	Psoriasis (p. 147)

*Refer to the Individual Health Concern for Complete Information

Who Is Likely to Be Deficient?

No deficiencies of fumaric acid have been reported; however, some doctors of natural medicine suggest that individuals with psoriasis may have a biochemical defect that interferes with adequate fumaric acid production in the skin.

How Much Is Usually Taken?

Only the esterified forms of fumaric acid are used therapeutically, such as fumaric acid monoethylester or fumaric acid di-methylester. Healthy people do not need to supplement with fumaric acid. Those using this substance (either orally or topically) should work with a dermatologist, since determining the optimal intake should be done on an individual basis. Even under these circumstances, supplementing should be started with small amounts (60–100 mg per day) and increased gradually over several weeks until an effect is noted.

Are There Any Side Effects or Interactions? Kidney disorders have been reported in people taking fumaric acid, possibly due to taking large amounts too quickly.[6,7] Most studies have reported gastrointestinal upset and skin flushing as common side effects; some have also found decreased white blood cell counts with prolonged use.[8,9]

Gamma Oryzanol

Gamma oryzanol is a mixture of sterols and ferulic acid esters. Some evidence suggests that it increases testosterone levels, the release of endorphins, and the growth of lean muscle tissue;[1] however, gamma oryzanol has been reported to not result in improved **exercise performance** (p. 20).[2]

Where Is It Found?

Gamma oryzanol is a natural component of rice bran, corn, and barley oils.

Who Is Likely to Be Deficient?

Since gamma oryzanol is not an essential nutrient, it is not associated with a deficiency state.

Gamma Oryzanol Has Been Used in Connection with the Following Condition*

Ranking	Health Concern
Primary	Gastritis (p. 71)

*Refer to the Individual Health Concern for Complete Information

How Much Is Usually Taken?

Much of the human research with gamma oryzanol uses 300 mg per day. Healthy people do not appear to need this supplement.

Are There Any Side Effects or Interactions? Some research suggests that gamma oryzanol taken in moderately high amounts (up to 600 mg per day) for several months can cause dry mouth, sleepiness, hot flushes, irritability, and light-headedness in some individuals.[3]

Glucosamine Sulfate

Glucosamine sulfate provides the joints with the building blocks they need to repair damage caused by **osteoarthritis** (p. 130) or injuries. Specifically, glucosamine sulfate provides the raw material needed by the body to manufacture a mucopolysaccharide (called glycosaminoglycan) found in cartilage. Glucosamine sulfate may also play a role in **wound healing** (p. 167).

Which Form Is Best?

Glucosamine is available in several forms. The glucosamine sulfate form (stabilized with a mineral salt) has been the primary form used in the controlled trials of people with osteoarthritis. For this reason, it is the preferred form.

Glucosamine sulfate is stabilized with one of two mineral salts: sodium chloride (NaCl) or potassium chloride (KCl).[1,2] Although they both appear to effectively stabilize glucosamine sulfate, the use of KCl as a stabilizer is preferable since the average Western diet already provides far too much salt (NaCl) and not enough **potassium** (p. 323).

Another form of glucosamine sulfate, N-acetyl glucosamine (NAG), has never been studied in people with osteoarthritis. In the only known study to investigate the effects of the form glucosamine hydrochloride (glucosamine HCl) in people with osteoarthritis, unpublished data from Canada have not shown any significant advantage for this supplement compared with placebo. Therefore, these forms cannot be recommended on the basis of available research at this time.

Where Is It Found?

Glucosamine sulfate does not appear in significant amounts in most diets. Supplemental sources are derived from seashells.

Who Is Likely to Be Deficient?

A glucosamine sulfate deficiency in humans has not been reported.

How Much Is Usually Taken?

Healthy people do not need to routinely supplement with glucosamine sulfate. Most research with people who have osteoarthritis uses 500 mg 3 times per day. Appropriate levels for other conditions remain unclear.

Glucosamine Sulfate Has Been Used in Connection with the Following Conditions*

Ranking	Health Concerns
Primary	Osteoarthritis (p. 130)
Other	Kidney stones (p. 111) Minor injuries (p. 122) and wound healing (p. 167)

*Refer to the Individual Health Concern for Complete Information

Are There Any Side Effects or Interactions? At the amount most frequently taken by adults—500 mg 3 times per day—toxicity has not been reported. Some glucosamine sulfate is processed with sodium chloride (table salt), which is restricted in some diets, particularly for people with **high blood pressure** (p. 544).

The hypothesis that glucosamine sulfate and **chondroitin sulfate** (p. 281) work synergistically in the support of osteoarthritis remains unproven. The fact that they are structurally similar suggests that they may act in similar ways.

Glutamic Acid

Glutamic acid is a nonessential **amino acid** (p. 265) that the body uses to build proteins. Although **glutamine** (p. 300) and glutamic acid have similar names, they are structurally different.

The fluid produced by the prostate gland contains significant amounts of glutamic acid, and this amino acid may play a role in normal function of the prostate. In one study, symptoms of **benign prostatic hyperplasia** (BPH) (p. 145) were improved in a group of forty-five men taking 780 mg of glutamic acid per day for 2 weeks and then 390 mg for the next 2½ months in combination with equal amounts of the

Glutamic Acid

amino acids **alanine** (p. 264) and **glycine** (p. 300),[1] an effect also reported by other researchers.[2]

Where Is It Found?

As with the other amino acids, excellent sources of glutamic acid include meat, poultry, fish, eggs, and dairy products. Some protein-rich plant foods also supply glutamic acid.

Glutamic Acid Has Been Used in Connection with the Following Condition*

Ranking	Health Concern
Secondary	Benign prostatic hyperplasia (p. 145)
*Refer to the Individual Health Concern for Complete Information	

Who Is Likely to Be Deficient?

Most food sources of protein supply glutamic acid, so only an individual deficient in protein would become deficient in glutamic acid.[3]

How Much Is Usually Taken?

Healthy people do not need to take glutamic acid as a supplement; for those who do use this amino acid, appropriate amounts should be determined with the consultation of a nutritionally oriented physician.

Are There Any Side Effects or Interactions? Glutamic acid is generally free of side effects for the vast majority of people who take it; however, individuals with kidney or liver disease should not consume high intakes of amino acids without consulting a health-care professional.

Glutamine

Glutamine is the most abundant **amino acid** (p. 265) (protein building block) in the body and is involved in more metabolic processes than any other amino acid. Glutamine is converted to glucose when more glucose is required by the body as an energy source. It serves as a source of fuel for cells lining the intestines. Without it, these cells waste away. It is also used by white blood cells and is important for **immune function** (p. 94). In animal research, glutamine has anti-inflammatory effects. Glutamine in combination with **N-acetyl cysteine** (p. 317) promotes the synthesis of glutathione, a naturally occurring **antioxidant** (p. 267) that is believed to be protective in people with **HIV infection** (p. 87).[1] Evidence indicates that critically ill people are more likely to survive with intravenous glutamine supplementation.[2]

Where Is It Found?

Glutamine is found in many foods high in protein, such as fish, meat, beans, and dairy products.

Glutamine Has Been Used in Connection with the Following Conditions*

Ranking	Health Concerns
Secondary	Athletic performance (p. 20) (for reducing risk of post-exercise infection) Immune function (for post-exercise infection prevention in endurance athletes) (p. 94)
Other	Alcohol withdrawal support (p. 6) Gastritis (p. 71) HIV support (p. 87) Peptic ulcer (p. 138) Ulcerative colitis (p. 158)
*Refer to the Individual Health Concern for Complete Information	

Who Is Likely to Be Deficient?

Few people are glutamine deficient, in part because the body makes its own. During fasting, starvation, cirrhosis, critical illnesses in general, and weight loss associated with **AIDS** (p. 87) and cancer, however, deficiencies often develop.

How Much Is Usually Taken?

Healthy people do not need to supplement glutamine. A nutritionally oriented physician should be consulted for the supplemental use of glutamine for the support of serious health conditions.

Are There Any Side Effects or Interactions? No clear toxicity has emerged in glutamine studies.

Glycine

Glycine is a nonessential **amino acid** (p. 265) used by the body to build proteins. It is present in considerable amounts in prostate fluid. Glycine may play a role in maintaining the health of the prostate, since a study of forty-five men with **benign prostatic hyperplasia** (BPH) (p. 145) found that 780 mg of glycine per day for 2 weeks and then 390 mg for the next 2½ months, taken in combination with equal amounts of the amino acids **alanine** (p. 264) and **glutamic acid** (p. 299), reduced symptoms of the condition.[1] This effect has been reported by others.[2]

Where Is It Found?

Glycine is found in many foods high in protein, such as fish, meat, beans, and dairy.

Glutamine

**Glycine Has Been Used in
Connection with the Following Condition***

Ranking	Health Concern
Secondary	Benign prostatic hyperplasia (p. 145)

*Refer to the Individual Health Concern for Complete Information

Who Is Likely to Be Deficient?

Few people are glycine deficient, in part because the body makes its own supply of the nonessential amino acids.

How Much Is Usually Taken?

Healthy people do not need to supplement glycine. A nutritionally oriented physician should be consulted for the supplemental use of glycine for the support of serious health conditions.

Are There Any Side Effects or Interactions? No clear toxicity has emerged from glycine studies; however, individuals with kidney or liver disease should not consume high intakes of amino acids without consulting a health-care professional.

Histidine

Histidine is called a semi-essential **amino acid** (p. 265) (protein building block) because adults generally produce adequate amounts but children may not. Histidine is also a precursor of histamine, a compound released by immune system cells during an **allergic reaction** (p. 8).

Where Is It Found?

Dairy, meat, poultry, and fish are good sources of histidine and the other amino acids.

Who Is Likely to Be Deficient?

According to limited research, many individuals with **rheumatoid arthritis** (p. 151) have low levels of histidine. Taking histidine supplements might improve arthritis symptoms in some individuals.[1]

How Much Is Usually Taken?

Most people do not need to supplement histidine. Optimal levels for others remain unknown. Human research has used between 1 gram and 8 grams per day.

Are There Any Side Effects or Interactions? No side effects have been reported with histidine; however, individuals with kidney or liver disease should not consume large amounts of amino acids without consulting a health-care professional.

**Histidine Has Been Used in
Connection with the Following Condition***

Ranking	Health Concern
Other	Rheumatoid arthritis (p. 151)

*Refer to the Individual Health Concern for Complete Information

HMB (Beta Hydroxy-Beta-Methylbutyrate)

HMB (beta hydroxy-beta-methylbutyrate) is a metabolite of the essential **amino acid** (p. 265) leucine (p. 274), one of the **branched-chain amino acids**. As with other amino acid—related substances, HMB appears to play a role in the synthesis of protein—including the protein that builds new muscle tissue.

Animal research suggests that HMB may improve the growth of lean muscle tissue,[1] but only preliminary and limited research in humans supports the potential link between HMB and enhanced muscle building in **athletes** (p. 20).[2] One study involving twenty-eight individuals involved in a regular weight-lifting program found that supplements of 3 grams of HMB, compared with no supplements, contributed to greater gains of muscle over the 7-week-long study.[3]

Where Is It Found?

Small amounts of HMB are present in many foods of animal and plant origin, especially **alfalfa** (p. 391) and catfish. The amino acid leucine is metabolized into a compound called alpha-ketoisocaproate (KIC), which is then turned into HMB by the body. Dietary supplements of HMB are also available.

**HMB Has Been Used in
Connection with the Following Condition***

Ranking	Health Concern
Other	Athletic performance (p. 20) (for strength and body composition)

*Refer to the Individual Health Concern for Complete Information

Who Is Likely to Be Deficient?

HMB is not an essential nutrient. The body creates HMB from leucine, so any diet containing sufficient amounts of leucine (most do) should lead to the adequate production of HMB. Limited evidence indicates that athletes may benefit from supplemental intake of HMB.

HMB

How Much Is Usually Taken?

Most individuals do not need to use HMB. For those involved in regular exercise who do choose to take this supplement, the research generally uses 3 grams of HMB per day in combination with resistive exercise, such as weight lifting.

Are There Any Side Effects or Interactions? No safety issues have been reported in the limited number of studies currently available.

Huperzine A

Huperzine A is a substance first found in Huperzia serrata, a Chinese medicinal herb. Huperzine A has been reported to prevent the breakdown of acetylcholine, an important substance needed by the nervous system to transmit information from cell to cell.[1] Animal research has suggested that huperzine A's ability to preserve acetylcholine may be greater than that of some prescription drugs.[2,3] Loss of acetylcholine function is a primary feature of several disorders of brain function, including **Alzheimer's disease** (p. 11). Huperzine A may also have a protective effect on brain tissue, further increasing its theoretical potential for helping reduce symptoms of some brain disorders.[4,5] In a well-designed placebo-controlled trial, 58% of people with Alzheimer's disease had significant improvement in memory and cognitive and behavioral functions after taking 200 mcg of huperzine A twice per day for 8 weeks—a statistically significant improvement over the 36% who responded to placebo.[6] Another double-blind report using injected huperzine A confirmed a positive effect in people with dementia, including, but not limited to, Alzheimer's disease.[7]

Where Is It Found?

Huperzine A is present in a type of moss known as *Huperzia serrata*, which has been used in a Chinese remedy called Qian Ceng Ta for centuries.

Who Is Likely to Be Deficient?

Huperzine A is not essential to the human body. However, people with certain neurological disorders related to insufficiency of acetylcholine function may respond to huperzine A.

How Much Is Usually Taken?

Human research on huperzine A has used 200 mcg taken twice per day. It is absorbed rapidly from the human digestive tract.[8]

Are There Any Side Effects or Interactions? Medications that prevent acetylcholine breakdown often

Huperzine A Has Been Used in Connection with the Following Condition*

Ranking	Health Concern
Secondary	Alzheimer's disease (p. 11)

| *Refer to the Individual Health Concern for Complete Information |

produce side effects, including nausea, vomiting, excess saliva and tear production, and sweating. However, while dizziness was reported in a few individuals in one study, no severe side effects have been reported in human trials.

(-)-Hydroxycitric Acid (HCA)

(-)-Hydroxycitric acid (HCA) is a fruit extract with a chemical composition similar to citric acid (the primary acid in citrus fruits). Preliminary research, based on laboratory experiments and animal research, suggests that HCA may be a useful **weight loss** (p. 165) aid.[1,2] HCA has been demonstrated in the laboratory (but not yet in trials with people) to reduce the conversion of carbohydrates into stored fat by inhibiting certain enzyme processes.[3,4] Animal research indicates that HCA suppresses appetite and induces weight loss.[5,6,7,8] One case report found that eating 1 gram of the fruit containing HCA before each meal resulted in the loss of 1 pound per day.[9]

A double-blind trial that provided either 1,500 mg of HCA or a placebo to 135 overweight men and women who also were on a calorie-restricted diet found after 12 weeks that the HCA supplementation did not produce a significant change in weight loss.[10] Uncontrolled and/or preliminary evidence from several other human trials suggest the possibility that weight loss might occur;[11] however, none of these studies is as methodologically strong as the negative trial previously mentioned.

Where Is It Found?

HCA is found in only a few plants, with the richest source being the rind of a little pumpkin-shaped fruit called *Garcinia cambogia,* native to Southeast Asia. Thai and Indian cuisines use this fruit (also called Malabar tamarind) as a condiment in dishes such as curry.

Who Is Likely to Be Deficient?

Since it is not an essential nutrient, HCA is not associated with a deficiency state.

HCA Has Been Used in Connection with the Following Condition*

Ranking	Health Concern
Other	Weight loss and obesity (p. 165)

*Refer to the Individual Health Concern for Complete Information

How Much Is Usually Taken?

Optimal levels of HCA remain unknown. Although dieters sometimes take 500 mg of HCA 3 times per day (before each meal), this amount is far below the levels used in animal research (figured on a per-pound body weight basis). The effect of HCA is enhanced when used in conjuncture with a lowfat diet, because HCA does nothing to reduce the caloric effects of dietary fat. HCA supplements are available in many forms, including tablets, capsules, powders, snack bars, and chewing gum.

Are There Any Side Effects or Interactions? HCA has not been linked to any adverse effects.

Inosine

Inosine is a nucleoside, one of the basic compounds comprising cells. It is a precursor to adenosine, an important energy molecule, and plays many supportive roles in the body, including releasing insulin, facilitating the use of carbohydrate by the heart, and, potentially, participating in oxygen metabolism and protein synthesis. Based upon anecdotal reports by Russian and Eastern European athletes, inosine has been investigated for ergogenic—**exercise boosting** (p. 20)—effects. Results of controlled studies have been disappointing, however, suggesting that inosine does not improve athletic performance and may even impair it.[1,2]

Where Is It Found?

Inosine is found in **brewer's yeast** (p. 275) and organ meats. It is also available as a supplement.

Who Is Likely to Be Deficient?

Inosine is not an essential nutrient, so deficiencies do not occur.

How Much Is Usually Taken?

Although a common amount of inosine taken by athletes is 5,000–6,000 mg per day, little scientific evidence supports the use of this supplement at any level.

Are There Any Side Effects or Interactions? No side effects have been reported with the use of inosine for 2 to 5 days in the limited research available. However, unused inosine is converted by the body to uric acid, which may be hazardous to people at risk for **gout** (p. 75).

Inositol

Inositol is required for proper formation of cell membranes. It affects nerve transmission and helps in transporting fats within the body.

Where Is It Found?

Nuts, beans, wheat and wheat bran, cantaloupe, and oranges are excellent sources of inositol. Most dietary inositol is in the form of phytate.

Who Is Likely to Be Deficient?

Clear deficiency of inositol has not been reported, although **diabetics** (p. 53) have increased excretion and may benefit from inositol supplementation.

Inositol Has Been Used in Connection with the Following Conditions*

Ranking	Health Concerns
Other	Anxiety (p. 14) Depression (p. 50) Diabetes (p. 53)

*Refer to the Individual Health Concern for Complete Information

How Much Is Usually Taken?

Most people do not need to take inositol. In addition, the small amounts commonly found in **multi-vitamin supplements** (p. 314) are probably unnecessary and ineffective. Nutritionally oriented doctors sometimes suggest 500 mg twice per day.

Are There Any Side Effects or Interactions? Toxicity has not been reported, although people with chronic renal failure show elevated levels.

Large amounts of phytate, the common dietary form of inositol, reduce the absorption of **calcium** (p. 277), **iron** (p. 304), and **zinc** (p. 346). However, supplemental inositol does not have this effect.

Iodine

Iodine is needed to make thyroid hormones, which are necessary for maintaining normal metabolism in all cells of the body. Reports suggest that iodine may have a number of important functions in the body

Iodine

IP-6 (Inositol Hexaphosphate, Phytate)

unrelated to thyroid function that might help people with a wide variety of conditions;[1] these other uses for iodine are only supported by minimal research.

Where Is It Found?

Seafood, iodized salt, and sea vegetables—for example, **kelp** (p. 306)—are high in iodine. Processed food may contain added iodized salt. Iodine is frequently found in dairy products. Vegetables grown in iodine-rich soil also contain this mineral.

Iodine Has Been Used in Connection with the Following Conditions*

Ranking	Health Concerns
Primary	Iodine deficiency-induced goiter
Secondary	Hypothyroidism (p. 93)
Other	Fibrocystic breast disease (p. 66)
*Refer to the Individual Health Concern for Complete Information	

Who Is Likely to Be Deficient?

People who avoid dairy, seafood, processed food, and iodized salt can become deficient. Iodine deficiency can cause low thyroid function, goiter, and cretinism; however, iodine deficiencies are now uncommon in Western societies.

How Much Is Usually Taken?

Since the introduction of iodized salt, iodine supplements are unnecessary and not recommended for most people. For strict vegetarians who avoid salt and sea vegetables, 150 mcg per day is more than adequate.

Are There Any Side Effects or Interactions? High doses (several milligrams per day) can interfere with normal thyroid function and should not be taken without consulting a nutritionally oriented doctor.[2] The average diet provides about four times the recommended amount of iodine, which may result in health problems.[3] In fact, goiter, traditionally a disease of iodine deficiency, is now linked sometimes to high iodine intake.[4] Also, speculations of an iodine link to thyroid cancer have been reported.[5] Some people react to supplemental iodine, the first symptom of which is usually an acne-like rash.

IP-6 (Inositol Hexaphosphate, Phytate)

IP-6 is a naturally occurring component of plant fiber that may possess **antioxidant** (p. 267),[1] anticancer,[2]

and other beneficial properties. For example, animal studies have shown that supplementation with large amounts of IP-6 provides substantial protection against colon cancer[3] and possibly breast cancer.[4,5] In one of these studies, the effect of pure IP-6 was significant, while an equivalent amount given as a wheat-bran breakfast cereal was not.[6] However, while some animals are able to digest and/or absorb IP-6, it is not known if this is true for humans.[7] This greatly limits the validity of this research for human health concerns, except possibly for colon cancer prevention, which may not depend on absorption. Unfortunately, human research to date has not found an association between higher levels of dietary IP-6 in the colon and reduced indicators of colon cancer risk.[8] Injections of IP-6 used to treat cancerous tumors in mice have been shown to cause partial regression of these tumors.[9]

IP-6 may have a beneficial effect on blood sugar control, similar to the effect of many dietary fibers.[10] However, no studies have been done to test this effect on people with blood sugar disorders.

Where Is It Found?

IP-6, also known as phytate, is associated with dietary fiber and thus is naturally present in a wide variety of plant foods, especially wheat bran, whole grains, and legumes. Usual dietary intakes range from 1–1.5 grams phytate per day.

Who Is Likely to Be Deficient?

While there is no dietary requirement for IP-6, people consuming diets low in dietary fiber, nuts, and seeds have the lowest intake.

How Much Is Usually Taken?

Virtually all research suggesting healthful effects from taking IP-6 involves animals and not people. It is not known whether IP-6 would be useful for humans or if so, what the optimal amount would be.

Are There Any Side Effects or Interactions? Phytate in foods has been associated with reduced mineral absorption,[11] but this effect may not be important except at very high intakes.

Iron

Iron is part of hemoglobin, the oxygen-carrying component of the blood. Iron-deficient people tire easily because their bodies are starved for oxygen. Iron is also part of myoglobin, which helps muscle cells store oxygen. Without enough iron, ATP (the fuel the body runs on) cannot be properly synthesized. As a result, some iron-deficient people become fatigued even when their hemoglobin levels are normal.

Although iron is part of the antioxidant enzyme catalase, iron is not generally considered an antioxidant, because too much iron can cause oxidative damage.

Where Is It Found?

The most absorbable form of iron, called "heme" iron, is found in oysters, meat, poultry, and fish. Non-heme iron is also found in these foods, as well as in dried fruit, molasses, leafy green vegetables, wine, and most iron supplements. Acidic foods (such as tomato sauce) cooked in an iron pan can also be a source of dietary iron.

Iron Has Been Used in Connection with the Following Conditions*

Ranking	Health Concerns
Primary	Athletic performance (p. 20) (for iron-deficiency anemia only) Celiac disease (p. 35) (for deficiency) Crohn's disease (p. 48) Depression (p. 50) (for deficiency) Iron-deficiency anemia (p. 107) Menorrhagia (heavy menstruation) (p. 120) (for deficiency)
Other	Canker sores (mouth ulcers) (p. 30) HIV support (p. 87) Infertility (female) (p. 102) (for deficiency) Restless legs syndrome (p. 149) (for deficiency)

*Refer to the Individual Health Concern for Complete Information

Who Is Likely to Be Deficient?

Vegetarians eat less iron than nonvegetarians, and the iron they eat is somewhat less absorbable. As a result, vegetarians are more likely to have reduced iron stores.[1] However, iron deficiency is not usually caused by a lack of iron in the diet alone; an underlying cause, such as iron loss in menstrual blood, often exists.

Pregnant women, marathon runners, people who take aspirin, and those who have **parasitic** (p. 137) infections, **hemorrhoids** (p. 77), **ulcers** (p. 158), **ulcerative colitis** (p. 158), **Crohn's disease** (p. 158), gastrointestinal cancers, or other conditions that cause blood loss or malabsorption are likely to become deficient.

Individuals who fit into one of these groups, even pregnant women, shouldn't automatically take iron supplements. Fatigue, the first symptom of iron deficiency, can be caused by many other things. A nutritionally oriented doctor should assess the need for iron supplements, since taking iron when it isn't needed does no good and may do some harm.

How Much Is Usually Taken?

If a nutritionally oriented doctor diagnoses iron deficiency, iron supplementation is essential. A common adult dose is 100 mg per day. When iron deficiency is diagnosed, the doctor must also determine the cause. Usually it's not serious (such as normal menstrual blood loss or blood donation). Occasionally, however, iron deficiency signals ulcers or even colon cancer.

Many premenopausal women become marginally iron deficient unless they supplement with iron. Even so, the 18 mg of iron present in most multiple-vitamin/mineral supplements is often adequate.

Are There Any Side Effects or Interactions? Huge overdoses (as when a child swallows an entire bottle of iron supplements) can be fatal. Keep iron-containing supplements out of a child's reach. Hemochromatosis, hemosiderosis, polycythemia, and iron-loading anemias (such as thalassemia and sickle cell anemia) are conditions involving excessive storage of iron. Supplementing iron can be quite dangerous for people with these diseases.

Supplemental amounts required to overcome iron deficiency can cause **constipation** (p. 44). Sometimes switching the form of iron, getting more exercise, or treating the constipation with **fiber** (p. 53) and fluids is helpful. Sometimes the amount of iron must be reduced if constipation occurs.

Some researchers have linked excess iron to **diabetes** (p. 53),[2] cancer,[3] increased risk of infection,[4] **systemic lupus erythematosus** (p. 115) (SLE),[5] exacerbation of **rheumatoid arthritis** (p. 151),[6] and **heart disease** (p. 32),[7,8,9] though a review of the best studies has found no link.[10] None of these links has been proven. Nonetheless, too much iron causes **free radical damage** (p. 267), which can cause or exacerbate most of these diseases. People who are not iron deficient should not supplement iron when potential risks might exist and no benefit can be found.

Caffeine, **high-fiber** (p. 293) foods, and **calcium** (p. 276) supplements reduce iron absorption. **Vitamin C** (p. 341) slightly increases iron absorption.[11] Taking **vitamin A** (p. 336) with iron helps treat iron deficiency, since vitamin A helps the body use iron stored in the liver.[12,13]

Deferoxamine is a drug that binds to some metals, including iron, and carries them out of the body. It is used to treat acute iron poisoning, chronic iron overload, and aluminum accumulation in people with kidney failure. People taking deferoxamine to treat iron overload must not take iron supplements, including the amounts found in many multivitamin/minerals.

Penicillamine binds metals (including **copper** [p. 285] and iron) and carries them out of the body. When penicillamine and iron are taken together,

Iron

penicillamine absorption and activity are reduced. Four cases of penicillamine-induced kidney damage were reported when concomitant iron therapy was stopped, which presumably led to increased penicillamine absorption and toxicity.[14]

Kelp

Kelp is a sea vegetable that is a concentrated source of minerals, including **iodine** (p. 303), **potassium** (p. 323), **magnesium** (p. 310), **calcium** (p. 277), and **iron** (p. 304).

Kelp as a source of iodine assists in making thyroid hormones, which are necessary for maintaining normal metabolism in all cells of the body.

Where Is It Found?

Kelp can be one of several brown-colored seaweed species called *Laminaria*.

Kelp Has Been Used in Connection with the Following Condition*

Ranking	Health Concern
Other	Iodine deficiency (p. 303)
*Refer to the Individual Health Concern for Complete Information	

Who Is Likely to Be Deficient?

People who avoid sea vegetables, as well as dairy, seafood, processed food, and the saltshaker, can become deficient in iodine. Although rare in Western societies, iodine deficiency can cause low thyroid function, goiter, and cretinism.

How Much Is Usually Taken?

Since the introduction of iodized salt, additional sources of iodine, such as kelp, are unnecessary. However, kelp can be consumed as a source of other minerals.

Are There Any Side Effects or Interactions? Extremely high intakes of kelp could provide too much iodine and interfere with normal thyroid function.

Lactase

Lactase is the enzyme in the small intestine that digests lactose (the naturally occurring sugar in milk). A few children and many people after childhood do not produce sufficient lactase, which impairs the body's ability to digest milk. These individuals are **lactose intolerant** (p. 114) and suffer from symptoms including cramps, gas, and **diarrhea** (p. 58).

A simple test for lactose intolerance is to drink at least two glasses of milk on an empty stomach and note any gastrointestinal symptoms that develop in the next 4 hours; repeat the test using several ounces of cheese (which does not contain much lactose). If symptoms result from milk but not cheese, then the person has lactose intolerance. If symptoms occur with both milk and cheese, the person may be allergic to dairy.

Where Is It Found?

Lactase is produced by the body. Dairy products have varying levels of lactose, which affects how much lactase is required for proper digestion. Milk, ice cream, and yogurt contain significant amounts of lactose—although for complex reasons yogurt often doesn't trigger symptoms in lactose-intolerant people.

Lactase Has Been Used in Connection with the Following Conditions*

Ranking	Health Concerns
Primary	Diarrhea (p. 58) (for lactose-intolerant people) Indigestion and heartburn (p. 99) (for lactose-intolerant people) Irritable bowel syndrome (p. 109) (for lactose-intolerant people) Lactose intolerance (p. 114)
*Refer to the Individual Health Concern for Complete Information	

Who Is Likely to Be Deficient?

Only one-third of all people retain the ability to digest lactose into adulthood. Most individuals of Asian, African, and Native American descent are lactose intolerant. In addition, half of Hispanics and about 20 percent of Caucasians do not produce lactase as adults.[1]

How Much Is Usually Taken?

Lactose-reduced milk is available and can be used in the same quantities as regular milk. Lactase drops can be added to regular milk 24 hours before drinking to reduce lactose levels. Lactase drops, capsules, and tablets can also be taken directly, as needed, immediately before a meal containing dairy products. The degree of lactose intolerance varies by individual, so a greater or lesser amount of lactase may be needed to eliminate symptoms of lactose intolerance.

Are There Any Side Effects or Interactions? Lactase is safe and does not produce side effects.

Kelp

Some, but not all, studies suggest that lactose-intolerant individuals absorb less **calcium** (p. 277).[2]

Lecithin/Phosphatidyl Choline/Choline

When medical researchers use the term "lecithin," they are referring to a purified substance called phosphatidyl choline (PC). Supplements labeled as "lecithin" usually contain 10–20% PC. Relatively pure PC supplements are generally labeled as "phosphatidyl choline." PC best duplicates supplements used in medical research.

Choline by itself (without the "phosphatidyl" group) is also available in food and supplements. In high amounts, however, pure choline can make people smell like fish, so it's rarely used, except in the small amounts found in **multivitamin supplements** (p. 314).

What Do They Do? PC acts as a supplier of choline. Choline is now considered an essential nutrient, needed for cell membrane integrity and to facilitate the movement of fats in and out of cells. It is also a component of the neurotransmitter acetylcholine and is needed for normal brain functioning, particularly in infants. For this reason, PC has been used in a number of preliminary studies for a wide variety of neurological and psychiatric disorders.[1] Choline participates in many functions involving cellular components called phospholipids.

Where Are They Found?

Choline, the major constituent of PC, is found in **soybeans** (p. 332), liver, oatmeal, cabbage, and cauliflower. Egg yolks, meat, and some vegetables contain PC. Lecithin (containing 10–20% PC) is added to many processed foods in small amounts, for the purpose of maintaining texture consistency.

Who Is Likely to Be Deficient?

Although choline deficiencies have been artificially induced in people, little is known about human deficiency in the real world.

How Much Is Usually Taken?

Small amounts of choline are present in most **B-complex** (p. 341) and **multivitamin** (p. 314) supplements. **Are There Any Side Effects or Interactions?** At several grams per day, some people will experience abdominal discomfort, **diarrhea** (p. 58), or nausea.

Phosphatidyl Choline Has Been Used in Connection with the Following Conditions*

Ranking	Health Concerns
Secondary	Gallbladder attacks (p. 68) High homocysteine (p. 84) Tardive dyskinesia (p. 157)
Other	Hepatitis (p. 77) High cholesterol (p. 79) Manic depression Liver support

*Refer to the Individual Health Concern for Complete Information

Supplementing straight choline (as opposed to phosphatidyl choline) in large amounts (over 1,000 mg per day) can lead to a fishy odor; PC does not have this effect.

The body uses both PC and **pantothenic acid** (p. 340) to form acetylcholine.

Lipase

Lipase is any enzyme that helps to digest dietary fats.

Where Is It Found?

Lipase is produced by the pancreas and released into the small intestine, where it helps digest fat. Pancreatin contains lipase along with two other groups of enzymes: proteases and amylase.

Lipase Has Been Used in Connection with the Following Conditions*

Ranking	Health Concerns
Primary	Indigestion and heartburn (p. 99) (for pancreatic insufficiency only)
Secondary	Cystic fibrosis
Other	Celiac disease (p. 35) Crohn's disease (p. 48)

*Refer to the Individual Health Concern for Complete Information

Who Is Likely to Be Deficient?

People with pancreatic insufficiency and cystic fibrosis frequently require supplemental lipase and other enzymes. Those with celiac disease or **Crohn's disease** (p. 48) and perhaps some people suffering from **indigestion** (p. 9XX) may be deficient in **pancreatic enzymes** (p. 289) including lipase.[1]

How Much Is Usually Taken?

Lipase, as a digestive aid, is generally accompanied by other enzymes that help digest carbohydrates and

Lipase

protein. In the U.S., pancreatin, which contains lipase, amylase, and proteases, is rated against a government standard. For example, "9X pancreatin" is nine times stronger than the government standard. Each "X" contains 25 USP units of amylase, 2 USP units of lipase, and 25 USP units of proteolytic enzymes. A dose of 1.5 grams of 9X pancreatin (or a higher dose at lower potencies) with each meal can help people with pancreatic insufficiency digest food.

Are There Any Side Effects or Interactions? Lipase does not generally cause any side effects at the amounts listed above.

Lipase or other supplemental enzymes should not be taken with **betaine HCl** (p. 269), or hydrochloric acid, which could destroy the enzymes.

Lutein

Lutein is an **antioxidant** (p. 267) in the carotenoid family (naturally occurring fat-soluble pigments found in plants). It is the primary carotenoid present in the central area of the retina called the macula. Lutein may act as a filter to protect the macula from potentially damaging forms of light. Consequently, lutein appears to be associated with protection from age-related **macular degeneration** (p. 118) (the leading cause of blindness in older adults).

Where Is It Found?

Spinach, kale, collard greens, romaine lettuce, leeks, and peas are good sources of lutein.

Lutein Has Been Used in Connection with the Following Conditions*

Ranking	Health Concerns
Secondary	Macular degeneration (p. 118)
Other	Cataracts (p. 34)
*Refer to the Individual Health Concern for Complete Information	

Who Is Likely to Be Deficient?

While a deficiency has not been identified, people who eat more lutein-containing foods appear to be at lower risk of macular degeneration. One study found that adults with the highest dietary intake of lutein had a 57% decreased risk of macular degeneration compared with those people with the lowest intake, and of the carotenoids, lutein/zeaxanthin are most strongly associated with this protection.[1] In at least one trial, a similar link was suggested between low dietary lutein and increased risk of **cataracts** (p. 34).[2]

How Much Is Usually Taken?

People showing protection from macular degeneration have been reported to have eaten about 6 mg of lutein per day from food. Lutein, in supplemental form, should be taken with food to improve absorption.

Are There Any Side Effects or Interactions? No lutein toxicity has been identified.

Lutein functions together with zeaxanthin, another antioxidant found in the same foods and supplements as lutein.

Lycopene

Lycopene, found primarily in tomatoes, is a member of the carotenoid family—including **beta-carotene** (p. 268) and similar compounds found naturally in food—and has potent **antioxidant** (p. 267) capabilities.

A study conducted by Harvard researchers examined the relationship between carotenoids and the risk of prostate cancer.[1] Of the carotenoids, only lycopene was clearly linked to protection. The men who had the greatest amounts of lycopene (6.5 mg per day) in their diet showed a 21% decreased risk of prostate cancer compared with those eating the least. This report suggests that lycopene may be an important tool in the prevention of prostate cancer.

This study also reported that those who ate more than ten servings per week of tomato-based foods had a 35% decreased risk of prostate cancer compared with those eating less than 1.5 weekly servings. When the researchers looked at only advanced prostate cancer, the high lycopene eaters had an 86% decreased risk (although this did not reach statistical significance due to the small number of cases).

Prior research has associated tomato intake with a reduced rate of prostate cancer.[2] Although lycopene has potentially been linked to reduced risk of prostate cancer, evidence doe not yet suggest it has any effect on **benign prostatic hyperplasia** (BPH) (p. 145). Lycopene is the most abundant carotenoid in the prostate,[3] and high blood levels of lycopene have been linked to prostate cancer prevention.[4] Lycopene is also a more potent inhibitor of human cancer cells than all other carotenoids.[5]

Another study found that for the 25% of people with the greatest tomato intake, the risk for cancers of the gastrointestinal tract was 30–60% lower compared with those who ate fewer tomatoes. These reduced risks were statistically significant.[6] A study of women found that the 75% who ate the least amount of tomatoes had between 3.5 and 4.7 times the risk for cervical intraepithelial neoplasia—precancerous changes of the cervix.[7] Other researchers have also reported evidence suggesting that high dietary lycopene may be linked to protection from **cervical dysplasia** (p. 136).[8] Preliminary evidence also links dietary lycopene with protection from breast cancer.[9]

In Europe, researchers have found a statistically significant association between high dietary lycopene and a 48% lower risk of **heart disease** (p. 32).[10] Lycopene supplementation has also boosted **immune function** (p. 94) in the elderly. In that trial, 15 mg of lycopene per day increased natural killer cell activity by 28% in 12 weeks.[11]

Where Is It Found?

Tomatoes and tomato-containing foods are high in lycopene. In the Harvard study, the only tomato-based food that did not correlate with protection was tomato juice. Evidence suggests that people inaccurately report their intake of juice; moreover, the lycopene in juice may not be well absorbed. Other foods, including watermelon and guava, also contain lycopene.

Lycopene Has Been Used in Connection with the Following Condition*

Ranking	Health Concern
Other	Cancer risk reduction
*Refer to the Individual Health Concern for Complete Information	

Who Is Likely to Be Deficient?

This is unknown, but people who do not eat diets high in tomatoes or tomato products are likely to consume less than optimal amounts.

How Much Is Usually Taken?

The ideal intake of lycopene is currently unknown; however, the men in the Harvard study with the greatest protection against cancer consumed at least 6.5 mg per day.

Are There Any Side Effects or Interactions? No adverse effects have been reported with the use of lycopene.

Lysine

Lysine is an essential **amino acid** (p. 265) needed for growth and to help maintain nitrogen balance in the body. Essential amino acids cannot be made in the body and must be supplied by the diet or supplements. Lysine appears to help the body absorb and conserve calcium (p. 277).[1] Linus Pauling believed that lysine helps maintain healthy blood vessels, an idea based on biochemistry and results from three people with **angina pectoris** (p. 13) who responded to lysine supplementation.[2,3]

Lysine has many functions in the body because it is incorporated into many proteins, each of which is used by the body for a variety of purposes. Lysine interferes with replication of herpesviruses and is therefore often prescribed by nutritionally oriented doctors to people with **cold sores** (p. 39) or genital herpes. A review of the research trials investigating the effects of lysine on people with cold sores shows that most though not all trials support the use of lysine.[4]

Where Is It Found?

Brewer's yeast, legumes, dairy, wheat germ, fish, and meat all contain significant amounts of lysine.

Lysine Has Been Used in Connection with the Following Condition*

Ranking	Health Concerns
Secondary	Cold sores (p. 39)
*Refer to the Individual Health Concern for Complete Information	

Who Is Likely to Be Deficient?

Most people, including vegans (vegetarians who also avoid dairy and eggs), consume adequate amounts of lysine. **Athletes** (p. 20) involved in frequent vigorous exercise have increased need for essential amino acids, although most diets meet these increased needs. The essential amino acid requirements of burn patients may exceed the amount of lysine in the diet.

How Much Is Usually Taken?

Most people do not require lysine supplementation. Nutritionally oriented doctors often suggest that people with recurrent herpes simplex infections take 1,000–3,000 mg of lysine per day.

Are There Any Side Effects or Interactions? In animals, high doses of lysine have been linked to increased risk of **gallstones** (p. 69)[5] and **elevated cholesterol** (p. 79).[6] At supplemental doses, no consistent problems have been reported in humans, though abdominal cramps and transient **diarrhea** (p. 58) have occasionally been reported at very high (15 to 40 grams per day) intakes.[7]

Lysine supplementation increases the aborption of calcium and may reduce its excretion.[8] As a result, some researchers believe that lysine may eventually be shown to have a role in the prevention and treatment of **osteoporosis** (p. 133).[9]

Lysine works with other essential amino acids to maintain growth, lean body mass, and the body's store of nitrogen.

Magnesium

Magnesium is needed for bone, protein, and fatty acid formation, making new cells, activating B vitamins, relaxing muscles, clotting blood, and forming ATP—the energy the body runs on. Insulin secretion and function also require magnesium.

Magnesium also acts in a way related to calcium channel blocker drugs. This effect may be responsible for the fact that under certain circumstances, magnesium has been found to potentially improve vision in people with glaucoma (p. 74) in preliminary research.[1] Similarly, this action might account for magnesium's ability to lower blood pressure (p. 89).[2]

Because magnesium has so many different actions in the body, the exact reasons for some of its clinical effects are difficult to determine. For example, magnesium has reduced hyperactivity (p. 26) in children in preliminary research.[3] Other research suggests that some children with ADD have lowered levels of magnesium. In a preliminary but controlled trial, fifty ADD children with low magnesium (as determined by red blood cell, hair, and serum levels of magnesium) were given 200 mg of magnesium per day for 6 months.[4] Compared with 25 other magnesium-deficient ADD children, those given magnesium supplementation had a significant decrease in hyperactive behavior.

Magnesium levels have been reported to be low in those with chronic fatigue syndrome (CFS) (p. 36), and magnesium injections have been reported to improve symptoms.[5] In another report, oral magnesium supplementation has also improved symptoms in people with CFS who had low magnesium levels, although magnesium injections were sometimes necessary.[6] However, other research reports no evidence of magnesium deficiency in people with CFS.[7,8] The reason for this discrepancy remains unclear. People with CFS considering magnesium supplementation should have their magnesium status checked beforehand by a nutritionally oriented doctor. Only people with magnesium deficiency appear to benefit from this therapy.

Where Is It Found?

Nuts and grains are good sources of magnesium. Beans, dark green vegetables, fish, and meat also contain significant amounts.

Magnesium Has Been Used in Connection with the Following Conditions*

Ranking	Health Concerns
Primary	Celiac disease (p. 35) (if deficient) Congestive heart failure (p. 43) Diabetes (p. 53) Mitral valve prolapse (p. 125)
Secondary	ADD (p. 26) Celiac disease (p. 35) High blood pressure (p. 89) (for people taking depleting diuretics) Migraine headaches (p. 121) Osteoporosis (p. 133) Premenstrual syndrome (p. 141)
Other	Alcohol withdrawal support (p. 6) Anxiety (p. 14) Asthma (p. 15) Athletic performance (p. 20) Autism (p. 27) Chronic fatigue syndrome (p. 36) Chronic obstructive pulmonary disease (COPD) (p. 45) Fibromyalgia (p. 68) Glaucoma (p. 74) High cholesterol (p. 79) Hypoglycemia (p. 92) Intermittent claudication (p. 106) Multiple sclerosis (p. 127) Raynaud's disease (p. 148) Retinopathy (p. 150)

*Refer to the Individual Health Concern for Complete Information

Who Is Likely to Be Deficient?

Magnesium deficiency is common in people taking "potassium-depleting" prescription drugs. Taking too many laxatives can also lead to deficiency. Alcoholism, severe burns, diabetes (p. 53), and heart failure are other potential causes of deficiency.

Almost two-thirds of people in intensive care hospital units have been found to be magnesium deficient.[9] Deficiency is also associated with chronic diarrhea (p. 58), pancreatitis, and other conditions associated with malabsorption.

Fatigue, abnormal heart rhythms, muscle weakness and spasm, depression (p. 50), loss of appetite, listlessness, and potassium (p. 323) depletion can all result from a magnesium deficiency.

Deficiencies of magnesium that are serious enough to cause symptoms should be treated by medical doctors, as they might require intravenous administration of magnesium.[10]

How Much Is Usually Taken?

Most people don't consume enough magnesium. Many nutritionally oriented doctors recommend 250–350 mg per day for adults.

Are There Any Side Effects or Interactions? Taking too much magnesium often leads to **diarrhea** (p. 58). For some people this can happen with amounts as low as 350–500 mg per day. More serious problems can develop with excessive magnesium intake from magnesium-containing laxatives; however, the amounts of magnesium found in nutritional supplements are unlikely to cause such problems. People with kidney disease should not take magnesium supplements without consulting a doctor.

Vitamin B6 (p. 340) increases the amount of magnesium that can enter cells. As a result, these two nutrients are often taken together. Magnesium may compete for absorption with other minerals, particularly **calcium** (p. 277). Taking a **multimineral supplement** (p. 314) avoids this potential problem.

Malic Acid

Malic acid is a naturally occurring organic acid that plays a role in the complex process of deriving ATP—the energy currency that runs the body—from food.

Although uncontrolled research had suggested that the combination of 1,200–2,400 mg per day of malic acid and 300–600 mg of **magnesium** (p. 310) for 8 weeks reduced symptoms of **fibromyalgia** (p. 68),[1] double-blind evidence has shown that malic acid plus magnesium fails to help people with this condition.[2]

Where Is It Found?

Malic acid is found in a wide variety of fruits and vegetables, but the richest source is apples, which is why malic acid is sometimes referred to as "apple acid."

Malic Acid Has Been Used in Connection with the Following Condition*

Ranking	Health Concern
Other	Fibromyalgia (p. 68)

*Refer to the Individual Health Concern for Complete Information

Who Is Likely to Be Deficient?

A deficiency in humans is unlikely, since the body can produce malic acid.

How Much Is Usually Taken?

Healthy people do not need to take malic acid as a supplement. Research has been conducted with 1,200–2,400 mg of malic acid in combination with 300–600 mg of elemental **magnesium** (p. 310).

Are There Any Side Effects or Interactions? Current research does not indicate any adverse effects from the use of malic acid in moderate amounts.

Manganese

Manganese is needed for healthy skin, bone, and cartilage formation, as well as glucose tolerance. It also helps activate superoxide dismutase (SOD)—an important **antioxidant** (p. 267) enzyme.

Where Is It Found?

Nuts, wheat germ, wheat bran, leafy green vegetables, beet tops, pineapple, and seeds are all good sources of manganese.

Manganese Has Been Used in Connection with the Following Conditions*

Ranking	Health Concerns
Secondary	Tardive dyskinesia (p. 157)
Other	Hypoglycemia (p. 92) Minor injuries (p. 122)

*Refer to the Individual Health Concern for Complete Information

Who Is Likely to Be Deficient?

Many people consume less than the 2.5–5 mg of manganese currently considered safe and adequate. Nonetheless, clear deficiencies are rare. Individuals with **osteoporosis** (p. 133) sometimes have low blood levels of manganese, suggestive of deficiency.[1]

How Much Is Usually Taken?

Whether most people would benefit from manganese supplementation remains unclear. The 5–15 mg often found in a high-potency **multivitamin/mineral supplement** (p. 314) is generally considered to be a reasonable level for those wishing to supplement manganese.

Are There Any Side Effects or Interactions? Amounts found in supplements (5–20 mg) have not been linked with any toxicity. Excessive intake of manganese can lead to the rare side effects of dementia and psychiatric symptoms. Preliminary research suggests that individuals with cirrhosis may not be able to properly excrete manganese; until more is known, these people should not supplement manganese.[2]

Several minerals, such as **calcium** (p. 277) and **iron** (p. 304), and possibly **zinc** (p. 346) reduce the absorption of manganese.[3] Zinc and **copper** (p. 285) work together with manganese to activate superoxide dismutase.

Medium Chain Triglycerides

Medium chain triglycerides (MCT) are a class of fatty acids. Their chemical composition is of a shorter length than the long-chain fatty acids present in most other fats and oils, which accounts for their name. They are also different from other fats in that they have a slightly lower calorie content[1] and they are more rapidly absorbed and burned as energy, resembling carbohydrate more than fat.[2]

MCT has been shown to increase calorie burning compared with other fats.[3,4] However, researchers estimate that half of the calories in the diet would have to be eaten as MCT for significant **weight loss** (p. 165) to occur.[5] A weight-loss study using MCT for 24% of total calories found no greater weight loss after 3 months than when regular fat was used.[6] Therefore, MCT does not appear to help people lose weight in any meaningful way.

Because MCT is more rapidly used for energy than other fats, some **athletes** (p. 20) have been interested in its use, especially during prolonged endurance exercise.[7] However, no effect on carbohydrate sparing or endurance exercise performance has been shown with moderate amounts of MCT (30–45 grams).[8,9] Trials using very large amounts (about 85 grams) have produced conflicting results. One study found increased performance when MCT was added to a 10% carbohydrate solution,[10] and another study actually reported decreased performance, probably due to gastrointestinal distress, in athletes using MCT.[11]

Because some short-term studies have shown that MCT lowers blood glucose levels, a group of researchers investigated the use of MCT to treat people with type II **diabetes** (p. 53) mellitus.[12] In nonhospitalized diabetics who consumed MCT for an average of 17.5% of their total calorie intake for 30 days, MCT did not improve diabetic control by most measures.[13]

Where Are They Found?

Medium chain triglycerides are found in coconut oil, palm kernel oil, and butter.

Who Is Likely to Be Deficient?

Most people consume adequate or excessive fat in their diets, so extra fat intake as medium chain triglycerides is unnecessary.

How Much Is Usually Taken?

The best amount of medium chain triglycerides to take is currently unknown. Athletes will not benefit from less than 50 grams during exercise; larger amounts may possibly help some, but may also impair performance if not combined with carbohydrate.

Are There Any Side Effects or Interactions? Consuming medium chain triglycerides on an empty stomach can lead to gastrointestinal upset. Anyone with cirrhosis or other liver problems should not use medium chain triglycerides. Two reports suggest that MCT may raise serum **cholesterol** (p. 79) and/or **triglycerides** (p. 85).[14,15]

Melatonin

Melatonin is a natural hormone that regulates the human biological clock. Double-blind research with young adults shows that melatonin facilitates **sleep** (p. 105).[1] Another study of healthy, young adults reports that melatonin significantly shortens the time needed to go to sleep, reduces the number of night awakenings, and improves sleep quality.[2] Other researchers report that the time needed to get to sleep is reduced with melatonin but other parameters of sleep do not improve.[3]

Melatonin is also helpful in relieving symptoms of **jet lag** (p. 111). One double-blind trial, involving fifty-two international flight crew members taking either melatonin or a placebo for 3 days before and 5 days after an international flight, found that the melatonin significantly reduced symptoms of jet lag and resulted in a quicker recovery of preflight energy levels and alertness.[4]

Less than 1 mg of melatonin has lowered pressure within the eyes of healthy people,[5] but studies have not yet been published on the effects of using melatonin with people who have **glaucoma** (p. 74). Melatonin might help some people suffering from **depression** (p. 50). Preliminary double-blind research suggests that low levels of melatonin (0.125 mg taken twice per day) may reduce winter depression.[6]

When some people take melatonin to treat sleep disorders, chronic tension headaches are relieved.[7] Melatonin has also relieved cluster headaches in double-blind research,[8] though how melatonin is helping these people remains unclear. Melatonin also regulates **immunity** (p. 94). One group of doctors reported two successfully treated cases of sarcoidosis that it attributed to immune modulation.[9] Also because of its effects on the immune system, melatonin has been given to people with cancer in many research trials. Low blood levels of melatonin are associated with an increased risk of uterine cancer.[10] Melatonin has significantly reduced the level of prostate specific antigen (a marker for cancer) in prostate cancer patients.[11] Melatonin inhibits breast cancer cells in test tubes[12] and has put some women with breast cancer into remission in preliminary research.[13] Melatonin supplementation has improved disease-free survival in people with melanoma[14] and increased survival in people with brain cancer[15] and lung cancer.[16]

In a double-blind trial, people who had difficulty sleeping as a result of **tinnitus** (p. 158) were better able to sleep if given 3 mg melatonin per night for 1 month rather than placebo.[17] Although melatonin did not reduce overall symptom scores for tinnitus, people in this trial with higher symptom scores did appear to obtain some benefit.

Where Is It Found?

Melatonin is produced by the pineal gland, located within the brain. Levels of melatonin in the body correspond with the cycles of night and day, with the highest melatonin levels produced at night. Melatonin appears in foods only in trace amounts.

Melatonin Has Been Used in Connection with the Following Conditions*

Ranking	Health Concerns
Primary	Jet lag (p. 111)
Secondary	Insomnia (p. 105) Tinnitus (p. 158) (insomnia associated)
Other	Glaucoma (p. 74)

*Refer to the Individual Health Concern for Complete Information

Who Is Likely to Be Deficient?

The body produces less melatonin with advancing age, which may explain why elderly people often have difficulty sleeping[18] and why melatonin supplements improve sleep in the elderly.[19] Adults with **insomnia** (p. 105) have lower melatonin levels.[20] Frequent travelers and shift workers are also likely to benefit from melatonin for the resynchronization of their sleep schedules,[21] though a melatonin "deficiency" as such does not exist for these people.

How Much Is Usually Taken?

Normally, the body makes melatonin for several hours per night—an effect best duplicated with timed-release supplements. Studies using timed-release melatonin have reported good results.[22] Many doctors of natural medicine suggest 1–3 mg of melatonin taken 1 to 2 hours before bedtime. Studies with people suffering from sarcoidosis or cancer have used very high amounts of melatonin—typically 20 mg per night.

Such levels should never be taken without the supervision of a doctor who uses natural medicine. Melatonin should not be taken during the day.

Are There Any Side Effects or Interactions? Melatonin is associated with few side effects; however, morning grogginess, undesired drowsiness, sleepwalking, and disorientation have been reported. Researchers have hypothesized that certain individuals should not use melatonin supplements, including pregnant or breast-feeding women, individuals with **depression** (p. 50) or schizophrenia, and those with autoimmune disease, including **lupus** (p. 115), at least until more is known.

In a group of children suffering from neurological disorders, 1–5 mg of melatonin per night led to an increase in the rate of seizures despite the fact that sleep improved.[23] Until more is known, children with neurological conditions should take melatonin only under medical supervision.

Although a wide variety of side effects have been attributed to melatonin, including inhibition of fertility and sex drive, damage to the eye, formation of rudimentary breasts in men, and even psychosis, these associations have not been supported by solid evidence.[24,25] Because none of these claims have been well documented or independently confirmed, these problems were likely not due to melatonin.

Though most research reports that melatonin improves the quality of sleep, at least one trial has found that four of fifteen men given melatonin had their sleep patterns disturbed by supplemental melatonin.[26]

Special United Kingdom considerations: Melatonin is either not available or may require a prescription. People should check with their nutritionally oriented physician.

Methionine

Methionine is one of the essential **amino acids** (p. 265) (building blocks of protein). It supplies **sulfur** (p. 334) and other compounds required by the body for normal metabolism and growth. Methionine also belongs to a group of compounds called lipotropics; others in this group include **choline** (p. 307), **inositol** (p. 303), and betaine.

Persons with **AIDS** (p. 87) have low levels of methionine. Some researchers suggest that this may explain some aspects of the disease process,[1,2,3] especially the deterioration that occurs in the nervous system that can cause symptoms including dementia.[4,5] A preliminary study has suggested that methionine (6 grams per day) may improve memory recall in persons with AIDS-related nervous system degeneration.[6]

Other preliminary studies have suggested that methionine (5 grams per day) may help treat some symptoms of Parkinson's disease.[7]

Methionine (2 grams per day) in combination with several antioxidants reduced pain and recurrences of attacks of pancreatitis in a small but well-controlled trial.[8]

Where Is It Found?

Meat, fish, and dairy are all good sources of methionine.

Methionine Has Been Used in Connection with the Following Conditions*

Ranking	Health Concerns
Secondary	Pancreatitis
Other	HIV support (p. 87) Liver support Parkinson's disease

*Refer to the Individual Health Concern for Complete Information

Who Is Likely to Be Deficient?

Most people consume plenty of methionine through a typical diet. Lower intakes during pregnancy have been associated with neural tube defects in newborns, but the significance of this is not yet clear.[9]

How Much Is Usually Taken?

Amino acid requirements vary according to body weight; however, average-size adults require approximately 800–1,000 mg of methionine per day—an amount exceeded by most Western diets. Therefore, most people would not benefit from methionine supplementation.

Are There Any Side Effects or Interactions? Animal studies suggest that diets high in methionine, in the presence of B vitamin deficiencies, may increase the risk for **atherosclerosis** (p. 17) (hardening of the arteries) by increasing blood levels of **cholesterol** (p. 79) and a compound called **homocysteine** (p. 84).[10] This idea has not yet been tested in humans. Excessive methionine intake, in the presence of inadequate intake of **folic acid** (p. 297), **vitamin B$_6$** (p. 340), and **vitamin B$_{12}$** (p. 337), can increase the conversion of methionine to homocysteine—a substance linked to **heart disease** (p. 32) and stroke. However, whether this relationship creates a significant hazard for humans taking supplemental methionine has not been established. Supplementation of up to 2 grams methionine daily for long periods of time has not produced any serious side effects.[11]

Molybdenum

Molybdenum is an essential trace mineral. It is needed for the proper function of certain enzyme-dependent processes, including the metabolism of **iron** (p. 304). Preliminary evidence indicates that molybdenum, through its involvement in detoxifying sulfites, might reduce the risk of sulfite-reactive **asthma** (p. 15) attacks.[1] However, a nutritionally oriented physician should be involved in the evaluation and treatment of sulfite sensitivity.

Where Is It Found?

The amount of molybdenum in plant foods varies significantly and is dependent upon the mineral content of the soil. The best sources of this mineral are beans, legumes, dark green leafy vegetables, and grains. Hard tap water can also supply molybdenum to the diet.

Molybdenum Has Been Used in Connection with the Following Condition*

Ranking	Health Concern
Other	Asthma (p. 15)

*Refer to the Individual Health Concern for Complete Information

Who Is Likely to Be Deficient?

Although molybdenum is an essential mineral, no deficiencies have been reported in humans.

How Much Is Usually Taken?

No recommended dietary allowance (RDA) has been established for molybdenum. The estimated range recommended by the Food and Nutrition Board as safe and adequate is 75–250 mcg per day for adults.

Are There Any Side Effects or Interactions? Molybdenum is considered safe through a wide range of intakes (up to 15 mg per day), but it can interfere with the absorption of **copper** (p. 255). Molybdenum is needed to convert purine to uric acid, and excessive intake could, in rare cases, cause **gout** (p. 75)-like symptoms, such as joint pain and swelling.

Multiple Vitamin/Mineral

Multiple vitamin/mineral (MVM) supplements contain a variable number of essential and/or non-essential nutrients. Their primary purpose is to provide a convenient way to take a variety of supplemental nutrients from a single product, in order to prevent vitamin or mineral deficiencies, as well as to achieve higher intakes of nutrients believed to be of benefit above typical dietary levels. Many of these nutrients will be briefly discussed here; however, for more information, refer to individual nutrient sections.

An MVM supplement should not take the place of a healthful, well-balanced diet, but it will help prevent deficiencies that often arise. People may consume diets that are deficient in one or more nutrients for a variety of reasons. The typical Western diet often provides less than adequate amounts of several essential vitamins and minerals.[1] **Weight-loss** (p. 165), pure vegetarian, macrobiotic, and several other diets can also place some people at risk of deficiencies that vary with the type of diet. Aging, some medications, and certain health conditions can affect appetite, which may reduce nutrient intake.

Many MVMs contain at least 100% of the U.S. Recommended Dietary Allowance (USRDA) of all vitamins that have been assigned an RDA value. Mineral levels may be lower, or in the case of high potency MVMs, most or all mineral levels may also be at 100% of USRDA. This will include vitamins **A** (p. 336), **B-complex** (p. 341), **C** (p. 341), **D** (p. 343), **E** (p. 344), **K** (p. 345) and the minerals **calcium** (p. 277), **magnesium** (p. 310), **zinc** (p. 346), **iodine** (p. 303), **selenium** (p. 331), and possibly **iron** (p. 304) (see below). Phosphorus is another essential dietary mineral, but it is so abundant in the human diet that deficiencies are virtually unknown and it does not need to be included in an MVM formula. Many essential nutrients for which RDAs have not been established should also be included in ranges considered to be adequate and safe. These would include **biotin** (p. 272) (30–100 mcg per day), **pantothenic acid** (p. 340) (4 to 7 mg per day), **copper** (p. 285) (1.5 to 3.0 mg per day), **manganese** (p. 311) (2 to 5 mg per day), **chromium** (p. 282) (50 to 200 mcg per day), and **molybdenum** (p. 314) (75 to 250 mcg per day).[2] **Potassium** (p. 323) is an unusual case, as adequate amounts of potassium cannot by law be sold in nonprescription products. Thus potassium, when included in an MVM formula, represents only a trivial amount.

MVMs that contain iron should be taken only by people who are known to be iron deficient or have a history of frequent past iron deficiencies. Iron deficiency is not uncommon among many groups of people, including the following:

- Some groups of vegetarians
- People with **parasitic infections** (p. 137)
- Premenopausal women
- **Marathon runners** (p. 20)
- People with **Crohn's disease** (p. 48) and other conditions causing malabsorption
- People who regularly take aspirin and related drugs
- People who have donated blood recently
- People with conditions that cause gastrointestinal bleeding such as inflammatory bowel disease, **peptic ulcer** (p. 138), and **hemorrhoids** (p. 77)

Nonetheless, many people in these groups are not iron deficient. Therefore, people should be tested for iron deficiency by a health-care professional before assuming that an iron-containing MVM is appropriate. Excessive iron intake has been associated in some studies with **heart disease** (p. 323),[3] some cancers,[4] **diabetes** (p. 53),[5] increased risk of **infection** (p. 101),[6] and exacerbation of **rheumatoid arthritis** (p. 151).[7] While none of these links has yet been proven, people should avoid iron-containing MVMs unless diagnosed with an iron deficiency.

Some nutrients may be beneficial at levels above what is possible to obtain from diet alone, and an MVM formula can provide these levels as well. For example, a **vitamin E** (p. 344) intake of 100 to 800 IU per day has been associated with prevention of **coronary artery disease** (p. 17),[8,9,10] but the average Western diet provides only about 10 to 15 IU per day. Other nutrients that may be useful to most people in larger amounts include **vitamin C** (p. 341), **folic acid** (p. 297), and **calcium** (p. 277). Large amounts of vitamins B_1 (p. 337), B_2 (p. 338), B_3 (p. 339), and **pantothenic acid** (p. 340) are usually included in MVM formulas because of their low cost, but there is no scientific justification for these high levels.

The common inclusion of the nonessential nutrient **beta-carotene** (p. 268) in MVMs remains speculative. The synthetic beta-carotene found in most MVMs clearly does not prevent cancer and may increase risk of lung cancer in smokers (see **Beta-Carotene** [p. 268]). Therefore, it should be avoided, at least until more is known, especially about its use by smokers. However, natural beta-carotene and several other carotenoids may be helpful in preventing certain diseases, including some cancers.[11,12,13] Beta-carotene also provides a nontoxic form of **vitamin A** (p. 336). Increasingly, natural beta-carotene and several other carotenoids are found in better MVMs.

Another class of nonessential nutrients is the **flavonoids** (p. 267), which have **antioxidant** (p. 267) and other properties that have been reported by some,[14] though not all,[15] researchers to be linked with a reduced risk of heart disease. MVM supplements also frequently include other nonessential nutrients of uncertain benefit in the amounts supplied, such as **choline** (p. 307), **inositol** (p. 303), and various **amino acids** (p. 265).

What About "One-Per-Day" Multiples?

One-per-day multiples are primarily **B-complex** (p. 341) vitamins, with **vitamin A** (p. 336) and **vitamin D** (p. 343) sometimes being high and other times being low potency. The rest of the formula tends to be low potency. It does not take much of some of the minerals—for example, **copper** (p. 285), **zinc** (p. 346), and **iron** (p. 304)—to offer 100% or more of what people normally require, so these minerals may appear at reasonable levels in a one-per-day MVM.

One-per-day MVMs do not provide significant amounts of most nutrients that people eating a Western diet are most likely to benefit from supplemental amounts of, such as vitamin E, **calcium** (p. 277), **magnesium** (p. 310), or vitamin C. One-per-day MVMs should therefore not be viewed as a way to "cover all bases" in the way that high potency MVMs requiring 6 or more pills per day are viewed.

How Many Tablets or Capsules Are Required?

Because one-per-day formulas are hard to balance with adequate minerals and the key **vitamin C** (p. 341) and **vitamin E** (p. 344), multiples requiring several capsules or tablets per day are preferable. A one-a-day MVM may appear convenient, but is not likely to provide all necessary nutrients at optimal amounts. A complete MVM formula will require a daily intake of several tablets because useful amounts of all important nutrients cannot fit into fewer pills. For example, the RDA for calcium is at least 800 mg per day, an amount that alone requires several tablets or capsules. In general, about 6 tablets or capsules are required to fit all that is in the one-per-day plus 800 to 1,000 mg of calcium, 350 to 500 mg of magnesium, and reasonable amounts of C (300 to 1,000 mg) and E (400 IU).

With 2 to 6 per day multiples, intake of pills should be spread out over the day, instead of taking them all at one sitting. The amount of vitamins and minerals can be easily increased or decreased by taking more or fewer of the multiple.

Which Is Better—Capsule or Tablet?

Multiples are available as a powder inside a hard-shell pull-apart capsule, as a liquid inside a soft-gelatin capsule, or as a tablet.

Most multiples have all the ingredients mixed together. Sometimes the B vitamins react with the rest of the ingredients in the capsule or tablet. This reaction, which is sped up in the presence of moisture or heat, can cause the B vitamins to "bleed" through the tablet or capsule, discoloring it and also making the multiple "smell." While the multiple is still safe and effective, the smell is off-putting and usually not very well tolerated. Liquid multiples in a soft-gel capsule—or tablets or capsules that are kept dry and cool—don't have this problem.

Some people find capsules easier to swallow. This is often a function of size. Capsules are usually not as large as a tablet.

Some people prefer vegetarian multiples. While some capsules are made from vegetarian sources, most come from animal gelatin. Vegetarians need to carefully read the label to ensure they are getting a vegetarian product.

One concern people have with tablets is whether they will break down. Properly made tablets and capsules will both dissolve readily in the stomach.

What About Timed Release?

Some multiples are in timed-release form. The theory is that releasing vitamins and minerals slowly into the body over a period of time is better than releasing all the nutrients at once. Except for work done on vitamin C—some of which showed timed-release C was better absorbed than non-timed-release—research on this question has been lacking.

What About Nutrient Interactions?

Another area of controversy is whether all the nutrients in a multiple would be better utilized if they were taken separately. While certain nutrients compete with each other for absorption, this is also the case when the nutrients are supplied in food. For example, **magnesium** (p. 310), **zinc** (p. 346), and **calcium** (p. 277) compete; **copper** (p. 285) and zinc also compete. However, the body is designed to cope with this problem, and taking many different pills at different times is awkward and unnecessary.

How About Chewables?

Unfortunately, multiples do not taste very good. In order to make chewable multiples palatable, whether for children or adults, some compromises must be made. First, bad-tasting ingredients must be reduced or eliminated. Second, the rest of the ingredients must be masked with a sweetener.

Unless an artificial sweetener like aspartame (Nutra Sweet) or saccharine is used, the only sweeteners available are sugars. Generally, sugar is sugar (sucrose in white table sugar or fructose from fruit), and not having it in a dietary supplement would be preferable. However, xylitol, a natural sugar rarely used in chewables because it is relatively expensive, does not cause tooth decay or other known problems.

Some chewables, such as **vitamin C** (p. 341), contain more sugar than any other ingredient. In such products, the sweetener should be listed as the first ingredient, but often isn't. This means care needs to be exercised when reading labels about chewable vitamins. If it tastes sweet, it contains sugar or a synthetic sweetener.

When Should I Take My Multiple?

The best time to take vitamins or minerals is with meals. Multiples taken between meals sometimes cause stomach upset and are likely not as well absorbed.

N-Acetyl Cysteine (NAC)

N-acetyl cysteine (NAC) is an altered form of the **amino acid** (p. 265) **cysteine** (p. 286), which is commonly found in food and synthesized by the body. NAC helps break down mucus. Double-blind research has found that NAC supplements improved symptoms in individuals with bronchitis.[1,2]

NAC helps the body synthesize glutathione—an important **antioxidant** (p. 267). In animals, the antioxidant activity of NAC protects the liver from exposure to several toxic chemicals. NAC also protects the body from acetaminophen toxicity and is used at very high levels in hospitals for that purpose.

Where Is It Found?

Cysteine, the amino acid from which NAC is derived, is found in most high-protein foods. NAC is not found in the diet.

Who Is Likely to Be Deficient?

Deficiencies of NAC have not been defined and may not exist. Deficiencies of the related amino acid cysteine have been reported in **HIV-infected** (p. 87) patients.[3]

How Much Is Usually Taken?

Healthy people do not need to supplement NAC. Optimal levels of supplementation remain unknown, though much of the research uses 250 to 1,500 mg per day.

N-Acetyl Cysteine Has Been Used in Connection with the Following Conditions*

Ranking	Health Concerns
Primary	Bronchitis Chronic obstructive pulmonary disease (p. 45)
Secondary	Emphysema Gastritis (p. 71) HIV support (p. 87)
*Refer to the Individual Health Concern for Complete Information	

Are There Any Side Effects or Interactions? When NAC is taken by mouth, one trial reported nausea, vomiting, headache, dry mouth, dizziness, or abdominal pain, in 19% of people in the study.[4] These symptoms have not been consistently reported by other researchers, however.

One small study found that daily amounts of 1.2 grams or more could lead to oxidative damage.[5] Extremely large amounts of cysteine, the amino acid from which NAC is derived, may be toxic to nerve cells in rats.

NAC may increase urinary zinc excretion.[6] Therefore, supplemental **zinc** (p. 346) and **copper** (p. 285) should be added when supplementing with NAC for extended periods.

NADH (Nicotinamide Adenine Dinucleotide)

NADH is the active coenzyme form of **vitamin B3** (p. 339). It plays an essential role in the energy production of every human cell. In the brain, increased NADH concentrations may result in improved production of essential neurotransmitters.[1]

Large uncontrolled studies using oral or injected NADH to treat Parkinson's disease showed reductions in physical disability and in the need for medication,[2,3] but a small, controlled, short-term trial using injections of NADH found no significant effects.[4] A small uncontrolled study showed that oral NADH improved mental function in people with **Alzheimer's disease** (p. 11).[5] Preliminary research suggests that NADH may also help people with **depression**[6] (p. 50) or **chronic fatigue syndrome** (p. 36).[7] These promising results come from research conducted by the inventor of the oral NADH supplement and require independent confirmation.

Where Is It Found?

NADH is found in the muscle tissue of fish, poultry, and cattle, as well as in food products made with

Octacosanol

NADH Has Been Used in Connection with the Following Conditions*

Ranking	Health Concerns
Other	Alzheimer's disease (p. 11) Chronic fatigue syndrome (p. 36) Depression (p. 50) Parkinson's disease

*Refer to the Individual Health Concern for Complete Information

yeast. It is also found as a supplement, although it is not widely available.

Who Is Likely to Be Deficient?

NADH deficiency is known to occur only in the presence of **vitamin B₃** (p. 339) deficiency, which is rare in Western society except in some alcoholics.

How Much Is Usually Taken?

To date, researchers have used 10 mg per day, taken with water only, on an empty stomach.

Are There Any Side Effects or Interactions? Clinical studies of NADH using oral or intravenous administration have reported no side effects with up to 1 year or more of use. Longer-term use has not been evaluated.

Octacosanol

Octacosanol is a waxy substance naturally present in some plant oils and is the primary component of sugar cane extract called policosanol. In several well-controlled studies from Cuba, policosanol, at 10 to 20 mg per day has been reported to lower **LDL cholesterol** (p. 79) (the "bad" cholesterol) levels 21 to 29% while raising HDL cholesterol (the "good" cholesterol) levels 8 to 15%, although it does not affect triglyceride levels.[1,2,3,4,5] Smaller amounts (5 mg per day) have produced similar effects on LDL but no effect on HDL.[6,7] Policosanol appears to work primarily by inhibiting the liver's production of cholesterol.[8] In addition, policosanol may help **atherosclerosis** (p. 17) that affects arteries of the neck.[9]

Octacosanol-containing wheat germ oil was investigated long ago as an ergogenic (**exercise performance** [p. 20] -promoting) agent. These preliminary studies found that octacosanol had promising effects on endurance, reaction time, and other measures of exercise capacity.[10] In a more recent controlled trial, 1,000 mcg per day of octacosanol for 8 weeks was found to improve grip strength and visual reaction time, but had no effect on chest strength, auditory reaction time, or endurance.[11]

Where Is It Found?

Octacosanol is a waxy substance found in vegetable oils and sugarcane *(Saccharum officinarum)*. Another compound, called policosanol, contains several similar compounds, including a large proportion of octacosanol.

Octacosanol Has Been Used in Connection with the Following Conditions*

Ranking	Health Concerns
Secondary	Atherosclerosis (p. 17) High cholesterol (p. 79)
Other	Athletic performance (p. 20)

*Refer to the Individual Health Concern for Complete Information

Who Is Likely to Be Deficient?

Because octacosanol is not an essential bodily constituent, deficiencies do not occur.

How Much Is Usually Taken?

When octacosanol is taken as part of policosanol, 5 to 10 mg of policosanol is taken twice each day with meals. For exercise performance, 1 mg per day of octacosanol has been used.

Are There Any Side Effects or Interactions? Long-term human studies using doses up to twice the typical therapeutic dose (that is, 20 mg each day) have not shown any negative effects.[12]

Ornithine

Ornithine, an **amino acid** (p. 265), is manufactured by the body when another amino acid, **arginine** (p. 268), is metabolized during the production of urea (a constituent of urine). Animal research has suggested that ornithine, along with arginine, may promote muscle-building activity in the body by increasing levels of anabolic (growth-promoting) hormones such as insulin and growth hormone. However, most human research does not support these claims at reasonable intake levels.[1,2,3] One study that did demonstrate increased growth hormone with oral ornithine used very high amounts (an average of 13 grams/day) and reported many gastrointestinal side effects.[4] One controlled study reported greater increases in lean body mass and strength after 5 weeks of intensive strength training in **athletes** (p. 20) taking 1 gram per day each of arginine and ornithine compared to a group doing the exercise but taking placebo.[5] These findings require independent confirmation.

Where Is It Found?

As with amino acids in general, ornithine is predominantly found in meat, fish, dairy, and eggs. Western diets typically provide 5 grams per day. The body also produces ornithine.

Ornithine Has Been Used in Connection with the Following Condition*

Ranking	Health Concerns
Other	Athletic performance (p. 20) (for body composition and strength)

*Refer to the Individual Health Concern for Complete Information

Who Is Likely to Be Deficient?

Since ornithine is produced by the body, a deficiency of this nonessential amino acid is unlikely, though depletion can occur during growth or pregnancy, and after severe trauma or malnutrition.[6]

How Much Is Usually Taken?

Most people would not benefit from ornithine supplementation. In human research involving ornithine, several grams are typically used per day, sometimes combined with arginine.

Are There Any Side Effects or Interactions? No side effects have been reported with the use of ornithine, except for gastrointestinal distress with intakes over 10 grams per day.

The presence of arginine is needed to produce ornithine in the body, so higher levels of this amino acid should increase ornithine production.

Ornithine Alpha-Ketoglutarate (OKG)

The amino acids **ornithine** (p. 265) and **glutamine** (p. 300) are combined to form ornithine alpha-ketoglutarate (OKG). OKG has been shown to improve protein retention, **wound repair** (p. 167), and **immune function** (p. 94) in hospitalized patients, partly by increasing levels of anabolic (growth-promoting) hormones such as insulin and growth hormone.[1] Nonhospitalized elderly persons have benefited from 10 grams per day of OKG as they recovered from various illnesses or surgery, showing improved appetite, weight gain, muscle growth, reduced need for medical care, and improved quality of life in a large, well-controlled trial.[2] No studies on muscle growth in athletes using OKG have been published.

Where Is It Found?

Although the amino acids that comprise OKG are present in protein foods such as meat, poultry, and fish, the OKG compound is found only in supplements.

OKG Has Been Used in Connection with the Following Condition*

Ranking	Health Concerns
Secondary	Wound healing (p. 167)

*Refer to the Individual Health Concern for Complete Information

Who Is Likely to Be Deficient?

A deficiency of OKG has not been reported.

How Much Is Usually Taken?

Optimal levels remain unknown, though 10 grams per day has been used in research studies.

Are There Any Side Effects or Interactions? No side effects have been reported with the use of OKG.

No clear interaction between OKG and any nutrients has been established.

PABA (Paraaminobenzoic Acid)

PABA is the abbreviation for paraaminobenzoic acid, a compound that is an essential nutrient for microorganisms and some animals, but has not yet been shown to be essential for people. PABA is loosely considered by some to be a member of the vitamin B-complex, though its actions differ widely from other B vitamins. PABA has been reported to enhance the effects of cortisone.[1] It may also prevent or even reverse accumulation of abnormal fibrous tissue.

An isolated trial published in 1942 reported that twelve of sixteen **infertile women** (p. 102) were able to become pregnant after supplementing with 100 mg of PABA taken 4 times per day for 3 to 7 months.[2] The effect of PABA on fertility has not been studied in modern research.

Researchers have attempted to discover whether large amounts of PABA would be helpful in various connective tissue disorders. Although uncontrolled studies have reported that PABA (12 grams per day) was helpful to people with scleroderma,[3,4,5] a placebo-controlled trial found supplementation with PABA did not lead to improvement.[6]

Older published reports of uncontrolled investigations suggest that PABA may be helpful in a variety of conditions, including dermatomyositis,[7] Peyronie's disease (accumulation of abnormal fibrous tissue in the penis),[8] pemphigus (a severe blistering disease),[9] and **vitiligo** (a disorder in which patches of skin lose their pigmentation) (p. 164).[10] However, PABA was reported to cause vitiligo in one report.[11]

Older preliminary reports found that PABA darkened gray hair in a minority of elderly (but not younger) individuals.[12] In these trials, between 200 and 600 mg of PABA was taken per day for several months, in some cases accompanied by other B vitamins. At least one study failed to show any effect of PABA on darkening gray hair.[13] Therefore, the evidence supporting the use of PABA as a way to return gray hair to its original color remains very weak.

Where Is It Found?

PABA is found in grains and foods of animal origin.

Who Is Likely to Be Deficient?

Deficiencies of PABA have not been described in humans, and most nutritionists do not consider it an essential nutrient.

PABA Has Been Used in Connection with the Following Conditions*

Ranking	Health Concerns
Other	Dermatomyositis
	Infertility (female) (p. 102)
	Pemphigus
	Peyronie's disease
	Scleroderma
	Vitiligo
*Refer to the Individual Health Concern for Complete Information	

How Much Is Usually Taken?

Small amounts of PABA are present in some **B-complex vitamins** (p. 341) and **multi-vitamin formulas** (p. 314). The amount of PABA used for the conditions described above ranges from 300 mg per day and up to 12 grams per day for autoimmune, connective tissue, or skin disorders. Anyone taking more than 400 mg of PABA per day should consult a nutritionally oriented physician.

Are There Any Side Effects or Interactions? No serious side effects have been reported with 300 to 400 mg per day. Larger amounts (such as 8 grams per day or more) may cause low blood sugar, rash, fever, and (on rare occasions) liver damage.[14] One report exists of vitiligo appearing after ingestion of large amounts of PABA,[15] and use of amounts over 20 grams per day in small children has resulted in deaths.[16]

No interactions between PABA and other nutrients have been reported. However, PABA interferes with sulfa drugs (a class of antibiotics) and therefore should not be taken when these medications are being used.

L-Phenylalanine and D, L-Phenylalanine (DLPA)

L-phenylalanine serves as a building block for the various proteins that are produced in the body. L-phenylalanine can be converted to **L-tyrosine** (p. 335) (another **amino acid** [p. 265]) and subsequently to L-dopa, norepinephrine, and epinephrine. L-phenylalanine can also be converted (through a separate pathway) to phenylethylamine, a substance that occurs naturally in the brain and appears to elevate mood.

D-phenylalanine is not normally found in the body and cannot be converted to **L-tyrosine** (p. 335), L-dopa, or norepinephrine. As a result, D-phenylalanine is converted primarily to phenylethylamine (the potential mood elevator). D-phenylalanine also appears to influence certain chemicals in the brain that relate to pain sensation.

DLPA is a mixture of the essential amino acid L-phenylalanine and its mirror image D-phenylalanine. DLPA (or the D- or L-form alone) has been used to treat **depression** (p. 50).[1,2] D-phenylalanine may be helpful for some individuals with Parkinson's disease.[3] D-phenylalanine has been used to treat chronic pain—including **osteoarthritis** (p. 130, 562) and **rheumatoid arthritis** (p. 151)—with both positive[4] and negative[5] results. For conditions where D-phenylalanine alone has been shown to be effective, DLPA should also work, as it contains 50% D-phenylalanine.

Where Are They Found?

L-phenylalanine is found in most foods that contain protein. D-phenylalanine does not normally occur in food. However, when phenylalanine is synthesized in the laboratory, half appears in the L-form and the other half in the D-form. These two compounds can be separated. However, the combination supplement (DLPA) is often used because both components exert different health-enhancing effects.

Who Is Likely to Be Deficient?

Individuals whose diets are very low in protein may develop a deficiency of L-phenylalanine, although this is believed to be very uncommon. However, one does not necessarily have to be deficient in L-phenylalanine in order to benefit from a DLPA supplement.

Phenylalanine or DLPA Have Been Used in Connection with the Following Conditions*

Ranking	Health Concerns
Secondary	Depression (p. 50) (phenylalanine and DLPA)
Other	Alcohol withdrawal support (p. 6) (DLPA) Osteoarthritis (p. 130) (D-phenylalanine) Rheumatoid arthritis (p. 157) (DLPA) Vitiligo

*Refer to the Individual Health Concern for Complete Information

How Much Is Usually Taken?

DLPA has been used in amounts ranging from 75 to 1,500 mg per day. As this compound can have powerful effects on mood and on the nervous system, DLPA should be taken only under medical supervision.

Are There Any Side Effects or Interactions?

The maximum amount of DLPA that is safe is unknown; however, consistent toxicity has not been reported with 1,500 mg per day or less of DLPA, except for occasional nausea, heartburn, or transient headaches.

L-phenylalanine competes with several other amino acids for attachment on a common amino acid carrier in the body. Therefore, it should not be taken with protein-containing foods. Individuals taking prescription or over-the-counter medications should consult a nutritionally oriented physician before taking DLPA.

Phosphatidylserine

Phosphatidylserine (PS) belongs to a special category of fat-soluble substances called phospholipids, which are essential components of cell membranes. PS is found in high concentrations in the brain and may help preserve, or even improve, some aspects of mental functioning in the elderly when taken in the amount of 300 mg per day for 3 to 6 months, according to double-blind research.[1,2]

Placebo-controlled[3] and double-blind studies have shown mild benefits from PS supplementation when used in the amount of 300 mg per day for 3 to 12 weeks in patients with early Alzheimer's disease (p. 11).[4,5] In one double-blind study, the improvement on standardized tests of mental functioning averaged approximately 15%.[6] Continued improvement has been reported up to 3 months beyond the end of the supplementation period.[7]

PS is not a cure for Alzheimer's disease. While it may reduce symptoms in the short term, at best PS probably slows the rate of deterioration rather than halting the progression altogether. For example, in a 6-month trial, benefits began to fade after the fourth month.[8] Preliminary research also suggests PS may be useful for the treatment of depression (p. 50) in the elderly.[9]

Is the Form of Phosphatidylserine Important?

Most research has been conducted with PS derived from bovine (cow) brain tissue. Due to concerns about the possibility of humans contracting infectious diseases, soy-based PS supplements have completely replaced bovine-based PS. The soy- and the bovine-derived PS, however, are not structurally identical.[10] Doctors and researchers have debated whether the structural differences could be important,[11,12] but so far only a few trials have studied the effects of soy-based PS.

Preliminary animal research shows that the soy-derived PS does have effects on brain function similar to effects from the bovine source.[13,14] An isolated unpublished double-blind human study used soy-derived PS in an evaluation of memory and mood benefits in non-demented, non-depressed elderly people with impaired memories and accompanying depression.[15] In that 3-month study, 300 mg per day of PS produced statistically significant benefits in the PS group compared with those taking placebo; however, the actual clinical improvement induced by taking soy-based PS was barely better than improvement seen in the placebo group. Science does not yet have an answer to the question of whether the benefits shown in research using PS from a bovine source will be seen in individuals taking the soy-based PS.

Where Is It Found?

PS is found in only trace amounts in a typical diet. Very small amounts are present in lecithin (p. 307). The body manufactures PS from phospholipid building blocks. PS research has used material derived from a bovine source. Currently, PS that is commercially available is derived from soy.

Phosphatidylserine Has Been Used in Connection with the Following Conditions*

Ranking	Health Concerns
Primary	Alzheimer's disease (p. 11)
Other	Age-associated memory impairment Depression (p. 50)

*Refer to the Individual Health Concern for Complete Information

Phosphatidylserine

Pollen

Who Is Likely to Be Deficient?

PS is not an essential nutrient, and therefore dietary deficiencies do not occur. Adults age 50 and older, especially those with age-related declines in mental function (such as memory loss), may not synthesize enough PS, and appear most likely to benefit from supplemental PS.

How Much Is Usually Taken?

Positive effects on mental function have been achieved using 200–500 mg per day of PS.

Are There Any Side Effects or Interactions? No significant side effects associated with PS have been consistently reported.

Pollen

Pollen, collected from the flowers of various plants, contains carbohydrate, fat, protein, and some vitamins and minerals.[1]

A commercial product known as Cernilton is an extract of several species of rye pollens. It has been shown to have anti-inflammatory properties,[2] to relax the muscles that surround the urethra,[3] and to inhibit growth of prostate cells.[4]

Cernilton has been reported to improve symptoms of chronic prostatitis in uncontrolled studies,[5,6,7] including a recent trial in which 3 tablets daily significantly reduced symptoms in 78% of those with uncomplicated prostatitis, compared with only one of eighteen with complications such as scar tissue and calcifications.[8]

Cernilton has also benefited men with **benign prostatic hyperplasia** (BPH) (p. 145) in uncontrolled trials.[9,10,11] In addition, two double-blind studies have reported positive results. One of these demonstrated that two capsules of Cernilton taken twice per day led to reduction in symptoms of BPH compared with the effects of placebo.[12] A multicenter trial in Germany produced comparable results.[13] Cernilton was shown to be comparable in effect to an amino acid mixture used for BPH in a double-blind study;[14] and recently, a double-blind comparison with Pygeum africanum resulted in significant subjective improvement in 78% of those given Cernilton compared with 55% using Pygeum.[15] The effect of pollens other than Cernilton in men with prostate conditions has not yet been studied.

Cernilton also appears capable of protecting the liver from the effects of some toxins, according to animal studies from Poland.[16,17] A preliminary report from Ukraine on the use of flower pollen in humans

with **rheumatoid arthritis** (p. 151) suggested positive effects on related disorders of the liver, gallbladder, stomach, and intestine.[18] Cernilton has also shown **cholesterol-lowering** (p. 79) and anti-**atherosclerosis** (p. 17) effects in animals,[19] but it remains unknown whether these effects can be reproduced in humans.

Pollen extracts have been used orally to desensitize people to plants they are allergic to.[20,21,22,23,24] For example, people with **hay fever** (p. 76) allergies to grass pollen were asked to place drops of liquid grass pollen extract under their tongue daily for 3 weeks using a gradually increasing concentration in a double-blind study. After the 3-week period, pollen was given twice per week at a "maintenance" level. During the next allergy season they had significantly less severe hay fever symptoms than a group given placebo drops.[25]

Where Is It Found?

Most noncultivated plants produce pollen. Commercial pollen is collected from bees returning to their hives (bee pollen) or may be directly harvested with machines (flower pollen). It is not clear which plants produce the most effective pollens. Some of the most common pollens used are timothy grass, corn, rye, and pine. Cernilton is an extract of several rye pollens, and it is also produced under the name Prostaphil.

Pollen Has Been Used in
Connection with the Following Conditions*

Ranking	Health Concerns
Primary	Benign prostatic hyperplasia (p. 145)
Other	Prostatitis
*Refer to the Individual Health Concern for Complete Information	

Who Is Likely to Be Deficient?

Because pollen is not an essential bodily constituent, deficiencies do not occur.

How Much Is Usually Taken?

The optimal intake of pollen is unknown. Some doctors of natural medicine recommend using 500 mg 2 to 3 times per day. Research on Cernilton has used 3 to 6 tablets or 4 capsules per day.

Are There Any Side Effects or Interactions? Many people have allergies to inhaled pollens, and reactions to ingested pollen (some of them quite serious) have been reported.[26,27,28] Otherwise, no significant adverse effects have been reported.

Potassium

Potassium is needed to regulate water balance, levels of acidity, blood pressure, and neuromuscular function. It's also required for carbohydrate and protein metabolism.

Where Is It Found?

Most fruits are excellent sources of potassium. Beans, milk, and vegetables contain significant amounts of potassium.

Potassium Has Been Used in Connection with the Following Conditions*

Ranking	Health Concerns
Primary	High blood pressure (p. 89) (for people not taking potassium-sparing diuretics)
Secondary	Congestive heart failure (p. 43)
*Refer to the Individual Health Concern for Complete Information	

Who Is Likely to Be Deficient?

So-called primitive diets provided much greater levels of potassium; modern diets may provide too little. Gross deficiencies, however, are rare except in cases of prolonged vomiting, diarrhea (p. 58), or use of "potassium depleting" diuretic drugs. People taking one of these drugs should be informed by their doctor to take potassium. Prescription levels of potassium are higher than the amount sold over the counter but not more than the amount found in several pieces of fruit.

How Much Is Usually Taken?

The best way to get extra potassium is to eat several pieces of fruit per day. The amount allowed in supplements—99 mg per tablet or capsule—is very low, considering that one banana can contain 500 mg. Multiple potassium pills should not be taken in an attempt to get a higher amount, because they can irritate the stomach—a problem not encountered with the potassium in fruit.

Are There Any Side Effects or Interactions? High potassium intake (several hundred milligrams at one time in tablet form) can produce stomach irritation. People using potassium-sparing drugs should avoid the use of potassium chloride-containing products, such as Morton Salt Substitute, No Salt, Lite Salt, and others. Even eating several pieces of fruit per day can sometimes cause problems for people taking potassium-sparing diuretics, due to the high potassium content of fruit.

Potassium and sodium work together in the body to maintain muscle tone, blood pressure, water balance, and other functions. Many researchers believe that part of the **blood pressure** (p. 89) problem caused by too much salt (which contains sodium) is made worse by too little dietary potassium.

Pregnenolone

The functions of pregnenolone in the body are not well known. Pregnenolone serves as a precursor to other hormones, including dehydroepiandrosterone (**DHEA** [p. 288]) and **progesterone** (p. 326).[1] It has been suggested that the role of pregnenolone in the body is to serve as a "mother-steroid" (precursor hormone), and that it has no function on its own. More research is needed to determine the functions (if any) of pregnenolone in the body.

Many effects of pregnenolone on the nervous system have been studied. Rat studies indicate powerful memory-enhancing effects,[2] far beyond that of other neuroactive substances.[3,4] In healthy men aged 20 to 30, administration of pregnenolone (1 mg daily) was found to improve **sleep** (p. 105) quality and decrease intermittent wakefulness.[5]

It has been suggested that this hormone may play a role in the neuroendocrine response to stress. During periods of stress, the output of adrenal steroids increases. The increased output of these steroids has been associated with increased fatigue in army pilots resulting in poor performance. In a study of pilots under stress, pregnenolone therapy (25 mg, twice daily) improved performance with no adverse side effects.[6] In a rat study of the stress response, an increase in **anxiety** (p. 14) was observed following administration of pregnenolone. It is suggested that this is a beneficial response during a stressful period and is initiated through the nervous system.[7]

In a rat model of spinal cord injury, pregnenolone administration in conjunction with an anti-inflammatory medication (indomethacin) and an immune-modulating medication (bacterial lipopolysaccharide) resulted in a statistically significant improvement in motor function relative to controls. The control groups included rats on other combinations of the medications and other anti-inflammatory medications.[8]

Pregnenolone appears to exhibit an antagonistic effect on the calming receptors in the brain (GABA receptors), resulting in an excitatory effect. It is possible that this alteration in nervous system transmission could contribute to seizure activity.[9,10]

It is known that steroid hormones affect mood and behavior through the nervous system. In individuals with either current **depression** (p. 532) or a history of depression, pregnenolone (in the cerebrospinal fluid) was found to be significantly lower than in healthy people. In addition, it was found that patients with active depression had lower levels of pregnenolone compared with those with a prior history of depression.[11]

In a double-blind placebo-controlled study of elderly women with wrinkles, daily application of a pregnenolone acetate (0.5 percent) cream improved the visible wrinkling of the skin. When the treatment was discontinued, the benefit was not maintained. Because the results were only temporary, it is suggested that the beneficial effect of the cream was due to improved hydration of the skin.[12]

Researchers have reported on the use of pregnenolone in a variety of rheumatologic diseases. In a study of pregnenolone therapy (intramuscular injection, 50 to 600 mg daily) for **rheumatoid arthritis** (p. 151), six of eleven individuals experienced moderate to marked improvement in symptoms of joint pain and joint mobility. The symptom improvement was apparent 2 to 4 days after therapy was initiated. In a study of thirteen adults with **osteoarthritis** (p. 130), pregnenolone therapy reduced the pain and improved the range of motion in seven of the study participants. Pain recurred when therapy was discontinued. In a person who suffered from gouty arthritis and was unresponsive to traditional medications, pregnenolone therapy resulted in a dramatic response within 3 days of initiating therapy. This patient received 300 mg daily of pregnenolone (by intramuscular injection) for 4 weeks, followed by 200 mg weekly of pregnenolone as a maintenance dose. This study of pregnenolone therapy in rheumatologic diseases also reports a substantial benefit in patients with **systemic lupus erythematosus** (SLE) (p. 115), **psoriasis** (p. 147), and scleroderma. Of the 59 individuals reported in this paper, the only adverse effect was redness or pain at the site of injection. No systemic adverse effects were reported.[13]

Where Is It Found?

The cells of the adrenal gland, as well as the central nervous system, synthesize pregnenolone. Human studies show that there are much higher concentrations of pregnenolone in the nervous tissue than in the bloodstream.[14] Animal studies indicate that pregnenolone is found in the brain in ten-fold larger concentrations than the other stress-related hormones (including DHEA).[15] Pregnenolone is present in the blood as both free pregnenolone and a more stable form, pregnenolone-sulfate.

How Much Is Usually Taken?

Pregnenolone is generally available in amounts of 10 to 30 mg. It is unknown what amount of pregnenolone is necessary for autoimmune diseases, preventive therapy, or memory enhancement, especially since studies were performed primarily on rats, and used an injectable form of the hormone.

Many studies have indicated a U-shaped distribution[16] in the therapeutic response to pregnenolone therapy. The U-shaped distribution describes a benefit of low-dose pregnenolone, a loss of effect with increasing dose of pregnenolone, and a second peak of benefit with higher doses of the steroid. It is unknown what dosage range is represented in either part of the U-shaped curve for humans, and whether or not this curve is altered by disease.

Are There Any Side Effects or Interactions? Due to its antagonistic effects on the GABA receptor in the central nervous system, pregnenolone therapy may be contraindicated in people with a history of seizures. Pregnenolone may inhibit drugs used to increase GABA activity (such as neurontin); these drugs are frequently used in the treatment of epilepsy and **depression** (p. 50). Pregnenolone supplementation may increase **progesterone** (p. 326) levels and consequently other hormones in the body (testosterone and estradiol). Pregnenolone may cause disturbances in the endocrine system, including changes in the menstrual cycle and problems with hormone-sensitive diseases, or it may interact with hormone therapy such as oral contraceptives. The side effects and interactions with other therapies are currently unknown.

Proanthocyanidins (Pycnogenol)

Proanthocyanidins—also called "OPCs" for oligomeric proanthocyanidins and "PCOs" for procyanicolic oligomers—are a class of nutrients belonging to the **bioflavonoid** (p. 271) family. Some researchers also call these molecules "pycnogenol." The main functions of proanthocyanidins are **antioxidant** (p. 267) activity, stabilization of collagen, and maintenance of elastin—two critical proteins in connective tissue, blood vessels, and muscle.[1,2] Possibly because of their effects on blood vessels, proanthocyanidins have been reported to reduce **edema** (p. 65) after face-lift surgery from 15.8 to 11.4 days in double-blind research.[3] Although proanthocyanidins appear to have antimutagenic activity,[4] this research remains very preliminary.

Proanthocyanidins have been shown to strengthen capillaries in double-blind research using as little as two 50 mg tablets per day.[5] In another double-blind trial, French researchers reported that women with **chronic venous insufficiency** (p. 38) were helped using a total of 150 mg per day.[6] Using a total of 300 mg per day (100 mg taken 3 times), yet another French double-blind trial has reported good effects in just 4 weeks.[7]

Proanthocyanidins (200 mg per day for 5 weeks) have improved aspects of vision (visual performance in the dark and after exposure to glare) in healthy people.[8,9] While the antioxidant function of proanthocyanidins has not been well researched, it may be the most important function separating this supplement from other bioflavonoids.[10]

Where Are They Found?

Proanthocyanidins can be found in many plants, most notably pine bark, grape seed, and grape skin. However, **bilberry** (p. 396), **cranberry** (p. 414), black currant, **green tea** (p. 430), black tea, and other plants also contain these flavonoids. Nutritional supplements containing extracts of proanthocyanidins from various plant sources are available, alone or in combination with other nutrients, in herbal extracts, capsules, and tablets.

Who Is Likely to Be Deficient?

Flavonoids and proanthocyanidins are not classified as essential nutrients, since their absence does not induce a deficiency state. However, proanthocyanidins may have many health benefits, and anyone not eating a wide variety of plants will not derive these benefits.

Proanthocyanidins Have Been Used in Connection with the Following Condition*

Ranking	Health Concerns
Primary	Chronic venous insufficiency (p. 38)
*Refer to the Individual Health Concern for Complete Information	

How Much Is Usually Taken?

Flavonoids (proanthocyanidins and others) are a significant source of antioxidants in the average diet. Proanthocyanidins at 50 to 100 mg per day is considered a reasonable supplemental level by some nutritionally oriented doctors, but optimal levels remain unknown.

Are There Any Side Effects or Interactions? Flavonoids, in general, and proanthocyanidins, specifically, are free of side effects. Since they are water-soluble nutrients, excess intake is simply excreted in the urine.

Since proanthocyanidins, like **vitamin C** (p. 341), perform antioxidant functions in the body, the body's stores of vitamin C might be preserved when proanthocyanidins are present.

Probiotics and FOS

Beneficial bacteria, such as Lactobacillus acidophilus and Bifidobacterium bifidum, are called probiotics. Probiotic bacteria favorably alter the intestinal microflora balance, inhibit the growth of harmful bacteria, promote good digestion, boost **immune function** (p. 94), and increase resistance to **infection** (p. 101).[1,2] Individuals with flourishing intestinal colonies of beneficial bacteria are better equipped to fight the growth of disease-causing bacteria.[3,4]

Acidophilus and bifidobacteria maintain a healthy balance of intestinal flora by producing organic compounds—such as lactic acid, hydrogen peroxide, and acetic acid—that increase the acidity of the intestine and inhibit the reproduction of many harmful bacteria.[5,6] Probiotic bacteria also produce substances called bacteriocins, which act as natural antibiotics to kill undesirable microorganisms.[7]

Regular ingestion of probiotic bacteria may help prevent **vaginal yeast infection** (p. 579).[8,9] A review of the research concluded that both topical and oral use of acidophilus can prevent yeast infection caused by candida overgrowth.[10]

Diarrhea (p. 533) flushes intestinal microorganisms out of the gastrointestinal tract, leaving the body vulnerable to opportunistic infections. Replenishing the beneficial bacteria with probiotic supplements can help prevent new infections. The incidence of "traveler's diarrhea," caused by pathogenic bacteria in drinking water or undercooked foods, can be reduced by the preventive use of probiotics.[11]

One probiotic, Saccharomyces boulardii, has prevented diarrhea in several human trials.[12] Double-blind research studying critically ill patients found this strain of yeast to prevent diarrhea when 500 mg is taken 4 times per day.[13]

Probiotics are also important in recolonizing the intestine during and after antibiotic use. Probiotic supplements replace the beneficial bacteria, preventing up to 50% of infections occurring after antibiotic use.[14]

Probiotics also promote healthy digestion. Enzymes secreted by probiotic bacteria aid digestion. Acidophilus is a source of **lactase** (p. 306), the enzyme needed to digest milk, which is lacking in **lactose-intolerant** (p. 114) individuals.[15]

Fructo-oligosaccharides (FOS) are naturally occurring carbohydrates that cannot be digested or absorbed by humans but support the growth of bifidobacteria, one of the beneficial bacterial strains.[16] As a result, some nutritionally oriented doctors recommend taking FOS to all patients who are supplementing bifidobacteria. Several trials have used 8 grams per day. However, a review of the research has suggested that 4 grams per day appears to be enough to significantly increase the number of bifidobacteria in the gut.[17] FOS have been reported to reduce blood sugar and **cholesterol** (p. 79) levels.[18] FOS also appear to increase absorption of **calcium** (p. 277) in humans.[19]

Where Are They Found?

Beneficial bacteria present in fermented dairy foods—namely live culture yogurt—have been used as a folk remedy for hundreds, if not thousands of years. Yogurt is the traditional source of beneficial bacteria; however, different brands of yogurt can vary greatly in their bacteria strain and potency. Some (particularly frozen) yogurts do not contain any live bacteria. Supplements in powder, liquid extract, capsule, or tablet form containing beneficial bacteria are a source of probiotics.

FOS occur naturally in many foods, such as Jerusalem **artichokes** (p. 393), bananas, barley, garlic, honey, onions, wheat, and tomatoes; however, nutritional supplements containing FOS provide a more concentrated source of this compound.

Probiotics and FOS Have Been Used in Connection with the Following Conditions*

Ranking	Health Concerns
Primary	Diarrhea (p. 58) Vaginitis (p. 162) Yeast infection (p. 169)
Secondary	Immune function (p. 94) Infection (p. 101) Mouth ulcers (canker sores) (p. 30)
Other	Indigestion and heartburn (p. 99)
*Refer to the Individual Health Concern for Complete Information

Who Is Likely to Be Deficient?

People using antibiotics, eating a poor diet, or suffering from **diarrhea** (p. 58) are more likely to have depleted colonies of friendly bacteria.

How Much Is Usually Taken?

The amount of probiotics necessary to replenish the intestine varies according to the extent of microbial depletion and the presence of harmful bacteria. One to two billion colony-forming units (CFUs) per day of acidophilus is considered to be the minimum beneficial amount for the healthy maintenance of intestinal microflora. FOS is generally taken in amounts of 4 to 8 grams per day. Some *Saccharomyces boulardii* research has used 500 mg taken 4 times per day.

Are There Any Side Effects or Interactions? No
side effects have been reported, even with large intakes of probiotic bacteria.

Acidophilus and bifidobacteria may produce B vitamins, including **niacin** (p. 339), **folic acid** (p. 297), **biotin** (p. 272), and **vitamin B₆** (p. 340).

Progesterone

The hormone progesterone is the natural equivalent of synthetic progestins and is closely related to estrogen. However, natural progesterone and synthetic progestins are structurally different and may have differing roles in the body. Progesterone is necessary for proper uterine and breast development and function. Progestins are recommended if estrogen is prescribed during or after **menopause** (p. 118), because prolonged estrogen replacement therapy without the addition of progestins increases the risk of uterine cancer.[1] Women who have had a hysterectomy—and therefore no longer have a uterus—are sometimes prescribed estrogens without progestins. Although natural progesterone is considered by some doctors of natural medicine to be safer and more effective for a variety of health problems, researchers have studied the effects of supplemental natural progesterone much less than the effects of synthetic progestins.

Preliminary evidence suggests that progesterone plays a role in bone metabolism that could help reduce the risk of **osteoporosis** (p. 133).[2] An uncontrolled study using topically applied natural progesterone cream in combination with diet and exercise, vitamin and **calcium** (p. 277) supplementation, and oral estrogen therapy reported consistent gains in bone density over a 3-year period in postmenopausal women, but no comparison was made to a similar program without progesterone.[3] However, at least one trial found that adding natural progesterone to estrogen therapy had no better effect on bone mass than estrogen therapy alone, suggesting that natural progesterone may not help protect against osteoporosis.[4]

Most well-controlled studies have not shown a significant benefit of vaginally applied natural progesterone on the symptoms of **premenstrual syndrome** (p. 141).[5] However, some doctors of natural medicine report that oral and rectal progesterone may be effective.[6]

Some studies link synthetic progesterone-like drugs to increased risk of breast cancer.[7] In contrast, topical progesterone has produced changes in breast tissue that may have a cancer prevention effect.[8,9] Other researchers, however, have reported essentially opposite effects, suggesting that natural progesterone may increase proliferation of breast cells.[10] A few doctors of natural medicine have concluded that natural progesterone may help protect against breast cancer.[11] The research, however, remains incomplete and inconsistent. In one trial, (natural) progesterone deficiency was linked with an increased risk, but only when the breast cancer was diagnosed before menopause.[12] Such a finding fits with the idea that natural progesterone might be protective. However, most breast cancer begins postmenopausally, and this same trial found that progesterone deficiency was associated with a large (though statistically insignificant) decreased risk of postmenopausal breast cancer. If duplicated by future research, this finding would not suggest protection, nor even necessarily safety.

Synthetic progesterone drugs have sometimes been linked to effects that might increase the risk of **heart disease** (p. 32).[13] However, vaginally applied natural progesterone has been reported to significantly enhance the benefits of estrogen replacement therapy on heart function in women with coronary artery disease, though oral synthetic progestin produced no improvement in the same trial.[14] More research is needed to evaluate the effects of natural progesterone on heart disease.

Where Is It Found?

Progesterone is produced in the female body in the ovaries and adrenal glands. Progesterone production is high during the luteal phase of the menstrual cycle and low during the follicular phase, as well as being low before puberty and after menopause.

Supplemental sources of progesterone are available in oral and cream forms, as well as lozenges, suppositories, and injectable forms. "Natural" progesterone refers to the type that matches exactly the substance produced in a woman's body, as opposed to related synthesized molecules.

Progestins are also found in oral contraceptive pills and used in conventional hormone replacement therapy.

Wild yam (p. 469) contains precursors to progesterone (such as diosgenin) that can be converted through an industrial process into progesterone—the exact same molecule made in the human body. For this reason, this synthetically derived product is widely called "natural progesterone." However, contrary to popular claims, wild yam root cannot be converted into progesterone in the body.[15,16] Women who require progesterone should consult their nutritionally oriented physician and not rely on wild yam or other herbs.

Pregnenolone (p. 323), another hormone produced by the body, is converted by the body into progesterone. However, the effects that supplemental sources of pregnenolone may have on progesterone production in the body remain unclear.

Progesterone Has Been Used in Connection with the Following Conditions*

Ranking	Health Concerns
Other	Cancer risk reduction Heart disease (p. 32) Menopause (p. 118) Osteoporosis (p. 277) Premenstrual syndrome (p. 141)

*Refer to the Individual Health Concern for Complete Information

Who Is Likely to Be Deficient?

Postmenopausal women have reduced production of progesterone. While this "deficiency" is normal, progesterone, including the natural forms of progesterone, has been found to relieve menopausal symptoms when used in combination with estrogen replacement therapy.[17]

How Much Is Usually Taken?

The proper amount of progesterone for a woman should be determined in consultation with a doctor of natural medicine. Some research with the natural, oral form of progesterone has used 200 mg per day.[18] Progesterone is used in much lower amounts—such as 20 to 70 mg per day—by most doctors who prescribe topical natural progesterone. However, the ability of skin-applied progesterone to achieve effective levels in the body is the source of considerable debate.[19]

Are There Any Side Effects or Interactions?

Progesterone is a hormone, and as such, concerns about its inappropriate use have been raised. A nutritionally oriented physician should be consulted before using this hormone as a supplement. Few side effects have been associated with topical progesterone creams but can include skin reactions. Effects of natural progesterone on breast cancer risk remain unclear, with

Progesterone

some research suggesting the possibility of increased or reduced risk.

Synthetic progestins have many well-known side effects, including the increase of **LDL cholesterol** (p. 79) (the "bad" cholesterol) and the decrease of HDL cholesterol (the "good" cholesterol). Other side effects reported with synthetic progestins include bloating, breast soreness, **depression** (p. 50), and mood swings. Natural progesterone has been shown to have no effect on HDL cholesterol.[20] Consequently, the natural forms of progesterone that might be relatively safer are preferred by many doctors of natural medicine.[21]

Pyruvate

Pyruvate (in the form pyruvic acid) is created in the body during the metabolism of carbohydrates and protein. Pyruvate may aid weight loss efforts.[1] A clinical trial found that pyruvate supplements enhance **weight loss** (p. 165) and also result in a greater reduction of body fat in overweight adults consuming a lowfat diet compared with placebo.[2] Animal studies suggest that pyruvate leads to weight loss by increasing the resting metabolic rate.[3] A few clinical trials also indicate that pyruvate supplements may improve exercise endurance.[4,5]

Preliminary research indicates that pyruvate functions as an **antioxidant** (p. 267), inhibiting the production of harmful free radicals.[6,7,8] Preliminary research with animals suggests that due to its potential antioxidant function, pyruvate may inhibit the growth of cancer tumors;[9] however, this effect has not been confirmed in human studies.

Where Is It Found?

In addition to being formed in the body during digestive processes, pyruvate is present in several foods, including red apples, cheese, dark beer, and red wine. Dietary supplements of pyruvate are also available.

Who Is Likely to Be Deficient?

Because it is not an essential nutrient, pyruvate is not associated with a deficiency state.

How Much Is Usually Taken?

Most human research with pyruvate and weight loss has used at least 30 grams per day. There is no evidence that taking less than this huge amount would have any effects.

Are There Any Side Effects or Interactions? High intakes of pyruvate can trigger gastrointestinal upset, such as gas, bloating, and **diarrhea** (p. 58).

Pyruvate Has Been Used in Connection with the Following Conditions*

Ranking	Health Concerns
Secondary	Weight loss and obesity (p. 165)
Other	Athletic performance (p. 20)

*Refer to the Individual Health Concern for Complete Information

Quercetin

Quercetin belongs to a class of water-soluble plant pigments called **bioflavonoids** (p. 267). Quercetin acts as an antihistamine and has anti-inflammatory activity. As an **antioxidant** (p. 267), it protects LDL cholesterol (the "bad" cholesterol) from becoming damaged. Cardiologists believe that damage to LDL cholesterol is an underlying cause of **heart disease** (p. 32). Quercetin blocks an enzyme that leads to accumulation of sorbitol, which has been linked to nerve, eye, and kidney damage in those with **diabetes** (p. 53). However, no human research has evaluated the possible beneficial effect of quercetin for diabetics.

Where Is It Found?

Quercetin can be found in onions, apples, and black tea. Smaller amounts are found in leafy green vegetables and beans.

Quercetin Has Been Used in Connection with the Following Conditions*

Ranking	Health Concerns
Primary	Capillary fragility (p. 32)
Other	Asthma (p. 15) Atherosclerosis (p. 17) Cataracts (p. 34) Diabetes (p. 53) Edema (water retention) (p. 65) Gout (p. 75) Hay fever (p. 76) High cholesterol (p. 79) Peptic ulcer (p. 138) Retinopathy (p. 150)

*Refer to the Individual Health Concern for Complete Information

Who Is Likely to Be Deficient?

No clear deficiency of quercetin has been established.

How Much Is Usually Taken?

Common supplemental intake of quercetin is 400 mg 2 to 3 times per day.

Are There Any Side Effects or Interactions? No clear toxicity has been identified. Early quercetin research suggested that large amounts of quercetin could cause cancer in animals.[1] Most,[2,3,4] but not all,[5] current research finds quercetin to be safe or actually linked to protection from cancer.

Since flavonoids help protect and potentiate **vitamin C** (p. 341), quercetin is often taken with vitamin C.

Resveratrol

Resveratrol, found primarily in red wine, is a naturally occurring **antioxidant** (p. 267) that decreases the "stickiness" of blood platelets and helps blood vessels remain open and flexible.[1,2,3] A series of laboratory experiments suggests that resveratrol inhibits the development of cancer in animals and prevents the progression of cancer.[4] However, human research is still needed in this area. In another set of animal studies, resveratrol was shown to inhibit both the acute and chronic phases of inflammation.[5]

Where Is It Found?

Resveratrol is present in a wide variety of plants—of the edible plants, mainly in grapes and peanuts.[6] Wine is the primary dietary source of resveratrol. Red wine contains much greater amounts of resveratrol than does white wine, since resveratrol is concentrated in the grape skin and the manufacturing process of red wine includes prolonged contact with grape skins.

Resveratrol Has Been Used in Connection with the Following Conditions*

Ranking	Health Concerns
Other	Atherosclerosis (p. 17) Cancer risk reduction
*Refer to the Individual Health Concern for Complete Information	

Who Is Likely to Be Deficient?

Since it is not an essential nutrient, resveratrol is not associated with a deficiency state.

How Much Is Usually Taken?

A glass of red wine provides approximately 640 mcg of resveratrol, while a handful of peanuts provides about 73 mcg of resveratrol. Resveratrol supplements (often found in combination with grape extracts or other antioxidants) are generally taken in the amount of 200 to 600 mcg per day. The amount used in animals to prevent cancer, however, would exceed

500 **mg** per human adult (far in excess of the microgram dose). Therefore, it is not reasonable to assume that the traces found in supplements or food would be protective. Ideal amounts are not known.

Are There Any Side Effects or Interactions? No side effects have been reported with the use of resveratrol.

Royal Jelly

Royal jelly is a complex mixture of flower nectar, sugars, proteins, vitamins, and bee glandular secretions made by worker bees primarily for developing and maintaining the queen bee. It is purported to have many actions, including beneficial effects for people with anorexia, fatigue, headaches, failure to thrive in children, inadequate lactation, **asthma** (p. 15), and debility from a variety of causes.[1] However, these claims remain either weakly substantiated or unsubstantiated.

Royal jelly is **antibacterial** (p. 101) in test tube studies.[2] Animals studies suggest that royal jelly may promote **wound healing** (p. 167),[3] stimulate or inhibit various aspects of **immune function** (p. 94),[4] and have moderate antitumor activity.[5]

Royal jelly has been shown in animal studies to help prevent the cholesterol-elevating effect of nicotine[6] and to lower blood **cholesterol levels** (p. 79).[7] In human studies, royal jelly (50 to 100 mg per day) has also significantly lowered cholesterol levels.[8,9,10]

Where Is It Found?

Worker bees make royal jelly, which is fed to the queen bee. Other larvae are also fed royal jelly until they begin to mature; only the queen is fed it throughout her life. It is available as a supplement.

Royal Jelly Has Been Used in Connection with the Following Condition*

Ranking	Health Concern
Other	High cholesterol (p. 79)
*Refer to the Individual Health Concern for Complete Information	

Who Is Likely to Be Deficient?

Because royal jelly is not an essential bodily constituent, deficiencies do not occur.

How Much Is Usually Taken?

Royal jelly in the amount of 50 to 100 mg per day has been used in most of the studies on cholesterol lowering.

Are There Any Side Effects or Interactions? People susceptible to allergies may develop sensitivity to royal jelly.[11] Occasionally, royal jelly can provoke a severe allergic reaction in a susceptible individual.[12,13,14,15] While royal jelly contains very little chemical or bacterial contamination, some concern has been raised over the lack of standardized testing for environmental contaminants in bee products.[16]

SAMe (S-Adenosyl-L-Methionine)

SAMe is an important biological agent in the human body, participating in over 40 essential biochemical reactions. SAMe participates in detoxification reactions and in the manufacture of brain chemicals, **antioxidants** (p. 267), joint tissue structures, and many other important components.[1,2]

SAMe appears to raise levels of dopamine, an important neurotransmitter in mood regulation,[3] and higher SAMe levels in the brain are associated with successful drug treatment of **depression** (p. 50).[4] Oral SAMe has been demonstrated to be an effective treatment for depression in some,[5,6,7,8] though not all,[9] double-blind studies. While it does not seem to be as powerful as full doses of antidepressant medications[10] or **St. John's wort** (p. 461), its effects are felt more rapidly, often within 1 week.[11]

SAMe possesses anti-inflammatory, pain-relieving, and tissue-healing properties that may help protect the health of joints.[12,13] Several double-blind studies have shown that SAMe is useful for people with **osteoarthritis** (p. 130), increasing the formation of healthy tissue[14] and reducing pain, stiffness, and swelling better than placebos and equal to drugs such as ibuprofen and naproxen.[15,16,17,18,19,20,21,22]

Intravenous SAMe given to **fibromyalgia** (p. 68) patients has reduced pain and depression in two double-blind studies,[23,24] but a short (10-day) trial had no effect.[25] Oral SAMe was tested in one double-blind study and had some significant beneficial actions, such as reduced pain, fatigue, and stiffness, and improved mood.[26]

Oral and intravenous treatment with SAMe replenishes important substances in damaged livers and improves the flow of bile.[27,28] Preliminary research has indicated SAMe may be helpful in a variety of liver conditions, including cholestasis, Gilbert's syndrome, alcoholic liver injury, cirrhosis, and other liver disorders.[29,30,31] Preliminary research also suggests oral SAMe may increase sperm activity in **infertile men** (p. 103)[32] and may be helpful in the treatment of **migraine** (p. 121) headaches.[33] One double-blind study found injections of SAMe significantly more helpful than placebo injections for reducing the symptoms of postconcussion syndrome.[34]

Where Is It Found?

SAMe is not abundant in the diet, though an essential precursor, the amino acid **methionine** (p. 313), is plentiful in most protein foods. Supplements of SAMe have been available since 1997.

SAMe Has Been Used in Connection with the Following Conditions*

Ranking	Health Concerns
Primary	Osteoarthritis (p. 130)
Secondary	Depression (p. 50)
Other	Fibromyalgia (p. 68) Infertility (male) (p. 103) Liver disorders Migraine headaches (p. 121) Postconcussion

*Refer to the Individual Health Concern for Complete Information

Who Is Likely to Be Deficient?

SAMe is normally produced in the liver from the amino acid methionine, which is abundant in most diets. **Folic acid** (p. 297) and **vitamin B$_{12}$** (p. 337) are necessary for the synthesis of SAMe, and deficiencies of these vitamins results in low concentrations of SAMe in the central nervous system.[35] Low blood or central nervous system levels of SAMe have been detected in people with cirrhosis of the liver,[36] coronary **heart disease** (p. 32),[37] **Alzheimer's disease** (p. 11), and **depression** (p. 50).[38]

How Much Is Usually Taken?

Healthy people do not need to take this supplement. Researchers working with people suffering from a variety of conditions have been using amounts of SAMe as indicated: depression, 1,600 mg per day; osteoarthritis, 800 to 1,200 mg per day; fibromyalgia, 800 mg per day; liver disorders, 1,200 mg per day; and migraine, 800 mg per day.

Are There Any Side Effects or Interactions? Clinical trials in thousands of people for up to 2 years have demonstrated that SAMe is very well tolerated, much better than the medications with which it has often been compared.[39,40] Occasional gastrointestinal upset may be experienced by some people. Researchers treating people with manic-depression (bipolar illness) have reported that SAMe could cause them to switch from depression to a manic episode.[41,42] SAMe has been used in a study of pregnant women and was found to be safe.[43]

Selenium

Selenium activates an **antioxidant** (p. 267) enzyme called glutathione peroxidase, which may help protect the body from cancer. Selenium has also induced "apoptosis" (programmed cell death) in cancer cells. A recent double-blind study following over 1,300 people found that those given 200 mcg of yeast-based selenium per day for 7 years had a 50% drop in the cancer death rate compared with the placebo group.[1] Another recent trial found that men exposed to the most dietary selenium (as indirectly measured by toenail selenium levels) developed 65% less advanced prostate cancer than did men with the lowest levels of selenium.[2]

Selenium is also essential for healthy **immune functioning** (p. 94). As a result, selenium supplementation has reduced the incidence of hepatitis in deficient populations.[3] Even in a nondeficient population of elderly people, selenium supplementation has been found to stimulate the activity of white blood cells—primary components of the immune system.[4] Selenium is also needed to activate thyroid hormones.

Although details are not understood, selenium supplementation has partially normalized the actions of sperm cells in **infertile** (p. 103) men in double-blind research.[5]

Where Is It Found?

Brazil nuts are the best source of selenium. Yeast, whole grains, and seafood are also good sources.

Who Is Likely to Be Deficient?

While most people probably don't take in enough selenium, gross deficiencies are rare in Western countries. Soils in some areas are selenium deficient, and people who eat foods grown primarily on selenium-poor soils are at risk for deficiency. People with **AIDS** (p. 87) have been reported to be depleted in selenium.[6] Similarly, limited research has reported an association between **heart disease** (p. 32) and depleted levels of selenium.[7]

How Much Is Usually Taken?

An adult intake of 200 mcg of selenium per day is recommended by many nutritionally oriented doctors.

Selenium Has Been Used in Connection with the Following Conditions*

Ranking	Health Concerns
Primary	Cancer risk reduction
Secondary	Asthma (p. 15) Atherosclerosis (p. 17) Hypothyroidism (p. 93)
Other	HIV support (p. 87) Macular degeneration (p. 118) Osgood-Schlatter disease (p. 130) Pap smear (abnormal) (p. 136) Retinopathy (p. 150) (combined with vitamin A [p. 336] and Vitamin E [p. 344])
*Refer to the Individual Health Concern for Complete Information	

Are There Any Side Effects or Interactions? Selenium is safe at the level people typically supplement (200 mcg); however, taking more than 1,000 mcg of selenium per day can cause loss of fingernails, skin rash, and changes in the nervous system. In the presence of iodine deficiency–induced goiter, selenium supplementation has been reported to exacerbate low thyroid function.[8]

Selenium enhances the antioxidant effect of **vitamin E** (p. 344).

Silicon

Silicon is a trace mineral. The functions of silicon are not well understood, although silicon probably plays a role in making and maintaining connective tissue. Silicon is present in areas of bone that are undergoing mineralization, which indicates that this mineral might be important for normal bone function; however, evidence for this has not been confirmed in humans.[1]

Where Is It Found?

Good dietary sources for silicon include whole-grain breads and cereals, root vegetables, and beer. A form of silicon called silicates is added to some processed foods.

Who Is Likely to Be Deficient?

Silicon is not an essential mineral. Deficiencies have not been reported.

How Much Is Usually Taken?

Because silicon has not been established as essential, a recommended intake has not been established. The average diet is estimated to provide 5 to 20 mg of

Silicon

Silicon Has Been Used in Connection with the Following Condition*

Ranking	Health Concern
Other	Minor injuries (p. 122)
*Refer to the Individual Health Concern for Complete Information	

silicon per day—an amount that appears adequate. When used as a supplement, common amounts range from 1 to 2 mg per day.

Are There Any Side Effects or Interactions? A high dietary intake of silicon is not associated with any toxic effects. Inhalation of large amounts of silicon (in an industrial setting) can cause the respiratory disease silicosis.

Soy

Soy, a staple food in many Asian countries, contains valuable constituents, including protein, isoflavones, saponins, and phytosterols. Soy protein provides essential **amino acids** (p. 265) and can be used as effectively as animal protein by adults. It's also low in fat and cholesterol-free. The isoflavones in soy, primarily genistein and daidzein, have been well researched by scientists for their **antioxidant** (p. 267) and phytoestrogenic properties.[1] Saponins enhance **immune function** (p. 94) and bind to cholesterol to limit its absorption in the intestine. Phytosterols and other components of soy have been reported to lower **cholesterol levels** (p. 79).

Isoflavones may reduce the risk of hormone-dependent cancers, such as breast and prostate cancer, as well as other cancers. One study of soy research found that 65% of 26 animal-based cancer studies showed a protective effect of soy or soy isoflavones.[2] Human research also suggests a protective role of soy against cancer.[3,4]

A meta-analysis study that pooled 38 trials for reanalysis reported that a soy diet led to **cholesterol** (p. 79) reductions in 89% of the studies. Increasing soy intake was associated with a 23 mg per deciliter drop in total cholesterol levels.[5] Exactly how soy lowers cholesterol remains in debate.[6]

The mild estrogen activity of soy isoflavones may ease **menopause** (p. 118) symptoms for some women, without creating estrogen-related problems. A group of 58 menopausal women, who experienced an average of 14 hot flashes per week, supplemented their diets with either wheat flour or soy flour every day for 3 months; the women taking the soy reduced their hot flashes by 40%.[7] In one double-blind trial, 60 grams

of soy protein led to a 33% decrease in the number of hot flashes after 4 weeks and a 45% reduction after 12 weeks.[8] In addition, soy may help regulate hormone levels in premenopausal women.[9]

Soy may also be beneficial in preventing **osteoporosis** (p. 133). Isoflavones from soy protect animals from bone loss.[10] Taking 40 grams of soy protein powder containing 90 mg isoflavones increased bone mineral density of the spine according to a double-blind trial.[11] Although the use of soy in the prevention of osteoporosis looks hopeful, knowing to what extent soy reduces bone loss will require further research.

Where Is It Found?

In addition to whole soybeans, foods derived from soy include tofu, tempeh, soy milk, textured and hydrolyzed vegetable protein, meat substitutes, soy flour, miso, and soy sauce. Soy is also available as a supplement, as soy protein or isoflavone in powder, capsule, or tablet form. High levels of soy-based isoflavones are in roasted soy nuts, tofu, tempeh, soy milk, and some soy protein isolates.

Soy Has Been Used in Connection with the Following Conditions*

Ranking	Health Concerns
Primary	High cholesterol (p. 79) Menopause (p. 118)
Secondary	Cancer risk reduction Osteoporosis (p. 133)
Other	Vaginitis (p. 162)
*Refer to the Individual Health Concern for Complete Information	

Who Is Likely to Be Deficient?

Although deficiency levels have not been defined, people who do not consume soy foods will not gain the benefits of soy.

How Much Is Usually Taken?

The ideal intake of soy is not known. Researchers suggest that the equivalent of one serving of soy foods per day supports good health, and the benefits increase as soy intake increases.[12] Soy isoflavone supplements are now available. Societies that eat a high intake of soy products derive between 50 and 100 mg per day of soy isoflavones.

Are There Any Side Effects or Interactions? Soy products and cooked soybeans are safe at a wide range of intakes; however, a small percentage of people have allergies to soybeans and thus should avoid soy products. Certain constituents in soy interfere with[13] or alternatively might increase[14] thyroid function; however, the clinical importance of this problem remains unclear.

Although occasional animal studies have reported cancer-enhancing effects from soy extracts,[15] most research, including animal studies, report anticancer effects.[16]

Soy contains a compound called phytic acid, which can interfere with mineral absorption.

Spirulina (Blue-Green Algae)

Blue-green algae, of which spirulina is a well-known example, is a group of 1,500 species of microscopic aquatic plants. The two most common species used for human consumption are Spirulina maxima and Spirulina platensis. Spirulina is particularly rich in protein and also contains carotenoids, vitamins, minerals, and essential fatty acids,[1] though its **vitamin B$_{12}$** (p. 337) content does not appear to be readily usable by people.[2] Most health benefits to humans claimed for spirulina and other blue-green algae supplementation come from anecdotes and not scientific research. Test tube and animal studies have demonstrated several properties of large amounts of spirulina or spirulina extracts, including **antioxidant** (p. 267),[3] antiviral,[4,5] anticancer,[6,7,8,9] **antiallergy** (p. 541),[10,11] **immune-enhancing** (p. 94),[12,13,14] liver-protecting,[15,16,17] blood vessel-relaxing,[18] and blood lipid-lowering[19,20] effects.

One controlled human study found that Spirulina fusiformis reversed precancerous lesions of the mouth (leukoplakia) in 45% of the group given 1 gram per day for 1 year, compared with only 7% of the group receiving placebo.[21] Another small, controlled study found **overweight** (p. 165) individuals taking 8.4 grams per day of spirulina lost an average of 3 pounds in 4 weeks compared with 1.5 pounds when taking placebo, though this difference was not significant and no effects on blood pressure or serum cholesterol were observed.[22] A later controlled but unblinded trial found a small **cholesterol-lowering** (p. 79) effect when 4.2 grams spirulina per day were taken for 8 weeks, but serum triglycerides, blood pressure, and body weight were unchanged.[23]

Where Is It Found?

Blue-green algae grows in some lakes, particularly those rich in salts, in Central and South America and Africa. It is also grown in outdoor tanks specifically to be harvested for nutritional supplements.

Blue-Green Algae Has Been Used in Connection with the Following Conditions*

Ranking	Health Concerns
Other	Oral leukoplakia Weight loss and obesity (p. 165)
*Refer to the Individual Health Concern for Complete Information	

Who Is Likely to Be Deficient?

As it is not an essential nutrient, blue-green algae is not associated with a deficiency state. However, individuals who do not consume several servings of vegetables per day could benefit from the carotenoids and other nutrients in blue-green algae. Since it is a complete protein, it can be used in place of some of the protein in a healthy diet. However, very large amounts are required to provide significant quantities of these nutrients from blue-green algae.

How Much Is Usually Taken?

Blue-green algae can be taken as a powder, flakes, capsules, or tablets. The typical manufacturer's recommended intake is 2,000 to 3,000 mg per day divided throughout the day. However, typical amounts shown to have helpful properties in animal studies would be equivalent to 34 grams per day or more for a 150-pound human.

Are There Any Side Effects or Interactions? No

side effects have been reported with blue-green algae. However, as blue-green algae can accumulate heavy metals from contaminated water, consuming blue-green algae from such areas can increase the body's load of lead, mercury, and cadmium,[24] though non-contaminated blue-green algae has been identified.[25] Samples of spirulina have also been found to be contaminated with animal hairs and insect fragments,[26] and another popular species, *Aphanizomenon flos-aquae*, has been found to produce toxins.[27] A few reports also describe allergic reactions to blue-green algae. Animal studies have found spirulina to be safe during pregnancy.[28,29,30]

Strontium

The mineral strontium is not classified as essential for the human body, although it has been shown in research to promote strong, **osteoporosis** (p. 133)-resistant bones,[1] lessen the risk of dental cavities,[2] and reduce the pain of bone lesions that occasionally develop in association with certain cancers.[3] The type of strontium used as a supplement is not the radioactive type.

Where Is It Found?

Strontium is widely distributed throughout nature; strontium levels in the soil determine how much strontium will be in the foods grown in particular areas. Areas with strontium-rich soils also tend to have higher levels of strontium in the drinking water.

Strontium Has Been Used in Connection with the Following Condition*

Ranking	Health Concern
Other	Dental cavities

*Refer to the Individual Health Concern for Complete Information

Who Is Likely to Be Deficient?

Strontium is not an essential mineral, so deficiencies are not seen with this mineral.

How Much Is Usually Taken?

No recommended intake levels have been established for strontium, because it is not considered essential for humans. However, preliminary research in humans suggests that 600 to 1,700 mg of strontium, taken as a supplement in the form of strontium salts, may increase bone mass in the vertebra of individuals with osteoporosis.[4]

Are There Any Side Effects or Interactions? No consistent toxicities from strontium supplements have been reported.

Sulfur

The mineral sulfur is needed for the manufacture of many proteins, including those forming hair, muscles, and skin. Sulfur contributes to fat digestion and absorption, because it is needed to make bile acids. Sulfur is also a constituent of bones, teeth, and collagen (the protein in connective tissue). As a component of insulin, sulfur is needed to regulate blood sugar. Many claims are being made regarding the use of a sulfur-containing supplement called methylsulfonylmethane (MSM) in the treatment of a wide variety of disorders. To date, none of these claims have been substantiated in clinical research published in medical journals.

Where Is It Found?

Most dietary sulfur is consumed as part of certain **amino acids** (p. 265) in protein-rich foods. Meat, organ meats, poultry, fish, eggs, beans, legumes, and dairy products are all good sources of sulfur-containing amino acids. Sulfur also occurs in **garlic** (p. 425) and onions and may be partially responsible for the health benefits associated with these items.[1] Sulfur in organic forms, such as certain amino acids or in the compound MSM, may be more readily absorbed and used.[2] Supplements of MSM are available.

Most of the body's sulfur is found in the sulfur-containing amino acids **methionine** (p. 313), cystine, and **cysteine** (p. 286). **Vitamin B$_1$** (p. 336), **biotin** (p. 272), and **pantothenic acid** (p. 340) contain small amounts of sulfur.

Who Is Likely to Be Deficient?

Deficiencies of sulfur have not been documented, although a protein-deficient diet could theoretically lead to a deficiency of sulfur. Low levels of cystine, and therefore possibly sulfur, were reported many years ago in people with arthritis, but this association is far from proven.[3]

How Much Is Usually Taken?

No recommended intake levels have been established for sulfur. Since most Western diets are high in protein, the majority of diets probably supply enough sulfur.

Are There Any Side Effects or Interactions? No side effects have been reported with the use of sulfur.

Taurine

Taurine is an **amino acid** (p. 265) (protein building block), as well as a component of bile acids, which are used to help absorb fats and fat-soluble vitamins. Taurine also regulates heartbeat, maintains cell membrane stability, and helps prevent brain cell over activity.

Where Is It Found?

Taurine is found mostly in meat and fish. Except for infants, the human body is able to make taurine from **methionine** (p. 313)—another amino acid.

Who Is Likely to Be Deficient?

Vegans (vegetarians who eat no dairy or eggs) consume virtually no taurine but usually make enough to avoid deficiency. Infants do not make enough, but taurine is found in human milk and most infant

**Taurine Has Been Used in
Connection with the Following Conditions***

Ranking	Health Concerns
Primary	Congestive heart failure (p. 43)
Other	Diabetes (p. 53) High blood pressure (p. 89) Epilepsy

*Refer to the Individual Health Concern for Complete Information

formulas. **Diabetics** (p. 53) have been reported to have lower blood levels of taurine.[1]

How Much Is Usually Taken?

Most people, even vegans, do not need taurine supplements. While infants do require taurine, the level in either human milk or formula is adequate. In dealing with people suffering from specific conditions, nutritionally oriented doctors typically recommend 2 grams taken 3 times per day for a total of 6 grams per day.
Are There Any Side Effects or Interactions? Taurine has not been consistently linked with any toxicity.

Tyrosine

Tyrosine is a nonessential **amino acid** (p. 265) (protein building block) that the body synthesizes from **phenylalanine** (p. 320), another amino acid. Tyrosine is important to the structure of almost all proteins in the body. It is also the precursor of several neurotransmitters, including L-dopa, dopamine, norepinephrine, and epinephrine. Tyrosine, through its effect on neurotransmitters, may affect several health conditions, including Parkinson's disease, **depression** (p. 50), and other mood disorders. Studies have suggested that tyrosine may help people with depression.[1] Preliminary findings indicate a beneficial effect of tyrosine, along with other amino acids, in people affected by dementia, including **Alzheimer's disease** (p. 11).[2] Tyrosine may also ease the adverse effects of environmental stress.[3]

Tyrosine is formed by skin cells into melanin, the dark pigment that protects against the harmful effects of ultraviolet light. Thyroid hormones, which have a role in almost every process in the body, also contain tyrosine as part of their structure.

People born with the genetic condition phenylketonuria (PKU) are unable to metabolize the amino acid phenylalanine. Mental retardation and other severe disabilities can result. While phenylalanine restriction prevents these problems, it also leads to low tyrosine levels in many (but not all) people with PKU. Tyrosine supplementation may be beneficial in some people with PKU, although the evidence[4] remains contradictory.

Where Is It Found?

Dairy products, meats, fish, wheat, oats, and many other foods contain tyrosine.

**Tyrosine Has Been Used in
Connection with the Following Conditions***

Ranking	Health Concerns
Secondary	Depression (p. 50)
Other	Alcohol withdrawal support (p. 6) Phenylketonuria (PKU)

*Refer to the Individual Health Concern for Complete Information

Who Is Likely to Be Deficient?

Some people affected by PKU are deficient in tyrosine. Tyrosine levels are sometimes low in depressed people.[5] Any person losing large amounts of protein, such as those with some kidney diseases, may be deficient in several amino acids, including tyrosine.[6]

How Much Is Usually Taken?

Most people should not supplement tyrosine. Some human research with people suffering from a variety of conditions use the equivalent of 7 grams per day. A useful amount in people with PKU remains uncertain. In that case, monitoring of blood levels by a nutritionally oriented physician is recommended.
Are There Any Side Effects or Interactions? Tyrosine is not generally associated with side effects.

Vitamin B$_6$ (p. 340), **folic acid** (p. 296), and **copper** (p. 285) are necessary for conversion of tyrosine into neurotransmitters.

Vanadium

Vanadium is an ultra-trace mineral found in the human diet and body. It is essential for some animals, and deficiency symptoms in these animals include growth retardation, bone deformities, and infertility. However, vanadium has not yet been proven to be an essential mineral for humans. Vanadium may play a role in building bones and teeth.

Vanadyl sulfate, a form of this mineral, may improve glucose control in individuals with non-insulin-dependent **diabetes** (p. 53) mellitus (NIDDM), according to a study of eight diabetics supplemented

Vanadium

with 100 mg of the mineral daily for 4 weeks.[1] However, the researchers of this study caution that the long-term safety of such large doses of vanadium remains unknown. Many doctors of natural medicine expect future research is likely to show that amounts this high will turn out to be unsafe.

Where Is It Found?

Vanadium is found in very small amounts in a wide variety of foods, including seafood, cereals, mushrooms, parsley, corn, soy, and gelatin.

Vanadium Has Been Used in Connection with the Following Condition*

Ranking	Health Concern
Other	Diabetes (p. 53)

*Refer to the Individual Health Concern for Complete Information

Who Is Likely to Be Deficient?

Deficiencies of the mineral vanadium have not been reported and appear unlikely.

How Much Is Usually Taken?

As yet, research indicates that most people would not benefit from vanadium supplementation. Optimal intake of vanadium is unknown. The estimated requirement is probably less than 10 mcg per day, while an average diet provides 15 to 30 mcg per day.

Are There Any Side Effects or Interactions? Information about vanadium toxicity is limited. Workers exposed to vanadium dust can develop toxic effects. High blood levels have been linked to manic-depressive mental disorders, but the meaning of this remains uncertain.[2] Vanadium sometimes inhibits, but at other times stimulates, cancer growth in animals. The effect in humans remains unknown.[3]

Vanadium is not known to interact with other nutrients.

Vitamin A

Vitamin A helps cells reproduce normally—a process called differentiation. Cells that have not properly differentiated are more likely to undergo precancerous changes. Vitamin A, by maintaining healthy cell membranes, helps prevent invasion by disease-causing microorganisms. Vitamin A also stimulates **immunity** (p. 94) and is needed for formation of bone, protein, and growth hormone. **Beta-carotene** (p. 268) is a substance from plants that the body can convert to vitamin A.

Where Is It Found?

Liver, dairy, and cod liver oil provide vitamin A. Vitamin A can also be found in supplements.

Vitamin A Has Been Used in Connection with the Following Conditions*

Ranking	Health Concerns
Primary	Celiac disease (p. 35) (for deficiency) Infection (p. 63) Night blindness (p. 129)
Secondary	Bronchitis Celiac disease (p. 35) Immune function (p. 94) Iron deficiency anemia (p. 107) (as an adjunct to supplemental iron) Menorrhagia (heavy menstruation) (p. 120) Minor injuries (p. 122) (for deficiency) Peptic ulcer (p. 138) Wound healing (p. 167)
Other	Acne (p. 5) Conjunctivitis/blepharitis (p. 44) Crohn's disease (p. 48) Diarrhea (p. 58) Gastritis (p. 71) HIV support (p. 87) Pap smear (p. 136) (abnormal) Premenstrual syndrome (p. 141) (see dosage warnings) Retinopathy (p. 150) (in combination with selenium [p. 331] and vitamin E [p. 344]) Urinary tract infection (p. 160) Vaginitis (p. 162)

*Refer to the Individual Health Concern for Complete Information

Who Is Likely to Be Deficient?

Individuals who limit their consumption of liver, dairy foods, and beta-carotene-containing vegetables can develop a vitamin A deficiency. The earliest deficiency sign is poor night vision. Deficiency symptoms can also include dry skin, increased risk of infections, and metaplasia (a precancerous condition). Severe deficiencies causing blindness are extremely rare in Western societies.

How Much Is Usually Taken?

In males and postmenopausal women, up to 25,000 IU (7,500 mcg) of vitamin A per day is considered safe. In women who could become pregnant, the safest intake level is being reevaluated; less than 10,000 IU (3,000 mcg) per day is widely accepted as safe. Whether the average person would benefit from vitamin A supplementation remains unclear.

Are There Any Side Effects or Interactions? Since a 1995 report from the *New England Journal of Medicine,*[1] women who are or could become pregnant have been told by doctors to take less than 10,000 IU (3,000 mcg) per day of vitamin A to avoid the risk of birth defects. A recent report studied several hundred women exposed to 10,000 to 300,000 IU (median exposure of 50,000 IU) per day.[2] Three major malformations occurred in this study, but all could have happened in the absence of vitamin A supplementation. Surprisingly, no congenital malformations happened in any of the 120 infants exposed to maternal intakes of vitamin A that exceeded 50,000 IU per day. In fact, the high-exposure group had a 50% decreased risk for malformations compared with infants not exposed to vitamin A. The authors note that previous trials based the link to birth defects on very few cases, didn't measure vitamin A intake, or found no link to birth defects whatsoever. A closer look at the recent study reveals a 32% higher than expected risk of birth defects in infants exposed to 10,000 to 40,000 IU of vitamin A per day, but paradoxically a 37% decreased risk for those exposed to even higher levels; this suggests that both "higher" and "lower" risks may have been due to chance. At present, the level at which birth defects might be caused by vitamin A supplementation is not known, though it may well be higher than 10,000 IU per day. Women who are or who could be pregnant should talk with a nutritionally oriented doctor before supplementing with more than 10,000 IU per day.

For other adults, intake above 25,000 IU (7,500 mcg) per day can—in rare cases—cause headaches, dry skin, hair loss, fatigue, bone problems, and liver damage.[3] At higher levels (for example 100,000 IU per day), these problems become more common.

Taking vitamin A and **iron** (p. 304) together helps overcome iron deficiency more effectively than iron supplementation alone.[4]

Vitamin B₁ (Thiamine)

Vitamin B₁ is needed to process carbohydrates, fat, and protein. Every cell of the body requires vitamin B₁ to form ATP—the fuel the body runs on. Nerve cells require vitamin B₁ in order to function normally.

Where Is It Found?

Wheat germ, whole wheat, peas, beans, so-called enriched flour, fish, peanuts, and meat are all good sources of vitamin B₁.

Who Is Likely to Be Deficient?

Deficiency is most commonly found in alcoholics, people with malabsorption conditions, and those eating a very poor diet.

Vitamin B₁ Has Been Used in Connection with the Following Conditions*

Ranking	Health Concerns
Secondary	Canker sores (mouth ulcers) (p. 30) Diabetes (p. 53)
Other	Fibromyalgia (p. 68) HIV support (p. 87) Minor injuries (p. 122) Multiple sclerosis (p. 127)

*Refer to the Individual Health Concern for Complete Information

How Much Is Usually Taken?

While ideal levels are somewhat uncertain, one study reports that the healthiest people eat more than 9 mg per day.[1] The amount found in many **multivitamin** (p. 314) supplements (20 to 25 mg) is more than adequate.

Can I take too much? Vitamin B₁ is nontoxic, even in very high amounts.

Are there any interactions with other nutrients? Vitamin B₁ works hand in hand with **vitamin B₂** (p. 338) and B₃ (p. 339). Therefore, nutritionists usually suggest that vitamin B₁ be taken as part of a **B-complex** (p. 341) vitamin or other multivitamin supplement.

Vitamin B₁₂ (Cobalamin)

Vitamin B₁₂ is needed for normal nerve cell activity, DNA replication, and production of the mood-affecting substance called **SAMe (S-adenosyl-L-methionine)** (p. 330). Vitamin B₁₂ works with **folic acid** (p. 297) to control homocysteine levels. An **excess of homocysteine** (p. 84), which is an amino acid (protein building block), may increase the risk of **heart disease** (p. 32), stroke, and perhaps **osteoporosis** (p. 133) and **Alzheimer's disease** (p. 11).

Vitamin B₁₂ deficiency can cause fatigue, and some research indicates that individuals who are not deficient in this vitamin have increased energy after injections of vitamin B₁₂.[1] In one unblinded trial, 2,500 to 5,000 mcg of vitamin B₁₂, given by injection every 2 to 3 days, led to improvement in 50 to 80% of a group of people with **chronic fatigue syndrome (CFS)** (p. 36), with most improvement appearing after several weeks of B₁₂ shots.[2] While the research in this area remains preliminary, people with CFS interested in considering a trial of vitamin B₁₂ injections should consult a nutritionally oriented doctor. Oral or sublingual B₁₂ supplements are unlikely to obtain the same results as injectable B_{12}, because the body's ability to absorb large amounts is relatively poor.

Where Is It Found?

Vitamin B_{12} is found in all foods of animal origin, including dairy, eggs, meat, fish, and poultry. Inconsistent but small amounts occur in seaweed (including **spirulina** [p. 333]) and tempeh.

Who Is Likely to Be Deficient?

Vegans (vegetarians who also avoid dairy and eggs) frequently become deficient, though the process may take many years. People with malabsorption conditions may suffer from vitamin B_{12} deficiency. Individuals suffering from pernicious anemia require high-dose supplements of vitamin B_{12}. Older people with urinary incontinence[3] and hearing loss[4] have been reported to be at increased risk of B_{12} deficiency.

Vitamin B_{12} Has Been Used in Connection with the Following Conditions*

Ranking	Health Concerns
Primary	Crohn's disease (p. 48) Depression (p. 50) High homocysteine (p. 84) Pernicious anemia
Secondary	Atherosclerosis (p. 17) Bursitis (p. 30) Chronic fatigue syndrome (p. 36) Infertility (male) (p. 103) (shots)
Other	Alzheimer's disease (p. 11) Asthma (p. 15) Diabetes (p. 53) Hepatitis (p. 77) High cholesterol (p. 79) (protection of LDL cholesterol) HIV support (p. 87) Minor injuries (p. 122) Retinopathy (p. 150) (associated with childhood diabetes) Shingles (herpes zoster)/postherpetic neuralgia (p. 155) Tinnitus (p. 158) Vitiligo (p. 164)

*Refer to the Individual Health Concern for Complete Information

How Much Is Usually Taken?

Most people do not require vitamin B_{12} supplements. However, vegans should take at least 2 to 3 mcg per day. Treatment for pernicious anemia includes supplements of 1,000 mcg of vitamin B_{12} per day or vitamin B_{12} injections. Despite the beliefs of many medical doctors, scientific proof indicates that oral supplementation (1,000 mg per day) provides successful

therapy and that vitamin B_{12} injections are not needed.[5,6,7,8,9] In addition, the elderly may benefit from 10 to 25 mcg per day of vitamin B_{12}.[10,11,12]

Are There Any Side Effects or Interactions?

Vitamin B_{12} supplements are not associated with side effects.

If a person is deficient in vitamin B_{12} and takes 1,000 mcg of **folic acid** (p. 297) per day or more, the folic acid can improve anemia caused by the B_{12} deficiency, but not affect neurological symptoms. This is not a toxicity but rather a partial solution to one of the problems caused by B_{12} deficiency. The other problems caused by a lack of vitamin B_{12} (mostly neurological) do not improve with folic acid supplements.

Vitamin B_{12} deficiencies often occur without anemia (even in people who don't take folic acid supplements). Some doctors do not know that the absence of anemia does not rule out a B_{12} deficiency. If this confusion delays diagnosis of a vitamin B_{12} deficiency, the patient could be injured, sometimes permanently. This problem is rare and should not happen with doctors knowledgeable in this area using correct testing procedures.

Anyone supplementing more than 1,000 mcg per day of folic acid needs to be initially evaluated by a doctor of natural medicine to avoid this potential problem.

Vitamin B_2 (Riboflavin)

Vitamin B_2 is needed to process amino acids and fats, activate **vitamin B_6** (p. 340) and **folic acid** (p. 297), and help convert carbohydrates into ATP, the fuel the body runs on. Under some circumstances, vitamin B_2 can act as an **antioxidant** (p. 267).

Where Is It Found?

Dairy, eggs, and meat contain significant amounts of vitamin B_2. Leafy green vegetables and whole and so-called enriched grains contain some vitamin B_2.

Who Is Likely to Be Deficient?

Vitamin B_2 deficiency can occur in alcoholics. Also, a deficiency may be more likely in people with **cataracts** (p. 34)[1,2] or sickle cell anemia.[3]

How Much Is Usually Taken?

Ideal levels remain unknown, but the recommended daily allowance might be higher than necessary. Vegans (vegetarians who eat no dairy or eggs) generally consume less than 1 mg per day of vitamin B_2, yet they do not usually show any signs of deficiency. The amounts found in many **multivitamin** (p. 314) supplements (20 to 25 mg) are more than adequate.

Vitamin B₂ Has Been Used in Connection with the Following Conditions*

Ranking	Health Concerns
Primary	Migraine headaches (p. 558)
Secondary	Canker sores (mouth ulcers) (p. 30) Cataracts (p. 34)
Other	Athletic performance (p. 20)
*Refer to the Individual Health Concern for Complete Information	

Are There Any Side Effects or Interactions? At supplemental and dietary levels, vitamin B₂ is nontoxic.

Vitamin B₂ works with **vitamins B₁** (p. 337), **B₃** (p. 339), and **B₆** (p. 340); consequently, vitamin B₂ should be taken as part of a **B-complex** (p. 341) supplement.

Vitamin B₃ (Niacin, Niacinamide)

The body uses vitamin B₃ in the process of releasing energy from carbohydrates. It's needed to form fat from carbohydrates and to process alcohol. The niacin form of vitamin B₃ also regulates **cholesterol** (p. 79), though niacinamide does not.

Vitamin B₃ comes in two basic forms—niacin (also called nicotinic acid) and niacinamide (also called nicotinamide). A variation on niacin, called inositol hexaniacinate, is also available in supplements. Because it has not been linked with any of the usual niacin toxicity in scientific research, inositol hexaniacinate is sometimes prescribed by European doctors for those who need high doses of niacin.

Where Is It Found?

The best food sources of vitamin B₃ are peanuts, **brewer's yeast** (p. 275), fish, and meat. Some vitamin B₃ is also found in whole grains.

Who Is Likely to Be Deficient?

Pellagra, the disease caused by a vitamin B₃ deficiency, is rare in Western societies. Symptoms include loss of appetite, skin rash, diarrhea, mental changes, beefy tongue, and digestive and emotional disturbance.

How Much Is Usually Taken?

In part because it is added to white flour, most people probably get enough vitamin B₃ from their diets; however, 10 to 25 mg of the vitamin can be taken as part of a **B-complex** (p. 341) or **multivitamin** (p. 314) supplement.

Vitamin B₃ Has Been Used in Connection with the Following Conditions*

Ranking	Health Concerns
Primary	Alcohol withdrawal support (p. 6) (niacinamide) High cholesterol (p. 79) High triglycerides (p. 85)
Secondary	Cataracts (p. 34) (niacinamide) High cholesterol (p. 79) (inositol hexaniacinate) Intermittent claudication (p. 106) (niacin—inositol hexaniacinate) Osteoarthritis (p. 130) (niacinamide) Painful menstruation (dysmenorrhea) (p. 61) Raynaud's disease (p. 148) (niacin—inositol hexaniacinate)
Other	Acne (p. 5) (topical niacinamide) Anxiety (p. 14) (niacinamide) Bursitis (p. 30) (niacinamide) Diabetes (p. 53) (niacinamide) Hypoglycemia (p. 92) (niacinamide) Hypothyroidism (p. 93) (nicotinic acid) Multiple sclerosis (p. 127) (niacin) Photosensitivity (p. 140) (niacinamide) Pregnancy and postpartum support (p. 143) Tardive dyskinesia (p. 157) (niacin or niacinamide)
*Refer to the Individual Health Concern for Complete Information	

Are There Any Side Effects or Interactions? Niacinamide is almost always safe to take, although rare liver problems have occurred at doses in excess of 1,000 mg per day. Niacin, in amounts as low as 50 to 100 mg, may cause flushing, headache, and stomachache in some people. Doctors sometimes prescribe very high amounts of niacin (as much as 3,000 mg per day or more) for certain health problems. These large amounts can cause liver damage, **diabetes** (p. 53), **gastritis** (p. 71), damage to eyes, and elevated blood levels of uric acid (which can cause **gout** [p. 75]), and should never be taken without consulting a nutritionally oriented doctor.

Although the inositol hexaniacinate form of niacin has not been linked with side effects, the amount of research studying the safety of this form of the vitamin remains quite limited. Therefore, people taking this supplement in large amounts (several thousand milligrams per day or more) should be followed by a nutritionally oriented doctor.

Vitamin B₃ works with **vitamin B₁** (p. 337) and **B₂** (p. 338) to release energy from carbohydrates. Therefore, these vitamins are often taken together in a **B-complex** (p. 341) or **multiple vitamin** (p. 314) supplement (although most B₃ research uses niacin or niacinamide by itself).

Vitamin B₅ (Pantothenic Acid, Panthethine)

Pantothenic acid, sometimes called vitamin B₅, is involved in the Kreb's cycle of energy production and is needed to make the neurotransmitter acetylcholine. It is also essential in producing, transporting, and releasing energy from fats. Synthesis of cholesterol (needed for **vitamin D** [p. 343] and hormone synthesis) depends on pantothenic acid. Pantothenic acid also activates the adrenal glands.[1] Pantethine—a variation of pantothenic acid—has been reported to lower blood levels of **cholesterol** (p. 79) and **triglycerides** (p. 85).

Where Is It Found?

Liver, yeast, and salmon have high levels of pantothenic acid, but most other foods, including vegetables, dairy, eggs, grains, and meat also provide some pantothenic acid.

Pantothenic Acid or Pantethine Have Been Used in Connection with the Following Conditions*

Ranking	Health Concerns
Primary	High cholesterol (p. 79) (pantethine) High triglycerides (p. 85) (pantethine)
Secondary	Rheumatoid arthritis (p. 151) (pantothenic acid)
Other	Acne (p. 5) (pantothenic acid) Athletic performance (p. 20) (pantothenic acid) Lupus (SLE) (p. 115) Sinusitis (p. 156)

*Refer to the Individual Health Concern for Complete Information

Who Is Likely to Be Deficient?

Pantothenic acid deficiencies may occur in people with alcoholism but are generally believed to be rare.

How Much Is Usually Taken?

Most people do not need to supplement with pantothenic acid. However, the 10 to 25 mg found in many **multivitamin** (p. 314) supplements might improve pantothenic acid status, as so-called primitive human diets provided greater amounts of this nutrient than is found in modern diets. Most cholesterol researchers using pantethine have given people 300 mg 3 times per day (total 900 mg).

Are There Any Side Effects or Interactions?
Toxicity has not been reported at supplemental doses. Very large amounts of pantothenic acid (several grams per day) can cause **diarrhea** (p. 533).

Pantothenic acid works together with vitamins **B₁** (p. 337), **B₂** (p. 338), and **B₃** (p. 338) to help make ATP—the fuel bodies run on.

Vitamin B₆ (Pyridoxine)

Vitamin B₆ is the master vitamin in the processing of **amino acids** (p. 265)—the building blocks of all proteins and some hormones. Vitamin B₆ helps to make and take apart many amino acids and is also needed to make serotonin, **melatonin** (p. 312), and dopamine. Vitamin B₆ also aids in the formation of several neurotransmitters and is therefore an essential nutrient in the regulation of mental processes and possibly mood. To some extent, vitamin B₆ lowers **homocysteine** (p. 84) levels—a substance that has been linked to **heart disease** (p. 32), stroke, **osteoporosis** (p. 133), and **Alzheimer's disease** (p. 11).

A link between vitamin B₆ deficiency and **carpal tunnel syndrome** (p. 33) has been reported in some,[1] but not all, research.[2,3]

Where Is It Found?

Potatoes, bananas, raisin bran cereal, lentils, liver, turkey, and tuna are all good sources of vitamin B6.

Who Is Likely to Be Deficient?

Vitamin B₆ deficiencies, although very rare, cause impaired immunity, skin lesions, and mental confusion. A marginal deficiency sometimes occurs in alcoholics, patients with kidney failure, and women using oral contraceptives. Many nutritionally oriented doctors believe that most diets do not provide optimal amounts of this vitamin.

How Much Is Usually Taken?

The most common supplemental intake is 10 to 25 mg per day; however, higher amounts (200 to 500 mg per day) may be recommended for certain conditions.

Are There Any Side Effects or Interactions?
Although side effects from vitamin B6 supplements

Vitamin B₆ Has Been Used in Connection with the Following Conditions*

Ranking	Health Concerns
Primary	Autism (p. 27) Celiac disease (p. 35) (if deficient) Depression (p. 50) (with oral contraceptives) High homocysteine (p. 84) Kidney stones (in the presence of elevated urinary oxalate) (p. 111) Morning sickness (p. 126)
Secondary	Asthma (p. 514) Atherosclerosis (p. 17) Canker sores (mouth ulcers) (p. 30) Carpal tunnel syndrome (p. 33) Celiac disease (p. 35) Depression (p. 50) (for premenstrual syndrome [p. 532]) Diabetes (p. 53) (gestational only) Kidney stones (p. 111) (in the absence of elevated urinary oxalate) MSG sensitivity (p. 129) Premenstrual syndrome (p. 141)
Other	Acne (p. 5) Alcohol withdrawal support (p. 6) Athletic performance (p. 20) Attention deficit disorder (p. 26) Fibrocystic breast disease (p. 66) High cholesterol (p. 79) (protection of LDL cholesterol) HIV support (p. 87) Hypoglycemia (p. 92) Minor injuries (p. 122) Photosensitivity (p. 140) Retinopathy (p. 150) Tardive dyskinesia (p. 157)

*Refer to the Individual Health Concern for Complete Information

are rare, at very high levels (200 mg or more per day) this vitamin can eventually damage sensory nerves, leading to numbness in the hands and feet as well as difficulty walking. Vitamin B₆ supplementation should be stopped if any of these symptoms begin to develop.

Pregnant and lactating women should not take more than 100 mg of vitamin B₆. For other adults, vitamin B₆ is usually safe in amounts of 200 to 300 mg per day,[4] although occasional problems have been reported in this range.[5] Any adult taking more than 100 to 200 mg of vitamin B₆ for more than a few months should consult a nutritionally oriented doctor. Side effects from vitamin B₆ are dependent on the level of intake. No one should ever take more than 500 mg per day,[6] even with clinical supervision.

Since vitamin B6 increases the bioavailability of **magnesium** (p. 310), these nutrients are sometimes taken together.

Vitamin B-Complex

The vitamin B complex refers to all of the known essential water-soluble vitamins except for **vitamin C** (p. 341). These include **thiamine** (p. 337) (vitamin B₁), **riboflavin** (p. 338) (vitamin B₂), **niacin** (p. 339) (vitamin B₃), **pantothenic acid** (p. 340) (vitamin B₅), pyridoxine (**vitamin B₆** [p. 340]), **biotin** (p. 272), **folic acid** (p. 297) and the cobalamins (**vitamin B₁₂** [p. 337]). "Vitamin B" was once thought to be a single nutrient that existed in extracts of rice, liver, or yeast. Researchers later discovered that these extracts contained several vitamins, which were given distinguishing numbers. Unfortunately, this has led to an erroneous belief among non-scientists that these vitamins have a special relationship to each other. Further adding to confusion has been the "unofficial" designation of other substances as members of the B-complex, such as choline, **inositol** (p. 303), and para-aminobenzoic acid (**PABA** [p. 319]), even though they are not essential vitamins.

Each member of the B-complex has a unique structure and performs unique functions in the human body. Vitamins B₁, B₂, B₃, and biotin participate in different aspects of energy production; vitamin B₆ is essential for amino acid metabolism; and vitamin B₁₂ and folic acid facilitate steps required for cell division. Each of these vitamins has many additional functions. However, contrary to popular belief, no functions require all B-complex vitamins simultaneously.

Human requirements for members of the B-complex vary considerably—from 3 mcg per day for vitamin B₁₂ to 18 mg per day for vitamin B₃ in adult males, for example. Therefore, taking equal amounts of each one—as provided in many B-complex supplements—makes little sense. Furthermore, no evidence supports the use of megadoses of B-complex vitamins to combat everyday stress, boost energy, or control food cravings, unless a person has a severe deficiency of one or more of them. Again contrary to popular belief, no evidence indicates that people should take all B vitamins to avoid an imbalance when one or more individual B vitamin is taken for a specific health condition.

Most **multiple vitamin/mineral** (p. 314) products contain the B-complex along with the rest of the essential vitamins and minerals. Because they are more complete, multiple vitamin/mineral supplements are recommended to improve overall micronutrient intake and prevent deficiencies.

Vitamin C (Ascorbic Acid)

Vitamin C is a water-soluble vitamin that functions as a powerful **antioxidant** (p. 267). Acting as an antioxidant, one of vitamin C's important functions is to protect LDL cholesterol from oxidative damage. (Only when LDL is damaged does cholesterol appear to lead to **heart disease** (p. 32), and vitamin C may be the most important antioxidant protector of LDL.)[1]

Vitamin C is needed to make collagen, the "glue" that strengthens many parts of the body, such as muscles and blood vessels. Vitamin C also plays important roles in **wound healing** (p. 167) and as a natural antihistamine. This vitamin also aids in the formation of liver bile and helps to fight viruses and to detoxify alcohol and other substances.

Although vitamin C appears to have only a small effect in preventing the **common cold** (p. 41), it reduces the duration and severity of a cold. Large amounts of vitamin C (for example, 1 to 8 grams daily) taken at the onset of a cold episode shorten the duration of illness by an average of 23%.[2]

Recently, researchers have shown that vitamin C improves nitric oxide activity.[3] Nitric acid is needed for the dilation of blood vessels, potentially important in lowering **blood pressure** (p. 89) and preventing spasm of arteries in the heart that might otherwise lead to heart attacks. Vitamin C has reversed dysfunction of cells lining blood vessels.[4] The normalization of the functioning of these cells may be linked to prevention of heart disease.

Evidence indicates that vitamin C levels in the eye decrease with age[5] and that supplementing with vitamin C prevents this decrease,[6] leading to a lower risk of developing **cataracts** (p. 34).[7,8] Healthy people have been reported to be more likely to take vitamin C and **vitamin E** (p. 344) supplements than are people with cataracts in some,[9] but not all, studies.[10]

Vitamin C has been reported to reduce activity of the enzyme aldose reductase in people.[11] Aldose reductase is the enzyme responsible for accumulation of sorbitol in eyes, nerves, and kidneys of people with **diabetes** (p. 53). This accumulation is believed to be responsible for deterioration of these parts of the body associated with diabetes. Therefore, interference

with the activity of aldose reductase theoretically helps protect people with diabetes.

There is some speculative evidence that vitamin C might help prevent gallstones;[12] however, supportive evidence remains preliminary.

Where Is It Found?

Broccoli, red peppers, currants, Brussels sprouts, parsley, rose hips, acerola berries, citrus fruit, and strawberries are good sources of vitamin C.

Who Is Likely to Be Deficient?

Although scurvy (severe vitamin C deficiency) is uncommon in Western societies, many nutritionally oriented doctors believe that most people consume less than optimal amounts. Fatigue, easy bruising, and bleeding gums are early signs of vitamin C deficiency that occur long before frank scurvy develops. Smokers have low levels of vitamin C and require a higher daily intake to maintain normal vitamin C levels.

How Much Is Usually Taken?

Doctors of natural medicine often recommend 500 to 1,000 mg per day. Most research uses levels that do not exceed 1,000 mg per day. However, even greater levels (up to 10,000 mg per day) are not uncommon. In terms of heart disease prevention, as little as 100 to 200 mg of vitamin C might be adequate.[13]

In contrast, current vitamin C researchers believe that 200 mg per day gets close to raising blood levels in healthy people about as high as they will go, and that supplementing more results in an excretion level almost identical to intake, meaning that more vitamin C does not stay in the body.[14] This suggests that levels above 200 mg per day may prove to be superfluous for healthy people. The same kinds of studies that have ascertained that 200 mg is approximately correct for healthy people have not yet been done with sick individuals.

Are There Any Side Effects or Interactions? Some individuals develop **diarrhea** (p. 58) after as little as a few thousand milligrams of vitamin C per day, while others are not bothered by ten times this amount. However, high levels of vitamin C can deplete the body of **copper** (p. 285)[15,16]—an essential nutrient. People should be sure to maintain adequate copper intake at higher intakes of vitamin C. Copper is found in many **multivitamin/mineral** (p. 314) supplements. Vitamin C probably increases the absorption of **iron** (p. 304), although this effect is mild. Vitamin C helps recycle the antioxidant **vitamin E** (p. 344).

People with the following conditions should consult their doctor before supplementing with vitamin C:

Vitamin C Has Been Used in Connection with the Following Conditions*

Ranking	Health Concerns
Primary	Athletic performance (p. 20) (for deficiency only) Bronchitis Bruising (p. 28) (for deficiency only) Capillary fragility (p. 32) Common cold/sore throat (p. 41) Gingivitis (periodontal disease) (p. 73) (for deficiency only) Glaucoma (p. 74) High cholesterol (p. 79) (protection of LDL cholesterol) Infection (p. 101) Infertility (male) (p. 103) (for sperm agglutination) Minor injuries (p. 122) (oral and topical for sunburn protection) Scurvy Wound healing (p. 167)
Secondary	Athletic performance (p. 20) (for exercise recovery) Autism (p. 27) Cataracts (p. 34) Diabetes (p. 53) Immune function (p. 94) Influenza (p. 104) Iron deficiency anemia (p. 107) (as an adjunct to supplemental iron) Minor injuries (p. 122)
Other	Alcohol withdrawal support (p. 6) Asthma (p. 15) Atherosclerosis (p. 17) Backache Chronic obstructive pulmonary disease (p. 45) Ear infections (recurrent) (p. 63) Eczema (p. 64) Gallstones (p. 69) Gastritis (p. 71) Gout (p. 75) Hay fever (p. 76) Hepatitis (p. 77) High blood pressure (p. 89) HIV support (p. 87) Hypoglycemia (p. 92) Macular degeneration (p. 118) Menopause (p. 118) Menorrhagia (heavy menstruation) (p. 120) Morning sickness (p. 126) Retinopathy (p. 150) Sinusitis (p. 156) Tardive dyskinesia (p. 157) Urinary tract infection (p. 160) Vitiligo (p. 164)

*Refer to the Individual Health Concern for Complete Information

- Glucose-6-phosphate dehydrogenase deficiency
- Iron overload (hemosiderosis or hemochromatosis)
- History of kidney stones
- Kidney failure

It has been suggested that people who form kidney stones should avoid vitamin C supplements because vitamin C can convert into oxalate and increase urinary oxalate.[17,18] Initially, these concerns were questioned because the vitamin C converted to oxalate *after* urine had left the body.[19,20] However, using newer methodology that rules out this problem, recent evidence shows that as little as 1 gram of vitamin C per day can increase the urinary oxalate levels in some people, even those without a history of kidney stones.[21,22] In one case, 8 grams per day of vitamin C led to dramatic increases in urinary oxalate excretion and kidney stone crystal formation causing bloody urine.[23] Until more is known, people with kidney stones or a history of stone formation should not take large amounts (1 gram per day) of supplemental vitamin C. Significantly lower amounts (100 to 200 mg per day) appear to be safe.

Vitamin D
(Cholecalciferol, irradiated ergosterol)

Vitamin D's most important role is maintaining blood levels of **calcium** (p. 277), which it accomplishes by increasing absorption of calcium from food and reducing urinary calcium loss. Both effects keep calcium in the body and therefore spare the calcium that is stored in the bones. When necessary, vitamin D transfers calcium from the bone into the bloodstream, which does not benefit bones. Although the overall effect of vitamin D on the bones is complicated, some vitamin D is necessary for healthy bones and teeth.

From animal and human population studies, researchers from the University of Wisconsin have hypothesized that vitamin D may protect people from **multiple sclerosis** (p. 127).[1]

Vitamin D plays a role in **immunity** (p. 94) and blood cell formation. Vitamin D also helps cells "differentiate"—a process that may reduce the risk of cancer. Vitamin D is also needed for adequate blood levels of insulin[2] and has been reported to help the body process sugar.[3]

Where Is It Found?

Cod liver oil is an excellent dietary source of vitamin D, as are vitamin D–fortified foods. Traces of vitamin D are found in egg yolks and butter. However, the majority of vitamin D in the body is created during a chemical reaction that starts with sunlight exposure to the skin. Cholecalciferol (vitamin D_3) is the animal form of this vitamin.

Vitamin D

Who Is Likely to Be Deficient?

Vitamin D deficiency, which causes abnormal bone formation, is more common after the winter due to restricted sunlight exposure in that season. Deficiencies are also more common in strict vegetarians (who avoid vitamin D–fortified dairy), dark-skinned individuals, people with malabsorption conditions, liver disease, or kidney disease, and alcoholics. People with liver and kidney disease can make vitamin D but cannot activate it.

One in seven adults has been reported to be vitamin D deficient.[4] In hospitalized patients under age 65, 42% were reported to be vitamin D deficient.[5] This same report found that 37% of the people studied were vitamin D deficient despite the fact that they were eating the currently recommended amount of this nutrient. Vitamin D deficiency is particularly common in the elderly.

Vitamin D Has Been Used in Connection with the Following Conditions*

Ranking	Health Concerns
Primary	Celiac disease (p. 35) (if deficient) Crohn's disease (p. 48) (Crohn's associated Osteomalacia [p. 154]) Rickets (p. 154)
Secondary	Osteoporosis (p. 133)
Other	Alcohol withdrawal support (p. 510) (nutrient depletion) Diabetes (p. 53) Migraine headaches (p. 121) Osteomalacia (p. 154)

*Refer to the Individual Health Concern for Complete Information

How Much Is Usually Taken?

People who get plenty of sun exposure don't require supplemental vitamin D. (Sunlight increases vitamin D synthesis when it strikes bare skin.) Otherwise, 400 IU per day is a safe adult dose.

Are There Any Side Effects or Interactions?

Individuals with sarcoidosis who have elevated blood levels of calcium, and people with hyperparathyroidism should not take vitamin D without consulting a physician. Too much vitamin D taken for long periods of time can lead to headaches, weight loss, and **kidney stones** (p. 111); and rarely to deafness, blindness, increased thirst, increased urination, **diarrhea** (p. 58), irritability, failure to gain weight in children, and even death. Most people take more than 400 IU per day (a safe amount for adults), although one study showed that 800 IU per day prevented bone loss more

effectively than 200 IU per day in postmenopausal women.[6] Anyone wishing to take more than 1,000 IU per day for long periods of time should consult a physician. People should remember that the total daily intake of vitamin D includes vitamin D from fortified milk and other fortified foods, **cod liver oil** (p.294), and supplements that contain vitamin D. In addition, people who receive adequate sunlight exposure do not need as much vitamin D in their diet as do people who receive minimal sunlight exposure.

Vitamin D increases both **calcium** (p. 277) and phosphorus absorption. Vitamin D has also been reported to increase absorption of aluminum. Increased blood levels of calcium (which can be a marker for vitamin D status) have been linked to **heart disease** (p. 32).[7] Some,[8] but not all,[9] research suggests that vitamin D may slightly raise blood levels of **cholesterol** (p. 79) in humans.

Vitamin E (Tocopherol)

Vitamin E is a powerful **antioxidant** (p. 267) that protects cell membranes and other fat-soluble parts of the body, such as LDL cholesterol (the "bad" cholesterol). Protection of LDL cholesterol may reduce the risk of **heart disease** (p. 32). Two studies published in the *New England Journal of Medicine* show that both men[1] and women[2] who supplement with at least 100 IU of vitamin E per day for at least 2 years have a 37 to 41% drop in the risk of heart disease. Even more impressive is the 77% drop in nonfatal heart attacks reported in the double-blind Cambridge Heart Antioxidant Study (CHAOS) study, in which people were given 400 to 800 IU vitamin E per day.[3]

What About the Different Kinds of Vitamin E?

The names of all types of vitamin E begin with either "d" or "dl," which refer to differences in chemical structure. The "d" form is natural and "dl" is synthetic. The natural form is more active. More synthetic vitamin E is added to supplements to compensate for the low level of activity. For example, 100 IU of vitamin E requires about 67 mg of the natural form but at least 100 mg of the synthetic. Little is known about how the synthetic "dl" form affects the body, though no clear toxicity has been discovered. Most doctors of natural medicine advise people to use only the natural ("d") form of vitamin E.

After the "d" or "dl" designation, often the Greek letter "alpha" appears, which also describes the

Vitamin E Has Been Used in Connection with the Following Conditions*

Ranking	Health Concerns
Primary	Atherosclerosis (p. 17) Diabetes (p. 53) High cholesterol (p. 79) (protection of LDL cholesterol) Immune function (for elderly people) (p. 94) Minor injuries (oral and topical for sunburn) (p. 122) Osteoarthritis (p. 562) Tardive dyskinesia (p. 157) Yellow nail syndrome (p. 28)
Secondary	Alzheimer's disease (p. 11) Angina (p. 13) Athletic performance (p. 20) (for exercise recovery and high-altitude exercise performance only) Bronchitis Cold sores (p. 543) Intermittent claudication (p. 106) Premenstrual syndrome (p. 141) Retinopathy (p. 150) (for retrolental fibroplasia) Rheumatoid arthritis (p. 571) Wound healing (p. 167)
Other	Abnormal Pap smear (p. 136) Alcohol withdrawal support (p. 6) (nutrient depletion) Burns (minor) (p. 29) Cataracts (p. 34) Dupuytren's contracture (p. 61) Fibrocystic breast disease (p. 66) Fibromyalgia (p. 68) Hepatitis (p. 77) High cholesterol (p. 79) (increasing HDL cholesterol) HIV support (p. 87) Hypoglycemia (p. 92) Infertility (female) (p. 102) Infertility (male) (p. 103) Lupus (SLE) (p. 115) Macular degeneration (p. 118) Menopause (p. 118) Menorrhagia (heavy menstruation) (p. 120) Minor injuries (p. 122) (for exercise-related muscle strain and topical for scars) Osgood-Schlatter disease (p. 130) Photosensitivity (p. 140) Restless legs syndrome (p. 149) Retinopathy (p. 150) (associated with abetalipoproteinemia) Retinopathy (p. 150) (associated with diabetic retinopathy; combined with selenium [p. 331] and vitamin A [p. 336]) Vaginitis (p. 162)

*Refer to the Individual Health Concern for Complete Information

structure. Synthetic "dl" vitamin E is found only in the alpha form—as in "dl-alpha tocopherol." Natural vitamin E can be found either as alpha (as in "d-alpha tocopherol") or in combination with beta, gamma, and delta (this combination is labeled "mixed," as in mixed natural tocopherols).

Human trials with vitamin E have almost always been done with the alpha (not gamma) form. Historically the synthetic "dl" form was used in most trials, but some trials are now using the natural form. The two reports mentioned above (men and women who supplement vitamin E have fewer heart attacks) measured alpha intake. The double-blind CHAOS trial mentioned above, showing a 77% reduction in nonfatal attacks, used alpha and not gamma. This strongly suggests that the alpha form is protective.

A group of researchers recently claimed that gamma might better protect against oxidative damage;[4] the evidence comes from a test tube study. As a result, some have hypothesized that alpha might interfere with the activity of gamma-tocopherol, a claim that remains unproven.

The issue of alpha versus gamma requires much more research before it can be fully understood. Almost all vitamin E research shows that positive results require hundreds of units per day—an amount easily obtained with supplements but impossible with food. Therefore, switching to food sources as suggested by some researchers is impractical. Until more is known, people seeking to add gamma tocopherol can find mixed natural tocopherol supplements. They contain a small amount of gamma, but the percentage remains much lower than that found in food.

Vitamin E forms are listed as either "tocopherol" or "tocopheryl" followed by the name of what is attached to it, as in "tocopheryl acetate." The two forms are not greatly different; however, tocopherol may absorb a little better, while tocopheryl forms may have slightly better shelf life. Both forms are active when taken by mouth. However, the skin cannot utilize the tocopheryl forms, so those planning to apply vitamin E to the skin should buy tocopherol. In health-food stores, the most common forms of vitamin E are d-alpha tocopherol and d-alpha tocopheryl (acetate or succinate). Both of these d (natural) alpha forms are frequently recommended by doctors of natural medicine.

Where Is It Found?

Wheat germ oil, nuts, seeds, vegetable oils, whole grains, egg yolks, and leafy green vegetables all contain vitamin E. However, the high levels found in supplements, often 100 to 800 IU per day, are not obtainable from eating food.

Vitamin E (Tocopherol)

Who Is Likely to Be Deficient?

Severe vitamin E deficiencies are rare.

How Much Is Usually Taken?

The most commonly recommended dose of vitamin E for adults is 400 to 800 IU per day. However, some leading researchers suggest taking only 100 to 200 IU per day, as studies that have explored the long-term effects of different supplemental levels suggest no further benefit beyond that amount. In addition, research reporting positive effects with 400 to 800 IU per day has not investigated the effects of lower intakes. [5]

Are There Any Side Effects or Interactions? Vitamin E toxicity is very rare; supplements are widely considered to be safe.

A diet high in unsaturated fat increases vitamin E requirements. Vitamin E and **selenium** (p. 331) work together to protect fat-soluble parts of the body.

Vitamin K (Phylloquinone)

Vitamin K is needed for proper **bone formation** (p. 133) and blood clotting, in both cases by helping the body transport calcium. Vitamin K is used by medical doctors when treating an overdose of the drug warfarin. Also, medical doctors prescribe vitamin K to prevent excessive bleeding in people taking warfarin who require surgery.

Where Is It Found?

Leafy green vegetables are the best source of vitamin K.

Vitamin K Has Been Used in Connection with the Following Conditions*

Ranking	Health Concerns
Primary	Celiac disease (p. 35) (if deficient)
Secondary	Osteoporosis (p. 133)
Other	Morning sickness (p. 126)
*Refer to the Individual Health Concern for Complete Information	

Who Is Likely to Be Deficient?

A vitamin K deficiency, which causes uncontrolled bleeding, is rare, except in individuals with certain malabsorption diseases. All newborn infants receive vitamin K to prevent deficiencies that sometimes develop in breast-fed infants.

How Much Is Usually Taken?

Many physicians suggest 65 to 80 mg per day, a level that can be achieved without supplementation by eating vegetables.

Are There Any Side Effects or Interactions? Vitamin K interferes with the action of some prescription blood thinners. People taking these drugs should never supplement vitamin K without consulting a physician. Phylloquinone—the natural vegetable form of vitamin K—has not been linked with any other side effects.

Vitamin K facilitates the effects of **calcium** (p. 277) in building bone and proper blood clotting.

Whey Protein

Whey protein is a dairy-based source of **amino acids** (p. 265) (protein building blocks). Whey protein provides the body with several amino acids, including **leucine** (p. 274), **isoleucine** (p. 274), and **valine** (p. 274)—branched-chain amino acids (BCAAs) (p. 274) needed for the maintenance of muscle tissue.[1]

Where Is It Found?

During the process of making milk into cheese, whey protein is separated from the milk. This whey protein is then incorporated into ice cream, bread, canned soup, infant formulas, and other food products. Supplements containing whey protein are also available.

Who Is Likely to Be Deficient?

Individuals who do not include dairy foods in their diets would not consume whey protein; however, the amino acids in whey protein are available from other sources, and a deficiency of these amino acids is unlikely. In fact, most Americans consume too much rather than too little protein.

How Much Is Usually Taken?

Most people do not require extra protein such as whey protein. However, athletes in training sometimes take approximately 25 grams of whey protein per day, but no evidence indicates that whey improves **athletic performance** (p. 20).

Are There Any Side Effects or Interactions? People who are allergic to dairy products could react to whey protein and should therefore avoid it. **Lactose-intolerant** (p. 114) people will also react to whey protein. As with protein in general, long-term, excessive intake may be associated with deteriorating kidney function and possibly **osteoporosis** (p. 133). However, neither kidney nor bone problems have been directly associated with whey protein, and the other dietary sources of protein typically contribute more protein to the diet than does whey protein.

Zinc

Zinc is a component of more than 300 enzymes that are needed to **repair wounds** (p. 167), maintain **fertility** (p. 103), synthesize protein, help cells reproduce, preserve vision, boost **immunity** (p. 94), and protect against **free radicals** (p. 267), among other functions.

Zinc lozenges shorten the duration of **cold** (p. 41) symptoms for adults in most double-blind studies using proper methodology,[1,2,3] though this effect has not been reported in children.[4] Most successful studies have used zinc gluconate or zinc gluconate-glycine lozenges containing 15 to 25 mg of zinc per lozenge.

Cold sufferers should avoid lozenges that contain citric acid[5] or tartaric acid, substances that may interfere with efficacy and have been used in most trials that fail to get good results.[6] With one exception,[7] trials using forms other than zinc gluconate or zinc gluconate-glycine have failed, as have trials that use insufficient amounts of zinc.[8] Therefore, until more is known, people should only use zinc gluconate or gluconate-glycine. Zinc lozenges are not to be taken long term, but rather only at the onset of a cold and stopped when symptoms have disappeared. The best effect is obtained when lozenges are used at the first sign of a cold: up to 10 lozenges per day can be taken for several days during the cold.

Where Is It Found?

Good sources of zinc include oysters, meat, eggs, seafood, black-eyed peas, tofu, and wheat germ.

Who Is Likely to Be Deficient?

Low-income pregnant women and pregnant teenagers are at risk for marginal zinc deficiencies. Supplementing with 25 to 30 mg per day improves pregnancy outcome in these groups.[9,10]

The average diet frequently provides less than the recommended daily allowance for zinc. A low-dose supplement (15 mg per day) can fill in dietary gaps. Zinc deficiencies are more common in alcoholics and individuals with sickle cell anemia, malabsorption problems, and chronic kidney disease.[11]

How Much Is Usually Taken?

Moderate intake of zinc, 15 to 25 mg, is adequate to prevent deficiencies. Higher levels (up to 50 mg taken 3 times per day) are reserved for treating certain health conditions, under the supervision of a nutritionally oriented doctor. For the alleviation of cold symptoms, lozenges providing 15 to 25 mg of zinc in the form zinc gluconate are generally used frequently throughout the day.

Are There Any Side Effects or Interactions? Zinc intake in excess of 300 mg per day has been reported to impair **immune function** (p. 94).[12] Some people report that zinc lozenges lead to stomachache, nausea, mouth irritation, and a bad taste. In topical form, zinc has no known side effects when used as recommended.

Zinc Has Been Used in Connection with the Following Conditions*

Ranking	Health Concerns
Primary	Celiac disease (p. 35) (for deficiency) Common cold/sore throat (p. 527) Infertility (male) (p. 103) (for deficiency) Minor injuries (p. 122) (for deficiency only) Night blindness (p. 129) Wilson's disease (p. 166) Wound healing (p. 167) (topical)
Secondary	Cold sores (p. 39) (oral and topical) Crohn's disease (p. 48) Infection (p. 63) Injuries (minor) (p. 122) (topical for skin wounds) Peptic ulcer (p. 138) Sickle cell anemia
Other	Acne (p. 5) Anorexia nervosa Athletic performance (p. 20) Benign prostatic hyperplasia (p. 145) Diarrhea (p. 58) Down's syndrome Ear infections (recurrent) (p. 63) Gastritis (p. 71) HIV support (p. 87) Hypoglycemia (p. 92) Hypothyroidism (p. 93) Immune function (p. 94) Macular degeneration (p. 118) Rheumatoid arthritis (p. 151)

*Refer to the Individual Health Concern for Complete Information

Preliminary research had suggested that people with **Alzheimer's disease** (p. 11) should avoid zinc supplements.[13] More recently, preliminary evidence in four patients actually showed improved mental function with zinc supplementation.[14] In a convincing review of the zinc/Alzheimer's disease research, perhaps the most respected zinc researcher in the world concluded that zinc does not cause or exacerbate Alzheimer's disease symptoms.[15]

Zinc inhibits **copper** (p. 285) absorption, which can lead to anemia and lower levels of HDL cholesterol (the "good" cholesterol).[16,17,18] Copper intake should be increased if zinc supplementation continues for more than a few days (except for individuals with **Wilson's disease** [p. 166]).[19] Many zinc supplements, to prevent copper inhibition, include copper in the formulation.

Zinc competes for absorption with **iron** (p. 304),[20,21] **calcium** (p. 276),[22] and **magnesium** (p. 310).[23] A **multimineral** (p. 314) supplement will prevent mineral imbalances that can result from taking high doses of zinc for extended periods of time.

N-acetyl cysteine (NAC) (p. 317) may increase urinary excretion of zinc.[24] Long-term users of NAC may consider adding supplements of zinc and copper.

Zinc

Part Two: References

Acetyl-L-Carnitine

1. Pettegrew JW, Klunk WE, Panchalingam K, et al. Clinical and neurochemical effects of acetyl-L-carnitine in Alzheimer's disease. *Neurobio Aging* 1995; 16: 1–4.

2. Sano M, Bell K, Cote L, et al. Double-blind parallel design pilot study of acetyl levocarnitine in patients with Alzheimer's disease. *Arch Neurol* 1992; 49: 1137–41.

3. Cucinotta D et al. Multicenter clinical placebo-controlled study with acetyl-L-carnitine (LAC) in the treatment of mildly demented elderly patients. *Drug Development Res* 1988; 14: 213–16.

4. Thal LJ, Carta A, Clarke WR, et al. A 1-year multicenter placebo-controlled study of acetyl-L-carnitine in patients with Alzheimer's disease. *Neurology* 1996; 47: 705–11.

5. Rai G, Wright G, Scott L, et al. Double-blind, placebo controlled study of acetyl-L-carnitine in patients with Alzheimer's dementia. *Curr Med Res Opin* 1990; 11: 638–47.

Adenosine Monophosphate (AMP)

1. Sklar SH, Blue WT, Alexander EJ, et al. Herpes zoster: The treatment and prevention of neuralgia with adenosine monophosphate. *JAMA* 1985; 253: 1427–30.

2. Gajdos A. AMP in porphyria cutanea tarda. *Lancet* 1974; I: 163 [letter].

3. Sklar SH. Herpes virus infection. *JAMA* 1977; 237: 871–72.

4. Sherlock CH, Corey L. Adenosine monophosphate for the treatment of varicella zoster infections: A large dose of caution. *JAMA* 1985; 253: 1444–45.

5. Gaby AR, Wright JV. *Nutritional Therapy in Medical Practice.* Seattle, WA, Oct 25–28, 1996, 33.

Alanine

1. Damrau F. Benign prostatic hypertrophy: Amino acid therapy for symptomatic relief. *J Am Geriatrics Soc* 1962; 10(5): 426–30.

2. Feinblatt HM, Gant JC. Palliative treatment of benign prostatic hypertrophy. Value of glycine-alanine-glutamic acid combination. *J Maine Med Assoc* Mar 1958.

3. Zello GA, Wykes LF, Ball RO, et al. Recent advances in methods of assessing dietary amino acid requirements for adult humans. *J Nutr* 1995; 125: 2907–15.

Alpha Lipoic Acid

1. Kagan V, Khan S, Swanson C, Shevedova A, Serbinova E, and Packer L. Antioxidant action of thioctic acid and dihydrolipoic acid. *Free Rad Biol Med* 1990; 9S: 15.

2. Packer L, Witt EH, Tritschler HJ. Alpha-lipoic acid as a biological antioxidant. *Free Rad Biol Med* 1995; 19: 227–50 [review].

3. Ziegler D, Ulrich H, Schatz H, et al. Effects of treatment with the antioxidant alpha-lipoic acid on cardiac autonomic neuropathy in NIDDM patients. *Diabetes Care* 1997; 20: 369–73.

4. Filina AA, Davydova NG, Endrikhovskii SN, et al. Lipoic acid as a means of metabolic therapy of open-angle glaucoma. *Vestn Oftalmol* 1995; 111: 6–8.

5. Baur A et al. Alpha-lipoic acid is an effective inhibitor of human immuno-deficiency virus (HIV-1) replication. *Klin Wochenschr* 1991; 69: 722–24.

6. Nichols TW Jr. Alpha-lipoic acid: biological effects and clinical implications. *Alt Med Rev* 1997; 2: 177–83 [review].

7. Zempleni J, Trusty TA, Mock DM. Lipoic acid reduces the activities of biotin-dependent carboxylases in rat liver. *J Nutr* 1997; 127: 1776–81.

Amino Acids

1. Young VR, Pellett PL. Plant proteins in relation to human protein and amino acid nutrition. *Am J Clin Nutr* 1994; 59(suppl): 1203S–12S.

2. Lemon P. Is increased dietary protein necessary or beneficial for individuals with a physically active life? *Nutr Rev* 1996; 54: S169–75.

3. Sitprija V, Suvanpha R. Low protein diet and chronic renal failure in Buddhist monks. *BMJ* 1983; 287: 469–71.

4. Heaney R. Protein intake and the calcium economy. *J Am Diet Assoc* 1993; 93(11): 1259–60.

5. Abelow BJ, Folford TR, Insogna KL. Cross-cultural association between dietary animal protein and hip fracture: a hypothesis. *Calcif Tiss Int* 1992; 50: 14–18.

6. Schürch MA, Rizzoli R, Slosman D, et al. Protein supplements increase serum insulin-like growth factor-I levels and attenuate proximal femur bone loss in patients with recent hip fracture. *Ann Intern Med* 1998; 128: 801–9.

Androstenedione (Andro)

1. Mahesh VB, Greenblatt RB. The in vivo conversion of dehydroepiandrosterone and androstene-

dione to testosterone in humans. *Acta Endocrinologica* 1962; 41: 400–406.

2. German patent number DE 42 14953 A1.

3. Lea CK, Moxham V, Reed MJ, Flanagan AM. Androstenedione treatment reduces loss of cancellous bone volume in ovariectomised rats in a dose-responsive manner and the effect is not mediated by oestrogen. *J Endocrinol* 1998; 156: 331–39.

4. Saden-Krehula M et al. Testosterone, epitestosterone and androstenedione in the pollen of Scotch Pine *P. Silvestris L. Experientia* 1993; 27: 108–9.

5. Longcope C. Androgen metabolism and the menopause. *Semin Reprod Endocrinol* 1998; 16(2): 111–15.

6. Jiroutek MR, Chen MH, Johnston CC, Longcope C. Changes in reproductive hormones and sex hormone-binding globulin in a group of postmenopausal women measured over 10 years. *Menopause* Summer 1998; 5(2): 90–94.

7. Szymczak J, Milewicz A, Thijssen JH, Blankenstein MA, Daroszewski J. Concentration of sex steroids in adipose tissue after menopause. *Steroids* May/Jun 1998; 63(5–6): 319–21.

8. De Lorenzo A, Lello S, Andreoli A, Guardianelli F, Romanini C. Body composition and androgen pattern in the early period of postmenopause. *Gynecol Endocrinol* Jun 1998; 12(3): 171–77.

9. Vilarinho ST, Costallat LT. Evaluation of the hypothalamic-pituitary-gonadal axis in males with systemic lupus erythematosus. *J Rheumatol* Jun 1998; 25(6): 1097–103.

Antioxidants and Free Radicals

1. Ames BN, Shigenaga MK, Hagen TM. Oxidants, antioxidants, and the degenerative diseases of aging. *Proc Natl Acad Sci* 1993; 90: 7915–7922.

Arginine

1. Besset A, Bonardet A, Rondouin G, et al. Increase in sleep related GH and Prl secretion after chronic arginine aspartate administra-tion in man. *Acta Endocrinologica* 1982; 99: 18–23.

2. Elam RP. Morphological changes in adult males from resistance exercise and amino acid supplementation. *J Sports Med Phys Fitness* 1988; 28: 35–39.

3. Schacter A, Goldman JA, Zukerman Z. Treatment of oligospermia with the amino acid arginine. *J Urol* 1973; 110: 311–13.

4. Pryor JP, Blandy JP, Evans P, et al. Controlled clinical trial of arginine for infertile men with oligozoospermia. *Br J Urol* 1978; 50: 47059.

5. Barbul A, Rettura G, Levenson SM, et al. Wound healing and thymotropic effects of arginine: a pituitary mechanism of action. *Am J Clin Nutr* 1983; 37: 786–94.

6. Kirk SJ, Hurson M, Regan MC, et al. Arginine stimulates wound healing and immune function in elderly human beings. *Surgery* 1993; 114: 155–60.

7. Kohls KJ, Kies C, Fox HM. Serum lipid levels of humans given arginine, lysine and tryptophan supplements without food. *Nutr Rep Internat* 1987; 35: 5–13.

8. Wolf A, Zalpour C, Theilmeier G, et al. Dietary L-arginine supplementation normalizes platelet aggregation in hypercholesterolemic humans. *J Am Coll Cardiol* 1997; 29: 479–85.

9. Smith SD, Wheeler MA, Foster HE Jr, Weiss RM. Improvement in interstitial cystitis symptom scores during treatment with oral K-arginine. *J Urol* 1997; 158: 703–8.

10. Park KGM. The immunological and metabolic effects of L-arginine in human cancer. *Proc Nutr Soc* 1993; 52: 387–401.

11. Takeda Y, Tominga T, Tei N, et al. Inhibitory effect of L-arginine on growth of rat mammary tumors induced by 7, 12, Dimethlybenz(a)-anthracine. *Cancer Res* 1975; 35: 390–93.

12. Park KGM. The immunological and metabolic effects of L-arginine in human cancer. *Proc Nutr Soc* 1993; 52: 387–401.

13. Brittenden J, Park KGM, Heys SD, et al. L-arginine stimulates host defenses in patients with breast cancer. *Surgery* 1994; 115: 205–12.

Beta-Carotene

1. Shekelle RB, Lepper M, Liu S, et al. Dietary vitamin A and risk of cancer in the Western Electric Study. *Lancet* 1981; ii: 1185–90.

2. Hennekens CH, Burning JE, Manson JE, et al. Lack of effect of long-term supplementation with beta carotene on the incidence of malignant neoplasms and cardiovascular disease. *N Engl J Med* 1996; 334: 11145–49.

3. Albanes D, Heinone OP, Taylor PR, et al. Alpha-tocopherol and beta-carotene supplements and lung cancer incidence in the Alpha-Tocopherol, Beta-Carotene Cancer Prevention Study: effects of base-line characteristics and study compliance. *J Natl Cancer Inst* 1996; 88: 1560–70.

4. Omenn GS, Goodman GE, Thornquist MD, et al. Effects of a combination of beta carotene and vitamin A on lung cancer and cardio-vascular disease. *N Engl J Med* 1996; 334: 1150–55.

5. Wang, X-D, Liu C, Bronson RT, et al. Retinoid signaling and activator protein-1 expression in ferrets given ß-carotene supplements and exposed to tobacco smoke. *J Natl Cancer Inst* 1999; 91: 60-6.

6. You C-S, Parker RS, Goodman KJ, et al. Evidence of cis-trans isomerization of 9-cis-beta-carotene during absorption in humans. *Am J Clin Nutr* 1996; 64: 177–83.

7. Tamai H, Morinobu T, Murata T, et al. 9-cis beta-carotene in human plasma and blood cells after ingestion of beta-carotene. *Lipids* 1995; 30: 493–98.

8. Ben-Amotz A, Levy Y. Bioavailability of a natural isomer mixture compared with synthetic all-trans beta-carotene in human serum. *Am J Clin Nutr* 1996; 63: 729–34.

9. Bitterman N, Melamed Y, Ben-Amotz A. Beta-carotene and CNS oxygen toxicity in rats. *J Appl Physiol* 1994; 76: 1073–76.

10. Ben-Amotz A, Levy Y. Bioavailability of a natural isomer mixture compared with synthetic all-trans beta-carotene in human serum. *Am J Clin Nutr* 1996; 63: 729–34.

11. Yeum K-J, Azhu S, Xiao S, et al. Beta-carotene intervention trial in

Part Two: References

premalignant gastric lesions. *J Am Coll Nutr* 1995; 14: 536 [abstr #48].

12. Xu MJ, Plezia PM, Alberts DS, et al. Reduction in plasma or skin alpha-tocopherol concentration with long-term oral administration of beta-carotene in humans and mice. *J Natl Cancer Inst* 1992; 84: 1559–65.

Betaine Hydrochloride (Hydrochloric Acid)

1. Giannella RA, Broitman SA, Zamcheck N. Influence of gastric acidity on bacterial and parasitic enteric infections. *Ann Int Med* 1973; 78: 271–76.

2. Giannella RA, Broitman SA, Zamcheck N. Influence of gastric acidity on bacterial and parasitic enteric infections. *Ann Int Med* 1973; 78: 271–76.

3. Kokkonen J, Simila S, Herva R. Impaired gastric function in children with cow's milk intolerance. *Eur J Pediatr* 1979; 132: 1–6.

4. Gillespie M. Hypochlorhydria in asthma with specific reference to the age incidence. *Quart J Med* 1935; 4: 397–405.

5. Fravel RC. The occurrence of hypochlorhydria in gall-bladder disease. *Am J Med Sci* 1920; 159: 512–17.

6. Murray MJ, Stein N. A gastric factor promoting iron absorption. *Lancet* 1968; 1: 614.

7. Russell RM et al. Correction of impaired folic acid (Pte Glu) absorption by orally administered HCl in subjects with gastric atrophy. *Am J Clin Nutr* 1984; 39: 656.

Beta-Sitosterol

1. Lees AM, Mok HYI, Lee RS, et al. Plant sterols as cholesterol-lowering agents: Clinical trials in patients with hypercholesterolemia and studies of sterol balance. *Atheroscler* 1977; 28: 325–38.

2. Pelletier X, Belbraouet S, Mirabel D, et al. A diet moderately enriched in phytosterols lowers plasma cholesterol concentrations in normocholesterolemic humans. *Ann Nutr Metab* 1995; 39: 291–95.

3. Grundy SM, Ahrens EH Jr, Davignon J. The interaction of choles-terol absorption and cholesterol synthesis in man. *J Lipid Res* 1969; 10: 304–15 [review].

4. Berges RR, Windeler J, Trampisch HJ, et al. Randomised, placebo-controlled, double-blind clinical trial of beta-sitosterol in patients with benign prostatic hyperplasia. *Lancet* 1995; 345: 1529–32.

5. Kiriakdis S, Stathi S, Jha HC, et al. Fatty acid esters of sitosterol 3β-glucoside from soybeans and tempeh (fermented soybeans) as antiproliferative substances. *J Clin Biochem Nutr* 1997; 22: 139–47.

6. Berges RR, Windeler J, Trampisch HJ, et al. Randomised, placebo-controlled, double-blind clinical trial of beta-sitosterol in patients with benign prostatic hyperplasia. *Lancet* 1995; 345: 1529–32.

7. Klippel KF, Hiltl DM, Schipp B. A multicentric, placebo-controlled, double-blind clinical trial of β-sitosterol (phytosterol) for the treatment of benign prostatic hyperplasia. *Br J Urol* 1997; 80: 427–32.

Bioflavonoids

1. Peterson J, Dwyer J. Taxonomic classification helps identify flavonoid-containing foods on a semiquantitative food frequency questionnaire. *J Am Dietet Assoc* 1998; 98: 682–85.

2. So FV, Guthrie N, Chambers AF, et al. Inhibition of human breast cancer cell proliferation and delay of mammary tumorigenesis by flavonoids and citrus juices. *Nutr Cancer* 1996; 26: 167–81.

3. Pamukcu AM, Yalciner S, Hatcher JF, Bryan GT. Quercetin, a rat intestinal and bladder carcinogen present in bracken fern (*Pteridium aquilinum*). *Cancer Res* 1980; 40: 3468–72.

4. Hirono I, Ueno I, Hosaka S, Takanashi H, et al. Carcinogenicity examination of quercetin and rutin in ACI rats. *Cancer Lett* 1981; 13: 15–21.

5. Saito D, Shirai A, Matsushima T, et al. Test of carcinogenicity of quercetin, a widely distributed mutagen in food. *Teratog Carcinog Mutagen* 1980; 1: 213–21.

6. Aeschbacher H-U, Meier H, Ruch E. Nonmutagenicity *in vivo* of the food flavonol quercetin. *Nutr Cancer* 1982; 2: 90.

7. Nishino H, Nishino A, Iwashima A, et al. Quercetin inhibits the action of 12-O-tetradecanoylphorbol-13-acetate, a tumor promoter. *Oncology* 1984; 41: 120–23.

8. Kuo SM. Antiproliferative potency of structurally distinct dietary flavonoids on human colon cancer cells. *Cancer Lett* 1996; 110: 41–48.

9. Knekt P, Jävinen R, Seppänen R, et al. Dietary flavonoids and the risk of lung cancer and other malignant neoplasms. *Am J Epidemiol* 1997; 146: 223–30.

10. Hertog M, Feskens EJM, Hollman PCH, et al. Dietary flavonoids and cancer risk in the Zutphen Elderly Study. *Nutr Cancer* 1994; 22: 175–84.

11. Stavric B. Quercetin in our diet: from potent mutagen to probable anticarcinogen. *Clin Biochem* 1994; 27: 245–48.

12. Vinson JA, Bose P. Comparative bioavailability to humans of ascorbic acid alone or in a citrus extract. *Am J Clin Nutr* 1988; 48: 601–4.

13. Vinson JA, Bose P. Comparative bioavailability of synthetic and natural vitamin C in Guinea pigs. *Nutr Rep Intl* 1983; 27 (4): 875.

Biotin

1. Said HM, Redha R, Nylander W. Biotin transport in the human intestine: Inhibition by anticonvulsant drugs. *Am J Clin Nutr* 1989; 49: 127–31.

2. Zempleni J, Mock DM. Biotin biochemistry and human requirements. *J Nutr Biochem* 1999; 10: 128–38 [review].

3. Zempleni J, Mock DM. Biotin biochemistry and human requirements. *J Nutr Biochem* 1999; 10: 128–38 [review].

4. Coggeshall JC et al. Biotin status and plasma glucose in diabetics. *Ann NY Acad Sci* 1985; 447: 389.

5. Koutsikos D, Agroyannis B, Tzanatos-Exarchou H. Biotin for diabetic peripheral neuropathy. *Biomed Pharmacother* 1990; 44: 511–14.

6. Hochman LG, Scher RK, Meyerson MS. Brittle nails: Responses to daily biotin supplementation. *Cutis* 1993; 51(4): 303–5.

7. Somer E. *The Essential Guide to Vitamins and Minerals*. New York: Harper, 1995, 70–72.

8. Zempleni J, Mock DM. Biotin biochemistry and human requirements. *J Nutr Biochem* 1999; 10: 128–38 [review].

Boric Acid

1. van Slyke RK, Michel VP, Rein MF. Treatment of vulvovaginal candidiasis with boric acid powder. *Am J Obstet Gynecol* 1981; 141: 145.

2. Jovanovic R et al. Antifungal agents vs. boric acid for treating chronic mycotic vulvovaginitis. *J Reprod Med* 1977; 36(8): 593–97.

3. Skinner GRB, Hartley CE, Millar D, Bishop E. Possible treatment for cold sores. *BMJ* 1979; 2(6192): 704.

4. Penna RP, Corrigan LL, Welsh J, et al. *Handbook of Nonprescription Drugs,* 6th ed. American Pharmaceutical Association, Washington, DC: 1979, 424 [review].

5. Penna RP, Corrigan LL, Welsh J, et al. *Handbook of Nonprescription Drugs,* 6th ed. American Pharmaceutical Association, Washington, DC: 1979, 424 [review].

Boron

1. Nielsen FH. Boron—an overlooked element of potential nutritional importance. *Nutr Today* 1988; 23: 4–7.

2. Nielsen FH. Facts and fallacies about boron. *Nutr Today* May/Jun 1992; 6–12.

3. Kelly GS. Boron: a review of its nutritional interactions and therapeutic uses. *Alt Med Rev* 1997; 2: 48–56 [review].

4. Nielsen FH. Ultratrace minerals: Boron. *In Modern Nutrition in Health and Disease,* by Shils ME, VR Young. Philadelphia: Lea & Febiger, 1988; 281–83 [review].

5. Hunt CD, Herbel JL, Nielsen FH. Metabolic responses of postmenopausal women to supplemental dietary boron and aluminum during usual and low magnesium intake: boron, calcium, and magnesium absorption and retention and blood mineral concentrations. *Am J Clin Nutr* 1997; 65: 803–13.

6. Nielsen FH, Hunt CD, Mullen LM, Hunt JR. Effect of dietary boron on mineral, estrogen, and testosterone metabolism in postmenopausal women. *FASEB J* 1987; 1: 394–97.

7. Hunt CD, Herbel JL, Nielsen FH. Metabolic responses of postmenopausal women to supplemental dietary boron and aluminum during usual and low magnesium intake: boron, calcium, and magnesium absorption and retention and blood mineral concentrations. *Am J Clin Nutr* 1997; 65: 803–13.

Branched-Chain Amino Acids (BCAAs)

1. Blomstrand E, Ek S, Newsholme EA. Influence of ingesting a solution of branched-chain amino acids on plasma and muscle concentrations of amino acids during prolonged submaximal exercise. *Nutrition* 1996; 12: 485–90.

2. MacLean DA, Graham TE, Satlin B. Branched-chain amino acids augment ammonia metabolism while attenuating protein breakdown during exercise. *Am J Physiol* 1994; 267: E1010–22.

3. Kelly GS. Sports nutrition: A review of selected nutritional supplements for bodybuilders and strength athletes. *Med Rev* 1997; 2: 184–201.

4. Van Hall G, Raaymakers JSH, Saris WHM, Wagenmakers AJM. Supplementation with branched-chain amino acids (BCAA) and tryptophan has no effect on performance during prolonged exercise. *Clin Sci* 1994; 87: 52 [abstract #75].

5. Blomstrand E, Hassmen P, Ek S, et al. Influence of ingesting a solution of branched-chain amino acids on perceived exertion during exercise. *Acta Physiol Scand* 1997; 159: 41–49.

6. Van Hall G, Raaymakers JSH, Saris WHM, Wagenmakers AJM. Supplementation with branched-chain amino acids (BCAA) and tryptophan has no effect on performance during prolonged exercise. *Clin Sci* 1994; 87: 52 [abstract #75].

7. Madsen K, MacLean DA, Kiens B, et al. Effects of glucose, glucose plus branched-chain amino acids, or placebo on bike performance over 100 km. *J Appl Physiol* 1996; 81: 2644–50.

8. Vukovich MD, Sharp RL, Kesl LD, et al. Effects of a low-dose amino acid supplement on adaptations to cycling training in untrained individuals. *Int J Sport Nutr* 1997; 7: 298–309.

9. Freyssenet D, Berthon P, Denis C, et al. Effect of a six-week endurance training program and branched-chain amino acid supplementation on histomorphometric characteristics of aged human muscle. *Arch Physiol Biochem* 1996; 104: 157–62.

10. Schena F, Guerrini F, Tregnaghi P, et al. Branched-chain amino acid supplementation during trekking at high altitude. The effects on loss of body mass, body composition, and muscle power. *Eur J Appl Physiol* 1992; 65: 394–98.

11. Mittleman KD, Ricci MR, Bailey SP. Branched-chain amino acids prolong exercise during heat stress in men and women. *Med Sci Sports Exerc* 1998; 30: 83–91.

12. Hassmén P, Blomstrand E, Ekblom B, Newshomle EA. Branched-chain amino acid supplementation during 30-km competitive run: mood and cognitive performance. *Nutrition* 1994; 10: 405–10.

13. Blomstrand E, Hassmen P, Ek S, et al. Influence of ingesting a solution of branched-chain amino acids on perceived exertion during exercise. *Acta Physiol Scand* 1997; 159: 41–49.

14. Blomstrand E, Hassmen P, Ekblom B, et al. Administration of branched-chain amino acids during sustained exercise—effects on performance and on plasma concentration of some amino acids. *Eur J Appl Physiol* 1991; 63: 83–88.

15. Plaitakis A, Smith J, Mandeli J, et al. Pilot trial of branched-chain amino acids in amyotrophic lateral sclerosis. *Lancet* May 7, 1988: 1015–18.

16. The Italian ALS Study Group. Branched-chain amino acids and amyotrophic lateral sclerosis: a treatment

failure? *Neurology* 1993; 43: 2466–70.

17. Tandan R, Bromberg MB, Forshew D, Fries TJ, Badger GJ, Carpenter J, Krusinski PB, Betts EF, Arciero K, Nau K. A controlled trial of amino acid therapy in amyotrophic lateral sclerosis: I. Clinical, functional, and maximum isometric torque data. *Neurology* 1996; 47: 1220–26.

18. MacLean D, Vissing J, Vissing SF, Haller RG. Oral branched-chain amino acids do not improve exercise capacity in McArdle disease. *Neurology* 1998; 51: 1456–59.

19. Mourier A, Gautier JF, De Kerviler E, et al. Mobilization of visceral adipose tissue related to the improvement in insulin sensitivity in response to physical training in NIDDM. Effects of branched-chain amino acid supplements. *Diabetes Care* 1997; 20: 385–91.

20. Maddrey WC. Branched chain amino acid therapy in liver disease. *J Am Coll Nutr* 1985; 4: 639–50 [review].

21. Wahren J, Denis J, Desurmont P, et al. Is intravenous administration of branched chain amino acids effective in the treatment of hepatic encephalopathy? A multicenter study. *Hepatology* 1983; 3(4): 475–80.

22. Egberts E-H, Schomerus H, Hamster W, Jürgens P. Branched chain amino acids in the treatment of latent portosystemic encephalopathy. *Gastroenterol* 1985; 88: 887–95.

23. Naylor CD, O'Rourke K, Detsky AS, et al. Parenteral nutrition with branched-chain amino acids in hepatic encephalopathy. A meta-analysis. *Gastroenterology* 1989; 97: 1033–42.

24. Chin SE, Sheperd RW, Thomas BJ, et al. Nutritional support in children with end-stage liver disease: a randomized crossover trial of a branched-chain amino acid supplement. *Am J Clin Nutr* 1992; 56: 158–63.

25. Kato M, Miwa Y, Tajika M, et al. Preferential use of branched-chain amino acids as an energy substrate in patients with liver cirrhosis. *Internal Med* 1998; 37: 429–34.

26. Soreide E, Skeie B, Kirvela O, Lynn R, Ginsberg N, Manner T, Katz DP, Askanazi J. Branched-chain amino acid in chronic renal failure patients: respiratory and sleep effects. *Kidney Int* 1991; 40: 539–43.

27. Berry HK, Brunner RL, Hunt MM, et al. Valine, isoleucine, and leucine. A new treatment for phenylketonuria. *Am J Dis Child* 1990; 144: 539–43.

28. Zello GA, Wykes LF, Ball RO, et al. Recent advances in methods of assessing dietary amino acid requirements for adult humans. *J Nutr* 1995; 125: 2907–15.

29. Young VR, Bier DM, Pellett PL. A theoretical basis for increasing current estimates of the amino acid requirements in adult man, with experimental support. *Am J Clin Nutr* 1989; 50: 80–92.

Bromelain

1. Izaka K, Yamada M, Kawano T, Suyama T. Gastrointestinal absorption and anti-inflammatory effect of bromelain. *Jpn J Pharmacol* 1972; 22: 519–34.

2. Balakrishnan V, Hareendran A, Nair CS. Double-blind cross-over trial of an enzyme preparation in pancreatic steatorrhea. *J Assoc Phys Ind* 1981; 29: 207–9.

3. Seligman B. Bromelain: An anti-inflammatory agent. *Angiology* 1962; 13: 508–10.

4. Cirelli MG. Treatment of inflammation and edema with bromelain. *Delaware Med J* 1962; 34(6): 159–67.

5. Masson M. Bromelain in the treatment of blunt injuries to the musculoskeletal system. A case observation study by an orthopedic surgeon in private practice. *Fortschr Med* 1995; 113(19): 303–6.

6. Seltzer AP. Minimizing postoperative edema and ecchymoses by the use of a&n oral enzyme preparation (bromelain). *EENT Monthly* 1962; 41: 813–17.

7. Howat RCL, Lewis GD. The effect of bromelain therapy on episiotomy wounds—a double blind controlled clinical trial. *J Obstet Gynaecol Br Commonwealth* 1972; 79: 951–53.

8. Zatuchni GI, Colombi DJ. Bromelains therapy for the prevention of episiotomy pain. *Obstet Gynecol* 1967; 29: 275–78.

9. Taub SJ. The use of Ananase in sinusitis. A study of 60 patients. *EENT Monthly* 1966; 45: 96–98.

10. Ryan RE. A double-blind clinical evaluation of bromelains in the treatment of acute sinusitis. *Headache* 1967; 7: 13–17.

11. Mori S, Ojima Y, Hirose T, et al. The clinical effect of proteolytic enzyme containing bromelain and trypsin on urinary tract infection evaluated by double blind method. *Acta Obstet Gynaecol Jpn* 1972; 19: 147–53.

12. Cohen A, Goldman J. Bromelains therapy in rheumatoid arthritis. *Pennsylvania Med J* 1964; 67: 27–30.

13. Heinicke R, van der Wal L, Yokoyama M. Effect of bromelain (Ananase) on human platelet aggregation. *Experientia* 1972; 28: 844–45.

14. Nieper HA. Effect of bromelain on coronary heart disease and angina pectoris. *Acta Med Empirica* 1978; 5: 274–78.

15. Seligman B. Oral bromelains as adjuncts in the treatment of acute thrombophlebitis. *Angiology* 1969; 20: 22–26.

16. Schafer A, Adelman B. Plasma inhibition of platelet function and of arachidonic acid metabolism. *J Clin Invest* 1985; 75: 456–61.

17. Kelly GS. Bromelain: a literature review and discussion of its therapeutic applications. *Alt Med Rev* 1996; 1: 243–57 [review].

18. Gaby AR. The story of bromelain. *Nutr Healing* May 1995: 3,4,11.

19. Gutfreund AE, Taussig SJ, Morris AK. Effect of oral bromelain on blood pressure and heart rate of hypertensive patients. *Hawaii Med J* 1978; 37: 143–46.

Calcium

1. Osborne CG, McTyre RB, Dudek J, et al. Evidence for the relationship of calcium to blood pressure. *Nutr Rev* 1996; 54: 365–81.

2. Barilla DE, Notz C, Kennedy D, Pak CYC. Renal oxalate excretion

Part Two: References

following oral oxalate loads in patients with ileal disease and with renal and absorptive hypercalciurias: effect of calcium and magnesium. *Am J Med* 1978; 64: 579–85.

3. Curhan GC, Willett WC, Rimm EB, Stampfer MJ. A prospective study of dietary calcium and other nutrients and the risk of symptomatic kidney stones. *N Engl J Med* 1993; 328: 833–83.

4. Bell L, Halstenson CE, Halstenson CJ, et al. Cholesterol-lowering effects of calcium carbonate in patients with mild to moderate hypercholesterolemia. *Arch Intern Med* 1992; 152: 2441–44.

5. Sheikh MS, Santa Ana CA, Nicar MJ, et al. Gastrointestinal absorption of calcium from milk and calcium salts. *N Engl J Med* 1987; 317: 532–36.

6. Levenson DI, Bockman RS. A review of calcium preparations. *Nutr Rev* 1994; 52: 221–32 [review].

7. Nicar MJ, Pak CYC. Calcium bioavailability from calcium carbonate and calcium citrate. *J Clin Endocrinol Metabol* 1985; 61: 391–93.

8. Harvey JA, Kenny P, Poindexter J, Pak CYC. Superior calcium absorption from calcium citrate than calcium carbonate using external forearm counting. *J Am Coll Nutr* 1990; 9: 583–87.

9. Sheikh MS, Santa Ana CA, Nicar MJ, et al. Gastrointestinal absorption of calcium from milk and calcium salts. *N Engl J Med* 1987; 317: 532–36.

10. Epstein O, Kato Y, Dick R, Sherlock S. Vitamin D, hydroxyapatite, and calcium gluconate in treatment of cortical bone thinning in postmenopausal women with primary biliary cirrhosis. *Am J Clin Nutr* 1982; 36: 426–30.

11. Heaney RP, Recker RR, Weaver CM. Absorbability of calcium sources: the limited role of solubility. *Calcif Tissue Int* 1990; 46: 300–4.

12. Deroisy R, Zartarian M, Meurmans L, et al. Acute changes in serum calcium and parathyroid hormone circulating levels induced by the oral intake of five currently available calcium salts in healthy male volun-

teers. *Clin Rheumatol* 1997; 16: 249–53.

13. Heaney RP, Recker RR, Weaver CM. Absorbability of calcium sources: the limited role of solubility. *Calcific Tissue Int* 1990; 46: 300–4.

14. Levenson DI, Bockman RS. A review of calcium preparations. *Nutr Rev* 1994; 52: 221–32 [review].

15. Burros M. Testing calcium supplements for lead. *New York Times* June 4,1997, B7.

16. Bourgoin BP, Evans DR, Cornett JR, et al. Lead content in 70 brands of dietary calcium supplements. *Am J Publ Health* 1993; 83: 1155–60.

17. Civitelli R, Villareal DT, Agnusdei D, et al. Dietary L-lysine and calcium metabolism in humans. *Nutrition* 1992; 8: 400–5.

18. Flodin NW. The metabolic roles; pharmacology, and toxicology of lysine. *J Am Coll Nutr* 1997; 16: 7–21 [review].

19. Kobrin SM, Goldstine SJ, Shangraw RF, Raja RM. Variable efficacy of calcium carbonate tablets. *Am J Kidney Dis* 1989; 14: 461–65.

20. R. Shangraw, chair, Dept. Pharm, U. of Maryland, quoted in: "Ask Dr Tastebud," *Nutr Action Healthletter*, Sep 1990, 13.

21. Mortensen L, Charles P. Bioavailability of calcium supplements and the effect of vitamin D: Comparisons between milk, calcium carbonate, and calcium carbonate plus vitamin D. *Am J Clin Nutr* 1996; 63: 354–57.

22. Sheikh M, Santa Ana C, Nicar M, et al. Gastrointestinal absorption of calcium from milk and calcium salts. *N Engl J Med* 1987; 317: 532–36.

23. Kohls K, Kies C. Calcium bioavailability: A comparison of several different commercially available calcium supplements. *J Appl Nutr* 1992; 44: 50–62.

24. Heaney RP, Dowell MS, Barger-Lux MJ. Absorption of calcium as the carbonate and citrate salts, with some observations on method. *Osteoporos Int 1999*; 9: 19–23.

25. Miller J, Smith D, Flora L, et al. Calcium absorption from calcium carbonate and a new form of calcium (CCM) in healthy male and female adolescents. *Am J Clin Nutr* 1988; 48: 1291–94.

26. Harvey JA, Kenny P, Poindexter J, Pak CYC. Superior calcium absorption from calcium citrate than calcium carbonate using external forearm counting. *J Am Coll Nutr* 1990; 9: 583–87.

27. Smith KT, Heaney RP, Flora L, Hinders SM. Calcium absorption from a new calcium delivery system (CCM). *Calcif Tiss Int* 1987; 41: 351–52.

28. Dawson-Hughes B, Dallal GE, Krall EA, et al. A controlled trial of the effect of calcium supplementation on bone density in postmenopausal women. *N Engl J Med* 1990; 323: 878–83.

29. Nicar MJ, Pak CYC. Calcium bioavailability from calcium carbonate and calcium citrate. *J Clin Endocrinol Metabol* 1985; 61: 391–93.

30. Harvey JA, Kenny P, Poindexter J, Pak CYC. Superior calcium absorption from calcium citrate than calcium carbonate using external forearm counting. *J Am Coll Nutr* 1990; 9: 583–87.

31. Sheikh MS, Santa Ana CA, Nicar MJ, et al. Gastrointestinal absorption of calcium from milk and calcium salts. *N Engl J Med* 1987; 317: 532–36.

32. Epstein O, Kato Y, Dick R, Sherlock S. Vitamin D, hydroxyapatite, and calcium gluconate in treatment of cortical bone thinning in postmenopausal women with primary biliary cirrhosis. *Am J Clin Nutr* 1982; 36: 426–30.

33. Rüegsegger P, Keller A, Dambacher MA. Comparison of the treatment effects of ossein-hydroxyapatite compound and calcium carbonate in osteoporotic females. *Osteoporosis Int* 1995; 5: 30–34.

34. Lloyd T, Andon MB, Rollings N, et al. Calcium supplementation and bone mineral density in adolescent girls. *JAMA* 1993; 270: 841–44.

35. Heaney RP, Recker RR, Weaver CM. Absorbability of calcium

sources: the limited role of solubility. *Calcif Tissue Int* 1990; 46: 300–4.

36. Deroisy R, Zartarian M, Meurmans L, et al. Acute changes in serum calcium and parathyroid hormone circulating levels induced by the oral intake of five currently available calcium salts in healthy male volunteers. *Clin Rheumatol* 1997; 16: 249–53.

37. Heaney RP, Recker RR, Weaver CM. Absorbability of calcium sources: the limited role of solubility. *Calcif Tissue Int* 1990; 46: 300–4.

38. Heaney RP, Smith KT, Recker RR, Hinders SM. Meal effects on calcium absorption. *Am J Clin Nutr* 1989; 49: 372–76.

39. Curhan GC, Willett WC, Rimm EB, Stampfer MJ. A prospective study of dietary calcium and other nutrients and the risk of symptomatic kidney stones. *N Engl J Med* 1993; 328: 833–38.

40. Blumsohn A, Herrington K, Hannon RA, et al. The effect of calcium supplementation on the circadian rhythm of bone reabsorption. *J Clin Endocrinol* 1994; 79: 730–35.

41. Ivanovich P, Fellows H, Rich C. The absorption of calcium carbonate. *Ann Intern Med* 1967; 9: 271–85.

42. Recker RR. Calcium absorption and achlorhydria. *N Engl J Med* 1985; 313: 70–73.

43. Bo-Linn GW, Davis GR, Buddrus DH, et al. An evaluation of the importance of gastric acid secretion in the absorption of dietary calcium. *J Clin Invest* 1984; 73: 640–47.

44. Serfaty-Lacrosniere C, Woods RJ, Voytko D, et al. Hypochlorhydria from short-term omeprazole treatment does not inhibit intestinal absorption of calcium, phosphorus, magnesium or zinc from food in humans. *J Am Coll Nutr* 1995; 14: 364–48.

45. Knox TA, Kassarhian Z, Dawson-Hughes B, et al. Calcium absorption in elderly subjects on high- and low-fiber diets: effect of gastric acidity. *Am J Clin Nutr* 1991; 53: 1480–86.

46. Eastell R, Vieira NE, Yergey AL, et al. Pernicious anaemia as a risk factor for osteoporosis. *Clin Sci* 1992; 82: 681–85.

L-Carnitine

1. Mancini M, Rengo F, Lingetti M, Sorrentino GP, Nolfe G. Controlled study on the therapeutic efficacy of propionyl-L-carnitine in patients with congestive heart failure. *Arzneimittelforschung* 1992; 42: 1101–4.

2. Giamberardino MA et al. Effects of prolonged L-carnitine administration on delayed muscle pain and CK release after eccentric effort. *Int J Sports Med* 1996; 17: 320–24.

3. Green RE, Levine AM, Gunning MJ. The effect of L-carnitine supplementation on lean body mass in male amateur body builders. *J Am Dietet Assoc* 1997; (suppl): A-72.

4. Murray MT. The many benefits of carnitine. *Am J Natural Med* 1996; 3: 6–14 [review].

5. Dal Negro R, Pomari G, et al. L-carnitine and rehabilitative respiratory physiokinesitherapy: metabolic and ventilatory response in chronic respiratory insufficiency. *Int J Clin Pharmacol Ther Toxicol* 1986; 24: 453–56.

6. Dal Negro R, Turco P, Pomari C, De Conti F. Effects of L-carnitine on physical performance in chronic respiratory insufficiency. *Int J Clin Pharmacol Ther Toxicol* 1988; 26: 269–72.

7. Dipalma JR. Carnitine deficiency. *Am Family Phys* 1988; 38: 243–51.

8. Kendler BS. Carnitine: an overview of its role in preventive medicine. *Prev Med* 1986; 15: 373–90.

9. Del Favero A. Carnitine and gangliosides. *Lancet* 1988; ii: 337 [letter].

10. Kobayashi A, Masumura Y, Yamazaki N. L-carnitine treatment for congestive heart failure—experimental and clinical study. *Jpn Circ J* 1992; 56: 86–94.

Cartilage (Bovine and Shark)

1. Prudden JF, Allen J. The clinical acceleration of healing with a cartilage application. *JAMA* 1965; 192: 352–56.

2. Prudden JF, Wolarsky E. The reversal by cartilage of the steroid-induced inhibition of wound healing. *Surg Gyn Obstet* 1967; 125(7): 109–13.

3. Prudden JF. The treatment of human cancer with agents prepared from bovine cartilage. *J Biol Res Mod* 1985; 4: 551–84.

4. Lee A, Langer R. Shark cartilage contains inhibitors of tumor angiogenesis. *Science* 1983; 221: 1185–87.

5. Lane AW, Contreras E Jr. High rate of bioactivity (reduction in gross tumor size) observed in advanced cancer patients treated with shark cartilage material. *J Naturopathic Med* 1992; 3: 86–88.

6. Prudden JF. The treatment of human cancer with agents prepared from bovine cartilage. *J Biol Resp Modif* 1985; 4: 551–84.

Chitosan

1. Koide SS. Chitin-chitosan: properties, benefits and risks. *Nutr Res* 1998; 18: 1091–101 [review].

2. Maezaki Y, Tsuji K, Nakagawa Y, et al. Hypocholesterolemic effect of chitosan in adult males. *Biosci Biotech Biochem* 1993; 57: 1439–44.

3. Jing SB, Li L, Ji D, et al. Effect of chitosan on renal function in patients with chronic renal failure. *J Pharm Pharmacol* 1997; 49: 721–23.

4. Deuchi K, Kanauchi O, Imasato Y, et al. Effect of the viscosity or deacetylation degree of chitosan on fecal fat excreted from rats fed on a high-fat diet. *Biosci Biotech Biochem* 1995; 59: 781–85.

5. Deuchi K, Kanauchi O, Imasato Y, et al. Decreasing effect of chitosan on the apparent fat digestibility by rats fed on a high-fat diet. *Biosci Biotech Biochem* 1994; 58: 1613–16.

6. Kanauchi O, Deuchi K, Imasato Y, et al. Increasing effect of a chitosan and ascorbic acid mixture on fecal dietary fat excretion. *Biosci Biotech Biochem* 1994; 58: 1617–20.

7. Deuchi K, Kanauchi O, Shizukuishi M, et al. Continuous and massive intake of chitosan affects mineral and fat-soluble vitamin status in rats fed on a high-fat diet. *Biosci Biotech Biochem* 1995; 59: 1211–16.

Part Two: References

8. Kato H, Taguchi T, Okuda H, et al. Antihypertensive effect of chitosan in rats and humans. *J Trad Medicine* 1994; 11: 198–205.

9. Terada A, Hara H, Sato D, et al. Effect of dietary chitosan on faecal microbiota and faecal metabolites of humans. *Microb Ecol Health Dis* 1995; 8: 15–21.

10. Bone E, Tamm A, Hill M. The production of urinary phenols by gut bacteria and their possible role in the causation of large bowel cancer. *Am J Clin Nutr* 1976; 29: 1448–54.

11. Koide SS. Chitin-chitosan: properties, benefits and risks. *Nutr Res* 1998; 18: 1091–101 [review].

Chlorophyll

1. Rudolph C. The therapeutic value of chlorophyll. *Clin Med Surg* 1930: 37; 119–21.

2. Chernomorsky SA, Segelman AB. Biological activities of chlorophyll derivatives. *N J Med* 1988: 85; 669–73.

3. Gruskin B. Chlorophyll—its therapeutic place in acute and suppurative disease. *Am J Surg* 1940: 49; 49–56.

4. Hayatsu H, Negishi T, Arimoto S, et al. Porphyrins as potential inhibitors against exposure to carcinogens and mutagens. *Mutat Res* 1993: 290; 79–85.

Chondroitin Sulfate

1. Moss M, Kruger GO, Reynolds DC. The effect of chondroitin sulfate on bone healing. *Oral Surg Oral Med Oral Pathol* 1965; 20: 795–801.

2. Kerzberg EM, Roldan EJA, Castelli G, Huberman ED. Combination of glycosaminoglycans and acetylsalicylic acid in knee osteoarthritis. *Scand J Rheum* 1987; 16: 377.

3. Rovetta G. Galactosaminoglycuronoglycan sulfate (Matrix) in therapy of tibiofibular osteoarthritis of the knee. *Drugs Exptl Clin Res* 1991; 17: 53–57.

4. Mazieres B, Loyau G, Menkes CJ, et al. Le chondroitine sulfate dans le traitement de la gonarthrose et de la coxarthrose. *Rev Rhum Mal Steoartic* 1992; 59: 466–72.

5. Izuka K, Murata K, Nakazawa K, et al. Effects of chondroitin sulfates on serum lipids and hexosamines in atherosclerotic patients: With special reference to thrombus formation time. *Jpn Heart J* 1968; 9: 453–60.

6. Morrison LM, Bajwa GS, Alfin-Slater RB, Ershoff BH. Prevention of vascular lesions by chondroitin sulfate A in the coronary artery and aorta of rats induced by a hypervitaminosis D, cholesterol-containing diet. *Atherosclerosis* 1972; 16: 105–18.

7. Morrison LM, Branwood AW, Ershoff BH, et al. The prevention of coronary arteriosclerotic heart disease with chondroitin sulfate A: Preliminary report. *Exp Med Surg* 1969; 27: 278–89.

8. Morrison LM, Enrick NL. Coronary heart disease: Reduction of death rate by chondroitin sulfate A. *Angiology* 1973; 24: 269–82.

9. Lenclud C, Chapelle P, van Mylem A, et al. Effects of chondroitin sulfate on snoring characteristics: a pilot study. *Curr Ther Res* 1998; 59: 234–43.

10. Baggio B, Gambaro G, Marchini F, et al. Correction of erythrocyte abnormalities in idiopathic calcium-oxalate nephrolithiasis and reduction of urinary oxalate by oral glycosaminoglycans. *Lancet* 1991; 338: 403–5.

11. Cao LC, Boevé ER, de Bruihn WC, et al. Glycosaminoglycans and semisynthetic sulfated polysaccharides: an overview of their potential application in treatment of patients with urolithiasis. *Urology* 1997; 50: 173–83 [review].

Chromium

1. Saner G, Yüzbasiyan V, Neyzi O, et al. Alterations of chromium metabolism and effect of chromium supplementation in Turner's syndrome patients. *Am J Clin Nutr* 1983; 38: 574–78.

2. Riales R, Albrink MJ. Effect of chromium chloride supplementation on glucose tolerance and serum lipids including high-density lipoprotein of adult men. *Am J Clin Nutr* 1981; 34: 2670–78.

3. Wang MM, Fox EZ, Stoecker BJ, et al. Serum cholesterol of adults supplemented with brewer's yeast or chromium chloride. *Nutr Res* 1989; 9: 989–98.

4. Page TG, Ward TL, and Southern LL. Effect of chromium picolinate on growth and carcass characteristics of growing-finishing pigs. *J Animal Sci* 1991; 69: 356.

5. Lefavi R, Anderson R, Keith R, et al. Efficacy of chromium supplementation in athletes: Emphasis on anabolism. *Int J Sport Nutr* 1992; 2: 111–22.

6. McCarty MF. The case for supplemental chromium and a survey of clinical studies with chromium picolinate. *J Appl Nutr* 1991; 43: 59–66.

7. Hallmark MA, Reynolds TH, DeSouza CA, et al. Effects of chromium and resistive training on muscle strength and body composition. *Med Sci Spt Ex* 1996; 28: 139–44.

8. Kaats GR, Blum K, Fisher JA, Adelman JA. Effects of chromium picolinate supplementation on body composition: a randomized, double-masked, placebo-controlled study. *Curr Ther Res* 1996; 57: 747–56.

9. Kaats GR, Blum K, Pullin D, Keither SC, Wood R. A randomized, double-masked, placebo-controlled study of the effects of chromium picolinate supplementation on body composition: a replication and extension of a previous study. *Curr Ther Res* 1998; 59: 379–88.

10. Sterns DM, Belbruno JJ, Wetterhahn KE. A prediction of chromium (III) accumulation in humans from chromium dietary supplements. *FASEB J* 1995; 9: 1650–57.

11. Sterns DM, Wise JP, Patierno SR, Wetterhahn KE. Chromium (III) picolinate produces chromosome damage in Chinese hamster ovary cells. *FASEB J* 1995; 9: 1643–49.

12. Garland M, Morris JS, Colditz GA, et al. Toenail trace element levels and breast cancer. *Am J Epidemiol* 1996; 144: 653–60.

13. Cerulli J, Grabe DW, Guathier I, et al. Chromium picolinate toxicity. *Ann Pharmacother* 1998; 32: 428–31.

14. Wasser WG, Feldman NS. Chronic renal failure after ingestion of over-the-counter chromium picoli-

nate. *Ann Intern Med* 1997; 126: 410 [letter].

15. Cerulli J, Grabe DW, Gauthier I, et al. Chromium picolinate toxicity. *Ann Pharmacother* 1998; 32: 428–31.

16. Offenbacher EG. Promotion of chromium absorption by ascorbic acid. *Trace Elements Electrolytes* 1994; 11: 178–81.

Coenzyme Q$_{10}$

1. Weber C, Jakobsen TS, Mortensen SA, et al. Antioxidative effect of dietary coenzyme Q$_{10}$ in human blood plasma. *Internat J Vit Nutr Res* 1994; 64: 311–15.

2. Kelly GS. Sport nutrition: a review of selected nutritional supplements for endurance athletes. *Alt Med Rev* 1997; 2: 282–95.

3. Tanimura J. Studies on arginine in human semen. Part III. The influences of several drugs on male infertility. *Bull Osaka Med School* 1967; 12: 90–100.

4. Gaby AR. Coenzyme Q$_{10}$. In *A Textbook of Natural Medicine,* by JE Pizzorno, MT Murray. Seattle: Bastyr University Press, 1998, V: CoQ$_{10}$; 1–8. [review].

5. Shigeta Y, Izumi K Abe H. Effect of coenzyme Q$_7$ treatment on blood sugar and ketone bodies of diabetics. *J Vitaminol* 1966; 12: 293–98.

6. Mortensen SA, Vadhanavikit S, Baandrup U, Folkers K. Long-term coenzyme Q$_{10}$ therapy: a major advance in the management of resistant myocardial failure. *Drug Exptl Clin Res* 1985; 11: 581–93.

7. Morisco C, Trimarco B, Condorelli M. Effect of coenzyme Q$_{10}$ in patients with congestive heart failure: a long-term multicenter randomized study. *Clin Invest* 1993; 71: S134–36.

8. Mortensen SA, Vadhanavikit S, Baandrup U, Folkers K. Long-term coenzyme Q$_{10}$ therapy: a major advance in the management of resistant myocardial failure. *Drug Exptl Clin Res* 1985; 11: 581–93.

9. Gaby AR. The role of coenzyme Q$_{10}$ in clinical medicine: part II. Cardiovascular disease, hypertension, diabetes mellitus and infertility. *Alt Med Rev* 1996; 1: 168–75 [review].

10. Fujioka T, Sakamoto Y, Mimura G. Clinical study of cardiac arrhythmias using a 24-hour continuous electrocardiographic recorder (5th report)—antiarrhythmic action of coenzyme Q$_{10}$ in diabetics. *Tohoku J Exp Med* 1983; 141(suppl): 453–63.

11. Kamikawa T, Kobayashi A, Yamashita T, et al. Effects of coenzyme Q$_{10}$ on exercise tolerance in chronic stable angina pectoris. *Am J Cardiol* 1985; 56: 247.

12. Mortensen SA. Perspectives on therapy of cardiovascular diseases with coenzyme Q$_{10}$ (ubiquinone). *Clin Invest* 1993; 71: s116–23 [review].

13. Tanaka J, Tominaga R, Yoshitoshi M, et al. Coenzyme Q$_{10}$: the prophylactic effect on low cardiac output following cardiac valve replacement. *Ann Thorac Surg* 1982; 33: 14551.

14. Folkers K, Wolaniuk J, Simonsen R, et al. Biochemical rationale and the cardiac response of patients with muscle disease to therapy with coenzyme Q$_{10}$. *Proc Natl Acad Sci* 1985; 82: 4513–16.

15. Imagawa M, Naruse S, Tsuji S, et al. Coenzyme Q$_{10}$, iron, and vitamin B$_6$ in genetically-confirmed Alzheimer's disease. *Lancet* 1992; 340: 671 [letter].

16. Folkers K, Shizukuishi S, Takemura K, et al. Increase in levels of IgG in serum of patients treated with coenzyme Q$_{10}$. *Res Comm Pathol Pharmacol* 1982; 38: 335–38.

17. Lockwood K, Moesgaard S, Yamamoto T, Folkers K. Progress on therapy of breast cancer with vitamin Q$_{10}$ and the regression of metastases. *Biochem Biophys Res Comm* 1995; 212: 172–77.

18. Digiesi V, Cantini F, Bisi G, et al. Mechanism of action of coenzyme Q$_{10}$ in essential hypertension. *Curr Ther Res* 1992; 51: 668–72.

19. Gaby AR. The role of coenzyme Q$_{10}$ in clinical medicine: part II. Cardiovascular disease, hypertension, diabetes mellitus and infertility. *Alt Med Rev* 1996; 1: 168–75 [review].

20. Weiss M, Mortensen SA, Rassig MR, et al. Bioavailability of four oral coenzyme Q$_{10}$ formulations in healthy volunteers. *Molec Aspects Med* 1994; 15: 273–80.

21. Kaikkonen J, Nyyssonen K, Porkkala-Sarataho E, et al. Effect of oral coenzyme Q$_{10}$ on the oxidation resistance of human VLDL + LDL fraction: absorption and antioxidative properties of oil and granule-based preparations. *Free Radic Biol Med* 1997; 22: 1195–1202.

22. Chopra RK, Goldman R, Sinatra ST, Bhagavan HN. Relative bioavailability of coenzyme Q$_{10}$ formulations in human subjects. *Internat J Vit Nutr Res* 1998; 68: 109–13.

23. Larsson O. Effects of isoprenoids on growth of normal human mammary epithelial cells and breast cancer cells *in vitro*. *Anticancer Res* 1994; 114: 123–28.

24. Lockwood K, Moesgaard S, Folkers K. Partial and complete regression of breast cancer in patients in relation to dosage of coenzyme Q$_{10}$. *Biochem Biophys Res Comm* 1994; 199: 1504–1508.

25. Lockwood K, Moesgaard S, Yamamoto T, Folkers K. Progress on therapy of breast cancer with vitamin Q$_{10}$ and the regression of metastases. *Biochem Biophys Res Comm* 1995; 212: 172–77.

26. Judy WV. Nutritional intervention in cancer prevention and treatment. American College for Advancement in Medicine Spring Conference, Ft. Lauderdale, FL. May 3, 1998.

Conjugated Linoleic Acid (CLA)

1. Cesano A, Visonneau S, Scimeca JA, et al. Opposite effects of linoleic acid and conjugated linoleic acid on human prostatic cancer in SCID mice. *Anticancer Res* 1998; 18(3A): 1429–34.

2. Thompson H, Zhu Z, Banni S, et al. Morphological and biochemical status of the mammary gland as influenced by conjugated linoleic acid: implication for a reduction in mammary cancer risk. *Cancer Res* 1997; 57: 5067–72.

3. Ip C. Review of the effects of *trans* fatty acids, oleic acid, n-3 polyunsaturated fatty acids, and conjugated linoleic acid on mammary carcinogenesis in animals. *Am J Clin Nutr* 1997; 66(suppl): 1523S–29S [review].

Part Two: References

4. Parodi PW. Cows' milk fat components as potential anticarcinogenic agents. *J Nutr* 1997; 127: 1055–60 [review].

5. West DB, Delany JP, Camet PM, et al. Effects of conjugated linoleic acid on body fat and energy metabolism in the mouse. *Am J Physiol* 1998; 275: R667–72.

6. Park Y, Albright KJ, Liu W, et al. Effect of conjugated linoleic acid on body composition in mice. *Lipids* 1997; 32: 853–58.

7. Sugano M, Tsujita A, Yamasaki M, et al. Conjugated linoleic acid modulates tissue levels of chemical mediators and immunoglobulins in rats. *Lipids* 1998; 33: 521–27.

8. Nicolosi RJ, Rogers EJ, Kritchevsky D, et al. Dietary conjugated linoleic acid reduces plasma lipoproteins and early aortic atherosclerosis in hypercholesterolemic hamsters. *Artery* 1997; 22: 266–77.

9. Lee KN, Kritchevsky D, Pariza MW, et al. Conjugated linoleic acid and atherosclerosis in rabbits. *Atherosclerosis* 1994; 108: 19–25.

10. Houseknecht KL, Vanden Heuvel JP, Moya-Camarena SY, et al. Dietary conjugated linoleic acid normalizes impaired glucose tolerance in the Zucker diabetic fatty fa/fa rat. *Biochem Biophys Res Commun* 1998; 244: 678–82.

11. Herbel BK, McGuire MK, McGuire MA, et al. Safflower oil consumption does not increase plasma conjugated linoleic acid concentrations in humans. *Am J Clin Nutr* 1998; 67: 332–37.

12. Thom E. A pilot study with the aim of studying the efficacy and tolerability of Tonalin CLA on the body composition in humans. Medstat Research Ltd., Lillestrom, Norway, July 1997 [unpublished].

Copper

1. Sandstead HH. Requirements and toxicity of essential trace elements, illustrated by zinc and copper. *Am J Clin Nutr* 1995; 61(suppl): 62S–64S.

2. Broun ER. Greist A, Tricot G, Hoffman R. Excessive zinc ingestion. A reversible cause of sideroblastic anemia and bone marrow depression. *JAMA* 1990; 264: 1441–43.

3. Jacob RA, Skala JH, Omaye ST, Turnlund JR. Effect of varying ascorbic acid intakes on copper absorption and ceruloplasmin levels of young men. *J Nutr* 1987; 117: 2109–15.

Creatine Monohydrate

1. Greenhaff PL, Bodin K, Soderlund K, et al. Effect of oral creatine supplementation on skeletal muscle phosphocreatine resynthesis. *Am J Physiol* 1994; 266: E725–30.

2. Greenhaff PL. Creatine and its application as an ergogenic aid. *Int J Sport Nutr* 1995; 5: 94–101.

3. Harris RC, Soderlund K, Hultman E. Elevation of creatine in resting and exercised muscle of normal subjects by creatine supplementation. *Clin Sci* 1992; 83: 367–74.

4. Green AL, Simpson EJ, Littlewood JJ, et al. Carbohydrate ingestion augments creatine retention during creatine feeding in humans. *Acta Physiol Scand* 1996; 158: 195–202.

5. Kreider RB, Ferreira M, Wilson M, et al. Effects of creatine supplementation on body composition, strength, and sprint performance. *Med Sci Sports Exerc* 1998; 30: 73–82.

6. Toler SM. Creatine is an ergogen for anaerobic exercise. *Nutr Rev* 1997; 55: 21–25.

7. Greenhaff PL. The nutritional biochemistry of creatine. *J Nutr Biochem* 1997; 8: 610–18.

8. Mujika I, Padilla S. Creatine supplementation as an ergogenic aid for sports performance in highly trained athletes: a critical review. *Int J Sports Med* 1997; 18: 491–96.

9. Grindstaff PD, Kreider R, Bishop R, et al. Effects of creatine supplemenation on repetitive sprint performance and body composition in competitive swimmers. *Int J Sports Nutr* 1997; 7: 330–46.

10. Peyrebrune MC, Nevill ME, Donaldson FJ, et al. The effects of oral creatine supplementation on performance in single and repeated sprint swimming. *J Sports Sci* 1998; 16: 271–79.

11. Balsom PD, Harridge SDR, Soderlund K, et al. Creatine supplementation per se does not enhance endurance exercise performance. *Acta Physiol Scand* 1993; 149: 521–23.

12. Stout JR, Eckerson J, Noonan D, et al. The effects of a supplement designed to augment creatine uptake on exercise performance and fat-free mass in football players. *Med Sci Sports Exerc* 1997; 29: S251.

13. Tarnopolsky MA, Roy BD, MacDonald JR. A randomized, controlled trial of creatine monohydrate in patients with mitochondrial cytopathies. *Muscle & Nerve* 1997; 20: 1502–9.

14. Sipila I, Rapola J, Simell O, et al. Supplementary creatine as a treatment for gyrate atrophy of the choroid and retina. *New Engl J Med* 1981; 304: 867–70.

15. Tarnopolsky M, Martin J. Creatine monohydrate increases strength in patients with neuromuscular disease. *Neurology* 1999; 52: 854–7.

16. Andrews R, Greenhaff P, Curtis S, et al. The effect of dietary creatine supplementation on skeletal muscle metabolism in congestive heart failure. *Eur Heart J* 1998; 19: 617–22.

17. Gordon A, Hultman E, Kaijser L, et al. Creatine supplementation in chronic heart failure increases skeletal muscle creatine phosphate and muscle performance. *Cardiovasc Res* 1995; 30: 413–18.

18. Earnest CP, Almada AL, Mitchell TL. High-performance capillary electrophoresis-pure creatine monohydrate reduces blood lipids in men and women. *Clin Sci* 1996; 91: 113–18.

19. Greenhaff PL. The nutritional biochemistry of creatine. *J Nutr Biochem* 1997; 8: 610–18.

20. Hultman E, Soderlund K, Timmons J, et al. Muscle creatine loading in man. *J Appl Physiol* 1996; 81: 232–37.

21. Green AL, Hultman E, Macdonald IA, et al. Carbohydrate ingestion augments skeletal muscle creatine accumulation during creatine supplementation in man. *Am J Physiol* 1996; 271: E821–26.

22. Feldman EB. Creatine: a dietary supplement and ergogenic aid. *Nutr Rev* 1999; 57: 45–50.

23. Vandenberghe K, Gills N, Van Leemputte M, et al. Caffeine counteracts the ergogenic action of muscle creatine loading. *J Appl Physiol* 1996; 80: 452–57.

24. Sewell DA, Robinson TM, Casey A, et al. The effect of acute dietary creatine supplementation upon indices of renal, hepatic and haematological function in human subjects. *Proc Nutr Soc* 1998; 57: 17A.

25. Poortmans JR, Auquier H, Renaut V, Durussel A, Saugy M, Brisson GR. Effect of short-term creatine supplementation on renal responses in men. *Eur J Appl Physiol Occup Physiol* 1997; 76: 566–67.

26. Earnest C, Almada A, Mitchell T. Influence of chronic creatine supplementation on hepatorenal function. *FASEB J* 1996; 10: 4588.

27. Almada A, Mitchell T, Earnest C. Impact of chronic creatine supplementation on serum enzyme concentrations. *FASEB J* 1996; 10: 4567.

28. Koshy KM, Griswold E, Schneeberger EE. Interstitial nephritis in a patient taking creatine. *N Engl J Med* 1999; 340: 814–5 [letter].

29. Pritchard NR, Kaira PA. Renal dysfunction accompanying oral creatine supplements. *Lancet* 1998; 351: 1252–53 [letter].

Cysteine

1. Salim AS. Sulfhydryl-containing agents in the treatment of gastric bleeding induced by nonsteroidal anti-inflammatory drugs. *Can J Surgery* 1993; 36: 53–58.

2. Droge W, Eck HP, Gander H, Mihm S. Modulation of lymphocyte functions and immune responses by cysteine and cysteine derivatives. *Am J Med* 1991; 91(suppl 3C): 140S–44S.

3. Eck HP, Gander H, Hartmann M, et al. Low concentrations of acid-soluble thiol (cysteine) in the blood plasma of HIV-1 infected patients. *Biol Chem Hoppe Seyler* 1989; 370: 101–8.

4. Droge W, Eck HP, Mihm S. HIV-induced cysteine deficiency and T-cell dysfunction—a rationale for treatment with N-acetylcysteine. *Immunol Today* 1992; 13: 211–14.

5. Droge W. Cysteine and glutathione deficiency in AIDS patients: A rationale for the treatment with N-acetyl-cysteine. *Pharmacol* 1993; 46: 61–65.

6. Kleinveld HA, Demacker PNM, Stalenhoef AFH. Failure of N-acetylcysteine to reduce low-density lipoprotein oxidizability in healthy subjects. *Eur J Clin Pharmacol* 1992; 639–42.

7. Olney JW, Ho O-L. Brain damage in infant mice following oral intake of glutamate, aspartate or cysteine. *Nature* 1970; 227: 609–10 [letter].

DHA (Docosahexaenoic Acid)

1. Davidson MH, Maki KC, Kalkowski J, et al. Effects of docosahexaenoic acid on serum lipoproteins in patients with combined hyperlipidemia: A randomized, double-blind, placebo-controlled trial. *J Am Coll Nutr* 1997; 16(3): 236–43.

2. Conquer JA, Holub BJ. Supplementation with an algae source of docosahexaenoic acid increases (n-3) fatty acid status and alters selected risk factors for heart disease in vegetarian subjects. *J Nutr* 1996; 126: 3032–39.

3. Nelson GJ, Schmidt PS, Bartolini GL, et al. The effect of dietary docosahexaenoic acid on platelet function, platelet fatty acid composition, and blood coagulation in humans. *Lipids* 1997; 32: 1129–36.

4. Gibson RA, Neumann MA, Makrides M. Effect of dietary docosahexaenoic acid on brain composition and neural function in term infants. *Lipids* 1996; 31: 177S–81S.

5. Makrides M, Neumann MA, Gibson RA. Is dietary docosahexaenoic acid essential for term infants? *Lipids* 1996; 31: 115–19.

6. Werkman SH, Carlson SE. A randomized trial of visual attention of preterm infants fed docosahexaenoic acid until nine months. *Lipids* 1996; 31: 91–97.

7. Hamazaki T, Sawazaki S, Itomura M, Asaoka E, et al. The effect of docosahexaenoic acid on aggression in young adults. A placebo-controlled double-blind study. *J Clin Invest* 1996; 97: 1129–33.

8. Crawford MA, Costeloe K, Ghebremeskel K, et al. Are deficits of arachidonic and docosahexaenoic acids responsible for the neural and vascular complications of preterm babies? *Am J Clin Nutr* 1997; 66(suppl): 1032S–41S.

9. Soderberg M, Edlund C, Kristensson K, et al. Fatty acid composition of brain phospholipids in aging and in Alzheimer's disease. *Lipids* 1991; 26: 421–25.

10. Stevens LJ, Zentall SS, Deck JL, et al. Essential fatty acid metabolism in boys with attention-deficit hyperactivity disorder. *Am J Clin Nutr* 1995; 62: 761–68.

11. Leaf A, Weber PC. Cardiovascular effects of n-3 fatty acids. *New Engl J Med* 1988; 318: 549–57.

12. Malasanos TH, Stacpoole PW. Biological effects of omega-3 fatty acids in diabetes mellitus. *Diabetes Care* 1991; 14: 1160–79.

13. Schectman G, Kaul S, Kassebah AH. Effect of fish oil concentrate on lipoprotein composition in NIDDM. *Diabetes* 1988; 37: 1567–73.

14. Toft I, Bonaa KH, Ingebretsen OC, et al. Effects of n-3 polyunsaturated fatty acids on glucose homeostasis and blood pressure in essential hypertension. *Ann Intern Med* 1995; 123: 911–18.

15. Harris WS, Zucker ML, Dujovne CA. Omega-3 fatty acids in type IV hyperlipidemia: Fish oils vs. methyl esters. *Am J Clin Nutr* 1987; 45(4): 858 [abstract].

16. Piche LA, Draper HH, Cole PD. Malondialdehyde excretion by subjects consuming cod liver oil vs. a concentrate of n-3 fatty acids. *Lipids* 1988; 23: 370–71.

17. Wander RC, Du S-H, Ketchum SO, Rowe KE. Effects of interaction of RRR-alpha-tocopheryl acetate and fish oil on low-density-lipoprotein oxidation in postmenopausal women with and without hormone-replacement therapy. *Am J Clin Nutr* 1996; 63: 184–93.

Part Two: References

18. Kubo K, Saito M, Tadokoro T, Maekawa A. Changes in susceptibility of tissues to lipid peroxidation after ingestion of various levels of docosahexaenoic acid and vitamin E. *Br J Nutr* 1997; 78: 655–69.

19. Luostarinen R, Wallin R, Wibell L, et al. Vitamin E supplementation counteracts the fish oil-induced increase of blood glucose in humans. *Nutr Res* 1995; 15: 953–68.

20. Dunstan DW, Burke V, Mori TA, et al. The independent and combined effects of aerobic exercise and dietary fish intake on serum lipids and glycemic control in NIDDM. *Diabetes Care* 1997; 20: 913–21.

21. Sheehan JP, Wei IW, Ulchaker M, Tserng K-Y. Effect of high fiber intake in fish oil-treated patients with non-insulin-dependent diabetes mellitus *Am J Clin Nutr* 1997; 66: 1183–87.

22. Adler AJ, Holub BJ. Effect of garlic and fish-oil supplementation on serum lipid and lipoprotein concentrations in hypercholesterolemic men. *Am J Clin Nutr* 1997; 65: 445–50.

DHEA
(Dehydroepiandrosterone)

1. Weksler ME. Hormone replacement for men. *Br Med J* 1996; 312: 859–60 [editorial].

2. Ebeling P, Koivisto VA. Physiological importance of dehydroepiandrosterone. *Lancet* 1994; 343: 1479–81.

3. Labrie F, Belanger A, Simard J, et al. DHEA and peripheral androgen and estrogen formation: Intracrinology. *Ann NY Acad Sci* 1995; 774: 16–28.

4. Reiter WJ, Pycha A, Schatzl G, et al. Dehydroepiandrosterone in the treatment of erectile dysfunction: a prospective, double-blind randomized, placebo-controlled study. *Urology* 1999; 53: 590–95.

5. Diamond P, Cusan L, Gomez J-L, et al. Metabolic effects of 12-month percutaneous dehydroepiandrosterone replacement therapy in postmenopausal women. *J Endocrinol* 1996; 150: S43–50.

6. Nestler JE, Barlasini CO, Clore JN, et al. Dehydroepiandrosterone reduces serum low density lipoprotein levels and body fat but does not alter insulin sensitivity in normal men. *J Clin Endocrinol Metabol* 1988; 66: 57–61.

7. Welle S, Jozefowicz R, Statt M. Failure of DHEA to influence energy and protein metabolism in humans. *J Clin Endocrinol Metabol* 1990; 71: 1259.

8. Usiskin KS, Butterworth S, Clore JN, et al. Lack of effect of dehydroepiandrosterone in obese men. *Int J Obesity* 1990; 14: 457–63.

9. Vogiatzi MG, Boeck MA, Vlachopapadoulou E, et al. Dehydroepiandrosterone in morbidly obese adolescents: effects on weight, body composition, lipids, and insulin resistance. *Metabolism* 1996; 45: 1101–15.

10. Yen SSC, Morales AJ, Khorram O. Replacement of DHEA in aging men and women. *Ann NY Acad Sci* 1995; 774: 128–42.

11. Diamond P, Cusan L, Gomez J-L, et al. Metabolic effects of 12-month percutaneous dehydroepiandrosterone replacement therapy in postmenopausal women. *J Endocrinol* 1996; 150: S43–50.

12. Yen SSC, Morales AJ, Khorram O. Replacement of DHEA in aging men and women. *Ann NY Acad Sci* 1995; 774: 128–42.

13. Mortola J, Yen SSC. The effects of dehydroepiandrosterone on endocrine-metabolic parameters in postmenopausal women. *J Clin Endocrinol Metabol* 1990; 71: 695–704.

14. Khorram O, Vu L, Yen SS. Activation of immune function by dehydroepiandrosterone (DHEA) in age-advanced men. *J Gerontol A Biol Sci Med Sci* 1997; 52: M1–7.

15. Casson PR, Andersen RN, Herrod HG, et al. Oral dehydroepiandrosterone in physiologic doses modulates immune function in postmenopausal women. *Am J Obstet Gynecol* 1993; 169: 1536–39.

16. Schaefer C, Friedman G, Ettinger B, et al. Dehydroepiandrosterone sulfate (DHEAS), angina, and fatal ischemic heart disease. *Am J Epidemiol* 1996; 143(11suppl): S69 [abstr #274].

17. Barrett-Connor E, Goodman-Gruen D. The epidemiology of DHEAS and cardiovascular disease. *Ann NY Acad Sci* 1995; 774: 259–70.

18. Jessee RL, Loesser K, et al. Dehydroepiandrosterone inhibits human platelet aggregation in vitro and in vivo. *Ann NY Acad Sci* 1995; 29: 281–90.

19. Mortola J, Yen SSC. The effects of dehydroepiandrosterone on endocrine-metabolic parameters in postmenopausal women. *J Clin Endocrinol Metabol* 1990; 71: 695–704.

20. Yen SSC, Morales AJ, Khorram O. Replacement of DHEA in aging men and women. *Ann NY Acad Sci* 1995; 774: 128–42.

21. Vogiatzi MG, Boeck MA, Vlachopapadoulou E, et al. Dehydroepiandrosterone in morbidly obese adolescents: effects on weight, body composition, lipids, and insulin resistance. *Metabolism* 1996; 45: 1101–15.

22. Lahita RG et al. Low plasma androgens in women with systemic lupus erythematosus. *Arthrit Rheum* 1987; 30: 241–48.

23. van Hollenhoven RF, Engleman EG, McGuire JL. Dehydroepiandrosterone in systemic lupus erythematosus. *Arthrit Rheum* 1995; 38: 1826–31.

24. van Hollenhoven RF, Morabito LM, Engleman EG, McGuire JL. Treatment of systemic lupus erythematosus with dehydroepiandrosterone: 50 patients treated up to 12 months. *J Rheumatol* 1998; 25: 285–89.

25. Araghiniknam J, Chung S, Nelson-White T, et al. Antioxidant activity of dioscorea and dehydroepiandrosterone (DHEA) in older humans. *Life Sci* 1996; 59: 147–57.

26. Ebeling P, Koivisto VA. Physiological importance of dehydroepiandrosterone. *Lancet* 1994; 343: 1479–81.

27. Weinstein RE, Lobocki CA, Gravett S, et al. Decreased adrenal sex steroid in the absence of glucocorticoid suppression in postmenopausal

asthmatic women. *J Allerg Clin Immunol* 1996; 97: 1–8.

28. Wolkowitz OM, Reus VI, Roberts E, et al. Antidepressant and cognition-enhancing effects of DHEA in major depression. *Ann NY Acad Sci* 1995; 774: 337–39.

29. Gaby AR. Research review. *Nutr Healing* Jun 1997: 8.

30. Louviselli A, Pisanu P, Cossu E, et al. Low levels of dehydroepiandrosterone sulfate in adult males with insulin-dependent diabetes mellitus. *Minerva Endocrinol* 1994; 19: 113–19.

31. Gaby AR. Dehydroepiandrosterone: biological effects and clinical significance. *Alt Med Rev* 1996; 1: 60–69 [review].

32. Gaby AR. Research review. *Nutr Healing* Jan 1996: 7.

33. Casson PR, Buster JE. DHEA replacement after menopause: HRT 200 or nostrum of the '90s? *Contemporary OB/GYN* Apr 1997: 119–33.

34. van Hollenhoven RF, Morabito LM, Engleman EG, McGuire JL. Treatment of systemic lupus erythematosus with dehydroepiandrosterone: 50 patients treated up to 12 months. *J Rheumatol* 1998; 25: 285–89.

35. Orner GA et al. Dehydroepiandrosterone is a complete hepatocarcinogen and potent tumor promoter in the absence of peroxisome proliferation in rainbow trout. *Carcinogenesis* 1995; 16: 2893–98.

36. Metzger C, Mayer D, et al. Sequential appearance and ultrastructure of amphophilic cell foci, adenomas, and carcinomas in the liver of male and female rats treated with dehydroepiandrosterone. *Taxicol Pathol* 1995; 23: 591–605.

37. Schwartz AG. Inhibition of spontaneous breast cancer formation in female C3H (A vy/a) mice by long-term treatment with dehydroepiandrosterone. *Cancer Res* 1979; 39: 1129–32.

38. McNeil C. Potential drug DHEA hits snags on way to clinic. *J Natl Cancer Inst* 1997; 89: 681–83.

39. Jones JA, Nguyen A, Strab M, et al. Use of DHEA in a patient with advanced prostate cancer: a case report and review. *Urology* 1997; 50: 784–88.

40. Zumoff B, Levin J, Rosenfeld RS, et al. Abnormal 24-hr mean plasma concentrations of dehydroisoandrosterone and dehydroisoandrosterone sulfate in women with primary operable breast cancer. *Cancer Res* 1981; 41: 3360–63.

41. Skolnick AA. Scientific verdict still out on DHEA. *JAMA* 1996; 276: 1365–67 [review].

42. Sahelian R. New supplements and unknown, long-term consequences. *Am J Natural Med* 1997; 4: 8 [editorial].

43. Casson PR, Santoro N, Elkind-Hirsch K, et al. Postmenopausal dehydroepiandrosterone administration increases free insulin-like growth factor-I and decreases high-density lipoprotein: a six-month trial. *Fertil Steril* 1998; 70: 107–10.

Digestive Enzymes

1. Oelgoetz AW, Oelgoetz PA, Wittenkind J. The treatment of food allergy and indigestion of pancreatic origin with pancreatic enzymes. *Am J Dig Dis Nutr* 1935; 2: 422–26.

2. McCann M. Pancreatic enzyme supplement for treatment of multiple food allergies. *Ann Allerg* 1993; 71: 269 [abstr #17].

3. Ambrus JL, Lassman HB, DeMarchi JJ. Absorption of exogenous and endogenous proteolytic enzymes. *Clin Pharmacol Ther* 1967; 8: 362–68.

4. Avakian S. Further studies on the absorption of chymotrypsin. *Clin Pharmacol Ther* 1964; 5: 712–15.

5. Izaka K, Yamada M, Kawano T, Suyama T. Gastrointestinal absorption and anti-inflammatory effect of bromelain. *Jpn J Pharmacol* 1972; 22: 519–34.

6. Deitrick RE. Oral proteolytic enzymes in the treatment of athletic injuries: a double-blind study. *Pennsylvania Med J* Oct 1965: 35–37.

7. Seligman B. Bromelain: an anti-inflammatory agent. *Angiology* 1962; 13: 508–10.

8. Cichoke AJ. The effect of systemic enzyme therapy on cancer cells and the immune system. *Townsend Letter for Doctors and Patients* Nov 1995: 30–32 [review].

9. Wolf M, Ransberger K. *Enzyme Therapy.* New York: Vantage Press 1972: 135–220 [review].

10. Kleine MW, Stauder GM, Beese EW. The intestinal absorption of orally administered hydrolytic enzymes and their effects in the treatment of acute herpes zoster as compared with those of oral acyclovir therapy. *Phytomedicine* 1995; 2: 7–15.

11. Gullo L. Indication for pancreatic enzyme treatment in non-pancreatic digestive diseases. *Digestion* 1993; 54(suppl 2): 43–47.

12. Nakamura T, Tandoh Y, Terada A, et al. Effects of high-lipase pancreatin on fecal fat, neutral sterol, bile acid, and short-chain fatty acid excretion in patients with pancreatic insufficiency resulting from chronic pancreatitis. *Internat J Pancreatol* 1998; 23: 63–70.

13. Layer P, Groger G. Fate of pancreatic enzymes in the human intestinal lumen in health and pancreatic insufficiency. *Digestion* 1993; 54(suppl 2): 10–14.

DMAE
(2-Dimethylaminoethanol)

1. Zahniser NR, Chou D, Hanin I. Is 2-dimethylaminoethanol (Deanol) indeed a precursor of brain acetylcholine? A gas chromatographic evaluation. *J Pharm Exp Ther* 1977; 200: 545–59.

2. Kazamutsuri H, Chien C, Cole JO. Therapeutic approaches to tardive dyskinesia. *Arch Gen Psych* 1972; 27: 491–99.

3. Alphs L, Davis JM. Noncatecholaminergic treatments of tardive dyskinesia. *J Clin Psychopharmacol* 1982; 2: 380–85 [review].

4. Ferris SH, Sathananthan G, Gershon S, et al. Senile dementia. Treatment with Deanol. *J Am Ger Soc* 1977; 25: 241–44.

5. Fisman M, Mersky H, Helmes E. Double-blind trial of 2-dimethylaminoethanol in Alzheimer's disease. *Am J Psych* 1981; 138: 970–72.

6. Casey DE, Denney D. Dimethylaminoethanol in tardive dyskinesia. *N Engl J Med* 1974; 291: 797.

7. Fisman M, Mersky H, Helmes E. Double-blind trial of 2-dimethylaminoethanol in Alzheimer's disease. *Am J Psych* 1981; 138: 970–72.

8. Sergio W. Use of DMAE (2-dimethylaminoethanol) in the induction of lucid dreams. *Med Hypoth* 1988; 26: 255–57.

DMSO (Dimethyl Sulfoxide)

1. American Medical Association. Dimethyl sulfoxide. Controversy and current status—1981. *JAMA* 1982; 248: 1369–71.

2. Jimenez RAH, Willkens RF. Dimethyl sulfoxide: A perspective of its use in rheumatic diseases. *J Lab Clin Med* 1982; 100: 489–500.

3. Swanson BN. Medical use of dimethyl sulfoxide (DMSO). *Rev Clin Basic Pharmacol* 1985; 5: 1–33.

4. Jacob SW, Wood DC. Dimethyl sulfoxide (DMSO). Toxicology, pharmacology, and clinical experience. *Am J Surg* 114: 414–26.

5. Eberhardt R, Zwingers T, Hofmann R. DMSO in patients with active gonarthrosis. A double-blind placebo-controlled phase II study. *Fortschritte Med* 1995; 113: 446–50 [in German].

6. Zuurmond WW, Langendijk PN, Bezemer PD, et al. Treatment of acute reflex sympathetic dystrophy with DMSO 50% in a fatty cream. *Acta Anaesthesiol Scand* 1996; 40: 364–67.

7. Kneer W, Kuhnau S, Bias P, et al. Dimethylsulfoxide (DMSO) gel in treatment of acute tendopathies. A multicenter, placebo-controlled, randomized study. *Fortschritte Med* 1994; 112: 142–46 [in German].

8. Carson JD, Percy EC. The use of DMSO in tennis elbow and rotator cuff tendinitis: a double-blind study. *Med. Sci Sports Exer* 1981; 13: 215–19.

9. Ozkaya-Bayazit E, Baykal C, Kavak A. Local DMSO treatment of macular and papular amyloidosis. *Hautarzt* 1997; 48: 31–37 [in German].

10. Hanno PM, Wein AJ. Medical treatment of interstitial cystitis (other than Rimso-50/Elmiron). *Urology* 1987; 29(suppl): 22–26.

11. Salim AS. The relationship between Helicobacter pylori and oxygen-derived free radicals in the mechanism of duodenal ulceration. *Internal Med* 1993; 32: 359–64.

Evening Primrose Oil

1. Joe LA, Hart LL. Evening primrose oil in rheumatoid arthritis. *Ann Pharmacother* 1993; 27: 1475–77 [review].

2. Dippneaar N, Booyens J, Fabbri D, Katzeff IE. The reversibility of cancer: evidence that malignancy in melanoma cells is gamma linolenic acid deficiency-dependent. *S Afr Med J* 1982; 62: 505–9.

3. Pritchard GA, Mansel RE. The effects of essential fatty acids on the growth of breast cancer and melanoma. In *Omega-6 Essential Fatty Acids: Pathophysiology and Roles in Clinical Medicine,* ed. DF Horrobin. New York: Alan R Liss, 1990, 379–90.

4. Lee JH, Sugano M. Effects of linoleic and gamma-linolenic acid on 7,12-dimethylbenz(a)anthracene-induced rat mammary tumors. *Nutr Rep Internat* 1986; 34: 1041.

5. Naidu MRC, Das UN, Kshan A. Intratumoral gamma-linolenic acid therapy of human gliomas. *Prostaglandins Leukotrienes Essential Fatty Acids* 1992; 45: 181–84.

6. Van der Merwe CF, Booyens J. Oral gamma-linolenic acid in 21 patients with untreatable malignancy: An ongoing pilot open clinical trial. *Br J Clin Pract* 1987; 41: 907–15.

7. McIllmurray MB, Turkie W. Controlled trial of gamma linolenic in Duke's C colorectal cancer. *Br Med J* 1987; 294: 1260.

8. Ishikawa T, Fujiyama Y, Igarashi O, et al. Effects of gammalinolenic acid on plasma lipoproteins and apolipoproteins. *Atherosclerosis* 1989; 75: 95–104.

9. Boberg M, Vessby B, Selinus I. Effects of dietary supplementation with n-6 and n-3 long-chain polyunsaturated fatty acids on serum lipoproteins and platelet function in hypertriglyceridaemic patients. *Acta Med Scand* 1986; 220: 153–60.

10. Horrobin DF. The importance of gamma-linolenic acid and prostaglandin E1 in human nutrition and medicine. *J Holistic Med* 1981; 3: 118–39.

11. Horrobin DF, Manku M, Brush M, et al. Abnormalities in plasma essential fatty acid levels in women with pre-menstrual syndrome and with non-malignant breast disease. *J Nutr Med* 1991; 2: 259–64.

12. Keen H, Payan J, Allawi J, et al. Treatment of diabetic neuropathy with gamma-linolenic acid. *Diabetes Care* 1993; 16: 8–15 [reviews].

13. Horrobin DF. Essential fatty acid metabolism in diseases of connective tissue with special reference to scleroderma and to Sjogren's syndrome. *Med Hypoth* 1984; 14: 233–47.

14. Horrobin DF, Campbell A. Sjogren's syndrome and the sicca syndrome: the role of prostaglandin E1 deficiency. Treatment with essential fatty acids and vitamin C. *Med Hypoth* 1980; 6: 225–32.

15. Vaddadi KS, Gilleard CJ. Essential fatty acids, tardive dyskinesia, and schizophrenia. In *Omega-6 Essential Fatty Acids: Pathophysiology and Roles in Clinical Medicine,* ed. DF Horrobin. New York: Alan R Liss, 1990, 333–43.

16. Manku MS, Horrobin, DF, Morse NL, et al. Essential fatty acids in the plasma phospholipids of patients with atopic eczema. *Br J Derm* 1984; 110: 643.

17. Horrobin DF. Essential fatty acids in clinical dermatology. *J Am Acad Dermatol* 1989; 20: 1045–53.

18. Mansel RE, Pye JK, Hughes LE. Effects of essential fatty acids on cyclical mastalgia and noncyclical breast disorders. In *Omega-6 Essential Fatty Acids: Pathophysiology and Roles in Clinical Medicine,* ed. DF Horrobin. New York: Alan R Liss, 1990, 557–66.

19. Keen H, Payan J, Allawi J, et al. Treatment of diabetic neuropathy with gamma-linolenic acid. *Diabetes Care* 1993; 16: 8–15.

20. Horrobin DF. Essential fatty acid metabolism in diseases of connective tissue with special reference to scleroderma and to Sjogren's syndrome. *Med Hypoth* 1984; 14: 233–47.

21. Vaddadi KS, Gilleard CJ. Essential fatty acids, tardive dyskinesia, and schizophrenia. In *Omega-6 Essential Fatty Acids: Pathophysiology and Roles in Clinical Medicine,* ed. DF Horrobin. New York: Alan R Liss, 1990, 333–43.

22. Schalin-Karrila M, Mattila L, Jansen CT, et al. Evening primrose oil in the treatment of atopic eczema: effect on clinical status, plasma phospholipid fatty acids and circulating blood prostaglandins. *Brit J Dermatol* 1987; 117: 11–19.

23. Glen AIM, Glen EMT, MacDonnell LEF, et al. Essential fatty acids in the management of withdrawal symptoms and tissue damage in alcoholics, presented at the 2nd International Congress on Essential Fatty Acids, Prostaglandins and Leukotrienes, London, Zoological Society. March 24–27, 1985, abstract 53.

Fiber

1. Todd PA, Befield P, Goa KL. Guar gum: a review of its pharmacological properties and use as a dietary adjunct in hypercholesterolemia. *Drugs* 1990; 39: 917–28.

2. Jenkins DJA, Kendall CWC, Ransom TPP. Dietary fiber, the evolution of the human diet and coronary heart disease. *Nutr Res* 1998; 18: 633–52 [review].

3. Anderson JW, Gustafson NS, Bryart CA, Tietyen-Clark J. Dietary fiber and diabetes. *J Am Diet Assoc* 1987; 87: 1189–97.

4. Nuttall FW. Dietary fiber in the management of diabetes. *Diabetes* 1993; 42: 503–8.

5. Salmeron J, Manson JAE, Stampfer MJ, et al. Dietary fiber, glycemic load, and risk of non-insulin-dependent diabetes mellitus in women. *JAMA* 1997; 277: 472–77.

6. Kritchevsky D. Protective role of wheat bran fiber: preclinical data. *Am J Med* 1999; 106(1A): 28S–31S.

7. Meüller-Lissner SA. Effect of wheat bran on weight of stool and gastrointestinal transit time: a meta analysis. *Br Med J* 1988; 296: 615–17.

8. Jacobs DR Jr, Marquart L, Slavin J, Kushi LH. Whole-grain intake and cancer: an expanded review and meta-analysis. *Nutr Cancer* 1998; 30: 85–96.

9. Earnest DL, Einspahr JG, Alberts DS. Protective role of wheat bran fiber: data from marker trials. *Am J Med* 1999; 106(1A): 32S–7S.

10. Fuchs CS, Giovannucci EL, Colditz GA, et al. Dietary fiber and the risk of colorectal cancer and adenoma in women. *N Engl J Med* 1999; 340: 169–76.

11. Hylander B, Rössner S. Effects of dietary fiber intake before meals on weight loss and hunger in a weight-reducing club. *Acta Med Scand* 1983; 213: 217–20.

12. Adlercreutz H, Fotsis T, Hekkinen R, et al. Excretion of the lignans enterolactone and enterodiol and of equol in omnivorous and vegetarian postmenopausal women and in women with breast cancer. *Lancet* 1982; ii: 1295–99.

13. Shah PJR. Unprocessed bran and its effect on urinary calcium excretion in idiopathic hypercalciuria. *Br Med J* 1980; 281: 426.

14. Ebisuno S, Morimoto S, Yoshida T, et al. Rice-bran treatment for calcium stone formers with idiopathic hypercalciuria. *Brit J Urol* 1986; 58: 592–95.

Fish Oil (EPA and DHA) and Cod Liver Oil

1. Mate J, Castanos R, Garcia-Samaniego J, Pajares JM. Does dietary fish oil maintain the remission of Crohn's disease: a case control study. *Gastroenterology* 1991; 100: A228 [abstract].

2. Donadio JV Jr, Bergstrahl EJ, Offord KP, et al. A controlled trial of fish oil in IgA nephrophathy. *N Engl J Med* 1994; 331: 1194–99.

3. Peck LW. Essential fatty acid deficiency in renal failure: can supplements really help? *J Am Dietet Assoc* 1997; 97: 5150–53.

4. Shahar E, Folsom AR, Melnick SL, et al. Dietary n-3 polyunsaturated fatty acids and smoking-related chronic obstructive pulmonary disease. Atherosclerosis risk in communities study investigators. *N Engl J Med* 1994; 331: 228–33.

5. DiGiacoma RA, Kremer JM, Shah DM. Fish-oil dietary supplementation in patients with Raynaud's phenomenon: A double-blind, controlled,

prospective study. *Am J Med* 1989; 86: 158–64.

6. Laugharne JDE, Mellor JE, Peet M. Fatty acids and schizophrenia. *Lipids* 1996; 31: S-163–65.

7. Braden LM, Carroll KK. Dietary polyunsaturated fat in relation to mammary carcinogenesis in rats. *Lipids* 1986; 21(4): 285.

8. O'Connor TP, et al. Effect of dietary intake of fish oil and fish protein on the development of L-azaserine-induced preneoplastic lesions in the rat pancreas. *J Natl Cancer Inst* 1985; 75(5): 959–62.

9. Gonzalez MJ. Fish oil, lipid peroxidation and mammary tumor growth. *J Am Coll Nutr* 1995; 14: 325.

10. Zhu ZR, Mannisto JAS, Pietinene P, et al. Fatty acid composition of breast adipose tissue in breast cancer patients and patients with benign breast disease. *Nutr Cancer* 1995; 24: 151–60.

11. Nair SSD, Leitch JW, Falconer J, Garg ML. Prevention of cardiac arrhythmia by dietary (n-3) polyunsaturated fatty acids and their mechanism of action. *J Nutr* 1997; 127: 383–93.

12. Alexander JW. Immunonutrition: the role of omega-3 fatty acids. *Nutr* 1998; 14: 627–33.

13. Belluzzi A, Brignola C, Campieri M, et al. Effects of new fish oil derivative on fatty acid phospholipid-membrane pattern in a group of Crohn's disease patients. *Dig Dis Sci* 1994; 39: 2589–94.

14. Leaf A, Weber PC. Cardiovascular effects of n-3 fatty acids. *N Engl J Med* 1988; 318: 549–57.

15. Malasanos TH, Stacpoole PW. Biological effects of omega-3 fatty acids in diabetes mellitus. *Diabetes Care* 1991; 14: 1160–79.

16. Schectman G, Kaul S, Kassebah AH. Effect of fish oil concentrate on lipoprotein composition in NIDDM. *Diabetes* 1988; 37: 1567–73.

17. Toft I, Bonaa KH, Ingebretsen OC, et al. Effects of n-3 polyunsaturated fatty acids on glucose homeostasis and blood pressure in essential hypertension. *Ann Intern Med* 1995; 123: 911–18.

18. Harris WS, Zucker ML, Dujovne CA. Omega-3 fatty acids in type IV hyperlipidemia: fish oils vs methyl esters. *Am J Clin Nutr* 1987; 45(4): 858 [abstr].

19. Clarke JTR, Cullen-Dean G, Reglink E, et al. Increased incidence of epistaxis in adolescents with familial hypercholesterolemia treated with fish oil. *J Pediatr* 1990; 116: 139–41.

20. Piche LA, Draper HH, Cole PD. Malondialdehyde excretion by subjects consuming cod liver oil vs a concentrate of n-3 fatty acids. *Lipids* 1988; 23: 370–71.

21. Wander RC, Du S-H, Ketchum SO, Rowe KE. Effects of interaction of RRR-α-tocopheryl acetate and fish oil on low-density-lipoprotein oxidation in post-menopausal women with and without hormone-replacement therapy. *Am J Clin Nutr* 1996; 63: 184–93.

22. Luostarinen R, Wallin R, Wibell L, et al. Vitamin E supplementation counteracts the fish oil-induced increase of blood glucose in humans. *Nutr Res* 1995; 15: 953–68.

23. Dunstan DW, Burke V, Mori TA, et al. The independent and combined effects of aerobic exercise and dietary fish intake on serum lipids and glycemic control in NIDDM. *Diabetes Care* 1997; 20: 913–21.

24. Sheehan JP, Wei IW, Ulchaker M, Tserng K-Y. Effect of high fiber intake in fish oil-treated patients with non-insulin-dependent diabetes mellitus *Am J Clin Nutr* 1997; 66: 1183–87.

25. Adler AJ, Holub BJ. Effect of garlic and fish-oil supplementation on serum lipid and lipoprotein concentrations in hypercholesterolemic men. *Am J Clin Nutr* 1997; 65: 445–50.

5-Hydroxytryptophan (5-HTP)

1. Guyton AC, Hall JE. *Textbook of Medical Physiology*, 9th ed. Philadelphia: W. B. Saunders, 1996.

2. van Praag HM, Lemus C. Monoamine precursors in the treatment of psychiatric disorders. *Nutrition and the Brain*, vol. 7, eds. RJ Wurtman, JJ Wurtman. New York: Raven Press, 1986 [review].

3. Russell IJ, Michalek JE, Vipraio GA, Fletcher EM, Javors MA, Bowden CA. Platelet 3H-imipramine uptake receptor density and serum serotonin levels in patients with fibromyalgia/fibrositis syndrome. *J Rheumatol* 1992; 19: 90–94.

4. Yunus MB, Dailey JW, Aldag JC, Masi AT, Jobe PC. Platelet 3H-imiprimine uptake receptor density and serum serotonin levels in patients with fibromyalgia/fibrositis syndrome. *J Rheumatol* 1992; 19: 104–09.

5. Wolfe F, Russell IJ, Vipraio G, Ross K, Anderson J. Serotonin levels, pain threshold, and fibromyalgia symptoms in the general population. *J Rheumatol* 1997; 24: 555–59.

6. Kimball RW, Friedman AP, Vallejo E. Effect of serotonin in migraine patients. *Neurology* 1960; 10: 107–11.

7. Schneider-Helmert D, Spinweber CL. Evaluation of L-tryptophan for treatment of insomnia: A review. *Psychopharmacology* (Berlin) 1986; 89: 1–7.

8. Caruso I, Sarzi Puttini P, Cazzola M, Azzolini V. Double-blind study of 5-hydroxytryptophan versus placebo in the treatment of primary fibromyalgia syndrome. *J Int Med Res* 1990; 18: 201–09.

9. De Benedittis G, Massei R. 5-HT precursors in migraine prophylaxis: A double-blind cross-over study with L-5-hydroxytryptophan versus placebo. *Clin J Pain* 1986; 3: 123–29.

10. Titus F, Davalos A, Alom J, Codina A. 5-hydroxytryptophan versus methysergide in the prophylaxis of migraine. *Eur Neurol* 1986; 25: 327–29.

11. Maissen CP, Ludin HP. Comparison of the effect of 5-hydroxytryptophan and propranolol in the interval treatment of migraine. *Schweizerische Medizinische Wochenschrift /Journal Suisse de Medecine* 1991; 121: 1585–90 [in German].

12. Mathew NT. 5-hydroxytryptophan in the prophylaxis of migraine. *Headache* 1978; 18: 111–13.

13. De Giorgis G, Miletto R, Iannuccelli M, Camuffo M, Scerni S. Headache in association with sleep disorders in children: A psychodiagnostic evaluation and controlled clinical study L-5-HTP versus placebo. *Drugs Exptl Clin Res* 1987; 13: 425–33.

14. Byerley WF, Judd LL, Reimherr FW, Grosser BI. 5-hydroxytryptophan: A review of its antidepressant efficacy and adverse effects. *J Clin Psychopharmacol* 1987; 7: 127–37 [review].

15. Zmilacher K, Battegay R, Gastpar M. L-5-hydroxytryptophan alone and in combination with a peripheral decarboxylase inhibitor in the treatment of depression. *Neuropsychobiology* 1988; 20: 28–35.

16. Poldinger W, Calanchini B, Schwarz W. A functional-dimensional approach to depression: Serotonin deficiency as a target syndrome in a comparison of 5-hydroxytryptophan and fluvoxamine. *Psychopathology* 1991; 24: 53–81.

17. Soulairac A, Lambinet H. Etudes cliniques de líaction du precurseur de la serotonine le L-5-hydroxy-tryptophane, sur les troubles du sommeil. *Schweiz Bundschau Med (PRAXIS)* 1998; 77(34a): 19–23 [in French].

18. Ceci F, Cangiano C, Cairella M, et al. The effects of oral 5-hydroxytryptophan administration on feeding behavior in obese adult female subjects. *J Neural Transmission* 1989; 76: 109–17.

19. Cangiano C, Ceci F, Cascino A, et al. Eating behavior and adherence to dietary prescriptions in obese adult subjects treated with 5-hydroxytryptophan. *Am J Clin Nutr* 1992; 56: 863–67.

20. Michelson D, Page SW, Casey R, et al. An eosinophilia-myalgia syndrome related disorder associated with exposure to L-5-hydroxytryptophan. *J Rheumatol* 1994; 21: 2261–65.

21. Williamson BL, Tomlinson AJ, Gleich GJ, et al. Problems with over-the-counter 5-hydroxytryptophan. *Nature Med* 1998; 4: 983.

22. Sternberg EM, Van Woert MH, Young SN, et al. Development of a scleroderma-like illness during therapy with L-5-hydroxytryptophan and carbidopa. *New Engl J Med* 1980; 303: 782–87.

Flaxseed Oil

1. De Lorgeril M, Renaud S, Maelle N, et al. Mediterranean alpha-linolenic acid-rich diet in secondary prevention of coronary heart disease. *Lancet* 1994; 343: 1454–59.

2. Rice RD. Mediterranean diet. *Lancet* 1994; 344; 893–94 [letter].

3. Kelley DS, Nelson GJ, Love JE, et al. Dietary a-linolenic acid alters tissue fatty acid composition, but not blood lipids, lipoproteins or coagulation status in humans. *Lipids* 1993; 28: 533–37.

4. Abbey M, Clifton P, Kestin M, et al. Effect of fish oil on lipoproteins, lecithin: cholesterol acyltransferase, and lipid transfer protein activity in humans. *Arterioscler* 1990; 10: 85–94.

5. Chan JK, Bruce VM, McDonald BE. Dietary a-linolenic acid is as effective as oleic acid and linoleic acid in lowering blood cholesterol in normolipidemic men. *Am J Clin Nutr* 1991; 53: 1230–34.

6. Singer P, Jaeger W, Berger I, et al. Effects of dietary oleic, linoleic and a-linolenic acids on blood pressure, serum lipids, lipoproteins and the formation of eicosanoid precursors in patients with mild essential hypertension. *J Human Hypertension* 1990; 4: 227–33.

7. Sanders TAB, Roshanai F. The influence of different types of omega 3 polyunsaturated fatty acids on blood lipids and platelet function in healthy volunteers. *Clin Sci* 1983; 64: 91.

8. Mantzioris E, James MJ, Gibson RA, Cleland LG. Dietary substitution with alpha-linolenic acid-rich vegetable oil increases eicosapentaenoic acid concentrations in tissues. *Am J Clin Nutr* 1994; 59: 1304–49.

9. Indu M, Ghafoorunissa. n-3 fatty acids in Indian diets: comparison of the effects of precursor (alpha-linolenic acid) vs product (long-chain n-3 polyunsaturated fatty acids). *Nutr Res* 1992; 12: 569–82.

10. Braden LM, Carroll KK. Dietary polyunsaturated fat in relation to mammary carcinogenesis in rats. *Lipids* 1986; 21: 285–88.

11. Giovannucci E, Rimm EB, Colditz GA, et al. A prospective study of dietary fat and risk of prostate cancer. *J Natl Cancer Inst* 1993; 85: 1571–79.

12. De Stefani E, Deneo-Pellegrini H, Mendilaharsu M, Ronco A. Essential fatty acids and breast cancer; a case-control study in Uruguay. *Int J Cancer* 1998; 76: 491–94.

13. Shields PG, Xu GX, Blot WJ, et al. Mutagens from heated Chinese and U.S. cooking oils. *J Natl Cancer Inst* 1995; 87: 836–41.

14. Bougnoix P. Alpha-linolenic acid content of adipose breast tissue: a host determinant of the risk of early metastasis in breast cancer. *Br J Cancer* 1994; 70: 330–40.

Folic Acid

1. Daly LE, Kirke PN, Molloy A, et al. Folate levels and neural tube defects. *JAMA* 1995; 274: 1698–1702.

2. Shaw GM, O'Malley CD, Wasserman CR, et al. Maternal periconceptional use of multivitamins and reduced risk for conotruncal heart defects and limb deficiencies among offspring. *Am J Med Genetics* 1995; 59: 536–45.

3. Tolarova M. Periconceptional supplementation with vitamins and folic acid to prevent recurrence of cleft lip. *Lancet* 1982; ii: 217 [letter].

4. Shaw GM, Lammer EJ, Wasserman CR, et al. Risks of orofacial clefts in children born to women using multivitamins containing folic acid periconceptionally. *Lancet* 1995; 345: 393–96.

5. Hayes C, Werler MM, Willett WC, Mitchell AA. Case-control study of periconceptional folic acid supplementation and oral clefts. *Am J Epidemiol* 1996; 143: 1229–34.

6. Russel RM. A minimum of 13,500 deaths annually from coronary artery disease could be prevented by increasing folate intake to reduce homocysteine levels. *JAMA* 1996; 275: 1828–29.

7. Houston DK, Johnson MA, Nozza RJ, et al. Age-related hearing loss, vitamin B-12, and folate in elderly women. *Am J Clin Nutr* 1999; 69: 564–71.

8. Butterworth CE Jr, Tamura T. Folic acid safety and toxicity: a brief review. *Am J Clin Nutr* 1989; 50: 353–58.

9. Wald NJ, Bower C. Folic acid, pernicious anaemia, and prevention of neural tube defects. *Lancet* 1994; 343: 307.

10. Russell RM, Golner BB, Krasinski SD, et al. Effect of antacid and H2 receptor antagonists on the intestinal absorption of folic acid. *J Lab Clin Med* 1988; 112: 458–63.

11. Russell RM, Dutta SK, Oaks EV, et al. Impairment of folic acid absorption by oral pancreatic extracts. *Dig Dis Sci* 1980; 25: 369–73.

Fumaric Acid

1. Kolbach DN, Nieboer C. Fumaric acid therapy in psoriasis: results and side effects of 2 years of treatment. *J Am Acad Dermatol* 1992; 27: 769–71.

2. Altmeyer PJ, Matthes U, Pawlak F, et al. Antipsoriatic effect of fumaric acid derivatives. *J Am Acad Dermatol* 1994; 30: 977–81.

3. Mrowietz U, Christophers E, Altmeyer P. Treatment of psoriasis with fumaric acid esters: results of a prospective multicentre study. German Multicentre Study. *Br J Dermatol* 1998; 138: 456–60.

4. Nugteren-Huying WM, van der Schroeff JG, Hermans J, et al. Fumaric acid therapy in psoriasis; a double-blind, placebo-controlled study. *Ned Tijdschr Geneeskd* 1990; 134: 2387–91 [in Dutch].

5. Nieboer C, de Hoop D, van Loenen AC, et al. Systemic therapy with fumaric acid derivates: new possibilities in the treatment of psoriasis. *J Am Acad Dermatol* 1989; 20: 601–8.

6. Dalhoff K, Faerber P, Arnholdt H, et al. Acute kidney failure during psoriasis therapy with fumaric acid derivatives. *Dtsch Med Wochenschr* 1990; 115: 1014–17 [in German].

7. Roodnat JI, Christiaans MH, Nugteren-Huying WM, et al. Acute kidney insufficiency in patients treated with fumaric acid esters for psoriasis. *Ned Tijdschr Geneeskd* 1989; 133: 2623–26 [in Dutch].

8. Kolbach DN, Nieboer C. Fumaric acid therapy in psoriasis: results and side effects of 2 years of treatment. *J Am Acad Dermatol* 1992; 27: 769–71.

9. Altmeyer P, Hartwig, R, Matthes U. Efficacy and safety profile of fumaric acid esters in oral long-term therapy with severe treatment

refractory of psoriasis vulgaris. A study of 83 patients. *Hautarzt* 1996; 47: 190–96.

Gamma Oryzanol

1. Rosenbloom C, Millard-Stafford M, Lathrop J. Contemporary ergogenic aids used by strength/power athletes. *J Am Diet Assoc* 1992; 92(10): 1264–65.

2. Fry AC, Bonner E, Lewis DL, et al. The effects of gamma-oryzanol supplementation during resistance exercise training. *Internat J Sport Nutr* 1997; 7: 318–29.

3. Takemoto T et al. Clinical trial of Hi-Z fine granules (gamma-oryzanol) on gastrointestinal symptoms at 375 hospitals (Japan). *Shinyaku To Rinsho* 1977; 26 [in Japanese].

Glucosamine Sulfate

1. Drovanti A, Bignamini AA, Rovati AL. Therapeutic activity of oral glucosamine sulfate in osteoarthritis: a placebo-controlled double-blind investigation. *Clin Ther* 1980; 3(4): 260–72.

2. Vaz AL. Double-blind clinical evaluation of the relative efficacy of ibuprofen and glucosamine sulphate in the management of osteoarthritis of the knee in out-patients. *Curr Med Res Opin* 1982; 8(3): 145–9.

Glutamic Acid

1. Damrau F. Benign prostatic hypertrophy: Amino acid therapy for symptomatic relief. *J Am Geriatr Soc* 1962; 10(5): 426–30.

2. Feinblatt HM, Gant JC. Palliative treatment of benign prostatic hypertrophy. Value of glycine-alanine-glutamic acid combination. *J Maine Med Assoc* March 1958.

3. Zello GA, Wykes LF, Ball RO, et al. Recent advances in methods of assessing dietary amino acid requirements for adult humans. *J Nutr* 1995; 125: 2907–15.

Glutamine

1. Robinson MK et al. Glutathione deficiency and HIV infection. *Lancet* 1992; 339: 1603–4.

2. Griffiths RD. Outcome of critically ill patients after supplementa-tion with glutamine. *Nutrition* 1997; 13: 752–54.

Glycine

1. Damrau F. Benign prostatic hypertrophy: Amino acid therapy for symptomatic relief. *J Am Geriatrics Soc* 1962; 10(5): 426–30.

2. Feinblatt HM, Gant JC. Palliative treatment of benign prostatic hypertrophy. Value of glycine-alanine-glutamic acid combination. *J Maine Med Assoc* Mar 1958.

Histidine

1. Gerber DA et al. Specificity of a low free histidine concentration for rheumatoid arthritis. *J Chron Dis* 1977; 30: 115.

HMB (Beta Hydroxy-Beta-Methylbutyrate)

1. Nissen SL, Morrical D, Fuller JC. Effects of the leucine catabolite beta-hydroxy-beta-methylbutyrate (HMB) on the growth and health of growing lambs. *J Animal Sci* 1994; 77: 243.

2. Nissen S, Panton L, Wilhelm R, et al. Effect of beta-hydroxy-beta-methylbutyrate (HMB) supplementa-tion on strength and body composi-tion of trained and untrained males undergoing intense resistance training. *FASEB J* 1996; 10: A287 [abstract].

3. Nissen S, Sharp R, Ray M, et al. Effect of leucine metabolite beta-hydroxy-beta-methylbutyrate on mus-cle metabolism during resistive-exer-cise training. *J Appl Phys* 1996; 81: 2095–104.

Huperzine A

1. Ashani Y, Peggins JO 3d, Doctor BP. Mechanism of inhibition of cholinesterases by huperzine A. *Biochem Biophys Res Commun* 1992; 184: 719–26.

2. Cheng DH, Tang XC. Comparative studies of huperzine A, E2020, and tacrine on behavior and cholinesterase activities. *Pharmacol Biochem Behav* 1998; 60: 377–86.

3. Cheng DH, Ren H, Tang XC. Huperzine A, a novel promising acetylcholinesterase inhibitor. *Neuroreport* 1996; 8: 97–101.

4. Ved HS, Koenig ML, Dave JR, et al. Huperzine A, a potential thera-peutic agent for dementia, reduces neuronal cell death caused by gluta-mate. *Neuroreport* 1997; 8: 963–68.

5. Skolnick AA. Old Chinese herbal medicine used for fever yields possible new Alzheimer's disease ther-apy. *JAMA* 1997; 277: 776 [News item].

6. Xu SS, Gao ZX, Weng Z, et al. Efficacy of tablet huperzine-A on memory, cognition, and behavior in Alzheimer's disease. *Chung Kuo Yao Li Hsueh Pao* 1995; 16: 391–95.

7. Zhang RW, Tang XC, Han YY, et al. Drug evaluation of huperzine A in the treatment of senile memory dis-orders. *Chung Kuo Yao Li Hsueh Pao* 1991; 12: 250–52 [in Chinese].

8. Qian BC, Wang M, Zhou ZF, et al. Pharmacokinetics of tablet huperzine A in six volunteers. *Chung Kuo Yao Li Hsueh Pao* 1995; 16: 396–98.

(-)-Hydroxycitric Acid (HCA)

1. Lowenstein JM. Effect of (-)-hydroxycitrate on fatty acid synthesis by rat liver in vivo. *J Biol Chem* 1971; 246(3): 629–32.

2. Triscari J, Sullivan AC. Comparative effects of (-)-hydroxyci-trate and (=)-allo-hydroxycitrate on acetyl CoA carboxylase and fatty acid and cholesterol synthesis in vivo. *Lipids* 1977; 12(4): 357–63.

3. Cheema-Dhadli S, Harlperin ML, Leznoff CC. Inhibition of enzymes which interact with citrate by (-)hydroxycitrate and 1,2,3,-tricar-boxybenzene. *Eur J Biochem* 1973; 38: 98–102.

4. Sullivan AC, Hamilton JG, Miller ON, et al. Inhibition of lipoge-nesis in rat liver by (-)-hydroxycitrate. *Arch Biochem Biophys* 1972; 150: 183–90.

5. Greenwood MRC, Cleary MP, Gruen R, et al. Effect of (-)-hydroxyc-itrate on development of obesity in the Zucker obese rat. *Am Phys J* 1981; 240: E72–78.

6. Sullivan AC, Triscari J. Metabolic regulation as a control for lipid disorders. *Am J Clin Nutr* 1977; 30: 767–76.

7. Sullivan AC, Triscari J, Hamilton JG, et al. Effect of (-)-hydroxycitrate upon the accumulation

of lipid in the rat: I. Lipogenesis. *Lipids* 1974; 9: 121–128.

8. Sullivan AC, Triscari J, Hamilton JG, et al. Effect of (-)-hydroxycitrate upon the accumulation of lipid in the rat. II. Appetite. *Lipids* 1974; 9(2): 129–34.

9. Sergio W. A natural food, malabar tamarind, may be effective in the treatment of obesity. *Med Hypothesis* 1988; 27: 40.

10. Heymsfield SB, Allison DB, Vasselli JR, et al. Garcinia cambogia (hydroxycitric acid) as a potential antiobesity agent. *JAMA* 1998; 280: 1596–1600.

11. Seroy S. Response to JAMA HCA report. *Townsend Letter for Doctors and Patients* Feb/Mar 1999: 120–21 [letter/review].

Inosine

1. Starling RD, Trappe TA, Short KR, et al. Effect of inosine supplementation on aerobic and anaerobic cycling performance. *Med Sci Sports Ex* 1996; 28(9): 1193–98.

2. Williams MH, Kreider RB, Hunter DW, et al. Effect of inosine supplementation on 3-mile treadmill run performance and VO2 peak. *Med Sci Sports Exerc* 1990 Aug; 22(4): 517–22.

Iodine

1. Kunin RA. Clinical uses of iodide and iodine. *Nutr Healing* Jul 1998: 7–10 [interview].

2. Mu L, Derun L, Chengyi Q, et al. Endemic goiter in central China caused by excessive iodine intake. *Lancet* 1987; ii: 257–59.

3. Pennington JA. A review of iodine toxicity reports. *J Am Dietet Assoc* 1990; 1571–81.

4. Barker DJP, Phillips DIW. Current incidence of thyrotoxicosis and past prevalence of goiter in 12 British towns. *Lancet* 1984; ii: 567–70.

5. Williams ED, Doniach I, Bjarnason O, et al. Thyroid cancer in an iodide rich area. *Cancer* 1977; 39: 215–22.

IP-6 (Inositol Hexaphosphate, Phytate)

1. Graf E, Eaton JW. Antioxidant functions of phytic acid. *Free Rad Biol Med* 1990; 8: 61–69 [review].

2. Shamsuddin AM, Vucenik I, Cole KE. IP-6: a novel anticancer agent. *Life Sci* 1997; 61: 343–54 [review].

3. Graf E, Eaton JW. Suppression of colonic cancer by dietary phytic acid. *Nutr Cancer* 1993; 19: 11–19 [review].

4. Vucenik I, Sakamoto K, Bansal M, et al. Inhibition of rat mammary carcinogenesis by inositol hexaphosphate (phytic acid). A pilot study. *Cancer Lett* 1993; 75: 95–102.

5. Vucenik I, Yang G, Shamsuddin AM. Comparison of pure inositol hexaphosphate and high-bran diet in the prevention of DMBA-induced rat mammary carcinogenesis. *Nutr Cancer* 1997; 28(1): 7–13.

6. Vucenik I, Yang G, Shamsuddin AM. Comparison of pure inositol hexaphosphate and high-bran diet in the prevention of DMBA-induced rat mammary carcinogenesis. *Nutr Cancer* 1997; 28(1): 7–13.

7. Harland BF, Morris ER. Phytate: a good or a bad food component? *Nutr Res* 1995; 15: 733–54 [review].

8. Owen RW, Weisgerber UM, Spiegelhalder B, et al. Faecal phytic acid and its relation to other putative markers of risk for colorectal cancer. *Gut* 1996; 38: 591–97.

9. Vucenik I, Zhang ZS, Shamsuddin AM. IP6 in treatment of liver cancer II. Intra-tumoral injection of IP6 regresses pre-existing human liver cancer xenotransplanted in nude mice. *Anticancer Res* 1998; 18: 4091–96.

10. Yoon JH, Thompson LU, Jenkins DJA. The effect of phytic acid on in vitro rate of starch digestibility and blood glucose response. *Am J Clin Nutr* 1983; 38: 835–42.

11. Morris ER. Phytate and dietary mineral bioavailability. In *Phytic Acid Chemistry and Applications*, E Graf, ed. Minneapolis: Pilatus Press, 1986, 57–76 [review].

Iron

1. Sullivan JL. Stored iron and ischemic heart disease. *Circulation* 1992; 86: 1036 [editorial].

2. Cutler P. Deferoxamine therapy in high-ferritin diabetes. *Diabetes* 1989; 38: 1207–10.

3. Stevens RG, Graubard BI, Micozzi MS, et al. Moderate elevation of body iron level and increased risk of cancer occurrence and death. *Int J Cancer* 1994; 56: 364–69.

4. Weinberg ED. Iron withholding: a defense against infection and neoplasia. *Am J Physiol* 1984; 64: 65–102.

5. Oh VMS. Iron dextran and systemic lupus erythematosus. *Br Med J* 1992; 305: 1000 [letter].

6. Dabbagh AJ, Trenam CW, Morris CJ, Blake DR. Iron in joint inflammation. *Ann Rheum Dis* 1993; 52: 67–73.

7. Salonen JU, Nyyssonen K, Korpela H, et al. High stored iron levels associated with excess risk of myocardial infarction in western Finnish men. *Circulation* 1992; 86: 8031–11.

8. Kechl S, Willeit J, Egger G, et al. Body iron stores and the risk of carotid atherosclerosis. *Circulation* 1997; 96: 3300–3307.

9. Tzonou A, Lagiou P, Trichopoulou A, Tsoutsos V, Trichopoulos D. Dietary iron and coronary heart disease risk: a study from Greece. *Am J Epidemiol* 1998; 147: 161–66.

10. Danesh J, Appleby P. Coronary heart disease and iron status. Meta-analyses of prospective studies. *Circulation* 1999; 99:852–54.

11. Hunt JR, Gallagher SK, Johnson LK. Effect of ascorbic acid on apparent iron absorption by women with low iron stores. *Am J Clin Nutr* 1994; 59: 1381–85.

12. Suharno D, West CE, Muhilal, et al. Supplementation with vitamin A and iron for nutritional anemia in pregnant women in West Java, Indonesia. *Lancet* 1993; 342: 1325–28.

13. Semba RD, Muhilal, West KP Jr, et al. Impact of vitamin A supplementation on hematological indicators of iron metabolism and protein status in children. *Nutr Res* 1992; 12: 469–78.

14. Harkness JAL, Blake DR. Penicillamine nephropathy and iron. *Lancet* 1982: ii: 1368–69.

Part Two: References

Part Two: References

Lactase

1. Gudmand-Hoyer E. The clinical significance of disaccharide maldigestion. *Am J Clin Nutr* 1994; 59(3): 735S–41S.

2. Wheadon M, Goulding A, Barbezat GO, et al. Lactose malabsorption and calcium intake as risk factors for osteoporosis in elderly New Zealand women. *NZ Med J* 1991; 104: 417–19.

Lecithin/Phosphatidyl Choline/Choline

1. Benjamin J, Levine J, Fux M, et al. Double-blind, placebo-controlled, crossover trial of inositol treatment for panic disorder. *Am J Psychiatry* 1995; 152: 1084–86.

Lipase

1. Hegnhoj J, Hansen CP, Rannem T, et al. Pancreatic function in Crohn's disease. *Gut* 1990; 31: 1076–9.

Lutein

1. Seddon JM, Ajani UA, Sperduto RD, et al. Dietary carotenoids, vitamins A, C, and E, and advanced age-related macular degeneration. *JAMA* 1994; 272: 1413–20.

2. Hankinson SE, Stampfer MJ, Saddon JM, et al. Nutrient intake and cataract extraction in women: A prospective study. *Br Med J* 1992; 305: 335–39.

Lycopene

1. Giovannucci E, Ascherio A, Rimm EB, et al. Intake of carotenoids and retinol in relation to risk of prostate cancer. *J Natl Cancer Inst* 1995; 87: 1767–76.

2. Mills PK, Beeson WL, Phillips RL, Fraser GE. Cohort study of diet, lifestyle, and prostate cancer in Adventist men. *Cancer* 1989; 64: 598–604.

3. Carter HB, Coffey DS. The prostate: an increasing medical problem. *Prostate* 1990; 16: 39–48.

4. Hsing AW, Comstock GW, Abbey H, Polk F. Serologic precursors of cancer. Retinol, carotenoids, and tocopherol and risk of prostate cancer. *J Natl Cancer Inst* 1990; 82: 941–46.

5. Levy J, Bosin E, Feldman B, Giat Y, et al. Lycopene is a more potent inhibitory of human cancer cell proliferation than either beta-carotene or beta-carotene. *Nutr Cancer* 1995; 24: 257–66.

6. Franceshci S, Bidoli E, La Vecchia C, et al. Tomatoes and risk of digestive-tract cancers. *Int J Cancer* 1994; 59: 181–84.

7. Van Eenwyk J, Davis FG, Bowne PE. Dietary and serum carotenoids and cervical intraepithelial neoplasia. *Int J Cancer* 1991; 48: 34–38.

8. Kanetsky PA, Gammon MD, Mandelblatt J, et al. Dietary intake and blood levels of lycopene: association with cervical dysplasia among non-hispanic, black women. *Nutr Cancer* 1998; 31: 31–40.

9. Dorgan JF, Sowell A, Swanson CA, et al. Relationships of serum carotenoids, retinol, alpha-tocopherol, and selenium with breast cancer risk: results from a prospective study in Columbia, Missouri. *Cancer Causes Control* 1998; 9: 89–97.

10. Kohlmeyer L, Kark JD, Gomez-Gracia E, et al. Lycopene and myocardial infarction risk in the EUROMIC study. *Am J Epidemiol* 1997; 146: 618–26.

11. Corridan BM, O'Donohue MP, Morrissey PA. Carotenoids and immune response in elderly people. *Proc Nutr Soc* 1998; 57: 3A [abstr].

Lysine

1. Civitelli R, Villareal DT, Agnusdei D, et al. Dietary L-lysine and calcium metabolism in humans. *Nutrition* 1992; 8: 400–404.

2. Pauling L. Case report: Lysine/ascorbate-related amelioration of angina pectoris. *J Orthomol Med* 1991; 6: 144–46.

3. Flodin NW. The metabolic roles, pharmacology, and toxicology of lysine. *J Am Coll Nutri* 1997; 16: 7–21 [review].

4. Flodin NW. The metabolic roles, pharmacology, and toxicology of lysine. *J Am Coll Nutri* 1997; 16: 7–21 [review].

5. Kritchevsky D, Weber MM, Klurfeld DM. Gallstone formation in hamsters: influence of specific amino acids. *Nutr Rep Internat* 1984; 29: 117.

6. Leszczynski DE, Kummerow FA. Excess dietary lysine induces hypercholesterolemia in chickens. *Experientia* 1982; 38: 266–67.

7. Flodin NW. The metabolic roles, pharmacology, and toxicology of lysine. *J Am Coll Nutri* 1997; 16: 7–21 [review].

8. Civitelli R, Villareal DT, Agnusdei D, et al. Dietary L-lysine and calcium metabolism in humans. *Nutrition* 1992; 8: 400–405.

9. Flodin NW. The metabolic roles, pharmacology, and toxicology of lysine. *J Am Coll Nutr* 1997; 16: 7–21 [review].

Magnesium

1. Gaspar AZ, Gasser P, Flammer J. The influence of magnesium on visual field and peripheral vasospasm in glaucoma. *Ophthalmologica* 1995; 209: 11–13.

2. Kawano Y, Matsuoka H, Takishita S, Omae T. Effects of magnesium supplementation in hypertensive patients. *Hypertension* 1998; 32: 260–65.

3. Starobrat-Hermelin B, Kozielec T. The effects of magnesium physiological supplementation on hyperactivity in children with attention deficit hyperactivity disorder (ADHD): Positive response to magnesium oral loading test. *Magnesium Res* 1997; 10: 149–56.

4. Starobrat-Hermelin B, Kozielec T. The effects of magnesium physiological supplementation on hyperactivity in children with attention deficit hyperactivity disorder (ADHD). Positive response to magnesium oral loading test. *Magnes Res* 1997; 10: 149–56.

5. Cox IM, Campbell MJ, Dowson D. Red blood cell magnesium and chronic fatigue syndrome. *Lancet* 1991; 337: 757–60.

6. Howard JM, Davies S, Hunnisett A. Magnesium and chronic fatigue syndrome. *Lancet* 1992; 340: 426.

7. Gantz NM. Magnesium and chronic fatigue. *Lancet* 1991; 338: 66 [letter].

8. Hinds G, Bell NP, McMaster D, McCluskey DR. Normal red cell magnesium concentrations and magnesium loading tests in patients with chronic fatigue syndrome. *Ann Clin Biochem* 1994; 31(Pt 5): 459–61.

9. Weisinger JR. Bellorin-font, E. Magnesium and phosphorus. *Lancet* 1998; 352: 391–96 [review].

10. Weisinger JR. Bellorin-font, E. Magnesium and phosphorus. *Lancet* 1998; 352: 391–96 [review].

Malic Acid

1. Abraham G, Flechas J. Management of fibromyalgia: Rationale for the use of magnesium and malic acid. *J Nutr Med* 1992; 3: 49–59.

2. Russell J, Michalek J, Flechas J, et al. Treatment of fibromyalgia syndrome with SuperMalic: A randomized, double-blind, placebo-controlled, crossover pilot study. *J Rheum* 1995; 22(5): 953–57.

Manganese

1. Raloff J. Reasons for boning up on manganese. *Science* Sep 1986, 199 [review].

2. Krieger D, Krieger S, Jansen O, et al. Manganese and chronic hepatic encephalopathy. *Lancet* 1995; 346: 270–74.

3. Freeland-Graves JH. Manganese: an essential nutrient for humans. *Nutr Today* 1989; 23: 13–19 [review].

Medium Chain Triglycerides

1. Bach AC, Ingenbleek Y, Frey A. The usefulness of dietary medium-chain triglycerides in body weight control: fact or fancy? *J Lipid Res* 1996; 37: 708–26.

2. Bach AS, Babayan VK. Medium-chain triglycerides—an update. *Am J Clin Nutr* 1982; 36: 950.

3. Scalfi L, Coltorti A, Contaldo F. Postprandial thermogenesis in lean and obese subjects after meals supplemented with medium-chain and long-chain triglycerides. *Am J Clin Nutr* 1991; 53: 1130–33.

4. Seaton TB, Welle SL, Warenko MK, et al. Thermic effect of medium-chain and long-chain triglycerides in man. *Am J Clin Nutr* 1986; 44: 630–34.

5. Bach AC, Ingenbleek Y, Frey A. The usefulness of dietary medium-chain triglycerides in body weight control: fact or fancy? *J Lipid Res* 1996; 37: 708–26.

6. Yost TJ, Eckel RH. Hypocaloric feeding in obese women: metabolic effects of medium-chain triglyceride substitution. *Am J Clin Nutr* 1989; 49: 326–30.

7. Jeukendrup AE, Saris WH, Schrauwen P, et al. Metabolic availability of medium-chain triglycerides coingested with carbohydrates during prolonged exercise. *J Appl Physiol* 1995; 79: 756–62.

8. Jeukendrup AE, Wagenmakers AJM, Brouns F, et al. Effects of carbohydrate (CHO) and fat supplementation on CHO metabolism during prolonged exercise. *Metabolism* 1996; 45: 915–21.

9. Satabin P, Portero P, Defer G, et al. Metabolic and hormonal responses to lipid and carbohydrate diets during exercise in man. *Med Sci Sports Exer* 1987; 19: 218–23.

10. van Zyl CG, Lambert EV, Hawley JA, et al. Effects of medium-chain triglyceride ingestion on carbohydrate metabolism and cycling performance. *J Appl Physiol* 1996; 80: 2217–25.

11. Jeukendrup AE, Thielen JJHC, Wagenmakers AJM, et al. Effect of medium-chain triacylglycerol and carbohydrate ingestion during exercise on substrate utilization and subsequent cycling performance. *Am J Clin Nutr* 1998; 67: 397–404.

12. Eckel RH, Hanson AS, Chen AY, et al. Dietary substitution of medium-chain triglycerides improves insulin-mediated glucose metabolism in non-insulin dependent diabetics. *Diabetes* 1992; 41: 641–47.

13. Trudy J, Yost RN, Erskine JM, et al. Dietary substitution of medium-chain triglycerides in subjects with non-insulin dependent diabetes mellitus in an ambulatory setting: impact on glycemic control and insulin-mediated glucose metabolism. *J Am Coll Nutr* 1994; 13: 615–22.

14. Cater NB, Heller HJ, Denke MA. *Am J Clin Nutr* 1997; 65: 41–45.

15. Hill JO, Peters LL, Swift D, et al. *J Lipid Res* 1990; 31: 407–16.

Melatonin

1. Zhadanova IV, Wurtman RJ, Lynch HJ, et al. Sleep-inducing effects of low doses of melatonin ingested in the evening. *Clin Pharmacol Ther* 1995; 57: 552–58.

2. Waldhauser F, Saletu B, Trinchard-Lugan I. Sleep laboratory investigations on hypnotic properties of melatonin. *Psychopharmacology* 1990; 100(2): 222–26.

3. Hughes RJ, Sack RL, Lewy AJ. The role of melatonin and circadian phase in age-related sleep maintenance insomnia: assessment in a clinical trial of melatonin replacement. *Sleep* 1998; 21: 52–68.

4. Petrie K, Dawson AG, Thompson L, et al. A double-blind trial of melatonin as a treatment for jet lag in international cabin crew. *Bio Psych* 1993; 33(7): 526–30.

5. Samples RJ, et al. Effect of melatonin on intraocular pressure. *Curr Eye Res* 1988; 7: 649–53.

6. Lewy AJ, Bauer VK, Cutler NL, Sack RL. Melatonin treatment of winter depression: a pilot study. *Psychiatr Res* 1998; 77: 57–61.

7. Nagtegaal JE, Smits MG, Swart ACW, et al. Melatonin-responsive headache in delayed sleep phase syndrome: preliminary observations. *Headache* 1998; 38: 303–7.

8. Leone M, D'Amico D, Moschiano F, et al. Melatonin versus placebo in the prophylaxis of cluster headache: a double-blind pilot study with parallel groups. *Cephalagia* 1996; 16: 494–96.

9. Cagnoni ML, Lomardi A, Cerinic MM, et al. Melatonin for treatment of chronic refractory sarcoidosis. *Lancet* 1995; 346: 1229–30 [letter].

10. Grin W, Grüberger W. A significant correlation between melatonin deficiency and endometrial cancer. *Gynecol Obstet Invest* 1998; 45: 62–65.

11. Lissoni P, Cazzaniga M, Tancini GE, et al. Reversal of clinical resistance to LHRH analogue in metastatic prostate cancer by the pineal hormone melatonin: efficacy of LHRH

Part Two: References

analogue plus melatonin in patients progressing on LHRH analogue alone. *Eur Urol* 1997; 31: 178–81.

12. Blask DE, Wilson ST, Zalatan F. Physiological melatonin inhibition of human breast cancer cell growth in vitro: evidence for a glutathione-mediated pathway. *Cancer Res* 1997; 57: 1909–14.

13. Lissoni P, Barni S, Meregalli S, et al. Modulation of cancer endocrine therapy by melatonin: a phase II study of tamoxifen plus melatonin in metastitic breast cancer patients progressing under tamoxifen alone. *Br J Cancer* 1995; 71: 854–56.

14. Lissoni P, Brivio O, Brivio F, et al. Adjuvant therapy with the pineal hormone melatonin in patients with lymph node relapse due to malignant melanoma. *J Pineal Res* 1996; 21: 239–42.

15. Lissoni P, Barni S, Ardizzoia A, et al. A randomized study with the pineal hormone melatonin versus supportive care alone in patients with brain metastasis due to solid neoplasms. *Cancer* 1994; 73: 699–701.

16. Lissoni P, Barni S, Ardizzoia A, et al. Randomized study with the pineal hormone melatonin versus supportive care alone in advanced nonsmall cell lung cancer resistant to a first-line chemotherapy containing cisplatin. *Oncology* 1992; 49: 336–39.

17. Rosenberg SI, Silverstein H, Rowan PT, Olds MJ. Effect of melatonin on tinnitus. *Laryngoscope* 1998; 108: 305–10.

18. Haimov I, Laudon M, Zisapel N, et al. Sleep disorders and melatonin rhythms in elderly people. *BMJ* 1994; 309: 167.

19. Singer C, McArthur A, Hughes R, et al. Melatonin and sleep in the elderly. *J Am Geriatr Soc* 1996; 44: 51 [abstr #A1].

20. Attenburrow MEJ, Dowling BA, Sharpley AL, Cowen PJ. Case-control study of evening melatonin concentration in primary insomnia. *BMJ* 1996; 312: 1263–64.

21. Folkard S, Arendt J, and Clark M. Can melatonin improve shift workers' tolerance of the night shift? Some preliminary findings. *Chronobio Intern* 1993; 10(5): 315–20.

22. Garfinkel D, Laudon M, Nof D, Zisapel N. Improvement of sleep quality in elderly people by controlled-release melatonin. *Lancet* 1995; 346: 541–44.

23. Sheldon SH. Pro-convulsant effects or oral melatonin in neurologically disabled children. *Lancet* 1998; 351: 1254.

24. Lamberg L. Melatonin potentially useful but safety, efficacy remain uncertain. *JAMA* 1996; 276: 1011–14.

25. Force RW, Hansen L, Badell M. Psychotic episode after melatonin. *Ann Pharmacother* 1997; 31: 1408 [letter].

26. Middleton B. Melatonin and fragmented sleep patterns. *Lancet* 1996; 348: 551–52 [letter].

Methionine

1. Muller F et al. Elevated plasma concentration of reduced homocysteine in patients with Human Immunodeficiency Virus infection. *Am J Clin Nutr* 1996; 242–46.

2. Revillard JP. Lipid peroxidation in Human Immunodeficiency Virus infection. *J Acquired Immunodef Synd* 1992; 5: 637–38.

3. Singer P et al. Nutritional aspects of the Acquired Immunodeficiency Syndrome. *Am J Gastroenterol* 1992; 87: 265–73.

4. Tan SV, Guiloff RJ. Hypothesis on the pathogenesis of vacuolar myelopathy, dementia, and peripheral neuropathy in AIDS. *J Neurol Neurosurg Psychiat* 1998 65: 23–28.

5. Keating JN et al. Evidence of brain methyltransferase inhibition and early brain involvement in HIV-positive patients. *Lancet* 1991; 337: 935–39.

6. Dorfman D, DiRocco A, Simpson D, et al. Oral methionine may improve neuropsychological function in patients with AIDS myelopathy: results of an open-label trial. *AIDS* 1997; 11: 1066–67.

7. Smythies JR, Halsey JH. Treatment of Parkinson's disease with l-methionine. *South Med J* 1984; 77: 1577.

8. Uden S, Bilton D, Nathan L, et al. Antioxidant therapy for recurrent

pancreatitis: placebo-controlled trial. *Aliment Pharmacol Ther* 1990; 4: 357–71.

9. Shaw GM, Velie EM, Schaffer DM. Is dietary intake of methionine associated with a reduction in risk for neural tube defect-associated pregnancies? *Teratology* 1997; 56: 295–99.

10. Toborek M, Hennig B. Is methionine an atherogenic amino acid? *J Optimalt Nutr* 1994; 3(2): 80–83.

11. Leach FN, Braganza JM. Methionine is important in treatment of chronic pancreatitis. *Br Med J* 1998; 316: 474 [letter].

Molybdenum

1. Johnson JL et al. Molybdenum cofactor deficiency in a patient previously characterized as deficient in sulfite oxidase. *Biochem Med Metabol Biol* 1988; 40: 86–93.

Multiple Vitamin/Mineral

1. Pao EM, Mickle SJ. Problem nutrients in the United States. *Food Technology* 1981; 35: 58–79.

2. Food and Nutrition Board, National Research Council. *Recommended Dietary Allowances*, 10th ed. Washington, DC: National Academy Press, 1989.

3. Sempos CT, Looker AC, Gillum RF. Iron and heart disease: the epidemiologic data. *Nutr Rev* 1996; 54: 73–84 [review].

4. Okada S. Iron-induced tissue damage and cancer: the role of reactive oxygen species-free radicals. *Pathol Int* 1996; 46: 311–32 [review].

5. Cutler P. Deferoxamine therapy in high-ferritin diabetes. *Diabetes* 1989; 38: 1207–10.

6. Weinberg ED. Iron withholding: a defense against infection and neoplasia. *Am J Physiol* 1984; 64: 65–102.

7. Blake DR, Bacon PA. Effect of oral iron on rheumatoid patients. *Lancet* 1982; i: 623 [letter].

8. Rimm EB, Stampfer MJ, Ascherio A, et al. Vitamin E consumption and the risk of coronary heart disease in men. *N Engl J Med* 1993; 328: 1450–56.

9. Stampfer MJ, Hennekens CH, Manson JE, et al. Vitamin E consump-

tion and the risk of coronary heart disease in women. *N Engl J Med* 1993; 328: 1444–49.

10. Stephens NG, Parsons A, Schofield PM, et al. Randomised controlled trial of vitamin E in patients with coronary disease: Cambridge Heart Antioxidant Study (CHAOS). *Lancet* 1996; 347: 781–86.

11. Shekelle RB, Lepper M, Liu S, et al. Dietary vitamin A and risk of cancer in the Western Electric Study. *Lancet* 1981; ii: 1185–90.

12. Giovannucci E, Ascherio A, Rimm EB, et al. Intake of carotenoids and retinol in relation to risk of prostate cancer. *J Natl Cancer Inst* 1995; 87: 1767–76.

13. Seddon JM, Ajani UA, Sperduto RD, et al. Dietary carotenoids, vitamins A, C, and E, and advanced age-related macular degeneration. *JAMA* 1994; 272: 1413–20.

14. Hollman PC, Katan MB. Absorption, metabolism and health effects of dietary flavonoids in man. *Biomed Pharmacother* 1997; 51: 305–10 [Review].

15. Hertog MGL, Sweetnam PM, Fehily AM, et al. Antioxidant flavonols and ischemic heart disease in a Welsh population of men: the Caerphilly Study. *Am J Clin Nutr* 1997; 65: 1489–94.

N-Acetyl Cysteine (NAC)

1. Boman G, Bäcker U, Larsson S, et al. Oral acetylcysteine reduces exacerbation rate in chronic bronchitis: a report of a trial organized by the Swedish Society for Pulmonary Diseases. *Eur J Respir Dis* 1983; 64: 405–15.

2. Multicenter Study Group. Long-term oral acetylcysteine in chronic bronchitis. A double-blind controlled study. *Eur J Respir Dis* 1980; 61: 111: 93–108.

3. de Quay B, Malinverni R, Lauterburg BH. Glutathione depletion in HIV-infected patients: role of cysteine deficiency and effect of oral N-acetylcysteine. *AIDS* 1992; 6: 815–19.

4. Tattersall AB, Bridgman KM, Huitson A. Acetylcysteine (Fabrol) in chronic bronchitis—a study in general practice. *J Int Med Res* 1983; 11: 279–84.

5. Kleinveld HA, Demacker PNM, Stalenhoef AFH. Failure of N-acetylcysteine to reduce low-density lipoprotein oxidizability in healthy subjects. *Eur J Clin Pharmacol* 1992; 43: 639–42.

6. Brumas V, Hacht B, Filella M, Berthon G. Can N-acetyl-L-cysteine affect zinc metabolism when used as a paracetamol antidote? *Agents Actions* 1992; 36: 278–88.

NADH (Nicotinamide Adenine Dinucleotide)

1. Kuhn W, Muller T, Winkel R, et al. Parenteral application of NADH in Parkinson's disease: Clinical improvement partially due to stimulation of endogenous levodopa biosynthesis. *J Neural Transmission* 1996; 103: 1187–93.

2. Birkmayer W, Birkmayer JGD, Vrecko K, et al. The clinical benefit of NADH as stimulator of endogenous L-Dopa biosynthesis in Parkinsonian patients. In *Advances in Neurology*, vol. 53 (Parkinsons Disease: Anatomy, Pathology, and Therapy), eds. MB Streifler, AD Korczyn, E. Melamed, et al. New York: Raven Press, 1990, 545–49.

3. Birkmayer JGD, Vrecko K, Birkmayer W, et al. Nicotinamide adenine dinucleotide (NADH), a new therapeutic approach to Parkinson's disease: Comparison of oral and parenteral application. *Acta Neurologica Scand* 1993; 87(Suppl 146): 32–35.

4. Dizdar N, Kagedal B, Lindvall B. Treatment of Parkinson's disease with NADH. *Acta Neurologica Scand* 1994; 90: 345–47.

5. Birkmayer JGD. Coenzyme nicotinamide adenine dinucleotide: New therapeutic approach for improving dementia of the Alzheimer type. *Ann Clin Lab Sci* 1996; 26: 1–9.

6. Birkmayer JGD, Birkmayer W. The coenzyme nicotinamide adenine dinucleotide (NADH) as biological antidepressive agent: Experience with 205 patients. *New Trends Clin Neuropharmacol* 1991; 5: 19–25.

7. Forsyth LM, MacDowell-Carnciro AL, Birkmayer GD, et al. The use of NADH as a new therapeutic approach in chronic fatigue syndrome. Presented at the annual meeting of the American College of Allergy, Asthma & Immunology,1998.

Octacosanol

1. Castano G, Canetti M, Moreira M, et al. Efficacy and tolerability of policosanol in elderly patients with type II hypercholesterolemia: A 12-month study. *Curr Ther Res* 1995; 56: 819–23.

2. Castano G, Tula L, Canetti M, et al. Effects of policosanol in hypertensive patients with type II hypercholesterolemia. *Curr Ther Res* 1996; 57: 691–95.

3. Aneiros E, Mas R, Calderon B, et al. Effect of policosanol in lowering cholesterol levels in patients with Type II hypercholesterolemia. *Curr Ther Res* 1995; 56: 176–82.

4. Castano G, Mas R, Nodarse M, et al. One-year study of the efficacy and safety of policosanol (5 mg twice daily) in the treatment of type II hypercholesterolemia. *Curr Ther Res* 1995; 56: 296–304.

5. Aneiros E, Calderon B, Mas R, et al. Effect of successive dose increases of policosanol on the lipid profile and tolerability of treatment. *Curr Ther Res* 1993; 54: 304–12.

6. Pons P, Rodriguez M, Mas R, et al. One-year efficacy and safety of policosanol in patients with type II hypercholesterolemia. *Curr Ther Res* 1994; 55: 1084–92.

7. Pons P, Mas R, Illnait J, et al. Efficacy and safety of policosanol in patients with primary hypercholesterolemia. *Curr Ther Res* 1992; 52: 507–13.

8. Menendez R, Arruzazabala L, Mas R, et al. Cholesterol-lowering effect of policosanol on rabbits with hypercholesterolaemia induced by a wheat starch-casein diet. *Br J Nutr* 1997; 77: 923–32.

9. Batista J, Stusser R, Penichet M, Uguet E. Dopper-ultrasound pilot study of the effects of long-term policosanol therapy on carotid-vertebral atherosclerosis. *Curr Ther Res* 1995; 56: 906–8.

10. Cureton TK. The physiological effects of wheat germ oil on

humans. In *Exercise*. Illinois: Charles C Thomas, 1972: 296–300.

11. Saint-John M, McNaughton L. Octacosanol ingestion and its effects on metabolic responses to sub-maximal cycle ergometry, reaction time and chest and grip strength. *Int Clin Nutr Rev* 1986; 6(2): 81–87.

12. Pons P, Rodriguez M, Robaina C, et al. Effects of successive dose increases of policosanol on the lipid profile of patients with type II hypercholesterolaemia and tolerability to treatment. *Int J Clin Pharm Res* 1994; 14: 27–33.

Ornithine

1. Bucci LR, Hickson JF, Wolinsky I, et al. Ornithine supplementation and insulin release in bodybuilders. *Int J Sport Nutr* 1992; 2: 287–91.

2. Fogelholm GM, Naveri HK, Kiilavuori KT, et al. Low-dose amino acid supplementation: no effects on serum human growth hormone and insulin in male weightlifters. *Int J Sport Nutr* 1993; 3: 290–97.

3. Lambert MI, Hefer JA, Millar RP, et al. Failure of commercial oral amino acid supplements to increase serum growth hormone concentrations in male body-builders. *Int J Sport Nutr* 1993; 3: 298–305.

4. Bucci L, Hickson JF et al. Ornithine ingestion and growth hormone release in bodybuilders. *Nutr Res* 1990; 10: 239–45.

5. Elam RP, Hardin DH, Sutton RA, et al. Effects of arginine and ornithine on strength, lean body mass and urinary hydroxyproline in adult males. *J Sports Med Phys Fitness* 1989; 29: 52–56.

6. Zieve L. Conditional deficiencies of ornithine or arginine. *J Am Coll Nutr* 1986; 5: 167–76 [review].

Ornithine Alpha-Ketoglutarate (OKG)

1. Le Boucher J, Cynober LA. Ornithine alpha-ketoglutarate: the puzzle. *Nutrition* 1998; 14: 870–73 [review].

2. Brocker P, Vellas B, Albarede J, et al. A two-centre, randomized, double-blind trial of ornithine oxoglutarate in 194 elderly, ambulatory, con-valescent subjects. *Age Aging* 1994; 23: 303–6.

PABA (Paraaminobenzoic Acid)

1. Wiesel LL et al. The synergistic action of para-aminobenzoic acid and cortisone in the treatment of rheumatoid arthritis. *Am J Med Sci* 1951; 222: 243–48.

2. Sieve BF. The clinical effects of a new B-complex factor, para-aminobenzoic acid, on pigmentation and fertility. *South Med Surg* 1942(March); 104: 135–39.

3. Zarafonetis CJD. The treatment of scleroderma: results of potassium para-aminobenzoate therapy in 104 cases. In Mills LC, Moyer JH (eds.), *Inflammation and Diseases of Connective Tissue*, W. B. Saunders Co., Philadelphia. 1961, 688–96.

4. Zarafonetis CJD et al. Retrospective studies in scleroderma: effect of potassium para-aminobenzoate on survival. *J Clin Epidemiol* 1988; 41: 193–205.

5. Zarafonetis CJ, Dabich L, Devol EB, et al. Retrospective studies in scleroderma: pulmonary findings and effect of potassium p-aminobenzoate on vital capacity. *Respiration* 1989; 56: 22–33.

6. Clegg DO, Reading JC, Mayes MD, et al. Comparison of aminobenzoate potassium and placebo in the treatment of scleroderma. *J Rheumatol* 1994; 21: 105–10.

7. Grace WJ et al. Therapy of scleroderma and dermatomyositis. *NY State J Med* 1963; 63: 140–44.

8. Zarafonetis CJD. Treatment of Peyronie's disease with potassium para-aminobenzoate. *J Urol* 1959; 81: 770–72.

9. Zarafonetis CJD, et al. Treatment of pemphigus with potassium para-aminobenzoate. *Am J Med Sci* 1956; 231: 30–50.

10. Sieve BF. Further investigations in the treatment of vitiligo. *Virginia Med Monthly* 1945(January): 6–17.

11. Hughes CG. Oral PABA and vitiligo. *J Am Acad Dermatol* 1983; 9: 770 [letter].

12. Gaby AR. The story of PABA. *Nutr Healing* 1997; March: 3–4,11 [review].

13. Zarafonetis CJD. Darkening of gray hair during para-amino-benzoic acid therapy. *J Invest Dermatol* 1950; 15: 399–401.

14. Kantor GR, Ratz JL. Liver toxicity from potassium para-aminobenzoate. *J Am Acad Dermatol* 1985; 13: 671–2.

15. Hughes CG. Oral PABA and vitiligo. *J Am Acad Dermatol* 1983; 9: 770 [letter].

16. Worobec S, LaChine A. Dangers of orally administered para-aminobenzoic acid. *JAMA* 1984; 251: 2348.

L-Phenylalanine and D,L-Phenylalanine (DLPA)

1. Sabelli HC. Clinical studies on the phenylethylamine hypothesis of affective disorder: urine and blood phenylacetic acid and phenylalanine dietary supplements. *J Clin Psychiatry* 1986; 47: 66–70.

2. Fischer E et al. Therapy of depression by phenylalanine. *Arzneimittelforsch* 1975; 25: 132.

3. Heller B et al. Therapeutic action of D-phenylalanine in Parkinson's disease. *Arzneimittelforsch* 1976; 26: 577–79.

4. Budd K. Use of D-phenylalanine, an enkephalinase inhibitor, in the treatment of intractable pain. *Adv Pain Res Ther* 1983; 5: 305–8.

5. Anonymous. Phenylalanine fails to help chronic back pain patients. *Family Pract News* 1987; 17(3): 37.

Phosphatidylserine

1. Crook TH, Tinklenberg J, Yesavage J, et al. Effects of phosphatidylserine in age-associated memory impairment. *Neurology* 1991; 41: 644–49.

2. Cenacchi T, Bertoldin T, Farina C, et al. Cognitive decline in the elderly: a double-blind, placebo-controlled multicenter study on efficacy of phosphatidylserine administration. *Aging (Milano)* 1993; 5: 123–33.

3. Crook T, Petrie W, Wells C, Massari DC. Effects of phosphatidylserine in Alzheimer's disease.

Part Two: References

Psychopharmacol Bull 1992; 28: 61–66.

4. Delwaide PJ, Gyselynck-Mambourg AM, Hurlet A, et al. Double-blind randomized controlled study of phosphatidylserine in senile demented patients. *Acta Neurol Scand* 1986; 73: 136–40.

5. Engel RR, Satzger W, Gunther W, et al. Double-blind cross-over study of phosphatidylserine vs. placebo in patients with early dementia of the Alzheimer type. *Eur Neuropsychopharmacol* 1992; 2: 149–55.

6. Fünfgeld EW, Baggen M, Nedwidek P, et al. Double-blind study with phosphatidylserine (PS) in Parkinsonian patients with senile dementia of Alzheimer's type (SDAT). *Prog Clin Biol Res* 1989; 317: 1235–46.

7. Amaducci L. Phosphatidylserine in the treatment of Alzheimer's disease: results of a multicenter study. *Psychopharmacol Bull* 1988; 24: 130–34.

8. Heiss WD, Kessler J, Mielke R, et al. Long-term effects of phosphatidylserine, pyritinol, and cognitive training in Alzheimer's disease. A neuropsychological, EEG, and PET investigation. *Dementia* 1994; 5: 88–98.

9. Maggioni M, Picotti GB, Bondiolotti GP, et al. Effects of phosphatidylserine therapy in geriatric patients with depressive disorders. *Acta Psychiatr Scand (DENMARK)* 1990; 81: 265–70.

10. Sakai M, Yamatoya H, Kudo S. Pharmacological effects of phosphatidylserine enzymatically synthesized from soybean lecithin on brain functions in rodents. *J Nutr Sci Vitaminol (Tokyo)* 1996; 42: 47–54.

11. Kidd PM. Don't believe everything you read . . . a sequel. Point. *Townsend Letter for Doctors Patients* 1997; July: 122–4 [editorial].

12. Gaby AR. Don't believe everything you read. CounterPoint. *Townsend Letter for Doctors Patients* 1997; July: 125–26 [editorial].

13. Furushiro M, Suzuki S, Shishido Y, et al. Effects of oral administration of soybean lecithin transphosphatidylated phosphatidylserine on impaired learning of passive avoidance in mice. *Jpn J Pharmacol* 1997; 75: 447–50.

14. Sakai M, Yamatoya H, Kudo S. Pharmacological effects of phosphatidylserine enzymatically synthesized from soybean lecithin on brain functions in rodents. *J Nutr Sci Vitaminol (Tokyo)* 1996; 42: 47–54.

15. Gindin J, Novikov M, Kedar D, et al. The effect of plant phosphatidylserine on age-associated memory impairment and mood in the functioning elderly. Rehovot, Israel: Geriatric Institute for Education and Research, and Department of Geriatrics, Kaplan Hospital, 1995.

Pollen

1. Stanley RG, Liskens HF. *Pollens*. New York: Springer-Verlag, 1974.

2. Loschen G, Ebeling L. Inhibition of arachidonic acid cascade by extract of rye pollen. *Arzneimittelforschung* 1991; 41: 162–67 [in German].

3. Nakase K, Takenaga K, Hamanaka T, et al. Inhibitory effect and synergism of cernitin pollen extract on the urethral smooth muscle and diaphragm of the rat. *Nippon Yakurigaku Zasshi* 1988 Jun; 91(6): 385–92 [in Japanese].

4. Habib FK, Ross M, Buck AC, et al. In vitro evaluation of the pollen extract, cernitin T-60, in the regulation of prostate cell growth. *Br J Urol* 1990; 66: 393–97.

5. Jodai A, Maruta N, Shimomae E, et al. A long-term therapeutic experience with Cernilton in chronic prostatitis. *Hinyokika Kiyo* 1988; 34: 561–68 [in Japanese].

6. Ohkoshi M, Kawamura N, Nagakubo I. Clinical evaluation of Cernilton in chronic prostatitis. *Jpn J Clin Urol* 1967; 21: 73–76.

7. Suzuki T, Kurokawa K, Mashimo T, et al. Clinical effect of Cernilton in chronic prostatitis. *Hinyokika Kiyo* 1992; 38: 489–94 [in Japanese].

8. Rugendorff EW, Weidner W, Ebeling L, et al. Results of treatment with pollen extract (Cernilton N) in chronic prostatitis and prostatodynia. *Br J Urol* 1993; 71: 433–38.

9. Horii A, Iwai S, Maekawa M, Tsujita M. Clinical evaluation of Cernilton in the treatment of the benign prostatic hypertrophy. *Hinyokika Kiyo* 1985; 31: 739–46 [in Japanese].

10. Ueda K. Jinno H. Tsujimura S. Clinical evaluation of Cernilton on benign prostatic hyperplasia. *Hinyokika Kiyo* 1985; 31: 187–91 [in Japanese].

11. Hayashi J, Mitsui H, Yamakawa G, et al. Clinical evaluation of Cernilton in benign prostatic hypertrophy. *Hinyokika Kiyo* 1986; 32: 135–41 [in Japanese].

12. Buck AC, Cox R, Rees RW, et al. Treatment of outflow tract obstruction due to benign prostatic hyperplasia with the pollen extract, Cernilton. A double-blind, placebo-controlled study. *Br J Urol* 1990; 66: 398–404.

13. Becker H, Ebeling L. Conservative therapy of benign prostatic hyperplasia (BPH) with Cernilton. *Urologe (B)* 1988; 28: 301–306 [in German].

14. Maekawa M, Kishimoto T, Yasumoto R, et al. Clinical evaluation of Cernilton on benign prostatic hypertrophy—a multiple center double-blind study with Paraprost. *Hinyokika Kiyo* 1990; 36: 495–516 [in Japanese].

15. Dutkiewicz S. Usefulness of Cernilton in the treatment of benign prostatic hyperplasia. *Int Urol Nephrol* 1996; 28: 49–53.

16. Juzwiak S. Experimental evaluation of the effect of pollen extract on the course of paracetamol poisoning. *Ann Acad Med Stetin* 1993; 39: 57–69 [in Polish].

17. Mysliwiec Z. Effect of pollen extracts (cernitin preparation) on selected biochemical parameters of liver in the course of chronic ammonium fluoride poisoning in rats. *Ann Acad Med Stetin* 1993; 39: 71–85 [in Polish].

18. Voloshyn OI, Pishak OV, Seniuk BP, et al. The efficacy of flower pollen in patients with rheumatoid arthritis and concomitant diseases of the gastroduodenal and hepatobiliary systems. *Likarska Sprava* 1998; 4: 151–54 [in Ukrainian].

19. Wojcicki J, Samochowiec L, Bartlomowicz B, et al. Effect of pollen

extract on the development of experimental atherosclerosis in rabbits. *Atherosclerosis* 1986; 62: 39–45.

20. Vourdas D, Syrigou E, Potamianou P, et al. Double-blind, placebo-controlled evaluation of sublingual immunotherapy with standardized olive pollen extract in pediatric patients with allergic rhinoconjunctivitis and mild asthma due to olive pollen sensitization. *Allergy* 1998; 53: 662–72.

21. Horak F, Stubner P, Berger UE, et al. Immunotherapy with sublingual birch pollen extract. A short-term double-blind placebo study. *J Investig Allergol Clin Immunol* 1998; 8: 165–71.

22. Ariano R, Panzani RC, Augeri G. Efficacy and safety of oral immunotherapy in respiratory allergy to Parietaria judaica pollen. A double-blind study. *J Investig Allergol Clin Immunol* 1998; 8: 155–60.

23. Clavel R, Bousquet J, Andre C. Clinical efficacy of sublingual-swallow immunotherapy: a double-blind, placebo-controlled trial of a standardized five-grass-pollen extract in rhinitis. *Allergy* 1998; 5: 493–98.

24. Litwin A, Flanagan M, Entis G, et al. Oral immunotherapy with short ragweed extract in a novel encapsulated preparation: a double-blind study. *J Allergy Clin Immunol* 1997; 100: 30–38.

25. Hordijk GJ, Antvelink JB, Luwema RA. Sublingual immunotherapy with a standardised grass pollen extract; a double-blind placebo-controlled study. *Allergol Immunopathol (Madr)* 1998; 26: 234–40.

26. Cohen SH et al. Acute allergic reaction after composite pollen ingestion. *J Allergy Clin Immunol* 1979; 64: 270.

27. Mansfield LE, Goldstein GB. Anaphylactic reaction after ingestion of local bee pollen. *Ann Allergy* 1981; 47: 154–56.

28. Noyes JH, Boyd GK, Settipane GA. Anaphylaxis to sunflower seed. *J Allergy Clin Immunol* 1979; 63: 242–44.

Pregnenolone

1. Akwa Y, Young J, Kabbadj K, et al. Neurosteroids: biosynthesis, metabolism and function of pregnenolone and dehydroepiandrosterone in the brain. *J Steroid Biochem Molec Biol* 1991; 40(1–3): 71–81.

2. Isaacson RL, Varner JA, Baars JM, de Wied D. The effects of pregnenolone sulfate and ethylestrenol on retention of a passive avoidance task. *Brain Res* 1995; 689: 79–84.

3. Flood JF, Morley JE, Roberts E. Pregnenolone sulfate enhances post-trianing memory processes when injected in very low doses into limbic system structures: The amygdala is by far the most sensitive. *Proc Natl Acad Sci* 1995; 92: 10806–810.

4. Flood JF, Morley JE, Roberts E. Memory-enhancing effects in male mice of pregnenolone and steroids metabolically derived from it. *Proc Natl Acad Sci* 1992; 89: 1567–71.

5. Steiger A, Trachsel L, Guldner J, et al. Neurosteroid pregnenolone induces sleep-EEG changes in man compatible with inverse agonistic GABAA-receptor modulation. *Brain Res* 1993; 615: 267–74.

6. Pincus G, Hoagland H. Effects of administered pregnenolone on fatiguing psychomotor performance. *Aviation Med* 1944; April: 98–115.

7. Melchior CL, Ritzmann RF. Pregnenolone and pregnenolone sulfate, alone and with ethanol, in mice on the plus-maze. *Pharmacol Biochem Behav* 1994; 48(4): 893–97.

8. Guth L, Zhang Z, Roberts E. Key role for pregnenolone in combination therapy that promotes recovery after spinal cord injury. 1994; 91: 12308–312.

9. Wu FS, Gibbs TT, Farb DH. Pregnenolone sulfate: a positive allosteric modulator at the N-methyl-D-aspartate receptor. *Mol Pharmacol* 1991; 40(3): 333–36.

10. Maione S, Berrino L, Vitagliano S, et al. Pregnenolone sulfate increases the convulsant potency of N-methyl-D-aspartate in mice. *Eur J Pharmacol* 1992; 219: 477–79.

11. George MS, Guidotti A, Rubinow D, et al. CSF neuroactive steroids in affective disorders: pregnenolone, progesterone and DBI. *Biol Psychiatry* 1994; 35(10): 775–80.

12. Sternberg TH, LeVan P, Wright ET. The hydrating effects of pregnenolone acetate on the human skin. *Curr Ther Res* 1961; 3(11): 469–71.

13. McGavack TH, Chevalley J, Weissberg J. The use of D5-pregnenolone in various clinical disorders. *J Clin Endocrinol* 1951; 11(6): 559–77.

14. Morfin R, Young J, Corpechot C, et al. Neurosteroids: pregnenolone in human sciatic nerves. *Proc Natl Acad Sci* 1992; 89: 6790–793.

15. Akwa Y, Young J, Kabbadj K, et al. Neurosteroids: biosynthesis, metabolism and function of pregnenolone and dehydroepiandrosterone in the brain. *J Steroid Biochem Molec Biol* 1991; 40(1–3): 71–81.

16. Isaacson RL, Varner JA, Baars JM, de Wied D. The effects of pregnenolone sulfate and ethylestrenol on retention of a passive avoidance task. *Brain Res* 1995; 689: 79–84.

Proanthocyanidins (Pycnogenol)

1. Mitcheva M, Astroug H, Drenska D, et al. Biochemical and morphological studies on the effects of anthocyans and vitamin E on carbon tetrachloride induced liver injury. *Cell Mol Bio* 1993; 39(4): 443–48.

2. Maffei F. et al. Free radical scavenging action and anti-enzyme activities of procyanidines from *Vitis vinifera*. A mechanism for their capillary protective action. *Arzn Forsch* 1994; 44: 592–601.

3. Baroch J. Effect of Endotelon in postoperative edema. Results of a double-blind study versus placebo in 32 female patients. *Ann Chir Polast Esthet* 1984; 29: 393–95 [in French].

4. Liviero L, Puglisis E. Antimutagenic activity of procyanidins from vitis vinfera. *Fitother* 1994; 65: 203–209.

5. Dartenuc JY, Marache P, Choussat H. Resistance Capillaire en Geriatrie Etude d'un Microangioprotecteur. *Bordeaux Médical* 1980; 13: 903–907 [in French].

6. Delacroix P. Etude en Double Avengle de l'Endotelon dans l'Insuffisance Veineuse Chronique. *Therapeutique, la Revue de Medicine* 1981; 27–28 Sept: 1793–1802 [in French].

7. Thebaut JF, Thebaut P, Vin F. Study of Endotelon in functional manifestations of peripheral venous insufficiency. *Gazette Medicale* 1985; 92: 96–100 [in French].

8. Corbe C, Boissin JP, Siou A. Light vision and chorioretinal circulation. Study of the effect of procyanidalic oligomers. *J Fr Ophtalmol* 1988; 11: 453–60.

9. Boissin JP, Corbe C, Siou A. Chorioretinal circulation and dazzling; use of procyanidolic oligomers. *Bull Soc Ophtalmol Fr* 1988; 88: 173–74, 177–79 [in French].

10. Masquellier J. Oligomeric proanthocyanidins (OPCs) are the heart of the French paradox. *Townsend Letter for Doctors and Patients,* Dec 1996, 46–47.

Probiotics and FOS

1. Smirnov VV, Reznik SR, V'iunitskaia VA, et al. The current concepts of the mechanisms of the therapeutic-prophylactic action of probiotics from bacteria in the genus bacillus. *Mikrobiolohichnyi Zhurnal* 1993; 55(4): 92–112.

2. Mel'nikova VM, Gracheva NM, Belikov GP, et al. The chemoprophylaxis and chemotherapy of opportunistic infections. *Antibiotiki i Khimioterapiia* 1993; 38: 44–48.

3. De Simone C, Vesely R, Bianchi SB, et al. The role of probiotics in modulation of the immune system in man and in animals. *Int J Immunother* 1993; 9: 23–28.

4. Veldman A. Probiotics. *Tijdschrift voor Diergeneeskunde* 1992; 117(12): 345–48.

5. Kawase K. Effects of nutrients on the intestinal microflora of infants. *Jpn J Dairy Food Sci* 1982; 31: A241–43.

6. Rasic JL. The role of dairy foods containing bifido and acidophilus bacteria in nutrition and health. *N Eur Dairy J* 1983; 4: 80–88.

7. Barefoot SF, Klaenhammer TR. Detection and activity of Lactacin B, a Bacteriocin produced by Lactobacillus acidophilus. *Appl Environ Microbiol* 1983; 45: 1808–15.

8. Hilton E, Isenberg HD, Alperstein P, et al. Ingestion of yogurt containing Lactobacillus acidophilus as prophylaxis for candidal vaginitis. *Ann Int Med* 1992; 116: 353–57.

9. Reid G et al. Implantation of Lactobacillus casei var rhamnosus into vagina. *Lancet* 1994; 344: 1229.

10. Elmer GW, Surawicz CM, McFarland LV. Biotherapeutic agents. *JAMA* 1996; 275(11): 870–76.

11. Scarpignato C, Rampal P. Prevention and treatment of traveler's diarrhea: A clinical pharmacological approach. *Chemotherapy* 1995; 41: 48–81.

12. Golledge CL, Riley TV. "Natural" therapy for infectious diseases. *Med J Austral* 1996; 164: 94–95 [review].

13. Bleichner G, Blehaut H, Mentec H, Moyse D. *Saccharomyces boulardii* prevents diarrhea in critically ill tube-fed patients. A multicenter, randomized, double-blind placebo-controlled trial. *Intensive Care Med* 1997; 23: 517–23.

14. Loizeau E. Can antibiotic-associated diarrhea be prevented? *Annales de Gastroenterologie et d Hepatologie* 1993; 29(1): 15–18.

15. McDonough FE, Hitchins AD, Wong NP, et al. Modification of sweet acidophilus milk to improve utilization by lactose-intolerant persons. *Am J Clin Nutr* 1987; 45: 570–74.

16. Williams CH, Witherly SA, Buddington RK. Influence of Dietary Neosugar on Selected Bacterial Groups of the Human Faecal Microbiota. *Microb Ecol Health Dis* 1994; 7: 91–97.

17. Bigson GR. Dietary modulation of the human gut microflora using prebiotics. *Br J Nutr* 1998; 80(Suppl 2): S209–S212.

18. Yamashita K, Kawai K, Itakura M. Effects of fructo-oligosaccharides on blood glucose and serum lipids in diabetic subjects. *Nutr Res* 1984; 4: 961–66.

19. van den Heuvel EGHM, Muys T, van Dokkum W, Schaafsma G. Oligofructose stimulates calcium absorption in adolescents. *Am J Clin Nutr* 1999; 69: 544–48.

Progesterone

1. Smith DC, Prentice R, Thompson DJ, et al. Association of exogenous estrogen and endometiral carcinoma. *N Engl J Med* 1975; 293: 1164–67.

2. Prior JC. Progesterone as a bone-trophic hormone. *Endocr Rev* 1990; 11: 386–98.

3. Lee JR. Osteoporosis reversal: the role of progesterone. *Int Clin Nutr Rev* 1990; 10: 384–91.

4. Riis BJ, Thomsen K, Strom V, Christiansen C. The effect of percutaneous estradiol and natural progesterone on postmenopausal bone loss. *Am J Obstet Gynecol* 1987; 156: 61–65.

5. Freeman E, et al. Ineffectiveness of progesterone suppository treatment for premenstrual syndrome. *JAMA* 1990; 264: 349–53.

6. Martorano JT, Ahlgrimm M, Colbert T. Differentiating between natural progesterone and synthetic progestins: clinical implications for premenstrual syndrome and perimenopause management. *Comp Ther* 1998; 24: 336–39.

7. Skegg DCG, Noonan EA, Paul C, et al. Depot medroxyprogesterone acetate and breast cancer; a pooled analysis of the World Health Organization and New Zealand studies. *JAMA* 1995; 273: 799–804.

8. Foidart JM, Colin C, Denoo X, et al. Estradiol and progesterone regulate the proliferation of human breast epithelial cells. *Fertil Steril* 1998; 69: 963–69.

9. Chang KJ, Fournier S, Lee TTY, et al. Influences of percutaneous administration of estradiol and progesterone on human breast epithelial cell cycle in vivo. *Fertil Steril* 1995; 63: 785–91.

10. Söderqvist G, Isaksson E, von Schoultz B, et al. Proliferation of breast epithelial cells in healthy women during the menstrual cycle. *Obstet Gynecol* 1997; 176: 123–28.

11. Lee JR. *Natural Progesterone.* Sebastopol, CA: BLL Publishing, 1993, 71–76.

Part Two: References

12. Cowan LD, Gordis L, Tonascia JA, Jones GS. Breast cancer incidence in women with a history of progesterone deficiency. *Am J Epidemiol* 1981; 114: 209–17.

13. Adams MR, Register TC, Golden DL, et al. Medroxy-progesterone acetate antagonizes inhibitory effects of conjugated equine estrogens on coronary artery athero-sclerosis. *Arterioscler Thromb Vasc Biol* 1997; 17: 217–21.

14. Rosano GMC. Presentation to the American Heart Association's Scientific Sessions. New Orleans, Louisiana, 1996.

15. Araghiniknam M, Chung S, Nelson-White T, et al. Antioxidant activity of dioscorea and dehy-droepiandrosterone (DHEA) in older humans. *Life Sci* 1996; 11: 147–57.

16. Dollbaum CM. Lab analyses of salivary DHEA and progesterone following ingestion of yam-containing products. *Townsend Letter for Doctors and Patients* Oct 1995; 104.

17. Hargrove JT, Maxson WS, Wentz AC, et al. Menopausal hor-mone replacement therapy with con-tinuous daily oral micronized estradiol and progesterone. *Obstet Gynecol* 1989; 73: 606–12.

18. Hargrove JT, Osteen KG. An alternative method of hormone replacement therapy using the natural sex steroids. *Infert Repro Med Clin N Am* 1995; 6: 653–74.

19. Cooper A, Spencer C, Whitehead MI, et al. Systemic absorp-tion of progesterone from Progest cream in postmenopausal women. *Lancet* 1998; 351: 1255–56 [letter] and *Lancet* 1998; 352: 905–906 [comments].

20. Ottosson UB, Johansson BG, von Schoultz B. Subfractions of high-density lipoprotein cholesterol during estrogen replacement therapy: a com-parison between progestogens and natural progesterone. *Am J Obstet Gynecol* 1985; 151: 746–50.

21. Hargrove JT, Osteen KG. An alternative method of hormone replacement therapy using the natural sex steroids. *Infert Repro Med Clin N Am* 1995; 6: 653–74.

Pyruvate

1. Stanko RT, Tietze DL, and Arch JE. Body composition, energy utilization, and nitrogen metabolism with a 4.25-MJ/d low-energy diet sup-plemented with pyruvate. *Am J Clin Nutr* 1992; 56(4): 630–35.

2. Stanko RT, Reynolds HR, Hoyson R, et al. Pyruvate supplemen-tation of a low-cholesterol, low-fat diety: Effects on plasma lipid concen-tration and body composition in hyperlipidemic patients. *Am J Clin Nutr* 1994; 59: 423–27.

3. Ivy JL, Cortez MY, Chandler RM, et al. Effects of pyruvate on the metabolism and insulin resistance of obese Zucker rats. *Am J Clin Nutr* 1994; 59: 331–37.

4. Stanko RT, Robertson RJ, Galbreath RW, et al. Enhanced leg exercise endurance with a high-carbo-hydrate diet and dihyroxyacetone and pyruvate. *J Appl Phys* 1990; 69(5): 1651–56.

5. Stanko RT, Robertson RJ, Spina RJ, et al. Enhancement of arm exercise endurance capacity with dihy-droxyacetone and pyruvate. *J Appl Phys* 1990; 68(1): 119–24.

6. Deboer LWV, Bekx PA, Han L, et al. Pyruvate enhances recovery of rat hearts after ischemia and reperfu-sion by preventing free radical genera-tion. *Am J Physiol* 1993; 265: H1571–76.

7. Cicalese L, Subbotin V, Rastellini C, et al. Acute rejection of small bowel allografts in rats: Protection afforded by pyruvate. *Trans Proc* 1996; 28(5): 2474.

8. Cicalese L, Lee K, Schraut W, et al. Pyruvate prevents ischemia-reperfusion mucosal injury of rat small intestine. *Am J Surg* 1996; 171: 97–101.

9. Stanko RT, Mullick P, Clarke MR, et al. Pyruvate inhibits growth of mammary adenocarcinoma 13762 in rats. *Cancer Res* 1994; 54: 1004–1007.

Quercetin

1. Ishikawa M, Oikawa T, Hosokawa M, et al. Enhancing effect of quercetin on 3-methylcholanthrene

carcinogenesis in C57B1/6 mice. *Neoplasma* 1985; 43: 435–41.

2. Hertog MGL, Feskens EJM, Hollman PCH, et al. Dietary flavonoids and cancer risk in the Zutphen elderly study. *Nutr Cancer* 1994; 22: 175–84.

3. Castillo MH, Perkins E, Campbell JH, et al. The effects of the bioflavonoid quercetin on squamous cell carcinoma of head and neck ori-gin. *Am J Surg* 1989; 351–55.

4. Stavric B. Quercetin in our diet: from potent mutagen to probably anticarcinogen. *Clin Biochem* 1994; 27: 245–48.

5. Barotto NN, López CB, Eyard AR, et al. Quercetin enhances pretu-mourous lesions in the NMU model of rat pancreatic carcinogenesis. *Cancer Letters* 1998; 129: 1–6.

Resveratrol

1. Bertelli AA, Giovanninni L, Bernini W, et al. Antiplatelet activity of cis-resveratrol. *Drugs Exp Clin Res* 1996; 22(2): 61–63.

2. Chen CK, Pace-Asciak CR.Vasorelaxing activity of resvera-trol and quercetin in isolated rat aorta. *Gen Pharm* 1996; 27(2): 363–66.

3. Pace-Asciak CR, Rounova O, Hahn SE, et al. Wines and grape juices as modulators of platelet aggregation in healthy human subjects. *Clin Chim Acta* 1996; 246(1–2): 163–82.

4. Jang M, Cai L, Udeani GO, et al. Cancer chemopreventive activity of resveratrol, a natural product derived from grapes. *Science* 1997; 275: 218–20.

5. Jang M, Cai L, Udeani GO, et al. Cancer chemopreventive activity of resveratrol, a natural product derived from grapes. *Science* 1997; 275: 218–20.

6. Soleas GJ, Diamandis EP, Goldberg DM. Resveratrol: A mole-cule whose time has come? And gone? *Clin Biochem* 1997; 30(2): 91–113.

Royal Jelly

1. Lakin A. Royal Jelly and its effi-cacy. *Int J Alternative Complementary Med* 1993; Oct: 19–22 [review].

2. Fujiwara S, Imai J, Fujiwara M, et al. A potent antibacterial protein

in royal jelly. Purification and determination of the primary structure of royalisin. *J Biol Chem* 1990; 265: 11333–37.

3. Fujii A, Kobayashi S, Kuboyama N, et al. Augmentation of wound healing by royal jelly (RJ) in streptozotocin-diabetic rats. *Jpn J Pharmacol* 1990; 53: 331–37.

4. Sver L, Orsolic N, Tadic Z, et al. A royal jelly as a new potential immunomodulator in rats and mice. *Comp Immunol Microbiol Infect Dis* 1996; 19: 31–38.

5. Tamura T, Fujii A, Kuboyama N. Antitumor effects of royal jelly (RJ). *Nippo Yakurigaku Z* 1987; 89: 73–80 [in Japanese].

6. Abou-Hozaifa BM, Badr El-Din NK. Royal jelly, a possible agent to reduce the nicotine-induced atherogenic lipoprotein profile. *Saudi Med J* 1995; 16: 337–42.

7. Abou-Hozaifa BM, Roston AAH, El-Nokaly FA. Effects of royal jelly and honey on serum lipids and lipoprotein cholesterol in rats fed cholesterol-enriched diet. *J Biomed Sci Ther* 1993; 9: 35–44.

8. Cho YT. Studies on royal jelly and abnormal cholesterol and triglycerides. *Am Bee J* 1977; 117: 36–39.

9. Liusov VA, Zimin IU. Experimental rational and trial of therapeutic use of bee raising product in cardiovascular diseases. *Kardiologia* 1983; 23: 105–109 [in Russian].

10. Vittek J. Effect of royal jelly on serum lipids in experimental animals and humans with atherosclerosis. *Experientia* 1995; 51: 927–35 [summary].

11. Leung R, Ho A, Chan J, et al. Royal jelly consumption and hypersensitivity in the community. *Clin Exp Allergy* 1997; 27: 333–36.

12. Thien FCK, Leung R, Baldo BA, et al. Asthma and anaphylaxis induced by royal jelly. *Clin Exp Allergy* 1996; 26: 216–22.

13. Lombardi C, Senna GE, Gatti B, et al. Allergic reactions to honey and royal jelly and their relationship with sensitization to compositae. *Allergol Immunopathol (Madr)* 1998; 26: 288–90.

14. Shaw D, Leon C, Kolev S, et al. Traditional remedies and food supplements. A 5-year toxicological study (1991–1995). *Drug Saf* 1997; 17: 342–56.

15. Yonei Y, Shibagaki K, Tsukada N, et al. Case report: haemorrhagic colitis associated with royal jelly intake. *J Gastroenterol Hepatol* 1997; 12: 495–99.

16. Fleche C, Clement MC, Zeggane S, et al. Contamination of bee products and risk for human health: situation in France. *Rev Sci Tech* 1997; 16: 609–19 [in French].

SAMe (S-adenosyl-L-methionine)

1. Chiang PK, Gordon RK, Tal J, et al. S-Adenosylmethionine and methylation. *FASEB J* 1996; 10(4): 471–80 [review].

2. Bottiglieri T, Hyland K, Reynolds EH. The clinical potential of ademetionine (S-adenosylmethionine) in neurological disorders. *Drugs* 1994; 48: 137–52 [review].

3. Fava M, Rosenbaum JF, MacLaughlin R, et al. Neuroendocrine effects of S-adenosyl-L-methionine, a novel putative antidepressant. *J Psychiatr Res* 1990; 24: 177–84.

4. Bell KM, Potkin SG, Carreon D, Plon L. S-adenosylmethionine blood levels in major depression: Changes with drug treatment. *Acta Neurol Scand* 1994; 154(suppl): 15–18.

5. Bell KM, Potkin SG, Carreon D, Plon L. S-adenosylmethionine blood levels in major depression: changes with drug treatment. *Acta Neurol Scand* 1994; 154(suppl): 15–18.

6. Bressa GM. S-adenosyl-l-methionine (SAMe) as antidepressant: Meta-analysis of clinical studies. *Acta Neurol Scand* 1994; 154(suppl): 7–14.

7. Salmaggi P, Bressa GM, Nicchia G, et al. Double-blind, placebo-controlled study of s-adenosyl-methionine in depressed post-menopausal women. *Psychotherapy & Psychosomatics* 1993; 59: 34–40.

8. Kagan BL, Sultzer DL, Rosenlicht N, et al. Oral S-adenosyl-methionine in depression: A randomized, double-blind, placebo-controlled trial. *Am J Psychiatr* 1990; 147: 591–95.

9. Fava M, Rosenbaum JF, Birnbaum R, et al. The thyrotropin-releasing hormone as a predictor of response to treatment in depressed outpatients. *Acta Psychiatr Scand* 1992; 86: 42–45.

10. De Vanna M, Rigamonti R. Oral S-adenosyl-L-methionine in depression. *Curr Ther Res* 1992; 52: 478–85.

11. Fava M, Giannelli A, Rapisarda V. Rapidity of onset of the antidepressant effect of parenteral S-adenosyl-L-methionine. *Psychiatr Res* 1995; 56: 295–97.

12. Schumacher HR. Osteoarthritis: The clinical picture, pathogenesis, and management with studies on a new therapeutic agent, S-adenosylmethionine. *Am J Med* 1987; 83(suppl 5A): 1–4 [review].

13. Harmand MF, Vilamitjana J, Maloche E, et al. Effects of S-adenosylmethionine on human articular chondrocyte differentiation: An in vitro study. *Am J Med* 1987; 83(suppl 5A): 48–54.

14. Konig H et al. Magnetic resonance tomography of finger polyarthritis: Morphology and cartilage signals after ademetionine therapy. *Aktuelle Radiol* 1995; 5: 36–40.

15. Domljan Z et al. A double-blind trial of ademetionine vs naproxen in activated gonarthrosis. *Int J Clin Pharmacol Ther Toxicol* 1989; 27: 329–33.

16. Muller-Fassbender H. Double-blind clinical trial of S-adenosylmethionine in versus ibuprofen in the treatment of osteoarthritis. *Am J Med* 1987; 83(suppl 5A): 81–83.

17. Vetter G. Double-blind comparative clinical trial with S-adenosylmethionine and indomethacin in the treatment of osteoarthritis. *Am J Med* 1987; 83(suppl 5A): 78–80.

18. Maccagno A. Double-blind controlled clinical trial of oral S-adenosylmethionine versus piroxicam in knee osteoarthritis. *Am J Med* 1987; 83(suppl 5A): 72–77.

19. Caruso I, Pietrogrande V. Italian double-blind multicenter study comparing S-adenosylmethionine, naproxen, and placebo in the treatment of degenerative joint disease. *Am J Med* 1987; 83(suppl 5A): 66–71.

20. Marcolongo R, Giordano N, Colombo B, et al. Double-blind multicentre study of the activity of s-adenosyl-methionine in hip and knee osteoarthritis. *Curr Ther Res* 1985; 37: 82–94.

21. Glorioso S, Todesco S, Mazzi A, et al. Double-blind multicentre study of the activity of S-adenosylmethionine in hip and knee osteoarthritis. *Int J Clin Pharmacol Res* 1985; 5: 39–49.

22. Montrone F, Fumagalli M, Sarzi Puttini P, et al. Double-blind study of S-adenosyl-methionine versus placebo in hip and knee arthrosis. *Clin Rheumatol* 1985; 4: 484–85.

23. Tavoni A, Jeracitano G, Cirigliano G. Evaluation of S-adenosylmethionine in secondary fibromyalgia: A double-blind study. *Clin Exp Rheumatol* 1998; 16: 106–107 [letter].

24. Tavoni A, Vitali C, Bombardieri S, et al. Evaluation of S-adenosylmethionine in primary fibromyalgia: A double-blind crossover study. *Am J Med* 1987; 83(suppl 5A): 107–10.

25. Volkmann H, Norregaard J, Jacobsen S, et al. Double-blind, placebo-controlled cross-over study of intravenous S-adenosyl-L-methionine in patients with fibromyalgia. *Scand J Rheumatol* 1997; 26: 206–11.

26. Jacobsen S, Danneskiold-Samsoe B, Andersen RB. Oral S-adenosylmethionine in primary fibromyalgia: Double-blind clinical evaluation. *Scand J Rheumatol* 1991; 20: 294–302.

27. Lieber CS. Herman Award lecture, 1993: a personal perspective on alcohol, nutrition, and the liver. *Am J Clin Nutr* 1993; 58: 430–42 [review].

28. Osman E, Owen JS, Burroughs AK. S-adenosyl-L-methionine—a new therapeutic agent in liver disease? *Aliment Pharmacol Ther* 1993; 7: 21–28 [review].

29. Angelico M et al. Oral S-adenosyl-L-methionine (SAMe) administration enhances bile salt conjugation with taurine in patients with liver cirrhosis. *Scand J Clin Lab Invest* 1994; 54: 459–64.

30. Frezza M et al. Oral S-adenosyl-methionine in the symptomatic treatment of intrahepatic cholestasis: A double-blind, placebo-controlled study. *Gastroenterology* 1990; 99: 211–15.

31. Bombardieri G et al. Effects of S-adenosyl-L-methionine (SAMe) in the treatment of Gilbert's syndrome. *Curr Ther Res* 1985; 37: 580–85.

32. Piacentino R, Malara D, Zaccheo F, et al. Preliminary study of the use of s. adenosyl methionine in the management of male sterility. *Minerva Ginecologica* 1991; 43: 191–93 [in Italian].

33. Gatto G et al. Analgesizing effect of à methyl donor (S-adenosyl-methionine) in migraine: an open clinical trial. *Int J Clin Pharmacol Res* 1986; 6: 15–17.

34. Ballerini FB, Anguera AL, Alcaraz P, et al. SAM in the management of postconcussional syndrome. *Med Clin (Barc)* 1983; 80: 161–64.

35. Bottiglieri T, Hyland K, Reynolds EH. The clinical potential of ademetionine (S-adenosylmethionine) in neurological disorders. *Drugs* 1994; 48: 137–52 [review].

36. Osman E, Owen JS, Burroughs AK. S-adenosyl-L-methionine—a new therapeutic agent in liver disease? *Aliment Pharmacol Ther* 1993; 7: 21–28 [review].

37. Loehrer FM, Angst CP, Haefeli WE, et al. Low whole-blood S-adenosylmethionine and correlation between 5-methyltetrahydrofolate and homocysteine in coronary artery disease. *Arterioscler Thromb Vasc Biol* 1996; 16: 727–33.

38. Bottiglieri T, Godfrey P, Flynn T, et al. Cerebrospinal fluid S-adenosylmethionine in depression and dementia: Effects of treatment with parenteral and oral S-adenosylmethionine. *J Neurol, Neurosurg Psychiat* 1990; 53: 1096–98.

39. Bressa GM. S-adenosyl-l-methionine (SAMe) as antidepressant: Meta-analysis of clinical studies. *Acta Neurol Scand* 1994; 154(suppl): 7–14.

40. Di Padova C. S-adenosylmethionine in the treatment of osteoarthritis: Review of the clinical studies. *Am J Med* 1987; 83(suppl 5A): 60–64.

41. Carney MWP, Chary TK, Bottiglieri T, et al. The switch mechanism and the bipolar/unipolar dichotomy. *Br J Psychiatr* 1989; 154: 48–51.

42. Carney MWP, Chary TK, Bottiglieri T, et al. Switch and S-adenosyl-methionine. *Alabama J Med Sci* 1988; 25: 316–19.

43. Cerutti R et al. Psychological distress during peurperium: A novel therapeutic approach using S-adenosyl-methionine. *Curr Ther Res* 1993; 53: 707–17.

Selenium

1. Clark LC, Combs GF, Turnbull BW, et al. Effects of selenium supplementation for cancer prevention in patients with carcinoma of the skin. *JAMA* 1996; 276: 1957–63.

2. Yoshizawa K, Willett WC, Morris SJ, et al. Study of prediagnostic selenium levels in toenails and the risk of advanced prostate cancer. *J Natl Cancer Inst* 1998; 90: 1219–24.

3. Yu S-Y, Li W-G, Zhu Y-J, et al. Chemoprevention trial of human hepatitis with selenium supplementation in China. *Biol Trace Element Res* 1989; 20: 15–20.

4. Peretz A, Néve J, Desmedt J, et al. Lymphocyte response is enhanced by supplementation of elderly subjects with selenium-enriched yeast. *Am J Clin Nutri* 1991; 53: 1323–28.

5. Scott R, Macpherson A, Yates RWS, et al. The effect of oral selenium supplementation on human sperm motility. *Br J Urol* 1998; 82: 76–80.

6. Dworkin BM. Selenium deficiency in HIV infection and the acquired immunodeficiency syndrome (AIDS). *Chem Biol Iteract* 1994; 91: 181–86.

7. Moore JA, Noiva R, Wells IC. Selenium concentrations in plasma of patients with arteriographically defined coronary atherosclerosis. *Clin Chem* 1984; 30: 1171–73.

8. Contempre B, Dumont JE, Ngo B, et al. Effects of selenium supplementation in hypothyroid subjects of an iodine and selenium deficient area: The possible danger of indiscriminate supplementation of iodine deficient subjects with selenium. *J Clin Endocrinol Metabol* 1991; 73: 213–15.

Silicon

1. Nielsen FH. How should dietary guidance be given for mineral elements with beneficial actions or suspected of being essential? *J Nutr* 1996; 126: S2377–85 [review].

Soy

1. Wei H, Bowen R, Cai Q, et al. Antioxidant and antipromotional effects of the soybean isoflavone genistein. *Proc Soc Exp Biol Med* 1995; 208: 124–29.

2. Messina MJ, Persky V, Setchell KD, Barnes S, Soy intake and cancer risk: a review of the in vitro and in vivo data. *Nutri Cancer* 1994; 21: 113–31.

3. Adlercreutz H, Markkanen H, Watanabe S. Plasma concentrations of phyto-oestrogens in Japanese men. *Lancet* 1993; 342: 1209–10.

4. Lee HP, Gourley L, Duffy SW, et al. Dietary effects on breast-cancer risk in Singapore. *Lancet* 1991; 337: 1197–200.

5. Anderson JW, Johnstone BM, Cook-Newell ME. Meta-analysis of the effects of soy protein intake on serum lipids. *New Engl J Med* 1995; 333: 276–82.

6. Potter SM. Overview of proposed mechanisms for the hypocholesterolemic effect of soy. *J Nutr* 1995; 125: 6065–115.

7. Murkies AL, Lombard C, Strauss BJ, et al. Dietary flour supplementation decreases post-menopausal hot flushes: Effect of soy and wheat. *Maturitas* 1995; 21(3): 189–95.

8. Albertazzi P, Pansini F, Bonaccorsi G, et al. The effect of dietary soy supplementation on hot flushes. *Obstet Gynecol* 1998; 91: 6–11.

9. Cassidy A, Bingham S, Setchell KDR. Biological effects of a diet of soy protein rich isoflavones on the menstrual cycle of premenopausal women. *Am J Clin Nutr* 1994; 60: 333–40.

10. Anderson JJB, Ambrose WW, Garner SC. Biphasic effects of genistein on bone tissue in the ovariectomized, lactating rat model (44243). *Proc Soc Exp Biol Med* 1998; 217: 345–50.

11. Potter SM, Baum JA, Teng H, et al. Soy protein and isoflavones: Their effects on blood lipids and bone density in postmenopausal women. *Am J Clin Nutr* 1998; 68(suppl): 1375S–79S.

12. Messina M. To recommend or not to recommend soy foods. *J Am Diet Assoc* 1994; 94: (11): 1253–54.

13. Divi RL, Chang HC, Doerge DR. Antithyroid isoflavones from soybean. *Biochem Pharmacol* 1997; 54: 1087–96.

14. Potter SM, Pertile J, Berber-Jimenez MD. Soy protein concentrate and isolated soy protein similarly lower blood serum cholesterol but differently affect thyroid hormones in hamsters. *J Nutr* 1996; 126: 2007–11.

15. Rao CV, Wang C-X, Simi B, et al. Enhancement of experimental colon cancer by genistein. *Cancer Res* 1997; 57: 3717–22.

16. Messina MJ, Persky V, Setchell KD, Barnes S. Soy intake and cancer risk: a review of the in vitro and in vivo data. *Nutri Cancer* 1994; 21: 113–31.

Spirulina (Blue-Green Algae)

1. Dillon JC, Phuc AP, Dubacq JP. Nutritional value of the alga Spirulina. *World Rev Nutr Diet* 1995; 77: 32–46.

2. Dagnelie PC, van Staveren WA, van den Berg H. Vitamin B-12 from algae appears not to be bioavailable. *Am J Clin Nutr* 1991; 53: 695–97.

3. Miranda MS, Cintra RG, Barros SB, et al. Antioxidant activity of the microalga Spirulina maxima. *Braz J Med Biol Res* 1998; 31: 1075–79 [in Spanish].

4. Ayehunie S, Belay A, Baba TW, et al. Inhibition of HIV-1 replication by an aqueous extract of Spirulina platensis (Arthrospira platensis). *J Acquir Immune Defic Syndr Hum Retrovirol* 1998; 18: 7–12.

5. Hayashi K, Hayashi T, Kojima I. A natural sulfated polysaccharide, calcium spirulan, isolated from Spirulina platensis: in vitro and ex vivo evaluation of anti-herpes simplex virus and anti-human immunodeficiency virus activities. *AIDS Res Hum Retroviruses* 1996 Oct; 12: 1463–71.

6. Mishima T, Murata J, Toyoshima M, et al. Inhibition of tumor invasion and metastasis by calcium spirulan (Ca-SP), a novel sulfated polysaccharide derived from a blue-green alga, Spirulina platensis. *Clin Exp Metastasis* 1998; 16: 541–50.

7. Chen F, Zhang Q. Inhibitive effects of spirulina on aberrant crypts in colon induced by dimethylhydrazine. *Chung Hua Yu Fang I Hsueh Tsa Chih* 1995; 29: 13–17 [in Chinese].

8. Schwartz J, Shklar G, Reid S, Trickler D. Prevention of experimental oral cancer by extracts of Spirulina-Dunaliella algae. *Nutr Cancer* 1988; 11: 127–34.

9. Schwartz J, Shklar G. Regression of experimental hamster cancer by beta carotene and algae extracts. *J Oral Maxillofac Surg* 1987; 45: 510–15.

10. Kim HM, Lee EH, Cho HH, et al. Inhibitory effect of mast cell-mediated immediate-type allergic reactions in rats by spirulina. *Biochem Pharmacol* 1998; 55: 1071–76.

11. Yang HN, Lee EH, Kim HM. Spirulina inhibits anaphylactic reaction. *Life Sci* 1997; 61: 1237–44.

12. Qureshi MA, Garlich JD, Kidd MT. Dietary Spirulina platensis enhances humoral and cell-mediated immune functions in chickens. *Immunopharmacol Immunotoxicol* 1996; 18: 465–76.

13. Qureshi MA, Ali RA. Spirulina platensis exposure enhances macrophage phagocytic function in cats. *Immunopharmacol Immunotoxicol* 1996; 18: 457–63.

14. Hayashi O, Katoh T, Okuwaki Y. Enhancement of antibody production in mice by dietary Spirulina platensis. *J Nutr Sci Vitaminol (Tokyo)* 1994; 40: 431–41.

15. Torres-Duran PV, Miranda-Zamora R, Paredes-Carbajal MC, et al. Spirulina maxima prevents

induction of fatty liver by carbon tetrachloride in the rat. *Biochem Mol Biol Int* 1998; 44: 787–93.

16. Vadiraja BB, Gaikwad NW, Madyastha KM. Hepatoprotective effect of C-phycocyanin: protection for carbon tetrachloride and R-(+)-pulegone-mediated hepatotoxicty in rats. *Biochem Biophys Res Commun* 1998; 249: 428–31.

17. Gonzalez de Rivera C, Miranda-Zamora R, Diaz-Zagoya JC, et al. Preventive effect of Spirulina maxima on the fatty liver induced by a fructose-rich diet in the rat, a preliminary report. *Life Sci* 1993; 53: 57–61.

18. Paredes-Carbajal MC, Torres-Duran PV, Diaz-Zagoya JC, et al. Effects of dietary Spirulina maxima on endothelium dependent vasomotor responses of rat aortic rings. *Life Sci* 1997; 61(15): PL 211–19.

19. Iwata K, Inayama T, Kato T. Effects of Spirulina platensis on plasma lipoprotein lipase activity in fructose-induced hyperlipidemic rats. *J Nutr Sci Vitaminol (Tokyo)* 1990; 36: 165–71.

20. Gonzalez de Rivera C, Miranda-Zamora R, Diaz-Zagoya JC, et al. Preventive effect of Spirulina maxima on the fatty liver induced by a fructose-rich diet in the rat, a preliminary report. *Life Sci* 1993; 53: 57–61.

21. Mathew B, Sankaranarayanan R, Nair PP, et al. Evaluation of chemoprevention of oral cancer with Spirulina fusiformis. *Nutr Cancer* 1995; 24: 197–202.

22. Becker EW, Jakober B, Luft D, et al. Clinical and biochemical evaluations of the alga Spirulina with regard to its application in the treatment of obesity. A double-blind crossover study. *Nutr Rep Intl* 1986; 33: 565–73.

23. Nakaya N, Homma Y, Goto Y. Cholesterol lowering effect of Spirulina. *Nutr Rep Intl* 1988; 37: 1329–37.

24. Johnson PE and Shubert LE. Accumulation of mercury and other elements by spirulina (cyanophyceae). *Nutr Rep Intl* 1986; 34(6): 1063–71.

25. Slotton DG, Goldman CR, Franke A. Commercially grown spirulina found to contain low levels of mercury and lead. *Nutr Rep Intl* 1989; 40: 1165.

26. Nakashima MJ, Angold S, Beavin BB, et al. Extraction of light filth from spirulina powders and tablets: collaborative study. *J Assoc Off Anal Chem* 1989; 72: 451–53.

27. Elder GH, Hunter PR, Codd GA. Hazardous freshwater cyanobacteria (blue-green algae). *Lancet* 1993; 341: 1519–20 [letter].

28. Salazar M, Chamorro GA, Salazar S, et al. Effect of Spirulina maxima consumption on reproduction and peri- and postnatal development in rats. *Food Chem Toxicol* 1996; 34: 353–59.

29. Kapoor R, Mehta U. Effect of supplementation of blue green alga (Spirulina) on outcome of pregnancy in rats. *Plant Foods Hum Nutr* 1993; 43: 29–35.

30. Chamorro G, Salazar M. Teratogenic study of Spirulina in mice. *Arch Latinoam Nutr* 1990; 40: 86–94 [in Spanish].

Strontium

1. Brandi ML. New treatment strategies: Ipriflavone, strontium, vitamin D metabolites and analogs. *Am J Med* 1993; 95: 69–74S [review].

2. Anttila A. Proton-induced X-ray emission analysis of Zn, Sr and Pb in human deciduous tooth enamel and its relationship to dental caries scores. *Arch Oral Biol* 1986; 31(11): 723–26.

3. Hansen DV, Holmes ER, Catton G, et al. Strontium-89 therapy for painful osseous metastatic prostate and breast cancer. *Am Family Physician* 1993; 47: 1795–1800.

4. Gaby AR. *Preventing and Reversing Osteoporosis.* Rocklin, CA: Prima Publishing, 1994, 85–92 [review].

Sulfur

1. Augusti KT. Therapeutic values of onion (Allium cepa L.) and garlic (Allium sativum L.). *Ind J Exp Biol* 1996; 34: 634–40.

2. Richmond VL. Incorporation of methylsulfonylmethane sulfur into guinea pig serum proteins. *Life Sci* 1986; 39: 263–68.

3. Sullivan MX, Hess WC. The cystine content of the finger nails in arthritis. *J Bone Joint Surg* 1935; 16: 185–88.

Taurine

1. Franconi F, Bennardini F, Mattana A, et al. Plasma and platelet taurine are reduced in subjects with insulin-dependent diabetes mellitus: effects of taurine supplementation. *Am J Clin Nutr* 1995; 61: 1115–19.

Tyrosine

1. Gelenberg AJ, Gibson CJ, Wojcik JD. Neurotransmitter precursors for the treatment of depression. *Psychopharmacol Bull* 1982; 18: 7–18.

2. Meyer JS, Welch KMA, Deshmuckh VD, et al. Neurotransmitter precursor amino acids in the treatment of multi-infarct dementia and Alzheimer's disease. *J Am Ger Soc* 1977; 7: 289–98.

3. Banderet LE, Lieberman HR. Treatment with tyrosine, a neurotransmitter precursor, reduces environmental stress in humans. *Brain Res Bull* 1989; 22: 759–62.

4. Koch R. Tyrosine supplementation for phenylketonuria treatment. *Am J Clin Nutr* 1996; 64: 974–75.

5. Chiaroni P, Azorin JM, Bovier P, et al. A multivariate analysis of red blood cell membrane transports and plasma levels of L-tyrosine and L-tryptophan in depressed patients before treatment and after clinical improvement. *Neuropsychobiol* 1990; 23: 1–7.

6. Alvestrand A, Ahlberg M, Forst P, Bergstrom J. Clinical results of long-term treatment with a low protein diet and a new amino acid preparation in patients with chronic uremia. *Clin Nephrol* 1983; 19: 67–73.

Vanadium

1. Boden G, Chen X, Ruiz J, et al. Effects of vanadyl sulfate on carbohydrate and lipid metabolism in patients with non-insulin-dependent diabetes mellitus. *Metab Clin Exp* 1996; 45(9): 1130–35.

2. Naylor GJ. Vanadium and manic depressive psychosis. *Nutr Health* 1984; 3: 79–85 [review].

3. Chakraborty A, Ghosh R, Roy K, et al. Vanadium: A modifier of drug metabolizing enzyme patterns and its critical role in cellular proliferation in transplantable murine lymphoma. *Oncology* 1995; 52: 310–14.

Vitamin A

1. Rothman KJ, Moore LL, Singer MR, et al. Teratogenicity of high vitamin A intake. *N Engl J Med* 1995; 333: 1369–73.

2. Mastroiacovo P, Mazzone T, Addis A, et al. High vitamin A intake in early pregnancy and major malformations: a multicenter prospective controlled study. *Teratology* 1999; 59: 7–11.

3. Bendich A, Langseth L. Safety of vitamin A. *Am J Clin Nutr* 1989; 49: 358–71.

4. Mejia LA, Chew F. Hematological effect of supplementing anemic children with vitamin A alone and in combination with iron. *Am J Clin Nutr* 1988; 48: 595–600.

Vitamin B₁ (Thiamine)

1. Cheraskin E, Ringsdorf WM, Medford FH, Hicks BS. The "ideal" daily vitamin B1 intake. *J Oral Med* 1978; 33: 77–79.

Vitamin B₁₂ (Cobalamin)

1. Ellis FR, Nasser S. A pilot study of vitamin B12 in the treatment of tiredness. *Br J Nutr* 1973; 30: 277–83.

2. Lapp CW, Cheney PR. The rationale for using high-dose cobalamin (vitamin B12). *CFIDS Chronicle Physicians' Forum*, 1993; Fall: 19–20.

3. Rana S, D'Amico F, Merenstein JH. Relationship of vitamin B12 deficiency with incontinence in older people. *J Am Geriatr Soc* 1998; 46: 931 [letter].

4. Houston DK, Johnson MA, Nozza RJ, et al. Age-related hearing loss, vitamin B-12, and folate in elderly women. *Am J Clin Nutr* 1999; 69: 564–71.

5. Goldberg TH. Oral vitamin B12 supplementation for elderly patients with B12 deficiency. *J Am Geriatr Soc* 1995; 43: SA73 [abstr #P258].

6. Lederle FA. Oral cobalamin for pernicious anemia—medicine's best kept secret? *JAMA* 1991; 265: 94–95 [commentary].

7. Kondo H. Haematological effects of oral cobalamin preparations on patients with megaloblastic anemia. *Acta Haematol* 1998; 99: 200–205.

8. Waif SO, Jansen CJ, Crabtree RE, et al. Oral vitamin B12 without intrinsic factor in the treatment of pernicious anemia. *Ann Intern Med* 1963; 58: 810–17.

9. Crosby WH. Oral cyanocobalamin without intrinsic factor for pernicious anemia. *Arch Intern Med* 1980; 140: 1582.

10. Kaufman W. The use of vitamin therapy to reverse certain concomitants of aging. *J Am Geriatr Soc* 1955; 3: 927–36.

11. Lindenbaum J, Rosenberg IH, Wilson PWF, et al. Prevalence of cobalamin deficiency in the Framingham elderly population. *Am J Clin Nutr* 1994; 60: 2–11.

12. Verhaeverbeke I, Mets T, Mulkens K, Vandewoulde M. Normalization of low vitamin B12 serum levels in older people by oral treatment. *J Am Geriatr Soc* 1997; 45: 124–25 [letter].

Vitamin B₂ (Riboflavin)

1. Bhat KS. Nutritional status of thiamine, riboflavin and pyridoxine in cataract patients. *Nutr Rep Internat* 1987; 36: 685–92.

2. Prchal JT, Conrad ME, Skalka HW. Association of presenile cataracts with heterozygosity for galactosaemic states and with riboflavin deficiency. *Lancet* 1978; 12–13.

3. Varma RN, Mankad VN, Phelps DD, et al. Depressed erythrocyte glutathione reductase activity in sickle cell disease. *Am J Clin Nutr* 1983; 38: 884–87.

Vitamin B₅ (Pantothenic Acid and Pantethine)

1. Fidanza A. Therapeutic action of pantothenic acid. *Int J Vit Nutr Res* 1983; suppl 24: 53–67 [review].

Vitamin B₆ (Pyridoxine)

1. Keniston RC, Nathan PA, Leklem JE, Lockwood RS. Vitamin B6, vitamin C, and carpal tunnel syndrome. *J Occup Environ Med* 1997; 39: 949–59.

2. Franzblau A, Rock CL, Werner RA, et al. The relationship of vitamin B6 status to median nerve function and carpal tunnel syndrome among active industrial workers. *J Occup Environ Med* 1996; 38: 485–91.

3. Smith GP, Rudge PJ, Peters TJ. Biochemical studies of pyridoxal and pyridoxal phosphate status and therapeutic trial of pyridoxine in patients with carpal tunnel syndrome. *Ann Neurol* 1984; 15: 104–107.

4. Gaby AR. Literature review & commentary. *Townsend Letter for Doctors* June 1990; 338–39.

5. Parry G, Bredesen DE. Sensory neuropath with low-dose pyridoxine. *Neurology* 1985; 35: 1466–68.

6. Schaumburg H, Kaplan J, Windebank A, et al. Sensory neuropathy from pyridoxine abuse. *N Engl J Med* 1983; 309(8): 445–48.

Vitamin C (Ascorbic Acid)

1. Balz F. Antioxidant vitamins and heart disease. Presented at the 60th Annual Biology Colloquium, Oregon State University, Corvallis, Oregon, February 25, 1999.

2. Hemilä H. Does vitamin C alleviate the symptoms of the common cold? A review of current evidence. *Scand J Infect Dis* 1994; 26: 1–6.

3. Taddei S, Virdis A, Ghaidoni L, et al. Vitamin C improves endotheoium-dependent vasodilation by restoring nitric oxide activity in essential hypertension. *Circulation* 1998; 97: 2222–29.

4. Chambers JC, McGregor A, Jean-Marie J, et al. Demonstration of rapid onset vascular endothelial dysfunction after hyperhomocysteinemia. An effect reversible with vitamin C therapy. *Circulation* 1999; 99: 1156–60.

5. Taylor A. Cataract: relationship between nutrition and oxidation. *J Am Coll Nutr* 1993; 12: 138–46 [review].

Part Two: References

6. Taylor A, Jacques PF, Nadler D, et al. Relationship in humans between ascorbic acid consumption and levels of total and reduced ascorbic acid in lens, aqueous humor, and plasma. *Curr Eye Res* 1991; 10: 751–59.

7. Jacques PF, Chylack LT Jr. Epidemiologic evidence of a role for the antioxidant vitamins and carotenoids in cataract prevention. *Am J Clin Nutr* 1991; 53: 352S–55S.

8. Jacques PF, Chylack LT, McGandy RB, Hartz SC. Antioxidant status in persons with and without senile cataract. *Arch Ophthalmol* 1988; 106: 337–40.

9. Robertson JM, Donner AP, Trevithick JR. Vitamin E intake and risk of cataracts in humans. *Ann NY Acad Sci* 1989; 570: 372–82.

10. Seddon JM, Christen WG, Manson JE, et al. The use of vitamin supplements and the risk of cataract among U.S. male physicians. *Am J Public Health* 1994; 84: 788–92.

11. Vincent TE, Mendiratta S, May JM. Inhibition of aldose reductase in human erythrocytes by vitamin C. *Diabetes Res Clin Pract* 1999; 43: 1–8.

12. Simon JA. Ascorbic acid and cholesterol gallstones. *Med Hypotheses* 1993; 40: 81–84.

13. Balz F. Antioxidant vitamins and heart Disease. Presented at the 60th Annual Biology Colloquium, Oregon State University, February 25, 1999.

14. Levine M, Conry-Cantilena C, Wang Y, et al. Vitamin C pharmacokinetics in healthy volunteers: evidence for a recommended dietary allowance. *Proc Natl Acad Sci U S A* 1996; 93: 3704–709.

15. Sandstead HH. Copper bioavailability and requirements. *Am J Clin Nutr* 1982; 35: 809–14 [review].

16. Finley EB, Cerklewski FL. Influence of ascorbic acid supplementation on copper status in young adult men. *Am J Clin Nutr* 1983; 37: 553–56.

17. Piesse JW. Nutritional factors in calcium containing kidney stones with particular emphasis on vitamin C. *Int Clin Nutr Rev* 1985; 5(3): 110–129 [review].

18. Ringsdorf WM, Cheraskin WM. Medical complications from ascorbic acid: a review and interpretation (part one). *J Holistic Med* 1984; 6(1): 49–63.

19. Hoffer A. Ascorbic acid and kidney stones. *Can Med Assoc J* 1985; 32: 320 [letter].

20. Wandzilak TR, D'Andre SD, Davis PA, Williams HE. Effect of high dose vitamin C on urinary oxalate levels. *J Urol* 1994; 151: 834–37.

21. Levine M. Vitamin C and optimal health. Presented at the February 25, 1999 60th Annual Biology Colloquium, Oregon State University, Corvallis, Oregon.

22. Levine M, Conry-Cantilena C, Wang Y, et al. Vitamin C pharmacokinetics in healthy volunteers: evidence for a recommended dietary allowance. *Proc Natl Acad Sci U S A* 1996; 93: 3704–709.

23. Auer BL, Auer D, Rodgers AL. Relative hyperoxaluria, crystalluria and haematuria after megadose ingestion of vitamin C. *Eur J Clin Invest* 1998; 28: 695–700.

Vitamin D

(Colecalciferol, irradiated ergosterol)

1. Hayes CE, Cantorna MT, Deluca HF. Vitamin D and multiple sclerosis. *Proc Soc Exper Biol Med* 1997; 216: 21–27 [review].

2. Labriji-Mestaghanmi H, Billaudel B, Garnier PE, Sutter BCJ. Vitamin D and pancreatic islet function. Time course for changes in insulin secretion and content during vitamin deprivation and repletion. *J Endocrine Invest* 1988; 11: 577–87.

3. Boucher BJ. Inadequate vitamin D status: does it contribute to the disorders comprising syndrome 'X'? *Br J Nutr* 1998; 79: 315–27.

4. Chapuy M-C, Preziosi P, Maamer M, et al. Prevalence of vitamin D insufficiency in an adult normal population. *Osteoporosis Int* 1997; 7: 439–43.

5. Thomas MK, Lloyd-Jones DM, Thadhani RI, et al. Hypovitaminosis D in medical inpatients. *N Engl J Med* 1998; 338: 777–83.

6. Dawson-Hughes B, Harris SS, Krall EA, et al. Rates of bone loss in postmenopausal women randomly assigned to one of two dosages of vitamin D. *Am J Clin Nutr* 1995; 61: 1140–45.

7. Lind L, Skarfors E, Berglund L, et al. Serum calcium: A new, independent prospective risk factor for myocardial infarction in middle-aged men followed for 18 years. *J Clin Epidemio* 1997; 50: 967–73.

8. Heikkinen A-M, Tuppurainen MT, Komulainen M, et al. Long-term vitamin D3 supplementation may have adverse effects on serum lipids during postmenopausal hormone replacement therapy. *Eur J Endocrinol* 1997; 137: 495–502.

9. Scragg R, Khaw K-T, Murphy S. Effect of winter oral vitamin D3 supplementation on cardiovascular risk factors in elderly adults. *Eur J Clin Nutr* 1995; 49: 640–46.

Vitamin E (Tocopherol)

1. Rimm EB, Stampfer MJ, Ascherio A, et al. Vitamin E consumption and the risk of coronary heart disease in men. *N Engl J Med* 1993; 328: 1450–56.

2. Stampfer MJ, Hennekens CH, Manson JE, et al. Vitamin E consumption and the risk of coronary heart disease in women. *N Engl J Med* 1993; 328: 1444–49.

3. Stephens NG, Parsons A, Schofield PM, et al. Randomised controlled trial of vitamin E in patients with coronary disease: Cambridge Heart Antioxidant Study (CHAOS). *Lancet* 1996; 347: 781–86.

4. Christen S, Woodall AA, Shigenaga MK, Southwell-Keely, Duncan MW, Ames BN. Gamma-tocopherol traps mutagenic electrophiles such as NO+ and complements alpha-tocopherol: physiological implications. *Proc Natl Acad Sci* 1997; 94: 3217–22.

5. Rimm E. Micronutrients, coronary heart disease and cancer: Should we all be on supplements? Presented at the 60th Annual Biology Colloquium,

Oregon State University, February 25, 1999.

Whey Protein

1. Kelly GS. Sports nutrition: a review of selected nutritional supplements for bodybuilders and strength athletes. *Alt Med Rev* 1997; 2: 184–201.

Zinc

1. Mossad SB, Macknin ML, Medendorp SV, et al. Zinc gluconate lozenges for treating the common cold. *Ann Int Med* 1996; 125: 81–88.

2. Anonymous. Zinc lozenges reduce the duration of common cold symptoms. *Nutr Rev* 1997; 55: 82–88 [review].

3. Garland ML, Hagmeyer KO. The role of zinc lozenges in treatment of the common cold. *Ann Pharmacother* 1998; 32: 93–69 [review].

4. Macknin ML, Piedmonte M, Calendine C, et al. Zinc gluconate lozenges for treating the common cold in children. A randomized controlled trial. *JAMA* 1998; 279: 1962–67.

5. Eby G. Where's the bias? *Ann Intern Med* 1998; 128: 75 [letter].

6. Garland ML, Hagmeyer KO. The role of zinc lozenges in treatment of the common cold. *Ann Pharmacother* 1998; 32: 63–69 [review].

7. Petrus EJ, Lawson KA, Bucci LR, Blum K. Randomized, double-masked, placebo-controlled clinical study of the effectiveness of zinc acetate lozenges on common cold symptoms in allergy-tested subjects. *Curr Ther Res* 1998; 59: 595–607.

8. Weismann K, Jakobsen JP, Weismann JE, et al. Zinc gluconate lozenges for common cold. A double-blind clinical trial. *Dan Med Bull* 1990; 37: 279–81.

9. Cherry FF, Sandstead HH, Rojas P, et al. Adolescent pregnancy: associations among body weight, zinc nutriture, and pregnancy outcome. *Am J Clin Nutr* 1989; 50: 945–54.

10. Goldenberg RL, Tamura T, Neggers Y, et al. The effect of zinc supplementation on pregnancy outcome. *JAMA* 1995; 274: 463–68.

11. Prasad A. Discovery of human zinc deficiency and studies in an experimental human model. *Am J Clin Nutr* 1991; 53: 403–12 [review].

12. Chandra RK. Excessive intake of zinc impairs immune responses. *JAMA* 1984; 252(11): 1443.

13. Bush AI, Pettingell WH, Multhaup G, et al. Rapid induction of Alzheimer A8 amyloid formation by zinc. *Science* 1994; 265: 1464–65.

14. Potocnik FCV, van Rensburg SJ, Park C, et al. Zinc and platelet membrane microviscosity in Alzheimer's disease. *S Afr Med J* 1997; 87: 1116–19.

15. Prasad AS. Zinc in human health: an update. *J Trace Elements Exper Med* 1998; 11: 63–87.

16. Broun ER, Greist A, Tricot G, Hoffman R. Excessive zinc ingestion—a reversible cause of sideroblastic anemia and bone marrow depression. *JAMA* 1990; 264: 1441–43.

17. Resiser S, et al. Effect of copper intake on blood cholesterol and its lipoprotein distribution in men. *Nutr Rep Internat* 1987; 36(3): 641–49.

18. Sandstead HH. Requirements and toxicity of essential trace elements, illustrated by zinc and copper. *Am J Clin Nutr* 1995; 61(suppl): 621S–24S [review].

19. Fischer PWF, Giroux A, Labbe MR. Effect of zinc supplementation on copper status in adult man. *Am J Clin Nutr* 1984; 40(4): 743–46.

20. Dawson EB, Albers J, McGanity WJ. Serum zinc changes due to iron supplementation in teenage pregnancy. *Am J Clin Nutr* 1990; 50: 848–52.

21. Crofton RW, Gvozdanovic D, Gvozdanovic S, et al. Inorganic zinc and the intestinal absorption of ferrous iron. *Am J Clin Nutr* 1989; 50: 141–44.

22. Argiratos V, Samman S. The effect of calcium carbonate and calcium citrate on the absorption of zinc in healthy female subjects. *Eur J Clin Nutr* 1994; 48: 198–204.

23. Spencer H, Norris C, Williams D. Inhibitory effects of zinc on magnesium balance and magnesium absorption in man. *J Am Coll Nutr* 1994; 13: 479–84.

24. Brumas V, Hacht B, Filella M, Berthon G. Can N-acetyl-L-cysteine affect zinc metabolisms when used as a paracetamol antidote? *Agents Actions* 1992; 36: 278–88.

Part Two: References

Part Three
Herbs

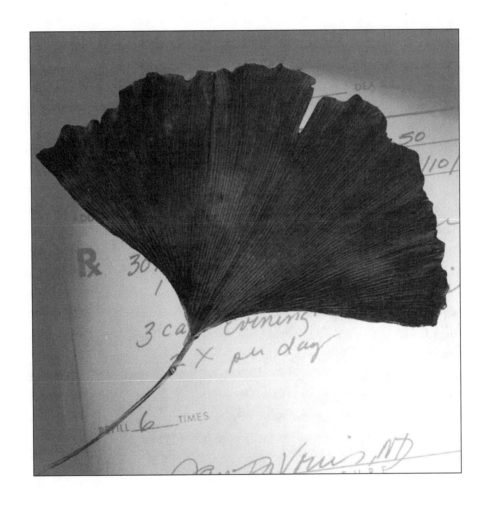

Part Three: Botanical (Latin) Names

Alfalfa
(Medicago sativa)

Parts Used and Where Grown: Alfalfa, also known as lucerne, is a member of the pea family and is native to western Asia and the eastern Mediterranean region. Alfalfa sprouts have become a popular food. Alfalfa herbal supplements primarily use the dried leaves of the plant.

In What Conditions Might Alfalfa Be Supportive?

Ranking	Health Concerns
Other	Menopause (p. 118) High cholesterol Poor appetite

Historical or Traditional Use

Early Chinese physicians used young alfalfa leaves to treat disorders of the digestive tract.[1] In India, Ayurvedic physicians prescribed the leaves and flowering tops for poor digestion. It was also considered therapeutic for **water retention** (p. 65) and arthritis. North American Indians recommended alfalfa to treat jaundice and to encourage blood clotting.

Although conspicuously absent from many classic textbooks on herbal medicine, alfalfa did find a home in the texts of the Eclectic physicians as a tonic for indigestion, dyspepsia, anemia, loss of appetite, and poor assimilation of nutrients.[2] The plant was also recommended to stimulate lactation in nursing mothers. The seeds have also been traditionally made into a poultice for the treatment of boils and insect bites.

Active Constituents

The constituents in alfalfa are well studied. The leaves contain about 2 to 3% saponins.[3] Animal studies indicate that these constituents block absorption of cholesterol and prevent the formation of atherosclerotic plaques.[4] Excess consumption of alfalfa seeds (80 to 100 grams per day) may potentially cause damage to red blood cells in the body. The leaves also contain flavones, isoflavones, sterols, and coumarin derivatives. The isoflavones are probably responsible for the estrogen-like effects in animals.[5] Although this has not been confirmed with human trials, it is used popularly to treat **menopause symptoms** (p. 118). Alfalfa contains protein and **vitamins A** (p. 336), **B₁** (p. 337), **B₆** (p. 340), **C** (p. 341), **E** (p. 344), and **K** (p. 345). Nutrient analysis demonstrates the presence of calcium (p. 277), potassium (p. 323), iron (p. 304), and zinc (p. 346).

How Much Is Usually Taken?

Dried alfalfa leaf is available as a bulk herb and in tablets or capsules. It is also available in liquid extracts. No therapeutic dose of alfalfa has been established for humans. Some experts recommend 500 to 1,000 mg of the dried leaf per day or 1 to 2 ml of tincture 3 times per day.[6]

Are There Any Side Effects or Interactions? Use of the dried leaves of alfalfa in the amounts listed above is usually safe. There have been isolated reports of persons allergic to alfalfa. Ingestion of very large amounts (the equivalent of several servings) of the seed and/or sprouts has been linked to the onset of **systemic lupus erythematosus (SLE)** (p. 115) in animal studies.[7] SLE is an autoimmune illness that is characterized by inflamed joints and potential kidney damage. The chemical responsible for this effect is believed to be canavanine. Persons with SLE or with a history of SLE should avoid the use of alfalfa products.

Aloe
(Aloe vera, Aloe barbadensis)

Parts Used and Where Grown: The aloe plant originally came from Africa. The leaves are used; they are long, green, fleshy, and have spikes along the edges. The fresh leaf gel and latex are used for many purposes. Aloe latex is the sticky residue left over after the liquid from cut aloe leaves has evaporated.

In What Conditions Might Aloe Be Supportive?

Ranking	Health Concerns
Primary	Constipation (p. 44)
Secondary	Burns (minor) (p. 29) Canker sores (mouth ulcers) (p. 30) Diabetes (p. 53) Injuries (minor) (p. 122) Wound healing (p. 167) Wound healing (topical) (p. 167)
Other	Crohn's disease (p. 48) Maintaining a healthy pancreas Ulcerative colitis (p. 158)

Historical or Traditional Use

Aloe has been historically used for many of the same conditions it is used for today—particularly constipation (p. 44) and **minor cuts and burns** (p. 122). In India, it was also used to treat intestinal infections and for suppressed menses. The root was used for **colic** (p. 40).

Active Constituents

The constituents that cause the cathartic laxative effects of aloe latex are known as anthraquinone glycosides. These molecules are split by the normal bacteria in the large intestines to form other molecules (aglycones), which exert the laxative action. Various constituents have been shown to have anti-inflammatory effects as well as to stimulate **wound healing** (p. 167).[1] Preliminary evidence also suggests an antibacterial effect.[2] Blood-sugar-lowering effects of aloe have been shown in **diabetic** (p. 53) mice[3] and confirmed in placebo-controlled human studies.[4] Aloe vera creams have been very effective in double-blind placebo-controlled studies in people with **psoriasis** (p. 147).[5] Numerous older case studies reported aloe gel applied topically could help heal radiation burns.[6] However, a large, modern, placebo-controlled study did not find aloe effective in this regard.[7] Most clinical studies suggest topical aloe gel for healing burns (p. 29). Early clinical reports suggest aloe gel may help with the healing of **ulcers** (p. 139) as well.[9]

How Much Is Usually Taken?

For constipation, a single 50 to 200 mg capsule of aloe latex can be taken each day for a maximum of 10 days.

Topically for minor burns, the stabilized aloe gel is applied to the affected area of skin 3 to 5 times per day. Treatment of more serious burns should only be done after first consulting a health-care professional. For internal use of aloe gel, 30 ml 3 times per day is used by some people for inflammatory bowel conditions such as **ulcerative colitis** (p. 158).

Are There Any Side Effects or Interactions?
Except in the rare person who is allergic to aloe, topical application of the gel is harmless. For any burn that blisters significantly or is otherwise severe, medical attention is absolutely essential. In some severe burns and wounds, aloe gel may actually impede healing.[10]

The latex form of aloe should not be used by anyone with intestinal diseases such as **Crohn's disease** (p. 48) or appendicitis. It should also not be used by children or by women during pregnancy.[11]

Laxative preparations, if used for more than 10 consecutive days, can aggravate constipation and cause dependency. Constipation that doesn't resolve within a few days of using laxatives may require medical attention.

Long-term use of latex aloe could result in a **potassium** (p. 323) deficiency.[12]

American Ginseng
(Panax quinquefolius)

Parts Used and Where Grown: Like its more familiar cousin, **Asian ginseng** *(Panax ginseng)* (p. 394), the root of American ginseng is used medicinally. The plant grows wild in shady forests of northern and central United States, as well as in parts of Canada. It is cultivated in the United States, China, and France.

In What Conditions Might American Ginseng Be Supportive?

Ranking	Health Concerns
Secondary	Athletic performance (p. 20)
Other	Infection (p. 63) Stress

Historical or Traditional Use

Many Native American tribes used American ginseng. Medicinal uses ranged from digestive disorders to sexual problems.[1] The Chinese began to use American ginseng after it was imported during the 1700s.[2] The traditional applications in China are significantly different from those for *Panax ginseng* (Asian ginseng). American ginseng is considered superior for gastrointestinal problems.[3]

Active Constituents

American ginseng contains ginsenosides, which stimulate the **immune system** (p. 94)[4] and fight fatigue and stress by supporting the adrenal glands and the use of oxygen by exercising muscles.[5] The type and ratio of ginsenosides are somewhat different in American and Asian ginseng. However, the extent to which this affects their medicinal properties is unclear. A recent study of healthy volunteers found no benefit in exercise performance after one week of taking American ginseng.[6] This study might have been too short to determine definitive results. Additional clinical trials are needed to determine American ginseng's medical uses. Refer to **Asian ginseng** (p. 394) for more information.

How Much Is Usually Taken?

Standardized extracts of American ginseng, unlike Asian ginseng, are not generally available. American ginseng can be taken in the amount of 1 to 2 grams

American Ginseng

per day in capsule or tablet form[7] or 3 to 5 ml of tincture 3 times per day.

Are There Any Side Effects or Interactions? Occasional cases of insomnia or agitation are reported with American ginseng use; these conditions are more likely when caffeine-containing foods and beverages are also being consumed.[8] Reducing intake of American ginseng or avoiding it later in the day can lessen the chances for adverse effects.

Artichoke
(Cynara scolymus)

Parts Used and Where Grown: This large thistle-like plant is native to the regions of southern Europe, North Africa, and the Canary Islands. The leaves of the plant are used medicinally; the roots and the immature flower heads may also contain beneficial compounds.[1]

In What Conditions Might Artichoke Be Supportive?

Ranking	Health Concerns
Primary	High cholesterol (p. 79)
Secondary	Indigestion (digestive aid) (p. 99) Liver protection
Other	Gallstones (p. 69)

Historical or Traditional Use

The artichoke is one of the world's oldest medicinal plants. The ancient Egyptians placed great value on the plant, as it is clearly seen in drawings involving fertility and sacrifice. Moreover, this plant was used by the ancient Greeks and Romans as a digestive aid. In sixteenth-century Europe, the artichoke was favored as a food by royalty.[2]

Active Constituents

Artichoke leaves contain a wide number of active constituents, including cynarin, 1,3-dicaffeoylquinic acid, 3-caffeoylquinic acid, and scolymoside.[3] The choloretic (bile-stimulating) action of the plant has been well documented in a placebo-controlled trial involving twenty healthy volunteers. After the administration of 1.92 grams of standardized artichoke extract, liver bile flow increased by 127.3% and 151.5% at the 30- and 60-minute mark, respectively.[4]

The plant has also been employed therapeutically in the treatment of elevated lipid levels, although with mixed results. For example, a research study in the late 1970s using cynarin at the 250 mg or 750 mg daily dose concluded that it did not alter **cholesterol** (p. 79) and **triglyceride** (p. 85) levels in people with familial high cholesterol, after 3 months of therapy.[5] In contrast, however, a recent European study suggests that artichoke is efficacious in altering lipid values. After using a standardized artichoke extract (320 mg/capsule) at a dose of 1 to 2 capsules 2 to 3 times per day for 6 weeks, total cholesterol and triglyceride values decreased significantly by an average of 12.78% and 8.79%, respectively. HDL-cholesterol levels did not rise significantly.[6]

While scientists are not certain how artichoke leaves lower cholesterol, test tube studies have suggested that the action may be due to an inhibition of cholesterol synthesis and/or the increased elimination of cholesterol because of the plant's choloretic action.[7] In test tube studies, the flavonoids from the artichoke (luteolin, for example) have been shown to prevent LDL-cholesterol oxidation.[8] Moreover, artichoke leaves may be liver protective, as test tube results have demonstrated its effectiveness against carbon tetrachloride induced toxicity.[9]

How Much Is Usually Taken?

Suggested adult dose of the standardized leaf extract is 320 mg 4 to 6 times daily for a minimum of 6 weeks.[10] Alternatively, if a standardized extract is not available, the crude dose of the leaves is 1 to 4 grams 3 times per day.[11]

Are There Any Side Effects or Interactions? At the recommended dose, and according to the German Commission E Monographs,[12] there are no known side effects or drug interactions. However, they also state that the use of artichoke is contraindicated in those who are allergic to artichokes and other members of the Compositae family (daisy, for example). In addition, those who have any obstruction of the bile duct (for example, as a result of **gallstones** [p. 69]) should not employ this plant therapeutically. There have been reports of kidney failure and/or toxicity from the use of artichoke leaves.[13] The plant's safety during pregnancy and lactation has not been established.

Ashwagandha
(Withania somnifera)

Parts Used and Where Grown: Ashwagandha, which belongs to the pepper family, is found in India and Africa. The roots of ashwagandha are used medicinally.

In What Conditions Might Ashwagandha Be Supportive?

Ranking	Nutritional Supplements
Secondary	Immune function (p. 94)
Other	Alzheimer's disease (p. 11) HIV support (p. 87) Infection (p. 101) Mental function Stress

Historical or Traditional Use

The health applications for ashwagandha in traditional Indian and Ayurvedic medicine are extensive. Of particular note is its use against tumors, inflammation (including arthritis), and a wide range of infectious diseases.[1] The shoots and seeds are also used as food and to thicken milk in India. Traditional uses of ashwagandha among tribal peoples in Africa include fevers and inflammatory conditions.[2] Ashwagandha is frequently a constituent of Ayurvedic formulas, including a relatively common one known as shilajit.

Active Constituents

Compounds known as withanolides are believed to account for the multiple medicinal applications of ashwagandha.[3] These molecules are steroidal and bear a resemblance, both in their action and appearance, to the active constituents of **Asian ginseng** (*Panax ginseng*) (p. 394) known as ginsenosides. Indeed, ashwagandha has been called "Indian ginseng" by some. Ashwagandha stimulates the activation of immune system cells, such as lymphocytes.[4] It has also been shown to inhibit inflammation[5] and improve memory.[6] Taken together, these actions support the traditional reputation of ashwagandha as a tonic or adaptogen[7]—an herb with multiple, nonspecific actions that counteract the effects of stress and generally promote wellness.

How Much Is Usually Taken?

Some experts recommend 1 to 2 grams of the whole herb, taken each day in capsule or tea form. To prepare a tea, 3 to 6 grams of ashwagandha roots are boiled for 15 minutes and cooled; 3 cups (750 ml) may be drunk daily. Tincture or fluid extracts can be used in the amount of 2 to 4 ml 3 times per day.

Are There Any Side Effects or Interactions? No significant side effects have been reported with ashwagandha. The herb has been used safely by children in India. Its safety during pregnancy and lactation are unknown.

Asian Ginseng
(Panax ginseng)

Common names: Korean ginseng, Chinese ginseng

Parts Used and Where Grown: Asian ginseng is a member of the Araliaceae family, which also includes the closely related **American ginseng**, *Panax quinquefolius* (p. 392), and less similar Siberian ginseng, *Eleutherococcus senticosus*, also known as **eleuthero** (p. 418). Asian ginseng commonly grows on mountain slopes and is usually harvested in the fall. The root is used, preferably from plants older than 6 years of age.

In What Conditions Might Asian Ginseng Be Supportive?

Ranking	Health Concerns
Primary	Diabetes (p. 53) Immune function (p. 94)
Secondary	Athletic performance (p. 20) Impotence (p. 98)
Other	Aerobic capacity Alzheimer's disease (p. 11) Common cold/sore throat (p. 41) Fibromyalgia (p. 68) HIV support (p. 87) Infection (p. 101) Influenza (flu) (p. 104) Stress

Historical or Traditional Use

Asian ginseng has been a part of Chinese medicine for over 2,000 years. The first reference to the health-enhancing use of Asian ginseng dates to the first century A.D., in which the writer mentions ginseng's use as follows: "It is used for repairing the five viscera, quieting the spirit, curbing the emotion, stopping agitation, removing noxious influence, brightening the eyes, enlightening the mind and increasing wisdom. Continuous use leads one to longevity with light weight." Ginseng was commonly used by elderly persons in the Orient to improve mental and physical vitality.

Active Constituents

Ginseng's actions in the body are due to a complex interplay of constituents. The primary group are the ginsenosides, which are believed to increase energy, counter the effects of stress, and enhance intellectual and physical performance. Thirteen ginsenosides have been identified in Asian ginseng. Ginsenosides Rg1 and Rb1 have received the most attention.[1] Other constituents include the panaxans, which help lower blood sugar, and the polysaccharides (complex sugar molecules), which support **immune function** (p. 94).[2,3]

Long-term intake may be linked to a reduced risk of cancer.[4] A double-blind study has confirmed Asian ginseng's blood-sugar-lowering effects in people with adult **diabetes** (p. 53).[5] Human studies have mostly failed to confirm the purported benefit of Asian ginseng for the enhancement of **athletic performance** (p. 20).[6] Some studies suggest it may help those in poor physical condition tolerate exercise better.[7] It does appear to effectively reduce fatigue in double-blind studies.[8] A double-blind study has confirmed it is helpful for relief of fatigue and possible stress.[9]

How Much Is Usually Taken?

The best researched form of ginseng is standardized herbal extracts that supply approximately 5 to 7% ginsenosides; more concentrated extracts may be less effective due to reduction of panaxan levels.[10] People often take 100 to 200 mg per day. Nonstandardized extracts require a higher intake, generally 1 to 2 grams per day for tablets, or 2 to 3 ml for dried root tincture 3 times per day. Ginseng is usually used for 2 to 3 weeks continuously, followed by a 1- to 2-week "rest" period before resuming.

Are There Any Side Effects or Interactions? Used in the recommended amounts, ginseng is generally safe. In rare instances, it may cause overstimulation and possibly insomnia.[11] Consuming caffeine with ginseng increases the risk of overstimulation and gastrointestinal upset. Persons with uncontrolled high blood pressure should not use ginseng. Long-term use of ginseng may cause menstrual abnormalities and breast tenderness in some women. Ginseng is not recommended for pregnant or lactating women.

Astragalus
(Astragalus membranaceus)

Common name: Huang qi
Parts Used and Where Grown: Astragalus is native to northern China and the elevated regions of the Chinese provinces Yunnan and Sichuan. The portion of the plant used medicinally is the 4- to 7-year-old dried root collected in the spring. While over 2,000 types of astragalus exist worldwide, the Chinese ver-

sion has been extensively tested, both chemically and pharmacologically.[1]

In What Conditions Might Astragalus Be Supportive?

Ranking	Health Concerns
Other	Alzheimer's disease (p. 11) Common cold/sore throat (p. 41) Immune function (p. 94) Infection (p. 101)

Historical or Traditional Use

Shen Nung, the founder of Chinese herbal medicine, classified astragalus as a superior herb in his classical treatise *Shen Nung Pen Tsao Ching* (circa A.D. 100). The Chinese name *huang qi* translates as "yellow leader," referring to the yellow color of the root and its status as one of the most important tonic herbs. Traditional Chinese medicine used this herb for night sweats, deficiency of chi (for example: fatigue, weakness, and loss of appetite), and diarrhea.[2]

Active Constituents

Astragalus contains numerous components, including flavonoids, polysaccharides, triterpene glycosides (such as astragalosides I to VII), amino acids, and trace minerals.[3] Preliminary test tube studies show that astragalus may help restore some **immune** (p. 94) activity in people with cancer.[4] It has shown efficacy as a diuretic and treatment for **congestive heart syndrome** (p. 43) in animal studies.[5]

How Much Is Usually Taken?

Textbooks on Chinese herbs recommend taking 9 to 15 grams of the crude herb per day in decoction form.[6] A decoction is made by boiling the root in water for a few minutes and then brewing the tea. Supplements typically contain 500 mg of astragalus. Two to three tablets or capsules or 3 to 5 ml of tincture 3 times per day are often recommended.

Are There Any Side Effects or Interactions? Astragalus has no known side effects when used as recommended.

Barberry
(Berberis vulgaris)

Parts Used and Where Grown: The root and stem bark contain the medicinally active components of barberry. The barberry bush also produces small red

Barberry

berries. Although this particular species is native to Europe, it now also grows throughout North America. A closely related species, **Oregon grape** (*Berberis aquifolium*) (p. 449), is native to North America.

In What Conditions Might Barberry Be Supportive?

Ranking	Health Concerns
Secondary	Bronchitis Diarrhea (berberine) (p. 58)
Other	Gallstones (p. 69) Gastritis (p. 71) Indigestion (p. 99) Psoriasis (p. 147) Vaginitis (p. 162)

Historical or Traditional Use

Traditionally, in European and American herbalism, barberry was used to treat a large number of conditions, particularly infections and stomach problems.[1] It has also been used internally to treat skin conditions.

Active Constituents

The alkaloid berberine receives the most research and widest acclaim as the active component of barberry and its relatives. Berberine is also a key constituent of **goldenseal** *(Hydrastis canadensis)* (p. 429). Berberine and its cousins (such as oxyacanthine) are antibacterial[2] and also kill amoeba in test tubes.[3] Berberine inhibits bacteria from attaching to human cells, which helps prevent an infection from occurring.[4] This compound treats **diarrhea** (p. 58) caused by bacteria, such as *E. coli*.[5] Berberine also stimulates some **immune system cells** (p. 94) to function better.[6] Berbamine is another alkaloid found in barberry. It helps reduce inflammation[7] and is an **antioxidant** (p. 266).[8]

The bitter compounds in barberry, including the alkaloids mentioned above, stimulate digestive function following meals.

How Much Is Usually Taken?

For digestive conditions, barberry is often combined with other bitter herbs, such as **gentian** (p. 426), in tincture form. Such mixtures are taken 15 to 20 minutes before a meal, usually 2 to 5 ml each time. As a tincture, 2 to 3 ml of barberry can be taken 3 times per day. Standardized extracts containing 5 to 10% alkaloids are preferable for preventing infections; with a total of approximately 500 mg of berberine

taken each day. Standardized extracts of **goldenseal** (p. 429) are a more common source of berberine, since it contains a higher concentration of this compound compared to barberry. An ointment made from a 10% extract of barberry can be applied topically 3 times per day. A tea/infusion can be prepared using 2 grams of the herb in a cup of boiling water. This can be repeated 2 to 3 times daily.[10]

Are There Any Side Effects or Interactions? Berberine alone has been reported to interfere with normal bilirubin metabolism in infants, raising a concern that it might worsen jaundice.[11] For this reason, berberine-containing plants, including barberry and goldenseal, should be used with caution in pregnancy and breastfeeding. Strong standardized extracts may cause stomach upset and should be used for no more than 2 weeks continuously. Other symptoms of excessive berberine intake include lethargy, nosebleed, skin and eye irritation, and kidney irritation.[12]

Bilberry
(Vaccinium myrtillus)

Parts Used and Where Grown: A close relative of **American blueberry** (p. 401), bilberry grows in northern Europe, Canada, and the United States. The ripe berries are used. The leaves may also contain beneficial compounds.

In What Conditions Might Bilberry Be Supportive?

Ranking	Health Concerns
Secondary	Diabetes (p. 53) Macular degeneration (p. 118) Retinopathy (p. 150)
Other	Atherosclerosis (p. 17) Diarrhea (p. 58) Cataracts (p. 34) Night blindness (p. 129) Varicose veins (p. 163)

Historical or Traditional Use

The dried berries and leaves of bilberry have been recommended for a wide variety of conditions, including scurvy, urinary tract infections, and kidney stones. Perhaps the most sound historical application is the use of the dried berries to treat **diarrhea** (p. 56). Modern research of bilberry was partly based on its use by British World War II pilots, who noticed that their night vision improved when they ate bilberry jam prior to night bombing raids.

Bilberry

Active Constituents

Anthocyanosides, the **bioflavonoid** (p. 271) complex in bilberries, are potent **antioxidants** (p. 267).[1] They support normal formation of connective tissue and strengthen capillaries in the body. Anthocyanosides may also improve capillary and venous blood flow. Preliminary human studies conducted in Europe show that bilberry may prevent **cataracts** (p. 34),[2] and even treat mild retinopathies (for example, **macular degeneration** [p. 118] and **diabetic retinopathy** [p. 150]).[3] Bilberry may also prevent blood vessel thickening due to **diabetes** (p. 53).[4]

Bilberry protects cholesterol from oxidizing in test tubes.[5] This may be part of how it helps people with **atherosclerosis** (p. 17).

How Much Is Usually Taken?

Bilberry herbal extract in capsules or tablets standardized to provide 25% anthocyanosides can be taken in the amount of 240 to 600 mg per day.[6] Traditional use is 1 to 2 ml 2 times per day in tincture form or 20 to 60 grams of the fruit daily.

Are There Any Side Effects or Interactions? In recommended amounts, side effects have been reported with bilberry extract. Bilberry is not contraindicated during pregnancy or lactation.

Bitter Melon
(Momordica charantia)

Parts Used and Where Grown: Bitter melon grows in tropical areas, including parts of East Africa, Asia, the Caribbean, and South America, where it is used as a food as well as a medicine. The fruit of this plant lives up to its name—it tastes very bitter. Although the seeds, leaves, and vines of bitter melon have all been used, the fruit is the safest and most prevalent part of the plant used medicinally.

In What Conditions Might Bitter Melon Be Supportive?

Ranking	Health Concerns
Secondary	Diabetes (p. 53)
Other	HIV support (p. 87)

Historical or Traditional Use

Being a relatively common food item, bitter melon was traditionally used for an array of conditions by people in tropical regions. Numerous infections, can-cer, and diabetes are among the most common conditions it was purported to improve.[1] The leaves and fruit have both been used occasionally to make teas and beer or to season soups in the Western world. The berries also produce wax, which can be made into candles.

Active Constituents

At least three different groups of constituents in bitter melon have been reported to have hypoglycemic (blood-sugar-lowering) actions of potential benefit in **diabetes mellitus** (p. 53). These include a mixture of steroidal saponins known as charantin, insulin-like peptides, and alkaloids. It is still unclear which of these is most effective, or if all three work together. Multiple controlled clinical studies have confirmed the benefit of bitter melon for people with diabetes.[2]

Two proteins, known as alpha- and beta-momor-charin, inhibit the **AIDS virus** (p. 87); however, this research has only been demonstrated in test tubes and not in humans.[3]

How Much Is Usually Taken?

For those with a taste or tolerance for bitter flavor, a small melon can be eaten as food, or up to 100 ml of a decoction or 2 ounces of fresh juice can be drunk per day.[4] Though still bitter, tinctures of bitter melon (5 ml 2 to 3 times per day) are also sometimes used.

Are There Any Side Effects or Interactions? Ingestion of excessive amounts of bitter melon juice (several times more than the amount recommended above) can cause abdominal pain and diarrhea.[5] Small children and anyone with hypoglycemia (low blood sugar) should not take bitter melon, because this herb could theoretically trigger or worsen the problem.

Black Cohosh
(Cimicifuga racemosa)

Parts Used and Where Grown: Black cohosh is a shrub-like plant native to the eastern deciduous forests of North America, ranging from southern Ontario to Georgia, north to Wisconsin and west to Arkansas. The dried root and rhizome are used medicinally.[1] When wild-harvested, the root is black in color. Cohosh, an Algonquin Indian word meaning "rough," refers to its gnarly root structure.[2]

Historical or Traditional Use

Native Americans valued the herb, using it for many conditions, ranging from gynecological problems to rattlesnake bites. Some nineteenth-century American physicians used black cohosh for fever, menstrual cramps, arthritis, and insomnia.[3]

In What Conditions Might Black Cohosh Be Supportive?

Ranking	Health Concerns
Primary	Menopause (p. 118)
Other	Menstruation, painful (dysmenorrhea) (p. 61) Osteoporosis (p. 133) Uterine spasms

Active Constituents

Black cohosh contains several important ingredients, including triterpene glycosides (e.g., acetin and cimicifugoside) and isoflavones (e.g., formononetin). Other constituents include aromatic acids, tannins, resins, fatty acids, starches, and sugars. Formononetin is a constituent in the herb that has been shown to bind to estrogen receptor sites in test tube studies. As a woman approaches **menopause** (p. 118), the signals between the ovaries and pituitary gland diminish, slowing down estrogen production and increasing luteinizing hormone (LH) secretions. Hot flashes can result from these hormonal changes. Clinical studies from Germany have demonstrated that an extract of black cohosh decreases LH secretions in menopausal women.[4] Black cohosh is therefore reserved for the symptomatic treatment of hot flashes associated with menopause. However, an estrogenic action has not been conclusively demonstrated in humans.

A recent study suggests black cohosh may protect animals from **osteoporosis** (p. 133).[5] Human studies have not confirmed this action.

How Much Is Usually Taken?

Black cohosh can be taken in several forms, including crude dried root or rhizome (300 to 2,000 mg per day) or as a solid dry powdered extract (250 mg 3 times per day). Standardized extracts of the herb are available. The recommended amount is 20 to 40 mg twice per day.[6] The best researched form provides 1 mg of deoxyactein per 20 mg of extract. Tinctures can be taken at 2 to 4 ml 3 times per day.[7] Black cohosh can be taken for up to 6 months, and then it should be discontinued.[8]

Are There Any Side Effects or Interactions? Black cohosh should not be used by pregnant or lactating women.[9] Very large amounts (over several grams daily) of this herb may cause abdominal pain, nausea, headaches, and dizziness. Women taking estrogen

therapy should consult a physician knowledgeable about herbs before using black cohosh. Black cohosh is not a substitute for hormone replacement therapy during menopause.

Blackberry
(Rubus fructicosus)

Common names: Dewberry, European blackberry
Parts Used and Where Grown: Blackberry leaf is more commonly used, but blackberry root also has medicinal value. Blackberries grow in wet areas across the United States and Europe. Several species of blackberry exist; some are native to the Americas and others are native to Europe. *Rubus fructicosus* is the most common European species and *Rubus canadensis* is a common North American species.

In What Conditions Might Blackberry Be Supportive?

Ranking	Health Concerns
Other	Common cold/sore throat (p. 41) Diarrhea (p. 58)

Historical or Traditional Use

Since ancient Greek physicians prescribed blackberry for gout, the leaves, roots, and even berries have been used as herbal medicines.[1] The most common uses were for treating diarrhea, sore throats, and wounds. These are similar to the uses of its close cousin, the **raspberry** (*Rubus idaeus*) (p. 454), and a somewhat more distant relative, the **blueberry** (*Vaccinium corymbosum*) (p. 401).

Active Constituents

The presence of large amounts of tannins give blackberry roots and leaves an astringent effect that is useful for treating **diarrhea** (p. 58).[2] These same constituents are also helpful for soothing **sore throats** (p. 41).

How Much Is Usually Taken?

The German Commission E monograph recommends 4.5 grams of blackberry leaf per day.[3] Blackberry tea is prepared by adding 10 to 15 ml of leaves or powdered root to 250 ml of boiling water and allowing it to steep for 10 to 15 minutes. Three or more cups per day should be drunk. Use 3 to 4 ml of tincture 3 times each day, or more for a more acute diarrhea problem.

Blackberry

Are There Any Side Effects or Interactions?
Tannins can cause nausea and even vomiting in people with sensitive stomachs. Individuals with chronic gastrointestinal problems might be particularly at risk for such reactions.

Blessed Thistle
(Cnicus benedictus)

Parts Used and Where Grown: Although native to Europe and Asia, blessed thistle is now cultivated in many areas of the world, including the United States. The leaves, stems, and flowers are all used in herbal preparations.

In What Conditions Might Blessed Thistle Be Supportive?

Ranking	Health Concerns
Other	Indigestion and heartburn (p. 99) Poor appetite

Historical or Traditional Use

Folk medicine used blessed thistle tea for digestive problems, including gas, constipation, and stomach upset. This herb was also used for liver and gallbladder diseases, in a similar way as its well-known relative **milk thistle** (p. 445).[1]

Active Constituents

The sesquiterpene lactones, such as cnicin, provide the main beneficial effects on digestion of blessed thistle. The bitterness of these compounds stimulates digestive activity, including the flow of saliva and secretion of gastric juice, which leads to improved appetite and digestion.[2] Some evidence indicates that blessed thistle also has anti-inflammatory properties.

How Much Is Usually Taken?

The German Commission E monograph recommends 4 to 6 grams of blessed thistle per day.[3] Some herbalists suggest 2 ml 3 times per day of blessed thistle tincture. Approximately 2 grams of the dried herb can also be added to 250 ml (1 cup) of boiling water and steeped 10 to 15 minutes to make a tea. Three cups can be drunk each day.

Are There Any Side Effects or Interactions?
Blessed thistle is generally safe and free from side effects. Anyone with allergies to plants in the daisy family should use blessed thistle cautiously.

Bloodroot
(Sanguinaria canadensis)

Parts Used and Where Grown: True to its name, bloodroot has a bright red root (technically, the red-colored underground part of this plant is the rhizome). A red dye is derived from bloodroot. The plant grows primarily in North America and also in India.

In What Conditions Might Bloodroot Be Supportive?

Ranking	Health Concerns
Secondary	Gingivitis (periodontal disease) (p. 73)
Other	Cough (p. 47)

Historical or Traditional Use

Native Americans employed bloodroot extensively in ritual and medicine. The dye was used as a body paint.[1] Sore throats, cough, rheumatic pains, and various types of cancer were all treated with bloodroot.

Active Constituents

Alkaloids—principally sanguinarine—constitute the primary active compounds in bloodroot. These are sometimes used in toothpaste and other oral hygiene products because they inhibit oral bacteria.[2,3] Test tube studies have shown a range of anticancer effects for bloodroot alkaloids; however, their safety and effectiveness remain unclear.

How Much Is Usually Taken?

Sanguinarine-containing toothpastes and mouth rinses can be used in the same way as other oral hygiene products. Bloodroot tincture is sometimes included in cough-relieving formulas, taken 3 times per day. However, bloodroot is rarely used alone for this purpose.

Are There Any Side Effects or Interactions? Long-term use of dental products containing sanguinarine is believed to be safe.[4] Only small amounts of bloodroot should be taken internally, since this herb can cause visual changes, stomach pain, vomiting, paralysis, fainting, and collapse. Long-term oral intake of bloodroot has been linked to glaucoma. Bloodroot is unsafe for use in children, as well as during pregnancy and lactation.

Bloodroot

Blue Cohosh
(Caulophyllum thalictroides)

Parts Used and Where Grown: The roots of this flower are used medicinally. Blue cohosh grows throughout North America. Blue cohosh is not related to **black cohosh** *(Cimicifuga racemosa)* (p. 397); however, both herbs are primarily used to treat women's health problems.

In What Conditions Might Blue Cohosh Be Supportive?

Ranking	Health Concerns
Other	Amenorrhea (lack of menstruation) Menstruation, painful (dysmenorrhea) (p. 61)

Historical or Traditional Use

Native Americans are believed to have used blue cohosh flowers to induce labor and menstruation.[1] Turn-of-the-century physicians in the United States who treated with natural remedies (known as Eclectic physicians) used blue cohosh for these same purposes and also to treat kidney infections, arthritis, and other ailments.

Active Constituents

A saponin from blue cohosh called caulosaponin is believed to stimulate uterine contractions.[2] Several other alkaloids may be active in this herb; however, current research about the active constituents of blue cohosh is insufficient.

How Much Is Usually Taken?

Blue cohosh is generally taken as a tincture and should be limited to no more than 1 to 2 ml taken 3 times per day. The average single amount of the whole herb is 300 to 1,000 mg.[3] Blue cohosh is generally used in combination with other herbs.

Are There Any Side Effects or Interactions? Large amounts of blue cohosh can cause nausea, headaches, and high blood pressure. Blue cohosh should only be used under medical supervision and in limited amounts. Use during pregnancy has been brought into question with a recent report of an infant born with congestive heart failure following use of blue cohosh by the mother.[4]

Blue Flag
(Iris versicolor)

Parts Used and Where Grown: The rhizome, or underground stem, of the aptly named blue flag (indi-cating its showy blue flowers) is used medicinally. Blue flag and closely related species (particularly *Iris missouriensis*, western blue flag) grow across North America.

In What Conditions Might Blue Flag Be Supportive?

Ranking	Health Concerns
Other	Impetigo (topical) Infections (p. 101) Malabsorption

Historical or Traditional Use

Based on Native American traditions, Eclectic physicians (turn-of-the-century doctors who relied on herbs) and herbalists used blue flag for a number of conditions. Of note was its use as a nonspecific **immune enhancer** (p. 94), as a cathartic, and to detoxify the intestinal tract.[1] In modern times, topical application of fresh, sliced rhizomes to the sores of impetigo (a common bacterial skin infection in children) has been recommended.[2] Blue flag is said to be a strong stimulant of bile production, and it has occasionally been used to stimulate the thyroid gland. Western blue flag is said to be more effective than blue flag.

Active Constituents

The resinous fraction of blue flag contains numerous phenolic glycosides. These appear to stimulate the parasympathetic nervous system, leading to production of bile, saliva, and sweat.[3] Modern research has not been conducted on blue flag or western blue flag.

How Much Is Usually Taken?

At most 10 drops of tincture of the dried rhizome should be taken 3 times per day.[4] The tea form is unlikely to be effective, since the active compounds in blue flag are not water soluble.

Are There Any Side Effects or Interactions? Blue flag, in excessive amounts, can cause nausea, vomiting, and loose stools.[5] People should not exceed the recommended amount given above. Fresh rhizome should only be applied topically and never taken internally, since it can irritate the mouth[6] and is much more likely to cause nausea and diarrhea. Blue flag should only be taken on the advice of a physician or herbalist trained in its use. Blue flag is unsafe for use during pregnancy or lactation. People should not give blue flag to children. Use of blue flag as a cathartic laxative is not recommended.

Blue Cohosh

Blueberry

(Vaccinium spp.)

Common name: Huckleberry

Parts Used and Where Grown: Blueberry leaves are the primary part of the plant used medicinally; however, the berries are occasionally used. Blueberry is related to the European **bilberry** *(Vaccinium myrtillus)* (p. 396). Several species of blueberries exist—including *V. globulare* and *V. corymbosum*—and grow throughout the United States.

In What Conditions Might Blueberry Be Supportive?

Ranking	Health Concerns
Other	Common cold/sore throat (p. 41) Diarrhea (p. 58)

Historical or Traditional Use

A tea made from blueberry leaves was traditionally considered helpful in diabetes, urinary tract infections, and poor appetite.[1] The berries were a prized commodity among the indigenous peoples of North America.

Active Constituents

Tannins make up as much as 10% of blueberry leaves. The astringent nature of tannins probably accounts for the usefulness of blueberry leaf in treating **diarrhea** (p. 58).[2] The astringent effect may also be soothing for sore throats.[3] The berries and leaves also contain anthocyanosides, which protect blood vessels.[4] Bilberry, blueberry's European cousin, is used primarily for maintaining blood vessels, particularly those in the eyes. Some preliminary evidence indicates that anthocyanosides may help people with **diabetes** (p. 53), particularly if they have damage to the retina (retinopathy). However, these studies are primarily based on a standardized extract from bilberry fruit.[5]

How Much Is Usually Taken?

A tea is prepared by combining 250 ml (1 cup) boiling water and 1 to 2 U.S. teaspoons (5 to 10 grams) of dried leaves and steeping for 15 minutes. As many as 6 cups each day may be drunk for diarrhea and 3 cups each day for diabetes. Alternatively, 5 ml of tincture can be used 3 times per day.

Are There Any Side Effects or Interactions? If the tea does not significantly reduce diarrhea within 2 to 3 days, consult with a health-care practitioner. Fresh

(but not dried) berries tend to be laxative and should be avoided in cases of diarrhea.[6]

Boldo

(Peumus boldus)

Parts Used and Where Grown: Boldo is an evergreen shrub or small tree that is native to Chile and is naturalized to the Mediterranean region of Europe. The leaves are used medicinally.[1]

In What Conditions Might Boldo Be Supportive?

Ranking	Health Concerns
Secondary	Indigestion (p. 99)
Other	Heartburn (p. 99)

Historical or Traditional Use

Boldo has a long history of use as a liver tonic and in the treatment of **gallstones** (p. 69) by the indigenous people of Chile.

Active Constituents

Boldo contains several types of primary constituents, including volatile oils (e.g., ascaridole, eucalyptol), flavonoids, and alkaloids. Boldine, which constitutes about one-fourth of the total number of alkaloids present, is said to be the major alkaloid.[2] Scientists believe that boldine is responsible for the plant's choloretic (bile stimulating) and diuretic actions.[3] In conjunction with other herbs, such as **cascara** (p. 407), rhubarb, and **gentian** (p. 426), boldo has been reported to improve symptoms related to loss of appetite.[4] Ascaridole, a compound found in the essential oil of the plant, has been used as an **antiparasitic** (p. 137) agent but has long fallen out of favor, as other compounds have lower toxicity levels.[5]

How Much Is Usually Taken?

Although the dried leaf can be used as an infusion at a dose of 3 grams per day, neither the infusion nor the tinctures and extracts are recommended due to the herb's high ascaridole content.[6,7]

Are There Any Side Effects or Interactions? The German Commission E monograph[8] on this herb suggests that only an ascaridole-free preparation should be used internally. Boldo contains terpene-4-ol, an ingredient similar to that found in **juniper** (p. 437), and should be avoided by individuals with a kidney disorder, as it could cause kidney irritation.[9] In addition, the herb should not be taken by those who are pregnant, nursing, have obstruction of the liver bile duct, or severe liver disease.[10] Excessive use of the herb over long time periods (over 3 to 4 weeks continuously) is not recommended.

Boneset
(Eupatorium perfoliatum)

Parts Used and Where Grown: Boneset's leaves and flowering tops are used medicinally. It belongs to the same botanical family as **echinacea** (p. 417) and Asteraceae (daisy). Boneset grows primarily in North America.

In What Conditions Might Boneset Be Supportive?

Ranking	Health Concerns
Other	Common cold/sore throat (p. 41) Influenza (p. 104)

Historical or Traditional Use

Native Americans pioneered the use of boneset as a treatment for a wide range of infectious, fever-related conditions. Europeans eventually adopted the use of the plant, and some claimed it was even occasionally effective in treating malaria.[1]

Active Constituents

Boneset contains sesquiterpene lactones, such as euperfolin, euperfolitin, and eufoliatin, as well as polysaccharides and flavonoids. In test tube and other studies, extracts of boneset have been shown to stimulate **immune cell function** (p. 94).[2] This may explain its ability to help fight off minor viral infections, such as **colds** (p. 41) and the **flu** (p. 104).

How Much Is Usually Taken?

Boneset is primarily used as a homeopathic remedy now.[3] Traditionally, boneset is taken as a tea or tincture. To prepare a tea, boiling water is added to 1 to 2 U.S. teaspoons (5 to 10 grams) of the herb and allowed to steep, covered, for 10 to 15 minutes. Three cups a day may be drunk (the tea is quite bitter). Tincture is often taken in a quantity of 2 to 3 ml 3 times per day.

Are There Any Side Effects or Interactions? A

small number of people experience nausea and/or vomiting when using boneset; the fresh plant is more likely than the dried herb to cause this. Although potentially liver-damaging chemicals called pyrro-

lizidine alkaloids are found in some plants similar to boneset, the levels are minimal in boneset and no liver damage has been reported.[4] Nevertheless, people with liver disease should avoid boneset, and no one should take it consistently for more than 6 months. Boneset is not recommended in pregnancy or lactation.

Borage
(Borago officinalis)

Parts Used and Where Grown: This large plant with blue, star-shaped flowers is found throughout Europe and North Africa. It is naturalized to North America. The plant's seed, leaves, and flowers are used medicinally.[1]

In What Conditions Might Borage Be Supportive?

Ranking	Health Concerns
Secondary	Eczema (p. 64) Infantile seborrheic dermatitis Rheumatoid arthritis (p. 151)

Historical or Traditional Use

Borage is an ancient herb widely used by the Greeks and Romans as a heart sedative. In addition, it was believed that Borage would instill the user with courage, as illustrated by the following phrase: *Ego Borago Doudia Semper Ago*, which translates as " I, borage, always bring courage." Throughout the Middle Ages, borage leaves steeped in wine were widely used to dispel the symptoms of melancholy.[2]

Active Constituents

Borage seed oil is the richest source of gamma linolenic acid (GLA) and contains 20 to 26% GLA.

While GLA from evening primrose oil has been widely researched, scientific evidence supporting the use of borage oil has been limited. People with **rheumatoid arthritis** (p. 151) who received either 1.4 grams of GLA daily from borage oil or placebo for 24 weeks experienced significant reductions in such symptoms as tender and swollen joints after utilizing the oil.[3]

Borage oil has also been employed for atopic dermatitis (**eczema** [p. 64]) in open clinical trials, with reductions in skin inflammation, dryness, scaliness, and itch without side effects being reported.[4] However, a controlled study using 360 mg of GLA daily from borage in people with atopic dermatitis (3 to 17 years of age) was unable to reproduce these results.[5] In another open pilot study, forty-eight children with infantile seborrheic dermatitis were treated with borage oil (0.5 ml) applied to the diaper region twice daily.[6] Within 10 to 12 days, all the children were free from skin lesions, even in the areas not treated with borage. Moreover, using the oil topically 2 to 3 times a week kept the seborrhea in remission until the children were 6 to 7 months old. There were no relapses after the oil was discontinued.

How Much Is Usually Taken?

For the treatment of rheumatoid arthritis, the adult dose of GLA from borage is 1.4 grams daily for at least 2 months.[7] Although one can try borage oil at a dose of 360 mg of GLA daily for eczema, research has not successfully supported its use for this condition.[8] Topically, 0.5 ml of borage oil can be applied to areas of seborrhea daily for 2 weeks and then 3 times a week until the condition is stable.[9]

Are There Any Side Effects or Interactions? Bor-

age seeds do contain small amounts of the liver toxins called pyrrolizidine alkaloids (PA). However, despite the fact that testing has demonstrated the presence of less than 5 mcg per gram of the alkaloid in the seed oil, the consumption of two to four 500 mg capsules of borage seed oil could result in an intake of such alkaloids approaching 5 to 10 micrograms per day. In the interests of public safety, borage oil should be PA free and follow the example set by the German Health Agency, which suggests that no more than 1 mcg of PA be consumed daily when the herb is taken as directed.[10,11] Although there are no known reports of health hazards when using GLA from borage, because it does contain small amounts of PA, its use during pregnancy and lactation is not recommended. One should contact the individual manufacturers of the oil to see if they assay for PA and to find out how much is present in their product. As with the use of GLA in **evening primrose oil** (p. 292), GLA from borage may potentially elicit temporal lobe epilepsy, especially in people with schizophrenic and/or those receiving medications such as phenothiazines. Minor side effects from borage oil use can include bloating, nausea, indigestion, and headache.[12]

Boswellia
(Boswellia serrata)

Common name: Salai guggal

Parts Used and Where Grown: Boswellia is a moderate to large branching tree found in the dry hilly areas of India. When the tree trunk is tapped, a gummy ole-

oresin is exuded. A purified extract of this resin is used in modern herbal preparations.

In What Conditions Might Boswellia Be Supportive?

Ranking	Health Concerns
Secondary	Osteoarthritis (p. 130)
	Rheumatoid arthritis (p. 151)
	Ulcerative colitis (p. 158)
Other	Bursitis (p. 30)

Historical or Traditional Use

In the ancient Ayurvedic medical texts of India, the gummy exudate from boswellia is grouped with other gum resins and referred to collectively as guggals. Historically, the guggals were recommended for a variety of conditions, including arthritis, diarrhea, dysentery, pulmonary disease, and ringworm.

Active Constituents

The gum oleoresin consists of essential oils, gum, and terpenoids. The terpenoid portion contains the boswellic acids that have been shown to be the active constituents in boswellia.[1] Today, extracts are typically standardized to contain 37.5 to 65% boswellic acids.

Studies have shown that the boswellic acids have an anti-inflammatory action[2]—much like the conventional nonsteroidal anti-inflammatory drugs (NSAIDs) used for inflammatory conditions. Boswellia inhibits pro-inflammatory mediators in the body, such as leukotrienes.[3] As opposed to NSAIDs, long-term use of boswellia does not lead to irritation or ulceration of the stomach. Controlled, double-blind studies have shown that boswellia extracts are very helpful for **ulcerative colitis** (p. 158).[4]

How Much Is Usually Taken?

The standardized extract of the gum oleoresin of boswellia is recommended by many herbalists. For **rheumatoid arthritis** (p. 158) or **osteoarthritis** (p. 130), boswellia can be taken in the amount of 150 mg 3 times per day.[5] As an example, if an extract contains 37.5% boswellic acids, 400 mg of the extract would be taken 3 times per day. Treatment with boswellia generally lasts 8 to 12 weeks.

Are There Any Side Effects or Interactions? Bos-

wellia is generally safe when used as directed. Rare side effects can include diarrhea, skin rash, and nausea. Any inflammatory joint condition should be closely monitored by a nutritionally oriented physician.

Buchu
(Agathosma betulina, A. crenultata)

Parts Used and Where Grown: Buchu is a low shrub native to the Cape region of South Africa. The dried leaves are harvested, and an essential oil is obtained by steam distillation. The two primary species of buchu used commercially are *Agathosma betulina* (syn. *Barosma betulina*) and *Agathosma crenulata* (syn. *Barosma crenultata*).

In What Conditions Might Buchu Be Supportive?

Ranking	Health Concerns
Other	Urinary tract infections and inflammation (p. 160)

Historical or Traditional Use

Buchu leaf preparations have a long history of use in traditional herbal medicine as a urinary tract disinfectant and diuretic.[1] It was used to treat **urinary tract infections** (p. 160) and inflammation as well as inflammation of the prostate. In Europe, it was also used to treat **gout** (p. 75).[2]

Active Constituents

The leaves of buchu contain 1.0 to 3.5% volatile oils as well as flavonoids.[3] The urinary tract antiseptic actions of buchu are thought to be due to the volatile oils and the anti-inflammatory effects due to the flavonoids. The primary volatile oil components thought to have antibacterial actions is the monoterpene disophenol. However, one test tube study using buchu oil found no significant antibacterial effect.[4]

How Much Is Usually Taken?

The German Commission E monograph on buchu concludes that there is insufficient evidence to support the modern use of buchu for the treatment of urinary tract infections or inflammation.[5] However, many traditional herbal practitioners continue to recommend the herb for these conditions. Traditional recommendations for the herb include the use of 1 to 2 grams of the dried leaf taken 3 times daily in capsules or in a tea.[6] Tinctures can be used at a dose of 2 to 4 ml 3 times per day.

Are There Any Side Effects or Interactions? Buchu
may cause the gastrointestinal irritation and should only be taken with meals. Pregnant or lactating women should not use it.

Bugleweed
(Lycopus virginicus)

Parts Used and Where Grown: The leaves and flowers of this plant from the mint family are used as medicine. Both it and its very similar European cousin, gypsywort *(Lycopus europaeus)*, grow in very wet areas.

In What Conditions Might Bugleweed Be Supportive?

Ranking	Health Concerns
Secondary	Thyroid conditions
Other	Breast pain

Historical or Traditional Use

The modern applications of bugleweed, unlike most other medicinal plants, do not match its traditional use. Historically, bugleweed and related species were used to treat coughs and as a sedative.[1] Today, the main use of this herb is for treating mild hyperthyroidism.

Active Constituents

Lithospermic acid and other organic acids are believed to be responsible for bugleweed's activity. These acids decrease levels of several hormones in the body, particularly thyroid-stimulating hormone[2] and the thyroid hormone thyroxine (T4).[3] Bugleweed inhibits the binding of antibodies to the thyroid gland.[4] These antibodies can cause the most common form of hyperthyroidism, Graves' disease. All these actions help explain bugleweed's benefit in people with overactive thyroids. Bugleweed also decreases production of the pituitary gland hormone known as prolactin,[5] an elevated level of which is associated with female reproductive difficulties and enlarged breasts in men (gynecomastia).

How Much Is Usually Taken?

Only small amounts are necessary for this plant to decrease thyroid function, however the optimal intake level is different for each individual. The German Commission E monograph recommends a daily dosage of 1 to 2 grams of the whole herb.[6] Intake of tincture should be limited to 1 to 2 ml 3 times a day. Bugleweed is often used in conjunction with other thyroid-suppressing herbs, including **lemon balm** *(Melissa officinalis)* (p. 440) and gromwell *(Lithospermum ruderale)*.

Are There Any Side Effects or Interactions? Excessive intake of bugleweed or use by healthy persons can detrimentally depress thyroid function. Thyroid disease is dangerous and should only be treated under the supervision of a health-care professional. However, long-term use of bugleweed is considered safe for individuals with hyperthyroidism.[7] Bugleweed should not be taken by people with **hypothyroidism** (p. 93). Bugleweed is unsafe during pregnancy and lactation.[8]

Burdock
(Arctium lappa)

Parts Used and Where Grown: Burdock is native to Asia and Europe. The root is the primary source of most herbal preparations. The root becomes very soft with chewing and tastes sweet, with a mucilaginous texture.

In What Conditions Might Burdock Be Supportive?

Ranking	Health Concerns
Other	Acne (p. 5) Psoriasis (p. 147) Rheumatoid arthritis (p. 151)

Historical or Traditional Use

In traditional herbal texts, burdock root is described as a "blood purifier" or "alterative,"[1] and was believed to clear the bloodstream of toxins. It was used both internally and externally for **eczema** (p. 64) and **psoriasis** (p. 147), as well as to treat painful joints and as a diuretic. In traditional Chinese medicine, burdock root in combination with other herbs is used to treat sore throats, tonsillitis, **colds** (p. 41), and even measles.[2] It is eaten as a vegetable in Japan and elsewhere.

Burdock root has recently become popular as part of a tea to treat cancer. To date, minimal research has substantiated this application.[3]

Active Constituents

Burdock root contains high amounts of inulin and mucilage. This may explain its soothing effects on the gastrointestinal tract. Bitter constituents in the root may also explain the traditional use of burdock to improve digestion. It also contains polyacetylenes that have been shown to have antimicrobial activity.[4] Burdock root and fruit also have the ability to mildly lower blood sugar (hypoglycemic effect). Even though test tube and animal studies have indicated some anti-tumor activity for burdock root, these results have not been duplicated in human studies.[5]

How Much Is Usually Taken?

Traditional herbalists recommend 2 to 4 ml of burdock root tincture per day.[6] For the dried root preparation in capsule form, the common amount to take is 1 to 2 grams 3 times per day. Many herbal preparations will combine burdock root with other alterative herbs, such as **yellow dock** (p. 472), **red clover** (p. 453), or **cleavers** (p. 412).

Are There Any Side Effects or Interactions? Use of burdock root at the dosages listed above is generally safe.

Butcher's Broom
(Ruscus aculeatus)

Parts Used and Where Grown: Butcher's broom is a spiny, small-leafed evergreen bush native to the Mediterranean region and Northwest Europe. It is a member of the lily family and is similar to asparagus in many ways. The roots and young stems of butcher's broom are used medicinally.

In What Conditions Might Butcher's Broom Be Supportive?

Ranking	Health Concerns
Other	Atherosclerosis (p. 17) Chronic venous insufficiency (p. 38) Hemorrhoids (p. 77) Varicose veins (p. 163)

Historical or Traditional Use

Butcher's broom is so named because the mature branches were bundled and used as brooms by butchers. The young shoots were sometimes eaten as food. Ancient physicians used the roots as a diuretic in the treatment of urinary problems.[1]

Active Constituents

Steroidal molecules called ruscogenins and neoruscogenins are responsible for the medicinal actions of butcher's broom.[2] Similar to diosgenins, found in **wild yam** (p. 469), ruscogenins decrease vascular permeability—which accounts for the anti-inflammatory activity of this herb. Butcher's broom also causes small veins to constrict.[3,4] Clinical studies, some double-blind, have confirmed the benefit of a combination of vitamin C (p. 341), **flavonoids** (p. 328), and butcher's broom for treatment of **chronic venous insufficiency** (p. 38).[5,6] An extract of butcher's broom combined with flavonoid derivatives has been shown to benefit people with **diabetes** (p. 53), by lowering cholesterol levels and improving glucose tolerance.[7]

How Much Is Usually Taken?

Ointments and suppositories including butcher's broom are typically used for **hemorrhoids** (p. 77). These are often applied or inserted at night before going to bed. Encapsulated butcher's broom extracts, sometimes combined with vitamin C or flavonoids, can be used for systemic venous insufficiency in the amount of 1,000 mg 3 times per day. Alternatively, standardized extracts providing 50 to 100 mg of ruscogenins per day can be taken.[8]

Are There Any Side Effects or Interactions? Butcher's broom has no significant side effects or problems if used in the amounts listed above. However, in rare cases butcher's broom can cause nausea.[9]

Calendula
(Calendula officinalis)

Common name: Marigold
Parts Used and Where Grown: Calendula grows as a common garden plant throughout North America and Europe. The golden-orange or yellow flowers of calendula have been used as medicine for centuries.

In What Conditions Might Calendula Be Supportive?

Ranking	Health Concerns
Secondary	Wound healing (topical) (p. 167)
Other	Burns (minor, including sunburn) (p. 29) Conjunctivitis/blepharitis (p. 44) Eczema (p. 64) Gastritis (p. 71) Injuries (minor) (p. 122) Peptic ulcer (p. 138) Ulcerative colitis (p. 158)

Historical or Traditional Use

Calendula flowers were historically considered beneficial for reducing inflammation, wound healing, and as an antiseptic. Calendula was used to treat various skin diseases, ranging from skin ulcerations to eczema.[1] Internally, the soothing effects of calendula have been used for stomach ulcers and inflammation. A sterile tea has also been applied in cases of conjunctivitis.

Active Constituents

Flavonoids, found in high amounts in calendula, account for much of its anti-inflammatory activity;[2] triterpene saponins may also be important.[3] Calendula also contains carotenoids.

Investigations into anticancer and antiviral actions of calendula are continuing. At this time insufficient evidence exists to recommend clinical use of calendula for cancer. Evidence suggests the use of calendula for some viral infections;[4,5] however, the constituents responsible for these actions are not clear.

How Much Is Usually Taken?

A tea of calendula can be made by pouring 200 ml of boiling water over 1 to 2 U.S. teaspoons (5 to 10 grams) of the flowers, which is steeped, covered for 10 to 15 minutes, strained, and then drunk.[6] At least 3 cups of tea are generally drunk per day. Tincture is similarly used 3 times a day, taking 1 to 2 ml each time. The tincture can be taken in water or tea. Prepared ointments are often useful for skin problems, although wet dressings made by dipping cloth into the tea (after it has cooled) are also effective. Home treatment for eye conditions is not recommended, as absolute sterility must be maintained.

Are There Any Side Effects or Interactions? Except for the very rare person who is allergic to calendula and therefore should not use it, no side effects or interactions are known to exist.

Carob
(Ceratonia siliqua)

Common name: St. John's bread
Parts Used and Where Grown: Carob is originally from the Mediterranean region and the western part of Asia. Today it is grown mostly in Mediterranean countries. The pods are used. Carob pods come from evergreen trees; the gum from carob seeds is called locust bean gum.

In What Conditions Might Carob Be Supportive?

Ranking	Health Concerns
Secondary	Diarrhea (p. 58)

Historical or Traditional Use

Carob has long been eaten as food. John the Baptist is said to have eaten it, and thus it is sometimes called St. John's bread. Carob pods have been used to treat diarrhea for centuries.

Active Constituents

The main constituents of carob are large carbohydrates (sugars) and tannins. The sugars make carob gummy and able to act as a thickener to absorb water and help bind together watery stools. Tannins from carob, being water insoluble, do not bind proteins as some tannins do. Carob tannins do bind to (and thereby inactivate) toxins and inhibit growth of bacteria—both of which are beneficial when it comes to **diarrhea** (p. 58). A double-blind clinical study has shown carob is useful for treating infants with diarrhea.[1] A less rigorous study showed it could help adults with traveller's diarrhea.[2] Dietary fiber and sugars may make food more viscous in the stomach and thus interfere with reflux of acid into the esophagus.[3]

How Much Is Usually Taken?

Commonly, 15 grams of carob powder is mixed with applesauce for children.[4] Adults should take at least 20 grams a day. The powder can be mixed in applesauce or with sweet potatoes. Carob should be taken with plenty of water. Please note that infant diarrhea must be monitored by a health-care professional and that proper hydration with a high electrolyte fluid is critical during acute diarrhea.

Are There Any Side Effects or Interactions? Carob is generally safe; only rarely have allergic reactions been reported.

Cascara

(Rhamnus purshiani cortex)

Common names: Cascara sagrada, sacred bark

Parts Used and Where Grown: Cascara is a small to medium-size tree native to the provinces and states of the Pacific coast, including British Columbia, Washington, Oregon, and northern California. The bark of the tree is removed, cut into small pieces, and dried for 1 year before being used medicinally. Fresh bark has an emetic or vomit-inducing property and therefore is not used.

In What Conditions Might Cascara Be Supportive?

Ranking	Health Concerns
Primary	Constipation (p. 44)

Historical or Traditional Use

Northern California Indians introduced this herb, which they called sacred bark, to sixteenth-century Spanish explorers. Being much milder in its laxative action than the herb buckthorn, cascara became popular in Europe as a treatment for constipation. Cascara has been part of the U.S. Pharmacopoeia since 1890.[1]

Active Constituents

Cascara bark is high in hydroxyanthraquinone glycosides called cascarosides. Resins, tannins, and lipids make up the bulk of the other bark ingredients. Cascarosides have a cathartic action, inducing the large intestine to increase its muscular contraction (peristalsis), resulting in bowel movement.[2]

How Much Is Usually Taken?

Only the dried form of cascara should be used. Capsules providing 20 to 30 mg of cascarosides per day can be used; however, the smallest amount necessary to maintain soft stool should be used.[3] As a tincture, 1 to 5 ml per day is generally taken. It is important to drink eight 6-ounce glasses of water throughout the day. Cascara should be taken for a maximum of 8 to 10 days.[4]

Are There Any Side Effects or Interactions? Women who are pregnant or lactating and children under the age of 12 should not use cascara without the advice of a physician. Those with an intestinal obstruction, **Crohn's disease** (p. 48), appendicitis, or abdominal pain should not employ this herb.[5] Long-term use or abuse of cascara may cause a loss of electrolytes (especially the mineral **potassium** [p. 323]) or weaken the colon. Loss of potassium may potentiate the action of digitalis-like medications with fatal consequences.

Catnip

(Nepeta cataria)

Parts Used and Where Grown: The catnip plant grows in North America and Europe. The leaves and flowers are used as medicine.

In What Conditions Might Catnip Be Supportive?

Ranking	Health Concerns
Other	Cough (p. 47) Insomnia (p. 105)

Historical or Traditional Use

Catnip is famous for inducing a delirious, stimulated state in felines. Throughout history, this herb has been used in humans to produce a sedative effect.[1] Catnip tea was a regular beverage in England before the introduction of tea from China.[2] Several other conditions (including cancer, toothache, corns, and hives) have been treated with catnip by traditional herbalists.

Active Constituents

The essential oil in catnip contains a monoterpene similar to the valepotriates found in **valerian** (p. 467), an even more widely renowned sedative.[3] Animal studies (except those involving cats) have found it to increase sleep.[4] The monoterpenes also help with **coughs** (p. 47).

How Much Is Usually Taken?

A catnip tea can be made by adding 250 ml (1 cup) of boiling water to 1 to 2 U.S. teaspoons (5 to 10 grams) of the herb; cover, then steep for 10 to 15 minutes. Drink 2 to 3 cups per day.[5] For children with coughs, 5 ml of tincture 3 times per day can be used. Adults may take twice this amount.

Are There Any Side Effects or Interactions? Using reasonable amounts, no side effects with catnip have been noted.

Cat's Claw
(Uncaria tomentosa)

Parts Used and Where Grown: Cat's claw grows in the rain forests of the Andes Mountains in South America, particularly in Peru. The root bark is used as medicine.

In What Conditions Might Cat's Claw Be Supportive?

Ranking	Health Concerns
Other	Injuries (minor) (p. 122) Immune function (p. 94)

Historical or Traditional Use

Cat's claw has been reportedly used by indigenous peoples in the Andes to treat inflammation, rheumatism, gastric ulcers, tumors, dysentery, and as birth control.[1] Cat's claw is popular in South American folk medicine for intestinal complaints, gastric ulcers, arthritis, and to promote wound healing.

Active Constituents

Oxyindole alkaloids appear to give cat's claw much of its activity, particularly to stimulate the **immune system** (p. 94).[2] The alkaloids and other constituents, such as glycosides, may account for the anti-inflammatory and antioxidant actions of this herb.[3,4]

Although cat's claw has become very popular in North America and is used for cancer and **HIV** (p. 87), little scientific evidence supports the use of cat's claw for these conditions.

How Much Is Usually Taken?

A cat's claw tea is prepared from 1 gram of root bark by adding 250 ml (1 cup) of water and boiling for 10 to 15 minutes. After cooling and straining, one cup is drunk 3 times per day. Alternatively, 1 to 2 ml of tincture can be taken up to 2 times per day or 20 to 60 mg of a standardized dry extract can be taken per day.[5]

Are There Any Side Effects or Interactions? No serious adverse effects have yet been reported. Cat's claw may be contraindicated in autoimmune illness, **multiple sclerosis** (p. 127), and tuberculosis. European practitioners avoid combining this herb with hormonal drugs, insulin, or vaccines. Cat's claw, until proven safe, should be taken only with great caution by pregnant or lactating women.

Cayenne
(Capsicum annuum, Capsicum frutescens)

Parts Used and Where Grown: Originally from South America, the cayenne plant has spread across the globe both as a food and as a medicine. Cayenne is very closely related to bell peppers, jalapeños, paprika, and other similar peppers. The fruit is used.

In What Conditions Might Cayenne Be Supportive?

Ranking	Health Concerns
Primary	Diabetes (topical for neuropathy) (p. 53) Osteoarthritis (topical, for pain only) (p. 133) Psoriasis (topical) (p. 147) Rheumatoid arthritis (topical) (p. 151) Shingles (herpes zoster)/postherpetic neuralgia (topical, for pain only) (p. 155)
Other	Bursitis (p. 30) Cluster headaches, Migraine headaches (p. 121)

Historical or Traditional Use

The potent, hot fruit of cayenne has been used as medicine for centuries. It was considered helpful for various conditions of the gastrointestinal tract, including stomachaches, cramping pains, and gas. Cayenne was frequently used to treat diseases of the circulatory system. It is still traditionally used in herbal medicine as a circulatory tonic (a substance believed to improve circulation). Rubbed on the skin, cayenne is a traditional, as well as modern, remedy for rheumatic pains and arthritis due to what is termed a counterirritant effect. A counterirritant is something that causes irritation to a tissue to which it is applied, thus distracting from the original irritation (such as joint pain in the case of arthritis).

Active Constituents

Cayenne contains a resinous and pungent substance known as capsaicin. This chemical relieves pain and itching by acting on sensory nerves. Capsaicin temporarily stimulates release of various neurotransmitters from these nerves, leading to their depletion. Without the neurotransmitters, pain signals can no longer be sent.[1] The effect is temporary. Capsaicin and other constituents in cayenne have been shown to have several other actions, including reducing platelet stickiness and acting as **antioxidants** (p. 267). Numerous double-blind studies have proven topically applied capsaicin creams are helpful for a range of conditions, including nerve pain in **diabetes** (diabetic neuropathy) (p. 53),[2,3] postsurgical pain,[4] **psoriasis** (p. 147),[5] muscle pain due to **fibromyalgia** (p. 68),[6] nerve pain after **shingles** (postherpetic neuralgia) (p. 155),[7] **osteoarthritis pain** (p. 133),[8,9] and **rheumatoid arthritis pain** (p. 151).[10]

With the aid of a health-care professional knowledgeable in nutritional medicine, capsaicin administered via the nose can also be a useful therapy for cluster headaches. This is supported by double-blind studies.[11] Weaker scientific support exists for the use of capsaicin for **migraines** (p. 121).[12]

How Much Is Usually Taken?

Creams containing 0.025 to 0.075% capsaicin are generally used.[13] A burning sensation may occur the first several times the cream is applied; however, this should gradually decrease with each use. The hands must be carefully and thoroughly washed after use, or gloves should be worn, to prevent the cream from accidentally reaching the eyes, nose, or mouth, which would cause a burning sensation. Do not apply the cream to areas of broken skin. A cayenne tincture can be used in the amount of 0.3 to 1 ml 3 times daily. An infusion can be made by pouring a cup of boiling water onto ½ to 1 tsp of cayenne powder and let set for 10 minutes. A teaspoon of this infusion can be mixed with water and drunk 3 to 4 times daily.

Are There Any Side Effects or Interactions? Besides causing a mild burning during the first few applications (or severe burning if accidentally placed in

sensitive areas, such as the eyes), no side effects accompany the use of cayenne (capsaicin cream).[14] As with anything applied to the skin, some people may have an allergic reaction to the cream, so the first application should be to a very small area of skin. Do not attempt to use capsaicin cream intranasally for headache treatment without professional support.

When consumed as food—one pepper per day for many years—cayenne may increase the risk of stomach cancer, according to one study.[15] A different human study found that people who ate the most cayenne actually had lower rates of stomach cancer.[16] Overall, the current scientific evidence is contradictory; thus, the relationship between cayenne consumption and increased risk of stomach cancer remains unclear.[17] Nevertheless, until more is known, no more than 1 ml of tincture 3 times per day should be used. Oral intake of even 1 ml 3 times per day can cause burning in the mouth and throat, and can cause the nose to run and eyes to water. Cayenne should be taken in amounts of less than 1 ml tincture 3 times daily, or less than 500 mg powder daily, by people with **ulcers** (p. 138), **heartburn** (p. 99), or **gastritis** (p. 71).

Chamomile
(Matricaria recutita)

Parts Used and Where Grown: Chamomile, a member of the daisy family, is native to Europe and western Asia. German chamomile is the most commonly used. The dried and fresh flowers are used medicinally.

In What Conditions Might Chamomile Be Supportive?

Ranking	Health Concerns
Secondary	Colic (p. 40) Gingivitis (periodontal disease) (p. 73)
Other	Anxiety (p. 14) Canker sores (mouth ulcers) (p. 30) Conjunctivitis/blepharitis (p. 44) Crohn's disease (p. 48) Diarrhea (p. 58) Eczema (p. 64) Gastritis (p. 71) Indigestion and heartburn (p. 99) Insomnia (p. 105) Irritable bowel syndrome (p. 109) Peptic ulcer (p. 138) Skin irritations Ulcerative colitis (p. 158) Wound healing (p. 167)

Historical or Traditional Use

Chamomile has been used for centuries as a medicinal plant, mostly for gastrointestinal complaints. This practice continues today.

Active Constituents

The flowers of chamomile provide 1 to 2% volatile oils containing alpha-bisabolol, alpha-bisabolol oxides A & B, and matricin (usually converted to chamazulene). Other active constituents include the **bioflavonoids** (p. 271) apigenin, luteolin, and **quercetin** (p. 328).[1] These active ingredients contribute to chamomile's anti-inflammatory, antispasmodic, and smooth-muscle relaxing action, particularly in the gastrointestinal tract.[2,3,4,5]

How Much Is Usually Taken?

Chamomile is often taken as a tea that can be drunk 3 to 4 times daily between meals.[6] Common alternatives are to use 2 to 3 grams of the herb in tablet or capsule form or 4 to 6 ml of tincture 3 times per day between meals.

Are There Any Side Effects or Interactions? Though rare, allergic reactions to chamomile have been reported.[7] These reactions have included bronchial constriction with internal use and allergic skin reactions with topical use. While such side effects are extremely uncommon, persons with allergies to plants of the Asteraceae family (ragweed, aster, and chrysanthemums) should avoid using chamomile. Chamomile is not contraindicated during pregnancy or lactation.

Chaparral
(Larrea tridentata)

Common name: Creosote bush

Parts Used and Where Grown: Chaparral takes its name from the area it grows in, the desert regions of the southwestern United States and northern Mexico known as the chaparral ecosystem. The leaves and flowers of this ancient plant are used as medicine.

In What Conditions Might Chaparral Be Supportive?

Ranking	Health Concerns
Other	Cold sores (p. 39) Dysmenorrhea (topical) (p. 61) Dyspepsia, Indigestion and heartburn (p. 99) Intestinal cramps (topical) Parasites (p. 137) Rheumatoid arthritis (topical) (p. 151) Wound healing (topical) (p. 167)

Historical or Traditional Use

Chaparral has been used for thousands of years by Native Americans for a variety of purposes. It has been employed primarily in tea form to help with cramping pains, joint pains, and allergic problems as well as to eliminate **parasites** (p. 137).[1,2] Externally it has been applied to aid inflammation, pain, and minor wounds.[3] In some cultures, bathing in chaparral once per year was customary to eliminate skin parasites and to detoxify.

Active Constituents

The major lignan in chaparral, known as nordihydroguaiaretic acid (NDGA), has potent anti-inflammatory activity, possibly due to its ability to block the actions of the enzyme lipoxygenase.[4] This enzyme creates pro-inflammatory chemicals known as prostaglandins; by blocking this process chaparral may be helpful for inflammatory conditions. At high doses NDGA also inhibits cyclooxygenase,[5] an enzyme similar to lipoxygenase. Chaparral also contains antioxidant flavonoids and has anti-amoeba activity in test tubes.[6] The potential of chaparral for cancer treatment has not been proven in human studies.[7]

How Much Is Usually Taken?

A tea can be prepared from 1 teaspoon of leaves and flowers by steeping it in 1 cup of hot water for 10 to 15 minutes.[8] People should drink 3 cups per day for a maximum of 2 weeks unless under the care of a physician expert in the use of botanical medicines. Or, 0.5 to 1 ml of tincture can be taken 3 times per day.[9] Topically, cloths can be soaked in oil preparations or tea of chaparral and applied several times per day (with heat if helpful) over the affected area. Powdered chaparral can be applied directly to **minor wounds** (p. 167). Capsules of chaparral should be avoided.

Are There Any Side Effects or Interactions? There have been sporadic reports of people developing liver or kidney problems after taking chaparral, particularly in capsules.[10] Almost all of these cases involved the use of capsules or excessive amounts of tea, or persons with previous liver disease were involved. Tea and tincture of chaparral have an extremely strong taste considered disagreeable by most persons, which restricts the amount they can tolerate before feeling nauseous. Capsules bypass this protective mechanism and should therefore be avoided. Because human studies have shown that large doses of chaparral tea and injections of NDGA in people with cancer do not cause liver or kidney problems,[11] it is likely the cases of toxicity represented individual reactions.[12] Nevertheless, chaparral should not be taken internally for more than 2 weeks consecutively unless prescribed by a doctor of natural medicine. It should be avoided for internal use during pregnancy and lactation. Chaparral is safe for topical use.

Chickweed
(Stellaria media)

Parts Used and Where Grown: The ubiquitous, small, green chickweed plant grows across the United States and originated in Europe. The leaves, stems, and flowers are used in botanical medicine.

In What Conditions Might Chickweed Be Supportive?

Ranking	Health Concerns
Other	Eczema (p. 64) Insect stings and bites

Historical or Traditional Use

Chickweed was reportedly used at times for food.[1] Chickweed enjoys a reputation in folk medicine for treating a wide spectrum of conditions, ranging from asthma and indigestion to skin diseases. Traditional Chinese herbalists used a tea made from chickweed for nosebleeds.

Active Constituents

The active constituents in chickweed are largely unknown. It contains relatively high amounts of vitamins and flavonoids, which may explain some of its activity. Although some older information suggests a possible benefit for chickweed in rheumatic conditions, this has not been validated in clinical studies.[2]

How Much Is Usually Taken?

Although formerly used as a tea, chickweed is mainly used today as a cream applied liberally several times each day to rashes and inflammatory skin conditions (e.g., eczema [p. 64]) to ease itching and inflammation.[3] As a tincture, 1 to 5 ml per day can be taken 3 times per day. Two teaspoonfuls of the dried herb may be used to make a tea. This may be drunk 3 times daily.
Are There Any Side Effects or Interactions? No side effects with chickweed have been reported.

Cinnamon
(Cinnamomum zeylanicum)

Parts Used and Where Grown: Most people are familiar with the sweet but pungent taste of the oil, powder, or sticks of bark from the cinnamon tree. Cinnamon trees grow in a number of tropical areas, including parts of India, China, Madagascar, Brazil, and the Caribbean.

In What Conditions Might Cinnamon Be Supportive?

Ranking	Health Concerns
Other	Heartburn (p. 99) Menorrhagia (heavy menstruation) (p. 120) Peptic ulcer (p. 138) Poor appetite Yeast infection (p. 169)

Historical or Traditional Use

Cinnamon is perhaps one of the oldest herbal medicines, having been mentioned in Chinese texts as long ago as 4,000 years. It has a broad range of historical uses in different cultures, including the treatment of diarrhea, arthritis, and various menstrual disorders.[1] The large number of applications for cinnamon indicates the widespread appreciation folk herbalists around the world have had for cinnamon as a medicine, although there is often no research to substantiate the health claims.

Active Constituents

Various terpenoids found in the essential oil are believed to account for cinnamon's medicinal effects. Important among these compounds are eugenol and cinnamaldehyde. Cinnamaldehyde and cinnamon oil vapors are potent antifungal compounds.[2] Preliminary human evidence confirms this effect in studies of people with AIDS who had oral candida (thrush) infections that improved with application of cinnamon oil.[3] Antibacterial actions have been demonstrated for cinnamon.[4] This antibacterial action has been extended recently to the bacterium that causes most **ulcers** (p. 138), *Helicobacter pylori.*[5] The diterpenes in the volatile oil have also shown antiallergic activity.[6] Water extracts may help reduce ulcers.[7]

How Much Is Usually Taken?

The German Commission E monograph suggests 2 to 4 grams of the powder daily.[8] A tea can be prepared from the powdered herb by boiling ½ U.S. teaspoon (2 to 3 grams) of the powder for 10 to 15 minutes, cooling, and then drinking. No more than a few drops of essential oil should be used and only for a few days at a time. Cinnamon tincture in the amount of 2 to 3 ml 3 times each day can also be used.
Are There Any Side Effects or Interactions? Some individuals develop allergies and dermatitis after

exposure to cinnamon.[9] Therefore, only small amounts should be used initially in persons who have not previously had contact with cinnamon, and anyone with a known allergy should avoid it. Chronic use may cause inflammation in the mouth. The concentrated oil is more likely to cause problems. According to the German Commission E monograph, cinnamon is not recommended for use by pregnant women.[10]

Cleavers
(Galium aparine)

Common names: Bedstraw, goose grass
Parts Used and Where Grown: The leaves and flowers of cleavers are used. It grows in wet areas of Britain, Europe, Asia, and North America. Cleavers grows small prickles on its leaves, causing it to have a sticky feeling and giving it its name.

In What Conditions Might Cleavers Be Supportive?

Ranking	Health Concerns
Other	Edema (p. 65) Urinary tract infection (p. 160)

Historical or Traditional Use

Cleavers is one of numerous plants considered diuretic in ancient times.[1] It was therefore used to relieve edema (p. 65) and to promote urine formation during bladder infections. It has also been used for people with lymph swellings, jaundice, and wounds.

Active Constituents

Galiosin, an anthraquinone glycoside, and other glycosides plus tannins and flavonoids may constitute the major active constituents of cleavers. Little research has been conducted on this plant, but preliminary lab experiments suggest it may have antispasmodic activity.[2]

How Much Is Usually Taken?

Cleavers tincture and tea are most widely recommended by herbal practitioners. Tincture in the amount of 3 to 5 ml can be taken 3 times per day. Tea is made by steeping 2 to 3 teaspoons of the herb in a cup of hot water for 10 to 15 minutes. People can drink 3 or more cups per day.

Are There Any Side Effects or Interactions? Cleavers has no known side effects and is thought to be safe for use in pregnant or nursing women and children.

Coltsfoot
(Tussilago farfara)

Parts Used and Where Grown: The flowers, leaves, and roots have been used. However, the roots are generally avoided now. It originates from Eurasia and North Africa and now also grows throughout damp areas of North America.

In What Conditions Might Coltsfoot Be Supportive?

Ranking	Health Concerns
Other	Cough (p. 47) Sore throat (p. 41)

Historical or Traditional Use

Coltsfoot historically has been used to alleviate **coughs** (p. 47) due to all manner of conditions. It is considered particularly useful for people with chronic coughs, such as those due to emphysema or silicosis.[1] Coltsfoot leaf was originally approved for the treatment of sore throats in the German Commission E monograph[2] but has since been banned in Germany for internal use.[3]

Active Constituents

Mucilage, bitter glycosides, and tannins are considered the major constituents of coltsfoot.[4] These appear to give the herb anti-inflammatory and antitussive (cough prevention and treatment) activity. Coltsfoot also contains pyrrolizidine alkaloids, discussed below.

How Much Is Usually Taken?

Internal use of coltsfoot root may be harmful due to the liver toxicity of the pyrrolizidine alkaloids. Internal use of the root is not recommended. Tea of coltsfoot leaf or flower is made by steeping 1 to 2 teaspoons in 1 cup hot water for 10 to 20 minutes.[5] Three cups per day can be drunk. Alternatively, 2 to 4 ml of tincture of the leaf or flower can be taken 3 times per day. Some doctors practicing herbal medicine have recommended having hot tea ready in a thermos to drink for morning coughs due to emphysema.[6] People should not use for more than 1 month consecutively unless on the advice of a doctor of natural medicine. Preparations guaranteed to be pyrrolizidine-free can be used indefinitely and are preferable.

Cleavers

Are There Any Side Effects or Interactions? Colts-foot contains potentially liver-damaging pyrrolizidine alkaloids. The root contains much higher levels than do the leaves or the flowers. Animal studies using amounts of coltsfoot hundreds of times higher than those used as medicine have shown these alkaloids can cause cancer in animals, but this is not applicable to usual amounts of coltsfoot used as medicine.[7] A single case of an infant who developed liver disease and died after the mother drank tea containing coltsfoot during pregnancy has been reported.[8] This eventually led to the banning of coltsfoot in Germany in 1992.

Leaf and flower preparations should not be taken for more than 1 month consecutively, and root products should not be used internally. Products guaranteed to be pyrrolizidine-free are preferable. Coltsfoot should not be taken during pregnancy or lactation.[9] Otherwise, coltsfoot is generally safe.[10]

Coltsfoot should be differentiated from the plant called western coltsfoot (*Petastites frigidus*) because western coltsfoot can contain even more pyrrolizidine alkaloids. Western coltsfoot should only be taken on the advice of a doctor knowledgeable in the use of botanical medicines.

Comfrey
(Symphytum officinale)

Common names: Knitbone, boneset
Parts Used and Where Grown: The leaf and root of comfrey have been employed medicinally for centuries. Originally from Europe and western Asia, it is now also grown in North America.

In What Conditions Might Comfrey Be Supportive?

Ranking	Health Concerns
Other	Broken bones (topical)
	Bruises (topical) (p. 28)
	Chronic skin ulcer (topical)
	Conjunctivitis/Blepharitis (p. 44)
	Cough (p. 47)
	Inflammatory bowel disease
	Minor injuries (p. 122)
	Peptic ulcer (p. 138)
	Sprains (topical) (p. 122)
	Thrombophlebitis (topical)
	Wound healing (topical) (p. 167)

Historical or Traditional Use

Comfrey has a long, consistent history of use as a topical agent for improving healing of wounds, skin ulcers, thrombophlebitis, strains, and sprains.[1,2] Also of note is the use of comfrey to promote more rapid repair of broken bones. Comfrey has a reputation as an anti-inflammatory for a variety of rashes. It was also used for persons with gastrointestinal problems, such as stomach **ulcers** (p. 138) and inflammatory bowel disease, and for lung problems.

Active Constituents

Mucilage and allantoin are considered the major compounds in comfrey that promote healing.[3] A water extract of comfrey has been shown to stimulate production of protective substances known as prostaglandins in the stomachs of experimental animals.[4] This may partially explain the historical use of comfrey to help heal ulcers.

How Much Is Usually Taken?

Fresh, peeled root (approximately 100 grams) or dried root is simmered in 1 pint (250 ml) water for 10 to 15 minutes to prepare comfrey for topical use.[5] Cloth or gauze is soaked in this liquid, then applied to the skin for at least 15 minutes. Fresh leaves can be ground up lightly and applied directly to the skin. Alternatively, creams or ointments made from root or leaf can be applied. All topical preparations should be applied several times per day. To aid the healing of a broken bone, a window would need to be left in the cast near the fracture site, and comfrey applied. However, this is not always possible.

Due to variations in pyrrolizidine alkaloid content, root preparations are unsafe for internal use unless they are guaranteed pyrrolizidine-free. Tea made from the leaf can generally be used safely for as long as a month. Tea is made by steeping 1 to 2 teaspoons of leaf in hot water for 15 minutes.[6] Three cups per day can be drunk. Alternatively, 2 to 4 ml of tincture of comfrey can be taken 3 times per day for no more than 1 month consecutively. Tinctures that are guaranteed pyrrolizidine-free are preferable and can be taken long-term.

Are There Any Side Effects or Interactions? Comfrey contains potentially dangerous compounds known as pyrrolizidine alkaloids. The roots contain higher levels of these compounds, and mature leaves contain very little if any of these alkaloids.[7,8] Fresh young leaves contain higher amounts (up to sixteen times more than mature leaves) and should be avoided.[9] Other related forms such as Russian comfrey (Symphytum x uplandicum) and prickly comfrey (Sympthytum asperum) are sometimes available or mistakenly sold as regular comfrey but contain higher levels and/or more toxic types of alkaloids.[10] One

Comfrey

study found that twenty-nine persons who had consumed comfrey from 1 to 20 years developed no sign of liver disease.[11] Nevertheless, several reports of individuals who developed liver disease or other serious problems from taking capsules or tea of comfrey have been reported over the years.[12] Because there is usually no indication on comfrey products whether they contain pyrrolizidine alkaloids, it is best to avoid internal use of products made from the root and to use products made from the mature leaf for no more than 1 month consecutively. Topical use of root or leaf is safe unless applied over broken skin, in which case comfrey should be used for no more than 3 days consecutively. Comfrey should not be taken internally during pregnancy or lactation.[13]

Cranberry
(Vaccinium macrocarpon)

Parts Used and Where Grown: Cranberry is a member of the same family as **bilberry** (p. 396). It is from North America and grows in bogs. The ripe fruit is used.

In What Conditions Might Cranberry Be Supportive?

Ranking	Health Concerns
Secondary	Urinary tract infection (p. 160)

Historical or Traditional Use

Cranberry has been used to prevent kidney stones and "bladder gravel" as well as to remove toxins from the blood. Cranberry has long been recommended for persons with recurrent urinary tract infections (UTIs).

Active Constituents

Cranberry prevents *E. coli,* the most common cause of UTIs and recurrent UTIs, from adhering to the cells lining the wall of the bladder. This antiadherence action renders the bacteria harmless in the urinary tract.[1,2] Recently, the proanthocyanidins in the berry were shown to have this antiadherence action.[3] Cranberry has been shown to reduce bacteria levels in the urinary bladders of older women significantly better than placebo, which may help to prevent future infections.[4] Other preliminary studies in humans suggest cranberry can help people with urostomies and enterocystoplasties to keep them clear of mucus buildup.[5]

How Much Is Usually Taken?

People often take one capsule or tablet of a concentrated cranberry juice extract (400 mg) 2 to 4 times per day.[6] Several glasses (16 ounces) of a high-quality cranberry juice each day can approximate the effect of the cranberry concentrate. Cranberry tincture, in the amount of 3 to 5 ml 3 times per day can also be taken.

Are There Any Side Effects or Interactions? Cranberry concentrate has no known side effects and is safe to use during pregnancy and lactation. Cranberry should not be used as a substitute for antibiotics during an acute urinary tract infection.

Cranesbill
(Geranium maculatum)

Parts Used and Where Grown: This plant originated in North America and is sometimes grown ornamentally in a variety of flower colors. The root is used primarily as a medicine, but the herb also has a few applications.

In What Conditions Might Cranesbill Be Supportive?

Ranking	Health Concerns
Other	Crohn's disease (p. 48) Diarrhea (p. 58)

Historical or Traditional Use

The Blackfoot used the root of cranesbill and closely related plants to stop bleeding.[1] Cranesbill has also been used by a number of the indigenous tribes of North America to treat diarrhea.

Active Constituents

Cranesbill is high in tannins, which accounts for its antidiarrheal activity.[2] Little scientific research exists to clarify cranesbill's constituents and actions.

How Much Is Usually Taken?

A tea can be prepared by boiling 1 to 2 U.S. teaspoons (5 to 10 grams) of the root for 10 to 15 minutes in 2 cups (500 ml) of water.[3] Three cups or more per day can be drunk. Cranesbill tincture in the amount of 3 ml 3 times per day is also commonly used, although generally this is in combination with other herbs and therapies for diarrhea.

Are There Any Side Effects or Interactions? The tea should not be used for more than 2 to 3 consecutive weeks. Some people could develop an upset stomach after using cranesbill.

Damiana
(Turnera diffusa)

Parts Used and Where Grown: The leaves of damiana were originally used as medicine by the indigenous cultures of Central America, particularly Mexico. Today the plant is found in hot, humid climates, including parts of Texas.

In What Conditions Might Damiana Be Supportive?

Ranking	Health Concerns
Other	Depression (p. 50) Impotence (p. 98)

Historical or Traditional Use

Damiana has been hailed as an aphrodisiac since ancient times, particularly by the native peoples of Mexico.[1] Other folk uses have included asthma, bronchitis, neurosis, and various sexual disorders.[2] It has also been promoted as a euphoria-inducing substance at various times.

Active Constituents

Most research has been done on the essential oil of damiana, which includes numerous small, fragrant substances called terpenes. As yet, it is unclear if the essential oil is truly the main active constituent of damiana. The leaves also contain the antimicrobial substances arbutin, alkaloids, and other potentially active compounds.[3] Damiana extracts have been shown, in the test tube, to weakly bind to progesterone receptors.[4] Damiana may thus be a potentially useful herb for some female health problems, though no human studies have investigated this possibility and it is not a strong traditional use.

How Much Is Usually Taken?

To make a tea, add 250 ml (1 cup) boiling water to 1 gram of dried leaves; allow to steep 10 to 15 minutes. Drink 3 cups per day. To use in tincture form, take 2 to 3 ml 3 times per day. Tablets or capsules may also be used in the amount of 400 to 800 mg 3 times per day. Damiana is not usually used alone; it is often more effective when combined with other herbs of similar or complementary activity. However, the German Commission

E monograph does not feel that traditional use of this herb is supported for modern use.[5]

Are There Any Side Effects or Interactions? The leaves have a minor laxative effect, which is more pronounced at higher intakes, and may cause loosening of stools.[6]

Dandelion
(Taraxacum officinale)

Parts Used and Where Grown: Closely related to chicory, dandelion is a common plant worldwide and the bane of those looking for the perfect lawn. The plant grows to a height of about 12 inches, producing spatula-like leaves and yellow flowers that bloom year-round. Upon maturation, the flower turns into the characteristic puffball containing seeds that are dispersed in the wind. Dandelion is grown commercially in the United States and Europe. The leaves and root are used in herbal supplements.

In What Conditions Might Dandelion Be Supportive?

Ranking	Health Concerns
Other	Alcohol withdrawal support (p. 6) Constipation (root) (p. 44) Edema (water retention) (leaves) (p. 65) Gallstones (root) (p. 69) Indigestion and heartburn (leaves and root) (p. 99) Liver support (root) Pregnancy and postpartum support (leaves and root) (p. 143)

Historical or Traditional Use

Dandelion is commonly used as a food. The leaves are used in salads and teas, while the roots are often used as a coffee substitute. Dandelion leaves and roots have been used for hundreds of years to treat liver, gallbladder, kidney, and joint problems. In some traditions, dandelion is considered a blood purifier and is used for ailments as varied as eczema and cancer. As is the case today, dandelion has also been used historically to treat poor digestion, water retention, and diseases of the liver, including hepatitis.

Active Constituents

The principal constituents responsible for dandelion's action on the digestive system and liver are the bitter principles. Previously referred to as taraxacin, these constituents are sesquiterpene lactones of the eudesmanolide and germacranolide type and are unique to dandelion.[1] Dandelion is also a rich source of vitamins and minerals. The leaves have a high content of **vitamin A** (p. 336) as well as moderate amounts of **vitamin D** (p. 343), **vitamin C** (p. 341), various B vitamins, **iron** (p. 304), **silicon** (p. 331), **magnesium** (p. 310), **zinc** (p. 346), and **manganese** (p. 311).[2]

Animal studies show, at high doses (2 grams per kg of body weight), the leaves possess diuretic effects comparable to the prescription diuretic frusemide (Lasix).[3] Since clinical data in humans is sparse, people should seek the guidance of a physician trained in herbal medicine before using dandelion leaves for **water retention** (p. 65).

The bitter compounds in the leaves and root help stimulate digestion and are mild laxatives.[4] These bitter principles also increase bile production in the gallbladder and bile flow from the liver.[5] For this reason dandelion is recommended by some herbalists for persons with sluggish liver function due to alcohol abuse or poor diet. The increase in bile flow may help improve fat (including cholesterol) metabolism in the body.

How Much Is Usually Taken?

As a general liver/gallbladder tonic and to stimulate digestion, 3 to 5 grams of the dried root or 5 to 10 ml of a tincture made from the root can be used 3 times per day.[6] Some experts recommend the alcohol-based tincture because the bitter principles are more soluble in alcohol.[7]

As a mild diuretic or appetite stimulant, 4 to 10 grams of dried leaves can be added to 250 ml (1 cup) of boiling water and drunk as a decoction;[8] or 5 to 10 ml of fresh juice from the leaves or 2 to 5 ml of tincture made from the leaves can be used, 3 times per day.

Are There Any Side Effects or Interactions?
Dandelion leaf and root should be used with caution by persons with **gallstones** (p. 69).[9] Persons with an obstruction of the bile ducts should avoid dandelion altogether. In cases of stomach **ulcer** (p. 138) or **gastritis** (p. 71), dandelion should be used cautiously, as it may cause overproduction of stomach acid. Those experiencing fluid or water retention should consult a nutritionally oriented doctor before taking dandelion leaves. The milky latex in the stem and leaves of fresh dandelion may cause an allergic rash in some individuals.

Devil's Claw
(Harpagophytum procumbens)

Parts Used and Where Grown: Devil's claw is a native plant of southern Africa, especially the Kalahari desert, Namibia, and the island of Madagascar. The name of devil's claw is derived from the herb's unusual fruits, which seem to be covered with numerous small hooks. The secondary storage roots, or tubers, of the plant are used in herbal supplements.[1]

In What Conditions Might Devil's Claw Be Supportive?

Ranking	Health Concerns
Secondary	Rheumatoid arthritis (p. 151)
Other	Indigestion and heartburn (p. 99) Lower back pain

Historical or Traditional Use

Numerous tribes native to southern Africa have used devil's claw for a wide variety of conditions, ranging from gastrointestinal difficulties to arthritic conditions.[2] Devil's claw has been widely used in Europe as a treatment for arthritis.

Active Constituents

Devil's claw tuber contains three important constituents belonging to the iridoid glycoside family: harpagoside, harpagide, and procumbide. The secondary tubers of the herb contain twice as much harpagoside as the primary tubers. As such, these secondary tubers contain the preferable concentration of active ingredients.[3] Harpagoside and other iridoid glycosides found in the plant may be responsible for the herb's anti-inflammatory and analgesic actions. However, research has not entirely supported the use of devil's claw in alleviating arthritic pain symptoms.[4,5] One double-blind study did find devil's claw capsules helpful for reducing low back pain.[6]

Devil's claw is also considered by herbalists to be a potent bitter. Bitter principles, like the iridoid glycosides found in devil's claw, stimulate the stomach to increase the production of acid, thereby helping to improve digestion.

How Much Is Usually Taken?

As a digestive stimulant, 1.5 to 2 grams per day of the powdered secondary tuber is used.[7] For tincture, the recommended amount is 1 to 2 ml 3 times per day. For arthritis, some herbalists suggest 4.5 to 10 grams per day. Again, recent studies do not support devil's claw as a treatment for arthritis.

Are There Any Side Effects or Interactions?
Since devil's claw promotes the secretion of stomach acid, anyone with gastric or duodenal **ulcers** (p. 138), **heartburn** (p. 99), **gastritis** (p. 71), or excessive stomach acid should not use the herb. Additionally, people

with **gallstones** (p. 69) should consult a physician before taking devil's claw.[8]

Dong Quai
(Angelica sinensis)

Parts Used and Where Grown: Dong quai is a member of the celery family. Greenish-white flowers bloom from May to August, and the plant is typically found growing in damp mountain ravines, meadows, river banks, and coastal areas. The root is used.

In What Conditions Might Dong Quai Be Supportive?

Ranking	Health Concerns
Other	Fibrocystic breast disease (p. 66) Painful menstruation (Dysmenorrhea) (p. 61) Premenstrual syndrome (p. 141)

Historical or Traditional Use

Also known as dang-gui in traditional Chinese medicine, dong quai is often referred to as the "female ginseng." In traditional Chinese medicine, dong quai is often included in prescriptions for abnormal menstruation, suppressed menstrual flow, painful or difficult menstruation, and uterine bleeding. Dong quai was traditionally used for hot flashes associated with perimenopause. It is also used for both men and women with cardiovascular disease, including high blood pressure and problems with peripheral circulation.[1]

Active Constituents

Traditionally, dong quai is believed to have a balancing or adaptogenic effect on the female hormonal system. Contrary to the opinion of several authors, dong quai does not qualify as a phytoestrogen or have any hormonelike actions in the body. This is supported by a double-blind study showing that dong quai capsules did not help women with menopausal symptoms.[2] A large part of its actions with regard to **premenstrual syndrome** (p. 141) may be related to its antispasmodic actions, particularly on smooth muscles.[3] Human research published in English is lacking to support any of the traditional uses of dong quai, though Chinese studies suggest it is beneficial for painful menses and **infertility** (p. 102).

How Much Is Usually Taken?

The powdered root can be used in capsules, tablets, tinctures, or as a tea.[4] Many women take 3 to 4 grams per day.

Are There Any Side Effects or Interactions? Dong quai is generally considered to be of extremely low toxicity.[5] It may cause some fair-skinned persons to become more sensitive to sunlight. Persons using it on a regular basis should limit prolonged exposure to the sun or other sources of ultraviolet radiation. Dong quai is not recommended for pregnant or lactating women.

Echinacea
(Echinacea purpurea, Echinacea angustifolia, Echinacea pallida)

Common name: Purple coneflower
Parts Used and Where Grown: Echinacea is a wildflower native to North America. While echinacea continues to grow and is harvested from the wild, the majority used for herbal supplements is from cultivated plants. The root or above-ground part of the plant during the flowering growth phase is used medicinally.

In What Conditions Might Echinacea Be Supportive?

Ranking	Health Concerns
Primary	Common cold/sore throat (for symptoms) (p. 41) Immune function (p. 94) Infection (p. 101) Influenza (flu) (p. 104)
Secondary	Bronchitis Common cold/sore throat (for prevention) (p. 41) Gingivitis (periodontal disease) (p. 73)
Other	Canker sores (mouth ulcers) (p. 30) Cold sores (p. 30) Crohn's disease (p. 48) Ear infections (recurrent) (p. 63) Pap smear (abnormal) (p. 136) Vaginitis (p. 162) Yeast infection (p. 169)

Historical or Traditional Use

Echinacea was used by Native Americans for a variety of conditions, including venomous bites and other external wounds. It was introduced into U.S. medical practice in 1887 and was touted for use in conditions ranging from colds to syphilis. Modern research started in the 1930s in Germany.

Active Constituents

Echinacea supports the immune system. Several constituents in echinacea team together to increase the production and activity of white blood cells

Echinacea

(lymphocytes and macrophages). The three major groups of constituents responsible are alkylamides/polyacetylenes, caffeic acid derivatives, and polysaccharides. Echinacea also increases production of interferon, an important part of the body's response to viral infection such as colds and the flu.[1] Echinacea is believed to work primarily by activating white blood cells, as mentioned above. It has been specifically shown to activate an important class of white blood cells known as natural killer cells.[2]

Several double-blind studies have confirmed the benefit of echinacea for treating and preventing **colds** (p. 41) and **flu** (p. 104).[3,4,5] Recent studies have suggested that echinacea is not effective for the prevention of colds and flu and should be reserved for use at the onset of these conditions.[6] In terms of other types of infections, research in Germany using injectable forms or an oral preparation of the herb along with a medicated cream reduced the recurrence of vaginal **yeast infections** (p. 169) compared to women given the cream alone.[7]

How Much Is Usually Taken?

At the onset of a cold or flu, 3 to 4 ml of echinacea in a liquid preparation can be taken every 2 hours for the first day of illness, and then 3 to 4 times per day for the next 10 to 14 days[8] or 300 mg of powdered echinacea in tablet or capsule form 3 times per day for the same period of time.

Are There Any Side Effects or Interactions? Echinacea is essentially nontoxic when taken orally.[9] People shouldn't take echinacea if they have an autoimmune illness, such as **lupus** (p. 115), or other progressive diseases, such as tuberculosis, **multiple sclerosis** (p. 127), or **HIV infection** (p. 87). Those who are allergic to flowers of the daisy family should not take echinacea. Echinacea is not contraindicated during pregnancy or lactation.

Elderberry
(Sambucus nigra)

Parts Used and Where Grown: Numerous species of elder or elderberry grow in Europe and North America. Only those with blue/black berries are medicinal. The flowers and berries are used. Species with red berries are not medicinal.

Historical or Traditional Use

Elderberries have long been used as food, particularly in the dried form. Elderberry wine, pie, and lemonade

are some of the popular ways to prepare this plant as food. The leaves were touted to be pain relieving and to promote healing of injuries when applied as a poultice.[1] Native Americans used the plant for infections, coughs, and skin conditions.

In What Conditions Might Elderberry Be Supportive?

Ranking	Health Concerns
Secondary	Bronchitis Common cold/sore throat (p. 41) Infection (p. 63) Influenza (p. 104)
Other	Cold sores (p. 39) Inflammation

Active Constituents

Flavonoids, including **quercetin** (p. 328), are believed to account for the therapeutic actions of the elderberry flowers and berries. According to laboratory research, an extract from the leaves, combined with **St. John's wort** (p. 461) and soapwort, inhibits the **influenza virus** (p. 104) and **herpes simplex virus** (p. 39).[2] A double-blind study in humans determined that an extract of elderberries is an effective treatment for influenza.[3] Animal studies have shown the flowers to have anti-inflammatory properties.[4]

How Much Is Usually Taken?

Liquid elderberry extract is taken in amounts of 5 ml (for children) to 10 ml (for adults) twice per day. A tea made from 3 to 5 grams of the dried flowers steeped in 250 ml (1 cup) boiling water for 10 to 15 minutes may also be drunk 3 times per day.[5]

Are There Any Side Effects or Interactions? No adverse reactions to elderberry are known to exist.

Elecampane
(Inula helenium)

Common name: Inula

Parts Used and Where Grown: Elecampane is indigenous to Europe and Asia and is now grown in the United States. The dried roots and rhizomes (branching part of the root) are collected in fall or early winter and used in herbal preparations.

Historical or Traditional Use

Traditionally, elecampane has been used to treat **coughs** (p. 47) and particularly coughs associated with bronchitis, **asthma** (p. 15), and whooping cough.[1] The herb has also been used to treat poor digestion and general complaints of the intestinal tract.

In What Conditions Might Elecampane Be Supportive?

Ranking	Health Concerns
Other	Asthma (p. 15)
	Bronchitis
	Chronic obstructive pulmonary disease (COPD) (p. 45)
	Cough (p. 47)
	Indigestion (p. 99)

Active Constituents

Elecampane root and rhizome contain approximately 1 to 4% volatile oils.[2] Most of these volatile oils are composed of sequiterpene lactones, of which alantolactone is a member. Elecampane is also very high in inulin (44%) as well as mucilage. Most herbal texts attribute the actions of elecampane to alantolactone. The antitussive (cough prevention and treatment) and carminative (soothing effect on the intestinal tract) effects of elecampane, however, may possibly be due to the inulin and mucilage content. Isolated alantolactone has been used to treat roundworm, threadworm, hookworm, and whipworm infection. This use is only by prescription and is only approved in some European countries.[3]

How Much Is Usually Taken?

The German Commission E monograph on elecampane states that the historical use of elecampane has not been adequately proven to recommend the use of the herb.[4] This is partially based on the potential side effects listed below. For traditional use, elecampane is typically recommended as a tea. Boiling water is poured over 1 gram of the ground root and rhizome and left to steep for 10 to 15 minutes after which it is strained. One cup of this preparation is drunk 3 to 4 times daily. Some texts recommend 3 to 5 ml of a tincture 3 times daily.[5]

Are There Any Side Effects or Interactions? Alantolactone can be an irritant to the intestinal tract and, along with other sesquiterpene lactones in elecampane, may cause localized irritation in the mouth and intestinal tract. Amounts several times larger than those stated above may cause vomiting, diarrhea, spasms, and signs of paralysis.[6] If these symptoms occur, people should contact their local poison control center. Pregnant or nursing women should not use elecampane.

Eleuthero (Siberian Ginseng)
(Eleutherococcus senticosus, Acanthopanax senticosus)

Common names: Siberian ginseng, ci wu jia

Parts Used and Where Grown: Eleuthero belongs to the Araliaceae family and is a distant relative of **Asian ginseng** *(Panax ginseng)* (p. 394). Also known commonly as touch-me-not and devil's shrub, eleuthero has been most frequently nicknamed Siberian ginseng in this country. Eleuthero is native to the Taiga region of the Far East (southeastern part of Russia, northern China, Korea, and Japan). The root and the rhizomes (underground stem) are used.

In What Conditions Might Siberian Ginseng Be Supportive?

Ranking	Health Concerns
Primary	Fatigue, Immune function (p. 94)
	Stress
Secondary	Athletic performance (p. 20)
Other	Alzheimer's disease (p. 11)
	Chronic fatigue syndrome (p. 36)
	Common cold/sore throat (p. 41)
	Diabetes (p. 53)
	Fibromyalgia (p. 68)
	HIV support (p. 87)
	Infection (p. 101)
	Influenza (p. 104)

Historical or Traditional Use

Although not as popular as Asian ginseng, eleuthero use dates back 2,000 years, according to Chinese medicine records. Referred to as ci wu jia in Chinese medicine, it was used to prevent respiratory tract infections as well as colds and flu. It was also believed to provide energy and vitality. In Russia, eleuthero was originally used by people in the Siberian Taiga region to increase performance and quality of life and to decrease infections.

In more modern times, eleuthero's ability to increase stamina and endurance led Soviet Olympic athletes to use it to enhance their training. Explorers, divers, sailors, and miners used eleuthero to prevent stress-related illness. After the Chernobyl accident, many Russian and Ukranian citizens were given eleuthero to counteract the effects of radiation.

Active Constituents

The constituents in eleuthero that have received the most attention are the eleutherosides.[1] Seven primary eleutherosides have been identified, with most of the research attention focusing on eleutherosides B and E.[2] Eleuthero also contains complex polysaccharides (complex sugar molecules).[3] These constituents play a critical role in eleuthero's ability to support **immune function** (p. 94).

As an adaptogen, eleuthero helps the body adapt to stress by supporting healthy adrenal gland function; it allows the glands to function optimally when challenged by stress.[4]

Eleuthero has been shown to enhance mental acuity and physical endurance without the letdown that comes with caffeinated products.[5] Research has shown that eleuthero improves the use of oxygen by the exercising muscle.[6] This means that a person is able to maintain aerobic **exercise** (p. 20) longer and recover from workouts more quickly.

Eleuthero also supports the body by helping the liver detoxify harmful toxins. It has shown a protective action in animal studies against chemicals such as ethanol, sodium barbital, tetanus toxoid, and chemotherapeutic agents.[7] Eleuthero also helps protect the body during radiation exposure.[8] Preliminary studies in Russia have confirmed the use of eleuthero for people undergoing chemotherapy and radiation therapy for cancer to help alleviate side effects and help the bone marrow recover more quickly.[9]

Eleuthero enhances and supports the immune response. Eleuthero may be useful as a preventive measure during **cold** (p. 41) and **flu** (p. 104) season. Preliminary evidence also suggests that eleuthero may prove valuable in the long-term management of various diseases of the immune system, including **HIV** (p. 187) infection and **chronic fatigue syndrome** (p. 36).[10] Healthy people taking 10 ml (2 U.S. teaspoons) of tincture 3 times daily have been shown to have increased numbers of immune cells (T lymphocytes).

How Much Is Usually Taken?

Dried, powdered root and rhizomes of 2 to 3 grams per day can be used.[11] Concentrated solid extract standardized on eleutherosides B and E, 300 to 400 mg per day, can also be used, as can alcohol-based extracts, 8 to 10 ml in 2 to 3 divided dosages. Historically, eleuthero is taken continuously for 6 to 8 weeks, followed by a 1- to 2-week break before resuming.

Are There Any Side Effects or Interactions? Reported side effects have been minimal with use of eleuthero.[12] Mild, transient diarrhea has been reported in a very small number of users. Eleuthero may cause insomnia in some people if taken too close to bedtime. Eleuthero is not recommended for individuals with uncontrolled high blood pressure. It can be used during pregnancy or lactation. However, pregnant or lactating women using eleuthero should avoid products that have been adulterated with Panax ginseng or other related species that are contraindicated.

Ephedra
(Ephedra sinica, Ephedra intermedia, Ephedra equisetina)

Common name: Ma huang

Parts Used and Where Grown: Ephedra is a shrublike plant found in desert regions throughout the world. It is distributed from northern China to Inner Mongolia. The dried green stems of the three Asian species (*E. sinica, E. intermedia, E. equisetina*) are used medicinally. The North American species of ephedra does not appear to contain the active ingredients of its Asian counterparts.

In What Conditions Might Ephedra Be Supportive?

Ranking	Health Concerns
Secondary	Asthma (p. 15) Cough (p. 47) Weight loss and obesity (p. 165)
Other	Chronic obstructive pulmonary disease (p. 45) Congestion Hay fever (p. 76)

Historical or Traditional Use

The Chinese have used ephedra medicinally for over 5,000 years. Ephedra is listed as one of the original 365 herbs from the classical first century A.D. text on Chinese herbalism by Shen Nong.[1] Ephedra's traditional medicinal uses include the alleviation of sweating, lung and bronchial constriction, and water retention. Coughing, shortness of breath, the common cold, and fevers without sweat are all indications for its use. While the active constituent, ephedrine, was isolated in 1887, the herb did not become popular with U.S. physicians until 1924 for its bronchodilating and decongesting properties.[2]

Active Constituents

Ephedra's main active medicinal ingredients are the alkaloids ephedrine and pseudoephedrine. The stem contains 1 to 3% total alkaloids, with ephedrine accounting for 30 to 90% of this total, depending on the plant species.[3] Both ephedrine and its synthetic counterparts stimulate the central nervous system, dilate the bronchial tubes, elevate blood pressure, and increase heart rate. Pseudoephedrine (the synthetic form) is a popular over-the-counter remedy for relief of nasal congestion. Little research has been done on the whole plant (compared to its isolated alkaloids) supporting its use for any condition.

How Much Is Usually Taken?

The crude powdered stems of ephedra (with less than 1% ephedrine) are used at 1.5 to 6 grams per day in tea form.[4] Tinctures of 1 to 4 ml 3 times per day can be taken. Over-the-counter drugs containing ephedrine can be safely used by adults at 12.5 to 25 mg every 4 hours. Adults should take no more than 150 mg every 24 hours. Pseudoephedrine is typically recommended at 60 mg every 6 hours.

Are There Any Side Effects or Interactions? Ephedra has a long history of safe use at the recommended amounts. However, abuse of ephedra (and particularly ephedrine)—especially for **weight loss** (p. 164) or as a recreational drug—can lead to amphetamine-like side effects, including elevated blood pressure, rapid heartbeat, nervousness, irritability, headache, urination disturbances, vomiting, muscle disturbances, insomnia, dry mouth, heart palpitations, and even death due to heart failure.[5] One study has shown that a single dose of ephedra caused mild elevation of heart rate but did not consistently affect blood pressure in otherwise healthy adults.[6] When taken at higher levels, ephedra can cause drastic increases in blood pressure, as well as cardiac arrhythmias. Ephedrine is considered potentially habituating, though it is unclear if whole herb ephedra is likely to do the same thing.[7]

Anyone with **high blood pressure** (p. 89), heart conditions, **diabetes** (p. 53), **glaucoma** (p. 74), hyperthyroidism, **anxiety** (p. 14) or restlessness, impaired circulation to the brain, **benign prostatic hyperplasia** (p. 145) with residual urine accumulation, pheochromocytoma, and those taking MAO-inhibiting antidepressants, digitoxin, or guanethidine should consult with a physician before using any type of product containing ephedra.[8] Pseudoephedrine can cause drowsiness and should be used with caution if driving or operating machinery. Ephedra-based products should be avoided during pregnancy and lactation and used with caution in children under the age of 6 years.

Special United Kingdom Consideration: Ephedra may be prescribed by a medical doctor or dispensed by a herbal practitioner at a maximum daily dose of 1,800 mg.

Eucalyptus
(Eucalyptus globulus)

Parts Used and Where Grown: Eucalyptus is an evergreen tree native to Australia but is cultivated worldwide. The plant's leaves—and the oil that is steam-distilled from them—are used medicinally.[1]

In What Conditions Might Eucalyptus Be Supportive?

Ranking	Health Concerns
Secondary	Insect repellant Tension headache
Other	Chronic obstructive pulmonary disease (COPD) (p. 45) Cold (p. 41) Cough (p. 47) Rheumatoid arthritis (topical) (p. 151) Sinusitis (p. 156) Snoring

Historical or Traditional Use

Eucalyptus was first employed by Australian aborigines, who not only chewed the roots for water in the dry outback but used the leaves as a remedy for fevers. In the 1800s crew members of an Australian freighter developed high fevers but were able to successfully cure their condition using eucalyptus tea. Thus, eucalyptus became well known throughout Europe and the Mediterranean as the Australian fever tree. The early nineteenth-century Eclectic physicians in the United States not only employed eucalyptus oil to sterilize instruments and wounds but recommended a steam inhalation of the vapor of the oil to help treat **asthma** (p. 15), bronchitis, whooping cough, and emphysema.[2]

Active Constituents

The key ingredient in eucalyptus leaves is a volatile oil known as eucalyptol (1,8-cineol). In order to provide an effective expectorant and antiseptic action, the leaf oil should contain approximately 70 to 85% eucalyptol.[3] Eucalyptus oil is said to function in a fashion similar to that of menthol by acting on receptors in the nasal mucosa, leading to a reduction in the symptoms of, for example, nasal stuffiness.[4] Moreover, eucalyptus species have been shown to possess in vitro (test tube) antibacterial actions against such organisms as *Bacillus subtilis*[5] as well as several strains of *Streptococcus*.[6]

Peppermint (p. 451) (10 grams) and eucalyptus (5 grams) oil in combination, applied topically to the forehead and temples for 3 minutes with a small sponge, have been shown to be helpful as a muscle relaxant (but not for pain relief) in individuals with tension headaches.[7] A eucalyptus oil extract containing 50% p-methane-3,8-diol (PMD) as the active ingredient has been shown to be effective in protecting human volunteers from various types of biting insects. On human forearms, it was determined that the eucalyptus extract was nearly as effective as a 20% solution of diethyltoluamine (used in many insect repellents) in repelling bites of the *Anopheles* mosquito (the insect that spreads malaria) for up to 5 hours. Moreover, the eucalyptus extract was also effective at repelling flies (94%) and midges (100%) for up to 6 hours.[8] Uncontrolled studies suggest that the combination of eucalyptus and menthol as a nasal inhalant is helpful in cases of mild to moderate snoring.[9]

How Much Is Usually Taken?

Eucalyptol or eucalyptus oil can be taken internally by adults at a dose of 0.05 to 0.2 ml daily.[10] For local applications, 30 ml of the oil can be mixed in 500 ml of lukewarm water and applied topically as an insect repellent or used over the temporal areas of the forehead for tension headaches. Eucalyptus oil needs to be used very cautiously since as little as 3.5 ml of the oil taken internally has proven fatal.[11] It is best for individuals to discuss internal use with a qualified healthcare professional.

Are There Any Side Effects or Interactions?

Side effects from its internal use can include nausea, vomiting, and diarrhea. Eucalyptus oil should not be used by infants and young children under the age of 2, especially near the face and nose, due to the risk of laryngeal spasm and subsequent respiratory arrest.[12] Moreover, the oil may aggravate bronchial spasms in asthmatics and should not be taken internally by those with severe liver diseases and inflammatory disorders of the gastrointestinal tract and kidney.[13,14] Although there are no known reports of drug interactions, the German Commission E monographs suggest that as eucalyptus oil activates certain enzyme systems in the liver, it can weaken or shorten the action of other types of medications including pentobarbital, aminopyrine, and amphetamine.[15,16] Moreover, eucalyptus should not be used in large doses by individuals with low blood pressure.[17] The safety of eucalyptus oil has not been established in pregnant or nursing women.

Eyebright
(Euphrasia officinalis)

Parts Used and Where Grown: Euphrasia officinalis refers to a vast genus containing over 450 species. European wild plants grow in meadows, pastures, and grassy places in Bulgaria, Hungary, and the former Yugoslavia. Eyebright is also grown commercially in Europe. The plant flowers in late summer and autumn. The whole herb is used in commercial preparations.

In What Conditions Might Eyebright Be Supportive?

Ranking	Health Concerns
Other	Conjunctivitis/blepharitis (p. 44) Hay fever (p. 76) Irritated eyes

Historical or Traditional Use

Eyebright was and continues to be used primarily as a poultice for the topical treatment of eye inflammations, including **blepharitis** (p. 44), **conjunctivitis** (p. 44), and sties. A compress made from a decoction of eyebright can give rapid relief from redness, swelling, and visual disturbances in acute and subacute eye infections.[1] A tea is usually given internally along with the topical treatment. It has also been used for the treatment of eye fatigue and disturbances of vision. In addition, herbalists have recommended eyebright for problems of the respiratory tract, including sinus infections, coughs, and sore throat.[2]

Active Constituents

Eyebright is high in iridoid glycosides, flavonoids, and tannins.[3] The plant has astringent properties that probably account for its usefulness as a topical treatment for inflammatory states and its ability to reduce mucous drainage.

How Much Is Usually Taken?

Traditional herbal texts recommend a compress made with 15 grams of the dried herb combined with 500 ml (2 cups) of water and boiled for 10 minutes.[4] The undiluted liquid is used as a compress after cooling. This was commonly combined with antimicrobial herbs, such as **goldenseal** (p. 429). The German Commission E monograph on eyebright does not support this application, due to possible impurities in non-pharmaceutical preparations.[5] Consult with a physician knowledgable in the use of herbs before applying eyebright to the eyes.

Internally, eyebright tea, made using the same formula above, can be drunk in the amount of 2 to 3 cups per day. Dried herb, as 2 to 4 grams 3 times per day, may be taken. The tincture is typically taken in 2 to 6 ml 3 times per day.

Are There Any Side Effects or Interactions? Due to limited information on the active constituents in eyebright and the need for sterility in substances used topically in the eyes, the traditional use of eyebright as a topical compress currently cannot be recommended without professional support. Used internally at the amounts listed above, eyebright is generally safe. However, its safety during pregnancy and lactation has not been proven.

False Unicorn
(Chamaelirium luteum)

Parts Used and Where Grown: False unicorn is native to Mississippi and continues to grow primarily in the southern parts of the United States. The roots of false unicorn contain the greatest amounts of the active constituents.

In What Conditions Might False Unicorn Be Supportive?

Ranking	Health Concerns
Other	Amenorrhea (lack of menstruation) Menorrhagia (heavy menstruation) (p. 120) Painful menstruation (dysmenorrhea) (p. 61) Premenstrual syndrome (p. 141)

Historical or Traditional Use

The medicinal use of false unicorn root is based in Native American tradition, where it was recommended for many women's health conditions, including lack of menstruation (amenorrhea), painful menstruation, and other irregularities of menstruation, as well as to prevent miscarriages.[1] It was also used as a remedy for **morning sickness** (p. 126).

Active Constituents

Steroidal saponins are generally credited with providing false unicorn root's activity.[2] Modern investigations have not confirmed this, and no research exists about the medical applications of this herb.

How Much Is Usually Taken?

Generally, false unicorn root is taken as a tincture in the amount of 2 to 5 ml 3 times per day.[3] The dried root may be used at a dose of 1 to 2 grams 3 times daily. It is almost always taken in combination with other herbs supportive of the female reproductive organs, particularly **vitex** (p. 467).

Are There Any Side Effects or Interactions? No adverse effects have been reported with the use of false unicorn. Its long history of use in pregnant women suggests it may be safe for these individuals, but no studies have confirmed this.

Fennel
(Foeniculum vulgare)

Parts Used and Where Grown: The fennel plant came originally from Europe, where it is still grown. Fennel is also cultivated in many parts of Asia and Egypt. Fennel seeds are used for medicinal purposes.

In What Conditions Might Fennel Be Supportive?

Ranking	Health Concerns
Secondary	Colic (p. 40) Indigestion and heartburn (p. 99)
Other	Irritable bowel syndrome (p. 109)

Historical or Traditional Use

One author reports that fennel may have bestowed immortality in the Greek legend of Prometheus.[1] Fennel seeds are a common cooking spice, particularly for use with fish. After meals, they are used in several cultures to prevent gas and upset stomach.[2] The seeds are also used in Latin America to increase the flow of breast milk. Fennel has also been used as a remedy for cough and colic in infants.

Active Constituents

The main active constituents, which include the terpenoid anethole, are found in the volatile oil. Anethole and other terpenoids may have mild estrogen-like activity[3] and inhibit spasms in smooth muscles,[4] such as those in the intestinal tract. Recent studies have found fennel to possess diuretic, choleretic (increase in production of bile), pain-reducing, fever-reducing, and antimicrobial actions.[5] Fennel was formerly an official drug in the United States and was listed as being used for **indigestion** (p. 99) and possibly for stimulating milk flow in women.[6]

How Much Is Usually Taken?

Whole seeds may be chewed or used in tea. The German Commission E monograph recommends 5 to 7 grams of seeds daily.[7] To make a tea, boil 2 to 3 grams of crushed seeds in 250 ml (1 cup) of water for 10 to 15 minutes, keeping the pot covered during the process. Cool, strain, and then drink 3 cups per day. As a tincture, 2 to 4 ml can be taken 3 times per day.

Are There Any Side Effects or Interactions? No significant adverse effects have been reported. However, in rare cases fennel can cause allergic reactions of the skin and respiratory tract.[8] Anyone with an estrogen-dependent cancer should avoid fennel in large quantities until the importance of its estrogen-like activity is clarified.

Fenugreek
(Trigonella foenum-graecum)

Parts Used and Where Grown: Although originally from southeastern Europe and western Asia, fenugreek grows today in many parts of the world, including India, northern Africa, and the United States. The seeds of fenugreek contain the most potent medicinal effects of the plant.

In What Conditions Might Fenugreek Be Supportive?

Ranking	Health Concerns
Primary	Atherosclerosis (p. 17) Diabetes (p. 53) High triglycerides (p. 85)
Other	Constipation (p. 44)

Historical or Traditional Use

A wide range of uses were found for fenugreek in ancient times. Medicinally it was used for the treatment of wounds, abscesses, arthritis, bronchitis, and digestive problems. Traditional Chinese herbalists used it for kidney problems and conditions affecting the male reproductive tract.[1] Fenugreek was, and remains, a food and a spice commonly eaten in many parts of the world.

Active Constituents

The steroidal saponins account for many of the beneficial effects of fenugreek, particularly the inhibition of cholesterol absorption and synthesis.[2] The seeds are rich in dietary fiber, which may be the main reason they can lower blood sugar levels in **diabetes** (p. 53).[3] One human study found that fenugreek can

help lower **cholesterol** (p. 79) and blood sugar levels in persons with moderate **atherosclerosis** (p. 17) and non-insulin-dependent diabetes.[4] Randomized and uncontrolled studies have confirmed fenugreek helps stabilize blood sugar control in people with insulin-dependent and non-insulin-dependent diabetes.[5,6,7] It helps lower elevated cholesterol and triglyceride levels in the blood,[8] including in those with diabetes,[9] according to several controlled studies. Generally fenugreek does not lower high-density lipoprotein (HDL) cholesterol levels. This type of cholesterol is believed to be beneficial.

How Much Is Usually Taken?

Due to the somewhat bitter taste of fenugreek seeds, debitterized seeds or encapsulated products are preferred. The German Commission E monograph recommends a daily intake of 6 grams.[10] The typical range of intake for diabetes or cholesterol-lowering is 5 to 30 grams with each meal or 15 to 90 grams all at once with one meal. As a tincture, 3 to 4 ml of fenugreek can be taken up to 3 times per day.

Are There Any Side Effects or Interactions? Use of more than 100 grams of fenugreek seeds daily can cause intestinal upset and nausea. Otherwise, fenugreek is extremely safe.

Feverfew
(Tanacetum parthenium)

Parts Used and Where Grown: Feverfew grows widely across Europe and North America. The leaves are used.

In What Conditions Might Feverfew Be Supportive?

Ranking	Health Concerns
Primary	Migraine headaches (p. 121)

Historical or Traditional Use

Feverfew was mentioned in Greek medical literature as a remedy for inflammation and for menstrual discomforts. Traditional herbalists in Great Britain used it to treat fevers, arthritis, and other aches and pains.

Active Constituents

Feverfew contains a range of compounds known as sesquiterpene lactones. Over 85% of these are a compound called parthenolide. Parthenolide helps prevent excessive clumping of platelets and inhibits the release of certain chemicals, including serotonin and some

Fenugreek

inflammatory mediators.[1,2] According to several double-blind studies involving people with migraine, feverfew reduces the severity, duration, and frequency of **migraine headaches** (p. 121).[3,4,5]

How Much Is Usually Taken?

Feverfew leaf products with at least 0.2% parthenolide content are generally used. Herbal products in capsules or tablets providing at least 250 mcg of parthenolide per day may be taken.[6] It may take 4 to 6 weeks before benefits are noticed. Alcohol extracts of feverfew have not proven effective in preventing migraines.[7]

Are There Any Side Effects or Interactions? Taken as recommended, standardized feverfew causes minimal side effects. Minor side effects include gastrointestinal upset and nervousness. Chewing feverfew leaves has been known to cause mouth ulcers.[8] Feverfew is not recommended during pregnancy or lactation and should not be used by children under the age of 2 years.

Fo-Ti
(Polygonum multiflorum)

Common name: He-shou-wu

Parts Used and Where Grown: Fo-ti is a plant native to China, where it continues to be widely grown. It also grows extensively in Japan and Taiwan. The unprocessed root is sometimes used; however, once it has been boiled in a special liquid made from black beans, it is considered a superior and rather different medicine according to traditional Chinese medicine. The unprocessed root is sometimes called white fo-ti and the processed root red fo-ti.

In What Conditions Might Fo-Ti Be Supportive?

Ranking	Health Concerns
Other	Atherosclerosis (p. 17) Constipation (p. 44) Fatigue High cholesterol (p. 79) Immune function (p. 94)

Historical or Traditional Use

The Chinese common name for fo-ti, he-shou-wu, was the name of a Tang dynasty man whose infertility was supposedly cured by fo-ti; in addition, his long life was attributed to the tonic properties of this herb.[1] Since then, traditional Chinese medicine has used fo-ti to treat premature aging, weakness, vaginal discharges, numerous infectious diseases, angina pec-

toris, and impotence. Fo-ti was a meaningless name created by an entrepreneur.

Active Constituents

The active constituents of fo-ti have yet to be determined. The whole root has been shown to lower cholesterol levels, according to animal and human research, as well as to decrease hardening of the arteries, or **atherosclerosis** (p. 17).[2,3] Other fo-ti research has investigated this herb's role in strong **immune function** (p. 94), red blood cell formation, and antibacterial action.[4] The unprocessed roots have a mild laxative action.

How Much Is Usually Taken?

The typical daily intake is 4 to 8 grams.[5] A tea can be made from processed roots by boiling ½ to 1 U.S. teaspoons (3 to 5 grams) in 250 ml (1 cup) of water for 10 to 15 minutes. Three or more cups are drunk each day. Fo-ti tablets (500 mg each) can be taken in the amount of five tablets 3 times per day.

Are There Any Side Effects or Interactions? The unprocessed roots may cause mild diarrhea.[6] Some people who are sensitive to fo-ti may develop a skin rash. Taking more than 15 grams of processed root powder may cause numbness in the arms or legs.

Garlic
(Allium sativum)

Parts Used and Where Grown: Garlic is closely related to onion and chives. The largest commercial garlic production is in central California. The bulb is used.

In What Conditions Might Garlic Be Supportive?

Ranking	Health Concerns
Primary	High blood pressure (p. 89) High triglycerides (p. 85) Intermittent claudication (p. 106)
Secondary	Atherosclerosis (p. 17) Athlete's foot (p. 20) Bronchitis High cholesterol (p. 79)
Other	Ear infections (recurrent) (p. 63) HIV support (p. 87) Infection (p. 63) Influenza (p. 104) Parasites (p. 137) Peptic ulcer (p. 138) Raynaud's disease (p. 148) Vaginitis (p. 162) Yeast infection (p. 169)

Historical or Traditional Use

Garlic is mentioned in the Bible and the Talmud. Hippocrates, Galen, Pliny the Elder, and Dioscorides all mention the use of garlic for many conditions, including parasites, respiratory problems, poor digestion, and low energy. Its use in China was first mentioned in A.D. 510. Louis Pasteur confirmed the antibacterial action of garlic in 1858.

Active Constituents

The sulfur compound allicin, produced by crushing or chewing fresh garlic, in turn produces other sulfur compounds: ajoene, allyl sulfides, and vinyldithiins.[1]

Cardiovascular Actions: Many publications have shown that garlic supports the cardiovascular system. It may mildly lower **cholesterol** (p. 79) and **triglyceride** (p. 85) levels in the blood, inhibit platelet stickiness (aggregation), and increase fibrinolysis[2]—which results in a slowing of blood coagulation. It is mildly **antihypertensive**[3] (p. 89) and has **antioxidant** (p. 267) activity.[4] Three reviews of double-blind studies in humans have found that garlic can lower blood cholesterol levels in adults by approximately 10%.[5,6,7] Garlic has been shown to be as effective as the drug bezafibrate in lowering cholesterol levels.[8] However, a recent placebo-controlled study found no effect for garlic on lowering cholesterol.[9] Several double-blind studies also suggest it can prevent **atherosclerosis** (p. 17).[10] Garlic is also helpful for persons with **intermittent claudication** (p. 106) (cramping in the lower legs secondary to poor blood flow), according to one controlled study.[11]

Antimicrobial Actions: Garlic has antibacterial, antiviral, and antifungal activity.[12] It may work against some intestinal **parasites** (p. 137). Garlic appears to have roughly 1% the strength of penicillin against certain types of bacteria. This means it is not a substitute for antibiotics but it can be considered as a support against some bacterial infections. *Candida albicans* growth is inhibited by garlic, and garlic has shown long-term benefit for recurrent **yeast infections** (p. 169). However, controlled human studies have yet to show garlic helps for yeast infections.

Anticancer Actions: Human population studies show that eating garlic regularly reduces the risk of esophageal, stomach, and colon cancer.[13] This is partly due to garlic's ability to reduce the formation of carcinogenic compounds. Animal and test tube studies also show that garlic and its sulfur compounds inhibit the growth of different types of cancer—especially breast and skin tumors.

How Much Is Usually Taken?

Some people chew one whole clove of raw garlic per day. For those who prefer it, odor-controlled, enteric-coated tablets or capsules with standardized allicin potential can be taken in amounts of 600 to 900 mg in 2 or 3 divided doses (providing up to 5,000 mcg of allicin potential).[14,15]

Are There Any Side Effects or Interactions? Most people enjoy garlic; however, some individuals who are sensitive to it may experience heartburn and flatulence. Because of garlic's anticlotting properties, persons taking anticoagulant drugs should check with their nutritionally oriented doctor before taking garlic.[16] Those scheduled for surgery should inform their surgeon if they are taking garlic supplements. Garlic is not contraindicated during pregnancy and lactation. In fact, two studies have shown that babies like breast milk better from mothers who eat garlic.[17,18]

Gentian
(Gentiana lutea)

Parts Used and Where Grown: This plant comes from meadows in Europe and Turkey. It is also cultivated in North America. The root is used medicinally.

In What Conditions Might Gentian Be Supportive?

Ranking	Health Concerns
Other	Indigestion (p. 90) Poor appetite

Historical or Traditional Use

Gentian root and other highly bitter plants have been used for centuries in Europe as digestive aids (the well-known Swedish bitters often contain gentian). Other folk uses included topical use on skin tumors, decreasing fevers, and treatment of diarrhea.[1] Its ability to increase digestive function, including production of stomach acid, has been validated in modern times.

Active Constituents

Gentian contains some of the most bitter substances known, particularly the glycosides gentiopicrin and amarogentin. The taste of these can be detected even when diluted 50,000 times.[2] Besides stimulating secretion of saliva in the mouth and hydrochloric acid in the stomach, gentiopicrin may protect the liver.[3] It is considered useful for poor appetite and **indigestion** (p. 99) according to the German government's Commission E monograph.[4]

How Much Is Usually Taken?

Gentian can be taken as a tincture (1 to 3 grams daily), as a fluid extract (2 to 4 grams daily), or as the whole root (2 to 4 grams daily).[5]

Are There Any Side Effects or Interactions? Gentian should not be used by people suffering from excessive stomach acid, **heartburn** (p. 99), **stomach ulcers** (p. 138), or **gastritis** (p. 71).[6]

Ginger
(Zingiber officinale)

Parts Used and Where Grown: Ginger is a perennial plant that grows in India, China, Mexico, and several other countries. The rhizome (underground stem) is used.

In What Conditions Might Ginger Be Supportive?

Ranking	Health Concerns
Primary	Morning sickness (p. 126) Motion sickness (p. 126) Nausea and vomiting following surgery
Other	Atherosclerosis (p. 17) Migraine headaches (p. 121) Rheumatoid arthritis (p. 151)

Historical or Traditional Use

Traditional Chinese medicine has recommended ginger for over 2,500 years. It is used for abdominal bloating, coughing, vomiting, diarrhea, and rheumatism. Ginger is commonly used in the Ayurvedic and Tibb systems of medicine for the treatment of inflammatory joint diseases, such as arthritis.

Active Constituents

The dried rhizome of ginger contains approximately 1 to 4% volatile oils. These are the medically active constituents of ginger, and they are also responsible for ginger's characteristic odor and taste. The aromatic principles include zingiberene and bisabolene, while the pungent principles are known as gingerols and shogaols.[1] The pungent constituents are credited with the antinausea and antivomiting effects of ginger.

Digestive System Actions: Ginger is a classic tonic for the digestive tract. Classified as an aromatic bitter, it stimulates digestion. It also keeps the intestinal muscles toned.[2] This action eases the transport of substances through the digestive tract, lessening irritation to the intestinal walls.[3] Ginger may protect the stomach from the damaging effect of alcohol and nonsteroidal anti-inflammatory drugs (such as ibuprofen) and may help prevent **ulcers** (p. 138).[4]

Antinausea/Antivomiting Actions: Research is inconclusive as to how ginger acts to alleviate nausea. Ginger may act directly on the gastrointestinal system, it may affect the part of the central nervous system that causes nausea,[5,6] it may exert a dual effect in reducing nausea and vomiting. Double-blind research has shown that ginger reduces nausea after surgery, although one study could not confirm this benefit.[7,8] However, the common antinausea drug droperidol was also ineffective in this study.[9] Other studies have found ginger helpful for preventing **motion sickness** (p. 126),[10] chemotherapy-induced nausea,[11] and nausea of **pregnancy** (p. 143).[12]

Circulatory Actions: Ginger also supports a healthy cardiovascular system. Like **garlic** (p. 425), ginger makes blood platelets less sticky and less likely to aggregate; however, not all human research has confirmed this. A high dose (10 grams) of ginger can inhibit excessive platelet aggregation in humans,[13] but lower doses taken for longer do not seem to have this effect.[14,15] This action reduces a major risk factor for **atherosclerosis** (p. 17).[16]

How Much Is Usually Taken?

Some herbalists suggest the use of 2 to 4 grams of the dried rhizome powder 2 to 3 times per day or a tincture of 1.5 to 3 ml 3 times daily. For treatment of nausea, approximately 250 to 500 mg should be taken every 2 to 3 hours. For prevention of motion sickness, ginger tablets, capsules, or liquid herbal extract should be taken 2 days before the planned trip. Pregnant women should not exceed 1 gram daily.[17]

Are There Any Side Effects or Interactions? Side effects of ginger are rare when used as recommended. However, some people may be sensitive to the taste or may experience heartburn. Persons with a history of **gallstones** (p. 69) should consult a nutritionally oriented doctor before using ginger.[18] Short-term use of ginger for nausea and vomiting during pregnancy appears to pose no safety problems; however, long-term use during pregnancy is not recommended. A doctor should be informed if ginger is used before surgery.

Ginkgo biloba

Common name: Maidenhair tree

Parts Used and Where Grown: Ginkgo biloba is the world's longest living species of tree; individual trees live as long as 1,000 years. Ginkgo grows most prominently in the southern and eastern United States and in China. The leaves of the tree are used.

Historical or Traditional Use

Medicinal use of ginkgo can be traced back almost 5,000 years in Chinese herbal medicine. The nuts of the tree were most commonly recommended and used to treat respiratory tract ailments. A tea of the leaves was occasionally used for elderly persons experiencing memory loss.

In What Conditions Might Ginkgo Biloba Be Supportive?

Ranking	Health Concerns
Primary	Age-related cognitive decline (p. 11) Alzheimer's disease (p. 11) Intermittent claudication (p. 106)
Secondary	Atherosclerosis (p. 17) Depression (for elderly persons) (p. 50) Impotence (of vascular origin) (p. 98) Macular degeneration (p. 118) Retinopathy (p. 150) Vertigo
Other	Asthma (p. 15) Depression (p. 50) Diabetes (p. 53) Migraine headaches (p. 121) Raynaud's disease (p. 148) Tinnitus (p. 158)

Active Constituents

The medical benefits of *Ginkgo biloba* extract (GBE) rely primarily on two groups of active components: the ginkgo flavone glycosides and the terpene lactones. The 24% ginkgo flavone glycoside designation on GBE labels indicates the carefully measured balance of **bioflavonoids** (p. 271). These bioflavonoids are primarily responsible for GBE's **antioxidant activity** (p. 267) and ability to inhibit platelet aggregation (stickiness). These two actions may help GBE prevent circulatory diseases such as **atherosclerosis** (p. 17) and support the brain and central nervous system.[1]

The unique terpene lactone components found in GBE, known as ginkgolides and bilobalide, typically make up 6% of the extract. They are associated with increased circulation to the brain and other parts of the body, as well as exertion of protective action on nerve cells.[2,3] Ginkgolides may improve circulation and inhibit platelet-activating factor (PAF). Bilobalide protects the cells of the nervous system. Recent animal studies indicate that bilobalide may help regenerate damaged nerve cells.

Circulatory Actions: GBE increases circulation to both the brain and extremities of the body. In addition to inhibiting platelet stickiness, GBE regulates the tone and elasticity of blood vessels.[4] In other words, it makes circulation more efficient. This improvement in circulation efficiency extends to both large vessels (arteries) and smaller vessels (capillaries) in the circulatory system.[5]

Cognitive Function: Recently, the ginkgo extract EGb 761 was found to increase alpha wave and decrease theta wave activity following oral intakes of 120 or 240 mg in healthy volunteers.[6] These brain wave changes indicate that EGb 761 is capable of improving cognitive function as demonstrated in increased mental sharpness, concentration, and memory. Three double-blind studies have now shown that GBE is helpful for persons in early stages of **Alzheimer's disease** (p. 11), as well as the closely related multi-infarct dementia.[7,8,9] People with other types of dementia also respond to GBE, including (as mentioned above) problems due to poor blood flow to the brain.

Antioxidant Properties: GBE has antioxidant actions in the brain, retina of the eye, and the cardiovascular system.[10] One double-blind study found that GBE could help people with **macular degeneration** (p. 118), an oxidation-related disorder causing decreased or lost vision.[11] Diabetic retinopathy is also improved by GBE, according to a double-blind study.[12] Its antioxidant activity in the brain and central nervous system may help prevent age-related declines in brain function. GBE's antioxidant activity in the brain is of particular interest. The brain and central nervous system are particularly susceptible to **free radical attack** (p. 267). Free radical damage in the brain is widely accepted as being a contributing factor in many disorders associated with aging, including Alzheimer's disease.[13]

Antidepressant Action: One double-blind study in Germany found that elderly depressed people (p. 50) with mild dementia (who were not responding to antidepressant medications) responded well to GBE supplementation.[14]

Nerve Protection and PAF Inhibition: One of the primary protective actions of the ginkgolides is their ability to inhibit the substance known as platelet-activating factor (PAF).[15] PAF is a mediator released from cells that causes platelets to aggregate (clump together). High amounts of PAF are associated with damage to nerve cells, poor blood flow to the central nervous system, inflammatory conditions, and bronchial constriction.[16] Much like free radicals, higher PAF levels are also associated with aging.[17] Ginkgolides and bilobalide protect nerve cells in the central nervous system from damage during periods of ischemia (lack of oxygen to tissues in the body).[18] This action may be supportive for persons who have suffered a stroke.

Tinnitus and Balance: Ginkgo may improve **tinnitus** (ringing in the ears) (p. 158) and balance problems related to the inner ear, an important part of maintaining balance. Double-blind studies have confirmed

Ginkgo biloba

the benefit of GBE for people with tinnitus or vertigo.[19,20]

How Much Is Usually Taken?

Most research studies have used between 120 to 240 mg of GBE, standardized to contain 6% terpene lactones and 24% flavone glycosides per day, generally divided into 2 or 3 portions.[21] Relatively high (240 mg per day) amounts have been used in reports studying people with age-associated memory loss, mild cognitive impairment, mild to moderate Alzheimer's disease, and resistant depression. GBE may need to be taken for 6 to 8 weeks before desired actions are noticed. Although non-standardized leaf and tinctures are available, there is no well-established dosage for these forms.

Are There Any Side Effects or Interactions? Ginkgo biloba extract is essentially devoid of any serious side effects.[22] Mild headaches lasting for a day or two and mild upset stomach have been reported in a very small percentage of people using GBE. GBE is not contraindicated for pregnant and lactating women.

Circulatory conditions in the elderly can involve serious disease. Individuals should seek proper medical care and accurate medical diagnosis prior to self-prescribing GBE.

Goldenseal
(Hydrastis canadensis)

Parts Used and Where Grown: Goldenseal is native to eastern North America and is cultivated in Oregon and Washington. It is seriously threatened in the wild by overharvesting. The dried root and rhizome are used.

In What Conditions Might Goldenseal Be Supportive?

Ranking	Health Concerns
Secondary	Bronchitis Diarrhea (berberine) (p. 58)
Other	Cold sores (p. 39) Common cold/sore throat (p. 41) Conjunctivitis/blepharitis (p. 44) Crohn's disease (p. 48) Gastritis (p. 71) Influenza (p. 104) Pap smear (abnormal) (p. 136) Parasites (p. 137) Urinary tract infection (p. 160) Vaginitis (p. 162)

Historical or Traditional Use

Goldenseal was used by the Native Americans as a treatment for irritations and inflammation of the mucous membranes of the respiratory, digestive, and urinary tracts. It was commonly used topically for skin and eye infections. Because of its antimicrobial activity, goldenseal has a long history of use for infectious diarrhea, upper respiratory tract infections, and vaginal infections. Goldenseal is often recommended in combination with **echinacea** (p. 417) for the treatment of colds and flu. Goldenseal was considered a critical remedy for stomach and intestinal problems of all kinds by turn-of-the-century physicians called the Eclectics.[1]

Active Constituents

The two primary alkaloids in goldenseal are hydrastine and berberine, along with smaller amounts of canadine. Little research has been done with goldenseal itself. Berberine, which ranges from 0.5 to 6.0% of the alkaloids present in goldenseal root and rhizome, has been the most extensively researched. It appears to have a wide spectrum of antibiotic activity against pathogens, such as *Chlamydia* species, *E. coli*, *Salmonella typhi,* and *Entamoeba histolytica*.[2] Human studies have used isolated berberine to treat **diarrhea** (p. 58) and gastroenteritis with good results.[3] The whole root has not been clinically studied.

How Much Is Usually Taken?

Powdered goldenseal root and rhizome can be used in the amount of 4 to 6 grams per day in tablet or capsule form.[4] For liquid herbal extracts, 2 to 4 ml 3 times per day are used. Standardized extracts supplying 8 to 1,290 alkaloids are available. Recommended dose is 250 to 500 mg 3 times per day. Continuous use should not exceed 3 weeks, with a break of at least 2 weeks between use. Goldenseal powder as a tea or tincture may soothe a sore throat. Due to environmental concerns of overharvesting,[5] many herbalists recommend alternatives to goldenseal, such as **Oregon grape** (p. 449) or goldenthread.

Are There Any Side Effects or Interactions? Taken as recommended, goldenseal is generally safe. However, as with all alkaloid-containing plants, high amounts may lead to gastrointestinal distress and possible nervous system effects.[6] Goldenseal is not recommended for pregnant or lactating women. Despite some traditional reports, goldenseal is not a substitute for antibiotics.

Goldenseal

Gotu Kola
(Centella asiatica)

Parts Used and Where Grown: This ground-hugging plant grows in a widespread distribution in tropical, swampy areas, including parts of India, Pakistan, Sri Lanka, Madagascar, and South Africa. It also grows in Eastern Europe. The roots and leaves are used medicinally.

In What Conditions Might Gotu Kola Be Supportive?

Ranking	Health Concerns
Secondary	Minor injuries (p. 122) Wound healing (p. 167)
Other	Burns (minor) (p. 29) Chronic venous insufficiency (p. 38) Scars Scleroderma Skin ulcers Varicose veins (p. 163)

Historical or Traditional Use

Gotu kola has been important in the medicinal systems of central Asia for centuries. It was purported in Sri Lanka to prolong life, as the leaves are commonly eaten by elephants. Numerous skin diseases, ranging from poorly healing wounds to leprosy, have been treated with gotu kola. Gotu kola also has a historical reputation for boosting mental activity and for helping a variety of systemic illnesses, such as high blood pressure, rheumatism, fever, and nervous disorders. Some of its common uses in Ayurvedic medicine include heart disease, water retention, hoarseness, bronchitis, and coughs in children and as a poultice for many skin conditions.[1]

Active Constituents

Saponins (also called triterpenoids) known as asiaticoside, madecassoside, and madasiatic acid are the primary active constituents.[2] These saponins beneficially affect collagen (the material that makes up connective tissue), for example, inhibiting its production in hyperactive scar tissue. One uncontrolled study in humans found that a gotu kola extract helped heal infected wounds (unless they had reached bone).[3] A review of French studies suggests that topical gotu kola can help **burns** (p. 29) and **wounds** (p. 167).[4] Double-blind studies have also shown it can help

those with **chronic venous insufficiency** (p. 38).[5,6] One study found gotu kola extract helpful for preventing and treating enlarged scars (keloids).[7]

How Much Should I Take?

Dried gotu kola leaf can be made into a tea by adding 1 to 2 U.S. teaspoons (5 to 10 grams) to 150 ml of boiling water and allowing it to steep for 10 to 15 minutes. Three cups are usually drunk per day. Tincture can also be used at a dose of 3 to 5 ml 3 times per day. Standardized extracts containing up to 100% total triterpenoids are generally taken as 60 mg once or twice per day.[8]

Are There Any Side Effects or Interactions? Except for the rare person who is allergic to gotu kola, no significant adverse effects are experienced with internal or topical use of this herb.[9]

Green Tea
(Camellia sinensis)

Parts Used and Where Grown: All teas (green, black, and oolong) are derived from the same plant, *Camellia sinensis.* The difference is in how the plucked leaves are prepared. Green tea, unlike black and oolong tea, is not fermented, so the active constituents remain unaltered in the herb. The leaves of the tea plant are used as both a social and medicinal beverage.

In What Conditions Might Green Tea Be Supportive?

Ranking	Health Concerns
Secondary	Gingivitis (periodontal disease) (p. 73)
Other	Cancer risk reduction Crohn's disease (p. 48) High triglycerides (p. 85) Immune function (p. 94) Infection (p. 101)

Historical or Traditional Use

According to Chinese legend, tea was discovered accidentally by an emperor 4,000 years ago. Since then, traditional Chinese medicine has recommended green tea for headaches, body aches and pains, digestion, depression, immune enhancement, detoxification, as an energizer, and to prolong life. Modern research has confirmed many of these health benefits.

Active Constituents

Green tea contains volatile oils, vitamins, minerals, and caffeine, but the active constituents are polyphenols, particularly the catechin called epigallocatechin gallate (EGCG). The polyphenols are believed to be responsible for most of green tea's roles in promoting good health.[1]

Research demonstrates that green tea mildly guards against cardiovascular disease in many ways. Green tea lowers total **cholesterol levels** (p. 79) and improves the cholesterol profile (the ratio of LDL cholesterol to HDL cholesterol), reduces platelet aggregation, and lowers **blood pressure** (p. 89).[2,3,4,5] However, not all studies have found that green tea intake lowers lipid levels.[6]

Green tea's effectiveness as an **antioxidant** (p. 267) remains unclear. While some studies show that green tea is an antioxidant in humans,[7] others have not been able to confirm that it protects LDL cholesterol from damage.[8] Oxidation of LDL cholesterol is thought to be important in causing or accelerating **atherosclerosis** (p. 17).

The polyphenols in green tea have also been shown to lessen the risk of cancers of several sites, stimulate the production of several **immune system** (p. 94) cells, and have antibacterial properties—even against the bacteria that cause dental plaque.[9,10,11]

One study found that intake of 10 cups or more of green tea per day improved blood test results, indicating protection against liver damage.[12] Further studies are needed to determine whether taking green tea helps those with liver diseases.

How Much Is Usually Taken?

Much of the research documenting the health benefits of green tea is based on the amount of green tea typically drunk in Asian countries—about 3 cups per day (providing 240 to 320 mg of polyphenols).[13] To brew green tea, 1 U.S. teaspoon (5 grams) of green tea leaves are combined with 250 ml (1 cup) of boiling water and steeped for 3 minutes. Decaffeinated tea is recommended to reduce the side effects associated with caffeine, including anxiety and insomnia. Tablets and capsules containing standardized extracts of polyphenols, particularly EGCG, are available; some provide up to 97% polyphenol content—which is equivalent to drinking 4 cups of tea. Many of these standardized products are decaffeinated.

Are There Any Side Effects or Interactions? Green tea is generally free of side effects; the most common adverse effects reported from consuming large amounts (several cups per day) of green tea are insomnia, anxiety, and other symptoms caused by the caffeine content in the herb.

Guaraná
(Paullinia cupana)

Parts Used and Where Grown: The vast majority of guaraná is grown in a small area in northern Brazil. Guaraná gum or paste is derived from the seeds and is used in herbal supplements.

In What Conditions Might Guaraná Be Supportive?

Ranking	Health Concerns
Other	Athletic performance (p. 20) Fatigue Weight loss and obesity (p. 165)

Historical or Traditional Use

The indigenous people of the Amazon rain forest used crushed guaraná seed as a beverage and a medicine. Guaraná was said to treat diarrhea, decrease fatigue, reduce hunger, and help arthritis.[1] It also has a history of use in treating hangovers from alcohol abuse, and headaches related to menstruation.

Active Constituents

Guaranine (which is nearly identical to caffeine) and the closely related alkaloids theobromine and theophylline make up the primary active agents in guaraná. Caffeine's effects (and hence those of guaranine) are well known and include stimulating the central nervous system, increasing metabolic rate, and having a mild diuretic effect.[2] One long-term study found no significant actions on thinking or mental function in humans taking guaraná.[3] Caffeine may have adverse effects on the blood vessels and other body systems, as well as on a developing fetus; presumably, guaranine would have similar effects. Guaraná also contains tannins, which act as astringents and may prevent **diarrhea** (p. 58).

How Much Is Usually Taken?

A cup of guaraná tea, prepared by adding 1 to 2 grams of crushed seed or resin to 250 ml (1 cup) of water and boiling for 10 minutes, can be drunk 3 times per day.[4] Each cup may provide up to 50 mg of guaranine.

Are There Any Side Effects or Interactions? As with any caffeinated product, guaraná may cause insomnia, trembling, anxiety, palpitations, urinary frequency, and hyperactivity.[5] Guaraná should be avoided during pregnancy and lactation.

Guggul
(Commiphora mukul)

Common names: Gugulipid, gum guggulu

Parts Used and Where Grown: The mukul myrrh *(Commiphora mukul)* tree is a small, thorny plant distributed throughout India. Guggul and gum guggulu are the names given to a yellowish resin produced by the stem of the plant. This resin has been used historically and is also the source of modern extracts of guggul.

In What Conditions Might Guggul Be Supportive?

Ranking	Health Concerns
Primary	Atherosclerosis (p. 17)
	High cholesterol (p. 79)
	High triglycerides (p. 85)

Historical or Traditional Use

The classical treatise on Ayurvedic medicine, Sushrita Samhita, describes the use of guggul for a wide variety of conditions, including arthritis and obesity. One of its primary indications was a condition known as *medoroga*. This ancient diagnosis is similar to the modern description of atherosclerosis. Guggul was primarily used to prevent this condition by lowering serum cholesterol and triglyceride levels.

Active Constituents

Guggul contains resin, volatile oils, and gum. The extract isolates ketonic steroid compounds known as guggulsterones. These compounds have been shown to provide the lipid-lowering actions noted for guggul.[1] Guggul significantly lowers serum **triglycerides** (p. 85) and **cholesterol** (p. 79) as well as LDL and VLDL cholesterols (the "bad" cholesterols).[2] At the same time, it raises levels of HDL cholesterol (the "good" cholesterol). As **antioxidants** (p. 267), guggulsterones keep LDL cholesterol from oxidizing which protects against **atherosclerosis** (p. 17).[3] Guggul has also been shown to reduce the stickiness of platelets—another effect that lowers the risk of coronary artery disease.[4] One study found guggul extract similar to the drug clofibrate for lowering cholesterol levels.[5] Clinical studies in India have consistently confirmed guggul extracts improve lipid levels in humans.[6]

How Much Is Usually Taken?

Daily recommendations for guggul are typically based on the amount of guggulsterones in the extract.[7] A common intake of guggulsterones is 25 mg 3 times per day. Most extracts contain 5 to 10% guggulsterones and can be taken daily for 12 to 24 weeks.

Are There Any Side Effects or Interactions? Early studies with the crude oleoresin reported numerous side effects, including diarrhea, anorexia, abdominal pain, and skin rash.[8] Modern extracts are more purified, and fewer side effects (such as mild abdominal discomfort) have been reported with long-term use. Guggul should be used with caution by persons with liver disease and in cases of inflammatory bowel disease and diarrhea. A physician should be consulted for any case of elevated cholesterol and triglycerides.

Gymnema
(Gymnema sylvestre)

Common names: Gurmarbooti, gurmar

Parts Used and Where Grown: Gymnema sylvestre is a woody climbing plant that grows in the tropical forests of central and southern India. The leaves are used in herbal medicine preparations. *G. sylvestre* is known as periploca of the woods in English and meshasringi (meaning "ram's horn") in Sanskrit. The leaves, when chewed, interfere with the ability to taste sweetness, which explains the Hindi name gurmar "destroyer of sugar."

In What Conditions Might Gymnema Be Supportive?

Ranking	Health Concerns
Secondary	Diabetes (p. 53)

Historical or Traditional Use

Gymnema has been used in India for the treatment of diabetes for over 2,000 years. The primary application was for adult-onset diabetes (NIDDM), a condition for which it continues to be recommended today in India. The leaves were also used for stomach ailments, constipation, water retention, and liver disease.

Active Constituents

The hypoglycemic (blood sugar-lowering) action of gymnema leaves was first documented in the late 1920s.[1] This action is gradual in nature, differing from the rapid effect of many prescription hypoglycemic drugs. Gymnema leaves raise insulin levels, according to research in healthy volunteers.[2] According to animal studies, this may be due to regeneration of the cells in the pancreas that secrete insulin.[3] The leaves are also noted for lowering serum **cholesterol** (p. 79) and **triglycerides** (p. 85).[4] While studies have shown that a water-soluble acidic fraction of the leaves provides hypoglycemic actions, the specific constituent in the leaves responsible for this action has not been clearly identified. Some researchers have suggested gymnemic acid as one possible candidate.[5] Further research is needed to clearly determine which constituent is responsible for this effect. Gurmarin, another constituent of the leaves, and gymnemic acid have been shown to block the ability to taste sweets in humans.[6]

How Much Is Usually Taken?

Recent studies in India have used 400 mg per day of a water-soluble acidic fraction of the gymnema leaves. In adult-onset diabetics, ongoing use for periods as long as 18 to 24 months has proven successful.[7] In people with IDDM (juvenile onset) diabetes, a similar amount has been used successfully as an adjunct to ongoing use of insulin.[8] The extract used in these studies contains approximately 2,990 gymnemic acids. Consult closely with a physician, as insulin doses may need to be lowered while taking gymnema. Traditionally, 2 to 4 grams of the leaf powder per day is used.

Are There Any Side Effects or Interactions? Used at the amounts suggested, gymnema is generally safe and devoid of side effects. The safety of gymnema during pregnancy and lactation has not yet been determined. Persons with NIDDM should only use gymnema to lower blood sugar under the clinical supervision of a health-care professional. Gymnema cannot be used in place of insulin to control blood sugar by persons with IDDM or NIDDM.

Hawthorn
(Crataegus laevigata, Crataegus oxyacantha, Crataegus monogyna)

Parts Used and Where Grown: Hawthorn is commonly found in Europe, western Asia, North America, and North Africa. Modern medicinal extracts use the leaves and flowers. Traditional preparations use the ripe fruit.

Historical or Traditional Use

Dioscorides, a Greek herbalist, used hawthorn in the first century A.D. Although numerous passing mentions are made for a variety of conditions, support for the heart is the main benefit of hawthorn.

In What Conditions Might Hawthorn Be Supportive?

Ranking	Health Concerns
Primary	Angina (p. 13) Congestive heart failure (p. 43)
Other	Atherosclerosis (p. 17)

Active Constituents

The leaves, flowers, and berries of hawthorn contain a variety of bioflavonoid-like complexes that appear to be primarily responsible for the cardiac actions of the plant. **Bioflavonoids** (p. 271) found in hawthorn include **oligomeric procyanidins** (OPCs [p. 324]), vitexin, **quercetin** (p. 328), and hyperoside. The action of these compounds on the cardiovascular system has led to the development of leaf and flower extracts, which are widely used in Europe.

Clinical Actions: Hawthorn has numerous beneficial actions on the heart and blood vessels. It may improve coronary artery blood flow[1] and the contractions of the heart muscle.[2] Also, it may mildly inhibit angiotensin-converting enzyme (ACE) and reduce production of the potent blood vessel-constricting substance angiotensin II. This reduces resistance in arteries and improves extremity circulation. The bioflavonoids in hawthorn are potent **antioxidants** (p. 267).[3] Hawthorn extracts may mildly lower **blood pressure** (p. 89) in some individuals with high blood pressure but should not be thought of as a substitute for cardiac medications for this condition. Clinical trials have confirmed hawthorn is beneficial for persons with stage II **congestive heart failure** (p. 43).[4,5] It has been shown to be as effective as the diuretic drug captopril for congestive heart failure.[6] Congestive heart failure is a serious medical condition that requires expert management rather than self-treatment. Other studies have shown it may help those with stable **angina** (p. 13).[7]

How Much Is Usually Taken?

Extracts of the leaves and flowers are most commonly used by nutritionally oriented doctors. Hawthorn extracts standardized for total bioflavonoid content (usually 2.2%) or oligomeric procyanidins (usually 18.75%) are often used. Many nutritionally oriented doctors recommend 80 to 300 mg of the herbal extract in capsules or tablets 2 to 3 times per day.[8] If traditional berry preparations are used, the

Hawthorn

recommendation is at least 4 to 5 grams per day or a tincture of 4 to 5 ml 3 times daily. Hawthorn may take 1 to 2 months for maximum effect and should be considered a long-term therapy.

Are There Any Side Effects or Interactions? Hawthorn is extremely safe for long-term use. People taking prescription cardiac medications should consult with their prescribing doctor or an herbally oriented doctor before using hawthorn-containing products. Hawthorn is not contraindicated during pregnancy or lactation.

Hops
(Humulus lupulus)

Parts Used and Where Grown: The hops plant, Humulus lupulus, is a climbing plant native to Europe, Asia, and North America. Hops are the cone-like, fruiting bodies (strobiles) of the plant and are typically harvested from cultivated female plants. Hops are most commonly used as a flavoring agent in beer.

In What Conditions Might Hops Be Supportive?

Ranking	Health Concerns
Other	Anxiety (p. 14)
	Insomnia (p. 105)

Historical or Traditional Use

Soothing the stomach and promoting healthy digestion have been the strongest historical use of this herb. Hops tea was also recommended as a mild sedative and remedy for insomnia, particularly for those with insomnia resulting from an upset stomach.[1] A pillow filled with hops was commonly used to encourage sleep. Traditionally, hops were also thought to have a diuretic effect and to treat sexual neuroses. A poultice of hops was used topically to treat sores and skin injuries and to relieve muscle spasms and nerve pain.[2]

Active Constituents

Hops are high in bitter substances. The two primary bitter principles are known as humulone and lupulone.[3] These bitter principles are thought to be responsible for the appetite-stimulating properties of hops. Hops also contain about 1 to 3% volatile oils. Hops have been shown to have mild sedative properties. Many herbal preparations for insomnia combine hops with more potent sedative herbs, such as **valerian**

(p. 467). Hops also contain phytoestrogens that bind estrogen receptors in cells but have only mild estrogen-like actions.[4]

How Much Is Usually Taken?

The German Commission E monograph recommends 500 mg for anxiety or insomnia.[5] This can be repeated 3 to 4 times daily. The dried fruits can be made into a tea by pouring 150 ml of boiling water over 1 to 2 U.S. teaspoons (5 to 10 grams) of the fruit. Steep for 10 to 15 minutes before drinking. Tinctures can be taken in amounts of 1 to 2 ml 2 or 3 times per day. Dried hops in tablet or capsule form can also be taken in amounts of 500 to 1,000 mg 2 or 3 times per day. As mentioned above, many herbal preparations use hops in combination with herbal sedatives, including valerian, **passion flower** (p. 449), and **scullcap** (p. 459).

Are There Any Side Effects or Interactions? Use of hops is generally safe and no contraindications or potential interactions with other medications are known. Some persons have been reported to experience an allergic skin rash after handling the dried flowers; this is most likely due to a pollen sensitivity.[6] Hops may worsen depression. Long-term exposure in male hops pickers causes gynecomastia (enlargement of breasts).

Horehound
(Marrubium vulgare)

Parts Used and Where Grown: Horehound is a perennial plant with small white flowers found growing in the wild throughout Europe and Asia. The entire pleasant-tasting herb is used medicinally.[1]

In What Conditions Might Horehound Be Supportive?

Ranking	Health Concerns
Other	Bronchitis
	Chronic obstructive pulmonary disease (COPD) (p. 45)
	Cough (p. 47)
	Indigestion (p. 99)
	Morning sickness (p. 126)

Historical or Traditional Use

Horehound was first employed in ancient Rome by the physician Galen, who recommended it as a therapy for coughs and other respiratory ailments. Like Galen, Nicholas Culpeper, the seventeenth-century

English herbalist, commented that it was helpful for a **cough** (p. 47) and was also useful in expectorating stubborn phlegm from the lung. Similarly, American Eclectic physicians of the nineteenth century remarked on its value as a medicinal plant not only for cough and **asthma** (p. 15) but also in menstrual complaints.[2]

Active Constituents

Horehound contains a number of constituents, including alkaloids, flavonoids, diterpenes (e.g., marrubiin), and trace amount of volatile oils.[3] The major active constituent is marrubiin and it, along with some of the volatile oils found in the herb, is believed to be responsible for expectorant action. In addition, marrubiin and possibly its precursor premarrubin are herbal bitters that increase the flow of saliva and gastric juice, thereby stimulating the appetite.[4]

How Much Is Usually Taken?

For adults, the German Commission E monograph recommends 4.5 grams of horehound per day or 2 to 6 tablespoons of the pressed juice.[5] Alternatively, horehound can be taken as a tea (1 to 2 grams of the crude dried herb) 3 times per day or as a liquid extract 2 to 4 ml 3 times per day.[6]

Are There Any Side Effects or Interactions? Because horehound acts as a bitter, individuals with stomach or intestinal ulcers should probably not use this herb. It is contraindicated during pregnancy.[7]

Horse Chestnut
(Aesculus hippocastanum)

Parts Used and Where Grown: The horse chestnut tree is native to Asia and northern Greece, but it is now cultivated in many areas of Europe and North America. The tree produces fruits that are made up of a spiny capsule containing one to three large seeds, known as horse chestnuts. Traditionally, many of the aerial parts of the horse chestnut tree, including the seeds, leaves, and bark, were used in medicinal preparations. Modern extracts of horse chestnut are usually extracts of the seeds that are high in the active constituent aescin.

Historical or Traditional Use

Horse chestnut leaves have been used as a cough remedy and to reduce fevers.[1] They were also believed to reduce pain and inflammation of arthritis and rheumatism. Poultices of the seeds were used topically to treat skin ulcers and skin cancer. Other uses include the internal and external application for problems of venous circulation, including varicose veins and hemorrhoids. The topical preparation was also used to treat phlebitis.

In What Conditions Might Horse Chestnut Be Supportive?

Ranking	Health Concerns
Primary	Chronic venous insufficiency (p. 38) Varicose veins (p. 163)
Secondary	Bruising (p. 28) Hemorrhoids (p. 77) Injuries (minor) (p. 122)
Other	Edema (water retention) (p. 65)

Active Constituents

Extracts of the seeds are the source of a saponin known as aescin, which has been shown to promote circulation through the veins.[2] Aescin promotes normal tone in the walls of the veins, thereby promoting return of blood to the heart. This has made both topical and internal horse chestnut extracts popular in Europe for the treatment of **chronic venous insufficiency** (p. 38) and **varicose veins** (p. 164). Aescin also possesses anti-inflammatory properties and has been shown to reduce **edema** (swelling with fluid) (p. 65) following trauma, particularly those following sports injuries, surgery, and head injury.[3] A topical aescin preparation is very popular in Europe for the treatment of acute sprains during sporting events. Horse chestnuts also contain flavonoids, sterols, and tannins.

Double-blind human studies have shown that oral horse chestnut extracts support people with chronic venous insufficiency.[5,6] Those suffering edema after surgery have also found relief from topical application of horse chestnut extracts, according to preliminary studies.[7]

How Much Is Usually Taken?

Traditionally, 0.2 to 1.0 grams of the dried seeds were used per day but are not recommended any more. Instead, horse chestnut seed extracts standardized for aescin content (16 to 21%) or isolated aescin preparations are often recommended in the amount of 50 to 75 mg of aescin twice per day.[8,9] Tincture can be used in the amount of 1 to 4 ml taken 3 times per day, though it is questionable whether a significant amount of aescin can be absorbed this way.[10] Topical aescin preparations are used in Europe for **hemorrhoids** (p. 77), skin ulcers, varicose veins, sports injuries, and trauma of other kinds. A gel of aescin is typically applied to the affected area 3 to 4 times per day. For hemorrhoids and varicose veins, **witch hazel** (p. 470) is often combined with horse chestnut.

Are There Any Side Effects or Interactions? Internal use of horse chestnut extracts standardized for aescin at recommended amounts is generally safe. However, in rare cases oral intake of horse chestnut may cause itching, nausea, and upset stomach.[11] Intravenous aescin given to persons with damaged kidneys can cause worsening of kidney function and death, though it appears to be safe when given to people with healthy kidneys.[12,13] When taken as advised here, oral horse chestnut products have not been associated with kidney damage. Horse chestnut should be avoided by anyone with liver or kidney disease unless under the supervision of a physician trained in botanical medicine. There is no known reason to avoid horse chestnut during pregnancy though it is best to avoid it unless recommended by a doctor of natural medicine.[14] Topically, horse chestnut has been associated with rare cases of allergic skin reactions. Circulation disorders and trauma associated with swelling may be the sign of a serious condition; therefore, a health-care professional should be consulted before self-treating with horse chestnut.

Horseradish
(Cochlearia armoracia)

Parts Used and Where Grown: Horseradish likely originated in Eastern Europe, but today it is cultivated worldwide. The root is used as food and medicine.

In What Conditions Might Horseradish Be Supportive?

Ranking	Health Concerns
Other	Bronchitis Common cold/sore throat (p. 41) Sinus congestion Urinary tract infection (p. 160)

Historical or Traditional Use

Horseradish, known for its pungent taste, has been used as a medicine and condiment for centuries in Europe. Its name is derived from the common practice of naming a food according to its similarity with another food (horseradish was considered a rough substitute for radishes).

Horseradish was used both internally and externally. Applied to the skin, it causes reddening and was used on arthritic joints or irritated nerves. Internally, it was considered primarily to be a diuretic and was used for kidney stones or edema. It was also recommended as a digestive stimulant. In addition, it was used to treat worms, coughs, and sore throats.[1]

Active Constituents

Horseradish contains many compounds similar to mustard, which is in the same botanical family. Among these constituents are volatile oil, isothiocyanates, and glycosides. Horseradish has antibiotic properties, which may account for its effectiveness in treating throat and upper respiratory tract infections.[2] The glycosides (e.g. glucosinolates) are responsible for the reddening effect on the skin (by increasing blood flow to the area) when horseradish is applied topically. Horseradish has been shown specifically to destroy the **influenza virus** (p. 104) in test tubes and to reduce the severity of influenza infections in animals.[3] At levels attainable in human urine after taking the essential oil of horseradish, the oil has been shown to kill bacteria that can cause **urinary tract infections** (p. 160),[4] and one early study found that horseradish extract may be a useful treatment for persons with urinary tract infections.[5] Further studies are necessary to confirm this.

How Much Is Usually Taken?

The German Commission E monograph suggests an average daily intake of 20 grams of the fresh root for adults.[6] The freshly grated root can be eaten in the amount of ½ to 1 U.S. teaspoon (3 to 5 grams) 3 times per day. Horseradish tincture is also available and can be used in the amount of 2 to 3 ml 3 times per day.

Are There Any Side Effects or Interactions? If used in amounts higher than recommended, horseradish can cause stomach upset,[7] vomiting, or excessive sweating. Direct application to the skin or eyes may cause irritation and burning. Horseradish should be avoided by people with **hypothyroidism** (p. 93), stomach or intestinal **ulcers** (p. 138), kidney disorders, and children under 4 years of age.[8]

Horsetail
(Equisetum arvense)

Common names: Shave grass, scouring rush

Parts Used and Where Grown: Horsetail is widely distributed throughout the temperate climate zones of the Northern Hemisphere, including Asia, North America, and Europe.[1] Horsetail is a unique plant with two distinctive types of stems. One variety of stem grows early in spring and looks like asparagus, except for its brown color and the spore-containing cones on top. The mature form of the herb, appearing in summer, has branched, thin, green, sterile stems and looks like a feathery tail.

In What Conditions Might Horsetail Be Supportive?

Ranking	Health Concerns
Other	Brittle nails (p. 28) Edema (water retention) (p. 65) Kidney stones (p. 111) Osteoarthritis (p. 130) Osteoporosis (p. 133) Rheumatoid arthritis (p. 151) Urinary tract infection (p. 160)

Historical or Traditional Use

Since recommended by the Roman physician Galen, several cultures have employed horsetail as a folk remedy for kidney and bladder troubles, arthritis, bleeding ulcers, and tuberculosis. Additionally, the topical use of horsetail is said to stop the bleeding of wounds and promote rapid healing. The use of this herb as an abrasive cleanser to scour pots or shave wood illustrates the origin of horsetail's common names—scouring rush and shave grass.[2]

Active Constituents

Horsetail is rich in silicic acid and silicates, which provide approximately 2 to 3% elemental **silicon** (p. 331). **Potassium** (p. 323), aluminum, and **manganese** (p. 311), along with fifteen different types of **bioflavonoids** (p. 271), are also found in the herb. The presence of these bioflavonoids is believed to cause the diuretic action, while the silicon content is said to exert a connective tissue strengthening and antiarthritic action.[3] Some experts have suggested that the element silicon is a vital component for bone and cartilage formation.[4] This would indicate that horsetail may be beneficial in preventing **osteoporosis** (p. 133). Anecdotal reports suggest that horsetail may be of some use in the treatment of **brittle nails** (p. 28).

How Much Is Usually Taken?

The German Commission E monograph suggests up to 6 grams of the herb daily for internal use.[5] This should be divided into 2 to 3 doses. A tincture can also be used at 2 to 6 ml 3 times per day.

Are There Any Side Effects or Interactions?

Horsetail is generally considered safe for nonpregnant adults. The only concern would be that the correct species of horsetail is used; Equisetum palustre is another species of horsetail, which contains toxic alkaloids and is a well-known livestock poison.

The Canadian Health Protection Branch requires supplement manufacturers to document that their products do not contain the enzyme thiaminase, found in crude horsetail, which destroys the B vitamin **thiamin** (p. 331). Since alcohol, temperature, and alkalinity neutralize this potentially harmful enzyme, tinctures, fluid extracts, or preparations of the herb subjected to 100°C temperatures during manufacturing are preferred for medicinal use.[6]

Juniper
(Juniperus communis)

Parts Used and Where Grown: Juniper, a type of evergreen tree, grows mainly in the plains regions of Europe as well as in other parts of the world. The medicinal portions of the plant are referred to as berries, but they are actually dark blue-black scales from the cones of the tree. Unlike other pine cones, the juniper cones are fleshy and soft.

In What Conditions Might Juniper Be Supportive?

Ranking	Health Concerns
Other	Edema (water retention) (p. 65) Urinary tract infection (p. 160)

Historical or Traditional Use

Aside from being used as the flavoring agent in gin, juniper trees have contributed to the making of everything from soap to perfume.[1] Medicinally, many conditions have been treated with juniper berries, including gout, warts and skin growths, cancer, upset stomach, and various urinary tract and kidney diseases.

Active Constituents

The volatile oils, particularly 4-terpineol, cause an increase in urine volume.[2] Some evidence suggests it may lower uric acid levels, although further study is required to confirm this action. Although juniper lignans inhibit the herpes simplex virus in laboratory studies, treatment for human herpes infections by juniper has yet to be proven.[3] Juniper contains bitter substances, at least partly accounting for its traditional use in digestive upset and related problems.

How Much Is Usually Taken?

The German Commission E monograph suggests 2 to 10 grams of the dried fruit daily.[4] This corresponds to 2 to 100 mg of the essential oil. To make a tea, 1 cup (250 ml) of boiling water is added to 1 U.S. teaspoon

Juniper

(5 grams) of juniper berries and allowed to steep for 20 minutes in a tightly covered container. One cup can be drunk each morning and night. Juniper is often combined with other diuretic and antimicrobial herbs. As a capsule or tablet, 1 to 2 grams can be taken 3 times per day, or 1 to 2 ml of tincture can be taken 3 times per day.

Are There Any Side Effects or Interactions? Due to potential damage to the kidneys, juniper should never be taken for more than 6 weeks continuously. Anyone with serious kidney diseases should not take juniper, although rats given very high amounts of juniper oil show no signs of kidney damage.[4] Application of the essential oil directly to skin can cause a rash. Pregnant women should avoid juniper until further information is available, as it may cause uterine contractions.

Kava
(Piper methysticum)

Parts Used and Where Grown: Kava is a member of the pepper family and is native to many Pacific Ocean islands. The rhizome (underground stem) is used.

In What Conditions Might Kava Be Supportive?

Ranking	Health Concerns
Primary	Anxiety (p. 14) Restlessness[1] Stress[2]

Historical or Traditional Use

A nonalcoholic drink made from the root of kava played an important role in a variety of ceremonies in the Pacific islands, including welcoming visiting royalty, at meetings of village elders, or as part of social gatherings. Kava was valued both for its mellowing effects and to encourage socializing. It was also noted for initiating a state of contentment, a greater sense of well-being, and enhanced mental acuity, memory, and sensory perception. Kava has also been used traditionally to treat pain.

Active Constituents

The kava-lactones, sometimes referred to as kava-pyrones, are important active constituents in kava herbal extracts. High-quality kava rhizome contains 5.5 to 8.3% kava-lactones.[3] Medicinal extracts used in Europe contain 30 to 70% kava-lactones. Kava-lactones may have antianxiety, mild analgesic (pain-

relieving), muscle-relaxing, and anticonvulsant effects.[4] Some researchers speculate that kava may directly influence the limbic system, the ancient part of the brain associated with emotions and other brain activities.[5] Double-blind studies have validated the effectiveness of kava for people with anxiety,[6,7] including **menopausal** women (p. 18).[8]

How Much Is Usually Taken?

Some doctors of natural medicine suggest the use of kava extracts supplying 200 to 250 mg of kava-lactones per day in 2 or 3 divided doses.[9] Alternatively (although it has not been researched), 1 to 3 ml of fresh liquid kava tincture can be taken 3 times per day. Kava should not be taken for more than 3 months without the advice of a physician, according to the German Commission E monograph.[10]

Are There Any Side Effects or Interactions? In recommended amounts, the only reported side effect from kava use is mild gastrointestinal disturbances in some people. Long-term consumption of very high doses of kava may turn the skin, nails, and hair yellow temporarily.[11] If this occurs, people should simply discontinue kava use. In rare cases, an allergic skin reaction, such as a rash, may occur. Enlargement of the pupils has also been reported after long-term use of kava.[12]

At the doses listed above, kava is not addictive.

Kava is not recommended for use by pregnant or lactating women. It should not be taken together with other substances that also act on the central nervous system, such as alcohol, barbiturates, antidepressants, and antipsychotic drugs. One study found that it was safe to drive after taking kava at the doses listed above.[13] However, the German Commission E monograph states that kava, when taken at the recommended levels, may adversely affect a person's ability to safely drive or operate heavy machinery.[14]

Kudzu
(Pueraria lobata)

Common name: Ge-gen

Parts Used and Where Grown: Kudzu is a coarse, high-climbing, twining, trailing, perennial vine. The huge root, which can grow to the size of a human body, is the source of medicinal preparations used in traditional Chinese medicine and modern herbal products. Kudzu grows in most shaded areas in mountains, fields, along roadsides, thickets, and thin forests throughout most of China and the southeastern United States. The root of another Asian species of kudzu, *Pueraria thomsonii*, is also used for herbal products.

In What Conditions Might Kudzu Be Supportive?

Ranking	Health Concerns
Other	Alcohol withdrawal support (p. 6) Angina (p. 13)

Historical or Traditional Use

Kudzu root has been known for centuries in traditional Chinese medicine as ge-gen. The first written mention of the plant as a medicine is in the ancient herbal text of Shen Nong (circa A.D. 100). In traditional Chinese medicine, kudzu root is used in prescriptions for the treatment of wei, or "superficial," syndrome (a disease that manifests just under the surface—mild, but with fever), thirst, headache, and stiff neck with pain due to high blood pressure.[1] It is also recommended for allergies, migraine headaches, and diarrhea. The historical application for drunkenness has become a major focal point of modern research on kudzu. It is also used in modern Chinese medicine as a treatment for angina pectoris.

Active Constituents

Kudzu root is high in isoflavones, such as daidzein, as well as isoflavone glycosides, such as daidzin and puerarin. Depending on its growing conditions, the total isoflavone content varies from 1.77 to 12.0%, with puerarin in the highest concentration, followed by daidzin and daidzein.[2]

As is the case with other flavonoid-like substances, the constituents in kudzu root are associated with improved microcirculation and blood flow through the coronary arteries. A widely publicized 1993 animal study showed that both daidzin and daidzein inhibit the desire for alcohol.[3] The authors concluded that the root extract may in fact be useful for reducing the urge for alcohol and as treatment for **alcoholism** (p. 6). This has not yet been proven in controlled clinical studies with humans.

How Much Is Usually Taken?

The 1985 *Chinese Pharmacopoeia* suggests 9 to 15 grams per day of kudzu root.[4] In China, tablets of the standardized root (10 mg of weight per tablet equivalent to 1.5 grams of the crude root) are used for angina pectoris. This would equate to 30 to 120 mg 2 to 3 times per day. Kudzu tincture can be used in the amount of 1 to 2 ml taken 3 to 5 times per day.

Are There Any Side Effects or Interactions? At the dosages recommended above, there have been no reports of kudzu toxicity in humans.

Lavender
(*Lavandula angustifolia*)

Parts Used and Where Grown: The fragrant flowers of lavender contain the medicinal compounds. Eastern European countries, particularly Bulgaria, as well as France, Britain, Australia, and Russia grow large quantities of lavender.

In What Conditions Might Lavender Be Supportive?

Ranking	Health Concerns
Secondary	Pregnancy and postpartum support (p. 143)
Other	Indigestion (p. 99) and heartburn (p. 99) Insomnia (p. 105) Stress

Historical or Traditional Use

Traditionally, herbalists used lavender for a variety of conditions of the nervous system, including depression and fatigue.[1] It has also been used for headache and rheumatism. Because of its delightful odor, lavender has found wide application in perfumes and cosmetics throughout history.

Active Constituents

The volatile or essential oil of lavender contains many medicinal components, including perillyl alcohol, linalool, and geraniol. The oil is calming[2] and thus can be helpful in some cases of insomnia. One study of elderly persons with sleeping troubles found that inhaling lavender oil was as effective as tranquilizers.[3] A large study found that although lavender oil added to a bath was not more effective than placebo for relieving perineal discomfort immediately after childbirth, pain was reduced 3 to 5 days afterward.[4] Linalool and other constituents of lavender tend to lower blood pressure in animals, but this has not been confirmed in humans.[5] Test tube studies suggest linalool, geraniol, and other parts of the oil have significant antibacterial and antifungal activity, but there are no studies in people to confirm these findings.[6]

How Much Is Usually Taken?

The German Commission E monograph suggests 1 to 2 teaspoons of the herb be taken as a tea.[7] The tea can be made by steeping 2 U.S. teaspoons (10 grams) of

Lavender

leaves in 1 cup (250 ml) boiling water for 15 minutes. Three cups can be drunk each day. For internal applications, 1 to 2 ml of tincture can be taken 2 to 3 times per day. Several drops of the oil can be added to a bath or diluted in vegetable oil for topical applications. The concentrated oil is not for internal use. Synthetic oils should be avoided, as they are less effective than true lavender oil.[8]

Are There Any Side Effects or Interactions? Internal use of the essential oil can cause severe nausea and other problems, and for this reason should be strictly avoided. Excessive intake (several times more than listed above) may cause drowsiness.[9] External use in reasonable amounts is safe during pregnancy and lactation.

Lemon Balm
(Melissa officinalis)

Parts Used and Where Grown: The lemon balm plant originated in southern Europe and is now found throughout the world. The lemony smell and pretty white flowers of the plant have led to its widespread cultivation in gardens. The leaves, stems, and flowers of lemon balm are used medicinally.

In What Conditions Might Lemon Balm Be Supportive?

Ranking	Health Concerns
Secondary	Cold sores (p. 39) Colic (p. 40)
Other	Graves' disease (hyperthyroidism) Indigestion and heartburn (p. 99) Insomnia (p. 105) Nerve pain

Historical or Traditional Use

Charlemagne once ordered lemon balm planted in every monastery garden, testifying to its importance and beauty.[1] It was used traditionally to treat gas, sleeping difficulties, and heart problems. In addition, topical applications to the temples were sometimes used for insomnia or nerve pain.

Active Constituents

The terpenes, part of the pleasant smelling essential oil from lemon balm, produce this herb's relaxing and gas-relieving effects. Flavonoids, polyphenolics, and other compounds appear to be responsible for lemon balm's anti-herpes and thyroid-regulating actions. These constituents block attachment to the thyroid

cells by the antibodies that cause Graves' disease.[2] The brain's signal to the thyroid (thyroid-stimulating hormone or TSH) is also blocked from further stimulating the excessively active thyroid gland in this disease.

How Much Is Usually Taken?

The German Commission E monograph suggests 1.5 to 4.5 grams of lemon balm in a tea several times daily.[3] A simple tea made from 2 U.S. tablespoons (30 grams) of the herb steeped for 10 to 15 minutes in 150 ml of boiling water, is often used. Tincture can also be used at 2 to 3 ml 3 times per day. Concentrated extracts are sometimes recommended for insomnia at a dose of 160 to 200 mg, 30 minutes to 1 hour before bed. Highly concentrated topical extracts for herpes can be applied 3 to 4 times per day to the herpes lesions to speed healing time, according to double-blind research.[4]

Lemon balm is frequently combined with other medicinal plants. For example, **peppermint** (p. 451) and lemon balm together are effective for calming an upset stomach. **Valerian** (p. 467) is often combined with lemon balm for insomnia and nerve pain. **Bugleweed** *(Lycopus virginicus)* (p. 404) and lemon balm are usually used together for Graves' disease.

Are There Any Side Effects or Interactions?
No significant adverse effects from lemon balm have been reported. Unlike sedative drugs, lemon balm is safe even while driving or operating machinery. Lemon balm's sedating effects are not intensified by alcohol. Persons with **glaucoma** (p. 74) should avoid lemon balm essential oil until human studies are conducted, as animal studies show that it may raise pressure in the eye.[5]

Licorice
(Glycyrrhiza glabra, Glycyrrhiza uralensis)

Parts Used and Where Grown: Originally from central Europe, licorice now grows all across Europe and Asia. The root is used medicinally.

Historical or Traditional Use

Licorice has a long and highly varied record of uses. It was and remains one of the most important herbs in traditional Chinese medicine. Among the most consistent and important uses are as a demulcent (soothing, coating agent) in the digestive and urinary tracts, to help with coughs, to soothe sore throats, and as a flavoring. It has also been used to treat conditions ranging from diabetes to tuberculosis.

In What Conditions Might Licorice Be Supportive?

Ranking	Health Concerns
Primary	Hepatitis (intravenous) (p. 77) Peptic ulcer (DGL) (p. 138)
Secondary	Bronchitis Canker sores (mouth ulcers) (DGL) (p. 30) Colic (p. 40) Eczema (p. 64) HIV support (p. 87)
Other	Asthma (p. 15) Chronic fatigue syndrome (p. 36) Crohn's disease (p. 48) Fibromyalgia (p. 68) Gastritis (p. 71) Cold sores (topical gel) (p. 39) Indigestion and heartburn (DGL) (p. 99) Menopause (p. 118) Shingles (herpes zoster)/postherpetic neuralgia (topical gel) (p. 155) Ulcerative colitis (p. 158)

Active Constituents

The two most important constituents of licorice are glycyrrhizin and flavonoids. Glycyrrhizin breaks down to glycyrrhizic or glycyrrhetinic acid; glycyrrhizin is an anti-inflammatory and inhibits the breakdown of the cortisol produced by the body.[1,2] It also has antiviral properties. Licorice flavonoids, as well as the closely related chalcones, help digestive tract cells heal. They are also potent **antioxidants** (p. 267) and work to protect the cells of the liver. In test tubes, the flavonoids have been shown to kill *Helicobacter pylori,* the bacteria that causes most **ulcers** (p. 138) and stomach inflammation.[3]

A single-blind study found that while the acid-blocking drug cimetidine (Tagamet) led to quicker symptom relief, chewable deglycyrrhizinated licorice (DGL) tablets (see How Much Is Usually Taken? below for an explanation of DGL) were just as effective at healing stomach ulcers and keeping them healed.[4] Chewable DGL is also helpful in treating ulcers of the duodenum, the first part of the small intestine.[5] Capsules of DGL may not work for ulcers; apparently DGL must mix with saliva to be activated.[6] One preliminary human study has found DGL helpful for canker sores as well.[7]

While DGL has not been studied on its own in people with heartburn, a very similar drug known as carbenoxolone has shown benefit when combined with antacids.[8] Studies are needed to determine whether DGL helps those with **heartburn** (p. 99).

People with **eczema** (p. 64) improved with application of ointment with pure glycyrrhetinic acid, which was as effective as hydrocortisone, according to one clinical study.[9] The **herpes virus** (p. 39) is inhibited by glycyrrhizic acid in test tubes,[10] and though many people use licorice extracts topically for herpes, controlled studies have not evaluated how effective these extracts are.

Viral hepatitis is frequently treated with injections of glycyrrhizic acid in Japan, and many studies have shown this to be effective.[11] However, the side effects are potentially severe. Whether orally administered licorice helps in other types of viral hepatitis has not been rigorously studied. **HIV** (p. 87) infection has also only been treated with injectable licorice compounds.[12] The usefulness of oral licorice is unknown.

How Much Is Usually Taken?

There are two types of licorice, "standard" licorice and "deglycyrrhizinated" licorice (DGL). Each type is suitable for different conditions. For respiratory infections, chronic fatigue syndrome, or herpes (topical), the standard licorice containing glycyrrhizin should be used. Licorice root capsules can be used in the amount of 5 to 6 grams per day. Concentrated extracts may be used in the amount of 250 to 500 mg 3 times per day. Alternatively, a tea can be made by boiling ½ ounce of root in 1 pint of water for 15 minutes, drinking 2 to 3 cups of this per day. Long-term (more than 2 to 3 weeks) internal use of high doses of glycyrrhizin-containing products should be attempted with caution and under the supervision of a nutritionally oriented doctor. Licorice creams or gels can be applied directly to herpes sores 3 to 4 times per day.

DGL is prepared without the glycyrrhizin in order to circumvent potential safety problems, as explained below, and is used for conditions of the digestive tract, such as ulcers. For best results, one 200 to 300 mg tablet is chewed 3 times per day before meals and before bed.[13] For mouth ulcers, 200 mg of DGL powder can be mixed with 200 ml warm water, swished in the mouth for 3 minutes, and then spit out. Licorice may also be taken as a tincture in the amount of 2 to 5 ml 3 times daily.

Are There Any Side Effects or Interactions? Licorice products that include glycyrrhizin may increase blood pressure and cause water retention.[14] Some people are more sensitive to this effect than others. Long-term (more than 2 to 3 weeks) intake of products containing more than 1 gram of glycyrrhizin (the amount in approximately 10 grams of root) daily is the usual amount required to cause these effects. As a result of these possible side effects, long-term intake of high

Licorice

levels of glycyrrhizin is discouraged and should only be undertaken if prescribed by a qualified health-care professional. According to the German Commission E monograph, licorice is contraindicated in pregnant women as well as in people with liver and kidney disorders.[15]

Deglycyrrhizinated licorice extracts do not cause these side effects because there is no glycyrrhizin in them.

Ligustrum

(Ligustrum lucidum)

Common name: Privet

Parts Used and Where Grown: The berry of ligustrum is used medicinally. The shrub is native to China and eastern Asia and is now grown ornamentally in the United States.

In What Conditions Might Ligustrum Be Supportive?

Ranking	Health Concerns
Secondary	Immune function (p. 94)
Other	Infection (p. 101)

Historical or Traditional Use

Since ancient times, ligustrum berries have been employed as a "yin" tonic in traditional Chinese medicine.[1] It was used for a wide range of conditions, including premature aging, ringing in the ears, and chronic toxicity.[2]

Active Constituents

The main active compound in the plant is ligustrin (oleanolic acid). Studies, mostly conducted in China, suggest that ligustrum stimulates the **immune system** (p. 94), quells inflammation, and protects the liver.[3] Ligustrum is often combined with **astragalus** (p. 395) in traditional Chinese medicine.

How Much Is Usually Taken?

Powdered, encapsulated berries can be used in the amount of 5 to 15 grams per day.[4] A similar amount of berries can be made into tea by adding ½ to 1 U.S. teaspoons (2 to 5 grams) of powdered or crushed berries to 1 cup (250 ml) of boiling water and steeping for 10 to 15 minutes. Alternatively, 3 to 5 ml of tincture 3 times per day can be taken.

Are There Any Side Effects or Interactions? No adverse effects have been reported.

Lobelia

(Lobelia inflata)

Common name: Indian tobacco

Parts Used and Where Grown: The leaves of lobelia are used primarily. The seeds and root may be more potent but also are more likely to cause side effects. Lobelia grows throughout North America.

In What Conditions Might Lobelia Be Supportive?

Ranking	Health Concerns
Other	Asthma (p. 15) Bronchitis Chronic obstructive pulmonary disease (COPD) (p. 45) Cough (p. 47) Intestinal cramps Poisoning (as an emetic) Smoking cessation

Historical or Traditional Use

Eclectic physicians, doctors at the turn of the century in North America who used herbs as their main medicine, considered lobelia to be one of the most important plant medicines.[1] It was used by Eclectics to treat **coughs** (p. 47) and spasms in the lungs from all sorts of causes, as well as spasms elsewhere in the body, including the intestines and ureters (passages from the kidney to the bladder).[2] It was also considered a useful pain reliever and in higher doses was used to induce vomiting in persons who had been poisoned.

Active Constituents

The alkaloid lobeline is responsible for most of lobelia's actions. Because lobeline is similar in structure to nicotine, it has been employed as an agent to help people stop smoking. Results of human trials with lobeline have been mixed and generally negative.[3] Preliminary uncontrolled studies suggest lobeline may improve lung function.[4]

How Much Is Usually Taken?

Eclectic physicians generally recommended using a tincture of lobelia made partially or entirely with vinegar instead of alcohol.[5] A vinegar extract is known as an acetract. At most 1 ml was given 3 times per day.

The absolute maximum amount to take should be that which causes no or minimal nausea. Lobelia ointment has also been used topically on the chest to relieve **asthma** (p. 15) and bronchitis. People should apply such ointments liberally several times per day.

Are There Any Side Effects or Interactions? Lobelia frequently causes nausea and vomiting when the amount used is too high. Generally, more than 1 ml of tincture or acetract taken at one time will cause nausea and possibly vomiting and should be avoided.[6] Though lobelia has a reputation for being toxic, a thorough review of the medical literature was unable to find any well-documented case of serious problems or death due to lobelia.[7] This may be because a toxic amount cannot be ingested without first causing vomiting. Signs of lobelia poisoning are said to include weakness, heartburn, weak pulse, difficulty breathing, and collapse.[8] Nevertheless, lobelia should not be used for more than 1 month consecutively and should be avoided during pregnancy and lactation.[9] This does not apply to its topical use on the cervix during delivery by trained practitioners of natural childbirth assistance. Due to its emetic actions, lobelia should be used cautiously with children under the age of 6 years.

Lomatium
(Lomatium dissectum)

Parts Used and Where Grown: The root of lomatium is used medicinally. The plant is native to and continues to grow in western North America.

In What Conditions Might Lomatium Be Supportive?

Ranking	Health Concerns
Other	Infection (p. 101)

Historical or Traditional Use

Native Americans of many tribes employed lomatium root to treat a wide variety of infections, particularly those affecting the lungs. Lomatium was used, particularly in the southwestern United States, during the influenza pandemic of 1917 with reportedly good results.

Active Constituents

Tetronic acids and a glucoside of luteolin appear to be the main antimicrobial agents in lomatium root.[1] Little is known about how these compounds act, or if

other ones might be as important. The resin fraction occasionally causes a whole-body rash in some people. There is not enough information at this time to determine if the resins are necessary for the medicinal action of lomatium. Another set of constituents, known as coumarins, may also contribute to the onset of rash.

How Much Is Usually Taken?

Lomatium extracts with the resins removed (often called lomatium isolates) can be used in the amount of 1 to 3 ml per day. Lomatium tincture, 1 to 3 ml 3 times per day, can also be used, but it may cause a rash in susceptible individuals. The tincture should not be used unless a very small amount of it is first tested for a reaction; however, even very small amounts can cause a reaction in sensitive persons.

Are There Any Side Effects or Interactions? Use of extracts containing the resin (and possibly the coumarins) can, in some people, cause a whole-body rash.[2] This herb may also lead to nausea in some people. The safety of lomatium during pregnancy and lactation is unknown and is therefore not recommended.

Maitake
(Grifola frondosa)

Parts Used and Where Grown: Maitake is a very large mushroom (the size of a basketball), which grows deep in the mountains of northeastern Japan, as well as North America and Europe. Famous for its taste and health benefits, maitake is also known as the "dancing mushroom."[1] Legend holds that those who found the rare mushroom began dancing with joy. Others attribute the name to the way the fruit bodies of the mushroom overlap each other, giving the appearance of dancing butterflies.

Maitake is extremely sensitive to environmental changes, which has presented many challenges to those cultivating this mushroom. Only recently have Japanese farmers succeeded in producing high-quality organic maitake mushrooms, allowing for wider availability both in Japan and the United States. The fruiting body and the mycelium of maitake are used.

In What Conditions Might Maitake Be Supportive?

Ranking	Health Concerns
Other	HIV support (p. 87) Immune function (p. 94) Infection (p. 63)

Maitake

Historical or Traditional Use

Historically, maitake has been used as a tonic and adaptogen. Along with other "medicinal" mushrooms, such as **shiitake** (p. 460) and **reishi** (p. 455), maitake was used as a food to help promote wellness and vitality. Traditionally, consumption of the mushroom was thought to prevent high blood pressure and cancer—two applications that have been the focal point of modern research.

Active Constituents

A common denominator among mushroom and herbal adaptogens is the presence of complex polysaccharides in their structure. These active components have the ability to act as immunomodulators and, as such, are researched for their potential role in cancer and **AIDS** (p. 87) treatment. The polysaccharides present in maitake have a unique structure and are among the most powerful studied to date.[2] The primary polysaccharide, beta-D-glucan, is well absorbed when taken orally and is currently under review for the prevention and treatment of cancer and as a supportive tool for HIV infection.[3,4] This research is still preliminary and requires confirmation.

How Much Is Usually Taken?

Maitake can be used as a food or tea and is also available as a capsule or tablet containing the whole fruiting body of maitake. What are normally called mushrooms are the fruiting bodies that grow above ground. The mycelium is a threadlike network that grows underground or in wood. For maitake, the fruit body is higher in polysaccharides than the mycelium, which is why it is recommended. Maitake supplements in the amount of 3 to 7 grams per day can be used.[5] A liquid product with a higher concentration of polysaccharides is available.

Are There Any Side Effects or Interactions? Used as recommended above, there have been no reports of side effects with maitake.

Marshmallow
(Althea officinalis)

Parts Used and Where Grown: The marshmallow plant loves water and grows primarily in marshes. Originally from Europe, it now grows in the United States as well. The root and leaves are used.

Historical or Traditional Use

Marshmallow (not to be confused with confectionery marshmallows, which are a product of the modern food industry) has long been used to treat coughs and sore throats.[1] Because of its high mucilage content, this plant is soothing to inflamed mucous membranes. Marshmallow is also used to treat chapped skin, chilblains, and minor wounds.

In What Conditions Might Marshmallow Be Supportive?

Ranking	Health Concerns
Other	Asthma (p. 15)
	Common cold/sore throat (p. 41)
	Cough (p. 47)
	Crohn's disease (p. 48)
	Diarrhea (p. 58)
	Gastritis (p. 71)
	Pap smear (abnormal) (p. 136)
	Peptic ulcer (p. 138)
	Ulcerative colitis (p. 158)

Active Constituents

The active constituents in marshmallow are large carbohydrate (sugar) molecules, which make up mucilage. This smooth, slippery substance can soothe and protect irritated mucous membranes. Although marshmallow has primarily been used for the respiratory and digestive tracts, its high mucilage content may also provide some minor relief for urinary tract and skin infections.[2]

How Much Is Usually Taken?

The German Commission E monograph suggests a daily dose of 6 grams of the root.[3] Marshmallow can be made into a hot or cold water tea. Often 2 to 3 teaspoons of the root and/or leaves are used per cup of water. Generally, a full day's amount is steeped overnight when making a cold water tea (6 to 9 teaspoons in 3 cups of water) or steep for 15 to 20 minutes in hot water. Drink 3 to 5 cups a day. Because the plant is so gooey, it does not combine well with other plants. Nevertheless, it can be found in some herbal cough syrups. Herbal extracts in capsules and tablets providing 5 to 6 grams of marshmallow per day can also be used, or it may be taken as a tincture in the amount of 5 to 15 ml 3 times daily.

Are There Any Side Effects or Interactions? Marshmallow is safe; only rare allergic reactions have been reported.

Meadowsweet
(Filipendula ulmaria)

Parts Used and Where Grown: Meadowsweet is found in northern and southern Europe, North America, and northern Asia. The flowers and flowering top are primarily used in herbal preparations, although there are some historical references to using the root.

In What Conditions Might Meadowsweet Be Supportive?

Ranking	Health Concerns
Other	Common cold (p. 41) Minor injuries (joint and muscle pain) (p. 122) Edema (p. 65)

Historical or Traditional Use

Meadowsweet was used historically for a wide variety of conditions including treating rheumatic complaints of the joints and muscles and even arthritis.[1] Culpeper mentions its use to help break fevers and promote sweating during a **cold** (p. 41) or **flu** (p. 104). Records also indicate its use as a diuretic for persons with poor urinary flow. It was also thought to have antacid properties and was used to treat stomach complaints, including heartburn.

Active Constituents

While the flowers are high in flavonoids, the primary constituents in meadowsweet are the salicylates, including salicin, salicylaldehyde, and methyl salicylate.[2] In the digestive tract, these compounds are oxidized into salicylic acid, a substance that is closely related to aspirin (acetylsalicylic acid). While not as potent as **white willow** (p. 468), which has a higher salicin content, the salicylates in meadowsweet do give it a mild anti-inflammatory effect and ability to reduce fevers during a cold or flu. However, this role is only based on historical use and knowledge of the chemistry of meadowsweet's constituents, and to date, no human studies have been completed with meadowsweet.

How Much Is Usually Taken?

The German Commission E monograph recommends daily doses of 2.5 to 3.5 grams of the flower or 4 to 5 grams of the herb—often in a tea or infusion.[3] Unfortunately, to achieve an aspirin-like effect, one would realistically need to consume about 50 to 60 grams of meadowsweet daily. This means that white willow bark extracts standardized to salicin are a far more practical herbal substitute for aspirin. Tinctures may be used at a dose of 2 to 4 ml 3 times daily.

Are There Any Side Effects or Interactions? People with sensitivity to aspirin should avoid the use of meadowsweet. It should not be used to lower fevers in children as it may lead to Reye's syndrome. One of the

historical recommendations for meadowsweet for children is **diarrhea** (p. 58); based on the salicylate content, this should be avoided—particularly during acute diarrhea with a fever.

Milk Thistle
(Silybum marianum)

Parts Used and Where Grown: Milk thistle is commonly found growing wild in a variety of settings, including roadsides. The seeds of the dried flower are used.

In What Conditions Might Milk Thistle Be Supportive?

Ranking	Health Concerns
Primary	Alcohol-related liver disease (p. 6)
Secondary	Cirrhosis of the liver Hepatitis (p. 77) Liver support
Other	Gallstones (p. 69) Psoriasis (p. 147)

Historical or Traditional Use

Medical use of milk thistle can be traced back more than 2,000 years. Culpeper, the well-known eighteenth-century herbalist, cited its use for opening "obstructions" of the liver and spleen and recommended it for the treatment of jaundice.

Active Constituents

Milk thistle seeds contain a bioflavonoid complex known as silymarin. This constituent is responsible for the medical benefits of the plant.[1] Silymarin is made up of three parts: silibinin, silidianin, and silicristin. Silibinin is the most active and is largely responsible for the benefits attributed to silymarin.[2]

Milk thistle extract may protect the cells of the liver by blocking the entrance of harmful toxins and helping remove these toxins from the liver cells.[3,4] As with other bioflavonoids, silymarin is a powerful **antioxidant** (p. 267).[5] Milk thistle also regenerates injured liver cells.[6] Milk thistle extract is most commonly recommended to counteract the harmful actions of alcohol on the liver.[7]

Long-term placebo-controlled double-blind studies have shown milk thistle extracts to be effective in people with liver cirrhosis,[8] chronic hepatitis,[9] and even **diabetes** (p. 53) due to cirrhosis.[10] However, there have also been studies that have shown no effect in people with cirrhosis.[11] Milk thistle alters bile makeup, thereby potentially reducing risk of gallstones (p. 69).[12] Combination of milk thistle with potentially liver-damaging drugs has been shown to protect the liver.[13]

How Much Is Usually Taken?

For liver disease and impaired liver function, some doctors of natural medicine suggest 420 mg of silymarin per day from an herbal extract of milk thistle standardized to 70 to 80% silymarin content.[14] According to research and clinical experience, improvement should be noted in about 8 to 12 weeks. Once that occurs, intake is sometimes reduced to 280 mg of silymarin per day. This lower amount may also be used for preventive purposes.

For those who prefer, 12 to 15 grams of milk thistle seeds can be ground and eaten or made into a tea. This should not be considered therapeutic for conditions of the liver, however.

Are There Any Side Effects or Interactions?
Milk thistle extract is virtually devoid of any side effects and may be used by most people, including pregnant and lactating women. In fact, it has been recommended as treatment for itching due to poor gallbladder function during pregnancy.[15] Since silymarin stimulates liver and gallbladder activity, it may have a mild, transient laxative effect in some individuals. This will usually cease within 2 to 3 days.

Mullein
(Verbascum thapsus)

Parts Used and Where Grown: In Europe, the flowers from *Verbascum phlomoides* or *Verbascum thapsiforme*, both close relatives of North American mullein, are the source of many mullein herbal products. The leaves and flowers of mullein are typically used in herbal preparations. The leaves are collected in late spring before flowering, the flowers between July and September, and the roots in March or October.

In What Conditions Might Mullein Be Supportive?

Ranking	Health Concerns
Other	Asthma (p. 15) Bronchitis Chronic obstructive pulmonary disease (p. 45) Common cold/sore throat (p. 41) Cough (p. 47) Ear infections (recurrent) (p. 63)

Historical or Traditional Use

Mullein is classified in herbal literature as an expectorant and demulcent herb. Historically, mullein has been used as a remedy for the respiratory tract, particularly in cases of irritating coughs with bronchial congestion.[1] As such, bronchitis sufferers often find relief with this herb, particularly when combined with **white horehound** (p. 434) and **lobelia** (p. 442). Some herbal texts extend the therapeutic use to pneumonia and asthma.[2] Because of its mucilage content, mullein has also been used topically as a soothing emollient for inflammatory skin conditions and burns.

Active Constituents

Mullein contains about 3% mucilage and small amounts of saponins and tannins.[3] The mucilaginous constituents are primarily responsible for the soothing actions on mucous membranes. The saponins may be responsible for the expectorant actions of mullein.[4]

How Much Is Usually Taken?

A tea of mullein is made by pouring 1 cup (250 ml) of boiling water over 1 to 2 U.S. teaspoons (5 to 10 grams) of dried leaves or flowers and steeping for 10 to 15 minutes. The tea can be drunk 3 to 4 times per day. For the tincture, 1 to 4 ml is taken 3 to 4 times per day. As a dried product, 3 to 4 grams is used 3 times per day.[5] As mentioned above, mullein is usually combined with other demulcent or expectorant herbs when used to treat coughs and bronchial irritation. For ear infections, modern naturopathic physicians apply an oil extract directly in the ear. If the eardrum has ruptured, nothing should be put directly in the ear; therefore, a qualified practitioner should always do an ear examination before mullein oil is placed in the ear.

Are There Any Side Effects or Interactions?
Mullein is generally safe except for rare reports of skin irritation. There are no known contraindications to its use during pregnancy or lactation.

Myrrh
(Commiphora molmol)

Parts Used and Where Grown: Myrrh grows as a shrub in desert regions, particularly in northeastern Africa and the Middle East. The resin obtained from the stems is used in medicinal preparations. It should not be confused with its close cousin, mukul (*Commiphora mukul*).

In What Conditions Might Myrrh Be Supportive?

Ranking	Health Concerns
Secondary	Gingivitis (periodontal disease) (p. 73)
Other	Athlete's foot (p. 20) Canker sores (mouth ulcers) (p. 30) Cold sores (p. 39) Common cold/sore throat (p. 41) Pap smear (abnormal) (p. 136) Ulcerative colitis (p. 158)

Historical or Traditional Use

In ancient times, the red-brown resin of myrrh was utilized in the preservation of mummies. It was also used as a remedy for numerous infections, including leprosy and syphilis. Myrrh was also recommended for relief from bad breath and for dental conditions.[1] In traditional Chinese medicine, it has been used for bleeding disorders and wounds.

Active Constituents

The three main constituents of myrrh are the resin, the gum, and the volatile oil. All are important in myrrh's activity as an herbal medicine. The resin has been shown to kill various microbes and to stimulate macrophages (a type of white blood cell).[2] Myrrh also has astringent properties and has a soothing effect on inflamed tissues in the mouth and throat. Studies continue on the potential anticancer and pain-relieving actions of myrrh resin.[3,4]

How Much Is Usually Taken?

The German Commission E monograph recommends that persons either dab the undiluted tincture in the mouth or gargle with 5 to 10 drops of tincture in a glass of water 3 times daily.[5] Tincture of myrrh is usually taken at a dose of 1 to 2 ml 3 times per day. The tincture can also be applied topically for canker sores and athlete's foot. Due to the gummy nature of the product, a tea cannot be made from myrrh. Capsules, containing up to 1 gram of resin taken 3 times per day, can also be used.

Are There Any Side Effects or Interactions? No adverse effects from myrrh usage have been reported.

Nettle
(Urtica dioica)

Parts Used and Where Grown: The Latin root of Urtica is uro, meaning "I burn," indicative of the small stings caused by the little hairs on the leaves of this plant when contact is made with the skin. The root and leaves are used.

In What Conditions Might Nettle Be Supportive?

Ranking	Health Concerns
Secondary	Benign prostatic hyperplasia (p. 145) Sinusitis (p. 156)
Other	Hay fever (p. 76) Kidney stones (p. 111) Pregnancy and postpartum support (p. 143) Urinary tract infection (p. 160)

Historical or Traditional Use

Nettle has a long history of use. The tough fibers from the stem have been used to make cloth, and cooked nettle leaves were eaten as vegetables. From ancient Greece to the present, nettle has been documented for its use in treating coughs, tuberculosis, and arthritis, and in stimulating hair growth.

Active Constituents

There has been a great deal of controversy regarding the identity of nettle's active constituents. Currently it is thought that polysaccharides (complex sugars) and lectins (large protein-sugar molecules) are probably the active constituents. The leaf has been shown to be anti-inflammatory by preventing the body from making inflammatory chemicals known as prostaglandins.[1] Nettle's root affects hormones and proteins that carry sex hormones (such as testosterone or estrogen) in the human body; this may explain why it helps **benign prostatic hyperplasia** (BPH [p. 145]).[2] This has been confirmed using extracts of the roots in double-blind studies.[3]

A preliminary study reported that capsules made from freeze-dried leaves had an **antiallergy** (p. 8) action in people.[4] Further studies are needed to confirm this finding.

How Much Is Usually Taken?

During the allergy season, two to three 300 mg nettle leaf capsules or tablets, or 2 to 4 ml tincture can be taken 3 times per day. For BPH, 240 mg per day of a concentrated root extract in capsules can be taken.[5] Many products for BPH will combine nettle root with **saw palmetto** (p. 457) or **pygeum** extracts (p. 453).

Are There Any Side Effects or Interactions? Nettle may cause mild gastrointestinal upset in some people. Although allergic reactions to nettle are rare, when contact is made with the skin, fresh nettles can cause a rash.[6]

Oak
(Quercus spp.)

Parts Used and Where Grown: The bark of the oak tree is used medicinally. There are several species of oak, and it is unclear which is most effective. Oak trees grow throughout North America and as far south as the Rio Grande. Some species of oak grow around the world, including China and the Middle East.

In What Conditions Might Oak Be Supportive?

Ranking	Health Concerns
Other	Crohn's disease (p. 48)
	Diarrhea (p. 58)
	Eczema (p. 64)

Historical or Traditional Use

Oak bark was utilized traditionally to treat hemorrhoids, varicose veins, diarrhea, and cancer. Tannic acid derived from oak trees has a long history of application in tanning hides and making ink.[1]

Active Constituents

Tannins are the main therapeutic component of oak bark.[2] These tannins are potent astringents, akin to those found in **witch hazel** *(Hamamelis virginiana)* (p. 470). Tannins bind liquids, absorb toxins, and soothe inflamed tissues. The oak tannin, known as ellagitannin, inhibits intestinal secretion,[3] which helps resolve **diarrhea** (p. 58). The nonirritating nature of oak is well regarded in Germany, where it is even recommended to treat mild, acute diarrhea in children (along with plenty of electrolyte-containing fluids).[4]

How Much Is Usually Taken?

The German Commission E monograph suggests a daily dose of 3 grams of the bark.[5] For eczema, oak is applied topically by first boiling 1 to 2 U.S. tablespoons (15 to 30 grams) of the bark for 15 minutes in 500 ml (2 cups) of water. After cooling, a cloth is dipped into the liquid and applied directly to the rash several times a day. The liquid prepared this way in the morning can be used throughout the day; unused portions should be discarded after that. Up to 5 cups of this same solution can be drunk each day in cases of diarrhea. Alternatively, a tincture of oak can be used in the amount of 2 to 3 ml 3 times per day.

Are There Any Side Effects or Interactions? Except for the occasional person reporting an upset stomach or constipation after drinking the tea, oak bark is very safe. There is no known direct problem during pregnancy or lactation, although oak can cause constipation. It is safe for use in children and infants. The German Commission E monograph warns against bathing in water with oak bark added if you have open sores or skin damage covering a large area or have a high fever or infection.[6]

Oats
(Avena sativa)

Parts Used and Where Grown: The common oat used in herbal supplements and foods is derived from wild species that have since been cultivated. For herbal supplements, the green or rapidly dried aerial parts of the plant are harvested just before reaching full flower. Many herbal texts refer to using the fruits (seeds) or green tops. Although some herb texts discuss oat straw, there is little medicinal action in this part of the plant. Oats are now grown worldwide.

In What Conditions Might Oats Be Supportive?

Ranking	Health Concerns
Primary	High triglycerides (p. 85)
Other	Anxiety (p. 14)
	Eczema (p. 64)
	High cholesterol (p. 79)
	Insomnia (p. 105)
	Nicotine withdrawal

Historical or Traditional Use

In folk medicine as well as among current herbalists, oats are used to treat nervous exhaustion, insomnia, and "weakness of the nerves." A tea made from oats was thought to be useful in rheumatic conditions and to treat water retention. A tincture of the green tops of oats was also used to help with withdrawal from tobacco addiction.[1] Oats were often used in baths to treat insomnia and anxiety as well as a variety of skin conditions, including burns and eczema.

Active Constituents

The fruits (seeds) contain alkaloids, such as gramine and avenine, as well as saponins, such as avenacosides A and B.[2] The seeds are also rich in **iron** (p. 304), **manganese** (p. 311), and **zinc** (p. 346). The straw is high in **silica** (p. 331). Oat alkaloids are believed to account for oats' relaxing action, but it should be noted that this action of oats continues to be debated in Europe; the German Commission E monographs do not endorse this herb as a sedative.[3] However, an alcohol-based tincture of the fresh plant has proven promising in cases of nicotine withdrawal.[4]

How Much Is Usually Taken?

Oats can be eaten as a morning breakfast cereal. A tea can be made from a heaping U.S. tablespoonful (30 grams) of oats brewed with 1 cup (250 ml) of boiling water; after cooling and straining, the tea can be drunk several times a day and shortly before going to bed.[5] As a tincture, oats are often taken at 3 to 5 ml 3 times per day. Encapsulated or tableted products can be used in the amount of 1 to 4 grams per day. A soothing bath to ease irritated skin can be made by running the bath water through a sock containing several tablespoons of oats.

Are There Any Side Effects or Interactions? Oats are not associated with any adverse effects.

Oregon Grape
(Berberis aquifolium)

Parts Used and Where Grown: Oregon grape is a close relative of **barberry** (p. 395) (Berberis vulgaris), and as with its cousin, the plant's medicinal portion is the root. Although Oregon grape originated in North America, it now also grows in Europe.

In What Conditions Might Oregon Grape Be Supportive?

Ranking	Health Concerns
Secondary	Diarrhea (berberine) (p. 58)
Other	Conjunctivitis/blepharitis (p. 44) Gallstones (p. 69) Infection (p. 101) Parasites (p. 137) Poor digestion (p. 99) Psoriasis (p. 147) Urinary tract infections (p. 160)

Historical or Traditional Use

Before European colonists arrived, the indigenous peoples of North America treated all manner of complaints with Oregon grape.[1] The berries were used for poor appetite. A tea made from the root was used to treat jaundice, arthritis, diarrhea, fever, and many other health problems.

Active Constituents

Alkaloids, including berbamine, canadine, hydrastine, and the most famous, berberine, account for the beneficial activity of Oregon grape. Berberine has been shown to effectively treat **diarrhea** (p. 58) in people infected with *E. coli*.[2] One of the ways berberine may ease diarrhea is by slowing the transit time in the intestine.[3] Berberine inhibits the ability of bacteria to attach to human cells, which helps prevent **infections** (p. 101), particularly in the throat, intestines, and urinary tract.[4] These actions, coupled with berberine's ability to enhance **immune cell function** (p. 94),[5] make Oregon grape possibly useful for mild infections.

An ointment of Oregon grape has been shown to effectively treat the skin disease **psoriasis** (p. 147) in a double-blind study.[6] Whole Oregon grape extracts were shown in one laboratory study to reduce inflammation (often associated with psoriasis) and to stimulate the white blood cells known as macrophages.[7] In this study, isolated alkaloids from Oregon grape did not have these actions. This suggests that something besides alkaloids are important to the properties of Oregon grape.

The bitter-tasting compounds as well as the alkaloids in Oregon grape root stimulate digestive function.

How Much Is Usually Taken?

A tea can be prepared by boiling 1 to 3 U.S. teaspoons (5 to 15 grams) of chopped roots in 500 ml (2 cups) of water for 15 minutes. After straining and cooling, 3 cups can be drunk per day. Tincture can also be used in the amount of 3 ml 3 times per day. Since berberine is not well absorbed, Oregon grape root might not provide adequate amounts of this compound to treat significant infections; standardized extracts containing 5 to 10% alkaloids, which supply 500 mg of berberine each day, can be used in these situations to ensure the necessary amount. A nutritionally oriented physician should be consulted in the case of infection. A 10% extract ointment applied 3 or more times daily might be useful for psoriasis.

Are There Any Side Effects or Interactions? Oregon grape is safe in the amounts indicated above. Long-term (more than 2 to 3 weeks) use of standardized extracts is not recommended. Berberine alone has been reported to interfere with normal bilirubin metabolism in infants, raising a concern that it might worsen jaundice.[8] For this reason, berberine-containing plants should be used with caution during pregnancy and breast-feeding.

Passion Flower
(Passiflora incarnata)

Parts Used and Where Grown: The beauty of the passion flower has made this plant very popular. The plant is native to North, Central, and South America. While primarily tropical, some of its 400 species can grow in colder climates. The name passion flower dates back to the seventeenth century. The mystery of the beautiful blossom out of the unassuming bud was compared to the Passion of Christ. The leaves, stems, and flowers are used for medicinal purposes.

In What Conditions Might Passion Flower Be Supportive?

Ranking	Health Concerns
Primary	Anxiety (p. 14)
Other	Insomnia (p. 105)

Historical or Traditional Use

The historical use of passion flower is not dissimilar to its current use as a mild sedative. Medical use of the herb did not begin until the late nineteenth century in the United States. Passion flower was used to treat nervous restlessness and gastrointestinal spasms. In short, the effects of passion flower were believed to be primarily on the nervous system, particularly for anxiety due to mental worry and overwork.[1]

Active Constituents

For many years, plant researchers believed that a group of harman alkaloids were the active constituents in passion flower. Recent studies, however, have pointed to the flavonoids in passion flower as the primary constituents responsible for its relaxing and antianxiety effects.[2] European pharmacopoeias typically recommend passion flower products containing no less than 0.8% total flavonoids. The European literature involving passion flower recommends it primarily for antianxiety treatment; in this context, it is often combined with **valerian** (p. 467), **lemon balm** (p. 440), and other herbs with sedative properties.

How Much Is Usually Taken?

The recommended intake of the dried herb is 4 to 8 grams 3 times per day.[3] To make a tea, 0.5 to 2.5 grams of the herb can be steeped with boiling water for 10 to 15 minutes and drunk 2 to 3 times per day. Alternatively, 2 to 4 ml of passion flower tincture can be taken per day. As mentioned above, many European products combine passion flower with other sedative herbs to treat mild to moderate anxiety.

Are There Any Side Effects or Interactions? Used in the amounts listed above, passion flower is generally safe and has not been found to negatively interact with other sedative drugs. However, some herbalists suggest not using passion flower with MAO-inhibiting antidepressant drugs.[4] Passion flower has not been proven to be safe during pregnancy and lactation.

Pau d'arco
(*Tabebuia avellanedae, Tabebuia impestiginosa*)

Common names: Lapacho, taheebo
Parts Used and Where Grown: Various related species of pau d'arco trees grow in rain forests throughout Latin America. The bark is used for medical purposes.

In What Conditions Might Pau d'arco Be Supportive?

Ranking	Health Concerns
Other	Infection (p. 101)
	Yeast infection (p. 169)

Historical or Traditional Use

Native peoples in Central and South America reportedly use pau d'arco bark to treat cancer, lupus, infectious diseases, wounds, and many other health conditions.[1] Caribbean folk healers use the leaf of this tree in addition to the bark for the treatment of backache, toothache, sexually transmitted diseases, and as an aphrodisiac.

Active Constituents

Lapachol and beta-lapachone (known collectively as naphthaquinones) are two primary active compounds in pau d'arco. According to laboratory tests, both have antifungal properties as potent or more so than ketaconazole, a common antifungal drug.[2] Although these compounds also have anticancer properties, the effective dosage for this effect is toxic.[3,4] Therefore, pau d'arco cannot currently be recommended as a treatment for cancer. Human studies are lacking to confirm the efficacy of pau d'arco.

How Much Is Usually Taken?

A traditional dosage is 2 to 3 U.S. teaspoons (15 to 20 grams) of the inner bark simmered in a pint of water for 15 minutes then taken in 3 daily doses.[5] Capsules or tablets providing 300 mg of powdered bark can be taken; usually 3 capsules are ingested 3 times per day. A tincture can be used in the amount of 0.5 to 1 ml 3 times per day.

Are There Any Side Effects or Interactions? High amounts (several grams daily over several days) of lapachol can cause uncontrolled bleeding, nausea, and vomiting.[6] Use of the whole bark is much safer than isolated lapachol—the whole bark has no known serious side effects.[7] Pregnant or lactating women should avoid use of pau d'arco.

Peppermint
(Mentha piperita)

Parts Used and Where Grown: Peppermint is a hybrid of water mint and spearmint and was first cultivated near London in 1750. Peppermint grows almost everywhere. The two main cultivated forms are the black mint, which has violet-colored leaves and stems and a relatively high oil content, and the white mint, which has pure green leaves and a milder taste. The leaves are used.

In What Conditions Might Peppermint Be Supportive?

Ranking	Health Concerns
Primary	Indigestion (p. 99)
Secondary	Colic (p. 40) Gallstones (p. 69) Gingivitis (periodontal disease) (p. 73) Irritable bowel syndrome (p. 109)
Other	Headache (tension)

Historical or Traditional Use

Recognized in the early eighteenth century, the historical use of peppermint is not dramatically different than its use in modern herbal medicine. Classified as a carminative herb, peppermint has been used as a general digestive aid and employed in the treatment of **indigestion** (p. 99) and intestinal colic.[1]

Active Constituents

Peppermint leaves contain about 0.5 to 4% volatile oil that is composed of 50 to 78% free menthol and 5 to 20% menthol combined with other constituents.[2] Peppermint oil is classified as a carminative,[3] meaning that it helps ease intestinal cramping and tone the digestive system. Peppermint oil or peppermint tea is often used to treat gas and indigestion. It may also increase the flow of bile from the gallbladder.[4]

Peppermint oil's relaxing action also extends to topical use. When applied topically, it acts as a coun-terirritant and analgesic with the ability to reduce pain and improve blood flow to the affected area.[5]

Enteric-coated peppermint oil has shown benefit for people with **irritable bowel syndrome** (p. 109), according to double-blind studies.[6,7] One double-blind study found that combining peppermint and caraway oils in an enteric-coated tablet was superior to placebo for people with irritable bowel syndrome.[8]

A tea of peppermint is a traditional therapy for **colic** (p. 40) in infants, and a double-blind study has confirmed its effectiveness.[9] The tea used in this study contained mint and also **licorice** (p. 440), vervain, **fennel** (p. 443), and **lemon balm** (p. 440). However, peppermint should be used cautiously in infants (see side effects below).

A study of topical peppermint oil applied to the temples of healthy volunteers (with or without **eucalyptus** oil [p. 421]) found that peppermint oil had a muscle-relaxing action and it also decreased tension. This may explain its usefulness in treating tension headaches.[10] Peppermint oil alone reduced pain as well.

How Much Is Usually Taken?

For internal use, a tea can be made by pouring 1 cup (250 ml) of boiling water over 1 heaped U.S. teaspoon (5 grams) of the dried leaves and steeping for 5 to 10 minutes. Drinking 3 to 4 cups daily between meals can relieve stomach and gastrointestinal complaints.[11] Peppermint leaf tablets, capsules, and liquid extracts are often taken at 3 to 6 grams per day. For treatment of irritable bowel syndrome, 1 to 2 capsules of the enteric-coated capsules containing 0.2 ml of peppermint oil taken 2 to 3 times per day may be preferable.

For headaches, a combination of peppermint oil and eucalyptus oil diluted with base oil can be applied to the temples at the onset of the headache and every hour after that or until symptom relief is noted.

Are There Any Side Effects or Interactions? Peppermint tea is generally considered safe for regular consumption. Peppermint oil can cause burning and gastrointestinal upset in some people.[12] It should be avoided by persons with chronic heartburn, severe liver damage, inflammation of the gallbladder, or obstruction of the bile ducts.[13] Some persons using the enteric-coated peppermint capsules may experience a burning sensation in the rectum. Rare allergic reactions have been reported with topical use of peppermint oil. Peppermint oil should not be applied to the face, in particular the nose, of children and infants.[14] Peppermint tea should be used with caution in infants and young children, as they may choke in reaction to the strong menthol; **chamomile** (p. 409) is usually a better choice for this group. People with **gallstones** (p. 69) should consult a physician before using peppermint leaf or peppermint oil.[15]

Phyllanthus
(Phyllanthus niruri)

Common names: Bahupatra, bhuiamla
Parts Used and Where Grown: Phyllanthus is an herb common to central and southern India. It can grow to 30 to 60 centimeters in height and blooms with many yellow flowers. All parts of the plant are employed therapeutically. Phyllanthus species are also found in other countries, including China (e.g., *Phyllanthus urinaria*), the Philippines, Cuba, Nigeria, and Guam.[1]

In What Conditions Might Phyllanthus Be Supportive?

Ranking	Health Concerns
Secondary	Hepatitis (p. 77)

Historical or Traditional Use

Phyllanthus has been used in Ayurvedic medicine for over 2,000 years and has a wide number of traditional uses: employing the whole plant for jaundice, gonorrhea, frequent menstruation, and diabetes and using it topically as a poultice for skin ulcers, sores, swelling, and itchiness. The young shoots of the plant are administered in the form of an infusion for the treatment of chronic dysentery.[2]

Active Constituents

Phyllanthus primarily contains lignans (e.g., phyllanthine and hypophyllanthine), alkaloids, and **bioflavonoids** (p. 271) (e.g., **quercetin** [p. 328]). While it remains unknown as to which of these ingredients has an antiviral effect, research shows that this herb acts primarily on the liver. This action in the liver confirms its historical use as a remedy for jaundice.

Phyllanthus blocks DNA polymerase, the enzyme needed for the hepatitis B virus to reproduce. In one study, 59% of those infected with chronic viral hepatitis B lost one of the major blood markers of HBV infection (e.g., hepatitis B surface antigen) after using phyllanthus for 30 days.[3] While clinical studies on the outcome of phyllanthus and HBV have been mixed, the species *P. urinaria* and *P. niruri* seem to work better than *P. amarus*.[4]

How Much Is Usually Taken?

Research has utilized the powdered form of phyllanthus in amounts ranging from 900 to 2,700 mg per day for 3 months.[5]

Are There Any Side Effects or Interactions? No side effects have been reported using phyllanthus as recommended in amounts above.

Psyllium
(Plantago ovata, Plantago ispaghula)

Common name: Plantago seed
Parts Used and Where Grown: Psyllium is native to Iran and India and is currently cultivated in these countries. The seeds are used. The seed husks are also sometimes used, but only to treat constipation; they are too irritating for other uses.

In What Conditions Might Psyllium Be Supportive?

Ranking	Health Concerns
Primary	Atherosclerosis (p. 17)
	Constipation (p. 44)
	Diabetes (p. 53)
	Hemorrhoids (p. 77)
	High cholesterol (p. 79)
	High triglycerides (p. 85)
	Irritable bowel syndrome (p. 109)
Secondary	Diarrhea (p. 58)
	Weight loss and obesity (p. 165)
Other	Psoriasis (p. 147)

Historical or Traditional Use

In addition to its traditional and current use for constipation, psyllium was also used topically to treat skin irritations, including poison ivy reactions and insect bites and stings. It has also been used in traditional herbal systems of China and India to treat diarrhea, hemorrhoids, bladder problems, and high blood pressure.

Active Constituents

Psyllium is a bulk-forming laxative and is high in both fiber and mucilage. Psyllium seeds contain 10 to 30% mucilage. The laxative properties of psyllium are due to the swelling of the husk when it comes in contact with water. This forms a gelatinous mass and keeps the feces hydrated and soft. The resulting bulk stimulates a reflex contraction of the walls of the bowel, followed by emptying.[1]

One observational study found that psyllium seeds sucessfully treated **constipation** (p. 44) due only to poor lifestyle (low fiber, low exercise, etc.), not when an actual disease was the cause.[2] Numerous double-blind studies confirm psyllium can lower total **cholesterol** (p. 79) levels, though high-density lipoprotein (HDL) cholesterol (a beneficial form of cholesterol) levels are not affected.[3] It is effective in children as well as adults.[4]

How Much Is Usually Taken?

The suggested daily dose for psyllium husks is 4 to 20 grams (1 U.S. teaspoon) or 10 to 20 grams (up to 2 U.S. teaspoons) of the powdered seeds. This is stirred into a large glass of water or juice and drunk immediately before it thickens.[5] It is best to follow label instructions on over-the-counter psyllium products for constipation. It is important to maintain adequate fluid intake when using psyllium.

Are There Any Side Effects or Interactions?
Using psyllium in recommended amounts is generally safe. People with chronic constipation should seek the advice of a health-care professional. Some people with **irritable bowel syndrome** (p. 109) feel worse when taking psyllium and may do better with soluble fiber, such as in fruit. Individuals with an obstruction of the bowel or **diabetics** (p. 53) who have difficulty regulating their disease should not use psyllium.[6] Side effects, such as allergic skin and respiratory reactions to psyllium dust, have largely been limited to people working in plants manufacturing psyllium products.

Pygeum
(Prunus africanum, Pygeum africanum)

Parts Used and Where Grown: Pygeum is an evergreen tree found in the higher elevations of central and southern Africa. The bark is used. These trees are environmentally threatened in the wild, so it is questionable whether this herb should be used for the time being. While some effort is being made to grow pygeum on plantations, not all companies are careful in choosing an ecologically sustainable supplier.

Historical or Traditional Use

The powdered bark was used as a tea for relief of urinary disorders. European scientists were so impressed with reports of pygeum's actions that they began laboratory investigations into the active constituents in the bark. This led to the development of the modern lipophilic (fat-soluble) extract used today.

In What Conditions Might Pygeum Be Supportive?

Ranking	Health Concerns
Primary	Benign prostatic hyperplasia (p. 145)

Active Constituents

Chemical analysis and pharmacological studies indicate that the lipophilic extract of pygeum bark has three categories of active constituents. The phytosterols, including **beta-sitosterol** (p. 270), have anti-inflammatory effects by interfering with the formation of pro-inflammatory prostaglandins that tend to accumulate in the prostate of men with benign prostatic hyperplasia (BPH). The pentacyclic terpenes have an anti-edema or decongesting effect. The last group is the ferulic esters. These constituents reduce levels of the hormone prolactin and also block cholesterol in the prostate. Prolactin increases uptake of testosterone in the prostate, and cholesterol increases binding sites for testosterone and its more active form dihydrotestosterone.[1] Pygeum alone has been shown in double-blind studies to help men with BPH.[2] It has also been used successfully in combination with **nettle** (p. 447) root.[3] However, long-term studies (6 months or greater) are lacking.

How Much Is Usually Taken?

The accepted form of pygeum used in Europe for treatment of BPH is a lipophilic extract standardized to 13% total sterols (typically calculated as beta-sitosterol).[4] The recommended dose is 50 to 100 mg 2 times per day. Pygeum should be monitored over at least a 6- to 9-month period to determine efficacy. As is the case with all BPH treatments, close medical supervision is important.

Are There Any Side Effects or Interactions?
Side effects to the lipophilic extract of pygeum are rare. In clinical studies, there were reports of mild gastrointestinal irritation in some people.

Red Clover
(Trifolium pratense)

Parts Used and Where Grown: This plant grows in Europe and North America. The flowering tops are used in botanical medicine. Another plant, white clover, grows in similar areas. Both have white arrow-shaped patterns on their leaves.

In What Conditions Might Red Clover Be Supportive?

Ranking	Health Concerns
Other	Cancer risk reduction Cough (p. 47) Eczema (p. 64) Menopause (p. 118)

Historical or Traditional Use

Traditional Chinese medicine and Western folk medicine used this plant for similar purposes. It was well regarded as a diuretic, a cough suppressant, and an alterative.[1] Alterative plants were considered beneficial for all manner of chronic conditions, particularly those afflicting the skin.

Active Constituents

Red clover contains high amounts of isoflavone compounds, such as genistein, which have weak estrogen properties.[2] Research on both red clover and **soy** (p. 332) isoflavones is currently looking at their action as potential alternatives to estrogen in **menopausal** (p. 118) women. Various laboratory studies show that these isoflavones may help prevent cancer.[3] In one case study, use of red clover by a man with prostate cancer led to noticeable anticancer effects in his prostate after the cancer was surgically removed.[4] Although the isoflavones in red clover may help prevent certain forms of cancer (e.g., breast and prostate), more clinical studies are needed before red clover is recommended for people with cancer. The mechanism of action and responsible constituents for its purported benefit in skin conditions is unknown.

How Much Is Usually Taken?

Usually red clover is taken as a tea, by adding 1 cup (250 ml) of boiling water to 2 to 3 U.S. teaspoons (10 to 15 grams) of dried flowers and steeping, covered, for 10 to 15 minutes.[5] Three cups can be drunk each day. Red clover can also be used in capsule or tablet form in the amount of 2 to 4 grams of the dried flowers or 2 to 4 ml of tincture 3 times per day. Dried red clover tops are also available in capsules, tablets, and tinctures.

Are There Any Side Effects or Interactions? Non-fermented red clover is relatively safe. However, fer-

mented red clover may cause bleeding and should be avoided.

Red Raspberry
(Rubus idaeus)

Parts Used and Where Grown: Although most well known for its delicious berries, raspberry's leaves are used in botanical medicine. Raspberry bushes are native to North America and are cultivated in Canada.

In What Conditions Might Red Raspberry Be Supportive?

Ranking	Health Concerns
Other	Common cold/sore throat (p. 41) Diarrhea (p. 58) Pregnancy and postpartum support (p. 143)

Historical or Traditional Use

Raspberry leaves, beyond their traditional use for diarrhea, have been connected to female health, including pregnancy. It was considered a remedy for excessive menstrual flow (menorrhagia) and as a "partus prepartor," or an agent used during pregnancy to help prevent complications.[1]

Active Constituents

Raspberry leaves are high in tannins and like its relative, blackberry, may relieve acute **diarrhea** (p. 58).[2] The constituents that affect the smooth muscles, such as in the uterus, have not yet been clearly identified.

How Much Is Usually Taken?

Traditionally, raspberry leaf tea is prepared by pouring 1 cup (250 ml) boiling water over 1 to 2 U.S. teaspoons (5 to 10 grams) of the herb and steeping for 10 to 15 minutes. Up to 6 cups per day may be necessary for acute problems such as diarrhea or sore throats due to a cold, while less (2 to 3 cups) is used for preventive use during pregnancy. By itself, raspberry is usually not a sufficient treatment for diarrhea. Tincture can be used in the amount of 4 to 8 ml 3 times per day. The German Commission E monograph has concluded that there is insufficient proof to recommend red raspberry in modern herbal medicine.[3]

Are There Any Side Effects or Interactions? Raspberry may cause mild loosening of stools and nausea.

Reishi
(Ganoderma lucidum)

Common names: Ling chih, ling zhi

Parts Used and Where Grown: Reishi mushrooms grow wild on decaying logs and tree stumps in the coastal provinces of China. The fruiting body of the mushroom is employed medicinally. Reishi grows in six different colors, but the red variety is most commonly used and commercially cultivated in North America, China, Taiwan, Japan, and Korea.[1]

In What Conditions Might Reishi Be Supportive?

Ranking	Health Concerns
Other	Altitude sickness
	Fatigue
	Hepatitis (p. 77)
	High triglycerides (p. 85)
	HIV support (p. 87)

Historical or Traditional Use

Reishi has been used in traditional Chinese medicine for more than 4,000 years.[2] The Chinese name *ling zhi* translates as the "herb of spiritual potency" and was highly prized as an elixir of immortality.[3] Its traditional Chinese medicine indications include treatment of general fatigue and weakness, asthma, insomnia, and cough.[4]

Active Constituents

Reishi contains several constituents, including sterols, coumarin, mannitol, polysaccharides, and triterpenoids called ganoderic acids. Ganoderic acids may **lower blood pressure** (p. 89) as well as decrease low-density lipoprotein (LDL [p. 79]) and **triglyceride** (p. 85) levels. These specific triterpenoids also help reduce blood platelets from sticking together—an important factor in lowering the risk for **coronary artery disease** (p. 17). While human research demonstrates some efficacy for the herb in treating altitude sickness and chronic hepatitis B, these uses still need to be confirmed.[5]

How Much Is Usually Taken?

Reishi can be taken as 1.5 to 9 grams per day of the crude dried mushroom, 1 to 1.5 grams per day in powder form, 1 ml per day of tincture, or as a tea.[6]

Are There Any Side Effects or Interactions?

Side effects from reishi can include dizziness, dry mouth and throat, nose bleeds, and abdominal upset; these rare effects may develop with continuous use over 3 to 6 months.[7] As it may increase bleeding time, reishi is not recommended for those taking anticoagulant (e.g., blood-thinning) medications. Pregnant or lactating women should consult a physician before taking reishi.

Rosemary
(Rosmarinus officinalis)

Parts Used and Where Grown: The rosemary plant originated in the countries surrounding the Mediterranean Sea; now it grows in North America as well. The leaf is employed medicinally.

In What Conditions Might Rosemary Be Supportive?

Ranking	Health Concerns
Other	Atherosclerosis (p. 17)
	Cancer risk reduction
	Infection (p. 101)
	Rheumatoid arthritis (topical) (p. 151)

Historical or Traditional Use

Throughout history, rosemary was used to preserve meats.[1] It has long played a role in European herbalism and popular folklore. Sprigs of rosemary were considered a love charm, a sign of remembrance, and a way to ward off the plague. Rosemary was used for headaches and topically for baldness in ancient China.[2]

Active Constituents

A number of constituents have shown activity in the test tube. The volatile oil, including eucalyptol (cineole), is considered to have potent antibacterial effects[3] and to relax smooth muscles in the lungs.[4] Rosmarinic acid has **antioxidant** (p. 267) activity.[5] Another ingredient of rosemary, known as carnosol, inhibits cancer formation in animal studies.[6] No human studies confirm rosemary's use for these conditions.

How Much Is Usually Taken?

The German Commission E monograph suggests a daily dose of 4 to 6 grams of rosemary leaf.[7] A tea can be prepared by adding 2 U.S. teaspoons (10 grams) of

Rosemary

herb to 1 cup (250 ml) boiling water and allowing it to steep in a covered container for 10 to 15 minutes. If tincture is preferred, 2 to 5 ml 3 times per day can be used. The concentrated essential oil should not be taken internally. Rosemary is often combined with other herbs.

Are There Any Side Effects or Interactions? There is no evidence to indicate that intermittent intake of moderate doses of rosemary poses any threat during pregnancy or lactation. However, internal intake of the oil should be avoided as it may act as an abortifacent.[8]

Sage
(Salvia officinalis)

Parts Used and Where Grown: The leaves of this common kitchen herb are used in medicine as well as in cooking. Sage originally came from the area around the Mediterranean but now also grows in North America.

In What Conditions Might Sage Be Supportive?

Ranking	Health Concerns
Other	Common cold/sore throat (p. 41)
	Gingivitis (periodontal disease) (p. 73)
	Menopause (p. 118)
	Pregnancy and postpartum support (p. 143)

Historical or Traditional Use

Sage has one of the longest histories of use as a medicinal herb. It has been employed to treat cancers and excessive perspiration and to dry up milk when a woman is no longer going to breastfeed.[1] Based on this antiperspiration and drying effect, sage is used for women who are sweating due to menopause.[2] Sage was also used, along with **rosemary** (p. 455) and **thyme** (p. 464), to preserve a number of foods, including meats and cheeses.

Active Constituents

The essential oil of sage contains active constituents, including ocimene, cineole, limonene, and terpinene. Several of these terpene compounds are **antioxidants** (p. 267)[3] and kill a variety of bacteria.[4] As yet, the mechanism of the plant in reducing lactation and sweating has not been investigated in depth.

How Much Is Usually Taken?

The German Commission E monograph suggests a daily dose of 4 to 6 grams of sage leaf.[5] A tea prepared

from 2 to 3 U.S. teaspoons (10 to 15 grams) of the herb is generally used. The tea is made by steeping sage leaves in hot water in a covered container for 15 minutes. This tea can be gargled for a sore throat, and then swallowed, or it can be swallowed for other purposes. Three cups a day should be drunk. Alternatively, 4 ml of the tincture 3 times per day can be used.

Are There Any Side Effects or Interactions? Women who are breastfeeding should only use sage in medicinal doses if they want to dry up the flow of milk. Pregnant women should not use the pure essential oil and alcoholic extracts of sage internally.[6] Sage should be avoided when fever is present.

Sandalwood
(Santalum album)

Parts Used and Where Grown: Sandalwood trees grow in India and Asia. The wood is renowned for carving and also yields the medicinal oil.

In What Conditions Might Sandalwood Be Supportive?

Ranking	Health Concerns
Other	Infection (p. 63)

Historical or Traditional Use

Sandalwood oil was used traditionally to treat skin diseases, acne, dysentery, gonorrhea, and a number of other conditions.[1] In traditional Chinese medicine, sandalwood oil is considered an excellent sedating agent.

Active Constituents

The essential oil contains high amounts of alpha- and beta-santalol. These small molecules possess antibacterial and sedative properties.[2,3] Synthetic sandalwood does not contain the active ingredients.

How Much Is Usually Taken?

The German Commission E monograph suggests 1 to 1.5 grams of the essential oil for the supportive treatment of **urinary tract infections** (p. 160).[4] This should only be done under the supervision of a doctor. Treatment should not exceed 6 weeks. Typically, a few drops of sandalwood oil are dissolved in 6 ounces of water and applied directly to the infected area of skin several times daily.

Are There Any Side Effects or Interactions? Some people may experience mild skin irritation from topical application of sandalwood oil.[5] Persons with kidney disease should not use sandalwood internally.

Sarsaparilla
(Smilax spp.)

Parts Used and Where Grown: Many different species are called by the general name sarsaparilla. Various species are found in Mexico, South America, and the Caribbean. The root is used therapeutically.

In What Conditions Might Sarsaparilla Be Supportive?

Ranking	Health Concerns
Other	Eczema (p. 64) Psoriasis (p. 147) Rheumatoid arthritis (p. 151)

Historical or Traditional Use

In Mexico, sarsaparilla was used for arthritis, cancer, skin diseases, and a host of other conditions.[1] At the turn of the century, there were reports of its use in the treatment of psoriasis and leprosy.[2] Sarsaparilla also has a tradition of use in various women's health concerns and was rumored to have a progesterone-like effect. Sarsaparilla was formerly a major flavoring agent in root beer.

Active Constituents

Sarsaparilla contains steroidal saponins, such as sarsasapogenin, which may mimic the action of some human hormones; this property remains undocumented. Sarsaparilla also contains phytosterols, such as **beta-sitosterol** (p. 270), which may contribute to the anti-inflammatory effect of this herb. Reports have shown anti-inflammatory[3] and liver-protecting[4] effects for this herb.

How Much Is Usually Taken?

Sarsaparilla is often taken in capsules at a dose of 2 to 4 grams 3 times daily.[5] A tincture may also be used in the amount of 2 to 4 ml 3 times daily. Sarsaparilla is usually used in conjunction with other therapeutic herbs.

Are There Any Side Effects or Interactions?

According to the German Commission E monograph, sarsaparilla may cause stomach irritation and temporary kidney irritation.[6] As sarsaparilla can increase absorption and/or elimination of digitalis and bismuth, such combinations are contraindicated.[7]

Saw Palmetto
(Serenoa repens, Sabal serrulata)

Parts Used and Where Grown: Saw palmetto (sometimes referred to as sabal in Europe) is a native of North America. The berries of the plant are used.

In What Conditions Might Saw Palmetto Be Supportive?

Ranking	Health Concerns
Primary	Benign prostatic hyperplasia (p. 145)

Historical or Traditional Use

In the early part of this century, saw palmetto berry tea was commonly recommended for benign enlargement of the prostate. It was also used to treat chronic urinary tract infections. Some believed that the berry increased sperm production and sex drive in men.

Active Constituents

The liposterolic (fat-soluble) extract of saw palmetto provides fatty acids, sterols, and esters. The extract is thought to reduce the amount of dihydrotesterone (an active form of testosterone) locally in the prostate.[1] Saw palmetto does not appear to inhibit production of this form of testosterone elsewhere in the body.[2] Saw palmetto also inhibits the actions of inflammatory substances that may contribute to **benign prostatic hyperplasia** (BPH [p. 145]). Contrary to some opinions, saw palmetto does not exert an estrogenic effect in men's bodies.

In Europe, herbal supplements have become one of the leading methods for managing early stages of BPH. Successful treatment of BPH is an ongoing process. Men with BPH will probably need to take one or a combination of these herbs indefinitely. Any nutritional support for BPH should be done after consulting a doctor.

Over the last decade, numerous clinical studies have proven that 320 mg per day of the liposterolic extract of saw palmetto berries is a safe and effective treatment for the symptoms of BPH. A recent review of studies completed by Harvard researchers concluded that saw palmetto extract was as effective as Proscar in the treatment of BPH.[3] Although some uncontrolled clinical studies have shown success over a 3-month period,[4,5,6] recent studies have demonstrated the effectiveness of saw palmetto in studies lasting 6 months to 3 years.

A 3-year study in Germany found that taking 160 mg of saw palmetto extract twice daily reduced nighttime urination in 73% of people and improved urinary flow rates significantly.[7] In a multicenter study at various sites in Europe, 160 mg of saw palmetto extract taken twice daily was found to treat BPH as effectively as Proscar without side effects such as loss of libido.[8] A 1-year study found that taking 320 mg once daily was as effective as 160 mg taken twice daily in the treatment of BPH.[9]

Saw palmetto extract has also been combined with a **nettle** root (p. 447) extract to successfully treat BPH. One study using a combination of saw palmetto extract (320 mg per day) and nettle root extract (240 mg per day) showed positive actions on symptoms of BPH over a 1-year treatment period.[10] Another study compared the same combination to Proscar for 1 year with positive results.[11]

How Much Is Usually Taken?

For early-stage benign prostatic hyperplasia (BPH), 320 mg per day of the liposterolic saw palmetto herbal extract—which is rich in fatty acids, sterols, and esters—can be taken.[12] It may take 4 to 6 weeks to see results with BPH; if improvement is noted, the saw palmetto should be used continuously. Although it has not been tested for efficacy, saw palmetto can also be used by making a tea with 5 to 6 grams of the powdered dried fruit. Liquid extracts of whole herb at 5 to 6 ml per day may also be used, but has not been specifically tested.

Are There Any Side Effects or Interactions? No significant side effects have been noted in clinical studies with saw palmetto extracts. However, in rare cases saw palmetto can cause stomach problems.[13] Saw palmetto extract does not interfere with accurate measuring of prostate-specific antigen—a marker for prostate cancer.[14] Saw palmetto is most effective in managing symptoms of BPH and has not been shown to aggressively shrink the size of the prostate. Please note that BPH can only be diagnosed by a physician; use of saw palmetto extract for this condition should only occur after a thorough workup and diagnosis by a doctor. There are no proven uses of saw palmetto for women.

Schisandra
(Schisandra chinensis)

Common name: Wu-wei-zi

Parts Used and Where Grown: Schisandra is a woody vine with numerous clusters of tiny, bright red berries. It is distributed throughout northern and northeast China and the adjacent regions of Russia and Korea.[1] The fully ripe, sun-dried fruit is used medicinally. It is purported to have sour, sweet, salty, hot, and bitter tastes. This unusual combination of flavors is reflected in schisandra's Chinese name wu-wei-zi, meaning "five taste fruit."

In What Conditions Might Schisandra Be Supportive?

Ranking	Health Concerns
Other	Common cold/sore throat (p. 41)
	Fatigue
	Hepatitis (p. 77)
	Infection (p. 63)
	Liver support
	Stress

Historical or Traditional Use

The classical treatise on Chinese herbal medicine, the *Shen Nung Pen Tsao Ching,* describes schisandra as a high-grade herbal drug useful for a wide variety of medical conditions—especially as a kidney tonic and lung astringent. In addition, other textbooks on traditional Chinese medicine note that schisandra is useful for coughs, night sweats, insomnia, thirst, and physical exhaustion.[2]

Active Constituents

Schisandra contains a number of compounds, including essential oils, numerous acids, and lignans. Lignans (schizandrin, deoxyschizandrin, gomisins, and pregomisin) are found in the seeds of the fruit and have a number of medicinal actions. Modern Chinese research suggests that lignans regenerate liver tissue damaged by harmful influences such as viral hepatitis and alcohol. Lignans lower blood levels of serum glutamic pyruvic transaminase (SGPT), a marker for infective hepatitis and other liver disorders.[3] Lignans also interfere with platelet-activating factor, a chemical that promotes inflammation in a number of conditions.[4] Standardized extracts of schisandra fruits have gained popularity for use in racehorses not running well in relation to elevated liver enzyme levels.[5]

Schisandra fruit may also have an adaptogenic action, much like the herb **ginseng** (p. 394), but with weaker effects. Laboratory work suggests that schisandra may improve work performance, build strength, and help to reduce fatigue.[6]

How Much Is Usually Taken?

Use of schisandra fruit ranges from 1.5 to 15 grams per day.[7] The tincture, in the amount of 2 to 4 ml 3 times per day, can also be used.

Are There Any Side Effects or Interactions? Side effects involving schisandra are uncommon but may include abdominal upset, decreased appetite, and skin rash.[8]

Scullcap
(Scutellaria lateriflora, Scutellaria baicalensis)

Parts Used and Where Grown: Scullcap is a member of the mint family. *Scutellaria lateriflora* grows in eastern North America and is most commonly used in U.S. and European herbal products containing scullcap. The aerial part of the plant is used in herbal preparations. *Scutellaria baicalensis* is grown in China and Russia. The root of this plant is used in traditional Chinese herbal medicines and has been the focus of most scientific studies on scullcap. American and Chinese scullcap are generally not interchangeable.

In What Conditions Might Scullcap Be Supportive?

Ranking	Health Concerns
Other	Anxiety (p. 14)
	Insomnia (p. 105)

Historical or Traditional Use

As is the case in modern herbal medicine, scullcap was used historically as a sedative for persons with nervous tension and insomnia. It was, and continues to be, commonly combined with **valerian** (p. 467) for insomnia.[1] It was also used as a remedy for epilepsy and nerve pain. Chinese scullcap is typically used in herbal combinations to treat inflammatory skin conditions, allergic diseases, high cholesterol and triglycerides, and high blood pressure.

Active Constituents

Few studies have been completed on the constituents of American scullcap. One of its constituents, scutellarian, has been shown to have mild sedative and antispasmodic actions.[2] Human studies have not yet been conducted to confirm the use of scullcap for **anxiety** (p. 14) or **insomnia** (p. 105). The root of Chinese scullcap also contains a flavonoid substance, baicalin, that has been shown to have protective actions on the liver. Antiallergy actions and the inhibition of bacteria and viruses in test tube studies has been documented with Chinese scullcap.[3] Clinical research is lacking to show efficacy for Chinese scullcap.

How Much Is Usually Taken?

A Chinese or American scullcap tea can be made by pouring 1 cup (250 ml) of boiling water over 1 to 2 U.S. teaspoons (5 to 10 grams) of the dried herb and steeping for 10 to 15 minutes; this tea may be drunk 3 times per day. As a tincture, American scullcap can be taken in the amount of 2 to 4 ml 3 times per day. For the dried herb, 1 to 2 grams 3 times per day is often used. In traditional Chinese herbal medicine, Chinese scullcap is typically recommended as a tea made from 3 to 9 grams of the dried root.[4]

Are There Any Side Effects or Interactions? Use of scullcap in the amounts listed above is generally safe. Due to limited information on the safety of scullcap during pregnancy and lactation, it should be avoided by pregnant or lactating women. Cases of liver damage have been reported in association with intake of scullcap. On closer examination, it appears that these scullcap products actually contained germander, an herb known to cause liver damage.[5]

Senna
(Cassia senna, Cassia angustifolia)

Parts Used and Where Grown: The senna shrub grows in India, Pakistan, and China. The leaves and pods are used medicinally.

In What Conditions Might Senna Be Supportive?

Ranking	Health Concerns
Primary	Constipation (p. 44)

Historical or Traditional Use

People in northern Africa and southwestern Asia have used senna as a laxative for centuries. It was considered a "cleansing" herb because of its cathartic effect. In addition, the leaves were sometimes made into a paste and applied to various skin diseases. Ringworm and acne were both treated in this way.

Active Constituents

Senna contains anthraquinone glycosides known as sennosides. These molecules are converted by the normal bacteria in the colon into rhein-anthrone, which in turn has two effects. It first stimulates colon activity and thus speeds bowel movements. Second, it increases fluid secretion by the colon.[1] Together, these actions work to get a sluggish colon functional again. Several controlled studies have confirmed the benefit of senna in treating **constipation** (p. 44).[2,3] Constipation induced by drugs such as the anti-diarrhea medicine Imodium (loperamide) has also been shown to be improved by senna in a clinical trial.[4]

How Much Is Usually Taken?

It's best to follow the instructions on the label of over-the-counter senna products. Some doctors of natural medicine suggest an herbal extract in capsules or tablets providing 20 to 60 mg of sennosides per day.[5] This can be continued for a maximum of 10 days maximum. Use beyond 10 days is strongly discouraged. If constipation is not alleviated within 10 days, individuals should seek the help of a health-care professional. Combination with herbal mint teas can help decrease cramping. Half the adult dose of senna can be safely used in children over the age of 6.

Are There Any Side Effects or Interactions? Senna can cause the colon to become dependent on it to move properly. Therefore, senna must not be used for more than 10 consecutive days. Chronic senna use can also cause loss of fluids, low **potassium** levels (p. 323), and **diarrhea** (p. 58), all of which can lead to dehydration and negative effects on the heart and muscles. Senna is safe for use during pregnancy and lactation but only under the supervision of a physician.[6,7] It is also safe for children over the age of 6. People with **Crohn's disease** (p. 48), appendicitis, intestinal obstructions, and abdominal pain should not supplement with senna.[8]

Shiitake
(Lentinus edodes)

Common name: Hua gu

Parts Used and Where Grown: Wild shiitake mushrooms are native to Japan, China, and other Asian countries and typically grow on fallen broadleaf trees. Shiitake is widely cultivated throughout the world, including the United States. The fruiting body is used medicinally.

In What Conditions Might Shiitake Be Supportive?

Ranking	Health Concerns
Other	Hepatitis (p. 77)
	HIV support (p. 87)

Historical or Traditional Use

Shiitake has been revered in Japan and China as both a food and medicinal herb for thousands of years. Wu

Ri, a famous physician from the Chinese Ming Dynasty (A.D. 1368 to 1644), wrote extensively about this mushroom, noting its ability to increase energy, cure colds, and eliminate worms.[1]

Active Constituents

Shiitake contains proteins, fats, carbohydrates, soluble fiber, vitamins, and minerals. In addition, shiitake's key ingredient—found in the fruiting body—is a polysaccharide called lentinan. Commercial preparations employ the powdered mycelium of the mushroom before the cap and stem grow; this is called LEM (lentinus edodes mycelium extract). LEM is also rich in polysaccharides and lignans.

Research indicates that lentinan injections may help some people with hepatitis.[2] A highly purified intravenous form of lentinan has been employed in Japan to increase survival in those with recurrent stomach cancer (particularly when used in combination with chemotherapy).[3] These effects may be due to shiitake's ability to stimulate specific types of white blood cells called T-lymphocytes. Case reports from Japan are also suggestive that lentinan is helpful in treating individuals with **HIV** (p. 87) infection. However, large-scale clinical trials to confirm this action have not yet been performed.[4]

How Much Is Usually Taken?

The traditional intake of the whole, dried shiitake mushroom, in soups or as a decoction, is 6 to 16 grams per day.[5] For LEM, the intake is 1 to 3 grams 2 to 3 times per day. As LEM is the more concentrated and hence more potent extract, it is preferred by many herbalists over the crude mushroom. Tincture, in the amount of 2 to 4 ml per day, can also be used.

Are There Any Side Effects or Interactions? Shiitake has an excellent record of safety but has been known to induce temporary diarrhea and abdominal bloating when used in high dosages (above 15 to 20 grams per day). Its safety during pregnancy has not yet been established.

Slippery Elm
(Ulmus rubra)

Parts Used and Where Grown: The slippery elm tree is native to North America, where it still primarily grows. The inner bark of the tree provides the greatest therapeutic benefit.

Historical or Traditional Use

Native Americans found innumerable medicinal and other uses for this tree. Canoes, baskets, and other household goods were made from the tree and its bark. Slippery elm was also used internally for everything from sore throats to diarrhea.[1] As a poultice, it was considered a remedy for almost any skin condition.

In What Conditions Might Slippery Elm Be Supportive?

Ranking	Health Concerns
Other	Common cold/sore throat (p. 41) Cough (p. 47) Crohn's disease (p. 48) Gastritis (p. 71)

Active Constituents

The mucilage of slippery elm gives it the soothing effect for which it is known.[2] The bark contains a host of other constituents, but the carbohydrates that comprise the mucilage are the most important.

How Much Is Usually Taken?

Two or more tablets or capsules (typically 400 to 500 mg each) can be taken 3 to 4 times per day. A tea is made by boiling ½ to 2 grams of the bark in 200 ml of water for 10 to 15 minutes, which is then cooled before drinking; 3 to 4 cups a day can be used.[3] Tincture, 5 ml 3 times per day, can be taken. Slippery elm is also an ingredient of some cough lozenges and cough syrups.

Are There Any Side Effects or Interactions? Slippery elm is quite safe. However, because it is so mucilaginous, it may interfere with the absorption of medicine taken at the same time.

St. John's Wort
(Hypericum perforatum)

Parts Used and Where Grown: St. John's wort is found in Europe and the United States; it is especially abundant in northern California and southern Oregon. The above-ground (aerial) parts of the plant are gathered during the flowering season. Similar species are found around the world.

Historical or Traditional Use

In ancient Greece, the herb was used to treat many ailments, including sciatica and poisonous reptile bites. In Europe, St. John's wort was, and continues to be, very popular for the topical treatment of wounds and burns. It is also a folk remedy for kidney and lung ailments as well as depression.

In What Conditions Might St. John's Wort Be Supportive?

Ranking	Health Concerns
Primary	Depression (p. 50)
Secondary	Anxiety (p. 14)
Other	Ear infections (recurrent) (p. 63) Cold sores (p. 41) Injuries (minor) (p. 122) Ulcerative colitis (p. 158) Vitiligo (p. 164) Wound healing (p. 167)

Active Constituents

St. John's wort has a complex diverse chemical make-up that includes hypericin and other dianthrones, flavonoids, xanthones, and hyperforin.[1] While it was previously thought that the antidepressant actions of St. John's wort were due to hypercin and inhibition of the enzyme monomine oxidase,[2] current research has challenged this belief. Recent studies have focused on other constituents, such as hyperforin, xanthones, and flavonoids.[3,4]

New research suggests that St. John's wort extracts exert their antidepressant actions by inhibiting the reuptake of the neurotransmitters serotonin, norepinephrine, and dopamine.[5] This action is possibly due to the constituent hyperforin.[6] By making more of these neurotransmitters available to the brain, St. John's wort is able to act as an antidepressant.

How Much Is Usually Taken?

The standard recommendation for mild to moderate depression is 300 mg of St. John's wort extract 3 times daily.[7] Higher intakes may be used, under the supervision of a health-care professional, for more severe depression. Results can be noted as early as 2 weeks, and length of use should be discussed with a health-care professional. Although research has used only standardized extracts, the German Commission E monograph suggests a daily amount of 2 to 4 grams of the whole herb.[8]

Are There Any Side Effects or Interactions? St. John's wort could, theoretically, make the skin more sensitive to sunlight, but this is rare when used at recommended levels.[9] However, fair-skinned individuals should be alert for any rashes or burns following exposure to the sun. Preliminary evidence suggests there may be a risk of St. John's wort interacting with selective serotonin reuptake inhibitor (SSRI) drugs, such as Prozac, and causing side effects known collectively as serotonin syndrome. For those taking an SSRI who wish to start St. John's wort, see a doctor first. While some research suggests St. John's wort is safe during pregnancy and lactation,[10] safety studies are lacking.

Stevia
(Stevia rebaudiana)

Common name: Sweetleaf

Parts Used and Where Grown: The leaf is utilized medicinally. The stevia plant originally came from the rain forests of Brazil and Paraguay. It is now grown in those areas, as well as in Japan, Korea, Thailand, and China. It is most widely used as a nonsugar sweetener in food and drink, particularly because it does not appear to have any of the side effects of sugar and is not broken down by heat.

Historical or Traditional Use

The native peoples in South America used stevia primarily as a sweetener, a practice adopted by European colonists in local regions. The indigenous tribes also used stevia to treat diabetes.[1] During World War II, stevia was grown in England as a sugar substitute. The greatest use of stevia today can be found in Japan.

Active Constituents

Various glycosides, particularly stevoside, give stevia its sweetness. Stevoside is somewhere between 100 and 200 times sweeter than sugar. Early reports suggested that stevia might reduce blood sugar (and therefore potentially help with **diabetes** [p. 53]),[2] although not all reports have confirmed this.[3] Even if stevia did not have direct antidiabetic effects, its use as a sweetener could reduce intake of sugars in people with diabetes. Other studies have shown stevia to dilate blood vessels in animals, which might reduce **high blood pressure** (p. 89).[4] The doses used were higher than those used for sweetening purposes, and this effect has not been proven in humans.

How Much Is Usually Taken?

Less than 1 gram per day can be used effectively as a sweetener. Usually, the powdered herb is added directly to tea or to food.

Are There Any Side Effects or Interactions? Extensive reviews of human and animal data indicate stevia to be safe.[5] Stevia accounts for nearly 40% of the sweetener market in Japan and is commonly used in various parts of South America.[6] Moderate intake of stevia is not believed to be harmful.

Sundew
(Drosera rotundifolia, D. ramentacea, D. intermedia, D. anglica)

Parts Used and Where Grown: Extracts from the carnivorous sundew *(Drosera rotundifolia, D. ramentacea)* as well as other species in the Droseracea family are made primarily from the roots, flowers, and fruit-like capsules.[1] The plants have their primary origins in East Africa and Madagascar but are cultivated throughout the world. The primary species originally used in cough preparations in Germany, *D. rotundifolia, D. intermedia,* and *D. anglica,* are rarely used currently due to threat of extinction. Instead, *D. ramentacea* and other *Drosera* species from Australia are employed.

In What Conditions Might Sundew Be Supportive?

Ranking	Health Concerns
Primary	Coughs (particularly dry and irritating) (p. 47)

Historical and Traditional Use

The historical use of sundew is similar to its use in modern herbal medicine. In 1685, Johann Schroder wrote in his book, *The Apothecary or a Treasure Chest of Valuable Medicines,* that sundew was a beneficial herb that "cures lung ailments and cures coughs." Sundew tea was specifically recommended in Europe for dry **coughs** (p. 47), bronchitis, whooping cough, **asthma** (p. 15), and "bronchial cramps."[2]

Active Constituents

The naphthaquinones are believed to give sundew the antispasmodic effects that have made it such a popular cough remedy in Europe.[3] These naphthaquinones include plumbagin, ramentone, ramentaceon, and biramentaceone. Pharmacological studies show a clear antispasmodic effect in the respiratory tract.[4] One naphthaquinone (referred to as C.O.N.) was found in an animal study to suppress the impulse to cough to a comparable degree as codeine. This finding has not been repeated in humans. Based on this effect, sundew is often referred to as an herbal antitussive (a substance capable of preventing or relieving coughing). Human studies have shown its value either alone or in combination with other herbs for the treatment of coughs associated with bronchitits, pharyngitis, laryngitis, and even whooping cough.[5]

How Much Is Usually Taken?

The average daily dose of sundew for adults and children older than 12 years of age is 3 grams.[6] To prepare tea, boiling water is poured over 1 to 2 grams (1 teaspoon or approximately 0.4 grams) of finely cut sundew root and above-ground parts, and strained after steeping for 10 minutes. One cup may be drunk 3 to 4 times daily. In Europe, liquid preparations of sundew are often combined with thyme, another antitussive, in cough syrups for adults and children. A tincture of sundew is sometimes used at a dose of 0.5 to 1.0 ml 3 times daily.

Are There Any Side Effects or Interactions?

At the amounts listed above, sundew is thought to be very safe.[7] Higher levels may lead to gastrointestinal irritation in some persons. Pregnant and lactating women should avoid use of sundew.

Sweet Annie

(Artemisia annua)

Common names: Qinghao, sweet wormwood

Parts Used and Where Grown: This inconspicuous herb originated in Europe and Asia and has since spread to North America. It is now a common weed around the world. The above-ground parts of the plant are used medicinally.

In What Conditions Might Sweet Annie Be Supportive?

Ranking	Health Concerns
Primary	Malaria (as prescription drug only)
Other	Fever Infectious diarrhea (p. 58) Intestinal parasites (p. 137)

Historical or Traditional Use

Ancient Chinese medical texts dating from around 150 B.C. suggest the use of sweet Annie for people with hemorrhoids (p. 77).[1] Other writings from A.D. 340 are the first known to mention sweet Annie as a treatment for people with fevers.[2] It has been used ever since for a variety of infections in Chinese traditional medicine.

Active Constituents

Artemisinin, called qinghaosu in China where it was first discovered, is thought to account for the antimalarial activity of the plant.[3,4] This compound is a sesquiterpene lactone and is believed to cause free radical damage to the organisms that cause malaria inside

of the red blood cells they infect. Numerous unblinded but randomized clinical studies, and some double-blind ones, have shown that injections or oral doses of artemisinin or similar compounds rapidly and effectively cure people with malaria.[5] Randomized, open, clinical studies have shown that artemisinin reduced mortality due to malaria by 50% compared with treatment with a standard quinoline anti-malarial drug.[6] Artemisinin-based drugs have not been studied for prevention of malaria. Test tube studies suggest artemisinin can kill other parasites and bacteria,[7] supporting the traditional notion of using it for **parasitic infections** (p. 137) of the gastrointestinal tract. Doctors of natural medicine use sweet Annie in combination with other antiparasitic herbs.

How Much Is Usually Taken?

Artemisinin-based drugs are not readily available in the United States or Europe and can be obtained only by prescription. Sweet Annie cannot be substituted for artemisinin as a drug and cannot be used to treat people with malaria, a potentially lethal disease requiring immediate antibiotic treatment. Traditionally 3 grams of powdered herb was taken each day.[8]

Are There Any Side Effects or Interactions?

No serious adverse effects have been seen in scores of clinical studies.[9] Upset stomach, loose stools, abdominal pain, and occasional fever may occur when taking artemisinin as a drug. The use of the whole herb is also not associated with side effects.

Tea Tree

(Melaleuca alternifolia)

Parts Used and Where Grown: The tea tree grows in Australia and Asia. This tall evergreen tree has a white, spongy bark. The oil from the leaves is used.

In What Conditions Might Tea Tree Be Supportive?

Ranking	Health Concerns
Primary	Acne (p. 5) Athlete's foot (p. 20)
Other	Injuries (minor) (p. 122) Vaginitis (p. 162) Yeast infection (p. 169)

Historical or Traditional Use

Australian aboriginals used the leaves to treat cuts and skin infections. They would crush the leaves and apply them to the affected area. Captain James Cook and his crew named the tree "tea tree," using its leaves as a substitute for tea as well as to flavor beer. Australian soldiers participating in World War I were given tea tree oil as a disinfectant, leading to a high demand for its production.

Active Constituents

The oil contains numerous chemicals known as terpenoids. Australian standards were established for the amount of one particular compound, terpinen-4-ol, which must make up at least 30% and preferably 40 to 50% of the oil for it to be medically useful. Another compound, cineole, should make up less than 15% and preferably 2.5% of the oil. The oil kills fungus and bacteria, including those resistant to some antibiotics.[1,2] A single-blind study has shown topical application of 5% tea tree oil in people with acne is as helpful as benzoylperoxide and has fewer side effects.[3]

A double-blind study found 100% tea tree oil applied topically was as effective as the antifungal medicine clotrimazole for people with **athlete's foot** (p. 20) fungus affecting the toe nails.[4] Another double-blind study found that 10% tea tree oil cream was as effective as antifungal medicine at improving symptoms associated with foot fungus, though it was not more effective than placebo for eliminating foot fungus.[5]

A single-blind study found that rinsing the mouth with 15 ml (1 U.S. tablespoon) tea tree oil solution 4 times daily effectively treated oral yeast (thrush) in people with **AIDS** (p. 87).[6] Solutions containing no more than 5% should be used orally and should never be swallowed.

How Much Is Usually Taken?

Oil at a strength of 70 to 100% should be applied moderately at least twice per day to the affected areas of skin or nail.[7] For topical treatment of acne, the oil is used at a dilution of 5 to 15%. Concentrations as strong as 40% may be used—with extreme caution and qualified advice—as vaginal douches. Oil diluted to 5% or less is used at a dose of 1 tablespoon 4 times daily for treatment of thrush in immune-compromised adults. Burning may occur when rinsing with tea tree oil. The solution is never swallowed after use.

Are There Any Side Effects or Interactions? While tea tree oil can be applied to minor cuts and scrapes, use caution for more extensive areas of broken skin or areas affected by rashes not due to fungus. The oil may burn if it gets into the eyes, nose, mouth, or other tender areas. Some people have allergic reactions, including rashes and itching, when applying tea tree

oil.[8] For this reason, only a small amount should be applied when first using it. Tea tree oil should never be swallowed, as it may cause nerve damage and other problems.

Thyme
(Thymus vulgaris)

Parts Used and Where Grown: The plant is indigenous to the Mediterranean region of Europe and is extensively cultivated in the United States. The dried or partially dried leaves and flowering tops are used.

In What Conditions Might Thyme Be Supportive?

Ranking	Health Concerns
Secondary	Bronchitis Cough (p. 47)
Other	Peptic ulcer (p. 138) Whooping cough

Historical or Traditional Use

Other than its use as a spice, thyme has a long history of use in Europe for the treatment of dry, spasmodic **coughs** (p. 47) as well as bronchitis.[1] Its antispasmodic actions have made it a common traditional recommendation for whooping cough. Thyme has also been used to ease an irritated gastrointestinal tract. The oil has been used to treat topical fungal infections and is also used in toothpastes to prevent **gingivitis** (p. 73).

Active Constituents

Many constituents in thyme team up to provide its antitussive (preventing and treating a cough), antispasmodic, and expectorant actions. The primary constituents are the volatile oils, which include the phenols thymol and carvacol.[2] These are complemented by the actions of flavonoids as well as saponins. Thyme, either alone or in combination with herbs such as sundew, continues to be one of the most commonly recommended herbs in Europe for the treatment of dry, spasmodic coughs as well as whooping cough.[3] Due to the low toxicity of the herb, it has become a favorite for treating coughs in small children.

How Much Is Usually Taken?

The German Commission E monograph recommends a cup of tea made from 1 to 2 grams of the herb taken several times daily as needed for a cough.[4] A fluid extract can be used in the amount of 1 to 4 ml 3 times daily. Another alternative is to use a tincture of thyme in the amount of 2 to 6 ml 3 times daily.

Are There Any Side Effects or Interactions? Used as listed above, thyme herbal preparations are generally very safe. However, a spasmodic cough, particularly in a young child, may be dangerous; a healthcare professional should be consulted before deciding on the proper course of treatment. There are no known contraindications to the use of thyme by pregnant or lactating women. Thyme oil should be reserved for topical use, as internally it may lead to dizziness, vomiting, and breathing difficulties.[5] Some persons may be sensitive to use of thyme oil topically on the skin or as a rinse in the mouth.

Turmeric
(Curcuma longa)

Parts Used and Where Grown: The vast majority of turmeric comes from India. Turmeric is one of the key ingredients in many curries, giving them color and flavor. The root and rhizome (underground stem) are used medicinally.

In What Conditions Might Turmeric Be Supportive?

Ranking	Health Concerns
Secondary	Indigestion and heartburn (p. 99) Rheumatoid arthritis (p. 151)
Other	Atherosclerosis (p. 17) Bursitis (p. 30) Gallstones (p. 69) Inflammation

Historical or Traditional Use

In Ayurvedic medicine (the traditional medicine of India), many different species similar to turmeric are used. It was prescribed for treatment of many conditions, including poor vision, **rheumatic pains,** coughs, and to increase milk production. Native peoples of the Pacific sprinkled the dust on their shoulders during ceremonial dances and used it for numerous medical problems ranging from constipation to skin diseases. Turmeric was used for numerous intestinal infections and ailments in Southeast Asia.

Active Constituents

The active constituent is known as curcumin. It has been shown to have a wide range of therapeutic actions. First, it protects against free radical damage because it is a strong **antioxidant** (p. 267).[1,2] Second, it reduces inflammation by lowering histamine levels and possibly by increasing production of natural cortisone by the adrenal glands.[3] Third, it protects the liver from a number of toxic compounds.[4] Fourth, it has been shown to reduce platelets from clumping together, which in turn improves circulation and helps protect against **atherosclerosis** (p. 17).[5] There are also numerous animal studies showing a cancer-preventing action of curcumin. This may be due to its antioxidant activity in the body. Curcumin inhibits **HIV** (p. 87) in test tubes, though human studies are needed to determine if it will be a useful therapy or not.[6]

Human studies are generally lacking for turmeric. A double-blind study in people with **rheumatoid arthritis** (p. 151) found curcumin extracted from turmeric to be less effective than the anti-inflammatory drug phenylbutazone, though independent observers of the study participants felt both agents were equally effective.[7] A separate double-blind trial found that curcumin was superior to placebo or phenylbutazone for alleviating postsurgical inflammation.[8]

While double-blind research has found turmeric helpful for people with **indigestion** (p. 99),[9] results in people with stomach or intestinal **ulcers** (p. 138) have not shown it to be superior to placebo and have shown it to be less effective than antacids.[10,11]

How Much Is Usually Taken?

A standardized extract of turmeric supplying 400 to 600 mg of curcumin can be taken 3 times per day in capsules or tablets.[12] Tincture can be used in the amount of 0.5 to 1.5 ml 3 times per day. Turmeric as a spice can also be incorporated into the diet.

Are There Any Side Effects or Interactions? Used in the recommended amounts, turmeric is generally safe. It has been used in large quantities as a condiment with no adverse reactions. However, persons with symptoms of **gallstones** (p. 69) or obstruction of bile passages should avoid turmeric.[13]

Usnea
(Usnea barbata)

Common name: Old man's beard

Parts Used and Where Grown: Usnea, also known as old man's beard, is not a plant but a lichen—a symbiotic relationship between an algae and a fungus. The entire lichen is used. Usnea looks like long, fuzzy strings hanging from trees in North American and European forests, where it grows.

In What Conditions Might Usnea Be Supportive?

Ranking	Health Concerns
Other	Common cold/sore throat (p. 41) Cough (p. 47) Infection (p. 101) Pap smear (abnormal) (p. 136)

Historical or Traditional Use

Because of its bitter taste, usnea stimulates digestion and was historically used to treat indigestion. It was also reportedly used over 3,000 years ago in ancient Egypt, Greece, and China to treat infections.[1]

Active Constituents

Usnic acid gives usnea its bitter taste and also acts as an antibiotic.[2] Usnea also contains mucilage, which can be helpful in easing irritating **coughs** (p. 47). Preliminary test tube studies suggested an anticancer activity for usnic acid; however, this action has not been sufficient to warrant further investigation.[3]

How Much Is Usually Taken?

Usnea, in capsule form, can be taken in the amount of 100 mg 3 times per day.[4] Tincture can be taken in the amount of 3 to 4 ml 3 times per day.

Are There Any Side Effects or Interactions? There are no known side effects of usnea. It is considered safe for use in children.

Uva Ursi
(Arctostaphylos uva-ursi)

Common name: Bearberry

Parts Used and Where Grown: The uva ursi plant is found in colder, northern climates. It has red berries, which bears are said to be fond of. The flowers are also red. The leaf is used.

Historical or Traditional Use

The leaves and berries were used by numerous indigenous people from northern latitudes. Native Americans sometimes combined uva ursi with tobacco and smoked it. It was also used as a beverage tea in some places in Russia. The berries were considered beneficial as a weight-loss aid. It was found in wide use for infections of all parts of the body because of its astringent, or "drying," action.

In What Conditions Might Uva Ursi Be Supportive?

Ranking	Health Concerns
Other	Urinary tract infection (p. 160)

Active Constituents

The glycoside arbutin is the active ingredient in uva ursi. Arbutin is present in fairly high amounts (up to 10%) in uva ursi. It has been shown to kill bacteria in the urine.[1] Arbutin undergoes a highly complex process in the body. It is split into a small sugar molecule and a hydroquinone in the intestines, then the liver hooks the hydroquinone to another molecule. This makes it water-soluble so it is easily carried via the blood to the kidney. There, if the urine is alkaline, the hydroquinone is released from its carrier. Hydroquinone is a powerful antimicrobial agent and is responsible for uva ursi's ability to treat urinary tract **infections** (p. 101). Arbutin has also been shown to increase the anti-inflammatory action of synthetic cortisone.[2] No human studies have been published confirming the role of uva ursi in people with urinary tract infections.

How Much Is Usually Taken?

The German Commission E monograph suggests 3 grams of uva ursi in 150 ml of water as an infusion to be taken 3 to 4 times daily.[3] For alcohol-based tinctures, 5 ml 3 times per day can be taken. Herbal extracts in capsules or tablets (containing 20% arbutin) in an amount of 250 to 500 mg 3 times per day can also be taken. Use of uva ursi should be limited to no more than 14 days. To ensure alkaline urine, 6 to 8 grams of sodium bicarbonate (baking soda) mixed in a glass of water can be drunk. Baking soda should not be taken for more than 14 days; as well, individuals with **high blood pressure** (p. 89) should not take baking soda. People should not use uva ursi to treat an infection without first consulting a physician.

Are There Any Side Effects or Interactions? Some people may experience nausea after taking uva ursi. Long-term (more than 2 to 3 weeks) use of uva ursi is not recommended, due to possible side effects from excessive levels of hydroquinone. People should avoid taking acidic agents, such as fruit juice (more than 16 ounces) or **vitamin C** (p. 341) (more than 500 mg), while using uva ursi. Uva ursi is contraindicated in pregnant or lactating women and should be used in young children only with the guidance of a health-care professional.

Uva Ursi

Valerian
(Valeriana officinalis)

Parts Used and Where Grown: Although valerian grows wild all over Europe, most of the valerian used for medicinal extracts is cultivated. The root is used.

In What Conditions Might Valerian Be Supportive?

Ranking	Health Concerns
Primary	Insomnia (p. 105)
Secondary	Anxiety (p. 14)

Historical or Traditional Use

The Greek physician Dioscorides recommended valerian for a host of medical problems, including digestive problems, nausea, liver problems, and even urinary tract disorders. Use of valerian for insomnia and nervous conditions has been common for many centuries. By the eighteenth century, it was an accepted sedative and was also used for nervous disorders associated with a restless digestive tract.

Active Constituents

Valerian root contains many different constituents, including essential oils that appear to contribute to the sedating properties of the herb. Central nervous system sedation is regulated by receptors in the brain known as GABA-A receptors. Valerian may weakly bind to these receptors to exert a sedating action.[1] This might explain why valerian can help some people deal with stress more effectively.[2]

Double-blind studies have repeatedly found that valerian is more effective than placebo and as effective as standard sleep medications for people with **insomnia** (p. 105).[3,4] Generally, valerian makes sleep more restful as well as making the transition to sleep easier, but does not tend to increase total time slept, according to these studies. Combining lemon balm and hops with valerian did not make it any more effective in another double-blind study involving people with difficulty sleeping.[5]

How Much Is Usually Taken?

For insomnia, some doctors of natural medicine suggest 300 to 500 mg of concentrated valerian root herbal extract (standardized to no less than 0.5% essential oils) in capsules or tablets 30 to 60 minutes before bedtime.[6] As an alcohol-based tincture, 5 ml can be taken before bedtime. Combination products

with **lemon balm** (p. 440), **hops** (p. 434), **passion flower** (p. 449), and **scullcap** (p. 459) can also be used. Children aged 6 to 12 often respond to half the adult dose.

Are There Any Side Effects or Interactions? Recent research indicates that valerian does not impair ability to drive or operate machinery.[7] Valerian does not lead to addiction or dependence. Valerian is not contraindicated during pregnancy or lactation.

Vitex
(Vitex agnus-castus)

Common names: Agnus-castus, chaste tree, monk's pepper

Parts Used and Where Grown: Vitex grows in the Mediterranean countries and central Asia. The dried fruit, which has a pepperlike aroma and flavor, is used.

In What Conditions Might Vitex Be Supportive?

Ranking	Health Concerns
Secondary	Infertility (female) (p. 102) Menstrual difficulties (Secondary amenorrhea) Premenstrual syndrome (p. 141)
Other	Acne (p. 5) Fibrocystic breast disease (p. 66) Menorrhagia (heavy menstruation) (p. 120)

Historical or Traditional Use

Hippocrates, Dioscorides, and Theophrastus mention the use of vitex for a wide variety of conditions, including hemorrhage following childbirth, and also to assist with the "passing of afterbirth." Decoctions of the fruit and plant were also used in sitz baths for diseases of the uterus. In addition, vitex was believed to suppress libido and inspire chastity, which explains one of its common names, chaste tree.

Active Constituents

The whole fruit extract, which contains several different components, is thought to be medicinally active.[1] Vitex does not contain hormones; its benefits stem from its actions upon the pituitary gland—specifically on the production of luteinizing hormone. This increases progesterone production and helps regulate a woman's cycle. Vitex also keeps prolactin secretion in check.[2] The ability to decrease excessive prolactin levels may benefit **infertile women** (p. 102).

A double-blind study found that women taking vitex had significantly greater relief from symptoms of **PMS** (p. 141), including breast tenderness, cramping, and headaches, than those taking **vitamin B**$_6$ (p. 339).[3] A review of other human studies suggests there is at least preliminary support that vitex should be considered for women with irregular periods, infertility, and mildly elevated prolactin levels.[4] Double-blind studies have confirmed the effectiveness of vitex at lowering prolactin levels in women[5] and men.[6] **Acne** (p. 5) associated with PMS is also reduced using vitex, according to one study.[7]

How Much Is Usually Taken?

Forty drops of the concentrated liquid herbal extract of vitex can be added to a glass of water and drunk in the morning.[8] Vitex is also available in powdered form in tablets and capsules, again to be taken once in the morning. The German Commission E monograph recommends a daily dose of 40 mg of the dried herb.

With its emphasis on long-term balancing of a woman's hormonal system, vitex is not a fast-acting herb. For premenstrual syndrome or frequent or heavy periods, vitex can be used continuously for 4 to 6 months. Women with amenorrhea and infertility can remain on vitex for 12 to 18 months, unless pregnancy occurs during treatment.

Are There Any Side Effects or Interactions? Side effects of using vitex are rare. Minor gastrointestinal upset and a mild skin rash with itching have been reported in less than 2% of the women monitored while taking vitex. Vitex is not recommended for use during pregnancy.

White Willow
(Salix alba)

Parts Used and Where Grown: The white willow tree grows primarily in central and southern Europe, although it is also found in North America. As with many medicinal trees, the bark of white willow contains the active constituents. Other species of willow may also be effective.

Historical or Traditional Use

White willow's Latin name is the source of the name for acetylsalicylic acid (aspirin), as well as the parent compound from which aspirin was eventually created. Willow bark was used traditionally for fever, headache, pain, and rheumatic complaints.[1]

In What Conditions Might White Willow Be Supportive?

Ranking	Health Concerns
Secondary	Osteoarthritis (p. 130)
Other	Bursitis (p. 130) Fever Headache (tension) Rheumatoid arthritis (p. 151)

Active Constituents

The glycoside salicin, from which the body can split off salicylic acid, is a source of the anti-inflammatory and pain-relieving actions of willow.[2] Other constituents may be just as important, however, and definitive proof of the importance of salicin is lacking. The analgesic actions of willow are typically slow acting but last longer than standard aspirin products. One study has found that a combination herbal product including 100 mg white willow bark improved functioning via pain relief in people with **osteoarthritis** (p. 130).[3]

How Much Is Usually Taken?

Willow extracts standardized for salicin content are available. The daily intake of salicin is typically 60 to 120 mg per day.[4] A white willow tea can be prepared from 1 to 2 grams of bark boiled in 200 ml of water for 10 minutes. Five or more cups of this tea can be drunk per day. Tincture is also used, commonly in the amount of 1 to 2 ml 3 times per day.

Are There Any Side Effects or Interactions? Some persons may experience gastrointestinal upset with willow. Although this is less likely compared to aspirin, persons with **ulcers** (p. 138) and **gastritis** (p. 71) should avoid use of willow.[5] As is the case with aspirin, willow should not be used to treat fevers in children.

Wild Cherry
(Prunus serotina)

Parts Used and Where Grown: Although native to North America, wild cherry trees now grow in many other countries. The bark of the wild cherry tree is used for medicinal preparations.

Historical or Traditional Use

Wild cherry syrup has been used traditionally to treat coughs and other lung problems. It has also been used to treat diarrhea and for relief of pain.[1]

In What Conditions Might Wild Cherry Be Supportive?

Ranking	Health Concerns
Secondary	Cough (p. 47)
Other	Chronic obstructive pulmonary disease (COPD) (p. 45)

Active Constituents

Wild cherry bark contains cyanogenic glycosides, particularly prunasin. These glycosides, once broken apart in the body, act by quelling spasms in the smooth muscles lining bronchioles, thereby relieving **coughs** (p. 47).[2]

How Much Is Usually Taken?

Wild cherry tincture or syrup can be used in the amount of 2 to 4 ml 3 to 4 times per day.[3]

Are There Any Side Effects or Interactions? Very large amounts (several times the recommended amount above) of wild cherry pose the theoretical risk of causing cyanide poisoning.[4] However, this has not been observed in clinical practice.

Wild Indigo
(Baptisia tinctoria)

Parts Used and Where Grown: The root of wild indigo is used medicinally. The plant is native to the midwestern United States and continues to grow primarily in this region.

In What Conditions Might Wild Indigo Be Supportive?

Ranking	Health Concerns
Other	Common cold/sore throat (p. 41) Crohn's disease (p. 48) Influenza (p. 104)

Historical or Traditional Use

Historically, the root of wild indigo was used to make blue dye as well as to treat several types of infections, including those affecting the mouth and gums, lymph nodes, throat, and ulcers.[1] In the past, wild indigo was used to treat more severe infections, such as typhus.

Active Constituents

The polysaccharides and proteins in wild indigo are believed to stimulate the **immune system** (p. 94), according to test tube experiments,[2] which might

account for its role against the **common cold** (p. 41) and **flu** (p. 104). The root also contains alkaloids, which may contribute to its medicinal actions.

How Much Is Usually Taken?

Wild indigo is rarely used alone and is instead used in combination with herbs such as **echinacea** (p. 417) and thuja. A tincture is used in the amount of 1 to 2 ml 3 times per day. When taking the whole herb, 500 to 1,000 mg is taken as a tea 3 times daily.[3]

Are There Any Side Effects or Interactions? Higher intakes (over 30 grams per day) of wild indigo can cause nausea and vomiting.[4] Long-term (more than 2 to 3 weeks) use is not recommended.

Wild Yam
(Dioscorea villosa)

Parts Used and Where Grown: Wild yam plants are found across the midwestern and eastern United States, Latin America (especially Mexico), and Asia. Several different species exist, all possessing similar constituents and properties. The root is used medicinally.

In What Conditions Might Wild Yam Be Supportive?

Ranking	Health Concerns
Other	Abdominal cramps, High cholesterol (p. 79) High triglycerides (p. 85) Menopause (p. 118) Muscle pain or spasms

Historical or Traditional Use

Wild yam has been used as an expectorant for people with coughs. It was also used for gastrointestinal upset, nerve pain, and morning sickness.[1] Eventually, it was discovered that the saponins from wild yam could be converted industrially into cortisone, estrogens, and progesterone-like compounds. Wild yam and other plants with similar constituents continue to be the main source of these drugs.

Active Constituents

The steroidal saponins (such as diosgenin) account for some of wild yam's activity. Another compound, dioscoretine, has been shown in animal studies to lower blood sugar levels.[2] An extract of wild yam was found to have **antioxidant** (p. 267) properties. It has also been shown to lower blood **triglycerides**

(p. 85) and to raise **HDL cholesterol** (p. 79) (the "good" cholesterol).[3] Wild yam is also considered to be a strong antispasmodic and is potentially anti-inflammatory.

Contrary to popular claims, wild yam roots do not contain and are not converted into **progesterone** (p. 326) or **dehydroepiandrosterone** (**DHEA** [p. 288]) in the body.[4,5] However, wild yam saponins or other constituents may have properties similar to these compounds. Pharmaceutical progesterone is made from wild yam using a chemical conversion process. This can lead to confusion—while wild yam can be a source of progesterone, it cannot be used without this pharmaceutical conversion, which cannot be duplicated by the body. Women who require progesterone should consult their nutritionally oriented physician and not rely solely on wild yam or other herbs.

How Much Is Usually Taken?

Up to 2 to 3 ml of wild yam tincture can be taken 3 to 4 times per day. Alternatively, 1 or 2 capsules or tablets of the dried root can be taken 3 times each day.[6]

Are There Any Side Effects or Interactions? Some people may experience nausea when taking large amounts of wild yam.

Witch Hazel
(Hamamelis virginiana)

Parts Used and Where Grown: Although native to North America, witch hazel now also grows in Europe. The leaves and bark of the tree are used as medicine.

In What Conditions Might Witch Hazel Be Supportive?

Ranking	Health Concerns
Secondary	Eczema (p. 64) Hemorrhoids (p. 77)
Other	Crohn's disease (p. 48) Injuries (minor) (p. 122) Skin ulcers Varicose veins (p. 163) Wound healing (p. 167)

Historical or Traditional Use

Native Americans utilized poultices of witch hazel leaves and bark to treat hemorrhoids, wounds, painful tumors, insect bites, and ulcers.[1]

Active Constituents

Tannins and volatile oils are the main active constituents in witch hazel, giving it a strong astringent effect. Witch hazel has also been shown to strengthen veins and to be anti-inflammatory.[2,3] Topical creams are currently used in Europe to treat inflammatory skin conditions, such as **eczema** (p. 64). One double-blind study found witch hazel ointment as effective as the topical anti-inflammatory drug bufexamac for people with eczema.[4] A different double-blind study was unable to confirm whether witch hazel was any better than placebo or hydrocortisone for people with eczema.[5]

How Much Is Usually Taken?

In combination with warm, moist compresses, witch hazel extracts can be applied liberally at least twice each day (in the morning and at bedtime) to hemorrhoids. For other skin problems, ointment or cream can be applied 3 or 4 times a day, or as needed.[6] For hemorrhoids and varicose veins, witch hazel is often combined with **horse chestnut** (p. 435).

Are There Any Side Effects or Interactions? This herb is not typically recommended for internal use, as it may cause stomach irritation.[7]

Wormwood
(Artemisia absinthium)

Parts Used and Where Grown: The wormwood shrub grows wild in Europe, North Africa, and western Asia. It is now cultivated in North America as well. The leaves and flowers, and the oil obtained from them, are used as medicine.

In What Conditions Might Wormwood Be Supportive?

Ranking	Health Concerns
Secondary	Indigestion and heartburn (p. 99)
Other	Gallbladder inflammation, Irritable bowel syndrome (p. 109) Parasites (p. 137) Poor appetite

Historical or Traditional Use

Wormwood is perhaps best known because of the use of its oil to prepare certain alcoholic beverages, most notably vermouth and absinthe. Absinthe, popular in the nineteenth century in Europe, caused several cases of brain damage and even death and was banned in most places in the early twentieth century.[1] Wormwood oil continues to be used as a flavoring agent for foods, although in much smaller amounts than were found in absinthe.

As a medicine, wormwood was traditionally used as a bitter to improve digestion, to fight worm infestations, and to stimulate menstruation.[2] Clinical studies are lacking to support these uses. It was regarded as a useful remedy for problems involving the liver and gallbladder.

Active Constituents

The aromatic oil of wormwood contains the toxins thujone and isothujone. Very little of this oil is present in ordinary wormwood teas or tinctures.[3] Although the oil destroys various types of worms, it may cause damage to the human nervous system. Also present in the plant are strong bitter agents known as absinthin and anabsinthin. These stimulate digestive function, including gall bladder function.[4]

How Much Is Usually Taken?

A wormwood tea can be made by adding ½ to 1 U.S. teaspoon (2.5 to 5 grams) of the herb to 1 cup (250 ml) of boiling water, allowing it to steep for 10 to 15 minutes.[5] Many doctors of natural medicine recommend drinking 3 cups each day. Tincture can be used, in the amount of 10 to 20 drops in water, taken 10 to 15 minutes before each meal.[6] Either preparation should not be used for more than 4 weeks consecutively.[7]

Are There Any Side Effects or Interactions?
Long-term (over 4 weeks) intake of the thujone-containing oil or alcoholic beverages (absinthe) made with the oil is strictly contraindicated—it is addictive and may cause brain damage, seizures, and even death.[8] Short-term (2 to 4 weeks) use of the wormwood tea or tincture has not resulted in any reports of significant side effects. Nevertheless, consult with a health-care professional knowledgeable in herbal medicine before taking wormwood. Longer-term (over 4 weeks) use or intake of amounts higher than those recommended can cause nausea, vomiting, insomnia, restlessness, vertigo, tremors, and seizures.[9] However, one study found that use of no more than 1 ml tincture 3 times per day for as long as 9 months to promote digestive function was associated with no side effects.[10] Wormwood is contraindicated during pregnancy and lactation.[11]

Yarrow
(Achillea millefolium)

Parts Used and Where Grown: The flowering tops of yarrow are used. This prolific plant grows in Europe, North America, and Asia. A number of species are used as garden ornamentals, but they are not potent medicines.

In What Conditions Might Yarrow Be Supportive?

Ranking	Health Concerns
Secondary	Colic (p. 40)
Other	Common cold/sore throat (p. 41) Crohn's disease (p. 48) Indigestion and heartburn (p. 99) Inflammation Injuries (minor) (p. 122) Menstruation, painful (dysmenorrhea) (p. 61) Pap smear (abnormal) (p. 136) Premenstrual syndrome (p. 141) Ulcerative colitis (p. 158)

Historical or Traditional Use

Traditional herbal medicine has used yarrow in three broad categories.[1] First, it was used to help stop minor bleeding and to treat wounds. Second, it was used to treat inflammation in a number of conditions, especially in the intestinal and female reproductive tracts. Third, it was utilized as a mild sedative. Some or all of these historical uses occurred in Europe, China, and India. The ancient Chinese fortune-telling system known as the I Ching apparently first used dried yarrow stems, then replaced them with coins.[2]

Active Constituents

A number of chemicals may contribute to yarrow's healing properties. The volatile oil, which is rich in sesquiterpene lactones, gives yarrow its anti-inflammatory activity.[3] Alkamides (which are also found in **echinacea [p. 417]**) may further reduce inflammation.[4] Animal studies have shown that this herb can reduce smooth muscle spasms, which might further explain its usefulness in gastrointestinal conditions.[5] The alkaloid obtained from yarrow, known as achilletin, reportedly stops bleeding in animals.[6] No clinical studies have confirmed the benefits of yarrow.

How Much Is Usually Taken?

The German Commission E monograph suggests 4.5 grams of yarrow daily or 3 teaspoons of the fresh pressed juice.[7] A tea can be prepared by steeping 1 to 2 U.S. teaspoons (5 to 10 grams) of yarrow in 1 cup (250 ml) boiling water for 10 to 15 minutes. Three cups a day can be drunk. If tincture is preferred, 3 to 4 ml can be taken 3 times per day. The tea, or cloths dipped in the tea, can be used topically as needed.

Are There Any Side Effects or Interactions?
People who take yarrow may occasionally develop an allergy

or rash.[8] Yarrow might increase sensitivity to sunlight. Yarrow should not be used to treat large, deep, or infected wounds, all of which require medical attention. Yarrow is not contraindicated during pregnancy or lactation.

Yellow Dock
(Rumex crispus)

Parts Used and Where Grown: The root of yellow dock is used as medicine. The plant is found in many places throughout North America.

In What Conditions Might Yellow Dock Be Supportive?

Ranking	Health Concerns
Other	Poor digestion (p. 99) Skin conditions

Historical or Traditional Use

Yellow dock has a long history of use as an alterative. Alterative herbs have nonspecific effects on the gastrointestinal tract and the liver. As a result, they are thought to treat skin conditions that are attributed to toxic metabolites from maldigestion and poor liver function.

Active Constituents

Yellow dock contains relatively small amounts of anthraquinone glycosides which contribute to its mild laxative effect.[1] It is also thought to stimulate bile production. It is often used as a digestive bitter for persons with poor digestion. No human studies have been done on its use as medicine.

How Much Is Usually Taken?

A tincture of yellow dock can be used in the amount of 1 to 2 ml 3 times per day.[2] Alternatively, a tea can be made by boiling 1 to 2 U.S. teaspoons (5 to 10 grams) of root in 2 cups (500 ml) water for 10 minutes and 3 cups each day may be drunk. Yellow dock is rarely used alone for any of its indications, due to the mild and general nature of its actions.

Are There Any Side Effects or Interactions?
Aside from mild diarrhea or loose stools in some persons, yellow dock is safe.[3]

Yohimbe
(Pausinystalia yohimbe)

Parts Used and Where Grown: The bark of this African tree is used medicinally. It still grows primarily in western Africa. Concerns have been raised that the tree may be endangered due to overharvesting for use as medicine. For this reason, yohimbe should perhaps only be used as a last resort until survival of the species can be guaranteed.

In What Conditions Might Yohimbe Be Supportive?

Ranking	Health Concerns
Primary	Impotence (p. 98)
Other	Depression (p. 50)

Historical or Traditional Use

Historically, yohimbe bark was used in western Africa for fevers, leprosy, and coughs.[1] It has also been used to dilate pupils, for heart disease, and as a local anesthetic. It has a more recent history of use as an aphrodisiac and a hallucinogen.

Active Constituents

The alkaloid known as yohimbine is the primary active constituent in yohimbe, although similar alkaloids may also play a role. Yohimbine blocks alpha-2 adrenergic receptors, part of the sympathetic nervous system.[2] It also dilates blood vessels. For these reasons, this herb has been used to treat male sexual dysfunction. Yohimbine inhibits monoamine oxidase (MAO) and therefore may be of benefit in depressive disorders. However, it does not have the clinical research of other herbs used for **depression** (p. 50), such as **St. John's wort** (p. 461).

Yohimbine has been shown in several double-blind studies to help treat men with **impotence** (p. 98);[3,4] negative studies have also been reported.[5,6]

How Much Is Usually Taken?

A tincture of the bark is often used in the amount of 5 to 10 drops 3 times per day. Standardized yohimbe products are also available for the treatment of impotence. A safe daily amount of yohimbine from any product is 15 to 30 mg.[7] Yohimbine should be used under the supervision of a physician.

Are There Any Side Effects or Interactions? People with kidney disease or **peptic ulcer** (p. 138), or pregnant or lactating women, should not use yohimbe.[8] Standard amounts may sometimes cause dizziness, nausea, insomnia, anxiety, increased blood pressure, and rapid heartbeat,[9] though all of these are rare.[10] Using more than 40 mg of yohimbine per day can cause dangerous side effects, including loss of muscle function, chills, and vertigo. Some people will also experience hallucinations when taking higher amounts of yohimbine.[11] Taking 200 mg yohimbine in one case led to only a brief episode of hypertension, palpitations, and anxiety.[12] Persons with post-traumatic stress disorder[13] and panic disorder[14] should avoid yohimbe.

Foods with high amounts of tyramine (such as cheese, red wine, and liver) should not be eaten while a person is taking yohimbe, as they may theoretically cause severe high blood pressure and other problems. Similarly, yohimbe should only be combined with other antidepressant drugs under the supervision of a physician, although at least one study suggests it may benefit those who aren't responding to serotonin reuptake inhibitors such as Prozac.[15]

Special United Kingdom Consideration: Yohimbe may be prescribed by a medical doctor or dispensed under the supervision of a pharmacist.

Yucca

(Yucca schidigera, Yucca spp.)

Parts Used and Where Grown: The stalk and root are used. This desert tree grows primarily in the southwestern United States and is related to the Joshua tree.

Historical or Traditional Use

Native Americans used the soapy leaves from yucca for numerous conditions. Poultices or baths were used for skin sores and other diseases as well as for sprains. Inflammation of all sorts, including joint inflammations, and bleeding were also treated with yucca. Some report that the Native Americans washed their hair with yucca to fight dandruff and hair loss.

In What Conditions Might Yucca Be Supportive?

Ranking	Health Concerns
Other	Osteoarthritis (p. 130) Rheumatoid arthritis (p. 151)

Active Constituents

The saponins from yucca are the main medicinal agents in the plant. They have both a water-soluble and fat-soluble end and therefore act like soap. The authors of the study looking at people with **osteoarthritis** (p. 130) and **rheumatoid arthritis** (p. 151) speculate that yucca saponins block release of toxins from the intestines that inhibit normal formation of cartilage.[1] An extract of one species of yucca has been found to fight melanoma cells in test tube studies.[2]

How Much Is Usually Taken?

Two capsules or tablets of yucca saponins can be taken per day.[3] Up to twice this dose has been used in some cases and may be required for more severe arthritis. Alternatively, one-quarter ounce of the root can be boiled in a pint of water for 15 minutes; and 3 to 5 cups of this tea may be drunk per day.[4]

Are There Any Side Effects or Interactions? Yucca can cause loose stools at higher doses.[5] Yucca and other saponins can cause red blood cells to burst (known as "hemolysis") in test tubes. The level to which this occurs when the saponins are taken by mouth, if it occurs at all, is unknown. However, yucca is approved for use in foods as a foaming agent (particularly in root beer). Since there have been no reports of problems with hemolysis in root beer drinkers, yucca herbal supplements are believed to be generally safe.[6] Use of yucca for more than 3 months consecutively is not recommended as it may interfere with absorption of fat-soluble vitamins.[7]

Part Three: References

Alfalfa

1. Briggs C. Alfalfa. *Canadian Pharm J* 1994; Mar: 84,85,115.

2. Castleman M. *The Healing Herbs.* Emmaus, PA: Rodale Press, 1991, 37–39.

3. Leung AY, Foster S. *Encyclopedia of Common Natural Ingredients Used in Food, Drugs, and Cosmetics,* 2d ed. New York: John Wiley & Sons, 1996, 13–15.

4. Story JA. Alfalfa saponins and cholesterol interactions. *Am J Clin Nutr* 1984; 39: 917–29.

5. Shemesh M, Lindrer HR, Ayalon N. Affinity of rabbit uterine oestradiol receptor for phyto-oestragens and its use in competitive protein-binding radioassay for plasma coumestrol. *J Reprod Fertil* 1972; 29: 1–9.

6. Foster S. *Herbs for Your Health.* Loveland, CO: Interweave Press, 1996, 2–3.

7. Malinow MR, Bardana EJ, Profsky B, et al. Systemic lupus erythematosus-like syndrome in monkeys fed alfalfa sprouts: Role of a nonprotein amino acid. *Science* 1982; 216: 415–17.

Aloe

1. Penneys NS. Inhibition of arachidonic acid oxidation in vitro by vehicle components. *Acta Derm Venerol Stockh* 1981; 62: 59–61.

2. Bruce W. Investigations of the antibacterial activity in the aloe. *S Afr Med J* 1967; 41: 984.

3. Ajabnoor M. Effect of aloes on blood glucose levels in normal and alloxan diabetic mice. *J Ethnopharmacol* 1990; 28: 215–20.

4. Bunyapraphatsara N, Yongchaiyudha S, Rungpitarangsi V, Chokechaijaroenposn O. Antidiabetic activity of *Aloe vera* L juice. II. Clinical trial in diabetes mellitus patients in combination with glibenclamide. *Phytomedicine* 1996; 3: 5–8.

5. Syed TA, Ahmad SA, Holt AH, et al. Management of psoriasis with *Aloe vera* extract in a hydrophilic cream: A placebo-controlled double-blind study. *Trop Med Int Health* 1996; 1: 505–9.

6. Loveman AB. Leaf of *Aloe vera* in treatment of Roentgen ray ulcers. *Arch Derm Syph* 1937; 36: 838–43.

7. Williams MS, Burk M, Loprinzi CL, et al. Phase III double-blind evaluation of an *Aloe vera* gel as a prophylactic agent for radiation-induced skin toxicity. *Int J Rad Oncol Biol Phys* 1996; 36: 345–49.

8. Visuthikosol V, Choucheun B, et al. Effect of *Aloe vera* to healing of burn wound: A clinical and histologic study. *J Med Assoc Thai* 1995; 78: 403–9.

9. Blitz J, Smith J, Gerard J. *Aloe vera* gel in peptic ulcer therapy: Preliminary report. *J Am Osteopathic Assoc* 1963; 62: 731–35.

10. Schmidt JM, Greenspoon JS. *Aloe vera* dermal wound gel is associated with a delay in wound healing. *Obstet Gynecol* 1991; 78: 115–17.

11. Blumenthal M, Busse WR, Goldberg A, et al. (eds). *The Complete Commission E Monographs: Therapeutic Guide to Herbal Medicines.* Boston, MA: Integrative Medicine Communications, 1998, 80–81.

12. Blumenthal M, Busse WR, Goldberg A, et al. (eds). *The Complete Commission E Monographs: Therapeutic Guide to Herbal Medicines.* Boston, MA: Integrative Medicine Communications, 1998, 80–81.

American Ginseng

1. Duke J. *Ginseng: A Concise Handbook.* Algonac, MI: Reference Publications, 1989, 36.

2. Bensky D, Gamble A, Kaptchuk T. *Chinese Herbal Medicine: Materia Medica.* Seattle: Eastland Press, 1993, 358–59.

3. Bensky D, Gamble A, Kaptchuk T. *Chinese Herbal Medicine: Materia Medica.* Seattle: Eastland Press, 1993, 358–59.

4. Foster S. *American Ginseng: Panax quinquefolius.* Austin, TX: American Botanical Council, 1991, 3–8.

5. Shibata S, Tanaka O, Shoji J, Saito H. Chemistry and pharmacology of *Panax. Econ Med Plant Res* 1: 218–84.

6. Morris AC, Jacobs I, McLellan TM, et al. No ergogenic effect on ginseng ingestion. *Int J Sport Nutr* 1996; 6: 263–71.

7. Foster S. *Herbs for Health.* Loveland, CO: Interweave Press, 1996, 48–49.

8. Yun TK, Choi Y. Preventive effect of ginseng intake against various human cancers: A case-control study on 1987 pairs. *Cancer Epidem Biomarkers Prev* 1995; 4: 401–8.

Artichoke

1. Brand N. *Cynara scolymus* L.—The artichoke. *Zeitschrift Phytother* 1990; 11: 169–75.

2. Brand N. *Cynara scolymus* L.—The artichoke. *Zeitschrift Phytother* 1990; 11: 169–75.

3. Leung AY, Foster S. *Encyclopedia of Common Natural Ingredients Used in Food, Drugs, and Cosmetics*, 2d ed. New York: John Wiley & Sons, 1996, 42–43.

4. Schulz V, Hansel R, Tyler VE. *Rational Phytotherapy*, 3rd ed. Berlin: Springer-Verlag, 1998, 174–75.

5. Heckers H, Dittmar K, Schmahl FW, Huth K. Inefficiency of cynarin as therapeutic regimen in familial type II hyperlipoproteinemia. *Atherosclerosis* 1977; 26: 249–53.

6. Fintelmann V. Antidyspeptic and lipid-lowering effect of artichoke leaf extract. *Zeitschrift fur Allgemeinmed* 1996; 72: 1–19.

7. Gebhardt R. New experimental results in the action of artichoke leaf extract. *Zeitschrift fur Allgemeinmed* 1996; 72: 20–23.

8. Brown JE, Rice-Evans CA. Luteolin rich artichoke extract protects low density lipoprotein from oxidation in vitro. *Free Radical Research* 1998; 29: 247–55.

9. Adzet T, Camarasa J, Laguna JC. Hepatoprotective effect of polyphenolic compounds from *Cynara scolymus* against CCL4 toxicity in isolated rat hepatocytes. *Journal of Natural Products* 1987; 50: 612–17.

10. Fintelmann V. Antidyspeptic and lipid-lowering effect of artichoke leaf extract. *Zeitschrift fur Allgemeinmed* 1996; 72: 1–19.

11. Newall CA, Anderson LA, Phillipson JD. *Herbal Medicines: A Guide for Health-Care Professionals*. London: The Pharmaceutical Press, 1996, 36.

12. Blumenthal M, Busse WR, Goldberg A, et al. (eds). *The Complete German Commission E Monographs: Therapeutic Guide to Herbal Medicines*. Austin: American Botanical Council and Boston: Integrative Medicine Communications, 1998: 84–85.

13. Farrell J, Campbell E, Walshe JJ. Renal failure associated with alternative medical therapies. *Renal failure* 1995; 17: 759–64.

Ashwagandha

1. Duke JA. *CRC Handbook of Medicinal Herbs*. Boca Raton, FL: CRC Press, 1985, 514–15.

2. Duke JA. *CRC Handbook of Medicinal Herbs*. Boca Raton, FL: CRC Press, 1985, 514–15.

3. Wagner H, Nërr H, Winterhoff H. Plant adaptogens. *Phytomed* 1994; 1: 63–76.

4. Wagner H, Nërr H, Winterhoff H. Plant adaptogens. *Phytomed* 1994; 1: 63–76.

5. Anabalgan K, Sadique J. Anti-inflammatory activity of *Withania somnifera*. *Indian J Exp Biol* 1981; 19: 245–49.

6. Bhattacharya SK, Kumar A, Ghosal S. Effects of glycowithanolides from *Withania somnifera* on an animal model of Alzheimer's disease and perturbed central cholinergic markers of cognition in rats. *Phytother Res* 1995; 9: 110–13.

7. Bone K. *Clinical Applications of Ayurvedic and Chinese Herbs*. Queensland, Australia: Phytotherapy Press, 1996, 137–41.

Asian Ginseng

1. Shibata S, Tanaka O, et al. Chemistry and pharmacology of *Panax*. In *Economic and Medicinal Plant Research*, vol 1, ed. H Wagner, H Hikino, NR Farnsworth. London: Academic Press, 1985, 217–84.

2. Tomoda M, Hirabayashi K, et al. Characterisation of two novel polysaccharides having immunological activities from the root of *Panax ginseng*. *Biol Pharm Bull* 1993; 16: 1087–90.

3. See DM, Broumand N, Sahi L, et al. In vitro effects of echinacea and ginseng on natural killer and antibody-dependent cell cytotoxicity in healthy subjects and chronic fatigue syndrome or acquired immunodeficiency syndrome patients. *Immunopharmacol* 1997; 35: 229–35.

4. Yun TK, Choi Y. Preventive effect of ginseng intake against various human cancers: A case-control study on 1987 pairs. *Cancer Epidem Biomarkers Prev* 1995; 4: 401–8.

5. Sotaniemi EA, Haapakoski E, Rautio A. Ginseng therapy in non-insulin-dependent diabetic patients. *Diabetes Care* 1995; 18: 1373–75.

6. Teves MA, Wright JE, Welch MJ, et al. Effects of ginseng on repeated bouts of exhaustive exercise. *Med Sci Sports Exerc* 1983; 15: 162.

7. Pieralisi G, Ripari P, Vecchiet L. Effects of a standardized ginseng extract combined with dimethylaminoethanol bitartrate, vitamins, minerals and trace elements on physical performance during exercise. *Clin Ther* 1991; 13: 373–82.

8. Le Gal M, Cathebras P, Struby K. Pharmaton capsules in the treatment of functional fatigue: A double-blind study versus placebo evaluated by a new methodology. *Phytother Res* 1996; 10: 49–53.

9. Caso Mardsco A, Vargas Ruiz R, Salas Villagomez A, Begona Infante C. Double-blind study of a multivitamin complex supplemented with ginseng extract. *Drugs Exp Clin Res* 1996; 22: 323–29.

10. Brown DJ. *Herbal Prescriptions for Better Health*. Rocklin, CA: Prima Publishing, 1996, 129–38.

11. Newall CA, Anderson LA, Phillipson JD. *Herbal Medicines: A Guide for Healthcare Professionals*. London: The Pharmaceutical Press, 1996, 145–50.

Astragalus

1. Leung AY, Foster S. *Encyclopedia of Common Natural Ingredients Used in Food, Drugs, and Cosmetics*, 2d ed. New York: John Wiley & Sons, 1996, 50–53.

2. Foster S, Yue CX. *Herbal Emissaries: Bringing Chinese Herbs to the West*. Rochester, VT: Healing Arts Press, 1992, 27–33.

3. Shu HY. *Oriental Materia Medica: A Concise Guide*. Palos Verdes, CA: Oriental Healing Arts Press, 1986, 521–23.

4. Chu D et al. Immunotherapy with Chinese medicinal herbs. I. Immune restoration of local xenogeneic graft-versus-host reaction in cancer patients by fractionated *Astragalus membranaceus* in vitro. *J Clin Lab Immunol* 1998; 25: 119–23.

5. Ma J, Peng A, Lin S. Mechanism of the therapeutic effect of

Astragalus membranaceus on sodium retention in experimental heart failure. *Clin Med J* 1998; 111: 17–23.

6. Foster S. *Herbs for Your Health.* Loveland, CO: Interweave Press, 1996, 6–7.

Barberry

1. Duke JA. *CRC Handbook of Medicinal Herbs.* Boca Raton, FL: CRC Press, 1985, 78.

2. Amin AH, Subbaiah TV, Abbasi KM. Berberine sulfate: Antimicrobial activity, bioassay and mode of action. *Can J Microbiol* 1969; 15: 1067–76.

3. Subbaiah TV, Amin AH. Effect of berberine sulphate on *Entamoeba histolytica. Nature* 1967; 215(100): 527–28.

4. Sun D, Courtney HS, Beachey EH. Berberine sulfate blocks adherence of *Streptococcus pyogenes* to epithelial cells, fibronectin, and hexadecane. *Antimicrob Agents Chemother* 1988; 32(9): 1370–74.

5. Rabbani GH, Butler T, Knight J, et al. Randomized controlled trial of berberine sulfate therapy for diarrhea due to enterotoxigenic *Escherichia coli* and *Vibrio cholerae. J Infect Dis* 1987; 155(5): 979–84.

6. Kumazawa Y et al. Activation of peritoneal macrophages by berberine-type alkaloids in terms of induction of cytostatic activity. *Int J Immunopharmacol* 1984; 6: 587–92.

7. Wong CW, Seow WK, O'Callaghan JW, Thong YH. Comparative effects of tetrandrine and berbamine on subcutaneous air pouch inflammation induced by interleukin-1, tumour necrosis factor and platelet-activating factor. *Agents Actions* 1992; 36(1–2): 112–18.

8. Ju HS, Li XJ, Zhao BL, et al. Scavenging effect of berbamine on active oxygen radicals in phorbol ester-stimulated human polymorphonuclear leukocytes. *Biochem Pharmacol* 1990; 39(11): 1673–78.

10. Gruenwald J, Brendler T, Jaenicke C, et al. (eds). *PDR for Herbal Medicines.* Montvale, NJ: Medical Economics, 1998, 688–90.

11. Chan E. Displacement of bilirubin from albumin by berberine. *Biol Neonate* 1993; 63: 201–8.

12. Blumenthal M, Busse WR, Goldberg A, et al. (eds). *The Complete Commission E Monographs: Therapeutic Guide to Herbal Medicines.* Boston, MA: Integrative Medicine Communications, 1998, 309–10.

Bilberry

1. Salvayre R, Braquet P, et al. Comparison of the scavenger effect of bilberry anthocyanosides with various flavonoids. *Proceed Intl Bioflavonoids Symposium,* Munich, 1981, 437–42.

2. Bravetti G. Preventive medical treatment of senile cataract with vitamin E and anthocyanosides: Clinical evaluation. *Ann Ottalmol Clin Ocul* 1989; 115: 109 [in Italian].

3. Perossini M, Guidi G, Chiellini S, Siravo D. Diabetic and hypertensive retinopathy therapy with *Vaccinium myrtillus* anthocyanosides (Tegens): Double-blind placebo-controlled clinical trial. *Ann Ottalmol Clin Ocul* 1987; 12: 1173–90 [in Italian].

4. Boniface R, Miskulin M, Robert AM. Pharmacological properties of myrtillus anthocyanosides: Correlation with results of treatment of diabetic microangiopathy. In *Flavonoids and Bioflavonoids,* eds. L Farkas, M Gabors, FL Kallay. Ireland: Elsevier, 1985, 293–301.

5. Francesca Rasetti M, Caruso D, Galli G, et al. Extracts of *Ginkgo biloba* L. leaves and *Vaccinium myrtillus* L. fruits prevent photo induced oxidation of low density lipoprotein cholesterol. *Phytomedicine* 1996/7; 3: 335–38.

6. Brown DJ. *Herbal Prescriptions for Better Health.* Rocklin, CA: Prima Publishing, 1996, 41–47.

Bitter Melon

1. Duke JA. *CRC Handbook of Medicinal Herbs.* Boca Raton, FL: CRC Press, 1985, 315–16.

2. Raman A, Lau C. Anti-diabetic properties and phytochemistry of *Momordica charantia* L (Curcur-

bitaceae). *Phytomed Res* 1996; 2: 349–62.

3. Zhang QC. Preliminary report on the use of *Momordica charantia* extract by HIV patients. *J Naturopathic Med* 1992; 3: 65–69.

4. Werbach MR, Murray MT. *Botanical Influences on Illness.* Tarzana, CA: Third Line Press, 1994, 139–41.

5. Brown DJ, Gaby A, Reichert R, Yarrell E. Phytotherapeutic and nutritional approaches to diabetes mellitus. *Quart Rev Nat Med* 1998; Winter: 329–54.

Black Cohosh

1. Leung AY, Foster S. *Encyclopedia of Common Natural Ingredients Used in Food, Drugs, and Cosmetics,* 2d ed. New York: John Wiley & Sons, 1996, 88–89.

2. Castleman M. *The Healing Herbs.* Emmaus, PA: Rodale Press, 1991, 75–78.

3. Foster S. *Herbs for Your Health.* Loveland, CO: Interweave Press, 1996, 12–13.

4. Düker EM, Kopanski L, Jarry H, Wuttke W. Effects of extracts from *Cimicifuga racemosa* on gonadotropin release in menopausal women and ovariectomized rats. *Planta Medica* 1991; 57: 420–24.

5. Kadota S, Li JX, Litt Y, et al. Effects of cimicifugae rhizome on serum calcium and phosphate levels in low calcium dietary rats and on bone mineral density in ovariectomized rats. *Phytomed* 1996/7; 3: 379–85.

6. Murray MT. *The Healing Power of Herbs.* Rocklin, CA: Prima Publishing, 1995, 376.

7. Bradley PR (ed). *British Herbal Compendium,* vol 1. Bournemouth, Dorset, UK: British Herbal Medicine Association, 1992, 34–36.

8. Blumenthal M, Busse WR, Goldberg A, et al. (eds). *The Complete Commission E Monographs: Therapeutic Guide to Herbal Medicines.* Boston, MA: Integrative Medicine Communications, 1998, 90.

9. Gruenwald J. Standardized black cohosh (*Cimicifuga*) extract clinical monograph. *Quart Rev Nat Med* 1998; Summer: 117–25.

Part Three: References

Blackberry

1. Castleman M. *The Healing Herbs.* New York: Bantam Books, 1991, 106–10.

2. Tyler V. *Herbs of Choice: The Therapeutic Use of Phytomedicinals.* New York: Pharmaceutical Products Press, 1994, 53.

3. Blumenthal M, Busse WR, Goldberg A, et al. (eds). *The Complete Commission E Monographs: Therapeutic Guide to Herbal Medicines.* Boston, MA: Integrative Medicine Communications, 1998, 91.

Blessed Thistle

1. Lust JB. *The Herb Book.* New York: Bantam Books, 1974, 343.

2. Bradley PR (ed). *British Herbal Compendium,* vol 1. Bournemouth, Dorset, UK: British Herbal Medicine Association, 1992, 126–27.

3. Blumenthal M, Busse WR, Goldberg A, et al. (eds). *The Complete Commission E Monographs: Therapeutic Guide to Herbal Medicines.* Boston, MA: Integrative Medicine Communications, 1998, 92.

Bloodroot

1. Duke JA. *CRC Handbook of Medicinal Herbs.* Boca Raton, FL: CRC Press, 1985, 424–25.

2. Dzink JL, Socransky SS. Comparative in vitro activity of sanguinarine against oral microbial isolates. *Antimicrob Agents Chemother* 1985; 27(4): 663–65.

3. Hannah JJ, Johnson JD, Kuftinec MM. Long-term clinical evaluation of toothpaste and oral rinse containing sanguinaria extract in controlling plaque, gingival inflammation, and sulcular bleeding during orthodontic treatment. *Am J Orthod Dentofacial Orthop* 1989; 96(3): 199–207.

4. Frankos VH, Brusick DJ, Johnson EM, et al. Safety of *Sanguinaria* extract as used in commercial toothpaste and oral rinse products. *J Can Dent Assoc* 1990; 56(suppl 7): 41–47.

Blue Cohosh

1. Castleman M. *The Healing Herbs.* New York: Bantam Books, 1991: 120–23.

2. Foster S. *Herbal Renaissance.* Salt Lake City: Gibbs-Smith Publisher, 1993: 48–50.

3. Greunwald J, Brendler T, Jaenicke C, et al. (eds). *PDR for Herbal Medicines.* Montvale, NJ: Medical Economics, 1998, 725–26.

4. Jones TK, Lawson BM. Profound neonatal congestive heart failure caused by maternal consumption of blue cohosh herbal medication. *J Pediatr* 1998; 132: 550–52.

Blue Flag

1. Ellingwood F. *American Materia Medica, Therapeutics and Pharmacognosy,* 11ᵗʰ ed. Sandy, OR: Eclectic Medical Publications, 1919, 312–13.

2. Moore M. *Medicinal Plants of the Mountain West.* Sante Fe: Museum of New Mexico Press, 1979, 39–40.

3. Moore M. *Medicinal Plants of the Mountain West.* Sante Fe: Museum of New Mexico Press, 1979, 39–40.

4. Ellingwood F. *American Materia Medica, Therapeutics and Pharmacognosy,* 11ᵗʰ ed. Sandy, OR: Eclectic Medical Publications, 1919, 312–13.

5. Ellingwood F. *American Materia Medica, Therapeutics and Pharmacognosy,* 11ᵗʰ ed. Sandy, OR: Eclectic Medical Publications, 1919, 312–13.

6. McGuffin M, Hobbs C, Upton R, Goldberg A (eds). *American Herbal Product Association's Herbal Safety Handbook.* Boca Raton, FL: CRC Press, 1997, 64.

Blueberry

1. Tilford GL. *Edible and Medicinal Plants of the West.* Missoula, MT: Mountain Press Publishing Company, 1997, 80–81.

2. Tyler V. *Herbs of Choice: The Therapeutic Use of Phytomedicinals.* New York: Pharmaceutical Products Press, 1994, 52–54.

3. Schilcher H. *Phytotherapy in Paediatrics.* Stuttgart, Germany: Medpharm Scientific Publishers, 1997, 126–27.

4. Leung AY, Foster S. *Encyclopedia of Common Natural Ingredients Used in Foods, Drugs, and Cosmetics,* 2d ed. New York: John Wiley & Sons, 1996, 84–85.

5. Passariello N, Bisesti V, Sgambato S. Influence of anthocyanosides on the microcirculation and lipid picture in diabetic and dyslipic subjects. *Gazz Med Ital* 1979; 138: 563–66.

6. Tyler V. *Herbs of Choice: The Therapeutic Use of Phytomedicinals.* New York: Pharmaceutical Products Press, 1994, 52–54.

Boldo

1. Leung AY, Foster S. *Encyclopedia of Common Natural Ingredients Used in Food, Drugs, and Cosmetics,* 2d ed. New York: John Wiley & Sons, 1996, 95–96.

2. Robbers JE, Tyler VE. *Tyler's Herbs of Choice: The Therapeutic Use of Phytomedicines.* New York: Haworth Press, 1999, 74–75.

3. Robbers JE, Tyler VE. *Tyler's Herbs of Choice: The Therapeutic Use of Phytomedicines.* New York: Haworth Press, 1999, 74–75.

4. Newall CA, Anderson LA, Phillipson JD. *Herbal Medicines: A Guide for Health-Care Professionals.* London: The Pharmaceutical Press, 1996: 46–47.

5. Newall CA, Anderson LA, Phillipson JD. *Herbal Medicines: A Guide for Health-Care Professionals.* London: The Pharmaceutical Press, 1996: 46–47.

6. Newall CA, Anderson LA, Phillipson JD. *Herbal Medicines: A Guide for Health-Care Professionals.* London: The Pharmaceutical Press, 1996: 46–47.

7. Blumenthal M, Busse WR, Goldberg A, et al. (eds). *The Complete German Commission E Monographs: Therapeutic Guide to Herbal Medicines.* Austin: American Botanical Council and Boston: Integrative Medicine Communications, 1998, 93–94.

8. Blumenthal M, Busse WR, Goldberg A, et al. (eds). *The Complete German Commission E Monographs: Therapeutic Guide to Herbal Medicines.* Austin: American Botanical Council and Boston: Integrative Medicine Communications, 1998, 93–94.

9. Newall CA, Anderson LA, Phillipson JD. *Herbal Medicines: A Guide for Health-Care Professionals.* London: The Pharmaceutical Press, 1996: 46–47.

10. Brinker F. *Herb Contraindications and Drug Interactions.* Sandy, OR: Eclectic Publications, 1997, 26.

Boneset

1. Castleman M. *The Healing Herbs.* New York: Bantam Books, 1991, 124–28.

2. Woerdenbag HJ, Bos R, Hendriks H. *Eupatorium perfoliatum* L.—the boneset. *Z Phytother* 1992; 13: 134–39 [review].

3. Greunwald J, Brendler T, Jaenicke C, et al. (eds). *PDR for Herbal Medicines.* Montvale, NJ: Medical Economics, 1998, 842–43.

4. Newall CA, Anderson LA, Phillipson JD. *Herbal Medicines: A Guide for Health-Care Professionals.* London: The Pharmaceutical Press, 1996, 48.

Borage

1. Wren RC. *Potter's New Cyclopedia of Botanical Drugs and Preparations.* Essex, England: C.W. Daniel and Co., 1988, 41.

2. Awang DVC. Borage. *Can Pharm J* 1990; 123: 121–23.

3. Leventhal LJ et al. Treatment of rheumatoid arthritis with gamma-linolenic acid. *Ann Intern Med* 1993; 119: 867–73.

4. Landi G. Oral administration of borage oil in atopic dermatitis. *J Appl Cosmetology* 1993; 11: 115–20.

5. Borreck S, Hildebrandt A, Forster J. Borage seed oil and atopic dermatitis. *Klinische Pediatrie* 1997; 203: 100–4.

6. Tolleson A, Frithz A. Borage oil, an effective new treatment for infantile seborrhoeic dermatitis. *Br J Dermatol* 1993; 25: 95.

7. Leventhal LJ, et al. Treatment of rheumatoid arthritis with gamma-linolenic acid. *Ann Intern Med* 1993; 119: 867–73.

8. Landi G. Oral administration of borage oil in atopic dermatitis. *J Appl Cosmetology* 1993; 11: 115–20.

9. Tolleson A, Frithz A. Borage oil, an effective new treatment for infantile seborrhoeic dermatitis. *Br J Dermatol* 1993; 25: 95.

10. DeSmet PAGM. Safety of borage seed oil. *Can Pharm J* 1991; 124: 5.

11. Robbers JE, Tyler VE. *Tyler's Herbs of Choice: The Therapeutic Use of Phytomedicinals.* New York: Haworth Press, 1999: 194.

12. Awang DVC. Borage. *Can Pharm J* 1990; 123: 121–23.

Boswellia

1. Safayhi H, Sailer ER, Amnon HPT. 5-lipoxygenase inhibition by acetyl-11-keto-b-boswellic acid. *Phytomed* 1996; 3: 71–72.

2. Safayhi H, Mack T, Saieraj J, et al. Boswellic acids: Novel, specific, nonredox inhibitors of 5-lipoxygenase. *J Pharmacol Exp Ther* 1992; 261: 1143–46.

3. Singh GB, Atal CK. Pharmacology of an extract of salai guggal ex-*Boswellia serrata,* a new non-steroidal anti-inflammatory agent. *Agents Actions* 1986; 18: 407–12.

4. Gupta I, Parihar A, Malhotra P, et al. Effects of *Boswellia serrata* gum resin in patients with ulcerative colitis. *Eur J Med Res* 1997; 2: 37–43.

5. Etzel R. Special extract of Boswellia serrata (H15) in the treatment of rheumatoid arthritis. *Phytomed* 1996; 3: 91–94.

Buchu

1. Leung AY, Foster S. *Encyclopedia of Common Natural Ingredients Used in Food, Drugs and Cosmetics.* New York: John Wiley & Sons, 1996, 104–5.

2. Gruenwald J, Brendler T, Jaenicke C, et al. (eds). *PDR for Herbal Medicines.* Montvale, NJ: Medical Economics, 1998, 686–87.

3. Wichtl M. *Herbal Drugs and Phytopharmaceuticals.* Boca Raton, FL: CRC Press, 1994, 102–3.

4. Didry N, Pinkas M. A propos du Buchu. *Plantes Méd et Phyothér* 1982; 16: 249–52.

5. Blumenthal M, Busse WR, Goldberg A, et al. (eds). *The Complete German Commission E Monographs: Therapeutic Guide to Herbal Medi-*cines. Austin: American Botanical Council and Boston: Integrative Medicine Communications, 1998, 317.

6. Bradley PR, ed. *British Herbal Compendium,* vol 1. Bournemouth, England: British Herbal Medicine Association, 1992, 43–45.

Bugleweed

1. Wren RC, Williamson EM, Evans FJ. *Potter's New Cyclopaedia of Botanical Drugs and Preparations.* Essex, UK: Saffron Walden, 1988, 47–48.

2. Wagner H, Horhammer L, Frank U. Lithospermic acid, the anti-hormonally active principle of *Lycopus europaeus* L. and *Symphytum officinale* L. *Arzneim Forsch* 1970; 20: 705–12.

3. Kohrle J, Auf'mkolk M, et al. Iodothyronine deiodinases: Inhibition by plant extracts. *Acta Endocrin Suppl* 1981; 16: 188–92.

4. Auf'mkolk M, Ingbar JC, et al. Extracts and auto-oxidized constituents of certain plants inhibit the receptor-binding and biological activity of Graves' disease immunoglobulins. *Endocrin* 1985; 116: 1687–93.

5. Sourgens H, Winteroff H, Gumbinger HG, Kemper FH. Anti-hormonal effects of plant extracts: TSH and prolactin-suppressing properties of *Lithospermum officinale* and other plants. *Planta Med* 1982; 45: 78–86.

6. Blumenthal M, Busse WR, Goldberg A, et al. (eds). *The Complete Commission E Monographs: Therapeutic Guide to Herbal Medicines.* Boston, MA: Integrative Medicine Communications, 1998, 98–99.

7. Weiss RF. *Herbal Medicine.* Beaconsfield, UK: Beaconsfield Publishers Ltd., 1988, 328–29.

8. Brinker F. Inhibition of endocrine function by botanical agents. I. Boraginaceae and Labiatae. *J Naturopathic Med* 1990; 1: 10–18.

Burdock

1. Hoffman D. *The Herbal Handbook: A User's Guide to Medical Herbalism.* Rochester, VT: Healing Arts Press, 1988, 23–24.

2. Leung AY, Foster S. *Encyclopedia of Common Natural Ingredients Used in Food, Drugs, and Cosmetics,* 2d ed. New York: John Wiley & Sons, 1996, 107–8.

3. Morita K, Kada T, Namiki M. A desmutagenic factor isolated from burdock *(Arctium lappa Linne). Mutation Res* 1984; 129: 25–31.

4. Wichtl M. *Herbal Drugs and Phytopharmaceuticals.* Boca Raton, FL: CRC Press, 1994, 99–101.

5. Newall CA, Anderson LA, Phillipson JD. *Herbal Medicines: A Guide for Health-Care Professionals.* London: The Pharmaceutical Press, 1996, 52–53.

6. Bradley DR, ed. *British Herbal Compendium, vol 1.* Bournemouth, England: British Herbal Medicine Association, 1992, 48–49.

Butcher's Broom

1. Grieve M. *A Modern Herbal,* vol I. New York: Dover Publications, 1971, 128–29.

2. Weiss RF. *Herbal Medicine.* Gothenburg, Sweden: Ab Arcanum, 1988, 117–18.

3. Bouskela E, Cyrino FZGA, Marcelon G. Inhibitory effect of the *Ruscus* extract and of the flavonoid heperidine methylchalcone on increased microvascular permeability induced by various agents in the hamster cheek pouch. *J Cardiovasc Pharmacol* 1993; 22: 225–30.

4. Bouskela E, Cyrino FZGA, Marcelon G. Effects of *Ruscus* extract on the internal diameter of arterioles and venules of the hamster cheek pouch microcirculation. *J Cardiovasc Pharmacol* 1993; 22: 221–24.

5. Capelli R, Nicora M, Di Perri T. Use of extract of *Ruscus aculeatus* in venous disease in the lower limbs. *Drugs Exp Clin Res* 1988; 14: 277–83.

6. Rudofski G, Diehm C, et al. Chronic venous insufficiency: Treatment with *Ruscus* extract and trimethylhesperidin chalcone. *MMW* 1990; 132: 205–10 [in German].

7. Archimowicz-Cyrylowska B et al. Clinical effect of buckwheat herb, *Ruscus* extract and Troxerutin on retinopathy and lipids in diabetic patients. *Phytother Res* 1996; 10: 659–62.

8. Capelli R, Nicora M, Di Perri T. Use of extract of *Ruscus aculeatus* in venous disease in the lower limbs. *Drugs Exp Clin Res* 1988; 14: 277–83.

9. Blumenthal M, Busse WR, Goldberg A, et al. (eds). *The Complete Commission E Monographs: Therapeutic Guide to Herbal Medicines.* Boston, MA: Integrative Medicine Communications, 1998, 99–100.

Calendula

1. Leung A, Foster S. *Encyclopedia of Common Natural Ingredients Used in Food, Drugs and Cosmetics,* 2d ed. New York: John Wiley & Sons, 1996, 113–14.

2. Weiss RF. *Herbal Medicine.* Gothenburg, Sweden: Ab Arcanum, 1988, 344.

3. Della Loggia R, Tubaro A, Sosa S, et al. The role of triterpenoids in the topical anti-inflammatory activity of *Calendula officinalis* flowers. *Planta Med* 1994; 60: 516–20.

4. Bogdanova WS, Nikolaeva IS, et al. Study of antiviral properties of *Calendula officinalis. Farmskolto Ksikol* 1970; 33: 349–55 [in Russian].

5. De Tommasi N, Conti C, Stein ML, et al. Structure and in vitro activity of triterpenoid saponins form *Calendula arvenis. Planta Med* 1991; 57: 250–53.

6. Wichtl M. *Herbal Drugs and Phytopharmaceuticals.* Boca Raton, FL: CRC Press, 1994, 118–20.

Carob

1. Leob H, Vandenplas Y, Wursch P, Guesry P. Tannin-rich carob pod for the treatment of acute-onset diarrhea. *J Pediatr Gastroent Nutr* 1989; 8: 480–85.

2. Hostettler M, Steffen R, Tschopp A. Efficacy of tolerability of insoluble carob fraction in the treatment of travellers' diarrhea. *J Diarr Dis Res* 1995; 13: 155–58.

3. Greally P, Hampton FJ, MacFadyen UM, Simpson H. Gaviscon and Carobel compared with cisapride in gastroesophageal reflux. *Arch Dis Child* 1992; 67: 618–21.

4. Brown DJ. *Herbal Prescriptions for Better Health.* Rocklin, CA: Prima Publishing, 1996, 206.

Cascara

1. Castleman M. *The Healing Herbs.* Emmaus, PA: Rodale Press, 1991, 99–100.

2. Leung AY, Foster S. *Encyclopedia of Common Natural Ingredients Used in Food, Drugs, and Cosmetics,* 2d ed. New York: John Wiley & Sons, 1996, 128–30.

3. Blumenthal M, Busse WR, Goldberg A, et al. (eds). *The Complete Commission E Monographs: Therapeutic Guide to Herbal Medicines.* Boston, MA: Integrative Medicine Communications, 1998, 104–5.

3. Bradley PR, ed. *British Herbal Compendium,* vol 1. Bournemouth, Dorset, UK: British Herbal Medicine Association, 1992, 52–54.

4. Blumenthal M, Busse WR, Goldberg A, et al. (eds). *The Complete Commission E Monographs: Therapeutic Guide to Herbal Medicines.* Boston, MA: Integrative Medicine Communications, 1998, 104–5.

Catnip

1. Tyler VE. *Herbs of Choice.* Binghamton, NY: Pharmaceutical Products Press, 1994, 120–21.

2. Duke JA. *CRC Handbook of Medicinal Herbs.* Boca Raton, FL: CRC Press, 1985, 325–26.

3. Weiss RF. *Herbal Medicine.* Gothenburg, Sweden: Ab Arcanum, 1988, 282.

4. Sherry CJ, Hunter PS. The effect of an ethanol extract of catnip *(Nepeta cataria)* on the behavior of the young chick. *Experientia* 1979; 35: 237–38.

5. Greunwald J, Brendler T, Jaenicke C, et al. (eds). *PDR for Herbal Medicines.* Montvale, NJ: Medical Economics, 1998, 991–92.

Cat's Claw

1. Foster S. *Herbs for Your Health.* Loveland, CO: Interweave Press, 1996, 18–19.

2. Keplinger H. Oxyindole alkaloids having properties stimulating the immunologic system and preparation

Part Three: References

containing same. US Patent no. 5,302,611, April 12, 1994.

3. Aquino R, De Feo V, De Simone F, et al. Plant metabolites, new compounds and antiinflammatory activity of *Uncaria tomentosa*. *J Nat Prod* 1991; 54: 453–59.

4. Rizzi R, Re F, Bianchi A, et al. Mutagenic and antimutagenic activities of *Uncaria tomentosa* and its extracts. *J Ethnopharmacol* 1993; 38: 63–77.

5. Foster S. *Herbs for Your Health*. Loveland, CO: Interweave Press, 1996, 18–19.

Cayenne

1. Lynn B. Capsaicin. Actions on nociceptive C-fibers and therapeutic potential. *Pain* 1990; 41: 61–69.

2. Capsaicin study group. Treatment of painful diabetic neuropathy with topical capsaicin. A multicenter, double-blind, vehicle-controlled study. The capsaicin study group. *Arch Int Med* 1991; 151: 2225–29.

3. Capsaicin study group. Effect of treatment with capsaicin on daily activities of patients with painful diabetic neuropathy. The capsaicin study group. *Diabet Care* 1992; 15: 159–65.

4. Ellison N, Loprinzi CL, Kugler J, et al. Phase III placebo-controlled trial of capsaicin cream in the management of surgical neuropathic pain in cancer patients. *J Clin Oncol* 1997; 15: 2974–80.

5. Bernstein JE, Parish LC, Rapaport M, et al. Effects of topically applied capsaicin on moderate and severe psoriasis vulgaris. *J Am Acad Dermatol* 1986; 15: 504–7.

6. McCarty DJ et al. Treatment of pain due to fibromyalgia with topical capsaicin: A pilot study. *Semin Arth Rhem* 1986; 23(suppl 3): 41–47.

7. Watson CP, Evans RJ, Watt VR, Birkett N. A randomized vehicle-controlled trial of topical capsaicin in the treatment of postherpetic neuralgia. *Clin Ther* 1993; 15: 510–23.

8. McCarthy GM, McCarty DJ. Effect of topical capsaicin in the therapy of painful osteoarthritis of the hands. *J Rheumatol* 1992; 19: 604–7.

9. Deal CL, Schnitzer TJ, Lipstein E, et al. Treatment of arthritis with topical capsaicin: A double-blind trial. *Clin Ther* 1991; 13(3): 383–95.

10. Deal CL, Schnitzer TJ, Lipstein E, et al. Treatment of arthritis with topical capsaicin: A double-blind trial. *Clin Ther* 1991; 13(3): 383–95.

11. Marks DR, Rapoport A, et al. A double-blind placebo-controlled trial of intranasal capsaicin for cluster headache. *Cephalalgia* 1993; 13: 114–16.

12. Levy RL. Intranasal capsaicin for acute abortive treatment of migraine without aura. *Headache* 1995; 35(5): 277 [letter].

13. Siften DW, ed. *Physicians' Desk Reference for Nonprescription Drugs*. Montvale, NJ: Medical Economics, 1998, 790–91.

14. Siften DW, ed. *Physicians' Desk Reference for Nonprescription Drugs*. Montvale, NJ: Medical Economics, 1998, 790–91.

15. Lopez-Carrillo L, Avila M, Dubrow R. Chili pepper consumption and gastric cancer in Mexico: A case-control study. *Amer J Epidem* 1994; 139(3): 263–71.

16. Buiatti E, Palli D, Decarli A, et al. A case-control study of gastric cancer and diet in Italy. *Int J Cancer* 1989; 44: 611–16.

17. Surh YJ, Lee SS. Capsaicin in hot chili pepper: Carcinogen, co-carcinogen or anticarcinogen? *Food Chem Toxic* 1996; 34: 313–16.

Chamomile

1. Wichtl M. *Herbal Drugs and Phytopharmaceuticals*. Boca Raton, FL: CRC Press, 1994, 322–25.

2. Jakolev V, Isaac O, et al. Pharmacological investigations with compounds of chamomile. II. New investigations on the antiphlogistic effects of (-)-a-bisabolol and bisabolol oxides. *Planta Med* 1979; 35: 125–40.

3. Jakolev V, Isaac O, Flaskamp E. Pharmacological investigations with compounds of chamomile. VI. Investigations on the antiphlogistic effects of chamazulene and matricine. *Planta Med* 1983; 49: 67–73.

4. Della Loggia R, Tubaro A, et al. The role of flavonoids in the antiin-flammatory activity of *Chamomilla recutita*. In *Plant Flavonoids in Biology and Medicine: Biochemical, Pharmacological, and Structure-Activity Relationships*, eds. V Cody, E Middleton, JB Harbone. New York: Alan R. Liss, 1986, 481–84.

5. Achterrath-Tuckerman U, Kunde R, et al. Pharmacological investigations with compounds of chamomile. V. Investigations on the spasmolytic effect of compounds of chamomile and Kamillosan on the isolated guinea pig ileum. *Planta Med* 1980; 39: 38–50.

6. Blumenthal M, Busse WR, Goldberg A, et al. (eds). *The Complete Commission E Monographs: Therapeutic Guide to Herbal Medicines*. Boston, MA: Integrative Medicine Communications, 1998, 107.

7. Brown DJ. *Herbal Prescriptions for Better Health*. Rocklin, CA: Prima Publishing, 1996, 49–56.

Chaparral

1. Brinker F. *Larrea tridentata* (D.C.) Coville (chaparral or creosote bush). *Br J Phytother* 1993/1994; 3(1): 10–31 [review].

2. Moore M. *Medicinal Plants of the Desert and Canyon West*. Santa Fe: Museum of New Mexico Press, 1989, 27–29.

3. Kay MA. *Healing with Plants in the American and Mexican West*. Tucson: University of Arizona Press, 1996, 178–81.

4. Bokoch G, Reed P. Evidence for inhibition of leukotriene A4 synthesis by 5,8,11,14-eicosatetraynoic acid in guinea pig polymorphonuclear leukocytes. *J Biol Chem* 1981; 256: 4156.

5. Salari H, Braquet P, Borgeat P. Comparative effects of indomethacin, acetylenic acids, 15-HETE, nordihydroguaiaretic acid and BW755C on the metabolism of arachidonic acid in human leukocytes and platelets. *Prostaglan Leukot Med* 1984; 13: 53–60.

6. Calzado-Flores C, Segura-Luna JJ, Guajardo-Touche EM. Effects of chaparrin, nordihydroguaiaretic acid and their structural analogues on *Entamoeba histolytica*

cultures. *Proc West Pharmacol Soc* 1995; 38: 105–6.

7. Smart CR, Hogle CR, Vogel H, et al. Clinical experience with nordihydroguaiaretic acid—"chapparel tea" [sic] in the treatment of cancer. *Rocky Mtn Med J* 1970; 67: 39–43.

8. Kay MA. *Healing with Plants in the American and Mexican West.* Tucson: University of Arizona Press, 1996, 178–81.

9. Moore M. *Medicinal Plants of the Desert and Canyon West.* Santa Fe: Museum of New Mexico Press, 1989, 27–29.

10. Sheikh NM, Philen RM, Love LA. Chaparral-associated hepatotoxicity. *Arch Int Med* 1997; 157: 913–19.

11. Smart CR, Hogle CR, Vogel H, et al. Clinical experience with nordihydroguaiaretic acid—"chapparel tea" [sic] in the treatment of cancer. *Rocky Mtn Med J* 1970; 67: 39–43.

12. McGuffin M, Hobbs C, Upton R, Goldberg A. *American Herbal Products Association's Botanical Safety Handbook.* Boca Raton, FL: CRC Press, 1997, 67.

Chickweed

1. Duke JA. *CRC Handbook of Medicinal Herbs.* Boca Raton, FL: CRC Press, 1985, 458–59.

2. Weiss RF. *Herbal Medicine.* Gothenburg, Sweden: Ab Arcanum, 1988, 265.

3. Hoffman D. *The Herbal Handbook.* Rochester, VT: Healing Arts Press, 1988, 64–65.

Cinnamon

1. Leung AY, Foster S. *Encyclopedia of Common Natural Ingredients Used in Foods, Drugs, and Cosmetics,* 2d ed. New York: John Wiley & Sons, 1996, 168–70.

2. Singh HB, Srivastava M, Singh AB, Srivastava AK. Cinnamon bark oil, a potent fungitoxicant against fungi causing respiratory tract mycoses. *Allergy* 1995; 50: 995–99.

3. Quale JM, Landman D, Zaman MM, et al. In vitro activity of *Cinnamomum zeylanicum* against azole resistant and sensitive *Candida* species and a pilot study of cinnamon for oral candidiasis. *Am J Chin Med* 1996; 24: 103–9.

4. Azumi S, Tanimura A, Tanamoto K. A novel inhibitor of bacterial endotoxin derived from cinnamon bark. *Biochem Biophys Res Commun* 1997; 234: 506–10.

5. Tabak M, Armon R, Potasman I, Neeman I. In vitro inhibition of *Helicobacter pylori* by extracts of thyme. *J Appl Bacteriol* 1996; 80(6): 667–72.

6. Nagai H, Shimazawa T, Matsuura N, Koda A. Immunopharmacological studies of the aqueous extract of *Cinnamomum cassia* (CCAq). I. Anti-allergic action. *Jpn J Pharmacol* 1982; 32: 813–22.

7. Akira T, Tanaka S, Tabata M. Pharmacological studies on the antiulcerogenic activity of Chinese cinnamon. *Planta Med* 1986; (6): 440.

8. Blumenthal M, Busse WR, Goldberg A, et al. (eds). *The Complete Commission E Monographs: Therapeutic Guide to Herbal Medicines.* Boston, MA: Integrative Medicine Communications, 1998, 110–11.

9. Blumenthal M, Busse WR, Goldberg A, et al. (eds). *The Complete Commission E Monographs: Therapeutic Guide to Herbal Medicines.* Boston, MA: Integrative Medicine Communications, 1998, 110–11.

10. Blumenthal M, Busse WR, Goldberg A, et al. (eds). *The Complete Commission E Monographs: Therapeutic Guide to Herbal Medicines.* Boston, MA: Integrative Medicine Communications, 1998, 110–11.

Cleavers

1. Mills SY. *Out of the Earth: The Essential Book of Herbal Medicine.* London: Viking Arkana, 1991, 493–94.

2. Mills SY. *Out of the Earth: The Essential Book of Herbal Medicine.* London: Viking Arkana, 1991, 493–94.

Coltsfoot

1. Weiss RF. *Herbal Medicine.* Gothenburg, Sweden: Ab Arcanum and Beaconsfield, UK: Beaconsfield Publishers Ltd., 1988, 196–97.

2. Blumenthal M, Busse WR, Goldberg A, et al. (eds). *The Complete German Commission E Monographs: Therapeutic Guide to Herbal Medicines.* Austin: American Botanical Council and Boston: Integrative Medicine Communications, 1998: 114–15.

3. Foster S. *Herbal Renaissance.* Salt Lake City: Gibbs-Smith Publisher, 1993, 74–78.

4. Weiss RF. *Herbal Medicine.* Gothenburg, Sweden: Ab Arcanum and Beaconsfield, UK: Beaconsfield Publishers Ltd., 1988, 196–97.

5. Weiss RF. *Herbal Medicine.* Gothenburg, Sweden: Ab Arcanum and Beaconsfield, UK: Beaconsfield Publishers Ltd., 1988, 196–97.

6. Weiss RF. *Herbal Medicine.* Gothenburg, Sweden: Ab Arcanum and Beaconsfield, UK: Beaconsfield Publishers Ltd., 1988, 196–97.

7. Weiss RF. *Herbal Medicine.* Gothenburg, Sweden: Ab Arcanum and Beaconsfield, UK: Beaconsfield Publishers Ltd., 1988, 196–97.

8. Roulet M, Laurini R, Rivier L, Calame A. Hepatic veno-occlusive disease in newborn infant of a woman drinking herbal tea. *J Pediatrics* 1988; 112: 433–36.

9. McGuffin M, Hobbs C, Upton R, Goldberg A. *American Herbal Products Association's Botanical Safety Handbook.* Boca Raton, FL: CRC Press, 1997, 117–18.

10. Weiss RF. *Herbal Medicine.* Gothenburg, Sweden: Ab Arcanum and Beaconsfield, UK: Beaconsfield Publishers Ltd., 1988, 196–97.

Comfrey

1. Mills SY. *Out of the Earth: The Essential Book of Herbal Medicine.* New York: Viking Arkana, 1991, 544–47.

2. Weiss RF. *Herbal Medicine.* Gothenburg, Sweden: Ab Arcanum and Beaconsfield, UK: Beaconsfield Publishers Ltd., 1988, 334–35.

3. Duke JA. *Handbook of Phytochemical Constituents of GRAS Herbs and Other Economic Plants.* Boca Raton, FL: CRC Press, 1992.

4. Stamford IF, Tavares IA. The effect of an aqueous extract of com-

frey on prostaglandin synthesis by rat isolated stomach. *J Pharm Pharmacol* 1983; 35: 816–17.

5. Weiss RF. *Herbal Medicine*. Gothenburg, Sweden: Ab Arcanum and Beaconsfield, UK: Beaconsfield Publishers Ltd., 1988, 334–35.

6. Mills SY. *Out of the Earth: The Essential Book of Herbal Medicine*. New York: Viking Arkana, 1991, 544–47.

7. Mills SY. *Out of the Earth: The Essential Book of Herbal Medicine*. New York: Viking Arkana, 1991, 544–47.

8. Winship KA. Toxicity of comfrey. *Adverse Drug React Toxicol Rev* 1991; 10: 47–59 [review].

9. Foster S. *Herbal Renaissance*. Salt Lake City: Gibbs-Smith Publisher, 1993, 74–78.

10. Foster S. *Herbal Renaissance*. Salt Lake City: Gibbs-Smith Publisher, 1993, 74–78.

11. Anderson PC, McLean AEM. Comfrey and liver damage. *Human Toxicol* 1989; 8: 68–69.

12. Stamford IF, Tavares IA. The effect of an aqueous extract of comfrey on prostaglandin synthesis by rat isolated stomach. *J Pharm Pharmacol* 1983; 35: 816–17.

13. McGuffin M, Hobbs C, Upton R, Goldberg A. *American Herbal Products Association's Botanical Safety Handbook*. Boca Raton, FL: CRC Press, 1997, 111–12.

Cranberry

1. Sobota AE. Inhibition of bacterial adherence by cranberry juice: Potential use for the treatment of urinary tract infections. *J Urol* 1984; 131: 1013–16.

2. Zafiri D, Ofek I, et al. Inhibitory activity of cranberry juice on adherence of type 1 and type P fimbriated *Esherichia coli* to eucaryotic cells. *Antimicrob Agents Chemother* 1989; 33: 92–98.

3. Howell AB, Vorsa N, Der Maderosian A. Inhibition of the adherence of P-fimbriated *Eshericia coli* to uroepithelial—all surfaces by proanthocyanidin extracts from cranberries. *New Engl J Med* 1998; 339: 1005–6.

4. Avorn J, Monane M, Gurwitz JH, et al. Reduction of bacteriuria and pyruria after ingestion of cranberry juice. *JAMA* 1994; 271: 751–54.

5. Leaver RB. Cranberry juice. *Prof Nurse* 1996; 11(8): 525–26 [review].

6. Brown DJ. *Herbal Prescriptions for Better Health*. Rocklin, CA: Prima Publishing, 1996, 57–61.

Cranesbill

1. Tilford GL. *Edible and Medicinal Plants of the West*. Missoula, MT: Mountain Press Publishing Company, 1997, 42–43.

2. Duke JA. *CRC Handbook of Medicinal Plants*. Boca Raton, FL: CRC Press, 1985, 209.

3. Hoffman D. *The Herbal Handbook*. Rochester, VT: Healing Arts Press, 1988, 43.

Damiana

1. Bradley PR, ed. *British Herbal Compendium*, vol 1. Bournemouth, Dorset, UK: British Herbal Medicine Association, 1992, 71–72.

2. Duke JA. *CRC Handbook of Medicinal Herbs*. Boca Raton, FL: CRC Press, 1985, 492.

3. Bradley PR, ed. *British Herbal Compendium*, vol 1. Bournemouth, Dorset, UK: British Herbal Medicine Association, 1992, 71–72.

4. Zava DT, Dollbaum CM, Blen M. Estrogen and progestin bioactivity of foods, herbs, and spices. *Proc Soc Exp Biol Med* 1998; 217: 369–78.

5. Blumenthal M, Busse WR, Goldberg A, et al. (eds). *The Complete Commission E Monographs: Therapeutic Guide to Herbal Medicines*. Boston, MA: Integrative Medicine Communications, 1998, 325–26.

6. Mills SY. *Out of the Earth: The Essential Book of Herbal Medicine*. Middlesex, UK: Viking Arkana, 1991, 516–17.

Dandelion

1. Wichtl M. *Herbal Drugs and Phytopharmaceuticals*. Boca Raton, FL: CRC Press, 1994, 486–89.

2. Bradley PR, ed. *British Herbal Compendium*, Vol 1. Bournemouth,

Dorset, UK: British Herbal Medicine Association, 1992, 73–75.

3. Racz-Kotilla E, Racz G, Solomon A. The action of *Taraxacum officinale* extracts on body weight and diuresis of laboratory animals. *Planta Med* 1974; 26: 212–17.

4. Kuusi T, Pyylaso H, Autio K. The bitterness properties of dandelion. II. Chemical investigations. *Lebensm-Wiss Technol* 1985; 18: 347–49.

5. Bëhm K. Choleretic action of some medicinal plants. *Arzneim-Forsch Drug Res* 1959; 9: 376–78.

6. Blumenthal M, Busse WR, Goldberg A, et al. (eds). *The Complete Commission E Monographs: Therapeutic Guide to Herbal Medicines*. Boston, MA: Integrative Medicine Communications, 1998, 119–20.

7. Foster S. *Herbs for Your Health*. Loveland, CO: Interweave Press, 1996, 26–27.

8. Blumenthal M, Busse WR, Goldberg A, et al. (eds). *The Complete Commission E Monographs: Therapeutic Guide to Herbal Medicines*. Boston, MA: Integrative Medicine Communications, 1998, 118–19.

9. Blumenthal M, Busse WR, Goldberg A, et al. (eds). *The Complete Commission E Monographs: Therapeutic Guide to Herbal Medicines*. Boston, MA: Integrative Medicine Communications, 1998, 118–20.

Devil's Claw

1. Tyler, VE. *The Honest Herbal*, 3d ed. Binghamton, NY: Pharmaceutical Products Press, 1993, 111–12.

2. Weiss RF. *Herbal Medicine*. Gothenburg, Sweden: Ab Arcanum, 1988, 238–39.

3. Leung AY, Foster S. *Encyclopedia of Common Natural Ingredients Used in Food, Drugs, and Cosmetics*, 2d ed. New York: John Wiley & Sons, 1996, 208–10.

4. Whitehouse LW, Znamirouska M, Paul CJ. Devil's claw (*Harpagophytum procumbens*) : no evidence for anti-inflammatory activity in the treatment of arthritic disease. *Can Med Assoc J* 1983; 129: 249–51.

5. Grahame R, Robinson BV. De-vil's claw (*Harpogophytum procumbens*):

pharmacological and clinical studies. *Ann Rheum Dis* 1981; 40: 632.

6. Chrubasik S, Zimpfer C, Schutt U, Ziegler R. Effectiveness of *Harpagophytum procumbens* in treatment of acute low back pain. *Phytomed* 1996; 3: 1–10.

7. Blumenthal M, Busse WR, Goldberg A, et al. (eds). *The Complete Commission E Monographs: Therapeutic Guide to Herbal Medicines.* Boston, MA: Integrative Medicine Communications, 1998, 120–21.

8. Blumenthal M, Busse WR, Goldberg A, et al. (eds). *The Complete Commission E Monographs: Therapeutic Guide to Herbal Medicines.* Boston, MA: Integrative Medicine Communications, 1998, 120–21.

Dong Quai

1. Foster S, Yue CX. *Herbal Emissaries.* Rochester, VT: Healing Arts Press, 1992, 65–72.

2. Hirata JD et al. Does dong quai have estrogenic effects in postmenopausal women? A double-blind, placebo-controlled trial. *Fertil Steril* 1997; 68: 981–86.

3. Qi-bing M, Jing-yi T, Bo C. Advance in the pharmacological studies of radix *Angelica sinensis* (Oliv) Diels (Chinese danggui). *Chin Med J* 1991; 104: 776–81.

4. Foster S. *Herbs for Your Health.* Loveland, CO: Interweave Press, 1996, 28–29.

5. Newall CA, Anderson LA, Phillipson JD. *Herbal Medicines: A Guide for Health-Care Professionals.* London: The Pharmaceutical Press, 1996, 28–29.

Echinacea

1. Leuttig B, Steinmuller C, et al. Macrophage activation by the polysaccharide arabinogalactan isolated from plant cell cultures of *Echinacea purpurea. J Natl Cancer Inst* 1989; 81: 669–75.

2. See DM, Broumand N, Sahl L, Tilles JG. In vitro effects of echinacea and ginseng on natural killer and antibody-dependent cell cytotoxicity in healthy subjects and chronic fatigue syndrome or acquired immunodefi-

ciency syndrome patients. *Immunpharmacol* 1997; 35: 229–35.

3. Melchart D, Linde K, et al. Immunomodulation with Echinacea —a systematic review of controlled clinical trials. *Phytomed* 1994; 1: 245–54.

4. Dorn M, Knick E, Lewith G. Placebo-controlled, double-blind study of *Echinacea pallida redix* in upper respiratory tract infections. *Comp Ther Med* 1997; 5: 40–42.

5. Hoheizel O, Sandberg M, Bertram S, et al. Echinacea shortens the course of the common cold: a double-blind, placebo-controlled clinical trial. *Eur J Clin Res* 1997; 9: 261–68.

6. Melchort D, Walther E, Linde K, et al. Echinacea root extracts for the prevention of upper respiratory tract infections: A double-blind, placebo-controlled randomized trial. *Arch Fam Med* 1998; 7: 541–45.

7. Coeugniet E, Kuhnast R. Recurrent candidiasis. Adjuvant immunotherapy with different formulations of Echinacea. *Therapiwoche* 1986; 36: 3352–58 [in German].

8. Brown DJ. *Herbal Prescriptions for Better Health.* Rocklin, CA: Prima Publishing, 1996, 63–68.

9. Blumenthal M, Busse WR, Goldberg A, et al. (eds). *The Complete Commission E Monographs: Therapeutic Guide to Herbal Medicines.* Boston, MA: Integrative Medicine Communications, 1998, 121–123.

Elderberry

1. Duke JA. *CRC Handbook of Medicinal Herbs.* Boca Raton, FL: CRC Press, 1985, 423.

2. Serkedjieva J, Manolova N, Zgórniak-Nowosielska I, et al. Antiviral activity of the infusion (SHS-174) from flowers of *Sambucus nigra* L., aerial parts of *Hypericum perforatum* L., and roots of *Saponaria officinalis* L. against influenza and herpes simplex viruses. *Phytother Res* 1990; 4: 97–100.

3. Zakay-Rones Z, Varsano N, Zlotnik M, et al. Inhibition of several strains of influenza virus in vitro and reduction of symptoms by an elderberry extract *(Sambucus nigra* L.) during

an outbreak of influenza B Panama. *J Alt Compl Med* 1995; 1: 361–69.

4. Mascolo N, Autore G, Capasso G, et al. Biological screening of Italian medicinal plants for anti-inflammatory activity. *Phytother Res* 1987; 1: 28–31.

5. Gruenwald J, Brendler T, Jaenicke C, et al. (eds). *PDR for Herbal Medicines.* Montvale, NJ: Medical Economics, 1998, 1116–17.

Elecampane

1. Leung AY, Foster S. *Encyclopedia of Common Natural Ingredients Used in Food, Drugs, and Cosmetics.* New York: John Wiley & Sons, 1996, 222–24.

2. Wichtl M. *Herbal Drugs and Phytopharmaceuticals.* Boca Raton, FL: CRC Press, 1994, 254–56.

3. Newall CA, Anderson LA, Phillipson JD. *Herbal Medicines: A Guide for Health-Care Professionals.* London: The Pharmaceutical Press, 1996, 106–7.

4. Blumenthal M, Busse WR, Goldberg A, et al. (eds). *The Complete German Commission E Monographs: Therapeutic Guide to Herbal Medicines.* Austin: American Botanical Council and Boston: Integrative Medicine Communications, 1998, 328–29.

5. Bradley PR, ed. *British Herbal Compendium,* vol. 1. Bournemouth, England: British Herbal Medicine Association, 1992, 87–88.

6. Gruenwald J, Brendler T, Jaenicke C, et al. (eds). *PDR for Herbal Medicines.* Montvale, NJ: Medical Economics, 1998, 912–13.

Eleuthero

1. Collisson RJ. Siberian ginseng *(Eleutherococcus senticosus). Brit J Phytother* 1991; 2: 61–71 [review].

2. Farnsworth NR, Kinghorn AD, Soejarto DD, Waller DP. Siberian ginseng *(Eleutherococcus senticosus):* Current status as an adaptogen. In *Economic and Medicinal Plant Research,* vol 1, eds. H Wagner, HZ Hikino, NR Farnsworth. London: Academic Press, 1985, 155–215 [review].

3. Hikino H, Takahashi M, et al. Isolation and hypoglycemic activity of eleutherans A, B, C, D, E, F and G: glycans of *Eleutherococcus senticosus* roots. *J Natural Prod* 1986; 49: 293–97.

4. Wagner H, Nörr H, Winterhoff H. Plant adaptogens. *Phytomed* 1994; 1: 63–76 [review].

5. Farnsworth NR, Kinghorn AD, Soejarto DD, Waller DP. Siberian ginseng *(Eleutherococcus senticosus)* : Current status as an adaptogen. In *Economic and Medicinal Plant Research*, vol 1, eds. H Wagner, HZ Hikino, NR Farnsworth. London: Academic Press, 1985, 155–215 [review].

6. Asano K, Takahashi T, Miyashita M, et al. Effect of *Eleutherococcus senticosus* extract on human working capacity. *Planta Medica* 1986; 37: 175–77.

7. Collisson RJ. Siberian ginseng *(Eleutherococcus senticosus)*. *Brit J Phytother* 1991; 2: 61–71 [review].

8. Ben-Hur E, Fulder S. Effect of *P. ginseng saponins* and *Eleutherococcus S.* on survival of cultured mammalian cells after ionizing radiation. *Am J Chin Med* 1981; 9: 48–56.

9. Kupin VI, Polevaia EB. Stimulation of the immunological reactivity of cancer patients by eleutherococcus extract. *Vopr Onkol* 1986; 32: 21–26 [in Russian].

10. Bohn B, Nebe CT, Birr C. Flow cytometric studies with *Eleutherococcus senticosus* extract as an immunomodulating agent. *Arzneim-Forsch Drug Res* 1987; 37: 1193–96.

11. Brown DJ. *Herbal Prescriptions for Better Health*. Rocklin, CA: Prima Publishing, 1996, 69–77.

12. McGuffin M, Hobbs C, Upton R, Goldberg A. *American Herbal Products Association's Botanical Safety Handbook*. Boca Raton, FL: CRC Press, 1997, 45.

Ephedra

1. Foster S. *Herbs for Your Health*. Loveland, CO: Interweave Press, 1996, 37–38.

2. Tyler, VE. *The Honest Herbal*, 3d ed. Binghamton, NY: Pharmaceutical Products Press, 1993, 119–21.

3. Leung AY, Foster S. *Encyclopedia of Common Natural Ingredients Used in Food, Drugs, and Cosmetics*, 2d ed. New York: John Wiley & Sons, 1996, 227–29.

4. Foster S. *Herbs for Your Health*. Loveland, CO: Interweave Press, 1996, 37–38.

5. Blumenthal M, Busse WR, Goldberg A, et al. (eds). *The Complete Commission E Monographs: Therapeutic Guide to Herbal Medicines*. Boston, MA: Integrative Medicine Communications, 1998, 125–26.

6. White LM, Gardner SF, Gurley BJ, et al. Pharmacokinetics and cardiovascular effects of ma-huang *(Ephedra sinica)* in normotensive adults. *J Clin Pharmacol* 1997; 37: 116–21.

7. Blumenthal M, Busse WR, Goldberg A, et al. (eds). *The Complete Commission E Monographs: Therapeutic Guide to Herbal Medicines*. Boston, MA: Integrative Medicine Communications, 1998, 125–26.

8. Blumenthal M, Busse WR, Goldberg A, et al. (eds). *The Complete Commission E Monographs: Therapeutic Guide to Herbal Medicines*. Boston, MA: Integrative Medicine Communications, 1998, 125–26.

Eucalyptus

1. Wren RC. *Potter's New Cyclopedia of Botanical Drugs and Preparations*. Essex, England: C.W. Daniel Co., 1988, 110–11.

2. Castleman M. *The Healing Herbs*. Emmaus, PA: Rodale Press, 1991, 162–63.

3. Robbers JE, Tyler VE. *Tyler's Herbs of Choice: The Therapeutic Use of Phytomedicines*. New York: Haworth Press, 1999, 123.

4. Schulz V, Hansel R, Tyler VE. *Rational Phytotherapy*, 3rd ed. Berlin, Germany: Springer-Verlag, 1998, 146–47.

5. Leung AY, Foster S. *Encyclopedia of Common Natural Ingredients Used in Food, Drugs, and Cosmetics*, 2d ed. New York: John Wiley & Sons, 1996, 232–33.

6. Newall CA, Anderson LA, Phillipson JD. *Herbal Medicines: A Guide for Health-Care Professionals*. London: The Pharmaceutical Press, 1996, 108.

7. Gobel H, Schmidt G, Dowarski M, et al. Essential plant oils and headache mechanisms. *Phytomed* 1995; 2: 93–102.

8. Trigg JK, Hill N. Laboratory evaluation of a eucalyptus-based insect repellent against four biting arthropods. *Phytother Res* 1996; 10: 313–16. Reviewed by Yarnell E. Selected herbal research summaries *QRNM* 1997; 116.

9. Ishizuka Y, Imamura Y, Tereshima K, et al. Effects of nasal inhalation capsule. *Oto-Rhino-Laryngology Tokyo* 1997; 40: 9–13.

10. Newall CA, Anderson LA, Phillipson JD. *Herbal Medicines: A Guide for Health-Care Professionals*. London: The Pharmaceutical Press, 1996, 108.

11. Leung AY, Foster S. *Encyclopedia of Common Natural Ingredients Used in Food, Drugs, and Cosmetics*, 2d ed. New York: John Wiley & Sons, 1996, 232–33.

12. Schulz V, Hansel R, Tyler VE. *Rational Phytotherapy*, 3rd ed. Berlin, Germany: Springer-Verlag, 1998, 146–47.

13. Blumenthal M, Busse WR, Goldberg A, et al. (eds). *The Complete German Commission E Monographs: Therapeutic Guide to Herbal Medicines*. Austin: American Botanical Council and Boston: Integrative Medicine Communications, 1998, 127–28.

14. Brinker F. *Herb Contraindications and Drug Interactions*. Sandy, OR: Eclectic Institute Publishers, 1997, 46–47.

15. Blumenthal M, Busse WR, Goldberg A, et al. (eds). *The Complete German Commission E Monographs: Therapeutic Guide to Herbal Medicines*. Austin: American Botanical Council and Boston: Integrative Medicine Communications, 1998, 127–28.

16. Brinker F. *Herb Contraindications and Drug Interactions*. Sandy, OR: Eclectic Institute Publishers, 1997, 46–47.

17. Brinker F. *Herb Contra-indications and Drug Interactions.* Sandy, OR: Eclectic Institute Publishers, 1997, 46–47.

Eyebright

1. Weiss RF. *Herbal Medicine.* Gothenburg, Sweden: Ab Arcanum, 1988, 339–40.

2. Hoffman D. *The Herbal Handbook: A User's Guide to Medical Herbalism.* Rochester, VT: Healing Arts Press, 1988, 136–37.

3. Wichtl M. *Herbal Drugs and Phytopharmaceuticals.* Boca Raton, FL: CRC Press, 1994, 195–96.

4. Weiss RF. *Herbal Medicine.* Gothenburg, Sweden: Ab Arcanum, 1988, 339–40.

5. Blumenthal M, Busse WR, Goldberg A, et al. (eds). *The Complete Commission E Monographs: Therapeutic Guide to Herbal Medicines.* Boston, MA: Integrative Medicine Communications, 1998, 329–30.

False Unicorn

1. Mills SY. *Out of the Earth: The Essential Book of Herbal Medicine.* Middlesex, UK: Viking Arkana, 1991, 520–22.

2. Mills SY. *Out of the Earth: The Essential Book of Herbal Medicine.* Middlesex, UK: Viking Arkana, 1991, 520–22.

3. Newall CA, Anderson LA, Phillipson JD. *Herbal Medicines: A Guide for Health-Care Professionals.* London: The Pharmaceutical Press, 1996, 116.

Fennel

1. Duke JA. *CRC Handbook of Medicinal Herbs.* Boca Raton, FL: CRC Press, 1985, 145–46.

2. Mills SY. *Out of the Earth: The Essential Book of Herbal Medicine.* Middlesex, UK: Viking Arkana, 1991, 424–26.

3. Albert-Puleo M. Fennel and anise as estrogenic agents. *J Ethnopharm* 1980; 2(4): 337–44.

4. Forster HB, Niklas H, Lutz S. Antispasmodic effects of some medicinal plants. *Planta Med.* 1980; 40(4): 303–19.

5. Tanira MOM, Shah AH, Mohsin A, et al. Pharmacological and toxicological investigations on *Foeniculum vulgare* dried fruit extract in experimental animals. *Phytother Res* 1996; 10: 33–36.

6. Hare HA, Caspari C, Rusby HH. *The National Standard Dispensatory.* Philadelphia: Lea & Febiger, 1916: 63,1129.

7. Blumenthal M, Busse WR, Goldberg A, et al. (eds). *The Complete Commission E Monographs: Therapeutic Guide to Herbal Medicines.* Boston, MA: Integrative Medicine Communications, 1998, 128–29.

8. Blumenthal M, Busse WR, Goldberg A, et al. (eds). *The Complete Commission E Monographs: Therapeutic Guide to Herbal Medicines.* Boston, MA: Integrative Medicine Communications, 1998, 128–29.

Fenugreek

1. Escot N. Fenugreek. *ATOMS* 1994/5; Summer: 7–12.

2. Sauvaire Y, Ribes G, Baccou JC, Loubatieres-Mariani MM. Implication of steroid saponins and sapogenins in the hypocholesterolemic effect of fenugreek. *Lipids* 1991; 26: 191–97.

3. Ribes G, Sauvaire Y, Da Costa C, et al. Antidiabetic effects of subfractions from fenugreek seeds in diabetic dogs. *Proc Soc Exp Biol Med* 1986; 182: 159–66.

4. Bordia A, Verma SK, Srivastava KC. Effect of ginger (*Zingiber officinale* Rosc) and fenugreek (*Trigonella foenumgraecum* L.) on blood lipids, blood sugar, and platelet aggregation in patients with coronary artery disease. *Prostagland Leukotrienes Essential Fatty Acids* 1997; 56: 379–84.

5. Sharma RD, Raghuram TC, Rao NS. Effect of fenugreek seeds on blood glucose and serum lipids in type I diabetes. *Eur J Clin Nutr* 1990; 44: 301–6.

6. Madar Z, Abel R, Samish S, Arad J. Glucose-lowering effect of fenugreek in non-insulin dependent diabetics. *Eur J Clin Nutr* 1988; 42: 51–54.

7. Raghuram TC, Sharma RD, Sivakumar B, Sahay BK. Effect of fenugreek seeds on intravenous glucose disposition in non-insulin dependent diabetic patients. *Phytother Res* 1994; 8: 83–86.

8. Sharma RD, Raghuram TC, Dayasagar Rao V. Hypolipidaemic effect of fenugreek seeds. A clinical study. *Phytother Res* 1991; 5: 145–47.

9. Sharma RD, Sarkar DK, Hazra B, et al. Hypolipidaemic effect of fenugreek seeds: A chronic study in non-insulin dependent diabetic patients. *Phytother Res* 1996; 10: 332–34.

10. Blumenthal M, Busse WR, Goldberg A, et al. (eds). *The Complete Commission E Monographs: Therapeutic Guide to Herbal Medicines.* Boston, MA: Integrative Medicine Communications, 1998, 130.

Feverfew

1. Makheja AN, Bailey JM. A platelet phospholipase inhibitor from the medicinal herb feverfew (*Tanacetum parthenium*). *Prostagland Leukotrienes Med* 1982; 8: 653–60.

2. Hepinstall S, White A, et al. Extracts of feverfew inhibit granule secretion in blood platelets and polymorphonuclear leukocytes. *Lancet* 1985; i: 1071–74.

3. Johnson ES, Kadan NP, Hylands DM, Hylands PJ. Efficacy of feverfew as prophylatic treatment of migraine. *Br Med J* 1985; 291: 569–73.

4. Murphy JJ, Heptinstall S, Mitchell JRA. Randomised double-blind placebo-controlled trial of feverfew in migraine prevention. *Lancet* 1988; ii: 189–92.

5. Palevitch D, Earon G, Carasso R. Feverfew (*Tanacetum parthenium*) as a prophylactic treatment for migraine: A double-blind placebo-controlled study. *Phytother Res* 1997; 11: 508–11.

6. Brown DJ. *Herbal Prescriptions for Better Health.* Rocklin, CA: Prima Publishing, 1996, 91–95.

7. De Weerdt CJ, Bootsma HPR, Hendriks H. Herbal medicines in migraine prevention. *Phytomed* 1996; 3: 225–30.

Part Three: References

8. Brown DJ. *Herbal Prescriptions for Better Health*. Rocklin, CA: Prima Publishing, 1996, 91–95.

Fo-Ti

1. Foster S, Yue CX. *Herbal Emissaries: Bringing Chinese Herbs to the West*. Rochester, VT: Healing Arts Press, 1992, 79–85.

2. Foster S, Yue CX. *Herbal Emissaries: Bringing Chinese Herbs to the West*. Rochester, VT: Healing Arts Press, 1992, 79–85.

3. Foster S. *Herbal Renaissance*. Layton, Utah: Gibbs-Smith Publisher, 1993, 40–41.

4. Foster S, Yue CX. *Herbal Emissaries: Bringing Chinese Herbs to the West*. Rochester, VT: Healing Arts Press, 1992, 79–85.

5. Bone K. *Clinical Applications of Ayurvedic and Chinese Herbs*. Warwick, Australia: Phytotherapy Press, 1996, 49–51.

6. Foster S. *Herbs for Your Health*. Loveland, CO: Interweave Press, 1996, 40–41.

Garlic

1. Koch HP, Lawson LD, eds. *Garlic: The Science and Therapeutic Application of Allium sativaum L and Related Species*, 2d ed. Baltimore: Williams and Wilkins, 1996, 62–4.

2. Legnani C, Frascaro M, et al. Effects of a dried garlic preparation on fibrinolysis and platelet aggregation in healthy subjects. *Arzneim-Forsch Drug Res* 1993; 43: 119–22.

3. Silagy C, Neil A. A meta-analysis of the effect of garlic on blood pressure. *J Hyperten* 1994; 12(4): 463–68.

4. Kleijnen J, Knipschild P, Ter Riet G. Garlic, onion and cardiovascular risk factors: A review of the evidence from human experiments with emphasis on commercially available preparations. *Br J Clin Pharmacol* 1989; 28: 535–44.

5. Warshafsky S, Kamer R, Sivak S. Effect of garlic on total serum cholesterol: A meta-analysis. *Ann Int Med* 1993; 119(7): 599–605.

6. Silagy C, Neil A. Garlic as a lipid-lowering agent—a meta-analysis. *J R Coll Phys* London 1994; 28(1): 39–45.

7. Neil HAW, Silagy CA, Lancaster T, et al. Garlic powder in the treatment of moderate hyperlipidaemia: A controlled trial and a meta-analysis. *J R Coll Phys* 1996; 30: 329–34.

8. Holzgartner H, Schmidt U, Kuhn U. Comparison of the efficacy and tolerance of a garlic preparation vs. bezafibrate. *Arzneim Forsch Drug Res* 1992; 42: 1473–77.

9. Isaacsohn JL, Moser M, Stein EA, et al. Garlic powder and plasma lipids and lipoproteins. *Arch Intern Med* 1998; 158: 1189–94.

10. Kleijnen J, Knipschild P, Ter Riet G. Garlic, onion and cardiovascular risk factors: A review of the evidence from human experiments with emphasis on commercially available preparations. *Br J Clin Pharmacol* 1989; 28: 535–44.

11. Kiesewetter H, Jung F, et al. Effects of garlic coated tablets in peripheral arterial occlusive disease. *Clin Invest* 1993; 71(5): 383–86.

12. Hughes BG, Lawson LD. Antimicrobial effects of *Allium sativum* L. (garlic), *Allium ampeloprasum* L. (elephant garlic) and *Allium cepa* L. (onion), garlic compounds and commercial garlic supplement products. *Phytother Res* 1991; 5: 154–58.

13. Dorant E, van der Brandt PA, et al. Garlic and its significance for the prevention of cancer in humans: A critical review. *Br J Cancer* 1993; 67: 424–29.

14. Brown DJ. *Herbal Prescriptions for Better Health*. Rocklin, CA: Prima Publishing, 1996, 97–109.

15. Blumenthal M, Busse WR, Goldberg A, et al. (eds). *The Complete Commission E Monographs: Therapeutic Guide to Herbal Medicines*. Boston, MA: Integrative Medicine Communications, 1998, 134.

16. Brown DJ. *Herbal Prescriptions for Better Health*. Rocklin, CA: Prima Publishing, 1996, 97–109.

17. Mennella JA, Beauchamp GK. Maternal diet alters the sensory qualities of human milk and the nursling's behavior. *Pediatr* 1991; 88: 737–44.

18. Mennella JA, Beauchamp GK. The effects of repeated exposure to garlic-flavored milk on the nursling's behavior. *Pediatr Res* 1993; 34: 805–8.

Gentian

1. Duke JA. *CRC Handbook of Medicinal Herbs*. Boca Raton, FL: CRC Press, 1985, 207–8.

2. Weiss RF. *Herbal Medicine*. Gothenburg, Sweden: Ab Arcanum, 1988, 40–42.

3. Kondo Y, Takano F, Hojo H. Suppression of chemically and immunologically induced hepatic injuries by gentiopicroside in mice. *Planta Med* 1994; 60: 414–16.

4. Schulz V, Hänsel R, Tyler VE. *Rational Phytotherapy: A Physician's Guide to Herbal Medicine,* 3rd ed. Berlin: Springer, 1988, 171.

5. Blumenthal M, Busse WR, Goldberg A, et al. (eds). *The Complete Commission E Monographs: Therapeutic Guide to Herbal Medicines*. Boston, MA: Integrative Medicine Communications, 1998, 135.

6. Blumenthal M, Busse WR, Goldberg A, et al. (eds). *The Complete Commission E Monographs: Therapeutic Guide to Herbal Medicines*. Boston, MA: Integrative Medicine Communications, 1998, 135.

Ginger

1. Tyler VE. *Herbs of Choice: The Therapeutic Use of Phytomedicinals*. Binghamton, NY: Pharmaceutical Products Press, 1994, 39–42.

2. Bradley PR, ed. *British Herbal Compendium*, vol 1. Bournemouth, Dorset, UK: British Herbal Medicine Association, 1992, 112–14.

3. Yamahara J, Huang Q, et al. Gastrointestinal motility enhancing effect of ginger and its active constituents. *Chem Pharm Bull* 1990; 38: 430–31.

4. Al-Yahya MA, Rafatullah S, et al. Gastroprotective activity of ginger in albino rats. *Am J Chinese Med* 1989; 17: 51–56.

5. Holtmann S, Clarke AH, et al. The anti-motion sickness mechanism of ginger. *Acta Otolaryngol (Stockh)* 1989; 108: 168–74.

6. Suekawa M, Ishige A, et al. Pharmacological studies on ginger. I. Pharmacological actions of pungent constituents, (6)-gingerol and (6)-shogaol. *J Pharm Dyn* 1984; 7: 836–48.

7. Bone ME, Wilkinson DJ, Young JR, et al. Ginger root—a new antiemetic: The effect of ginger root on postoperative nausea and vomiting after major gynaecological surgery. *Anaesthesia* 1990; 45: 669–71.

8. Phillips S, Ruggier R, Hutchingson SE. *Zingiber officinale* (ginger)—an antiemetic for day case surgery. *Anaesthesia* 1993; 48: 715–17.

9. Visalyaputra S, Petchpaisis N, Somcharoen K, Choavaratana R. The efficacy of ginger root in the prevention of postoperative nausea and vomiting after outpatient gynaecological laparoscopy. *Anaesthesia* 1998; 53: 506–10.

10. Grontved A, Brask T, Kambskard J, Hentzer E. Ginger root against seasickness. *Acta Otolaryngol* 1988; 105: 45–49.

11. Meyer K, Schwartz J, Craer D, Keyes B. *Zingiber officinale* (ginger) used to prevent 8-Mop associated nausea. *Dermatol Nursing* 1995; 7: 242–44.

12. Langner E, Greifenberg S, Gruenwald J. Ginger: History and use. *Adv Ther* 1998; 15: 25–44 [review].

13. Bordia A, Verma SK, Srivastava KC. Effect of ginger (*Zingiber officinale* Rosc) and fenugreek (*Trigonella foenumgraecum* L.) on blood lipids, blood sugar, and platelet aggregation in patients with coronary artery disease. *Prostagland Leukotrienes Essential Fatty Acids* 1997; 56: 379–84.

14. Lumb AB. Effect of dried ginger on human platelet function. *Thromb Haemost* 1994; 7: 110–11.

15. Janssen PLTMK, Meyboom S, van Staveren WA, et al. Consumption of ginger (*Zingiber officinale* Roscoe) does not affect ex vivo platelet thromboxane production in humans. *Eur J Clin Nutr* 1996; 50: 772–74.

16. Verma SK, Singh J, et al. Effect of ginger on platelet aggrega-tion in man. *Indian J Med Res* 1994; 98: 240–42.

17. Brown DJ. *Herbal Prescriptions for Better Health.* Rocklin, CA: Prima Publishing, 1996, 111–18.

18. Blumenthal M, Busse WR, Goldberg A, et al. (eds). *The Complete Commission E Monographs: Therapeutic Guide to Herbal Medicines.* Boston, MA: Integrative Medicine Communications, 1998, 135–36.

Ginkgo biloba

1. Drieu K. Preparation and definition of *Ginkgo biloba* extract. In: *Rokan (Ginkgo biloba): Recent Results in Pharmacology and Clinic,* ed. EW Fünfgeld. Berlin: Springer-Verlag, 32–36.

2. Krieglstein J. Neuroprotective properties of *Ginkgo biloba*—constituents. *Zeitschrift Phytother* 1994; 15: 92–96.

3. Bruno C, Cuppini R, et al. Regeneration of motor nerves in bilobalide-treated rats. *Planta Medica* 1993; 59: 302–7.

4. Clostre F. From the body to the cellular membranes: The different levels of pharmacological action of *Ginkgo biloba* extract. In *Rokan (Ginkgo biloba): Recent Results in Pharmacology and Clinic,* ed. EW Fünfgeld. Berlin: Springer-Verlag, 1988, 180–98.

5. Jung F, Mrowietz C, et al. Effect of *Ginkgo biloba* on fluidity of blood and peripheral microcirculation in volunteers. *Arzneim-Forsch Drug Res* 1990; 40: 589–93.

6. Itil TM, Eralp E, Tsambis E, et al. Central nervous system effects of *Ginkgo biloba*, a plant extract. *Am J Therapeutics* 1996; 3: 63–73.

7. Le Bars PL, Katz MM, Berman N, et al. A placebo-controlled, double-blind, randomized trial of an extract of *Ginkgo biloba* for dementia. North American EGb Study Group. *JAMA* 1997; 278: 1327–32.

8. Hofferberth B. The efficacy of EGb 761 in patients with senile dementia of the Alzheimer type, a double-blind, placebo-controlled study on different levels of investigation. *Human Psychopharmacol* 1994; 9: 215–22.

9. Kanowski S, Herrmann W, Stephan K, et al. Proof of efficacy of the *Ginkgo biloba* special extract EGb 761 in outpatients suffering from mild to moderate primary degenerative dementia of the Alzheimer type or multi-infarct dementia. *Pharmacopsychiatry* 1996; 29: 47–56.

10. Ferrandini C, Droy-Lefaix MT, Christen Y, eds. *Ginkgo biloba Extract (EGb 761) as a Free Radical Scavenger.* Paris: Elsevier, 1993.

11. Lebuisson DA, Leroy L, Rigal G. Treatment of senile macular degeneration with *Ginkgo biloba* extract. A preliminary double-blind, drug versus placebo study. *Presse Med* 1986; 15: 1556–58 [in French].

12. Lanthony P, Cosson JP. Evolution of color vision in diabetic retinopathy treated by extract of *Ginkgo biloba. J Fr Ophthalmol* 1988; 11: 671–74 [in French].

13. Harman D. Free radical theory of aging: a hypothesis on pathogenesis of senile dementia of the Alzheimer's type. *Age* 1993; 16: 23–30.

14. Schubert H, Halama P. Depressive episode primarily unresponsive to therapy in elderly patients: Efficacy of *Ginkgo biloba* extract (EGb 761) in combination with antidepressants. *Geriatr Forsch* 1993; 3: 45–53.

15. Lamant V, Mauco G, et al. Inhibition of the metabolism of platelet activating factor (PAF-acether) by three specific antagonists from *Ginkgo biloba. Biochem Pharmacol* 1987; 36: 2749–52.

16 Kroegel C. The potential pathophysiological role of platelet-activating factor in human disease. *Klin Wochenschr* 1988; 66: 373–78.

17. Kroegel C, Kortsik C, et al. The pathophysiological role and therapeutic implications of platelet activating factor in diseases of aging. *Drugs Aging* 1992; 2: 345–55.

18. Krieglstein J. Neuroprotective properties of *Ginkgo biloba*—constituents. *Zeitschrift Phytother* 1994; 15: 92–96.

19. Haguenauer JP, Cantenot F, Koskas H, Pierart H. Treatment of equilibrium problems with extract of

Ginkgo biloba. Multicenter, double-blind, placebo-controlled study. *Presse Med* 1986; 15: 1569–72 [in French].

20. Meyer B. A multicenter, double-blind, drug versus placebo study of *Ginkgo biloba* extract in the treatment of tinnitus. *Press Med* 1986; 15: 1562–64 [in French].

21. Blumenthal M, Busse WR, Goldberg A, et al. (eds). *The Complete Commission E Monographs: Therapeutic Guide to Herbal Medicines.* Boston, MA: Integrative Medicine Communications, 1998, 136–38.

22. Blumenthal M, Busse WR, Goldberg A, et al. (eds). *The Complete Commission E Monographs: Therapeutic Guide to Herbal Medicines.* Boston, MA: Integrative Medicine Communications, 1998, 136–38.

Goldenseal

1. Ellingwood F. *American Materia Medica, Therapeutics and Pharmacognosy.* 1919. Reprint, Sandy, OR: Eclectic Medical Publications, 1998.

2. Hahn FE, Ciak J. Berberine. *Antibiotics* 1976; 3: 577–88.

3. Bhakat MP, Naudi N, et al. Therapeutic trial of berberine sulfate in non-specific gastroenteritis. *Ind Med J* 1974; 68: 19–23.

4. Murray, MT. *The Healing Power of Herbs.* Rocklin, CA: Prima Publishing. 1995, 162–72.

5. Bannerman JE. Goldenseal in world trade: Pressures and potenials. *HerbalGram* 1997; 41: 51–52.

6. Newall CA, Anderson LA, Phillipson JD. *Herbal Medicines: A Guide for Health-Care Professionals.* London: The Pharmaceutical Press, 1996, 151–52.

Gotu Kola

1. Duke JA. *CRC Handbook of Medicinal Herbs.* Boca Raton, FL: CRC Press, 1985, 110–11.

2. Kartnig T. Clinical applications of *Centella asiatica* (L.) Urb. In *Herbs, Spices, and Medicinal Plants: Recent Advances in Botany, Horticulture, and Pharmacology,* vol. 3., eds. LE Craker, JE Simon. Phoenix, AZ: Oryx Press, 1986, 145–73.

3. Morisset R, Cote NG, Panisset JC, et al. Evaluation of the healing activity of hydrocotyle tincture in the treatment of wounds. *Phytother Res* 1987; 1: 117–21.

4. Kartnig T. Clinical applications of *Centella asiatica* (L.) Urb. In *Herbs, Spices, and Medicinal Plants: Recent Advances in Botany, Horticulture, and Pharmacology,* vol. 3., eds. LE Craker, JE Simon. Phoenix, AZ: Oryx Press, 1986, 145–73.

5. Mahajani SS, Oberai C, Jerajani H, Parikh KM. Study of venodynamic effect of an Ayurvedic formulation of *Centella asiatica* using venous occlusion plethysmography (VOP) and laser-Doppler velocimetry (LVD). *Can J Physiol Pharmacol* 1994; 72(suppl 1): 180.

6. Pointel JP, Boccalon H, Cloarec M, et al. Titrated extract of *Centella asiatica* (TECA) in the treatement of venous insufficiency of the lower limbs. *Angiology* 1986; 37(5): 420–21.

7. Bossé JP, Papillon J, Frenette G, et al. Clinical study of a new antikeloid drug. *Ann Plastic Surg* 1979; 3: 13–21.

8. Murray MT. *The Healing Power of Herbs.* Rocklin, CA: Prima Publishing, 1995, 171–83.

9. Murray MT. *The Healing Power of Herbs.* Rocklin, CA: Prima Publishing, 1995, 171–83.

Green Tea

1. Graham HN. Green tea composition, consumption, and polyphenol chemistry. *Prev Med* 1992; 21: 334–50.

2. Kono S, Shinchi K, Ikeda N, et al. Green tea consumption and serum lipid profiles: A cross-sectional study in Northern Kyushu, Japan. *Prev Med* 1992; 21: 526–31.

3. Yamaguchi Y, Hayashi M, Yamazoe H, et al. Preventive effects of green tea extract on lipid abnormalities in serum, liver and aorta of mice fed an atherogenic diet. *Nip Yak Zas* 1991; 97(6): 329–37.

4. Sagesaka-Mitane Y, Milwa M, Okada S. Platelet aggregation inhibitors in hot water extract of green tea. *Chem Pharm Bull* 1990; 38(3): 790–93.

5. Stensvold I, Tverdal A, Solvoll K, et al. Tea consumption. Relationship to cholesterol, blood pressure, and coronary and total mortality. *Prev Med* 1992; 21: 546–53.

6. Tsubono Y, Tsugane S. Green tea intake in relation to serum lipid levels in middle-aged Japanese men and women. *Ann Epidemiol* 1997; 7: 280–84.

7. Serafini M, Ghiselli A, Ferro-Luzzi A. In vivo antioxidant effect of green tea in man. *Eur J Clin Nutr* 1996; 50: 28–32.

8. van het Hof KH, de Boer HSM, Viseman SA, et al. Consumption of green or black tea does not increase resistance of low-density lipoprotein to oxidation in humans. *Am J Clin Nutr* 1997; 66: 1125–32.

9. Stoner GD, Mukhtar H. Polyphenols as cancer chemopreventive agents. *J Cell Bioch* 1995; 22: 169–80.

10. You SQ. Study on feasibility of Chinese green tea polyphenols (CTP) for preventing dental caries. *Chin J Stom* 1993; 28(4): 197–99.

11. Hamilton-Miller JM. Antimicrobial properties of tea (*Camellia sinensis* L.). *Antimicro Agents Chemother* 1995; 39(11): 2375–77.

12. Imai K, Nakachi K. Cross sectional study of effects of drinking green tea on cardiovascular and liver diseases. *BMJ* 1995; 310: 693–96.

13. Murray MT. *The Healing Power of Herbs.* Rocklin, CA: Prima Publishing, 1995, 192–96.

Guaraná

1. Duke JA. *CRC Handbook of Medicinal Herbs.* Boca Raton, FL: CRC Press, 1985, 349.

2. Leung A Y, Foster S. *Encyclopedia of Common Natural Ingredients Used in Food, Drugs, and Cosmetics,* 2d ed. New York: John Wiley & Sons, 1996, 293–94.

3. Galduroz JC, Carlini EA. The effects of long-term administration of guarana on the cognition of normal, elderly volunteers. *Rev Paul Med* 1996; 114: 1073–78.

4. Duke JA. *CRC Handbook of Medicinal Herbs*. Boca Raton, FL: CRC Press, 1985, 349.

5. Greunwald J, Brendler T, Jaenicke C, et al. (eds). *PDR for Herbal Medicines*. Montvale, NJ: Medical Economics, 1998, 1017–18.

Guggul

1. Satyavati GV. Gum guggul *(Commiphora mukul)*—The success of an ancient insight leading to a modern discovery. *Indian J Med* 1988; 87: 327–35.

2. Nityanand S, Kapoor NK. Hypocholesterolemic effect of *Commiphora mukul* resin (Guggal). *Indian J Exp Biol* 1971; 9: 367–77.

3. Singh K, Chander R, Kapoor NK. Guggulsterone, a potent hypolipidaemic, prevents oxidation of low density lipoprotein. *Phytother Res* 1997; 11: 291–94.

4. Mester L, Mester M, Nityanand S. Inhibition of platelet aggregation by guggulu steroids. *Planta Med* 1979; 37: 367–69.

5. Malhotra SC, Ahuja MMS, Sundarum KR. Long-term clinical studies on the hypolipidemic effect of *Commiphora mukul* (guggul) and clofibrate. *Ind J Med Res* 1977; 65: 390–95.

6. Nityanand S, Srivastava JS, Asthana OP. Clinical trials with gugulipid—a new hypolipidemic agent. *J Assoc Phys India* 1989; 37: 323–28.

7. Brown D, Austin S. *Hyperlipidemia and Prevention of Coronary Artery Disease*. Seattle, WA: NPRC, 1997, 4–6.

Gymnema

1. Mhasker KS, Caius JF. A study of Indian medicinal plants. II. *Gymnema sylvestre* R.Br. *Indian J Med Res Memoirs* 1930; 16: 2–75.

2. Shanmugasundaram KR, Panneerselvam C, Sumudram P, Shanmugasundaram ER. Insulinotropic activity of *G. sylvestre,* R. Br. and Indian medicinal herb used in controlling diabetes mellitus. *Pharmacol Res Commun* 1981; 13: 475–86.

3. Shanmugasundaram ER, Gopinath KL, Radha Shanmugasundaram K, Rajendran VM. Possible regeneration of the islets of Langerhans in streptozotocin diabetic rats given *Gymnema sylvestre* leaf extracts. *J Ethnopharmacol* 1990; 30: 265–79.

4. Bishayee A, Chatterjee M. Hypolipidemic and antiatherosclerotic effects of oral *Gymnema sylvestre* R.Br. leaf extract in albino rats fed on a high fat diet. *Phytother Res* 1994; 8: 118–20.

5. Gymnema. *Lawrence Review of Natural Products*. Aug 1993 (monograph).

6. Fushiki T, Kojima A, Imoto T, et al. An extract of *Gymnema sylvestre* leaves and purified gymnemic acid inhibits glucose-stimulated gastric inhibitory peptide secretion in rats. *J Nutr* 1992; 122: 2367–73.

7. Baskaran K, Ahmath BK, Shanmugasundaram KR, Shanmugasundaram ERB. Antidiabetic effect of a leaf extract from *Gymnema sylvestre* in non-insulin-dependent diabetes mellitus patients. *J Ethnopharmacol* 1990; 30: 295–305.

8. Shanmugasundaram ER, Rajeswari G, Baskaran K, et al. Use of *Gymnema sylvestre* leaf extract in the control of blood glucose in insulin-dependent diabetes mellitus. *J Ethnopharmacol* 1990; 30: 281–94.

Hawthorn

1. Rewerski VW, Piechoscki T, et al. Some pharmacological properties of oligomeric procyanidin isolated from hawthorn *(Crataegus oxyacantha)*. *Arzneim-Forsch Drug Res* 1967; 17: 490–91.

2. Weikl A, Noh HS. The influence of *Crataegus* on global cardiac insufficiency. *Herz Gefabe* 1993; 11: 516–24.

3. Bahorun T, Trotin F, et al. Antioxidant activities of *Crataegus monogyna* extracts. *Planta Med* 1994; 60: 323–28.

4. Weihmayr T, Ernst E. Therapeutic effectiveness of *Crataegus*. *Fortschr Med* 1996; 114(1–2): 27–29 [in German].

5. Schmidt U, Kuhn U, Ploch M, Hübner W-D. Efficacy of the Hawthorn *(Crataegus)* preparation LI 132 in 78 patients with chronic congestive heart failure defined as NYHA functional class II. *Phytomed* 1994; 1(1): 17–24.

6. Tauchert M, Ploch M, Hubner WD. Effectiveness of hawthorn extract LI 132 compared with the ACE inhibitor Captopril: Multicenter double-blind study with 132 patients NYHA stage II. *Münch Med Wochenschr* 1994; 132(suppl): S27–33.

7. Hanack T, Brückel M-H. The treatment of mild stable forms of angina pectoris using Crataegutt (R) Novo. *Therapiewoche* 1983; 33: 4331–33 [in German].

8. Brown DJ. *Herbal Prescriptions for Better Health*. Rocklin, CA: Prima Publishing, 1996, 139–44.

Hops

1. Weiss RF. *Herbal Medicine*. Gothenburg, Sweden: Ab Arcanum, 1988, 285–86.

2. Foster S. *Herbs for Your Health*. Loveland, CO: Interweave Press, 1996, 56–57.

3. Wichtl M. *Herbal Drugs and Phytopharmaceuticals*. Boca Raton, FL: CRC Press, 1994, 305–8.

4. Eagon CL, Elm MS, Eagon PK. Estrogenicity of traditional Chinese and Western herbal remedies. *Proc Annu Meet Am Assoc Cancer Res* 1996; 37: A1937 [abstract].

5. Blumenthal M, Busse WR, Goldberg A, et al. (eds). *The Complete Commission E Monographs: Therapeutic Guide to Herbal Medicines*. Boston, MA: Integrative Medicine Communications, 1998, 147.

6. Foster S. *Herbs for Your Health*. Loveland, CO: Interweave Press, 1996, 56–57.

Horehound

1. Wren RC. *Potter's New Cyclopedia of Botanical Drugs and Preparations*. Essex, England: C.W. Daniel Co., 1988, 146.

2. Castleman M. *The Healing Herbs*. Emmaus, PA: Rodale Press, 1991, 216–17.

3. Leung AY, Foster S. *Encyclopedia of Common Natural Ingredients Used in Food, Drugs, and Cosmetics,* 2d ed. New York: John Wiley & Sons, 1996, 303.

4. Bradley PR. *British Herbal Compendium,* vol 1. Great Britain: British Herbal Medicine Association, 1990, 218–19.

5. Blumenthal M, Busse WR, Goldberg A, et al. (eds). *The Complete German Commission E Monographs: Therapeutic Guide to Herbal Medicines.* Austin: American Botanical Council and Boston: Integrative Medicine Communications, 1998, 127–28.

6. Newall CA, Anderson LA, Phillipson JD. *Herbal Medicines: A Guide for Health-care Professionals.* London: The Pharmaceutical Press, 1996, 165.

7. Brinker F. *Herb Contraindications and Drug Interactions.* Sandy, OR: Eclectic Publishers, 1997, 54.

Horse Chestnut

1. Chandler RF. Horse chestnut. *Canadian Pharm J* Jul/Aug 1993: 297, 300.

2. Guillaume M, Padioleau F. Venotonic effect, vascular protection, anti-inflammatory and free radical scavenging properties of horse chestnut extract. *Arzneim-Forsch Drug Res* 1994; 44: 25–35.

3. Guillaume M, Padioleau F. Venotonic effect, vascular protection, anti-inflammatory and free radical scavenging properties of horse chestnut extract. *Arzneim-Forsch Drug Res* 1994; 44: 25–35.

4. Calabrese C, Preston P. Report of the results of a double-blind, randomized, single-dose trial of a topical 2% escin gel versus placebo in the acute treatment of experimentally-induced hematoma in volunteers. *Planta Med* 1993; 59: 394–97.

5. Dittler MH, Ernst E. Horse Chestnut seed extract for chronic venous insufficiency: A criteria-based systematic review. *Arch Dermatol* 1998; 134: 1356–60.

6. Diehm C, Trampish HJ, Lange S, Schmidt C. Comparison of leg compression stocking and oral horse chestnut seed extract therapy in patients with chronic venous insufficiency. *Lancet* 1996; 347: 292–94.

7. Wilhelm K, Felmeier C. Thermometric investigations about the efficacy of beta-escin to reduce postoperative edema. *Med Klin* 1977; 72(4): 128–34 [in German].

8. Tyler VE. *Herbs of Choice: The Therapeutic Use of Phytomedicinals.* Binghamton, NY: Pharmaceutical Products Press, 1994, 112–13.

9. Blumenthal M, Busse WR, Goldberg A, et al, eds. *The Complete Commission E Monographs: Therapeutic Guide to Herbal Medicines.* Boston, MA: Integrative Medicine Communications, 1998, 148–49.

10. Weiss RF. *Herbal Medicine.* Gothenburg, Sweden: Ab Arcanum and Beaconsfield, UK: Beaconsfield Publishers Ltd., 1988: 188–89.

11. Blumenthal M, Busse WR, Goldberg A, et al. (eds). *The Complete Commission E Monographs: Therapeutic Guide to Herbal Medicines.* Boston, MA: Integrative Medicine Communications, 1998, 148–49.

12. Hellberg K, Ruschewski W, de Vivie R. Medikamentoes bedingtes post-operatives Nierenversagen nach herzchirurgischen Eingriffen. *Thoraxchirurgie* 1975; 23: 396–99.

13. Wilhelm K, Feldmeier C. Postoperative und posttraumatische Oedemprophylaxe und -therapie. Laborchemische Untersuchungen ueber die Nierenvertraeglichkeit von beta-Aescin. *Med Klin* 1975; 70: 2079–83.

11. Blumenthal M, Busse WR, Goldberg A, et al. (eds). *The Complete Commission E Monographs: Therapeutic Guide to Herbal Medicines.* Boston, MA: Integrative Medicine Communications, 1998, 148–49.

Horseradish

1. Grieve M. *A Modern Herbal,* vol 2. New York: Dover Publications, 1971, 417–19.

2. Weiss RF. *Herbal Medicine.* Gothenburg, Sweden: Ab Arcanum, 1988, 207.

3. Esanu V, Prahoveanu E. The effect of an aqueous horse-radish extract, applied as such or in association with caffeine, on experimental influenza in mice. *Virologie* 1985; 36(2): 95–98.

4. Kienholz VM, Kemkes B. The anti-bacterial action of ethereal oils obtained from horse radish root (*Cochlearia armoracia* L.). *Arzneim Forsch* 1961; 10: 917–18 [in German].

5. Schindler VE, Zipp H, Marth I. Comparative clinical investigations of an enzyme glycoside mixture obtained from horse radish roots (*Cochlearia armoracia* L). *Arzneim Forsch* 1961; 10: 919–21 [in German].

6. Blumenthal M, Busse WR, Goldberg A, et al. (eds). *The Complete Commission E Monographs: Therapeutic Guide to Herbal Medicines.* Boston, MA: Integrative Medicine Communications, 1998, 150.

7. Blumenthal M, Busse WR, Goldberg A, et al. (eds). *The Complete Commission E Monographs: Therapeutic Guide to Herbal Medicines.* Boston, MA: Integrative Medicine Communications, 1998, 150.

8. Blumenthal M, Busse WR, Goldberg A, et al. (eds). *The Complete Commission E Monographs: Therapeutic Guide to Herbal Medicines.* Boston, MA: Integrative Medicine Communications, 1998, 150.

Horsetail

1. Leung AY, Foster S. *Encyclopedia of Common Natural Ingredients Used in Foods, Drugs, and Cosmetics,* 2nd ed. New York: John Wiley & Sons, 1996, 306–8.

2. Castleman M. *The Healing Herbs.* Emmaus, PA: Rodale Press, 1991, 219–21.

3. Weiss RF. *Herbal Medicine.* Gothenburg Sweden: Ab Arcanum, 1988, 238–39.

4. Seaborn CD, Nielsen FH. Silicon: a nutritional beneficence for bones, brains and blood vessels? *Nutr Today* 1993; 28: 13–18.

5. Blumenthal M, Busse WR, Goldberg A, et al. (eds). *The Complete Commission E Monographs: Therapeutic Guide to Herbal Medicines.* Boston, MA: Integrative Medicine Communications, 1998, 150–51.

6. Fabre B, Geay B, Beaufils P. Thiaminase activity in *Equisetum arvense* and its extracts. *Plant Med Phytother* 1993; 26: 190–97.

Juniper

1. Duke JA. *CRC Handbook of Medicinal Herbs*. Boca Raton, FL: CRC Press, 1985, 256.

2. Tyler VE. *Herbs of Choice: The Therapeutic Use of Phytomedicinals*. Binghamton, NY: Pharmaceutical Products Press, 1994, 76–77.

3. Markkanen T, Markinen ML, Nikoskelainen J, et al. Antiherpetic agent from juniper tree *(Juniperus communis)*, its purification, identification and testing in primary human amnion cell cultures. *Drugs Exptl Clin Res* 1981; 7: 691–97.

4. Blumenthal M, Busse WR, Goldberg A, et al. (eds). *The Complete Commission E Monographs: Therapeutic Guide to Herbal Medicines*. Boston, MA: Integrative Medicine Communications, 1998, 155–56.

5. Schilcher H, Leuschner F. The potential nephrotoxic effects of essential juniper oil. *Arzneim Forsch* 1997; 47: 855–58 [in German].

Kava

1. Blumenthal M, Busse WR, Goldberg A, et al. (eds). *The Complete Commission E Monographs: Therapeutic Guide to Herbal Medicines*. Boston, MA: Integrative Medicine Communications, 1998, 156–57.

2. Blumenthal M, Busse WR, Goldberg A, et al. (eds). *The Complete Commission E Monographs: Therapeutic Guide to Herbal Medicines*. Boston, MA: Integrative Medicine Communications, 1998, 156–57.

3. Bone K. Kava: A safe herbal treatment for anxiety. *Br J Phytother* 1994; 3: 145–53.

4. Buckley JP, Furgiulel AR, O'Hara MJ. Pharmacology of kava. In *Ethnopharmacoligical Search for Psychoactive Drugs,* eds. DH Efron, B Holmstedt, NS Kline. New York: Raven Press, 1979, 141–51.

5. Holm E, Staedt U, et al. Studies on the profile of the neurophysiological effects of D,L-kavain: Cerebral sites of action and sleep-wakefulness rhythm in animals. *Arzneim-Forsch Drug Res* 1991; 41: 673–83.

6. Lehmann EE, Kinzler J, Friedmann J. Efficacy of a special kava extract *(Piper methysticum)* in patients with states of anxiety, tension and excitedness of non-mental origin. A double-blind placebo-controlled study of four weeks treatment. *Phytomedicine* 1996; 3: 113–19.

7. Volz HP, Kieser M. Kava-kava extract WS 1490 versus placebo in anxiety disorders. A randomized placebo-controlled 25-week outpatient trial. *Pharmacopsychiatry* 1997; 30: 1–5.

8. Warnecke G. Psychosomatic dysfunctions in the female climacteric. Clinical effectiveness and tolerance of kava extract WS 1490. *Fortschr Med* 1991; 119–22 [in German].

9. Brown DJ. *Herbal Prescriptions for Better Health*. Rocklin, CA: Prima Publishing, 1996, 145–50.

10. Blumenthal M, Busse WR, Goldberg A, et al. (eds). *The Complete Commission E Monographs: Therapeutic Guide to Herbal Medicines*. Boston, MA: Integrative Medicine Communications, 1998, 156–57.

11. Blumenthal M, Busse WR, Goldberg A, et al. (eds). *The Complete Commission E Monographs: Therapeutic Guide to Herbal Medicines*. Boston, MA: Integrative Medicine Communications, 1998, 156–57.

12. Blumenthal M, Busse WR, Goldberg A, et al. (eds). *The Complete Commission E Monographs: Therapeutic Guide to Herbal Medicines*. Boston, MA: Integrative Medicine Communications, 1998, 156–57.

13. Herberg KW. Driving ability after intake of kava special extract WS 1490. *Z Allgemeinmed* 1993; 69; 271–77.

14. Blumenthal M, Busse WR, Goldberg A, et al. (eds). *The Complete Commission E Monographs: Therapeutic Guide to Herbal Medicines*. Boston, MA: Integrative Medicine Communications, 1998, 156–57.

Kudzu

1. Foster S. Kudzu root monograph. *Quart Rev Nat Med* 1994; Winter: 303–8.

2. Zhao SP, Zhang YZ. Quantitative TLC-densitometry of isoflavones in *Pueraria lobata* (Willd.) Ohwi. *Yaoxue Xuebao* 1985; 20: 203.

3. Keung WM, Vallee BL. Daidzin and daidzein suppress free-choice ethanol intake by Syrian Golden hamsters. *Proc Natl Acad Sci USA* 1993; 90: 10008–12.

4. Leung AY, Foster S. *Encyclopedia of Common Natural Ingredients Used in Food, Drugs, and Cosmetics*, 2d ed. New York: John Wiley & Sons, 1996, 333–36.

Lavender

1. Hoffmann D. *The New Holistic Herbal*, 2d ed. Rockport, MA: Element, 1990, 210.

2. Buchbauer G, Jirovetz L, Jager W, et al. Aromatherapy: Evidence for sedative effects of the essential oil of lavender after inhalation. *Z Naturforsch [C]* 1991; 46: 1067–72.

3. Hardy M, Kirk-Smith MD, Stretch DD. Replacement of drug therapy for insomnia by ambient odour. *Lancet* 1995; 346: 701 [letter].

4. Dale A, Cornwell S. The role of lavender oil in relieving perineal discomfort following childbirth: A blind randomized trial. *J Adv Nursing* 1994; 19: 89–96.

5. Tisserand R, Balacs T. *Essential Oil Safety: A Guide for Health Care Professionals*. Edinburgh, UK: Churchill Livingstone, 1995, 65.

6. Pattnaik S, Subramanyam VR, Bapaji M, Kole CR. Antibacterial and antifungal activity of aromatic constituents of essential oils. *Microbios* 1997; 89: 39–46.

7. Blumenthal M, Busse WR, Goldberg A, et al. (eds). *The Complete Commission E Monographs: Therapeutic Guide to Herbal Medicines*. Boston, MA: Integrative Medicine Communications, 1998, 159–60.

8. Dale A, Cornwell S. The role of lavender oil in relieving perineal discomfort following childbirth: A blind randomized trial. *J Adv Nursing* 1994; 19: 89–96.

9. Leung AY, Foster S. *Encyclopedia of Common Natural Ingredients Used in Food, Drugs, and*

Part Three: References

Cosmetics. New York: John Wiley & Sons, 1996, 339–42.

Lemon Balm

1. Weiss RF. *Herbal Medicine.* Gothenburg, Sweden: Ab Arcanum, 1988, 31, 286.

2. Auf'mkolk M, Ingbar JC, Kubota K, et al. Extracts and auto-oxidized constituents of certain plants inhibit the receptor-binding and the biological activity of Graves' immunoglobulins. *Endocrinol* 1985; 116(5): 1687–93.

3. Blumenthal M, Busse WR, Goldberg A, et al. (eds). *The Complete Commission E Monographs: Therapeutic Guide to Herbal Medicines.* Boston, MA: Integrative Medicine Communications, 1998, 160–61.

4. Wëhlbling RH, Leonhardt K. Local therapy of herpes simplex with dried extract of *Melissa officinalis.* *Phytomedicine* 1994; 1(1): 25–31.

5. Leach EH, Lloyd JPF. Experimental ocular hypertension in animals. *Trans Ophthalm Soc UK* 1956; 76: 453–60.

Licorice

1. Steinberg D, Sgan-Cohen HD, Stabholz A, et al. The anticariogenic activity of glycyrrhizin: Preliminary clinical trials. *Isr J Dent Sci* 1989; 2: 153–55.

2. Soma R, Ikeda M, Morise T, et al. Effect of glycyrrhizin on cortisol metabolism in humans. *Endocrin Regulations* 1994; 28: 31–34.

3. Beil W, Birkholz C, Sewing KF. Effects of flavonoids on parietal cell acid secretion, gastric mucosal prostaglandin production and *Helicobacter pylori* growth. *Arzneim Forsch* 1995; 45: 697–700.

4. Morgan AG, McAdam WAF, Pacsoo C, Darnborough A. Comparison between cimetidine and Caved-S in the treatment of gastric ulceration, and subsequent maintenance therapy. *Gut* 1982; 23: 545–51.

5. Kassir ZA. Endoscopic controlled trial of four drug regimens in the treatment of chronic duodenal ulceration. *Irish Med J* 1985; 78: 153–56.

6. Bardhan KD, Cumberland DC, Dixon RA, Holdsworth CD. Clinical trial of deglycyrrhizinised liquorice in gastric ulcer. *Gut* 1978; 19: 779–82.

7. Das SK, Das V, Gulati AD, Singh VP. Deglycyrrhizinated licorice in aphthous ulcers. *J Assoc Physicians India* 1989; 37: 647.

8. Reed PI, Davies WA. Controlled trial of a carbenoxolone/alginate antacid combination in reflux oesophagitis. *Curr Med Res Opin* 1978; 5: 637–44.

9. Evans FQ. The rational use of glycyrrhetinic acid in dermatology. *Br J Clin Pract* 1958; 12: 269–74.

10. Pompei R, Flore O, Marccialis MA, et al. Glycyrrhizic acid inhibits virus growth and inactivates virus particles. *Nature* 1979; 281: 689–90.

11. Abe Y, Ueda T, Kato T, et al. Effectiveness of interferon, glycyrrhizin combination therapy in patients with chronic hepatitis C. *Nippon Rinsho* 1994; 52: 1817–22 [in Japanese].

12. Hattori I, Ikematsu S, Koito A, et al. Preliminary evidence for inhibitory effect of glycyrrhizin on HIV replication in patients with AIDS. *Antivir Res* 1989; 11: 255–62.

13. Murray MT. *The Healing Power of Herbs.* Rocklin, CA: Prima Publishing, 1995, 228–39.

14. Blumenthal M, Busse WR, Goldberg A, et al. (eds). *The Complete Commission E Monographs: Therapeutic Guide to Herbal Medicines.* Boston, MA: Integrative Medicine Communications, 1998, 161–62.

15. Blumenthal M, Busse WR, Goldberg A, et al. (eds). *The Complete Commission E Monographs: Therapeutic Guide to Herbal Medicines.* Boston, MA: Integrative Medicine Communications, 1998, 161–62.

Ligustrum

1. Benksy D, Gamble A, Kaptchuk T. *Chinese Herbal Medicine: Materia Medica.* Seattle: Eastland Press, 1993, 366.

2. Leung AY, Foster S. *Encyclopedia of Common Natural Ingredients Used in Foods, Drugs, and Cosmetics,* 2d ed. New York: John Wiley & Sons, 1996, 350–52.

3. Leung AY, Foster S. *Encyclopedia of Common Natural Ingredients Used in Foods, Drugs, and Cosmetics,* 2d ed. New York: John Wiley & Sons, 1996, 350–52.

4. Foster S, Yue CX. *Herbal Emissaries: Bringing Chinese Herbs to the West.* Rochester, VT: Healing Arts Press, 1992, 227–32.

Lobelia

1. Felter HW, Lloyd JU. *King's American Dispensatory,* 18th ed. Sandy, OR: Eclectic Medical Publications, 1898, 1983, 1199–1205.

2. Ellingwood F. *American Materia Medica, Therapeutics and Pharmacognosy,* 11th ed. Sandy, OR: Eclectic Medical Publications, 1919, 1998, 235–42.

3. Davison GC, Rosen RC. Lobeline and reduction of cigarette smoking. *Psychol Reports* 1972; 31: 443–56.

4. Pocta J. *Therapeutic* use of lobeline Spofa. *Cas Lek Cesk* 1970; 109(36): 865 [in Czech].

5. Felter HW, Lloyd JU. *King's American Dispensatory,* 18th ed. Sandy, OR: Eclectic Medical Publications, 1898, 1983, 1199–1205.

6. Felter HW, Lloyd JU. *King's American Dispensatory,* 18th ed. Sandy, OR: Eclectic Medical Publications, 1898, 1983, 1199–1205.

7. Bergner P. Is lobelia toxic? *Medical Herbalism* 1998; 10(1,2): 1,15–32 [review].

8. Ellingwood F. *American Materia Medica, Therapeutics and Pharmacognosy,* 11th ed. Sandy, OR: Eclectic Medical Publications, 1919, 1998, 235–42.

9. McGuffin M, Hobbs C, Upton R, Goldberg A. *American Herbal Products Association's Botanical Safety Handbook.* Boca Raton, FL: CRC Press, 1997, 71.

Lomatium

1. Vanwagenen BC, Cardellina JH. Native American food and medicinal plants. 7. Antimicrobial tetronic acids from *Lomatium dissectum.* *Tetrahedron* 1986; 42: 1117.

Part Three: References

2. Moore M. *Medicinal Plants of the Pacific West.* Santa Fe: Red Crane Books, 1993, 61–71.

Maitake

1. Hobbs C. *Medicinal Mushrooms.* Santa Cruz, CA: Botanica Press, 1995, 110–15.

2. Nanba H, Hamaguchi AM, Kuroda H. The chemical structure of an antitumor polysaccharide in fruit bodies of *Grifola frondosa* (maitake). *Chem Pharm Bull* 1987; 35: 1162–68.

3. Yamada Y, Nanba H, Kuroda H. Antitumor effect of orally administered extracts from fruit body of *Grifola frondosa* (maitake). *Chemotherapy* 1990; 38: 790–96.

4. Nanba H. Immunostimulant activity in vivo and anti-HIV activity in vitro of 3 branched b-1-6-glucans extracted from maitake mushrooms *(Grifola frondosa).* VIII International Conference on AIDS, Amsterdam, 1992 [abstract].

5. Hobbs C. *Medicinal Mushrooms.* Santa Cruz, CA: Botanica Press, 1995, 110–15.

Marshmallow

1. Nosal'ova G, Strapkova A, Kardosova A, et al. Antitussive action of extracts and polysaccharides of marsh mallow (*Althea offcinalis* L., var. robusta). *Pharmazie* 1992; 47: 224–26 [in German].

2. Tomoda M, Shimizu N, Oshima Y, et al. Hypoglycemic activity of twenty plant mucilages and three modified products. *Planta Med* 1987; 53: 8–12.

3. Blumenthal M, Busse WR, Goldberg A, et al. (eds). *The Complete Commission E Monographs: Therapeutic Guide to Herbal Medicines.* Boston, MA: Integrative Medicine Communications, 1998, 166–67.

Meadowsweet

1. Zeylstra H. *Filipendila ulmaria. Br J Phytotherapy* 1998; 5: 8–12.

2. Newall CA, Anderson LA, Phillipson JD. *Herbal Medicines: A Guide for Health-Care Professionals.* London: The Pharmaceutical Press, 1996, 191–92.

3. Blumenthal M, Busse WR, Goldberg A, et al. (eds). *The Complete German Commission E Monographs: Therapeutic Guide to Herbal Medicines.* Austin: American Botanical Council and Boston: Integrative Medicine Communications, 1998, 169.

Milk Thistle

1. Wagner H, Horhammer L, Munster R. The chemistry of silymarin (silybin), the active principle of the fruits of *Silybum marianum* (L.) Gaertn. *Arzneim-Forsch Drug Res* 1968; 18: 688–96.

2. Hikino H, Kiso Y, et al. Antihepatotoxic actions of flavonolignans from *Silybum marianum* fruits. *Planta Medica* 1984; 50: 248–50.

3. Faulstich H, Jahn W, Wieland T. Silibinin inhibition of amatoxin uptake in the perfused rat liver. *Arzneim-Forsch Drug Res* 1980; 30: 452–54.

4. Tuchweber B, Sieck R, Trost W. Prevention by silibinin of phalloidin induced hepatotoxicity. *Toxicol Appl Pharmacol* 1979; 51: 265–75.

5. Feher J, Lang I, et al. Free radicals in tissue damage in liver diseases and therapeutic approach. *Tokai J Exp Clin Med* 1986; 11: 121–34.

6. Sonnenbichler J, Zetl I. Stimulating influence of a flavonolignan derivative on proliferation, RNA synthesis and protein synthesis in liver cells. In *Assessment and Management of Hepatobiliary Disease,* eds. L Okolicsanyi, G Csomos, G Crepaldi. Berlin: Springer-Verlag, 1987, 265–72.

7. Leng-Peschlow E. Alcohol-related liver diseases—use of Legalon. *Z Klin Med* 1994; 2: 22–27.

8. Ferenci P, Dragosics B, Dittrich H, et al. Randomized controlled trial of silymarin treatment in patients with cirrhosis of the liver. *J Hepatol* 1989; 9: 105–13.

9. Lirussi F, Okolicsanyi L. Cytoprotection in the nineties: Experience with ursodeoxycholic acid and silymarin in chronic liver disease. *Acta Phys Hungarics* 1992; 80: 1–4.

10. Velussi M, Cernigo AM, Viezzoli L, et al. Silymarin reduces hyperinsulinemia, malondialdehyde

levels and daily insulin need in cirrhotic diabetic patients. *Curr Ther Res* 1993; S3: S33–45.

11. Pares A, Plancs R, Torres M, et al. Effects of silymarin in alcoholic patients with cirrhosis of the liver: results of a controlled, double-blind, randomized and multicenter trial. *J Hepatol* 1998; 28: 615–21.

12. Nassuato G, Iemnolo RN, et al. Effect of silibinin on bilary lipid composition. Experimental and clinical study. *J Hepatol* 1991; 12: 290–95.

13. Palasciano G, Portinascasa P, et al. The effect of silymarin on plasma levels of malondialdehyde in patients receiving long-term treatment with psychotropic drugs. *Curr Ther Res* 1994; S5: S37–45.

14. Brown DJ. *Herbal Prescriptions for Better Health.* Rocklin, CA: Prima Publishing, 1996, 151–58.

15. Reyes H. The spectrum of liver and gastrointestinal disease seen in cholestasis of pregnancy. *Gastroert Clin N Am* 1992; 21: 905–21.

Mullein

1. Hoffman D. *The Herbal Handbook: A User's Guide to Medical Herbalism.* Rochester, VT: Healing Arts Press, 1988, 67.

2. Grieve M. *A Modern Herbal,* vol 2. New York: Dover Publications, 1971, 562–66.

3. Wichtl M. *Herbal Drugs and Phytopharmaceuticals.* Boca Raton, FL: CRC Press, 1994, 18–19.

4. Tyler VE. *The Honest Herbal,* 3d ed. Binghamton, NY: Pharmaceutical Products Press, 1993, 219–20.

5. Blumenthal M, Busse WR, Goldberg A, et al. (eds). *The Complete Commission E Monographs: Therapeutic Guide to Herbal Medicines.* Boston, MA: Integrative Medicine Communications, 1998, 173.

Myrrh

1. Leung AY, Foster S. *Encyclopedia of Common Natural Ingredients Used in Food, Drugs, and Cosmetics,* 2d ed. New York: John Wiley & Sons, 1996, 382–83.

2. Mills SY. *Out of the Earth: The Essential Book of Herbal Medicine.*

Middlesex, UK: Viking Arkana, 1991, 500–2.

3. Al-Harbi MM, Qureshi S, Raza M, et al. Anticarcinogenic effect of *Commiphora molmol* on solid tumors induced by Ehrlich carcinoma cells in mice. *Chemotherapy* 1994; 40: 337–47.

4. Dolara P, Luceri C, Ghelardini C, et al. Analgesic effects of myrrh. *Nature* 1996; 376: 29.

5. Blumenthal M, Busse WR, Goldberg A, et al. (eds). *The Complete Commission E Monographs: Therapeutic Guide to Herbal Medicines.* Boston, MA: Integrative Medicine Communications, 1998, 173–74.

Nettle

1. Obertreis B, Giller K, Teucher T, et al. Antiphlogistic effects of *Urtica dioica folia* extract in comparison to caffeic malic acid. *Arzneim Forsch Drug Res* 1996; 46: 52–56.

2. Hirano T, Homma M, Oka K. Effects of stinging nettle root extracts and their steroidal components on the Na+,K+-ATPase of the benign prostatic hyperplasia. *Planta Med* 1994; 60: 30–33.

3. Vontobel H, Herzog R, Rutishauser G, Kres H. Results of a double-blind study on the effectiveness of ERU (extractum radicis urticae) capsules in conservative treatment of benign prostatic hyperplasia. *Urologe* 1985; 24(1): 49–51 [in German].

4. Mittman P. Randomized, double-blind study of freeze-dried *Urtica dioica* in the treatment of allergic rhinitis. *Planta Med* 1990; 56: 44–47.

5. Brown D, Austin S, Reichert R. *Benign Prostatic Hyperplasia and Prostate Cancer Prevention.* Seattle: NPRC, 1997, 9–10.

6. Blumenthal M, Busse WR, Goldberg A, et al. (eds). *The Complete Commission E Monographs: Therapeutic Guide to Herbal Medicines.* Boston, MA: Integrative Medicine Communications, 1998, 216–17.

Oak

1. Leung AY, Foster S. *Encyclopedia of Common Natural Ingredients Used in Foods, Drugs, and Cosmetics,* 2d ed. New York: John Wiley & Sons, 1996, 485–87.

2. Weiss RF. *Herbal Medicine.* Beaconsfield, UK: Beaconsfield Publishers Ltd., 1988, 328–29.

3. Konig M, Scholz E, Hartmann R, Lehmann W, Rimpler H. Ellagitannins and complex tannins from *Quercus petraea* bark. *J Nat Prod* 1994; 57(10): 1411–15.

4. Schilcher H. *Phytotherapy in Paediatrics.* Stuttgart, Germany: Medpharm Scientific Publishers, 1997, 49–50.

5. Blumenthal M, Busse WR, Goldberg A, et al. (eds). *The Complete Commission E Monographs: Therapeutic Guide to Herbal Medicines.* Boston, MA: Integrative Medicine Communications, 1998, 175–76.

6. Blumenthal M, Busse WR, Goldberg A, et al. (eds). *The Complete Commission E Monographs: Therapeutic Guide to Herbal Medicines.* Boston, MA: Integrative Medicine Communications, 1998, 175–76.

Oats

1. Weiss RF. *Herbal Medicine.* Gothenburg, Sweden: Ab Arcanum, 1988, 287–88.

2. Mills SY. *Out of the Earth: The Essential Book of Herbal Medicine.* Middlesex, UK: Viking Arcana, 1991, 510–12.

3. Wichtl M. *Herbal Drugs and Phytopharmaceuticals.* Boca Raton, FL: CRC Press, 1994, 96–98.

4. Anand CL. Effect of *Avena sativa* on cigarette smoking. *Nature* 1974; 233: 496.

5. Wichtl M. *Herbal Drugs and Phytopharmaceuticals.* Boca Raton, FL: CRC Press, 1994, 96–98.

Oregon Grape

1. Duke JA. *CRC Handbook of Medicinal Herbs.* Boca Raton, FL: CRC Press, 1985, 287–88.

2. Rabbani GH, Butler T, Knight J, et al. Randomized controlled trial of berberine sulfate therapy for diarrhea due to enterotoxigenic *Escherichia coli* and *Vibrio cholerae. J Infect Dis* 1987; 155(5): 979–84.

3. Eaker EY, Sninsky CA. Effect of berberine on myoelectric activity and transit of the small intestine in rats. *Gastroenterol* 1989; 96: 1506–13.

4. Sun D, Courtney HS, Beachey EH. Berberine sulfate blocks adherence of *Streptococcus pyogenes* to epithelial cells, fibronectin, and hexadecane. *Antimicrob Agents Chemother* 1988; 32(9): 1370–74.

5. Kumazawa Y, et al. Activation of peritoneal macrophages by berberine-type alkaloids in terms of induction of cytostatic activity. *Int J Immunopharmacol* 1984; 6: 587–92.

6. Wiesenauer M, Lüdtke R. *Mahonia aquifolium* in patients with psoriasis vulgaris—an intraindividual study. *Phytomedicine* 1996; 3: 231–35.

7. Galle K, Müller-Jakic B, Proebstle A, et al. Analytical and pharmacological studies on *Mahonia aquifolium. Phytomedicine* 1994; 1: 59–62.

8. Chan E. Displacement of bilirubin from albumin by berberine. *Biol Neonate* 1993; 63: 201–8.

Passion Flower

1. Foster S. *Herbs for Your Health.* Loveland, CO: Interweave Press, 1996, 68–69.

2. Meier B. *Passiflora incarnata* L.—Passion flower: Portrait of a medicinal plant. *Zeitschrift Phytother* 1995; 16: 115–26.

3. Wichtl M. *Herbal Drugs and Phytopharmaceuticals.* Boca Raton, FL: CRC Press, 1994, 363–65.

4. Newall CA, Anderson LA, Phillipson JD. *Herbal Medicines: A Guide for Health-Care Professionals.* London: The Pharmaceutical Press, 1996, 206–7.

Pau d'arco

1. Duke JA. *CRC Handbook of Medicinal Herbs.* Boca Raton, FL: CRC Press, 1985, 470–71.

2. Guiraud P, Steiman R, Campos-Takaki GM, et al. Comparison of antibacterial and antifungal activities of lapachol and beta-lapachone. *Planta Med* 1994; 60: 373–74.

3. Tyler VE. *Herbs of Choice: The Therapeutic Use of Phytomedicinals.* Binghamton, NY: Pharmaceutical Products Press, 1994, 180.

4. Oswald EH. Lapacho. *Br J Phytother* 1993/4; 3: 112–17.

5. Foster S. *Herbs for Your Health*. Loveland, CO: Interweave Press, 1996, 70–71.

6. Duke JA. *CRC Handbook of Medicinal Herbs*. Boca Raton, FL: CRC Press, 1985, 470–71.

7. Oswald EH. Lapacho. *Br J Phytother* 1993/4; 3: 112–17.

Peppermint

1. Foster S. *Herbs for Your Health*. Loveland, CO: Interweave Press, 1996, 72–73.

2. Bradley PR, ed. *British Herbal Compendium*, vol 1. Bournemouth, Dorset UK: British Herbal Medicine Association, 1992, 174–76.

3. Tyler VE. *Herbs of Choice: The Therapeutic Use of Phytomedicinals*. Binghamton, NY: Pharmaceutical Products Press, 1994, 56–57.

4. Trabace L, et al. Choleretic activity of some typical components of essential oils. *Planta Med* 1992; 58: A650–51.

5. Gëbel H, Schmidt G, Dwoshak M, et al. Essential plant oils and headache mechanisms. *Phytomedicine* 1995; 2: 93–102.

6. Rees W, Evans B, Rhodes J. Treating irritable bowel syndrome with peppermint oil. *Br Med J* 1979; ii: 835–36.

7. Pittler MH, Ernst E. Peppermint oil for irritable bowel syndrome: A critical review and meta-analysis. *Am J Gastroenterol* 1998; 93: 1131–35.

8. May B, Kuntz HD, Kieser M, Kohler S. Efficacy of a fixed peppermint/caraway oil combination in non-ulcer dyspepsia. *Arzneim Forsch Drug Res* 1996; 46: 1149–53.

9. Weizman Z, Alkrinawi S, Goldfarb D, Bitran C. Efficacy of herbal tea preparation in infantile colic. *J Pediatr* 1993; 122: 650–52.

10. Gëbel H, Schmidt G, Soyka DS. Effect of peppermint and eucalyptus oil preparations on neurophysiological and experimental algesimetric headache parameters. *Cephalalgia* 1994; 14: 228–34.

11. Wichtl M. *Herbal Drugs and Phytopharmaceuticals*. Boca Raton, FL: CRC Press, 1994, 336–38.

12. Sigmund DJ, McNally EF. The action of a carminative on the lower esophageal sphincter. *Gastroent* 1969; 56: 13–18.

13. Blumenthal M, Busse WR, Goldberg A, et al. (eds). *The Complete Commission E Monographs: Therapeutic Guide to Herbal Medicines*. Boston, MA: Integrative Medicine Communications, 1998, 180–82.

14. Blumenthal M, Busse WR, Goldberg A, et al. (eds). *The Complete Commission E Monographs: Therapeutic Guide to Herbal Medicines*. Boston, MA: Integrative Medicine Communications, 1998, 180–82.

15. Blumenthal M, Busse WR, Goldberg A, et al. (eds). *The Complete Commission E Monographs: Therapeutic Guide to Herbal Medicines*. Boston, MA: Integrative Medicine Communications, 1998, 180–82.

Phyllanthus

1. Bharatiya VB. *Selected Medicinal Plants of India*. Bombay: Tata Press, 1992, 235–37.

2. Nadkarmi KM. *India Materia Medica*, vol 1. Bombay: Popular Prakashan Private Ltd., 1993, 947–48.

3. Thyagarajan SP, Subramanian S, Thirunalasundar T, et al. Effect of *Phyllanthus amarus* on chronic carriers of hepatitis B virus. *Lancet* 1988: ii: 764–66.

4. Meixa W, Haowei C, Yanjin L, et al. Herbs of the genus *Phyllanthus* in the treatment of chronic hepatitis B: observation with three preparations from different geographic sites. *J Lab Clin Med* 1995; 126: 350–52.

5. Reichert R. Phytotherapeutic alternatives for chronic hepatitis. *Quart Rev Natural Med* 1997; Summer: 103–8.

Psyllium

1. Leung AY, Foster S. *Encyclopedia of Common Natural Ingredients Used in Food, Drugs, and Cosmetics*, 2d ed. New York: John Wiley & Sons, 1996, 427–29.

2. Voderholzer WA, Schatke W, Mühldorfer BE, et al. Clinical response to dietary fiber treatment of chronic constipation. *Am J Gastroenterol* 1997; 92: 95–98.

3. Oson BH, Anderson SM, Becker MP, et al. Psyllium-enriched cereals lower blood total cholesterol and LDL cholesterol, but not HDL cholesterol, in hypercholesterolemic adults: Results of a meta-analysis. *J Nutr* 1997; 127: 1973–80.

4. Davidson MH, Dugan LD, Burns JH, et al. A psyllium-enriched cereal for the treatment of hypercholesterolemia in children: A controlled, double-blind, crossover study. *Am J Clin Nutr* 1996; 63(1): 96–102.

5. Foster S. *Herbs for Your Health*. Loveland, CO: Interweave Press, 1996, 74–75.

6. Blumenthal M, Busse WR, Goldberg A, et al. (eds). *The Complete Commission E Monographs: Therapeutic Guide to Herbal Medicines*. Boston, MA: Integrative Medicine Communications, 1998, 190–92.

Pygeum

1. Murray MT. *The Healing Power of Herbs*. Rocklin, CA: Prima Publishing, 1995, 286–93.

2. Barlet A, Albrecht J, Aubert A, et al. Efficacy of *Pygeum africanum* extract in the treatment of micturational disorders due to benign prostatic hyperplasia. Evaluation of objective and subjective parameters. A multicenter, randomized, double-blind trial. *Wein Klin Wochenschr* 1990; 102: 667–73.

3. Krzeski T, Kazón M, Borkowski A, et al. Combined extracts of *Urtica dioica* and *Pygeum africanum* in the treatment of benign prostatic hyperplasia: Double-blind comparison of two doses. *Clin Ther* 1993; 15: 1011–20.

4. Murray MT. *The Healing Power of Herbs*. Rocklin, CA: Prima Publishing, 1995, 286–93.

Red Clover

1. Leung AY, Foster S. *Encyclopedia of Common Natural Ingredients Used in Food, Drugs, and Cosmetics,*

2d ed. New York: John Wiley & Sons, 1996, 177–78.

2. Leung AY, Foster S. *Encyclopedia of Common Natural Ingredients Used in Food, Drugs, and Cosmetics*, 2d ed. New York: John Wiley & Sons, 1996, 177–78.

3. Yanagihara K, Toge T, Numoto M, et al. Antiproliferative effects of isoflavones on human cancer cell lines established from the gastrointestinal tract. *Cancer Res* 1993; 53: 5815–21.

4. Stephens FO. Phytoestrogens and prostate cancer. Possible preventive role. *Med J Australia* 1997; 167: 138–40.

5. Foster S. *Herbs for Your Health*. Loveland, CO: Interweave Press, 1996, 76–77.

Red Raspberry

1. Lust JB. *The Herb Book*. New York: Bantam Books, 1974, 328–29.

2. Tyler VE. *Herbs of Choice: The Therapeutic Use of Phytomedicinals*. Binghamton, NY: Pharmaceutical Products Press, 1994, 52,139.

3. Blumenthal M, Busse WR, Goldberg A, et al. (eds). *The Complete Commission E Monographs: Therapeutic Guide to Herbal Medicines*. Boston, MA: Integrative Medicine Communications, 1998, 366.

Reishi

1. Leung AY, Foster S. *Encyclopedia of Common Natural Ingredients Used in Foods, Drugs, and Cosmetics*, 2d ed. New York: John Wiley & Sons, 1996, 255–60.

2. Jones K. *Reishi: Ancient Herb for Modern Times*. Issaquah, WA: Sylvan Press, 1990, 6.

3. Willard T. *Reishi Mushroom: Herb of Spiritual Potency and Wonder*. Issaquah, WA: Sylvan Press, 1990, 11.

4. Shu HY. *Oriental Materia Medica: A Concise Guide*. Palos Verdes, CA: Oriental Healing Arts Press, 1986, 640–41.

5. Hobbs C. *Medicinal Mushrooms*. Santa Cruz, CA: Botanica Press, 1995, 96–107.

6. Hobbs C. *Medicinal Mushrooms*. Santa Cruz, CA: Botanica Press, 1995, 96–107.

7. McGuffin M, Hobbs C, Upton R, Goldberg A, eds. *American Herbal Products Association's Botanical Safety Handbook*. Boca Raton, FL: CRC Press, 1997, 55.

Rosemary

1. Castleman M. *The Healing Herbs*. New York: Bantam Books, 1991, 452–56.

2. Leung AY, Foster S. *Encyclopedia of Common Natural Ingredients Used in Foods, Drugs, and Cosmetics*, 2d ed. New York: John Wiley & Sons, 1996, 446–48.

3. Huhtanen C. Inhibition of *Clostridium botulinum* by spice extract and aliphatic alcohols. *J Food Protect* 1980; 43: 195–96.

4. Aqel MB. Relaxant effect of the volatile oil of *Rosmarinus officinalis* on tracheal smooth muscle. *J Ethnopharmacol* 1991; 33: 57–62.

5. Leung AY, Foster S. *Encyclopedia of Common Natural Ingredients Used in Foods, Drugs, and Cosmetics*, 2d ed. New York: John Wiley & Sons, 1996, 446–48.

6. Singletary K, MacDonald C, Wallig M. Inhibition by rosemary and carnosol of 7,12-dimethyl-benz[a]anthracene (DMBA)-induced rat mammary tumorigenesis and in vivo DMBA-DNA adduct formation. *Cancer Lett* 1996; 104: 43–48.

7. Blumenthal M, Busse WR, Goldberg A, et al. (eds). *The Complete Commission E Monographs: Therapeutic Guide to Herbal Medicines*. Boston, MA: Integrative Medicine Communications, 1998, 197.

8. Newall CA, Anderson LA, Phillipson JD. *Herbal Medicine: A Guide for Health-Care Professionals*. London: The Pharmaceutical Press, 1996, 229–30.

Sage

1. Duke JA. *CRC Handbook of Medicinal Herbs*. Boca Raton, FL: CRC Press, 1985, 420–21.

2. Weiss RF. *Herbal Medicine*. Beaconsfield, UK: Beaconsfield Publishers Ltd., 1988, 229–30.

3. Schwarz K, Ternes W. Antioxidative constituents of *Rosmarinus officinalis* and *Salvia*

officinalis. I. Determination of phenolic diterpenes with antioxidative activity amongst tocochromanols using HPLC. *Z Lebsnm Unters Forsch* 1992; 195(2): 95–98.

4. Masterova I, Misikova E, Sirotkova L, Vaverkova S, Ubik K. Royleanones in the roots of *Salvia officinalis* L. of domestic provenance and their antimicrobial activity. *Ceska Slov Farm* 1996; 45(5): 242–45.

5. Blumenthal M, Busse WR, Goldberg A, et al. (eds). *The Complete Commission E Monographs: Therapeutic Guide to Herbal Medicines*. Boston, MA: Integrative Medicine Communications, 1998, 198.

6. Blumenthal M, Busse WR, Goldberg A, et al. (eds). *The Complete Commission E Monographs: Therapeutic Guide to Herbal Medicines*. Boston, MA: Integrative Medicine Communications, 1998, 198.

Sandalwood

1. Duke JA. *CRC Handbook of Medicinal Herbs*. Boca Raton, FL: CRC Press, 1985, 426–27.

2. Okazai K, Oshima S. Antibacterial activity of higher plants. XXIV. Antimicrobial effect of essential oils (5). *J Pharm Soc Japan* 1953; 73: 344–47.

3. Okugawa H, Ueda R, Matsumoto K, et al. Effect of alpha-santalol and beta-santalol from sandalwood on the central nervous system in mice. *Phytomedicine* 1995; 2: 119–26.

4. Blumenthal M, Busse WR, Goldberg A, et al. (eds). *The Complete Commission E Monographs: Therapeutic Guide to Herbal Medicines*. Boston, MA: Integrative Medicine Communications, 1998, 199.

5. Blumenthal M, Busse WR, Goldberg A, et al. (eds). *The Complete Commission E Monographs: Therapeutic Guide to Herbal Medicines*. Boston, MA: Integrative Medicine Communications, 1998, 199.

Sarsaparilla

1. Duke JA. *CRC Handbook of Medicinal Herbs*. Boca Raton, FL: CRC Press, 1985, 446.

2. Bradley PR, ed. *British Herbal Compendium*, vol 1. Bournemouth, Dorset, UK: British Herbal Medicine Association, 1992, 194–96.

3. Ageel AM, Mossa JS, Al-Yahya MA, et al. Experimental studies on antirheumatic crude drugs used in Saudi traditional medicine. *Drugs Exp Clin Res* 1989; 15: 369–72.

4. Rafatullah S, Mossa JS, Ageel AM, et al. Hepatoprotective and safety evaluation studies on sarsaparilla. *Int J Pharmacognosy* 1991; 29: 296–301.

5. Blumenthal M, Busse WR, Goldberg A, et al. (eds). *The Complete Commission E Monographs: Therapeutic Guide to Herbal Medicines*. Boston, MA: Integrative Medicine Communications, 1998, 372–73.

6. Blumenthal M, Busse WR, Goldberg A, et al. (eds). *The Complete Commission E Monographs: Therapeutic Guide to Herbal Medicines*. Boston, MA: Integrative Medicine Communications, 1998, 372–73.

7. Bradley PR, ed. *British Herbal Compendium*, vol 1. Bournemouth, Dorset, UK: British Herbal Medicine Association, 1992, 194–96.

Saw Palmetto

1. Di Silverio F, Monti S, Sciarra A, et al. Effects of long-term treatment with Serenoa repens (Permixon) on the concentrations and regional distribution of androgens and epidermal growth factor in benign prostatic hyperplasia. *Prostate* 1998; 37: 77–83.

2. Strauch G, Perles P, Vergult G, et al. Comparison of finasteride (Proscar) and *Serenoa repens* (Permixon) in the inhibition of 5-alpha reductase in healthy male volunteers. *Eur Urol* 1994; 26: 247–52.

3. Wilt TJ, Ishani A, Stark G, et al. Saw palmetto extracts for treatment of benign prostatic hyperplasia. *JAMA* 1998; 280: 160–69.

4. Braeckman J. The extract of *Serenoa repens* in the treatment of benign prostatic hyperplasia: multicenter open study. *Curr Ther Res* 1994; 55: 776–85.

5. Redecker KD, Hëlscher U. Extractum *Sabal fructus* in benign prostatic hyperplasia (BPH)—clinical

trial in BPH stages I and II according to Alken. *Extracta Urologica* 1998; 21: 23–25.

6. Ziegler, K, Hëlscher U. Efficacy of special extract WS 1473 from saw palmetto fruit in patients with BPH (stage I and II according to Alken). *Jatros Uro* 1998; 3: 36–43.

7. Bach D, Ebeling L. Long-term drug treatment of benign prostatic hyperplasia)—results of a prospective 3-year multicenter study using Sabal extract IDS 89. *Phytomedicine* 1996; 3: 105–11 (originally published in *Urologe [B]* 1995; 35: 178–83).

8. Carraro JC, Raynaud JP, Koch G, et al. Comparison of phytotherapy (Permixon) with finasteride in the treatment of benign prostate hyperplasia: A randomized international study of 1,098 patients. *Prostate* 1996; 29: 231–40.

9. Braeckman J, Bruhwyler J, Vandekerckhove K, Géczy J. Efficacy and safety of the extract of *Serenoa repens* in the treatment of benign prostatic hyperplasia: Therapeutic equivalence between twice and once daily dosage forms. *Phytotherapy Res* 1997; 11: 558–63.

10. Metzker H, Kieser M, Hëlscher U. Efficacy of a combined Sabal-Urtica preparation in the treatment of benign prostatic hyperplasia (BPH). *Urologe [B]* 1996; 36: 292–300.

11. Sëkeland J, Albrecht J. A combination of Sabal and Urtica extracts versus finasteride in BPH (stage I and II according to Alken): a comparison of therapeutic efficacy in a one-year double-blind study. *Urolge [A]* 1997; 36: 327–33.

12. Brown DJ. *Herbal Prescriptions for Better Health*. Rocklin, CA: Prima Publications, 1996, 167–72.

13. Blumenthal M, Busse WR, Goldberg A, et al. (eds). *The Complete Commission E Monographs: Therapeutic Guide to Herbal Medicines*. Boston, MA: Integrative Medicine Communications, 1998, 201.

14. Carraro JC, Raynaud JP, Koch G, et al. Comparison of phytotherapy (Permixon) with finasteride in the treatment of benign prostate hyperplasia: A randomized interna-

tional study of 1,098 patients. *Prostate* 1996; 29: 231–40.

Schisandra

1. Leung AY, Foster S. *Encyclopedia of Common Natural Ingredients Used in Food, Drugs, and Cosmetics*, 2d ed. New York: John Wiley & Sons, 1996, 469–72.

2. Shu HY. *Oriental Materia Medica: A Concise Guide*. Palos Verdes, CA: Oriental Healing Arts Press, 1986, 624–25.

3. Bao TR, Xu GF, Liu GT, et al. Comparison of the pharmacological effects of seven constituents isolated from the fruits of schisandra. *Acta Pharm Sinica* 1979; 14: 1–7 [in Chinese].

4. Jung KY, Lee IS, Oh SR, et al. Lignans with platelet activating factor antagonist activity from *Schisandra chinensis* (Turcz) Baill. *Phytomedicine* 1997; 4: 229–31.

5. Hancke J, Burgos R, Cáceres D, et al. Reduction of serum hepatic transaminases and CPK in sport horses with poor performance treated with a standardized *Schizandra chinensis* fruit extract. *Phytomedicine* 1996; 3: 237–40.

6. Foster S, Yue CX. *Herbal Emissaries: Bringing Chinese Herbs to the West*. Rochester, VT: Healing Arts Press, 1992, 146–52.

7. Foster S, Yue CX. *Herbal Emissaries: Bringing Chinese Herbs to the West*. Rochester, VT: Healing Arts Press, 1992, 146–52.

8. McGuffin M, Hobbs C, Upton R, Goldberg A. *American Herbal Product Association's Botanical Safety Handbook*. Boca Raton, FL: CRC Press, 1997, 104.

Scullcap

1. Hoffman D. *The Herbal Handbook: A User's Guide to Medical Herbalism*. Rochester, VT: Healing Arts Press, 1988, 77.

2. Foster S. *Herbs for Your Health*. Loveland, CO: Interweave Press, 1996, 86–87.

3. Newall CA, Anderson LA, Phillipson JD. *Herbal Medicines: A Guide for Health-Care Professionals*. London: The Pharmaceutical Press, 1996, 239–40.

4. Foster S. *Herbs for Your Health*. Loveland, CO: Interweave Press, 1996, 86–87.

5. McGuffin M, Hobbs C, Upton R, Goldberg A. *American Herbal Product Association's Botanical Safety Handbook*. Boca Raton, FL: CRC Press, 1997, 105.

Senna

1. Leng-Peschlow E. Dual effect of orally administered sennosides on large intestinal transit and fluid absorption in the rat. *J Pharm Pharmacol* 1986; 38: 606–10.

2. Passmore AP, Davies KW, Flanagan PG, et al. A comparison of Agiolax and Lactulose in elderly patients with chronic constipation. *Pharmacol* 1993; 47(suppl 1): 249–52.

3. Kinnunen O, Winblad I, Koistinen P, Salokannel J. Safety and efficacy of a bulk laxative containing senna versus lactulose in the treatment of chronic constipation in geriatric patients. *Pharmacol* 1993; 47(suppl 1): 253–55.

4. Ewe K, Ueberschaer B, Press AG. Influence of senna, fibre, and fibre+senna on colonic transit in loperamide-induced constipation. *Pharmacol* 1993; 47(suppl 1): 242–48.

5. Gruenwald J, Brendler T, Jaenicke C. *PDR for Herbal Medicines*. Montvale, NJ: Medical Economics, 1998, 722–24.

6. Mengs U. Reproductive toxicological investigations with sennosides. *Arzneim Forsch Drug Res* 1986; 36: 1355–58.

7. Faber P, Strenge-Hesse A. Relevance of rhein excretion into breast milk. *Pharmacol* 1988; 36(suppl 1): 212–20.

8. Blumenthal M, Busse WR, Goldberg A, et al. (eds). *The Complete Commission E Monographs: Therapeutic Guide to Herbal Medicines*. Boston, MA: Integrative Medicine Communications, 1998, 204–8.

Shiitake

1. Jones K. *Shiitake: The Healing Mushroom*. Rochester, VT: Healing Arts Press, 1995.

2. Lin Y, et al. A double-blind treatment of 72 cases of chronic hepatitis with lentinan injection. *News Drugs and Clin Remedies* 1987; 6: 362–63 [in Chinese].

3. Taguchi I. Clinical efficacy of lentinan on patients with stomach cancer: End point results of a four-year follow-up survey. *Cancer Detect Prevent Suppl* 1987; 1: 333–49.

4. Hobbs C. *Medicinal Mushrooms*. Santa Cruz, CA: Botanica Press, 1995, 125–28.

5. Hobbs C. *Medicinal Mushrooms*. Santa Cruz, CA: Botanica Press, 1995, 125–28.

Slippery Elm

1. Duke JA. *CRC Handbook of Medicinal Herbs*. Boca Raton, FL: CRC Press, 1985, 495–96.

2. Wren RC, Williamson EM, Evans FJ. *Potter's New Cyclopedia of Botanical Drugs and Preparations*. Essex, UK: CW Daniel Company, 1988, 252.

3. Foster S. *Herbs for Your Health*. Loveland, CO: Interweave Press, 1996, 88–89.

St. John's Wort

1. Gruenwald J. Standardized St. John's wort clinical monograph. *Quart Rev Nat Med* 1997; Winter: 289–99.

2. Suzuki O, Katsumata Y, Oya M. Inhibition of monoamine oxidase by hypericin. *Planta Med* 1984; 50: 272–74.

3. Holzl J, Demisch L, Gollnik B. Investigations about antidepressive and mood changing effects of *Hypericum perforatum*. *Planta Med* 1989; 55: 643.

4. Chatterjee SS, Koch E, Noldner M, et al. Hyperforin with hypericum extract: Interactions with some neurotransmitter systems. *Quart Rev Nat Med* 1997; Summer: 110.

5. Müller WE, Rolli M, Schäfer C, Hafner U. Effects of hypericum extract (LI 160) in biochemical models of antidepressant activity. *Pharmacopsychiatry* 1997; 30(suppl):102–7.

6. Müller WE, Singer A, Wonnemann M, et al. Hyperforin represents the neurotransmitter reuptake inhibiting constituent of hypericum extract. *Pharmacopsychiatry* 1998; 31(suppl): 16–21.

7. Brown DJ. *Herbal Prescriptions for Better Health*. Rocklin, CA: Prima Publishing, 1996, 159–65.

8. Blumenthal M, Busse WR, Goldberg A, et al. (eds). *The Complete Commission E Monographs: Therapeutic Guide to Herbal Medicines*. Boston, MA: Integrative Medicine Communications, 1998, 214–15.

9. Brockmëller J, Reum T, Bauer S, et al. Hypericin and pseudohypericin: Pharmacolinetics and effects on photosensitvity in humans. *Pharmacopsychiatry* 1997; 30(suppl): 94–101.

10. Monograph, *Hyperici herba* (St. John's wort), *Bundesanzeiger* Dec 5, 1984.

Stevia

1. Leung AY, Foster S. *Encyclopedia of Common Natural Ingredients Used in Foods, Drugs, and Cosmetics*, 2d ed. New York: John Wiley & Sons, 1996, 478–80.

2. Curi R, Alvarez M, Bazotte RB, et al. Effect of *Stevia rebaudiana* on glucose tolerance in normal adult humans. *Braz J Med Biol Res* 1986; 19(6): 771–74.

3. White JR Jr, Kramer J, Campbell RK, Bernstein R. Oral use of a topical preparation containing an extract of *Stevia rebaudiana* and the chrysanthemum flower in the management of hyperglycemia. *Diabetes Care* 1994; 17: 940.

4. Melis MS. A crude extract of *Stevia rebaudiana* increases the renal plasma flow of normal and hypertensive rats. *Braz J Med Biol Res* 1996; 29(5): 669–75.

5. Leung AY, Foster S. *Encyclopedia of Common Natural Ingredients Used in Foods, Drugs, and Cosmetics*, 2d ed. New York: John Wiley & Sons, 1996, 478–80.

6. Blumenthal M. FDA rejects AHPA stevia petition. *Whole Foods* Apr 1994: 61–64.

Sundew

1. Wichtl M. *Herbal Drugs and Phytopharmaceuticals*. Boca Raton, FL: CRC Press, 1994, 178–81.

2. Schilcher H, Elzer M. *Drosera* (Sundew): A proven antitussive.

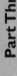

Zeitschrift Phytotherapie 1993; 14: 50–54.

3. Luckner R, Luckner M. Naphthaquinone derivative from *Drosera ramentacea* Burch. *Ex harv. Et ond. Pharmazie* 1970; 25: 261–65.

4. Krahl R. An effective principle from *Drosera rotundifolia*. *Arzneim-Forsch Drug Res* 1956; 6: 617–19.

5. Schilcher H, Elzer M. *Drosera* (Sundew): A proven antitussive. *Zeitschrift Phytotherapie* 1993; 14: 50–54.

6. Blumenthal M, Busse WR, Goldberg A, et al. (eds). *The Complete German Commission E Monographs: Therapeutic Guide to Herbal Medicines*. Austin: American Botanical Council and Boston: Integrative Medicine Communications, 1998, 217–18.

7. Newall CA, Anderson LA, Phillipson JD. *Herbal Medicines: A Guide for Health-Care Professionals*. London: The Pharmaceutical Press, 1996, 100.

Sweet Annie

1. Foster S, Yue CX. *Herbal Emissaries: Bringing Chinese Herbs to the West*. Rochester, VT: Healing Arts Press, 1992, 322.

2. Foster S, Yue CX. *Herbal Emissaries: Bringing Chinese Herbs to the West*. Rochester, VT: Healing Arts Press, 1992, 322.

3. Hien TT, White NJ. Qinghaosu. *Lancet* 1993; 341: 603–608 [review].

4. Tang W, Eisenbrand G. *Chinese Drugs of Plant Origin*. Berlin: Springer-Verlag, 1992, 160–74.

5. Hien TT, White NJ. Qinghaosu. *Lancet* 1993; 341: 603–608 [review].

6. Hien TT, White NJ. Qing-haosu. *Lancet* 1993; 341: 603–608 [review].

7. Bone K, Morgan M. *Clinical Applications of Ayurvedic and Chinese Herbs: Monographs for the Western Herbal Practitioner*. Warwick, Australia: Phytotherapy Press, 1992, 7–12.

8. Foster S, Yue CX. *Herbal Emissaries: Bringing Chinese Herbs to*

the West. Rochester, VT: Healing Arts Press, 1992, 322.

9. Hien TT, White NJ. Qinghaosu. *Lancet* 1993; 341: 603–608 [review].

Tea Tree

1. Carson CF, Riley TV. Antimicrobial activity of the essential oil of *Melaleuca alternifolia*—A review. *Lett Appl Microbiol* 1993; 16: 49–55.

2. Carson CF, Cookson BD, Farrelly HD, Riley T. Susceptibility of methicillin-resistant *Staphylococcus aureus* to the essential oil of *Melaleuca alternifolia*. *J Antimicrobial Chemother* 1995; 35: 421–24.

3. Bassett IB, Pannowitz DL, Barnetson RS. A comparative study of tea-tree oil versus benzoylperoxide in the treatement of acne. *Med J Austral* 1990; 153: 455–58.

4. Buck DS, Nidorf DM, Addino JG. Comparison of two topical preparations for the treatment of onychomycosis: *Melaleuca alternifolia* (tea tree) oil and clotrimazole. *J Garm Pract* 1994; 38: 601–5.

5. Tong MM, Altman PM, Barnetson RS. Tea tree oil in the treatment of tinea pedis. *Austral J Dermatol* 1992; 33: 145–49.

6. Jandourek A, Vaishampayan JK, Vazquez JA. Efficacy of melaleuca oral solution for the treatment of fluconazole refractory oral candidiasis in AIDS patients. *AIDS* 1998; 12: 1033–37.

7. Brown DJ. Phytotherapeutic approaches to common dermatological conditions. *Quart Rev Natural Med* 1998; Summer: 161–73.

8. Knight TE, Hansen BM. Melaleuca oil (tea tree oil) dermatitis. *Med J Australia* 1994; 30: 423–27.

Thyme

1. Leung AY, Foster S. *Encyclopedia of Common Natural Ingredients Used in Food, Drugs, and Cosmetics*. New York: John Wiley & Sons, 1996, 492–95.

2. Gruenwald J, Brendler T, Jaenicke C. *PDR for Herbal Medicines*. Montvale, NJ: Medical Economics, 1998, 1184–85.

3. Weiss RF. *Herbal Medicine*. Gothenburg, Sweden: Ab Arcanum and Beaconsfield, UK: Beaconsfield Publishers Ltd., 1988, 208–9.

4. Blumenthal M, Busse WR, Goldberg A, et al. (eds). *The Complete German Commission E Monographs: Therapeutic Guide to Herbal Medicines*. Austin: American Botanical Council and Boston: Integrative Medicine Communications, 1998, 219–20.

5. Newall CA, Anderson LA, Phillipson JD. *Herbal Medicines: A Guide for Health-Care Professionals*. London: The Pharmaceutical Press, 1996, 256–57.

Turmeric

1. Sreejayan N, Rao MNA. Free radical scavenging activity of curcuminoids. *Arzneim Forsch Drug Res* 1996; 46: 169–71.

2. Ramirez-Boscá A, Soler A, Gutierrez MAC, et al. Antioxidant curcuma extracts decrease the blood lipid peroxide levels of human subjects. *Age* 1995; 18: 167–69.

3. Arora RB, Basu N, Kapoor V, Jain AP. Anti-inflammatory studies on *Curcuma longa* (turmeric). *Ind J Med Res* 1971; 59: 1289–95.

4. Kiso Y, Suzuki Y, Watanbe N, et al. Antihepatotoxic principles of *Curcuma longa* rhizomes. *Planta Med* 1983; 49: 185–87.

5. Srivastava R, Dikshit M, Srimal RC, Dhawan BN. Anti-thrombotic effect of curcumin. *Thromb Res* 1985; 40: 413–17.

6. Barthelemy S, Vergnes L, Moynier M, et al. Curcumin and curcumin derivatives inhibit Tat-mediated transactivation of type 1 human immunodeficiency virus long terminal repeat. *Res Virol* 1998; 149: 43–52.

7. Deodhar SD, Sethi R, Srimal RC. Preliminary studies on antirheumatic activity of curcumin (diferuloyl methane). *Ind J Med Res* 1980; 71: 632–34.

8. Satoskar RR, Shah SJ, Shenoy SG. Evaluation of anti-inflammatory property of curcumin (diferuloyl methane) in patients with postoperative inflammation. *Int J Clin Pharmacol Ther Toxicol* 1986; 24: 651–54.

9. Thamlikitkul V, Bunyapra-phathara N, Dechatiwongse T, et al. Randomized double-blind study of *Curcuma domestica* Val for dyspepsia. *J Med Assoc Thai* 1989; 72: 613–20.

10. Van Dau N, Ngoc Ham N, Huy Khac D, et al. The effects of tra-ditional drug, turmeric *(Curcuma longa),* and placebo on the healing of duodenal ulcer. *Phytomedicine* 1998; 5: 29–34.

11. Kositchaiwat C, Kositchaiwat S, Havanondha J. *Curcuma longa* Linn in the treatment of gastric ulcer comparison to liquid antacid: A con-trolled clinical trial. *J Med Assoc Thai* 1993; 76: 601–5.

12. Murray MT. *The Healing Power of Herbs.* Rocklin, CA: Prima Publishing, 1995, 327–35.

13. Blumenthal M, Busse WR, Goldberg A, et al. (eds). *The Complete Commission E Monographs: Thera-peutic Guide to Herbal Medicines.* Boston, MA: Integrative Medicine Communications, 1998, 222.

Usnea

1. Tilford GL. *Edible and Medi-cinal Plants of the West.* Missoula, MT: Mountain Press Publishing Company, 1997, 148–49.

2. Weiss RF. *Herbal Medicine.* Beaconsfield, UK: Beaconsfield Pub-lishers Ltd., 1988, 49.

3. Evans WC. *Trease and Evans' Pharmacognosy,* 13th ed. London: Baillière Tindall, 1989, 643.

4. Gruenwald J, Brendler T, Jaenicke C, et al. (eds). *PDR for Herbal Medicines.* Montvale, NJ: Medical Economics, 1998, 1199–200.

Uva Ursi

1. Jahodar L, Jilek P, Pakova M, Dvorakova V. Antimicrobial effect of arbutin and an extract of the leaves of *Arctostaphylos uva-ursi* in vitro. *Ceskoslov Farm* 1985; 34: 174–78.

2. Matsuda H, Nakamura S, Tanaka T, Kubo M. Pharmacological studies on leaf of *Arctostaphylos uva-ursi* (L.) Spreng. V. Effect of water extract from *Arctostaphylos uva-ursi* (L.) Spreng (bearberry leaf) on the antiallergic and antiinflammatory activities of dexamethasone ointment.

J Pharm Soc Japan 1992; 112: 673–77.

3. Blumenthal M, Busse WR, Goldberg A, et al. (eds). *The Complete Commission E Monographs: Thera-peutic Guide to Herbal Medicines.* Boston, MA: Integrative Medicine Communications, 1998, 224–25.

Valerian

1. Mennini T, Bernasconi P, et al. In vitro study on the interaction of extracts and pure compounds from *Valeriana officinalis* roots with GABA, benzodiazepine and barbitu-rate receptors. *Fitoterapia* 1993; 64: 291–300.

2. Kohnen R, Oswald WD. The effects of valerian, propranolol and their combination on activation per-formance and mood of healthy volun-teers under social stress conditions. *Pharmacopsychiatry* 1988; 21 447–48.

3. Leathwood PD, Chauffard F, Heck E, Munoz-Box R. Aqueous extract of valerian root (*Valeriana officinalis* L.) improves sleep quality in man. *Pharmacol Biochem Behav* 1982; 17: 65–71.

4. Leathwood PD, Chauffard F. Aqueous extract of valerian reduces latency to fall asleep in man. *Planta Med* 1985; 51: 144–48.

5. Lindahl O, Lindwall L. Double-blind study of a valerian preparation. *Pharmacol Biochem Behav* 1989; 32: 1065–66.

6. Brown DJ. *Herbal Pres-criptions for Better Health.* Rocklin, CA: Prima Publishing, 1996, 173–78.

7. Albrecht M, Berger W, et al. Psychopharmaceuticals and safety in traffic. *Zeits Allgemeinmed* 1995; 71: 1215–21 [in German].

Vitex

1. Blumenthal M, Busse WR, Goldberg A, et al. (eds). *The Complete Commission E Monographs: Thera-peutic Guide to Herbal Medicines.* Boston, MA: Integrative Medicine Communications, 1998, 108.

2. Sliutz G, Speiser P, et al. *Agnus castus* extracts inhibit prolactin secre-tion of rat pituitary cells. *Horm Metab Res* 1993; 25: 253–55.

3. Lauritzen C, Reuter HD, Repges R, et al. Treatment of premen-strual tension syndrome with *Vitex agnus-castus.* Controlled, double-blind study versus pyridoxine. *Phyto-med* 1997; 4(3): 183–89.

4. Bone K. *Vitex agnus-castus:* Scientific studies and clinical applica-tions. *Eur J Herbal Med* 1994; 1: 12–15.

5. Milewicz A, Gejdel E, Sworen H, et al. *Vitex agnus castus* extract for the treatment of menstrual irregulari-ties due to latent hyperprolactinemia. *Arzneim Forsch* 1993; 43: 752–56 [in German].

6. Merz PG, Gorkow C, Schrëdter A, et al. The effects of a spe-cial *Agnus castus* extract (BP1095E1) on prolactin secretion in healthy male subjects. *Exp Clin Endocrinol Diabetes* 1996; 104: 447–53.

7. Amann W. Improvement of acne vulgaris with *Agnus castus* (Agnolyt TM). *Ther d Gegenw* 1967; 106: 124–26 [in German].

8. Blumenthal M, Busse WR, Goldberg A, et al. (eds). *The Complete Commission E Monographs: Thera-peutic Guide to Herbal Medicines.* Boston, MA: Integrative Medicine Communications, 1998, 108.

White Willow

1. Weiss RF. *Herbal Medicine.* Gothenburg, Sweden: Ab Arcanum, 1988, 31,303.

2. Bradley PR, ed. *British Herbal Compendium,* vol 1. Bournemouth, Dorset, UK: British Herbal Medicine Association, 1992, 224–26.

3. Mills SY, Jacoby RK, Chacksfield M, Willoughby M. Effect of a proprietary herbal medicine on the relief of chronic arthritic pain: A double-blind study. *Br J Rheum* 1996; 35: 874–78.

4. Blumenthal M, Busse WR, Goldberg A, et al. (eds). *The Complete Commission E Monographs: Thera-peutic Guide to Herbal Medicines.* Boston, MA: Integrative Medicine Communications, 1998, 230.

5. Blumenthal M, Busse WR, Goldberg A, et al. (eds). *The Complete Commission E Monographs: Thera-peutic Guide to Herbal Medicines.*

Boston, MA: Integrative Medicine Communications, 1998, 230.

Wild Cherry

1. Leung AY, Foster S. *Encyclopedia of Common Natural Ingredients Used in Food, Drugs, and Cosmetics,* 2d ed. New York: John Wiley & Sons, 1996, 155–56.

2. Mills SY. *Out of the Earth: The Essential Book of Herbal Medicine.* Middlesex, UK: Viking Arkana, 1991, 314.

3. Wren RC. *Potter's New Cyclopaedia of Botanical Drugs and Preparations.* Essex, England: CW Daniel Company, 1975, 320.

4. McGuffin M, Hobbs C, Upton R, Goldberg A. *American Herbal Products Association's Botanical Safety Handbook.* Boca Raton, FL: CRC Press, 1997, 92.

Wild Indigo

1. Hoffmann D. *The New Holistic Herbal.* Shaftsbury, Dorset, UK and Rockport, MA: Element, 1990, 241.

2. Beuscher N, Kopanski L. Stimulation of immunity by the contents of *Baptisia tinctoria. Planta Med* 1985; 5: 381–84.

3. Gruenwald J, Brendler T, Jeanicke C, et al. (eds). *PDR for Herbal Medicines.* Montvale, NJ: Medical Economics, 1998, 684–85.

4. Gruenwald J, Brendler T, Jeanicke C, et al. (eds). *PDR for Herbal Medicines.* Montvale, NJ: Medical Economics, 1998, 684–85.

Wild Yam

1. Lust JB. *The Herb Book.* New York: Bantam Books, 1974, 401.

2. Iwu MM, Okunji CO, Ohiaeri GO, et al. Hypoglycaemic activity of dioscoretine from tubers of *Dioscorea dumetorum* in normal and alloxan diabetic rabbits. *Planta Med* 1990; 56: 264–67.

3. Araghiniknam M, Chung S, Nelson-White T, et al. Antioxidant activity of dioscorea and dehydroepiandrosterone (DHEA) in older humans. *Life Sci* 1996; 11: 147–57.

4. Araghiniknam M, Chung S, Nelson-White T, et al. Antioxidant activity of dioscorea and dehydroepiandrosterone (DHEA) in older humans. *Life Sci* 1996; 11: 147–57.

5. Dollbaum CM. Lab analyses of salivary DHEA and progesterone following ingestion of yam-containing products. *Townsend Letter for Doctors and Patients* Oct 1995: 104.

6. Bertram T. *Encyclopedia of Herbal Medicine.* Dorset, England: Grace Publishers, 1995, 454.

Witch Hazel

1. Duke JA. *CRC Handbook of Medicinal Herbs.* Boca Raton, FL: CRC Press, 1985, 221.

2. Bernard P, Balansard P, Balansard G, Bovis A. Venotonic pharmacodynamic value of galenic preparations with a base of *hamamelis* leaves. *J Pharm Belg* 1972; 27: 505–12.

3. Korting HC, Schafer-Korting M, Hart H, et al. Anti-inflammatory activity of *Hamamelis* distillate applied topically to the skin. *Eur J Clin Pharmacol* 1993; 44: 315–18.

4. Swoboda M, Meurer J. Treatment of atopic dermatitis with *Hamamelis* ointment. *Br J Phytother* 1991/2; 2(3): 128–32.

5. Korting HC, Schafer-Korting M, Klovekorn W, et al. Comparative efficacy of *hamamelis* distillate and hydrocortisone cream in atopic eczema. *Eur J Clin Pharmacol* 1995; 48(6): 461–65.

6. Blumenthal M, Busse WR, Goldberg A, et al. (eds). *The Complete Commission E Monographs: Therapeutic Guide to Herbal Medicines.* Boston, MA: Integrative Medicine Communications, 1998, 231.

7. McGuffin M, Hobbs C, Upton R, Goldberg A. *American Herbal Products Association's Botanical Safety Handbook.* Boca Raton, FL: CRC Press, 1997, 105.

Wormwood

1. Leung AY, Foster S. *Encyclopedia of Common Natural Ingredients Used in Food, Drugs, and Cosmetics,*

2d ed. New York: John Wiley & Sons, 1996, 1–3.

2. Leung AY, Foster S. *Encyclopedia of Common Natural Ingredients Used in Food, Drugs, and Cosmetics,* 2d ed. New York: John Wiley & Sons, 1996, 1–3.

3. Weiss RF. *Herbal Medicine.* Gothenburg, Sweden: Ab Arcanum, 1988, 79–81.

4. Blumenthal M, Busse WR, Goldberg A, et al. (eds). *The Complete Commission E Monographs: Therapeutic Guide to Herbal Medicines.* Boston, MA: Integrative Medicine Communications, 1998, 232–33.

5. Weiss RF. *Herbal Medicine.* Gothenburg, Sweden: Ab Arcanum, 1988, 79–81.

6. Weiss RF. *Herbal Medicine.* Gothenburg, Sweden: Ab Arcanum, 1988, 79–81.

7. McGuffin M, Hobbs C, Upton R, Goldberg A. *American Herbal Products Association's Botanical Safety Handbook.* Boca Raton, FL: CRC Press, 1997, 15.

8. McGuffin M, Hobbs C, Upton R, Goldberg A. *American Herbal Products Association's Botanical Safety Handbook.* Boca Raton, FL: CRC Press, 1997, 15.

9. Leung AY, Foster S. *Encyclopedia of Common Natural Ingredients Used in Food, Drugs, and Cosmetics,* 2d ed. New York: John Wiley & Sons, 1996, 1–3.

10. Yarnell E, Heron S. Retrospective analysis of the safety of bitter herbs with an emphasis on *Artemisia absinthium* L. (wormwood). *J Naturopathic Med* 1999; 9: in press.

11. McGuffin M, Hobbs C, Upton R, Goldberg A. *American Herbal Products Association's Botanical Safety Handbook.* Boca Raton, FL: CRC Press, 1997, 15.

Yarrow

1. Castleman M. *The Healing Herbs.* New York, Bantam Books, 1991, 550–54.

2. Castleman M. *The Healing Herbs.* New York, Bantam Books, 1991, 550–54.

Part Three: References

3. Zitterl-Eglseer K, Jurenitsch J, et al. Sesquiterpene lactones of *Achillea setacea* with antiphlogistic activity. *Planta Med* 1991; 57(5): 444–46.

4. Muller-Jakic B, Breu W, Probstle A, et al. In vitro inhibition of cyclooxygenase and 5-lipoxygenase by alkamides from *Echinacea* and *Achillea* species. *Planta Med* 1994; 60(1): 37–40.

5. Tewari JP, Srivastava MC, Bajpai JL. Pharmacologic studies of *Achillea millefolium* Linn. *Indian J Med Sci* 1994; 28(8): 331–36.

6. Duke JA. *CRC Handbook of Medicinal Herbs*. Boca Raton, FL: CRC Press, 1985, 10–11.

7. Blumenthal M, Busse WR, Goldberg A, et al. (eds). *The Complete Commission E Monographs: Therapeutic Guide to Herbal Medicines*. Boston, MA: Integrative Medicine Communications, 1998, 233–34.

8. McGuffin M, Hobbs C, Upton R, Goldberg A. *American Herbal Products Association's Botanical Safety Handbook*. Boca Raton, FL: CRC Press, 1997, 3.

Yellow Dock

1. Hoffman D. *The Herbal Handbook: A User's Guide to Medical Herbalism*. Rochester, VT: Healing Arts Press, 1988, 40.

2. Newall CA, Anderson LA, Phillipson JD. *Herbal Medicines: A Guide for Health-Care Professionals*. London: The Pharmaceutical Press, 1996, 274.

3. Newall CA, Anderson LA, Phillipson JD. *Herbal Medicines: A Guide for Health-Care Professionals*. London: The Pharmaceutical Press, 1996, 274.

Yohimbe

1. Duke J. *CRC Handbook of Medicinal Herbs*. Boca Raton, FL: CRC Press, 1985, 351.

2. Riley AJ. Yohimbine in the treatment of erectile disorder. *Br J Clin Pract* 1994; 48: 133–36.

3. Ernst E, Pittler MH. Yohimbine for erectile dysfunction: A systematic review and meta-analysis of randomized clinical trials. *J Urol* 1998; 159: 433–36.

4. Carey MP, Johnson BT. Effectiveness of yohimbine in the treatment of erectile disorder: Four meta-analytic integrations. *Arch Sex Behav* 1996; 25: 341.

5. Kunelius P, Häkkinen J, Lukkarinen O. Is high-dose yohimbine hydrochloride effective in the treatment of mixed-type impotence? A prospective, randomized, controlled double-blind crossover study. *Urol* 1997; 49: 441–44.

6. Mann K, Klingler T, Noe S, et al. Effect of yohimbine on sexual experiences and nocturnal tumescence and rigidity in erectile dysfunction. *Arch Sex Behav* 1996; 25: 1–16.

7. Goldberg KA. Yohimbine in the treatment of male erectile sexual dysfunction—a clinical review. *Today's Ther Trends J New Dev Clin Med* 1996; 14: 25–33.

8. *Drug Facts and Comparisons*. St. Louis: Facts and Comparisons, 1998, 3659.

9. Blumenthal M, Busse WR, Goldberg A, et al. (eds). *The Complete Commission E Monographs: Therapeutic Guide to Herbal Medicines*. Boston, MA: Integrative Medicine Communications, 1998, 382–83.

10. Goldberg KA. Yohimbine in the treatment of male erectile sexual dysfunction—a clinical review. *Today's Ther Trends J New Dev Clin Med* 1996; 14: 25–33.

11. *Drug Facts and Comparisons*. St. Louis: Facts and Comparisons, 1998, 3659.

12. Friesen K, Palatnick W, Tenenbein M. Benign course after massive ingestion of yohimbine. *J Emerg Med* 1993; 11: 287–88.

13. Bremner JD, Innis RB, Ng CK, et al. Positron emission tomography measurement of cerebral metabolic correlates of yohimbine administration in combat-related post-traumatic stress disorder. *Arch Gen Psychiatry* 1997; 54: 246–54.

14. Charney DS, Woods SW, Goodman WK, Heninger GR. Neurobiological mechanisms of panic anxiety: Biochemical and behavioral correlates of yohimbine-induced panic attacks. *Am J Psychiatry* 1987; 144: 1030–36.

15. Cappiello A, McDougle CJ, Maleson RT, et al. Yohimbine augmentation of fluvoxamine in refractory depression: A single-blind study. *Biol Psychol* 1995; 38: 765–67.

Yucca

1. Bingham R, Bellew BA, Bellew JG. Yucca plant saponin in the management of arthritis. *J Appl Nutr* 1975; 27: 45–50.

2. Foster S, Duke JA. *A Field Guide to Medicinal Plants: Eastern and Central North America*. Boston: Houghton Mifflin Co., 1990; 18, 228.

3. Bingham R, Bellew BA, Bellew JG. Yucca plant saponin in the management of arthritis. *J Appl Nutr* 1975; 27: 45–50.

4. Moore M. *Medicinal Plants of the Desert and Canyon West*. Santa Fe: Museum of New Mexico Press, 1989, 134–35.

5. Moore M. *Medicinal Plants of the Desert and Canyon West*. Santa Fe: Museum of New Mexico Press, 1989, 134–35.

6. McGuffin M, Hobbs C, Upton R, Goldberg A. *American Herbal Products Association's Botanical Safety Handbook*. Boca Raton, FL: CRC Press, 1997, 124.

7. Moore M. *Medicinal Plants of the Desert and Canyon West*. Santa Fe: Museum of New Mexico Press, 1989, 134–35.

Part Three: References

Part Four

Homeopathic Remedies

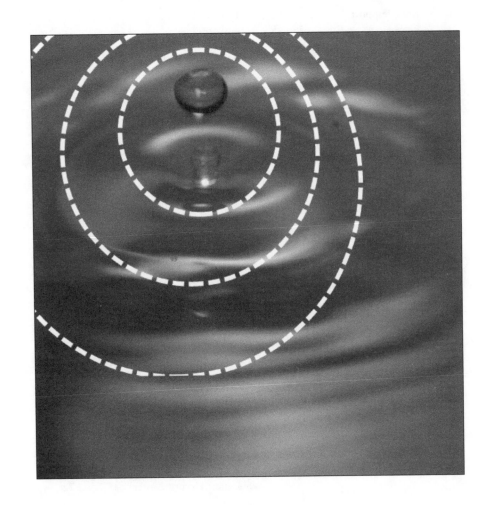

What Is Homeopathy?

Homeopathy is a nontoxic system of medicine used to treat illness and relieve discomfort in a wide variety of health conditions. It is practiced by licensed physicians and other qualified prescribers in many regions of the world, including Europe, Asia, the U.K., and the U.S. Information on the use of several hundred remedies has been collected for nearly two centuries by homeopathic practitioners, through research studies known as "provings," as well as documented clinical cases and recent scientific trials.[1,2,3]

The Law of Similars and Potentization

Two important ideas on which the science of homeopathy is based are the Law of Similars and Potentization. Simply expressed, the Law of Similars states that since exposure to a substance can cause specific symptoms in a healthy person, that substance—when correctly prepared as a homeopathic remedy—can stimulate the body's curative powers to overcome similar symptoms during illness. For example: A person who chops an onion can develop watery eyes, a runny nose, sneezing, coughing, and throat irritation from exposure to the onion's active substances. The homeopathic remedy, *Allium cepa,* made of potentized red onion, can help the body overcome a cold or allergy attack in which the person has similar symptoms (watery eyes, runny nose, sneezing, coughing, or throat irritation). The actual symptoms of the illness were not caused by exposure to an onion, but the remedy made from the onion can help the body overcome them, because the symptoms are similar.

Potentization is a process that involves a series of precise dilutions and succussions (succussion is a vigorous shaking action). A substance has to undergo this process to be useful as a homeopathic remedy. Potentization is very important because the repeated process of dilution and succussion brings about an energetic change that gives the substance a deeper curative effect. Repeated dilution removes the risk of chemical toxicity, allowing the homeopathic use of many substances that would otherwise not be safe to take as medicine.

The safety and nontoxicity of homeopathic remedies is reassuring; however, they still must be chosen carefully on the basis of specific information—and used correctly—or they may affect the symptoms only superficially, or have no effect at all. Homeopathic remedies are not selected simply to treat an isolated symptom or a named disease. To work correctly, they must be chosen to match the way an individual's system expresses its unique response to the current stress and illness. Even within the same diagnosis, different people respond to different remedies.

How to Use Homeopathic Remedies

Self-care with homeopathy for moderate, short-term illnesses and injuries can be rewarding. A correctly chosen remedy can work gently and efficiently to relieve discomfort and help the body heal itself without toxicity or side effects. If an illness or condition is chronic or serious, it is best to consult an experienced prescriber for a remedy that more deeply suits the person's needs. (See **Using Homeopathy with Professional Guidance** on the next page.)

- Observe the person, taking special note of the strongest and most unusual symptoms, as well as the way the individual responds to the stress of illness—things that relieve or aggravate the symptoms (motion, temperature, light, noise) and the person's emotional and mental state.
- Choose the remedy whose description most closely matches the symptoms the person is expressing. When a remedy's pattern of action is similar to the person's response to the stress or illness, it can help the natural defenses more efficiently overcome the problems and return the person to a better state of health.
- Take one dose of the selected remedy, then wait for a response to show. If relief of important symptoms is noted—or if the person starts to improve in general—the remedy is acting. Continue to wait and let it do its work. Do not give another dose unless improvement stops. (Unnecessary repetitions can interfere with or slow down a remedy's action.)
- Further doses of the remedy should be given according to how the person is responding, not on a pre-set schedule. Intense or painful situations may require more frequent repetitions. For instance, in severe discomfort (as with a burn or throbbing headache) a dose may be needed every few minutes to an hour. In moderate conditions, such as flu or indigestion, a dose once every few hours may be indicated. In many situations, one dose of a correctly chosen remedy will be enough to stimulate the body to heal itself.
- If no response is evident after a reasonable amount of waiting, give another dose and wait again. If no response is seen after several repetitions, review the important symptoms and choose another closely indicated remedy.

Lower potencies of a remedy are most appropriate for the non-professional self-care situations. A higher potency will often act more quickly and deeply than a lower one and need fewer repetitions—but, the higher the potency, the more precise the remedy choice must be to bring results. High potencies should only be used by those with formal homeopathic training, as a more developed knowledge of the remedies is needed to make an accurate prescription and to monitor results. (See also **Understanding Homeopathic Potency** below.)

Using Homeopathy with Professional Guidance

Homeopathic remedies can also be helpful in complex or even serious conditions—although self-prescribing is not appropriate in such cases. To correctly select the remedy and monitor the healing process, an experienced physician who is trained in homeopathy should be involved, for the following reasons:

- Medical knowledge is needed to assess complex or serious conditions. Professional diagnostic tests may be necessary, as well.
- Using a remedy that covers isolated symptoms superficially, but does not fit the person on deeper levels, may change or suppress the symptoms, yet not be deeply curative.
- Even with a correctly chosen remedy, a temporary aggravation of symptoms may occur as part of the healing process. Training and experience are required to distinguish a helpful aggravation from an intensification of symptoms that occurs because a remedy has not acted and the illness is progressing.
- An inexperienced or impatient person might be tempted to repeat the remedy unnecessarily, or change to other remedies at times when waiting is appropriate.

If an illness or condition is chronic or deep-seated, it is best to consult an experienced homeopathic practitioner, for a "constitutional" remedy that fits the characteristic symptoms of the case and matches the person's physical condition and individual nature in a more comprehensive way. At a typical first visit, a homeopath interviews a patient for at least an hour—to take a careful history and elicit information about many aspects of the person's state of health—before choosing a remedy.

How Does Homeopathy Work?

Within the limitations of available scientific funding, interesting research is being undertaken to understand how and why such highly diluted remedies have pro-

found and curative effects. Formal studies published in current medical journals show that homeopathic remedies, when used correctly, are significantly more effective than placebo.[1,2,3] Researchers theorize that, during potentization, an energetic change occurs in the remedy substance and its medium of dilution (usually water), enabling them to stimulate a person's system to deal with stress and illness more efficiently. Homeopathic remedies do not have chemical action in the body, and thus work differently than nutrients or drugs—which has made it difficult for some researchers who are accustomed to assessing drugs to adequately consider them. Since the body is clearly affected by many forces that have no chemical content (such as electricity, radiation, thermal energy), it is reasonable to think that research designed to observe nonchemical effects will yield more useful information.

(References to the meta-analyses of results of over 100 clinical studies assessing effects of homeopathic medicines can be found in Part Four: References [page 581].)

Understanding Homeopathic Potency

Homeopathic remedies are prepared through a process called *potentization*. Potentization involves a series of systematic dilutions and succussions (a forceful shaking action). Potentization is important because it removes all risk of chemical toxicity while activating a remedy substance and enabling it to affect the body therapeutically.

Homeopathic pharmacies operate according to strict guidelines, to ensure that the remedies and potencies are consistent and reliable. The first step in producing a homeopathic remedy is acquiring a pure preparation of the original substance in its natural form (such as a solution of a mineral salt or a "mother tincture" of a plant). The original substance is then put through a measured series of dilutions, alternating with succussions, until the desired potency is made.

Homeopathic potencies are designated by the combination of a number and a letter (for example, 6X or 30C). The number refers to the number of dilutions the tincture has undergone within a series to prepare that remedy. The letter refers to the proportions used in each dilution of the series (the Roman numeral X means 10; and the Roman numeral C means 100), as well as to the number of succussions the vial of solution undergoes in each successive stage. For example: To prepare a 6X potency of *Ledum palustre*, one part of the *Ledum* mother tincture is combined in a vial

Understanding Homeopathic Potency

with nine parts of the carrier liquid (usually water or alcohol), and the vial is succussed ten times. This makes a 1X solution. One part of the 1X solution is then combined with nin parts of the carrier liquid, and succussed ten times again, making a 2X solution. The process is repeated four more times, for a total of six dilutions and succussions—and the final result is a 6X potency of *Ledum*. (To make a 30C, one part of the tincture would be combined with ninety-nine parts of the carrier liquid and succussed 100 times in each of 30 steps.) Pellets, tablets, or powders are then medicated with the potentized liquid, or drops of the remedy are taken in liquid form.

The more dilutions and succussions a substance undergoes, the higher the homeopathic potency will be. Higher potencies of homeopathic remedies (anything higher than 12C) have been diluted past the point that molecules of the original substance would be measurable in the solution. This is a major stumbling block for skeptics when it comes to understanding and accepting the idea of homeopathy. Homeopathic remedies, when correctly chosen, clearly work—but not in the way that drugs do (through chemical actions that affect the body processes). It is not completely understood why potentized remedies can work so deeply and specifically, but many likely theories have arisen through research and observation. It appears that they function on an energetic level to stimulate the body to heal itself more efficiently.

Homeopathy: Dosage Directions

Select the remedy that most closely matches the symptoms. In conditions where self-treatment is appropriate, unless otherwise directed by a physician, a lower potency (6X, 6C, 12X, 12C, 30X, or 30C) should be used. In addition, instructions for use are usually printed on the label.

Many homeopathic physicians suggest that remedies be used as follows: Take one dose and wait for a response. If improvement is seen, continue to wait and let the remedy work. If improvement lags significantly or has clearly stopped, another dose may be taken. The frequency of dosage varies with the condition and the individual. Sometimes a dose may be required several times an hour; other times a dose may be indicated several times a day; and in some situations, one dose per day (or less) can be sufficient.

If no response is seen within a reasonable amount of time, select a different remedy.

For more information, see **What Is Homeopathy?** (p. 507), and **Understanding Homeopathic Potencies** (p. 508), and **Part Four: References** (p. 581).

Remedies for Acne

Acne vulgaris (p. 5), although most common during adolescence, can occur at other times in life, especially during times of hormonal shifts. Blackheads or pimples may be a problem on the face, neck, chest, and back when pores become infected or clogged with oil. The bacteria involved are always present on normal skin, so improving the skin's resistance to infection is important. Most cases of acne can be resolved through hygiene and nutrition. Remedies may be helpful during flare-ups, but a constitutional remedy, prescribed by an experienced homeopath, is the most appropriate way to deal with severe or persistent skin problems.

Antimonium tartaricum

This remedy may be helpful for acne with large pustules that are tender to touch, with bluish-red marks that remain on the skin after active infection has passed. The person may be irritable, with low resistance to illness.

Calcarea carbonica

If a person with frequent pimples and skin eruptions is chilly with clammy hands and feet, easily tired by exertion, and flabby or overweight, this remedy may help improve the skin's resistance to infection. People who need this remedy are often very anxious when overworked, and have cravings for sweets and eggs.

Hepar sulphuris calcareum

This remedy may be indicated when the skin is easily infected, slow to heal, and painful eruptions like boils appear. The pimples are very sensitive to touch and slow to come to a head; eventually, offensive-smelling pus may form. A person who needs *Hepar sulph* will usually be chilly, sensitive to cold in any form, and feel irritable and touchy.

Pulsatilla

This remedy can be helpful if acne becomes worse after eating rich or fatty foods, and is aggravated by warmth or heat. It is indicated especially around the time of puberty, or when acne breaks out near menstrual periods. The person often has a fair complexion and is inclined toward childish emotions and moodiness, feeling worse in warm or stuffy rooms and better in fresh air.

Silicea (*also called* Silica)

A person with deep-seated acne, along with a general low immune resistance, swollen lymph nodes, and a

Acne

tendency toward fatigue and nervousness, may benefit from this remedy. Infected spots are slow to come to a head, and also slow to resolve, so may result in scarring. A person who needs this remedy is generally very chilly but inclined to sweat at night.

Sulphur

Itching, sore, inflamed eruptions with reddish or dirty-looking skin often indicate a need for *Sulphur*. Itching may be worse from scratching, and worse from any form of heat—especially bathing or washing. Individuals who need this remedy are often inclined toward convoluted mental notions and tend to give order and neatness a low priority.

See p. 509 for Homeopathy: Dosage Directions.

Remedies for Alcohol Withdrawal Support

Withdrawal from the use of **alcohol** (p. 6) can be a complicated matter. Guidance from a professional can be both physically and emotionally supportive. The following remedies may ease some difficulties during the time that stressful changes are taking place.

Aconitum napellus

If the person is very fearful while going through a withdrawal period, this remedy may be indicated—especially if intense palpitations are experienced, making the person even more frightened and anxious.

Arsenicum album

A person who feels exhausted and extremely chilly, yet is driven by anxiety to move restlessly from place to place, may benefit from this remedy. A person who needs *Arsenicum* may also be obsessive about small details and feel afraid to be alone.

Aurum metallicum

This remedy may be helpful during the withdrawal process, especially for individuals who feel disgusted with themselves, believe they have failed in life, or have become depressed and hopeless. Serious, work-oriented people who have turned to alcohol or other addictive substances as a tension outlet are especially likely to respond to *Aurum*.

Carbo vegetabilis

When withdrawal symptoms include fatigue and faintness, with a lot of gas and belching, this remedy can bring relief. The person may feel weak and very cold (especially in the extremities), yet still has a desperate craving for fresh or moving air. This remedy is often helpful for regaining energy after long-term illnesses or health problems.

Chamomilla

If a person is hypersensitive, and finds discomfort unbearable to the point of seeming irritable and angry, this remedy may help. The person will feel worse from heat and worse at night. Relief from motion, especially vigorous rocking, is a strong indication for *Chamomilla*.

Coffea cruda

This remedy is often helpful when a person's mind is active and excitable. Sleeplessness is a common problem. The person is very sensitive to noise or any distraction. Neuralgic pains or headaches can occur, and may be soothed by cold applications.

Nux vomica

A person who needs this remedy is nervous, irritable, impatient, easily offended, and oversensitive to light, noise, touch, and odors. Chilliness, cramps, and digestive upsets, with an urge to vomit or move the bowels (with limited results) are other indications. *Nux vomica* is known for its beneficial effects on conditions—acute or chronic—related to overuse of alcohol and drugs.

Staphysagria

This remedy may be helpful to a person who has had an abusive relationship or childhood, with deeply suppressed emotions, and has subsequently turned to alcohol. Habitually meek and mild-natured, and very sensitive to humiliation or embarrassment, the person may have started letting the anger out—to the point of throwing things or flying into rages. *Staphysagria* may help a person stay in balance without suppressing feelings.

See p. 509 for Homeopathy: Dosage Directions.

Remedies for Allergies and Sensitivities

Allergy or sensitivity (p. 8) to foods or chemicals can result in fatigue, confusion, anxiety, dizziness, muscle tension, digestive problems, inflammation of mucous membranes, itching, and other discomforts because of an exaggerated immune response. Remedies mentioned here, when they fit the individual, may gradually help a person overcome imbalances. A constitutional remedy, chosen by an experienced homeopath, is usually the best approach.

Arsenicum album

This remedy is useful for people who are highly sensitive to many foods and substances, and respond to them by feeling restless, ill, and exhausted. Asthma and digestive disorders (such as vomiting and diarrhea) are common reactions. Burning sensations relieved by warmth, and thirst for frequent small sips of water can also suggest this remedy. A person who needs *Arsenicum* tends toward strong anxiety, and may have excessive concern over neatness, details, and order.

Calcarea carbonica

This remedy is often helpful to responsible, steady people who become fatigued and overwhelmed. Anxiety may develop, sometimes with fear of heights or claustrophobia. The person is typically chilly, with clammy hands and feet, and has low stamina. Digestive troubles with gas and heartburn are common, especially after eating wheat or dairy products. Swollen lymph nodes and tonsils, head sweats during sleep, shortness of breath from exertion, back pain, dizziness, nightmares, and strong cravings for sweets are often seen. Individuals who need this remedy are sometimes oversensitive to aspirin.

Calcarea phosphorica

Irritability, headaches, stomach and abdominal pains, and a craving for "junk food" are all indications for this remedy. Stiffness in the neck and back, leg cramps, and aggravation from cold are also likely. The person may seem dissatisfied, with a strong desire for travel or a change of circumstances and a tendency to complain when fatigue and health problems interfere. This remedy is often helpful to restless, whiny children who have growing pains, get headaches from school, and have picky appetites with many food problems.

Carbo vegetabilis

A person who reacts to foods or substances with weakness, faintness, chilliness, and indigestion may be helped by this remedy. Bloating, flatulence, and a frequent need to burp are often seen. Breathing may be difficult and, even when feeling very cold, the person has a strong desire for fresh and moving air. Feeling insecure because of weakness, the person may be cross and demanding toward family members. Problems typically are worse in the evening and from talking, eating, or lying down.

Gelsemium

Allergy reactions with flu-like symptoms—weakness, trembling, aching muscles, droopy-looking eyes, and chills along the spine—may indicate a need for this remedy. Headaches in the back of the head and involving the muscles of the neck are common. A person who needs this remedy may seem ill and weak, with a feeling of internal shakiness. Being under pressure to perform (exams, public speaking, etc.) or hearing distressing news can often make things worse both mentally and physically.

Hepar sulphuris calcareum

People who need this remedy are oversensitive to stimuli and substances of many kinds, and can be extremely irritable and touchy, often feeling worse from even slight exposure to cold or drafts. Skin problems, ear infections, or respiratory problems with yellow discharge and offensive sour or cheese-like odors often occur as results of allergy. Because these people feel so deeply vulnerable, they may develop a fear of going out in public. Discouragement about their health can lead to angry outbursts or despair.

Ignatia amara

This remedy is indicated for sensitive, emotional, defensive, idealistic people with a tendency toward mood swings and cramping pains. Cramps are often felt in the stomach and abdomen or in the neck and back. Headaches may feel like a nail driven into the side of the head. A heavy feeling in the chest is often present, and the person may frequently sigh or yawn. People who need this remedy often have "paradoxical" symptoms (such as heartburn improved by eating onions, sore throats improved by swallowing, or joint inflammations improved by touch).

Lycopodium

Food allergy problems with heartburn, gas, and rumbling in the abdomen may indicate a need for this remedy. The person may feel ravenous hunger yet quickly get bloated from eating a very small amount. Fatigue or drowsiness develop after eating, but the person also feels weak from missing meals. Problems are typically the worst in late afternoon and evening. The person may have a chronic worried look, a craving for sweets, a preference for warm drinks, and discomfort felt mostly on the right side of the body.

Allergies and Sensitivties

Natrum carbonicum

This remedy can be helpful to people who have trouble digesting and assimilating many foods and have to stay on restricted diets. Indigestion, heartburn, and ulcers can occur if offending foods are eaten. Milk or dairy products can lead to flatulence or sputtery diarrhea that leaves an empty feeling in the stomach. Cravings for potatoes and sweets are common; also milk, but it makes these people sick, so they usually learn to avoid it. They are sensitive to weather changes and temperatures, as well as foods, and (although they make an effort to be cheerful and considerate) often feel weak and want to be alone to rest.

Natrum muriaticum

A person who needs this remedy can react to allergens in many ways—with headaches, mouth sores, hay fever symptoms, respiratory problems, back pain, or fatigue. Headaches may tend to be worse in late morning and early afternoon, and asthma may be worse in the early evening. Staying in the sun too long can also lead to headache or weakness. These people usually seem reserved, disliking consolation when ill or upset, yet often have deep feelings. A craving for salt and very strong thirst may help to confirm the choice of this remedy.

Nux moschata

If a person reacts to chemical or allergen exposure with an overwhelming feeling of sleepiness—or seems dizzy, giddy, or absent-minded—this remedy should be considered. A very dry mouth, dry eyes, a feeling of weight in the chest, and numbness in the extremities are other indications. Joint pains that move from place to place and stubborn constipation are also possible.

Nux vomica

Irritability, cramping pains, and chilliness are typical when this remedy is needed. Oversensitivity to substances can lead to many ailments—headaches, runny nose, tight breathing, heartburn, stomach problems, constipation, back pain, and insomnia. People who need this remedy are often irritable, impatient, easily angered or frustrated, and have a lot of trouble relaxing. They tend to crave stimulants, alcohol, tobacco, sweets, and strong foods, and feel worse from having them. They are also very sensitive to odors, light, and noise.

Petroleum

A person needing this remedy can be extremely sensitive to fumes from traffic or industry, reacting with headaches, chilliness, diarrhea, and nausea with an empty feeling inside. The person may feel confused, disoriented, or anxious when exposed to toxins. Individuals who need this remedy sometimes develop eczema with inflamed and cracking skin, especially on the palms and fingertips.

Phosphorus

People who need this remedy are usually excitable, imaginative, and sensitive to impressions, having strong anxieties and fears. They react to many foods and substances by becoming tired, "spaced-out," and dizzy, and may have headaches, nosebleeds, respiratory problems, nausea, or diarrhea. The person feels worse from missing meals and better from eating and sleeping well. A strong desire for ice cold drinks, ice cream, and refreshing things can help to confirm the choice of *Phosphorus*.

Silicea (*also called* Silica)

This remedy can be helpful to individuals who have low stamina, are prone to fatigue, and are very sensitive to substances. Resistance to infection may be low and the person may have frequent colds, sore throats, and swollen lymph nodes. Fine hair and skin, weak or brittle nails, and offensive perspiration (especially on the feet) are often seen. People who need this remedy are usually nervous, shy, refined, and fragile, yet also capable and quietly stubborn internally. A strong desire for sweets, and a tendency to be energized by moderate exercise are other traits that fit this remedy.

Sulphuricum acidum

People with intense sensitivity to fumes and environmental toxins may benefit from this remedy. The person has a frantic, hurried feeling and can be scatter-brained and forgetful. Trembling, cold sweat, and headache may also occur. Deep fatigue and a tendency toward easy bruising or bleeding are other indications for this remedy.

See p. 509 for Homeopathy: Dosage Directions.

Remedies for Anxiety

Short periods of **anxiety** (p. 14) are experienced by almost everyone, but some individuals are more inclined to be troubled with this problem. A sensation of discomfort or apprehension is experienced (both emotional and physical) and, although the person may be aware of a reason for feeling insecure or worried, the cause is sometimes difficult to identify. Some individuals experience "panic attacks"—very distressing episodes accompanied by breathing problems, palpitations, and intense (but temporary) feelings of both agitation and helplessness. Homeopathic remedies can often help to soothe anxiety and bring a person's system into better balance.

Aconitum napellus

A panic attack that comes on suddenly with very strong fear (even fear of death) may indicate this remedy. A state of immense anxiety may be accompanied by strong palpitations, shortness of breath, and flushing of the face. Sometimes a shaking experience will be the underlying cause. Strong feelings of anxiety may also occur when a person is just beginning to come down with a flu or cold.

Argentum nitricum

This remedy can be helpful when anxiety develops before a big event: an exam, an important interview, a public appearance or social engagement. Dizziness and diarrhea may also be experienced. People who need this remedy are often enthusiastic and suggestible, with a tendency toward peculiar thoughts and impulses. They often crave sweets and salt (which usually make their symptoms worse).

Arsenicum album

People who are deeply anxious about their health, and extremely concerned with order and security, often benefit from this remedy. Obsessive about small details and very neat, they may feel a desperate need to be in control of everything. Panic attacks often occur around midnight or the very early hours of the morning. The person may feel exhausted yet still be restless—fidgeting, pacing, and anxiously moving from place to place. These people may also have digestive problems or asthma attacks accompanied by anxiety.

Calcarea carbonica

This remedy is usually indicated for dependable, solid people who become overwhelmed from physical illness or too much work and start to fear a breakdown. Their thoughts can be muddled and confused when tired, which adds to the anxiety. Worry and bad news may agitate them, and a nagging dread of disaster (to themselves or others) may develop. Fear of heights and claustrophobia are also common. A person who needs this remedy is often chilly and sluggish, has a craving for sweets, and is easily fatigued.

Gelsemium

Feelings of weakness, trembling, and mental dullness (being "paralyzed by fear") suggest a need for this remedy. It is often helpful when a person has stage fright about a public performance or interview, or feels anxious before a test, a visit to the dentist, or any stressful event. Chills, perspiration, diarrhea, and headaches will often occur with nervousness. Fear of crowds, a fear of falling, and even a fear that the heart might stop are other indications for *Gelsemium*.

Ignatia amara

A sensitive person who is anxious because of grief, loss, disappointment, criticism, loneliness (or any stressful emotional experience) may benefit from this remedy. A defensive attitude, frequent sighing, and mood swings are other indications. The person may burst unexpectedly into either tears or laughter. Headaches that feel like a nail driven into the side of the head, and cramping pains in the abdomen or back, are often seen when this remedy is needed.

Kali phosphoricum

When a person has been exhausted by overwork or illness and feels a deep anxiety and inability to cope, this remedy may help. The person is jumpy and oversensitive, and may be startled by ordinary sounds. Hearing unpleasant news or thinking of world events can aggravate the problems. Insomnia and an inability to concentrate may develop, increasing the sense of nervous dread. Eating, warmth, and rest often bring relief. Headaches, backaches, and nervous digestive upsets are often seen when this remedy is needed.

Lycopodium

Individuals likely to respond to this remedy feel anxiety from mental stress and suffer from a lack of confidence. They can be self-conscious and feel intimidated by people they perceive as powerful (yet may also swagger or be domineering toward those with whom they feel more comfortable). Taking on responsibility can cause a deep anxiety and fear of failure, although the person usually does well, once started on a task. Claustrophobia, irritability, digestive upsets with gas and bloating, and a craving for sweets are often seen when this remedy is needed.

Natrum muriaticum

Deep emotions and a self-protective shyness can make these people seem reserved, aloof, and private. Even when feeling lonely, they tend to stay away from social situations, not knowing what to say or do. (Inhibitions sometimes leave completely if they turn to alcohol, which makes them feel embarrassed afterwards.) Easily hurt and offended, they can brood, bear grudges, dwell on unhappy feelings, and isolate themselves—refusing consolation even when they

Anxiety

want it. However, they are often sympathetic listeners to other people's problems. Claustrophobia, anxiety at night (with fears of robbers or intruders), migraines, and insomnia are often seen when this remedy is needed.

Phosphorus

People who need this remedy are open-hearted, imaginative, excitable, easily startled, and full of intense and vivid fears. Strong anxiety can be triggered by thinking of almost anything. Nervous and sensitive to others, they can overextend themselves with sympathy to the point of feeling exhausted and "spaced out" or even getting ill. They want a lot of company and reassurance, often feeling better from conversation or a back rub. Easy flushing of the face, palpitations, thirst, and a strong desire for cold, refreshing foods are other indications for *Phosphorus*.

Pulsatilla

People who need this remedy often express anxiety as insecurity and clinginess, with a need for constant support and comforting. The person may be moody, tearful, whiny, even emotionally childish. (*Pulsatilla* is a very useful remedy for children.) Getting too warm or being in a stuffy room often increases anxiety. Fresh air and gentle exercise can bring relief. Anxiety around the time of hormonal changes (puberty, menstrual periods, or menopause) often is helped with *Pulsatilla*.

Silicea (*also called* Silica)

People who need this remedy are capable and serious, yet are also nervous, shy, and subject to bouts of temporary loss of confidence. Anxiety can be extreme when they are faced with a public appearance, interview, examination, or any new job or task. Worry and overwork can bring on headaches, difficulty concentrating, and states of exhaustion, oversensitivity, and dread. Responsible and diligent, they often overreact and devote attention to tiny details—making their worries (and their work) more difficult. They often have low stamina and come down with colds, sore throats, or other illnesses after working hard or being under stress.

See p. 509 for Homeopathy: Dosage Directions.

Remedies for Asthma

People suffering from **asthma** (p. 15) often have allergic tendencies; a genetic predisposition is common. Constitutional homeopathic care (with the guidance of an experienced professional) can help to improve a person's general health on deeper levels and possibly reduce the tendency toward asthma. Correctly chosen remedies can help reduce distress during asthma attacks; however, emergency medical care must be sought in any serious attack. If a person has great difficulty breathing, looks very pale, has bluish lips, or seems to be very weak or in danger of losing consciousness, seek a doctor's help immediately.

Arsenicum album

A person needing this remedy can feel exhausted, yet be very restless and anxious. Breathing problems tend to be worse while lying down, better when sitting up, and may begin, or be the most intense, between midnight and 2:00 A.M. Dry wheezing may progress to a cough that brings up frothy whitish fluid. The person can be thirsty, taking frequent tiny sips. General chilliness is usually seen, with burning pains in the chest and heat in the head. Warmth often brings improvement.

Carbo vegetabilis

This remedy may be indicated when a person feels weak or faint with a hollow sensation in the chest. Coughing jags can lead to gagging. The person may be very cold (especially hands and feet), yet feel a need for moving air, wanting to sit beside a fan or open window. Gas and digestive upset are also likely, and sitting up and burping offers some relief. Feeling worse in the evening, and worse from talking, eating, or lying down are other indications for this remedy.

Chamomilla

Asthma with a dry, hard, irritating cough that starts after being exposed to wind, or after becoming overexcited and angry, may be helped with this remedy. The cough is often worse around 9:00 P.M., and may continue into the night. The person seems hypersensitive and may be extremely irritable and agitated. (Children may even shriek and hit, though they often calm down if someone carries them.)

Ipecacuanha

Coughing spasms that lead to retching or vomiting strongly indicate this remedy. Wheezing can come on suddenly with a feeling of suffocation and heaviness in the chest. Mucus collects in breathing tubes, but the person has difficulty coughing much out. The person may sweat a lot and feel clammy or nauseous, be worse from motion, and sometimes worse from warmth.

Natrum sulphuricum

This remedy is sometimes indicated when asthma attacks are brought on by exposure to mold and dampness. The person may hold the chest while coughing, because it feels so weak. Wheezing and breathing difficulties are aggravated by exertion, and episodes tend to be worse in the very early morning.

Nux vomica

Indications for this remedy include a tense, constricted feeling in the chest during asthma attacks, with pressure in the stomach. Problems are often worse in the morning. Overindulgence in stimulants, alcohol, sweets, or strong spicy food can bring on or aggravate an episode. Both physical effort and mental exertion can make things worse, and warmth and sleep often bring relief. A person needing this remedy is typically very irritable and impatient, with a general feeling of chilliness.

Pulsatilla

Wheezing that starts when a person gets too warm (especially in a stuffy room), or after eating rich food, can indicate this remedy. Coughing brings up yellow-colored mucus, with gagging and choking. Tightness in the chest tends to be worse in the evening and at night, and is relieved by cool fresh air. A person who needs this remedy is likely to be changeable and emotional, wanting a lot of attention and comforting. (*Pulsatilla* is often useful in children's illnesses.)

Spongia tosta

A hard or "barking" cough during an asthma attack is a strong indication for this remedy. Breathing can be labored, with a sawing sound, and not much mucus is produced. The person may feel best when sitting up and tilting the head back, or when leaning forward. Warm drinks may be helpful. The problems often start while the person is asleep (typically before midnight). *Spongia* is often used in croup, as well.

See p. 509 for Homeopathy: Dosage Directions.

Remedies for Athletic Performance/Injury Support

During **athletic training** (p. 20), development of stamina and skill can be encouraged by a constitutional remedy—chosen by an experienced homeopath to fit the individual and to help the body work effi-ciently. Remedies listed here may help prevent and ease the aches and pains of physical exertion, and are useful as first aid for injuries. If any pain or injury seems serious, a medical practitioner should be consulted.

Arnica montana

Homeopathic *Arnica* is helpful for bruising, tissue-damage, shock, and soreness. If taken shortly after an injury occurs, both pain and swelling may be reduced, and healing can take place more quickly and efficiently. Conditions needing *Arnica* are usually worse from touch and heat. For sprains or deeper injuries that require days or weeks to heal, another remedy may follow *Arnica*. (Some athletes take *Arnica* "preventively" before a workout, to reduce the tendency toward soreness. Gels and ointments containing the herbal form or very low dilutions may be soothing to sore muscles.)

Bellis perennis

This remedy is often indicated for injuries resulting from collisions, falls, and twisting or wrenching motions that occur in active sports. It is especially indicated for bruising injuries involving the abdomen, trunk, and pelvis or deeper body areas. *Bellis perennis* may also be given for bruising, sprains, or strains when *Arnica* has been tried without significant result. Aggravation from soaking, or from wet applications, is another indication for this remedy.

Hypericum performatum

Injuries to nerve-rich parts of the body (such as smashed fingertips or toes, a blow to the back, or a fall on the tailbone) often are relieved by this remedy. Shooting pains and muscle cramping may be felt around the injured area.

Ledum palustre

This remedy is indicated for sprains and other injuries with pain and puffy swelling that are greatly relieved by ice, cold soaks, or cold applications. Ankles injured in the past that swell from overuse may also be helped with *Ledum*.

Rhus toxicodendron

This remedy is very useful for limbering up after overuse of joints and muscles. The area feels extremely stiff and painful on initial movement, improving as motion continues. Warm applications and hot baths or showers also bring relief. *Rhus tox* is usually indicated for injuries in later stages, after acute inflammation and swelling have passed.

Athletic Performance/Injury Support

Ruta graveolens

This remedy is indicated when overuse of muscles and tendons leads to remarkable stiffness. Injuries involving tendons, ligaments, and periosteum (the tissue that covers the bones) are likely to respond. It should be considered for injuries of elbows, wrists, and knees that feel stiff and sore and are slow to heal. Repeated injury or overuse that has led to thickening or even hardened growths on connective tissues, may also be helped with *Ruta*.

Sarcolactic acid

This remedy is sometimes used to ease muscular soreness and fatigue caused by overexertion. It may also help to relieve the cramps or spasms that occur after intense exercise.

See p. 509 for Homeopathy: Dosage Directions.

Remedies for Backache

Many different factors can contribute to back pain. Injury, overwork, emotional and mental stress, menstrual tension, prostate conditions, and problems with posture or weight are common causes. Homeopathy can offer safe and effective pain relief for many kinds of backaches. If problems are extreme, consult a licensed health-care professional with experience in spinal care.

Aesculus hippocastanum

Pain in the very low back (the sacral or sacroiliac areas) that feels worse when standing up from a sitting position, and worse from stooping, may be eased with this remedy. *Aesculus* is especially indicated for people with low back pain who also have a tendency toward venous congestion and hemorrhoids.

Arnica montana

When back pain results from a strain or injury, *Arnica* should usually be taken first. The affected area feels bruised and sore, and tissues around the joints may be tender or swollen. Cold applications may help to bring relief. Soreness related to heavy lifting, engaging in active sports, or any unaccustomed physical exertion may also respond to this remedy. (Ointments and gels made with Arnica, in herbal form or low dilutions, can also be soothing when applied to injured areas; topical Arnica should not be used on scraped or broken skin.)

Bryonia

This remedy is indicated when back pain is worse from even the slightest motion. Changing position, coughing, turning, or walking may bring on sharp, excruciating pain. This remedy can be helpful for back pain after injury and backaches during illness.

Calcarea carbonica

This remedy is often useful for low back pain and muscle weakness, especially in a person who is chilly, flabby or overweight, and easily tired by exertion. Chronic low back pain and muscle weakness may lead to inflammation and soreness that are aggravated by dampness and cold.

Calcarea phosphorica

Stiffness and soreness of the spinal muscles and joints, especially in the neck and upper back, may be relieved by this remedy. The person feels worse from drafts and cold, as well as from exertion. Aching in the bones and feelings of weariness and dissatisfaction are often seen in people who need this remedy.

Cimicifuga
(*also called* Actaea racemosa)

Severe aching and stiffness in the upper back and neck, as well as the lower back—with pains that extend down the thighs or across the hips—may be eased with this remedy. It is often helpful for back pain during menstrual periods, with cramping, heaviness, and soreness. A person who needs this remedy typically is talkative and energetic, becoming agitated or depressed when ill.

Dulcamara

If back pain sets in during cold damp weather, along with catching a cold, or after getting wet and chilled, this remedy may be indicated. Stiffness and chills can be felt in the back, and pain is usually worse from stooping.

Ignatia amara

Back pains related to emotional upsets—especially grief—will often respond to this remedy. The person may have spasms in the muscles of the lower back and twitches, drawing pains, and cramps often occur in other areas.

Kali carbonicum

This remedy may be indicated if low back pain drives the person out of bed at night, making it necessary to get up to be able to turn over. Pain is usually worse on the right side of the lower back, worse around the menstrual period, and aggravated by sitting and by walking. Pressure on the area often brings relief.

Natrum muriaticum

Back pain that improves from lying on something hard or pressing a hard object (such as a block or book) against the painful area suggests a need for this remedy. The person often seems reserved or formal, but has strong emotions that are kept from others. Back pain from suppressed emotions, especially hurt or anger, may respond to *Natrum muriaticum*.

Nux vomica

When this remedy is indicated, muscle cramps or constricting pains may be felt in the back. Discomfort is made worse by cold and relieved by warmth. Pain will usually be worse at night, and the person may have to sit up in bed to turn over. Backache is also worse during constipation, and the pain is aggravated when the person feels the urge to move the bowels.

Rhus toxicodendron

This remedy can be useful for pain in the neck and shoulders as well as the lower back, when the pain is worse on initial movement and improves with continued motion. Even though in pain, the person finds it hard to lie down or stay still for very long, and often restlessly paces about. Aching and stiffness are aggravated in cold damp weather and relieved by warm applications, baths or showers, and massage.

Ruta graveolens

This remedy is indicated when tremendous stiffness is felt in the muscles or joints, especially after sprains or twisting injuries. The person feels lame and sore, and experiences relief from lying down.

Sulphur

This remedy is often indicated when a person with back pain has a slouching posture. The back is weak and the person feels much worse from standing up for any length of time. Pain is also worse from stooping. Warmth may aggravate the pain and inflammation.

See p. 509 for Homeopathy: Dosage Directions.

Remedies for Bell's Palsy

When Bell's palsy occurs, one side of the face becomes paralyzed, flat, and rigid; as a result, the other side (not paralyzed) may feel twisted and uncomfortable. The cause is not well understood, but a person with these symptoms should be examined by a physician, to rule out other neurological problems. Although uncomfortable and disconcerting, this condition usually resolves itself in time, although it may take many months. Homeopathic remedies can sometimes bring relief. For a remedy that suits the situation more specifically, see a homeopathic physician.

Aconitum napellus

When one side of a person's face becomes paralyzed, especially after being exposed to wind or cold air, this remedy may be helpful. A feeling of fear and agitation and a sudden onset of symptoms are strong indications for *Aconitum napellus*.

Agaricus

This remedy may be indicated in Bell's palsy when the facial muscles on one side are stiff, and grimacing or twitching occurs in other parts of the face. People who need this remedy are often excitable, with senses that are overly acute. Many people who need this remedy have deep anxiety about their health.

Cadmium sulphuratum

Facial paralysis (usually left-sided) that starts after exposure to wind, and is accompanied by chilliness or overwhelming weakness, suggests a need for this remedy. The person's mouth may look distorted, and it is often impossible to completely close one of the eyes.

Causticum

This remedy can be helpful when facial paralysis has developed gradually (most often on the right side). Opening and closing the mouth can be difficult, and the person may accidentally bite the tongue or the inside of the cheek. The person may be weak but restless, and tends to feel best when keeping warm.

Cocculus

One-sided facial paralysis, with pain or tension felt in the other cheek, especially when opening the mouth, suggests a need for this remedy. Weakness, dizziness, or numbness are other indications. The person may feel worse from lack of sleep or from being emotionally upset.

Dulcamara

This remedy may be indicated when a person has one-sided facial paralysis that makes it difficult to speak. *Dulcamara* is indicated in many conditions that develop after exposure to cold and dampness, especially after chills in rainy weather. People who need this remedy are often inclined toward sinusitis, allergies, and back pain.

Nux vomica

One-sided facial paralysis (more often on the left) in a person who is irritable, impatient, and hypersensitive to odors, sounds, and light may indicate a need for this remedy. Cramping and constricting sensations may be felt, and problems may be worse from cold.

Platina (*also called* Platinum)

This remedy may be indicated for painless paralysis of the face, with facial distortion that raises one eyebrow or creates a "haughty" look. The person may also experience numbness in the lips and cheeks, or other body parts.

See p. 509 for Homeopathy: Dosage Directions.

Remedies for Boils

A boil is an inflamed, hard, tender, infected lump or pocket that forms in the skin or underlying tissue. Bacteria that are present on healthy skin are usually involved—which means a person with boils has low resistance to infection. Homeopathic remedies can be useful for reducing the discomfort and promoting healing. If infection is severe or spreads, the person should seek a doctor's care.

Arsenicum album

This remedy is useful for deeply infected boils with intensely burning pain and offensive discharge. Warmth and hot applications will usually be soothing. The person may feel exhausted and ill, yet anxiety and discomfort also make them restless.

Belladonna

This remedy is often indicated in early stages of inflammation, before much pus has formed. The area is red, hot, throbbing, and tender, often with intense or stabbing pains. Jarring or touch may increase discomfort. The person may also feel excitable or feverish.

Calendula

This remedy is often helpful as a topical application for boils and infected sores. It can be used in herbal form or in low dilution as a tincture, ointment, or compress. Taken internally, *Calendula* can help the body overcome infection.

Echinacea angustifolia

This well-known herb is often used to help the immune system overcome infection. In homeopathic form, it will sometimes help a person with recurring boils. People who need this remedy typically feel sickly, lethargic, achy, and chilly.

Hepar sulphuris calcareum

When a boil is extremely tender and sensitive to touch, this remedy can be helpful. A splinter-like, sticking pain is often felt. The boil may produce deep pockets of offensive pus or be slow to heal. This remedy is also indicated when boils seem to be spreading. A person who needs this remedy will usually be vulnerable and touchy, with extreme sensitivity to cold.

Mercurius solubilis

This remedy is indicated when boils are very sensitive with advanced development of pus. The person may have moist or greasy-looking skin, with swollen lymph nodes and offensive breath, and be very sensitive to changes in temperature. Warmth may aggravate the pain.

Silicea (*also called* Silica)

Boils that form hard lumps and are slow to come to a head and slow to heal suggest a need for this remedy. If many boils form at once, or boils frequently recur, it is often very useful. People who need this remedy are sensitive and nervous, inclined toward colds and swollen glands, and easily fatigued.

Tarentula cubensis

This remedy may be indicated when a boil is sore and swollen with stinging, burning pain, and purplish or bluish discoloration of surrounding tissues. A person who needs this remedy may also have restless feet and difficulty sleeping.

See p. 509 for Homeopathy: Dosage Directions.

Remedies for Broken Bone Support

If an injury involving a bone is very painful, and the person has difficulty moving the body part or bearing weight on it, the bone could be fractured. A doctor's care should always be sought because correct assessment and proper setting of a fracture is very important for healing. Homeopathic remedies can ease the pain and swelling associated with broken bones, as well as help to accelerate the healing process.

Arnica montana

This remedy is useful for reducing the pain and swelling that accompany any new injury, and should be taken as soon as possible after a break occurs. It may also be helpful in calming the person, since breaking a bone is traumatic as well as painful. Doses may be taken frequently, according to how the person feels. *Arnica* may be used for several days while pain and soreness are prominent. Another remedy may be indicated later, to encourage proper healing of the bones and surrounding tissues.

Bryonia

This remedy may help to bring relief if excruciating pain results from even the slightest motion. The person usually wants to remain completely still and not be touched or interfered with.

Calcarea phosphorica

This is a useful remedy for aching and soreness in bones and joints, especially when the area feels cold and numb. It can help relieve the pain of fractures and bone bruises, and encourages repair and strengthening if a fracture is slow to heal.

Eupatorium perfoliatum

This remedy is well known for its use in flu and fever when the bones are extremely painful ("as if broken") and is also useful to relieve the deep or aching pain of actual broken bones.

Hypericum perforatum

This remedy is very useful for crushing injuries to body areas that are well supplied with nerves. If smashed fingertips or toes are severe enough to traumatize the bones, *Hypericum* can be a welcome form of pain relief.

Ruta graveolens

This remedy is known for its effect on bone bruises and on injuries to the periosteum (the covering of the bones); both of these types of trauma are involved when a fracture of a bone occurs. *Ruta* is also indicated when the pain around a fracture is extreme, and the person feels lame or weak. This remedy is also helpful in many cases when pain persists after taking *Arnica*.

Symphytum officinale

This remedy is best known for helping broken bones rejoin and heal. It should be taken after a bone is set to ensure proper joining of the bone. (A common recommendation is to take it several times in the first few days, then once a week while the bone is healing.) It is also useful in many cases when pain persists in old, healed fractures.

See p. 509 for Homeopathy: Dosage Directions.

Remedies for Bronchitis

Bronchitis occurs when the mucous membranes that line the upper breathing tubes become inflamed. Acute bronchitis often follows a viral illness such as a cold or flu, and can last for several weeks. Chronic bronchitis may develop if a person has repeated bouts of illness that are not well cared for, or if other factors such as smoking, exposure to polluted air, and allergies have lowered the person's resistance and made the lungs susceptible. Homeopathic remedies may help relieve discomfort caused by coughing and help the body overcome infection. Serious or prolonged bronchitis requires a physician's attention.

Antimonium tartaricum

When this remedy is indicated, the person has a feeling of wet mucus in the chest, and breathing can make a bubbly, rattling sound. The cough takes effort and is often not quite strong enough to bring the mucus up, although burping and spitting may be of help. The person may feel drowsy or dizzy, and feel better when lying on the right side or sitting up.

Bryonia

This remedy is often indicated when a cough is dry and very painful. The person feels worse from any movement, and may even need to hold his or her sides or press against the chest to keep it still. The cough can make the stomach hurt, and digestion may be upset. A very dry mouth is common, and the person may be thirsty. A person who wants to be left alone when ill, and not talked to or disturbed, is likely to need *Bryonia*.

Calcarea carbonica

This remedy is often indicated for bronchitis after a cold. The cough can be troublesome and tickling, worse from lying down or stooping forward, worse from getting cold, and worse at night. Children may have fever, sweaty heads while sleeping, and be very tired. Adults may feel more chilly and have clammy hands and feet, breathing problems when walking up slopes or climbing stairs, and generally poor stamina.

Causticum

Bronchitis with a deep, hard, racking cough can indicate a need for this remedy. The person feels that mucus is stuck in the throat and upper chest, and may cough continually to try to loosen it. A feeling of rawness and soreness can develop, or a sensation as if a rock is stuck inside. Chills can occur along with fever. Exposure to cool air aggravates the cough, but drinking something cold can help. The person may feel worse when days are cold and clear, and better in wet weather.

Dulcamara

When a person easily gets ill after being wet and chilled (or when the weather changes from warm and dry to wet and cool), this remedy may be indicated. The cough can be tickly, hoarse, and loose, and worse from physical exertion. Tendencies toward allergies (to cats or pollen, for example) may increase the person's susceptibility to bronchitis.

Hepar sulphuris calcareum

The cough that fits this remedy is usually hoarse and rattling, with yellow mucus coming up. The person can be extremely sensitive to cold—even a minor draft or an arm out from under the covers may set off jags of coughing. Cold food or drink can make things worse. A person who needs this remedy feels vulnerable both physically and emotionally, and may act extremely irritable and out of sorts.

Kali bichromicum

A metallic, brassy, hacking cough that starts with a troublesome tickling in the upper air tubes and brings up strings of sticky yellow mucus can indicate this remedy. A sensation of coldness may be felt inside the chest, and coughing can lead to pain behind the breast bone or extending to the shoulders. Breathing may make a rattling sound when the person sleeps. Problems are typically worse in the early morning, after eating and drinking, and from exposure to open air. The person may feel best just lying in bed and keeping warm.

Pulsatilla

Bronchitis with a feeling of weight in the chest, and a cough with choking and gagging that brings up thick yellow mucus, may respond to this remedy. The cough tends to be dry and tight at night, and loose in the morn-

ing. The fever may be worse in the evening and at night. Feeling too warm or being in a stuffy room tends to make the person worse, and open air brings improvement. Thirst is usually low. A person who needs this remedy will often be moody and emotional, wanting much attention and sympathy. (This remedy is often helpful to children who are tearful when not feeling well and want to be held and comforted.)

Silicea (*also called* Silica)

A person who needs this remedy can have bronchitis for weeks at a stretch, or even all winter long. The cough takes effort and may bring up yellow or greenish mucus, or little granules that have an offensive smell. Stitching pains may be felt in the back when the person is coughing. Chills are felt more than heat during fever, and the person is likely to sweat at night. A person who needs this remedy is usually sensitive and nervous, with low stamina, swollen lymph nodes, and poor resistance to infection.

Sulphur

This remedy can be indicated when a person has had many bouts of bronchitis. (Sometimes the resistance has been weakened by taking antibiotics too often for minor complaints.) The cough feels irritating, burning, and painful; yellow or greenish mucus may be produced. Problems can be worse if the person gets too warm in bed, and breathing problems at night may wake the person up. Redness of the eyes and mucous membranes, and foul-smelling breath and perspiration are often seen when a person needs this remedy.

See p. 509 for Homeopathy: Dosage Directions.

Remedies for Bruising

Homeopathic remedies, used as first aid, can soothe the pain and soreness of **bruising** (p. 28) that comes from injury, reduce swelling and fluid leakage into surrounding tissues, and generally encourage healing. A carefully chosen remedy may also help correct a person's tendency toward easy bruising and soreness. (Frequent bruising or easy bleeding can sometimes occur in a serious illness or disorder.)

Arnica montana

This is the primary remedy for new, traumatic injuries—including bruises caused by impact with blunt objects (from simple contusions to concussions), early stages of sprains and strains, and bruise-like soreness after muscular exertion (such as physically taxing work, athletic activity, or childbirth). The symptoms typically feel worse from touch and motion. *Arnica* is also helpful for controlling soreness, bleeding, and tissue bruising related to surgery and dental work.

Bellis perennis

This remedy is helpful for injuries and bruises, especially those caused by trauma to the trunk or in deeper tissues—for example, internal soreness after an accident or surgery. When a bruised and injured area develops a feeling of stiffness or coldness, *Bellis perennis* is strongly indicated. It may also be effective for bruises (in any area) that do not respond to *Arnica*.

Calcarea phosphorica

This remedy is often indicated for bone bruises, as well as other kinds of pain and soreness in the bones, especially when the area feels cold and numb. This remedy is also used when fractures are slow to heal.

Hypericum perforatum

This remedy is best for bruising or crushing injuries to body areas containing many nerves—smashed fingertips and toes, injuries to the spine or genitals, bruising or displacement of the tailbone (from falls or during childbirth), and injuries to the eyeball. Nerve pain after root canals may also be helped with *Hypericum*.

Ledum palustre

This remedy is indicated when bruises or bruise-type injuries such as sprains and strains become very puffy and swollen, and cold applications such as ice packs or cold soaks bring some relief. Black eyes (which usually meet those two criteria) often respond to *Ledum*.

Millefolium

This remedy is indicated when bruising is followed by persistent bleeding. It is often useful for nosebleeds after injury, as well as for bleeding in other parts of the body. (Any condition involving serious bleeding should be treated by a physician.)

Phosphorus

This remedy may be indicated when small wounds bleed easily and profusely, or when a person has a tendency to bruise from minor injuries. Tiny red dots may be seen beneath the skin on arms and legs or other areas. (If these have recently appeared or if bleeding is significant, the person should see a physician.)

Ruta graveolens

This remedy is helpful for bone bruises when the area is very sensitive to touch. The bone aches and may

seem lame, and the person can feel weak. *Ruta* is useful after *Arnica* in many injuries affecting the joints and bone coverings.

Symphytum officinale

This remedy is well known for its healing effect on broken bones, and is also good for bone bruises. *Symphytum* is valuable when the eyeball has been injured by a blow from any blunt object—such as a stick, a rock, or a flying ball. (Any injury to the eye should be examined by a doctor.)

Sulphuricum acidum

When a person feels tired after a bruising injury, this remedy may be indicated. A professional homeopath may consider it for a person who tends toward easy bruising and is extra-sensitive to fumes and environmental toxins. (Any person with a tendency toward unusual bruising and bleeding should consult a physician.)

See p. 509 for Homeopathy: Dosage Directions.

Remedies for Burns

Homeopathic remedies can help to soothe the pain of **burns** (p. 29) and reduce the chance of blistering. Burns require immediate attention to prevent further tissue damage, so cold applications and natural remedies should always be close at hand. Burns—even minor ones—can cause some degree of shock, and care should be taken that the person rests. Any serious burn should have emergency attention from a physician. (Remedies can be used while en route to medical care.)

Arnica montana

This is a valuable first-aid remedy to help reduce pain and swelling and prevent the onset of shock after any injury. Another remedy that is more specific to the burn should be considered after *Arnica*.

Cantharis

This remedy is indicated for extreme burning pain, when the person is very intense and restless. It is often useful in reducing or preventing blister formation. *Cantharis* can help with any burn, but is most often indicated for severe ones (second or third degree).

Causticum

If a burn is intensely painful and blisters seem to be forming, this remedy may help to bring relief. The person often feels more sad than restless from the pain. Rawness and soreness may develop in the injured area. *Causticum* is also helpful when pain remains in older burns, or when burns have not completely healed.

Hepar sulphuris calcareum

This remedy is helpful for treating very sensitive and painful burns in people who are prone to infection. The person may feel extremely vulnerable and irritable, and may have chills or be very sensitive to cold.

Hypericum perforatum

This remedy is often helpful when the pain of a burn is intense and the nerves are extremely sensitive. Along with the usual discomfort of a burn, stabbing or shooting pains may be felt in the injured area.

Phosphorus

This remedy may be useful for the pain of electrical burns, taken on the way to medical care. (When electrical burns occur, the damaged area may look small on the surface, but can be more extensive underneath. Electrical burns should always be examined by a doctor.)

Urtica urens

When a burn is mild and the primary symptoms are redness and stinging pain, this remedy often brings relief. It is often useful for sunburn when the pain is prickly and stinging.

Calendula and Hypericum Tinctures

These tinctures (used topically in unpotentized herbal form) often are helpful in soothing burns and promoting tissue healing. Ten drops of either Calendula or Hypericum tincture, or both, may be mixed in an ounce of water and applied to the area several times per day.

See p. 509 for Homeopathy: Dosage Directions.

Remedies for Bursitis

Bursitis (p. 30) is painful inflammation of a bursa (a fluid-filled sac that cushions a body site that is subject to pressure and friction). It is most often seen in the shoulder, but is also common in elbows, knees, hips, heels, and other areas. The cause of bursitis is often overuse, but injury or infection may also be involved. Homeopathic remedies often help to ease discomfort.

Arnica montana

This remedy is especially useful when bursitis is related to traumatic injury or strain. The affected area feels bruised and sore, and the person tries to avoid being touched, because of pain.

Belladonna

Bursitis with a sensation of heat and throbbing, along with intense discomfort caused by jarring and touch, suggests a need for this remedy. The area often is red and swollen, and the overlying skin feels hot.

Bryonia

When bursitis pain has a stitching or tearing quality and is worse from even the slightest motion, this remedy is a likely choice. The affected area is hot and swollen, feeling worse from warmth.

Ferrum phosphoricum

Inflammation, especially in the right shoulder—with pain that extends to the wrist, or sometimes to the neck—may be soothed by this remedy. Gentle motion and cool applications often bring relief. The person's face may be flushed and pinkish.

Kalmia latifolia

Pain that starts in a higher joint (especially the hip or shoulder), and shoots or travels downward, suggests a need for this remedy. Right shoulder bursitis is common and extends to the elbow, wrist, or hand. Pain and inflammation may come on suddenly, and often shift around. Discomfort is worse from motion, worse at night, and has a neuralgic character.

Rhus toxicodendron

This remedy is helpful to those who experience stiffness and pain on initial movement, gradually improving as motion continues—although too much motion can also aggravate the pain. Pain is often worse during sleep and on waking in the morning. Cold, damp weather can increase the problems, and warm applications and baths bring relief.

Ruta graveolens

If bursitis is acute—with swelling, great stiffness, and aching pain—this remedy may be indicated. Problems can be aggravated by stretching, and the person often feels fatigued or weak. Cold and dampness make things worse, and lying down to rest may help. This remedy is often useful for bursitis after injuries.

Sanguinaria canadensis

This remedy is often indicated for bursitis in the shoulder—especially the right shoulder. Raising the arm is difficult, and pain can extend down the arm if the shoulder is moved. Discomfort may be worse at night in bed, from lying on the affected part, and also when turning over. Flushing of the face and a tendency toward allergies or migraines are often seen in people who need *Sanguinaria*.

Sulphur

This remedy may be indicated for bursitis—especially on the left side—with inflammation and burning pain. Symptoms will be aggravated by warmth and bathing. A person needing *Sulphur* often has a slouching posture and feels worse from standing up for extended lengths of time.

See p. 509 for Homeopathy: Dosage Directions.

Remedies for Canker Sores

Painful mouth ulcers (also called canker sores) often break out during times of stress. They may be related to nutritional deficiencies or allergies to foods and other substances. Homeopathic remedies can ease the pain of canker sores, reduce inflammation, and help the tissues heal.

Arsenicum album

A person who breaks out in burning, painful mouth sores, and also feels anxious and tired, is likely to benefit from this remedy. Hot drinks often ease the pain, and the person feels best when keeping warm. People who need this remedy often have unhealthy, easily bleeding gums, and tend to be extremely neat and tense.

Borax

This remedy is often helpful when canker sores feel hot and sensitive. Acidic foods—especially citrus fruits—may be irritating. Sores may break out on the inside of the cheeks, on the gums, and on the tongue. The person may produce profuse saliva, yet still feel dry inside the mouth. People needing *Borax* are often very sensitive to noise and inclined toward motion sickness.

Calcarea carbonica

This remedy is often indicated when infants and small children have recurring canker sores. A child who needs this remedy may also have head sweats during sleep, and be slow to teethe or learn to walk. *Calcarea carbonica* may help with canker sores in adults who are chilly, stout, and easily fatigued.

Hepar sulphuris calcareum

If a person develops painful mouth sores that become infected—with pus formation, extreme sensitivity, and aggravation from cold drinks—this remedy may be indicated. A person needing *Hepar sulph* often feels extremely chilly, vulnerable, and oversensitive.

Mercurius solubilis

Bleeding gums, a swollen coated tongue, and offensive breath are seen along with canker sores when this remedy is needed. The painful, burning sores feel worse at night, and salivation is profuse, with drooling during sleep. The person tends to sweat at night and is very sensitive to any change in temperature.

Natrum muriaticum

Pearly sores that erupt inside the mouth, especially on the gums or tongue, may respond to this remedy. The mouth feels dry, and the tongue may have a tingling feeling. People who need this remedy often are troubled by cold sores around the corners of the mouth or chin, and have chapped or cracking lips. A craving for salt, strong thirst, and a tendency to feel worse from being in the sun are other indications for *Natrum muriaticum*.

Nux vomica

A person who needs this remedy may break out in canker sores after overindulging in sweets, strong spicy foods, stimulants, or alcoholic beverages. The sores are often small, and the person may have swollen gums, a coated tongue, and bloody salivation. Irritability, impatience, and a general chilliness are often seen when this remedy is needed.

Sulphur

This remedy may be helpful for sores that are painful, red and inflamed, with burning pain that is worse from warm drinks and aggravated by heat of any kind. The mouth may have a bitter taste, and the gums can be swollen and throbbing. A person who needs this remedy often has reddish lips and mucous membranes, and a tendency toward itching and skin irritations.

See p. 509 for Homeopathy: Dosage Directions.

Canker Sores

Remedies for Carpal Tunnel Syndrome

Carpal tunnel syndrome is a condition of the forearm and wrist that comes from overuse or stress, causing nerve compression that leads to weakness, pain, and restricted movement. Working at a keyboard, typing, carpentry, and other tasks that require repetitive motions of the wrists and hands are common causes. Sensations of numbness, tingling, and burning may be felt, and pain or weakness can affect the arm and neck. Homeopathic remedies often help to relieve discomfort and limitation.

Arnica montana

This remedy can be used for flare-ups of inflammation or new injuries caused by repetitive use of the fingers and wrists. The area feels bruised and sore, and cramping may occur. External application of herbal Arnica lotion or ointment may help to ease the swelling and soreness, while other remedies are used internally.

Calcarea phosphorica

When this remedy is indicated, pain is felt in the bones and nerves of the wrists and arms, and stiffness and discomfort may also involve the neck. Cold and drafts often aggravate discomfort. The person may feel irritable and sensitive, or weak from overwork and pain.

Causticum

This remedy is useful when carpal tunnel syndrome is long-lasting or recurring. The area feels bruised, with drawing, burning pains. Stiffness and a feeling of weakness and contraction may be felt in the muscles of the hand and forearm. The condition is worse from getting cold and improved by warm applications. People who need this remedy often feel best in rainy weather.

Guaiacum

This remedy is indicated in carpal tunnel syndrome when the wrists (especially the left) are stiff with burning pain, and significantly relieved by applying ice or ice-cold water. Because of so much tightness, the person may feel a need to stretch the wrist, despite the pain.

Hypericum perforatum

This remedy may be useful if sharp or shooting pains are felt extending from the wrist. *Hypericum* is known for its soothing effect when body parts containing many nerves are injured, as well as in other traumatic nerve conditions.

Rhus toxicodendron

This remedy is useful when stiffness and pain are worse on initial motion and improve as movement continues. Overuse may lead to soreness, pain, and further stiffening. Discomfort is relieved by warmth and worse in cold, damp weather.

Ruta graveolens

This remedy is indicated when overuse of joints and irritation of nerves lead to tremendous stiffness. A feeling of bruising and lameness may be present, even when the wrist is allowed to rest. Weakness in the arms and wrists, especially after repetitive tasks causing wear and tear on the joints and nerves, often indicates *Ruta*.

Viola odorata

This remedy is useful for many conditions that involve the wrist and hand, especially the right. Pain and numbness may extend from the wrist through the hand and into the fingers, and the hands and arms may tremble. Symptoms are worse from getting cold.

See p. 509 for Homeopathy: Dosage Directions.

Remedies for Cataracts

Cataracts (p. 34) are caused by oxidative changes in the lens of the eye, which can lead to gradual clouding and impairment of vision. Cataracts are mostly seen in older people, although exposure to radiation, excessive sunlight, pollutants, and certain medications can increase the risk for anyone. Remedies below have been helpful in many cases of cataracts, and are mentioned here to introduce a few of the possibilities homeopathy can offer, not as suggestions for self-care. A constitutional remedy chosen by an experienced prescriber is the most appropriate way to help a person with deep-seated or chronic conditions.

Calcarea carbonica

This remedy may be indicated when a person developing cataracts has the feeling of looking through a mist. A person needing this remedy tends to be a responsible type, but feels overwhelmed when under stress and fears breakdown or disease. Chilliness, swollen glands, weight problems, and easy tiring from exertion are other indications for *Calcarea carbonica*.

Calcarea fluorica

This remedy is often indicated when tissues harden or thicken abnormally. A person needing this remedy may also have a tendency toward hard swollen lymph nodes, joint pains, fibrous growths, or bone spurs. The person generally feels worse during weather changes and improved by warmth.

Causticum

This remedy has been helpful in some cases when the person developing cataracts also has problems moving the eyes, as if the muscles around the eyeballs were stiff or weak—especially after getting cold in the wind or open air. The person may have a feeling of sand in the eyes. A person who needs this remedy may tend to have muscular stiffness in many body areas. They are generally worse from cold and improved by warmth, and often feel best in damp or rainy weather.

Natrum muriaticum

This remedy may be indicated when cataracts begin to develop. The muscles around the eyes can feel bruised and weak, especially when the person looks down. The person may have a feeling of gauze across the eyes, and parts of the field of vision may be hard to focus on. A person who needs this remedy usually craves salt, feels worse from being in the sun, and has deep emotions yet appears to be reserved.

Phosphorus

People who need this remedy may have a feeling that dust or mist in the eyes is obscuring vision, or may experience soreness that feels like eyestrain after very little use. They sometimes see little bright dots of colored light when the eyes are closed. People who need this remedy are usually sympathetic and fond of company, but can tire easily. An active imagination (including many fears) and a strong desire for cold drinks and refreshing things are other indications for *Phosphorus*.

Silicea (*also called* Silica)

This remedy has been helpful to some individuals who developed cataracts after extended periods of eyestrain, or after perspiration of the feet had been suppressed. People needing this remedy tend to be chilly (although they often sweat at night) and often have low resistance to infection. Fine hair, weak nails, easy tiredness, and swollen lymph nodes are other signs suggesting *Silicea*.

See p. 509 for Homeopathy: Dosage Directions.

Remedies for Chemotherapy Support

People undergoing chemotherapy and experiencing side effects may find some relief in homeopathic reme-

dies. These remedies are not intended as substitutes for treatment, nor should they be considered part of the therapy. Homeopathic remedies are safe, nontoxic, and will not interfere with the treatment.

Cadmium sulphuratum

This remedy may be helpful to a person with debilitating nausea and vomiting after chemotherapy. A person who needs this remedy usually feels extremely chilly and exhausted.

Gelsemium

This remedy is often helpful when a person feels ill from anxiety or nervous anticipation of a stressful event or outcome. Weakness and trembling may occur, and the person may have chills and headache.

Ipecacuanha

Persistent nausea and violent vomiting that does not relieve the discomfort suggest a need for this remedy. The person may also salivate profusely. Lying down and resting may offer little or no relief.

Kali phosphoricum

This remedy can be helpful for exhaustion and weakness after any kind of illness or extended stress. The person may be oversensitive to light and noise, and feel deeply chilly. Mental dullness, depression, and a feeling of inability to cope are often seen when this remedy is needed.

Nux vomica

A person who experiences nausea but has difficulty vomiting may find relief in this remedy. Headache and great sensitivity (to odors, noise, and light) are also likely. Chilliness, irritability, and impatience are often present when *Nux vomica* is needed.

Sepia

This remedy may be indicated if nausea is severe and debilitating, with a headache (especially left-sided) and a dragged-out feeling of weariness. The person may have a strong desire to be left alone and not be expected to interact with others.

(Note: The homeopathic remedy *Cadmium iodatum* has been used by some physicians to counteract unpleasant side effects of radiation therapy.)

See p. 509 for Homeopathy: Dosage Directions.

Remedies for Chicken Pox

Chicken pox is a common childhood viral illness. Many cases are mild; however, those that are

Chicken Pox

uncomfortable can often be helped with homeopathy. Fatigue and low fever typically begin 10 days to 3 weeks from the time of exposure. A flat red rash comes out, transforms into pimples, then develops into blisters that eventually break and harden into itchy crusts. If fever is very high and persistent, or if a person seems to be extremely ill, it is best to consult a physician.

Antimonium tartaricum

This remedy may be indicated when eruptions are large and slow to emerge. The child feels sweaty, fussy, and may be nauseous with a white-coated tongue. If chest congestion with a rattling cough develops, or a bubbly sound on breathing, *Antimonium tart* is likely to be the appropriate remedy.

Antimonium crudum

A child who needs this remedy usually is irritable and may object to being touched or looked at. The eruptions can be sore, and touching them may bring on shooting pains.

Apis mellifica

When this remedy is indicated, the skin around the eruptions is pink and puffy and very itchy, with stinging pains. The eyelids may also be swollen. The person feels worse from warmth, is irritable, and usually is not thirsty.

Belladonna

This remedy is indicated when a child is hot and feverish, with a red-flushed face, and eyes that are sensitive to light. A pounding headache may be felt, accompanied by either restlessness or drowsiness. The rash usually is red, with a feeling of heat and throbbing.

Bryonia

When fever persists for several days during chicken pox, and a dry nagging cough develops, this remedy may be useful. The person's mouth is dry, with thirst for long cold drinks. The person may be very grumpy, feel worse from motion, and dislike being interfered with in any way.

Mercurius solubilis

This remedy may be indicated if eruptions are large and become infected. The child is very sensitive to temperature changes and feels worse at night. Perspiration and drooling during sleep, swollen lymph nodes, and offensive breath are strong indications for *Mercurius*.

Pulsatilla

A child who needs this remedy is often sweet and tearful when ill and wants a lot of attention and comforting. Itching and other discomforts are worse from

warmth and in stuffy rooms, and improved by cool fresh air. The person is rarely thirsty, even during fever.

Rhus toxicodendron

This remedy is useful in cases of chicken pox with tremendous itching that is worse from scratching and relieved by warm baths or applying heat. The child may be very restless, both physically and mentally. The eyes may become inflamed and sticky. Muscles can ache and feel very stiff, also relieved by warmth and gentle motion. (Some homeopathic physicians recommend *Rhus tox* to people who have been exposed to chicken pox, to help prevent infection.)

Sulphur

If itching is so severe that the person finds it impossible to keep from scratching—or if eruptions have a nagging, burning pain—this remedy may bring relief. The symptoms (and the person) become worse from warmth and aggravated after bathing. Both heat and chills are felt during fever. The person may feel drowsy in the afternoon and restless and hot at night.

Urtica urens

Eruptions with stinging, burning pain and itching may be relieved by this remedy. Symptoms are aggravated by exertion and from overheating.

See p. 509 for Homeopathy: Dosage Directions.

Remedies for Colic

Colic (p. 40) is defined as acute abdominal pain with intense spasmodic cramping. Infants with colic become upset and cry as if in pain, at the same time every evening. Abdominal discomfort appears to be the cause of colicky babies' suffering—but, since babies are too young to talk, it is hard to know exactly what distresses them. Homeopathic remedies are often very soothing, both to babies and adults, during colic episodes. If symptoms of illness are present (fever, chills, diarrhea, vomiting, oddly colored urine or bowel movements) or if pain appears to be unusually severe, a physician should be consulted.

Belladonna

Sudden onset of intense, cutting, clutching pain may signal a need for this remedy. The upper abdomen may look tense and swollen, and jarring or light touch can make discomfort worse. Some relief may come from pressing firmly on the area or bending forward. The person may either seem excitable with dilated eyes, or woozy with discomfort.

Bryonia

Extreme stitching pain in the abdomen that is worse from the slightest motion suggests a need for this remedy. The abdomen may seem bloated and tender to touch, and talking or breathing can increase discomfort. Keeping warm and lying completely still may bring relief.

Carbo vegetabilis

This remedy is often indicated when a person has a distended abdomen with colicky pain and belching. The face may look very pale, and the hands and feet are cold. Faintness, weakness, and a strong desire for moving air are other indications for *Carbo vegetabilis*.

Chamomilla

This remedy is indicated when a person is hypersensitive to pain. It is especially helpful to colicky babies who desperately scream or shriek and want to be constantly rocked and carried. The abdomen may be distended with gas, and pain can be focused in the navel region. Hot perspiration and facial flushing (sometimes only one cheek) are other indications for *Chamomilla*.

Colocynthis

Cramping, cutting pain that makes the person double over is a strong indication for this remedy. Pressing hard against the abdomen will usually bring relief. Babies who need this remedy look extremely anxious and often feel relief when carried tummy-down on someone's arm. Adults who experience painful colic after feeling angry or indignant (especially if suppressing it) may also benefit from *Colocynthis*.

Cuprum metallicum

If intense abdominal pain with violent spasms and cramping occurs at intervals, this remedy may bring relief. The abdomen feels tender, tight, and hot, and drinking cold water may bring improvement. The person's face may look extremely tense, or even contorted, with pain.

Dioscorea

Abdominal pain that feels better from bending backward is often relieved by this remedy. Babies may arch their backs and try to stay in that position. Pain comes in paroxysms, often with gas and burping, or with nausea.

Magnesia phosphorica

Colicky pain that is relieved by warmth and pressure will often respond to this remedy. Hot water bottles, heating pads, or drinking something warm can soothe discomfort, and rubbing the abdomen may also help.

The person (often a baby) may seem nervous from the pain, and can be irritable or fearful.

Nux vomica

This remedy is helpful for tense and impatient people when colicky pains result from overeating or from overindulgence in coffee, alcohol, and other strong or stimulating substances. The abdomen feels tight, and constricting pains press upward, making breathing difficult. Warm applications and warm drinks may bring relief. Infants who need this remedy often arch their backs, and seem impatient and angry.

See p. 509 for Homeopathy: Dosage Directions.

Remedies for the Common Cold

Colds (p. 41) are viral infections that take hold when the body's resistance is low because of fatigue, nutritional deficiencies, or stress. Typical symptoms include a stuffy or runny nose, sneezing, watery eyes, moderate fever, achiness or lethargy, and often sore throat or coughing. Homeopathic remedies can help relieve these symptoms and encourage the body's healing response.

Aconitum napellus

This remedy can be indicated in the early stages of a cold, if symptoms are intense and come on suddenly. Exposure to cold and wind, or a stressful or traumatic experience may precipitate the illness. Symptoms include a dry stuffy nose with a hot thin discharge, tension in the chest, a scratchy throat, and choking cough. The person often feels thirsty, chilly, anxious, and agitated.

Allium cepa

This remedy is often indicated when a person has watery eyes that sting, a teasing cough, much sneezing, and a runny nose with clear discharge that irritates the nostrils and upper lip. The nose is inclined to run when the person is indoors and stops in open air.

Arsenicum album

A person who has frequent colds, sore throats, and chest problems—with burning pain and feelings of weakness, restlessness, and anxiety—may benefit from this remedy. The person's head may feel hot while the rest of the body is cold, and problems can be worse near midnight. The nose often feels stopped up, and the person may sneeze repeatedly, without relief. White, thin, burning mucus may be produced.

Common Cold

Baryta carbonica

This remedy is indicated for people who frequently catch colds from getting chilled. A runny nose and swollen upper lip, and swollen lymph nodes, tonsils, and adenoids are typical symptoms. This remedy is often helpful to children who are bashful and slow to develop.

Belladonna

Sudden onset of a cold—with fever, flushed face, and restlessness—strongly indicates this remedy. Symptoms may include a hot dry feeling in the nose with watery discharge, and a nagging tickle in the throat. A hard or nagging cough, bright red sore throat, and throbbing pain in the head or ears are often seen. The person may be sensitive to light and either drowsy or delirious with the fever.

Dulcamara

When a person comes down with a cold after getting wet and chilled, or if colds come on when the weather changes, this remedy should come to mind. A stopped-up nose and face pain are likely. A person who needs *Dulcamara* may also tend to have allergies.

Euphrasia officinalis

Red, watery, irritated eyes; frequent sneezing; and a mild, clear nasal discharge suggest a need for this remedy. The person may cough from irritation and from phlegm collecting in the throat. Symptoms can be worse at night, and the person tends to feel better from eating and lying down.

Ferrum phosphoricum

This remedy often stops a cold from developing if taken right away when symptoms start. It is also helpful during colds that are more advanced, when the person feels very weary, with a moderate fever, rosy cheeks, sneezing, and a short hard cough.

Gelsemium

Lethargy and aching, with headache and droopy eyes, often indicate this remedy. Fever and chills run up and down the spine, and heat or pressure may be felt in the face and nose. A person who needs *Gelsemium* may tend to tremble and feel shaky or seem dull and apathetic. This remedy is often helpful for colds that come on in hot weather.

Kali bichromicum

This remedy is usually indicated for later stages of a cold with thick, stringy mucus that is difficult to clear from the nose and throat. The person may experience pain at the root of the nose or hoarse coughing with tenacious expectoration. The person often feels better from resting and keeping warm.

Mercurius solubilis

A person who needs this remedy can be extremely sensitive to temperatures, and may experience night sweats and drooling during sleep. Swollen lymph nodes and bad breath are other indications. The person's nose may feel raw, and the tonsils or ears often become infected.

Natrum muriaticum

Colds with clear nasal discharge like egg-white, sneezing (which is often worse in the morning), headache, and a diminished sense of smell or taste may respond to this remedy. The person may develop cold sores around the mouth, and the lips can be chapped and cracked.

Nux vomica

Colds with a stuffy head at night and runny nose in the daytime, rough throat, harsh cough, and chilliness suggest a need for this remedy. A person who needs *Nux vomica* is usually very irritable, impatient, and sensitive to odors, sounds, and light.

Phosphorus

This remedy may be helpful to a person who feels weak, "spaced out," or anxious when ill with colds that tend to go easily to the chest. One nostril may be blocked while the other runs. Hoarseness, laryngitis, and nosebleeds are other likely symptoms. The person is often thirsty for cold drinks and feels better from massage.

Pulsatilla

Colds producing thick, bland, yellow or greenish mucus suggest a need for this remedy. The nose feels stuffed indoors and runs in open air. The person feels worse in warm or stuffy rooms, with improvement from going outdoors. Congestion and fever often are worse in the evening. A person who needs *Pulsatilla* tends to want a lot of attention and comforting when ill, and children may be tearful.

Rhus toxicodendron

If a cold begins with stiffness and body aches, especially during cool damp weather or weather changes, and leads to nasal congestion or sore throat, this remedy should come to mind. The person may feel extremely restless and even pace or fidget. Warmth and motion bring relief, both physically and mentally.

See p. 509 for Homeopathy: Dosage Directions.

Remedies for Conjunctivitis

Conjunctivitis (p. 44), or "pinkeye" is an inflammation of the membrane that lines the eyelids and covers the whites of the eyes. The cause is usually viral (if bacteria are involved, the discharge will be thick and yellow-green). Conjunctivitis can also be caused by allergy, irritation from pollutants, windburn, or exposure to too much sun. Homeopathic remedies can help to reduce inflammation and ease discomfort in conjunctivitis. If significant improvement does not take place within a week, consult a doctor.

Apis mellifica

Puffy, pink, watery swelling that feels better from cold applications is a strong indication for this remedy. Stinging, burning pain may be experienced, and the eyelids may stick together. A person who needs this remedy often feels irritable, disliking interference.

Argentum nitricum

Swelling with yellowish or pus-like discharge, and redness and inflammation of the whites and inner corners of the eyes, suggest the use of this remedy. The person's eyes may be tired and achy, worse from light and warmth, and better from cool water, cold compresses, and fresh air. People who need this remedy often have a strong desire for both salt and sweets.

Hepar sulphuris calcareum

When the eyes feel sore or bruised, with inflammation and burning pain, or a feeling as if the eyeballs are being pulled back into the head, this remedy may be indicated. Yellow discharge can stick the eyelids shut, especially in the morning. Warm compresses, and warmth in general, often ease discomfort. Extreme sensitivity to cold, as well as to light and noise, is often seen. The person may be very irritable and touchy.

Mercurius solubilis

People needing this remedy often feel ill and tired, with erratic body temperature and sensitivity both to heat and cold. Discharge is greenish-yellow and can irritate the lids and margins of the eyes. A person who needs this remedy often has swollen glands, offensive breath, and excessive salivation.

Natrum muriaticum

Swollen lids with burning tears and a feeling that the eyes are bruised suggest a need for this remedy. Mucus or pus can form and make the eyelids stick together.

People who need this remedy may often feel sad and tired, acting irritable if someone shows them sympathy.

Pulsatilla

Conjunctivitis with thick, yellow, itchy discharge (often accompanying a cold or the measles) suggests a need for this remedy. The person tends to be emotional and sensitive, feeling worse from warmth and in stuffy rooms, and relieved by cool fresh air.

Sulphur

This remedy may be helpful if the eyes are very red and irritated, with burning, smarting, sticking pains and a nagging itch. The whites of the eyes look red and bloodshot, and the tears feel hot. Symptoms are worse from heat, and light will hurt the eyes. The eyelids may look contracted, especially in the morning.

See p. 509 for Homeopathy: Dosage Directions.

Remedies for Constipation

Diet, exercise, and lifestyle factors are often the key to **constipation** (p. 44). Homeopathic remedies can also help the body work efficiently. Long-standing cases of constipation, or those involving great discomfort, may be best addressed with a constitutional remedy and the guidance of a homeopathic practitioner.

Bryonia

This remedy is indicated for constipation with a feeling of dryness in the rectum and large dry stools that are hard to push out, with sticking or tearing pains. The person may feel grouchy or out of sorts, and may be tense from business-related worries.

Calcarea carbonica

People who need this remedy often feel more stable when constipated, and experience discomfort and fatigue when the bowels have moved. Large stools are hard at first, then sticky, then liquid. The person may feel chilly and sluggish, have clammy hands and feet, crave sweets, and feel weak and anxious when ill or overworked.

Causticum

This remedy may be helpful when stool is difficult to pass, with lots of painful straining. The person's face may turn red from effort, and more success may come from standing up. When it finally emerges, the stool will often be narrow and full of mucus.

Constipation

Graphites

This remedy is indicated when large stools look like "sheep dung" or little balls stuck together with mucus. Aching often is felt in the anus after the bowels have moved. People who need this remedy are slow to become alert in the morning, usually stout, and may have a tendency toward eczema.

Lycopodium

A person who needs this remedy has frequent indigestion with gas and bloating, and many problems involving the bowels. Rubbing the abdomen or drinking something warm may help to relieve the symptoms. A craving for sweets and an energy slump in late afternoon and early evening are strong indications for *Lycopodium*.

Nux vomica

"Wants to but can't" is a phrase that brings *Nux vomica* to mind. This remedy is often helpful to people who are impatient, tense, and ambitious—who work too hard and exercise too little, indulge in stimulants or alcohol, and are partial to sweets and spicy food. Headaches, chilliness, and constricting pains in the bowels or rectal area often accompany constipation when *Nux vomica* is needed.

Sepia

A heavy sensation in the rectum, remaining after a bowel movement, may indicate a need for this remedy. Stools can be hard and difficult to pass, although they may be small. The person often has cold hands and feet and a tendency to be weary and very irritable. Exercise may bring improvement, both to constipation and to mood and energy level. (*Sepia* is often useful to women who develop constipation just before or just after a menstrual period.)

Silicea (*also called* Silica)

When this remedy is indicated, the person may strain for long periods without success. A "bashful" stool might begin to come out, but eventually retreat. People who need this remedy are typically nervous and mentally acute, but also chilly, physically frail, and easily fatigued.

Sulphur

Dry, hard stools with reddish inflammation of the anus and offensive flatulence suggest a need for this remedy. Constipation may also alternate with diarrhea. People who need this remedy are often "characters" with unusual mental notions, slouching posture, and very little interest in tidiness.

See p. 509 for Homeopathy: Dosage Directions.

Remedies for Cough

Coughing (p. 47) is the body's way of removing irritating substances, excess secretions, and foreign objects from air passages. This is important, both as a protective mechanism and for the healing process—which is why a cough should not be artificially suppressed with drugs. When a cough is painful, too intense, or prevents good rest, the use of remedies can gently relieve discomfort and help with recovery. Coughing can accompany a wide variety of illnesses or conditions. If a person has serious difficulty breathing, coughs up blood or abnormal discharge, or seems very ill in other ways, professional help should be sought.

Aconitum napellus

This remedy is indicated when a cough has come on suddenly—often from exposure to cold wind, or after a traumatic experience. The cough is likely to be sharp, short, dry, and constant. It may begin during sleep and wake the person up, or can start when the person goes from a cool place into a warmer one. Restlessness and fear are typical when this remedy is needed. It is often used in early stages of croup and asthma.

Belladonna

A cough that comes on suddenly, often with the feeling of a speck or tickle in the throat, is a strong indication for this remedy. The cough is intense and nagging and the person may feel as if the head is about to burst. Sensations of heat, a reddened face, and dilated pupils are often seen when this remedy is needed.

Bryonia

This remedy is indicated when a cold goes into the chest and the cough is very painful and dry. The person feels worse from any movement, and may even need to hold his or her sides or press against the chest to keep it still. The cough can also make the head or stomach hurt, and digestion may be upset. The mouth can be dry and the person may be thirsty. If someone is very grumpy when ill and wants to be left alone, not talked to or disturbed, *Bryonia* is likely to be the remedy.

Chamomilla

A dry, hard, irritating cough that starts after being exposed to wind, or after being overexcited and angry, can indicate this remedy. The cough is often worse around 9:00 in the evening and may continue into the night. The nervous system is hypersensitive, and the person can be extremely irritable and agitated.

Cough

(Children may even shriek and hit, though they often calm down if someone carries them.) This remedy is also useful in asthma attacks, especially those brought on by anger.

Ferrum phosphoricum

This is an excellent remedy for the early stages of many inflammatory conditions, especially colds and allergy attacks. The cough is typically short and tickling, and may be painful. Things are worse in cold air, at night, and in the early morning. The person feels weary, and often has a moderate fever and lightly flushed cheeks.

Hepar sulphuris calcareum

This remedy is very helpful when a cough is loose, rattling and gagging, and brings up yellow mucus. It also can relieve long, dry coughing jags. Extreme sensitivity to all sensations—especially cold—suggests a need for this remedy. Cold in any form (even food or drink) can set off a bout of coughing, and make the person feel more ill. A person who needs this remedy feels both physically and emotionally vulnerable, and can be irritable and touchy. This remedy is often indicated in bronchitis and croup.

Ipecacuanha

A violent cough that comes with every breath, and long spasmodic bouts of coughing that end in gagging or vomiting, are indications for this remedy. The person may have a clean, uncoated tongue and experience tightness in the throat and chest, or an aggravating tickle. Warm, humid air or changes in the weather tend to make problems worse. *Ipecacuanha* is often used during asthma attacks.

Nux vomica

Indications for this remedy include a tight sensation in the chest with a dry, hacking, teasing cough—often causing soreness or a feeling that something has been torn inside. Long coughing jags can end in stomach pain and retching, and may make the person's head ache. A person who needs this remedy is likely to be impatient, irritable, and oversensitive to everything. A feeling of chilliness is typical, and problems are often worse from exertion (both mental and physical) and worse in the morning.

Phosphorus

This remedy is indicated when a person experiences hoarseness and a tickly cough that hurts the throat, or a cold that travels quickly to the chest. The cough can be aggravated by talking, laughing, and exposure to cold air. The person may feel heaviness or tightness. A thirst for cold drinks (that may cause nausea after warming up in the stomach) is another indication for *Phosphorus*. A person who needs this remedy is typically imaginative and fearful, and likes the company of others, but tires very easily. This remedy is often used for loss of the voice and laryngitis.

Pulsatilla

Coughs that are dry in the evening and loose in the morning, worse in a stuffy room or when the person feels too warm, and improved in open air may indicate this remedy. The chest will often have a feeling of pressure and soreness, and thick yellow mucus may be coughed up with gagging and choking. A person who needs this remedy usually likes attention and company. It is often given to children who tend toward tears when ill and want to be held and comforted.

Rumex crispus

A teasing, hacking cough that is triggered by a tickle in the pit of the throat is a strong indication for this remedy; even touching the base of the throat can set off coughing. The cough is often dry, but frothy or stringy mucus may come up. Coughing may begin when the person goes outside or changes from a warm place to a cool one. The cough can keep the person from sleeping, and the center and left side of the chest are likely to be sore.

Spongia tosta

This remedy is indicated when a cough is loud, harsh, dry, and sounds like barking or sawing wood. The person may wake up feeling suffocated, as if the throat is plugged or the breathing passages are dry. Problems are usually made worse from being in a room that is too warm, or from lying down with the head too low. Talking aggravates the cough, and so does exposure to cold air and smoke. Sitting up usually helps, and drinking something warm or eating small amounts brings some relief. This remedy is often helpful during croup and asthma.

Sulphur

This remedy is indicated for burning, irritating coughs that get worse at night in bed, as well as for breathing problems during sleep. It can also be useful when a mild cough drags on for a week or more without getting worse, but without much improvement. Burning sensations, redness of eyes and mucous membranes, foul odors, and an aggravation from bathing are often seen in a person who needs this remedy.

See p. 509 for Homeopathy: Dosage Directions.

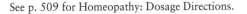

Remedies for Dental Support

Homeopathic remedies can be helpful in many ways, both before and after dental work—to ease anxiety before a visit, reduce the tendency toward bruising and tissue damage during procedures, and to relieve discomfort afterward.

Arnica montana

This is a useful first-aid remedy for any situation involving bruising and tissue damage. Some dentists recommend that patients take it both before and after stressful dental work, including dental surgery. *Arnica* may be used as long as soreness lasts, or followed by another remedy aimed at more specific symptoms.

Calendula

This remedy can help the body overcome inflammation, infection, and abscess. It can be taken internally in potentized form, or used as an herbal tincture. Applied to injured gums and areas around the teeth, the tincture can help reduce the chance of infection, and help the tissues heal after being cut or bruised.

Chamomilla

This remedy is often helpful when a person is hypersensitive to pain and the aftermath of dental work seems intolerable. *Chamomilla* sometimes works when pain medications have little or no effect, by helping the person's nerve response become more balanced.

Gelsemium

This remedy can help to ease the apprehension and anxiety that often precede a visit to the dentist. The person may tremble and feel weak from dread, develop a headache (in the back of the head and the muscles of the neck), or feel mentally dull and lethargic.

Hypericum perforatum

This remedy is known for its soothing effect when nerves or nerve-filled body areas are injured. Shooting, jabbing pains are often felt. *Hypericum* is very useful after oral surgery, especially root canals.

Mercurius solubilis

A person with a tendency toward tender, bleeding, swollen gums and teeth that easily loosen and decay may benefit from this remedy. Offensive breath, excessive salivation, and swollen glands are other indications. Symptoms are worse at night, and the person is very sensitive to temperatures, both cold and hot.

See p. 509 for Homeopathy: Dosage Directions.

Remedies for Depression

When a person feels depressed, something needs attention. Too much stress can make it hard to cope, and important feelings may be suppressed or turned inside. A major loss or grief requires time and emotional support for real recovery—and even a buildup of minor stresses (disappointments, setbacks, trouble in relationships, or work-related problems) can contribute to **depression** (p. 50). Dietary deficiencies, allergies and sensitivities, hormonal imbalances, or biochemical conditions may also be involved. A person going through a period of mild sadness or depression may find relief through homeopathy. The guidance of an experienced homeopath is often valuable, to choose a remedy that fits the situation best. Any person with deep, long-lasting, or recurring depression should seek the care of a licensed mental health professional.

Arsenicum album

Anxious, insecure, and perfectionistic people who need this remedy may set high standards for themselves and others and become depressed if their expectations are not met. Worry about material security sometimes borders on despair. When feeling ill, these people can be demanding and dependent, even suspicious of others, fearing their condition could be serious.

Aurum metallicum

This remedy can be helpful to serious people, strongly focused on work and achievement, who become depressed if they feel they have failed in some way. Discouragement, self-reproach, humiliation, and anger can lead to feelings of emptiness and worthlessness. The person may feel worse at night, with nightmares or insomnia.

Calcarea carbonica

A dependable, industrious person who becomes overwhelmed from too much worry, work, or physical illness may benefit from this remedy. Anxiety, fatigue, confusion, discouragement, self-pity, and a dread of disaster may develop. A person who needs this remedy often feels chilly and sluggish and easily tires from exertion.

Causticum

A person who feels depressed because of grief and loss (either recent or over time) may benefit from this remedy. Frequent crying or a feeling of mental dullness and forgetfulness (with anxious checking to see if the door is locked, if the stove is off, etc.) are other indications. People who need this remedy are often deeply sympathetic toward others and, having a strong sense of justice, can be deeply discouraged or angry about the world.

Cimicifuga

A person who needs this remedy can be energetic and talkative when feeling well, but upset and gloomy when depressed—with exaggerated fears (of insanity, of being attacked, of disaster). Painful menstrual periods and headaches that involve the neck are often seen when this remedy is needed.

Ignatia amara

Sensitive people who suffer grief or disappointment and try to keep the hurt inside may benefit from this remedy. Wanting not to cry or appear too vulnerable to others, they may seem guarded, defensive, and moody. They may also burst out laughing, or into tears, for no apparent reason. A feeling of a lump in the throat and heaviness in the chest with frequent sighing or yawning are strong indications for *Ignatia*. Insomnia (or excessive sleeping), headaches, and cramping pains in the abdomen and back are also often seen.

Kali phosphoricum

If a person feels depressed after working too hard, being physically ill, or going through prolonged emotional stress or excitement, this remedy can be helpful. Exhausted, nervous, and jumpy, they may have difficulty working or concentrating—and become discouraged and lose confidence. Headaches from mental effort, easy perspiration, sensitivity to cold, anemia, insomnia, and indigestion are often seen when this remedy is needed.

Natrum carbonicum

Individuals who need this remedy are usually mild, gentle, and selfless—making an effort to be cheerful and helpful, and avoiding conflict whenever possible. After being hurt or disappointed, they can become depressed, but keep their feelings to themselves. Even when feeling lonely, they withdraw to rest or listen to sad music, which can isolate them even more. Nervous and physically sensitive (to sun, to weather changes, and to many foods, especially milk), they may also get depressed when feeling weak or ill.

Natrum muriaticum

People who need this remedy seem reserved, responsible, and private—yet have strong inner feelings (grief, romantic attachment, anger, or fear of misfortune) that they rarely show. Even though they want other people to feel for them, they can act affronted or angry if someone tries to console them, and need to be alone to cry. Anxiety, brooding about past grievances, migraines, back pain, and insomnia can also be experienced when the person is depressed. A craving for salt and tiredness from sun exposure are other indications for this remedy.

Pulsatilla

People who need this remedy have a childlike softness and sensitivity—and can also be whiny, jealous, and moody. When depressed, they are sad and tearful, wanting a lot of attention and comforting. Crying, fresh air, and gentle exercise usually improve their mood. Getting too warm or being in a stuffy room can increase anxiety. Depression around the time of hormonal changes (puberty, menstrual periods, or menopause) can often be helped with *Pulsatilla*.

Sepia

People who feel weary, irritable, and indifferent to family members, and worn out by the demands of everyday life, may respond to this remedy. They want to be left alone and may respond in an angry or cutting way if anyone bothers them. They often feel better from crying, but would rather have others keep their distance and not try to console them or cheer them up. Menstrual problems, a sagging feeling in internal organs, sluggish digestion, and improvement from vigorous exercise are other indications for this remedy.

Staphysagria

Quiet, sensitive, emotional people who have difficulty standing up for themselves may benefit from this remedy. Hurt feelings, shame, resentment, and suppressed emotions can lead them to depression. If under too much pressure, they can sometimes lose their natural inhibition and fly into rages or throw things. A person who needs this remedy may also have insomnia (feeling sleepy all day, but unable to sleep at night), toothaches, headaches, stomachaches, or bladder infections that are stress-related.

See p. 509 for Homeopathy: Dosage Directions.

Remedies for Diarrhea

Diarrhea (p. 58) is the body's cleansing response, removing unwanted substances by way of the

Diarrhea

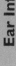

digestive tract. Looseness of the bowels can be caused by allergens, contaminated food, toxins, viral and bacterial illness, or occur during times of emotional stress. Some babies have diarrhea during teething, and many people experience diarrhea as a physical overreaction to nervousness.

Argentum nitricum

If a person has diarrhea when anticipating a stressful event (such as giving a speech or a public performance, taking a test, or attending a party), this remedy should come to mind. Bloating and flatulence are usually apparent, pain may be felt in the region of the groin, and the diarrhea may look green. Diarrhea that occurs immediately after eating or drinking, or after eating too much sugar, will often respond to *Argentum nitricum*.

Arsenicum album

Diarrhea accompanied by anxiety, restlessness, and exhaustion suggests a need for this remedy. Burning pain is felt in the digestive tract, and the person may be thirsty for frequent small sips of tea or water. The stools may be watery and have a putrescent odor. Simultaneous diarrhea and vomiting can be another strong indication. *Arsenicum* is often useful when diarrhea has been caused by spoiled or tainted food.

Bryonia

This remedy is often helpful for diarrhea during flu (especially when the person feels grumpy and wants to lie still and be left alone). It may also be helpful for diarrhea that occurs when a person gets overheated, then drinks a lot of cold water. Symptoms often are worse in the morning. The person's mouth may be very dry.

Chamomilla

Hot, green, watery diarrhea with abdominal pain and gas suggests a need for this remedy. The person's face can be red and flushed (sometimes only on one side) and problems may be worse from warmth. Children who need this remedy will often seem extremely angry, and scream or hit. Adults may be more irritable and hypersensitive.

Colocynthis

Cutting and cramping pains in the abdomen precede the diarrhea when this remedy is indicated. The person feels relief from doubling over, or from putting hard pressure on the abdomen. This remedy is often helpful when diarrhea follows anger (especially if the feelings were not expressed).

Gelsemium

This remedy is often indicated if trembling and weakness accompany diarrhea, especially when nervous-

ness, fear, or emotional upset is the cause. *Gelsemium* is also useful during flu with diarrhea, droopy lethargy, fever, chills, and headache.

Ipecacuanha

If a person has diarrhea accompanied by extreme or constant nausea, this remedy may bring relief. Cutting, clutching pains are worse around the navel, and the diarrhea looks frothy or green.

Phosphorus

This remedy can be soothing if a person has a weak or empty feeling in the abdomen, followed by diarrhea that runs out "like an open faucet." People who need this remedy are often thirsty, and may be fearful when ill.

Podophyllum

Profuse, gushing, watery diarrhea that is usually not accompanied by pain suggests the use of this remedy. The abdomen rumbles and gurgles before the diarrhea passes, and urging may soon be felt again. Bouts of diarrhea are often worse in the morning, and also in hot weather.

Pulsatilla

If diarrhea occurs after eating rich and fatty foods, this remedy can be helpful. Queasiness and abdominal pain are likely to occur, and the diarrhea has a changeable appearance. The person will usually not be thirsty, feels worse from being warm or in a stuffy room, and is better in open air. A need for attention, sympathy, and comforting is a strong indication for *Pulsatilla* (a very useful remedy for children).

Sulphur

Urgent, hot diarrhea that occurs in the early morning, making the person rush to the bathroom, suggests a need for this remedy. Burning is often felt in the digestive tract, and the anus can be itchy, red, and irritated. The person may also have hemorrhoids that burn and itch.

See p. 509 for Homeopathy: Dosage Directions.

Remedies for Ear Infections

Small children often develop middle ear infections (otitis media) during colds; however, **ear infections** (p. 63) can occur at any age. Allergy or swelling of the tonsils and adenoids may block the eustachian tubes and sinus passages, and inflammation and fluid can increase in the middle ear, causing pressure, pain, and sometimes even a ruptured eardrum and discharge. A different kind of ear infection (otitis externa) affects the outer ear and the sensitive skin inside the ear canal; it often starts with a scratch that gets infected by bacteria or fungus (swimmer's ear), becoming swollen, inflamed, and very painful.

Aconitum napellus

This remedy is indicated if an earache comes on suddenly with cutting, throbbing pain—often after exposure to cold and wind, or after a shaking experience. The person can be fearful, agitated, and restless. Fever may be high and thirst is strong. Symptoms are often worse near midnight, and can even wake the person up.

Belladonna

Intense bouts of earache that come and go very suddenly, with heat and inflammation, suggest a need for this remedy. Pain can be pounding or throbbing, and may be worse from jarring. The person usually has a fever, a flushed red face, eyes that are sensitive to light, and skin that is hot to touch. The right ear is most often affected. A child needing *Belladonna* may feel drowsy with the fever, or be restless and have nightmares.

Chamomilla

Paroxysms of pain that seem intolerable suggest a need for this remedy. Children may seem angry and beside themselves, and often scream and hit. They may feel better from being carried constantly and vigorously walked around or rocked. Ear pain and other symptoms are worse from heat and wind, and the cheeks (often only one) may be hot and red.

Ferrum phosphoricum

This remedy can soothe the ache and inflammation of an ear infection—or even stop it, if given when the symptoms have just begun to show. The person looks pink and flushed, with fever and a feeling of weariness. The outer ear may look warm and pink, and the eardrum can slightly bulge.

Hepar sulphuris calcareum

This remedy is indicated when an earache is very painful or infection is advanced (with a bulging eardrum or pus formation). Stabbing, sticking pains "like a splinter being driven in" are a likely indication. The person is very sensitive to everything, especially cold and drafts, and may feel extremely vulnerable and touchy.

Magnesia phosphorica

An earache that feels much better when warmth and pressure are applied suggests a need for this remedy. The pain may be mostly neuralgic, with little evidence of fluid or infection.

Mercurius solubilis

This remedy may be helpful if an ear infection is advanced, with pus formation, shooting pains, and roaring in the ear. A person who needs this remedy is often very sensitive to temperatures (both hot and cold), with swollen lymph nodes, offensive breath, a puffy tongue, and sweat and drooling during sleeping.

Pulsatilla

This remedy is often indicated for ear infections that follow or accompany a cold. (Cold symptoms include a stuffy nose, especially indoors, and large amounts of yellow or greenish mucus.) The ear may be hot and swollen, with a feeling that something is pressing out. Pain can be worse in the evening and at night, as well as worse from heat, with a pulsing sensation. Deep itching may be felt inside, especially if ear infections are chronic. A child needing *Pulsatilla* usually is sad and tearful, wanting to be held and comforted.

See p. 509 for Homeopathy: Dosage Directions.

Remedies for Eczema

Eczema (p. 64) is the common term for atopic dermatitis—a chronic, allergic skin irritation. An itchy, flaking rash may appear on the inner surface of elbows and knees, the backs of the upper arms, wrists, cheeks, scalp, or eyelids. From the homeopathic point of view, the suppression of skin eruptions (especially with cortisone or other drugs) can lead to deeper health problems. Homeopathic and herbal remedies can be soothing during flare-ups—but for deeper treatment, a constitutional remedy should be chosen by an experienced practitioner, to fit a person on many levels, and bring the body into better balance.

Antimonium crudum

People likely to respond to this remedy have eczema with thick, cracked skin and are also prone to indigestion. They are usually sensitive and sentimental, love to eat (craving pickles, vinegar, and other sour things), and may be overweight. Children can be shy and irritable, insisting that they not be touched or looked at. Itching can be worse from warmth and sun exposure. *Antimonium crudum* is often indicated for impetigo, plantar warts, and calluses, as well as eczema.

Arsenicum album

People who need this remedy usually are anxious, restless, and compulsively neat and orderly. The skin is dry, with intense itching and burning. Scratching can make the itching worse, and applying heat will

Eczema

bring relief. Indigestion with burning pain and a general feeling of chilliness are often seen when *Arsenicum* is indicated.

Arum triphyllum

This remedy can be useful when allergic skin eruptions are focused on the lower part of the face, especially around the mouth. The chin may look chapped and feel hot and irritated. The lips are cracked (and usually raw from the person picking them) and the nostrils may be sore. People who need this remedy are often inclined toward throat irritation and hoarseness.

Calcarea carbonica

This remedy is suited to people who are chilly with clammy hands and feet, and tend to develop eczema and cracking skin that is worse in the wintertime. They are easily fatigued by exertion, and feel anxious and overwhelmed if ill or overworked. Cravings for sweets and eggs, a sluggish metabolism, and a tendency toward weight problems are other indications for *Calcarea*.

Calendula

This remedy (in potentized homeopathic form) can be helpful if the irritated skin has a tendency to get infected. Topical use of the unpotentized herb in lotion, gel, or tincture form is soothing to irritated skin, and can often ease inflammation and prevent infection without artificially suppressing it.

Graphites

People likely to respond to this remedy have tough or leathery skin with cracks and soreness, and often have a long-term history of skin disorders (such as impetigo or herpes). The areas behind the ears, around the mouth, or on the hands are often cracked, with a golden oozing discharge that hardens into crusts. Itching is worse from getting warm in bed, and the person will often scratch the irritated places till they bleed. Difficulty concentrating, especially in the morning, is often seen in a person who needs *Graphites*.

Hepar sulphuris calcareum

This remedy may be helpful to very sensitive, chilly people whose eczema is extremely sore and becomes infected easily. The skin, especially on the hands and feet, may look chapped and deeply cracked and be very slow to heal. The person usually feels vulnerable and irritable, with a low resistance to illness and infection.

Mezereum

A person who needs this remedy often has strong anxiety, felt physically in the stomach. Intensely itching eruptions start as blisters, then ooze and form thick crusts, and scratching can lead to thickened skin. Cold applications often help the itch (although the person is chilly in general). A craving for fat and a tendency to feel better in open air are other indications for *Mezereum*.

Petroleum

This remedy is indicated for individuals whose skin is extremely dry and tends to crack, especially on the fingertips and palms. Eczema is worse in winter, with deep, sore cracks that often bleed. The person feels a cold sensation after scratching. Itching is worse at night and from getting warm in bed. The skin is easily infected, and may get tough and leathery from chronic irritation.

Rhus toxicodendron

A person whose eczema has blister-like eruptions that look red and swollen, itch intensely, and are soothed by hot applications may respond to this remedy. The person is restless from discomfort and often is very irritable and anxious. Muscle stiffness, relieved by warmth and motion, is also likely. A person who needs *Rhus tox* will often crave cold milk.

Sulphur

Intensely burning, itching, inflamed eruptions that are worse from warmth and worse from bathing suggest a need for this remedy. Affected areas may be red, with scaling or crusted skin. Eruptions can be either dry or moist. This remedy is sometimes helpful to people who have repeatedly used medications and ointments on their eczema without success.

See p. 509 for Homeopathy: Dosage Directions.

Remedies for Edema (Water Retention)

Swelling and puffiness in the ankles (or around the eyes and other body areas) are sometimes caused by minor stresses, such as standing for long periods of time, unaccustomed heavy exercise, hot weather, a change in salt intake, premenstrual stress, or minor conditions involving circulation. **Edema** (p. 65) can also occur in serious conditions such as heart disease, kidney disorders, liver problems, or complications during pregnancy—all of which require a physician's care. Homeopathic remedies may be used when the cause is obviously minor, but any extreme or long-lasting edema should have a physician's attention and diagnosis.

Apis mellifica

This remedy may be indicated when puffy swelling develops below the eyes or in the extremities. The area can feel tight and numb, or tender with stinging sensations. Cold soaks and cold applications help, while warmth and touch can make things worse. A person who needs this remedy typically has low thirst, dislikes interference, and feels irritable.

Calcarea carbonica

A person who develops swelling in the lower extremities, especially around the knees, may be helped with this remedy. Symptoms can be worse from sitting, unless the legs are supported. The person may have a tendency toward weight problems, get tired easily, and feel worse from exertion. Hands and feet are often cold and clammy (although the feet may heat up at night).

Bovista

Puffiness can be seen in various parts of the body when this remedy is needed. The person may feel awkward and even drop things because the hands feel weak or numb. *Bovista* is often helpful to women with water-retention around the time of the menstrual period, especially if diarrhea also occurs.

Ferrum metallicum

This remedy may be indicated if swelling in the extremities comes on after fluid loss (such as heavy sweating or loss of blood). Things may improve with walking slowly or other gentle motion. People needing this remedy tend to feel tired and be anemic, although they may look robust to others—being sturdily built, with a face that flushes easily.

Graphites

This remedy may be indicated if swelling of the lower extremities develops in a person who is stout and has a tendency toward skin problems (such as cracks behind the ears or on the fingertips). Pain in the lower back and trouble becoming alert after waking in the morning are other indications for *Graphites*.

Kali carbonicum

A "bag-like" swelling above the eyes is a strong indication for this remedy. Sensitive soles of the feet and swelling in the lower extremities (only one foot, at times) may also be seen. Gently moving around may bring improvement.

Ledum palustre

This remedy may be indicated if the ankles and soles of the feet are swollen and tender. The problems are worse from being warm, and cold soaks and cold applications bring relief. *Ledum* is most often used for injuries (sprains, black eyes, or puncture wounds) and insect bites, when swelling is relieved by cold.

Lycopodium

If swelling is seen in a person inclined toward abdominal bloating and digestive problems, this remedy may be helpful. Numbness or heaviness in the extremities, and a feeling of one foot being warm and the other cold are other indications. Problems may be worse in the late afternoon and evening. Cravings for sweets and warm drinks, and an inner lack of confidence, are often seen in people needing *Lycopodium*.

Natrum muriaticum

If swelling occurs around the eyes because of allergy, or if a person develops swollen extremities after sun exposure, this remedy may be needed. An emotional nature with an outer appearance of reserve, a craving for salt, marked thirst, and a tendency to feel tired or ill from being in the sun are other indications for *Natrum muriaticum*.

Pulsatilla

Swelling that involves the knees, ankles, feet, or hands and is accompanied by a feeling of heaviness or weariness suggests the use of this remedy—especially if it occurs premenstrually or after overindulging in rich foods. Problems are worse when the extremities are hanging down, worse from warmth, and improved by gentle motion. A person needing this remedy will often be changeable, emotional, and moody—with low thirst and a tendency to feel better in fresh air.

See p. 509 for Homeopathy: Dosage Directions.

Remedies for Eye Injuries/Eyestrain

Long hours staring at a computer screen, reading, writing, doing beadwork, sewing, tying flies, repairing electronics equipment, or any close and detailed work can lead to eye strain from overuse. Soreness of the muscles around the eyeballs, weak or blurry vision,

Eye Injuries/Eyestrain

burning, watering, and oversensitivity to light are common symptoms. Discomfort from minor eye irritations (from smoke, pollutants, smog, or pollens), slight abrasions (from contact lenses, sand, or dirt), or bruising injuries can also often be relieved with homeopathy. If an eye has undergone a traumatic injury, or if any symptoms are unusual or distressing, see a physician right away.

Aconitum napellus

This remedy may bring relief when foreign matter gets into the eye and causes irritation. The person can feel very fearful and agitated—with eye pain, heavy watering, and heightened sensitivity to light.

Apis mellifica

This remedy can be helpful if the eyelids and surrounding areas get very puffy and tender, with burning or stinging pain that cold applications partially relieve. *Apis* can also be useful after overexposure to very bright light (such as looking at snow in bright sunlight or sun reflecting off the water for long periods, or driving into the sun) when the eyes feel sore and oversensitive.

Argentum nitricum

Aching from overuse or detailed work, relieved by closing the eyes or pressing on them, suggests a need for this remedy. The muscles around the eyes feel weak and the person is unable to keep them focused and steady. The whites or corners often look inflamed. Being in an overheated room may aggravate the symptoms.

Arnica montana

This remedy can bring relief to a person with a bruised, sore feeling in the eyes after closely focused work or from looking into the distance (such as sightseeing or watching movies). The person may feel a need to keep the eyes open, getting dizzy when closing them.

Kali phosphoricum

This remedy can be helpful when exhaustion from illness, overwork, or stress has led to eyestrain. The eyes feel very tired and the vision seems blurred and weak. A person who needs this remedy often startles easily and may be oversensitive to light.

Kalmia latifolia

Great stiffness felt in the eyes and eyelids, worse when moving the eyes, suggests a need for this remedy. The vision may seem to be impaired or weak. A person who needs this remedy may also have nerve pains in the face and teeth, or joint and muscle stiffness that shifts from place to place.

Natrum muriaticum

This remedy may be useful if extended periods of reading or doing schoolwork have led to a weak, bruised feeling in the eyes. The muscles around the eyeballs can feel weak and stiff, and the letters on a page may appear to run together. The eyelids feel heavy, and the person may be inclined toward headaches.

Ruta graveolens

This remedy is often indicated for eyestrain caused by overuse. Stiffness and pain can lead to headaches, and soreness and pressure are felt behind the eyeballs. The eyes may become inflamed and swollen, with heavy watering and oversensitivity to light. The person may also have problems with focusing the eyes or accommodating to changes in brightness.

Symphytum officinale

This is an important remedy when the eyeball has been bruised or injured by a blow from a blunt object (for example a tool-handle, baseball, or rock). Injuries to the eyeball can be serious, and should always be examined by a doctor.

See p. 509 for Homeopathy: Dosage Directions.

Remedies for Fibromyalgia

Homeopathy can often provide relief from the unpredictable, sometimes debilitating, aches and pains of **fibromyalgia** (p. 68). Nutritional supplements, dietary monitoring, special types of exercise, and other natural approaches are also helpful and may be used along with remedies.

Arnica montana

This remedy is indicated when any body area feels bruised and sore, after exertion, overuse of muscles, or injury. Sometimes *Arnica* is enough to soothe a chronic condition; often, other remedies will follow *Arnica*.

Bryonia

A person who needs this remedy will try to stay as still as possible, since even the slightest motion aggravates the pain. People who need this remedy often feel extremely irritable and grumpy, not wanting to be touched or interfered with. Warmth often makes things worse and cool applications may be soothing.

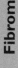

Fibromyalgia

Pressure on the painful parts (or lying on them) often helps, because it minimizes movement.

Calcarea carbonica

Muscle soreness and weakness that are worse from exertion, and worse from getting cold and damp, may be relieved by this remedy. The person often is chilly with clammy hands and feet, is easily fatigued, and has a tendency to feel overwhelmed and anxious. Cravings for sweets and eggs often confirm the choice of this remedy.

Causticum

Soreness, weakness, and stiffness in the muscles—worse from being cold and worse from overuse—suggest a need for this remedy. The forearms often feel stiff, unsteady, and very weak. The muscles of the legs can feel contracted and sore, and the person may have restless legs at night. Problems tend to be worse when the weather is dry, and better in rainy weather (although getting wet may aggravate the pain and stiffness). Warm applications and warming up in bed often relieve discomfort.

Cimicifuga (also called Actaea racemosa)

People who need this remedy are often energetic and talkative, becoming depressed or fearful when physical problems trouble them. Soreness and stiffness of muscles may be accompanied by shooting pains and are usually aggravated by getting cold. The neck and spinal muscles can be very tight, and the person may have headaches and other problems during menstrual periods.

Kalmia latifolia

Severe pain in the muscles, extending from higher areas to lower ones, will often respond to this remedy. Shooting pains may occur, along with stiffness, neuralgia, and numbness or a cold sensation. Pains can come on suddenly, and often shift around, being worse from motion and worse at night.

Ranunculus bulbosus

This remedy is often helpful with fibrositis and muscle stiffness, especially when the neck and back muscles are involved. Stabbing pains and soreness may be felt near the spine and shoulder blades, especially on the left. Problems may be aggravated by cold damp weather, walking, and alcoholic beverages.

Rhus toxicodendron

If a person feels very restless, with stiffness and soreness that find relief in warmth and motion, this reme-

dy should be considered. Problems are often brought on by cold, damp weather. Stiffness and pain are worse on waking in the morning, and after periods of rest.

Ruta graveolens

Tremendous stiffness of the muscles, with lameness, pain, and weakness (especially after overuse) may be soothed with this remedy. The legs and hips are sore and weak, and the person may find it difficult to stand after sitting in a chair. Muscles in the back and neck feel bruised, the tendons may be sore, and the wrists and hands feel painful and contracted.

See p. 509 for Homeopathy: Dosage Directions.

Remedies for Gallstones

Small stones in the gall bladder are common, and many people are not aware they have them until a distressing episode occurs. If a **gallstone** (p. 69) moves into the duct that carries bile, and stretches it or gets stuck, distressing symptoms (such as abdominal pain, nausea, vomiting, fever, chills, even jaundice) can result. Some remedies may be helpful as first aid for pain relief, but medical care is required in these situations. Remedies below have been helpful to some people with gallstones. They are mentioned here to introduce a few of the possibilities homeopathy can offer, and not as recommendations for self-treatment. A constitutional remedy chosen by an experienced prescriber is a more appropriate way to treat deep-seated, serious, or chronic conditions.

Berberis vulgaris

This remedy may be indicated when stitching pains extend from the gallbladder region to the stomach and sometimes to the shoulder. Sharp twinges radiating outward can be felt in the groin and pelvic bones and may seem to come from the lower back. Pain can be worse when the person is standing up, and from changing position. The person may be constipated and have a tendency toward gout or joint pains. Rapidly changing states (sudden thirst, then lack of thirst; hunger, then loss of appetite) can point to this remedy.

Calcarea carbonica

When a person needing this remedy has gallbladder problems, the abdomen may feel swollen on the right and be very sensitive to pressure, with cutting pains that extend to the chest and are worse from stooping.

The person feels worse from standing, worse from exertion, and better from lying on the painful side. *Calcarea carbonica* is often indicated for people who tire easily, feel cold and sluggish with clammy hands and feet, crave sweets, and tend to feel anxious and overwhelmed when ill.

Chelidonium majus

This remedy is often indicated when pain extends to the back, right shoulder, and shoulder blade. The abdomen is distended, with a constricting feeling as if a string were pulled across it. Pain is worse from motion, and lying on the left with the legs drawn up may help. The person may feel nauseous, especially after eating fat or drinking something cold (warm drinks stay down more easily). The person may feel tired, worse from being cold, and worse in the early morning.

Colocynthis

Cutting, cramping pains that make a person double over or want to lie down and put hard pressure on the abdomen may indicate a need for this remedy. Pain in the upper right abdomen, extending to the shoulder, may also be seen. A person needing this remedy may have aggravated physical symptoms after feeling angry or emotional, especially after suppressing those feelings.

Dioscorea

This remedy is indicated when abdominal pain from gallstones is relieved by bending backward, and is worse when the person is bending forward or lying flat. Standing up and moving around in open air can also bring improvement. Pains can spread to the back, chest, and arms, or may shift around. The person tends to feel worse in the evening and at night, and also when lying down.

Lycopodium

This remedy is often indicated for people who have chronic digestive problems with abdominal bloating, flatulence, and discomfort. Problems are worse from eating, and the pains may extend from the right side to the left. A person who needs this remedy typically craves sweets, prefers warm drinks, and may feel worse in the late afternoon and evening.

Nux vomica

Constricting pains that travel upward, stitching pains, and a swollen feeling in the upper right part of the abdomen suggest a need for this remedy. Digestive cramps and nausea, along with a general feeling of

chilliness, are likely. The person may crave fats, strong spicy foods, alcohol, coffee and other stimulants, and feel worse from having them. Irritability and impatience are usually pronounced when this remedy is needed.

Podophyllum

This remedy is sometimes indicated in liver and gallbladder problems when soreness is felt in the upper right part of the abdomen along with a feeling of weakness, sinking, or emptiness. Heat may also be felt in the area. Constipation with clay-colored stools that are dry and hard to pass may alternate with watery diarrhea.

See p. 509 for Homeopathy: Dosage Directions.

Remedies for Gout

Gout (p. 75) is a painful condition resulting from the buildup of uric acid crystals in or around a joint. Diet, genetics, and certain medications may be contributing factors. Homeopathic remedies can provide a measure of relief during painful attacks of joint pain and inflammation. A constitutional remedy prescribed by an experienced homeopath may help to reduce the likelihood of further episodes.

Arnica montana

Although this remedy usually comes to mind for injuries, it can also be very helpful for discomfort that comes with gout. Pain is sore and bruise-like, and it hurts to walk. The person may be afraid to be approached or touched, because of pain.

Belladonna

Sudden onset, swelling, throbbing, heat, and intensity are symptoms that suggest this remedy. The joints look red, inflamed, and shiny—with sharp or violent pains that are worse from touch and jarring. The person may feel restless, flushed, and hot.

Berberis vulgaris

Twinges of pain in gouty joints, or stitching pains that are aggravated by changing position or walking, may indicate a need for this remedy. *Berberis* is often indicated for people who ache all over; some have nagging back pain or a tendency toward kidney stones.

Bryonia

When this remedy is needed, tearing pain is worse from the slightest movement, and the joints are swollen and hot. Areas with swelling and inflammation are painful to touch. The knees can be very stiff and the feet may swell. When *Bryonia* is indicated, the person is irritable and self-protective, not wanting to be touched or interfered with.

Calcarea fluorica

When this remedy is indicated, the finger joints may become enlarged because of gout, and the knees and toes may be involved. Stabbing pain is experienced, and the joints may make a cracking sound on movement. Discomfort is worse during weather changes, and warmth may bring relief.

Colchicum autumnale

Gout in the big toe or heel—so painful the person finds both motion and touch unbearable—suggests a need for this remedy. The joints are swollen, red and hot. Pain is often worse in the evening and at night. Flare-ups may occur in the springtime or with weather changes. Individuals who need this remedy often have a feeling of internal coldness and may be very tired.

Ledum palustre

When this remedy is indicated, the foot and big toe can be extremely swollen. Shooting pains are felt all through the foot and ankle, moving upward to the knee. This remedy is especially indicated when cold applications relieve both the swelling and the pain.

Rhododendron

This remedy can be useful for gouty swelling of the big toe joint that flares up before a storm. Other joints may ache and swell, especially on the right side of the body. Pain usually is worse toward early morning and after staying still too long. The person may feel better from warmth and after eating.

Rhus toxicodendron

This remedy can be helpful for joints that are hot, stiff, painful, and swollen. Symptoms are often worse in cold, damp weather and improved by warmth and gentle motion.

Sulphur

Painful gouty joints that itch, along with a burning feeling in the feet, suggest the use of this remedy. The knees and other joints may be involved. Problems can be aggravated by heat in any form, and are often worse in damp weather and in springtime.

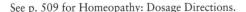

See p. 509 for Homeopathy: Dosage Directions.

Remedies for Hay Fever

Acute attacks of **hay fever** (p. 76) often respond to homeopathic remedies. Allergies are usually deep-seated problems, and are often best addressed with a constitutional remedy and the guidance of an experienced practitioner.

Allium cepa

Indications for this remedy include watery eyes and a clear nasal discharge that irritates the upper lip, along with sneezing and a tickling cough. The person may be thirsty, and feel worse indoors (especially when rooms are warm) and better in fresh air.

Arsenicum album

A burning, watery, runny nose with a stuffy, tickling feeling during allergy attacks suggests a need for this remedy. Swelling below the eyes and a wheezy cough are common. The person may feel chilly, restless, anxious, and is often very tired.

Euphrasia officinalis

This remedy can be helpful if the eyes are swollen and irritated with acrid tears or pus. The nose also runs, but with a discharge that is more bland. Symptoms are often worse in the daytime and worse from warmth, and the eyes may hurt from too much light. The person can also have a cough in the daytime, which improves at night.

Ferrum phosphoricum

This is a very useful remedy in the early stages of any inflammation. Taken when allergy symptoms start, it often slows or stops an episode. Symptoms include runny eyes with a burning or gritty feeling, facial flushing, watery nose, and short, hard, tickling cough.

Gelsemium

A tired, droopy feeling during allergies with a flushed and heavy-feeling face suggest a need for this remedy. A sensation of dryness or of swollen membranes may be felt inside the nose—or the nose may run with irritating watery discharge, with the person sneezing frequently. Aching in the back of the head and neck, a trembling feeling, and chills along the spine are often seen when a person needs *Gelsemium*.

Natrum muriaticum

Allergy attacks with sneezing, watery eyes, clear nasal discharge that resembles egg white, and a loss of taste and smell will all suggest a need for this remedy. The person may have dark circles under the eyes, be thirsty, feel withdrawn and sad, and act irritable if sympathy is offered.

Nux vomica

If the nose is alternately stuffed up (especially outdoors or at night) and running (indoors and in the daytime), this remedy may bring relief. Other symptoms include a teasing cough, a scraped or tickly feeling in the throat, and headache. A person who needs this remedy often feels impatient, irritable, and chilly.

Sabadilla

Long paroxysms of sneezing, itching in the nose with irritating runny discharge, a feeling of a lump in the throat, and watery eyes will all suggest a need for this remedy. The person may feel nervous during allergy attacks, and trying to concentrate can bring on drowsiness or headache.

Wyethia

Intolerable itching felt on the roof of the mouth and behind the nose—sometimes extending into the throat and ears—strongly suggests the use of this remedy. Everything in the person's head feels dry and irritated, but the nose may still be runny.

See p. 509 for Homeopathy: Dosage Directions.

Remedies for Hemorrhoids

Hemorrhoids (p. 77) (also called "piles") are troublesome varicose veins in the rectal and anal region, which can lead to protrusion, pain, and bleeding after bowel movements. This condition can occur at any age, and the symptoms can come and go unpredictably. **Constipation** (p. 44), overeating, and inadequate exercise may contribute to the problem. Homeopathic remedies can offer gentle, safe relief. (A constitutional homeopathic remedy chosen by an experienced practitioner may help a person overcome the tendency toward hemorrhoids.) If hemorrhoids are very sore and congested, ulcerated, or bleed profusely, medical care should be sought.

Aesculus hippocastanum

When this remedy is needed, hemorrhoids are sore and aching, with a swollen feeling. Pain may last for hours after the bowels have moved. People who need this remedy often have the sensation of a lump, or a feeling that a lot of small sharp sticks are inside the rectum, poking them. Sharp and shooting pains may be felt in the rectum and back. A person who needs this remedy may also have low back problems.

Aloe socotrina

This remedy may help if hemorrhoids are swollen and protrude "like a bunch of grapes" and are soothed by cold soaks or compresses. Hemorrhoids may alternate with diarrhea, and the person may have a lot of flatulence.

Arnica montana

Sore, bruised-feeling hemorrhoids may be relieved with this remedy, especially when straining or overexertion (for instance, childbirth or heavy lifting) has brought on the hemorrhoids.

Calcarea fluorica

This remedy may be indicated for hemorrhoids with bleeding and itching in the anal region, or internal hemorrhoids causing soreness in the very low back and sacrum. The person may also have problems with flatulence and constipation.

Graphites

Burning hemorrhoids with soreness, cracks, and itching in the anal region suggest a need for this remedy. A person who needs *Graphites* is often overweight, has difficulty concentrating, and tends toward skin eruptions.

Hamamelis virginiana

A raw, sore feeling in the anus, with bleeding hemorrhoids, indicates a need for this remedy. Pulsation may be felt in the rectum, and the lower back often aches. Symptoms may be worse from warmth.

Ignatia amara

Hemorrhoids accompanied by spasms and stabbing pain in the rectum suggest a need for this remedy— especially if the person is sensitive and emotional. Stitching pains can be felt in the rectal area when coughing. Bleeding and pain are often worse when the stool is loose, and rectal prolapse sometimes follows bowel movements.

Nux vomica

Itching, painful hemorrhoids, a feeling of constriction in the rectum, and chronic constipation with ineffectual urging are indications for this remedy. People who need *Nux vomica* are usually impatient, tense, and irritable, and often have a tendency toward heavy use of stimulants, strong foods, and alcohol or drugs.

Pulsatilla

When this remedy is indicated, hemorrhoids are itchy and uncomfortable, with sticking pains. They are likely to protrude, with improvement after lying down. Warmth often aggravates the symptoms. This is a very helpful remedy for hemorrhoids that appear during pregnancy or around the menstrual period.

Sulphur

Itching, burning, oozing hemorrhoids accompanied by a feeling of fullness and pressure in the abdomen suggest a need for this remedy. The anus is inflamed and red and may protrude significantly. The person may feel worse from warmth and bathing, and have flatulence with a strong, offensive odor.

See p. 509 for Homeopathy: Dosage Directions.

Remedies for Herpes Simplex (Cold Sores; Genital Herpes)

Herpes is a common virus that causes painful **cold sores** (p. 39) around the mouth. Genital herpes infection is a related condition and potentially can be treated in much the same way. A burning or itching sensation may precede the outbreak by several days. Eruptions are most likely to come out in times of stress and tend to reappear in the same locations. Constitutional homeopathic care with the guidance of an experienced practitioner may help to raise a person's resistance to cold sores.

Apis mellifica

When a herpes outbreak is accompanied by stinging pain and the area looks red and swollen, this remedy can be helpful. The sores are tender to touch, and ice or cold compresses are soothing.

Arsenicum album

Eruptions with burning pain relieved by applying heat suggest a need for this remedy. The person may feel anxious, restless, chilly, and exhausted.

Borax

This remedy can be useful for herpes eruptions in any area, with tense-feeling inflammation. Sensitivity to noise and a fear of falling are other indications for *Borax*.

Dulcamara

This remedy is often helpful if herpes sores have appeared with a change to rainy weather, or break out when a person has gotten wet and chilled and is coming down with a cold.

Graphites

Herpes eruptions, with oozing of honey-like discharge and crusting and cracking of the skin, suggest a need for this remedy. The person may tend toward many problems with the skin, be stout, and have trouble concentrating.

Hepar sulphuris calcareum

Herpes sores that are very sensitive to touch and worse from any form of cold suggest a need for this remedy. A person who needs *Hepar sulph* is extremely sensitive to cold, and often has a low resistance to infection.

Mercurius solubilis

This remedy may be indicated for sore, infected eruptions—especially if the person has swollen lymph nodes and offensive breath, is extremely sensitive to temperatures, and tends to sweat at night.

Natrum muriaticum

This remedy sometimes stops a herpes outbreak if taken in the early, tingling stage. It is also helpful for raw, red cold sores that develop on the lips and corners of the mouth, as well as the nostril area, face, and chin. Eruptions may also appear in the genital area. Eating too much salt (which the person craves) and being in the sun sometimes aggravate the symptoms.

Petroleum

This remedy may be helpful for genital herpes that spread to the anal area and thighs. People who need this remedy have a tendency toward many skin problems, with rough, dry skin that cracks and bleeds.

Rhus toxicodendron

Herpes simplex outbreaks in any location, especially around the lips, the corners of the mouth, or on and near the genitals and inner thighs, may respond to this remedy. Eruptions are red and swollen with burning pain and itching, relieved by hot water or warm applications. The person may be very restless, and often paces or feels a constant need to move around.

See p. 509 for Homeopathy: Dosage Directions.

Remedies for High Blood Pressure (Hypertension)

Hypertension (p. 89) is sometimes very serious, since the risk of stroke, as well as heart and kidney problems, can increase if the blood pressure gets too high. Stressful episodes of nervousness or worry may raise the blood pressure temporarily, but long-term resting elevated blood pressure is more dangerous and should be monitored. A constitutional remedy chosen by an experienced prescriber is more appropriate than self-care in deep-seated, serious, or chronic conditions. Some remedies may be useful as first aid in intense situations, but medical care should also be sought immediately. Remedies below have been helpful to some people with hypertension. They are mentioned here to introduce a few of the possibilities homeopathy can offer, and not as recommendations for self-treatment.

Argentum nitricum

If blood pressure rises with anxiety and nervousness, this remedy may be indicated. "Stage fright" or anticipation of a stressful event can bring on dizziness, headache, diarrhea, and a pounding pulse. People who need this remedy are typically warm-blooded, imaginative, impulsive, claustrophobic, and have strong cravings for sweets and salt.

Aurum metallicum

This remedy is sometimes indicated for serious people, focused on career and accomplishment, with blood pressure problems related to stress. Worry, depression, or anger may occur, especially when these people feel they have made a mistake or failed in some way. A general tendency to feel worse at night, and a strong desire for alcohol, sweets, bread, and pastries are other indications for *Aurum*.

Belladonna

This remedy is indicated when symptoms come on suddenly, with great intensity and heat. The person's face is flushed, with dilated pupils; and pulsations and throbbing may be felt in various parts of the body. Despite the general heat, the person's hands and feet may be cold. Vertigo and pounding headaches, worse from jarring and worse from light, may also occur.

Calcarea carbonica

This remedy is often helpful to people with high blood pressure who easily tire and have poor stamina. They are typically responsible types, who feel overwhelmed when ill and fear a breakdown. Palpitations and breathing problems can be worse from walking up a slope or stairs, and also when lying down. A general chilliness with clammy hands and feet (the feet may heat up in bed at night) and sweat on the head during sleep are other indications. The person may have cravings for sweets and eggs, and tend toward weight problems.

Glonoinum

A flushed face with a pounding headache and visible throbbing in the blood vessels of the neck may indicate a need for this remedy. The chest can feel congested or hot, with a pounding or irregular heartbeat. The person is worse from moving around, after heat and sun exposure, and after drinking alcohol. A feeling of "being lost in a familiar place" is a strong indication for this remedy.

Lachesis

A person who needs this remedy typically is intense and talkative, with inner passion and agitation that need an outlet—a "pressure-cooker." The person may have a strong fear of disease, and feelings of suspicion, revenge, or jealousy are common. The person may also have heart or artery problems, look flushed or purplish, and feel constriction in the chest, with pulsations in many areas. Feeling worse after taking a nap or on waking in the morning, and a strong intolerance of clothing around the neck (or any kind of restriction), are other indications for *Lachesis*.

Natrum muriaticum

A person who needs this remedy seems reserved and responsible, but may have very strong feelings (of grief, disappointment, anger, lingering grudges, a fear of misfortune) inside. Headaches and palpitations are common, as well as a feeling of tension (even coldness) in the chest. The person may feel worse from being in the sun, worse around mid-morning, and better from being alone in a quiet place. A craving for salt and strong thirst can help to confirm the choice of this remedy.

Nux vomica

A person who needs this remedy is usually impatient and driven—easily frustrated, angered, and offended. A strong desire for coffee and other stimulants, sweets, strong foods, and alcohol or drugs may aggravate blood pressure problems. Palpitations, constricting feelings in the chest, constipation, and hemorrhoids are often seen. The person is typically sensitive to light, noise, odors, and interference.

Phosphorus

A person who needs this remedy usually is sensitive, suggestible, and sympathetic, with a tendency toward weakness, dizziness, a "spaced-out" feeling, and fearfulness. Nosebleeds, facial flushing, palpitations, a feeling of heaviness or pain in the chest, and left-sided problems are often seen. A strong desire for cold drinks and cool or refreshing foods, and a marked improvement after eating and sleeping are other indications for *Phosphorus*.

Plumbum

This remedy is indicated for people with degenerative problems of the nerves and hardening of the arteries. Chest tightness and palpitations are often worse when lying on the left side. Contractures, paralysis, and nerve or muscle problems are also likely. The person may have a history of heavy drinking and "high living"—becoming apathetic or depressed when physical debility and memory problems develop.

Sanguinaria canadensis

A feeling that blood is rushing to the head, with flushed red cheeks and pulsing in the neck, may indicate this remedy. The person may have headaches or migraines (usually on the right and worse from light and noise). Right-sided neck and shoulder problems, allergies, heartburn, and digestive problems are often seen, and burning pains are typical. Symptoms are worse from motion, and relief may come from being in the dark and sleeping. A craving for spicy food and a tendency to feel worse from eating sweets are other indications for *Sanguinaria*.

See p. 509 for Homeopathy: Dosage Directions.

Remedies for IBS (Irritable Bowel Syndrome)

Irritable bowel syndrome (p. 109) is a chronic problem with varying symptoms, including abdominal pain and bloating, alternating diarrhea and constipation, flatulence, back pain, and fatigue. The cause is not clearly understood; however, since no significant tissue changes in the bowel are evident on medical examination, some speculation indicates that allergies and emotional stress may contribute to this condition. Remedies listed here may help bring some relief in moderate situations. A constitutional remedy prescribed by an experienced professional is often helpful in restoring balance to a person's system.

Argentum nitricum

Digestive upsets accompanied by nervousness and anxiety suggest the use of this remedy. Bloating, rumbling flatulence, nausea, and greenish diarrhea can be sudden and intense. Diarrhea may come on immediately after drinking water. Eating too much sweet or salty food (which the person often craves) may also lead to problems. A person who needs this remedy tends to be expressive, impulsive, and claustrophobic, and may have blood sugar problems.

Asafoetida

A feeling of constriction all along the digestive tract (especially if muscular contractions in the intestines and esophagus seem to be moving in the wrong direction) strongly indicates this remedy. The person may have a feeling that a bubble is stuck in the throat, or that a lump is moving up from the stomach. The abdomen feels inflated, but the person finds it hard to pass gas in either direction to get relief. Constipation brings on griping pains. Diarrhea can be explosive, and the person may even regurgitate food in small amounts. The person may exhibit a strong emotional or "hysterical" element when this remedy is needed.

Colocynthis

This remedy is indicated when cutting pains and cramping occur, making the person bend double or need to lie down and press on the abdomen. Cramps may be felt in the area of the pubic bone. Pain is likely to be worse just before the diarrhea passes, and after eating fruit or drinking water. Problems tend to be aggravated by emotions, especially if indignation or anger has been felt but not expressed. Back pain, leg pain, and gall bladder problems are sometimes seen when this remedy is needed.

Lilium tigrinum

When this remedy is indicated, the person may make frequent unsuccessful efforts to move the bowels all day and have sudden diarrhea the following morning. A feeling of a lump in the rectum, worse when standing up, is common. Hemorrhoids may develop. Constricting feelings are often felt in the chest. The person is likely to be worse from excitement and strong emotions, and may tend toward irritability or even rage.

Lycopodium

This remedy is often indicated for people with chronic digestive discomforts and bowel problems. Bloating and a feeling of fullness come on early in a meal or shortly after, and a large amount of gas is usually produced. Heartburn and stomach pain are common, and the person may feel better from rubbing the abdomen. Things are typically worse between 4:00 and 8:00 P.M. Despite so many digestive troubles, the person can have a ravenous appetite, and may even get up in the middle of the night to eat. Problems with self-confidence, a worried facial expression, a craving for sweets, and a preference for warm drinks are other indications for *Lycopodium*.

Natrum carbonicum

This remedy is often indicated for mild people who have trouble digesting and assimilating many foods and have to stay on restricted diets. Indigestion, heartburn, and even ulcers may occur if offending foods are eaten. The person often is intolerant of milk, and drinking it or eating dairy products can lead to gas and sputtery diarrhea with an empty feeling in the stomach. The person may have cravings for potatoes and for sweets (and sometimes also milk, but has learned to avoid it). A person who needs this remedy usually makes an effort to be cheerful and considerate but, when feeling weak and sensitive, wants to be alone to rest.

Nux vomica

Abdominal pains and bowel problems accompanied by tension, constricting sensations, chilliness, and irritability can indicate a need for this remedy. Soreness in the muscles of the abdominal wall, as well as painful gas and cramps, are common. Firm pressure on the abdomen brings some relief. When constipated, the person has an urge to move the bowels, but only small amounts come out. The person may experience a constant feeling of uneasiness in the rectum. After diarrhea has passed, the pain may be eased for a little while. A person who needs this remedy often craves strong spicy foods, alcohol, tobacco, coffee, and other stimulants—and usually feels worse from having them.

Podophyllum

This remedy is indicated when abdominal pain and cramping with a gurgling, sinking, empty feeling are followed by watery, offensive-smelling diarrhea—alternating with constipation, or pasty yellow bowel movements containing mucus. Things tend to be worse in the very early morning, and the person may feel weak and faint or have a headache afterward. Rubbing the abdomen (especially on the right) may help relieve discomfort. A person who needs this remedy may also experience stiffness in the joints and muscles.

Sulphur

This remedy is often indicated when a sudden urge toward diarrhea wakes the person early in the morning (typically 5:00 A.M.) and makes them hurry to the bathroom. Diarrhea can come on several times a day. The person may, at other times, be constipated and have gas with an offensive and pervasive smell. Oozing around the rectum, as well as itching, burning, and red irritation may also be experienced. A person who needs this remedy may tend to have poor posture and back pain, and feel worse from standing up too long.

See also Remedies for **Allergies and Sensitivities** (p. 510).

See p. 509 for Homeopathy: Dosage Directions.

Remedies for Impotence

Impotence (p. 98) is the inability to maintain an erection long enough to engage in normal sexual intercourse. Many factors can contribute, including emotional issues, dietary factors, use of alcohol or drugs, and level of physical fitness. Homeopathic remedies sometimes help with temporary difficulties. If the problem is constant or recurrent, a doctor should be consulted to check for physical, hormonal, or nervous system problems. A constitutional remedy and the guidance of an experienced practitioner may help bring balance to a person's system, both emotionally and physically.

Agnus castus

This remedy may be helpful if problems with impotence develop after a man has led a life of intense and frequent sexual activity for many years. A cold sensation felt in the genitals is a strong indication for *Agnus castus*. People who need this remedy are often very anxious about their health and loss of abilities, and may have problems with memory and concentration.

Argentum nitricum

This remedy may be helpful if a man's erection fails when sexual intercourse is attempted, especially if thinking about the problem makes it worse. People who need this remedy are often nervous and imaginative. A person who needs *Argentum nitricum* is usually warm-blooded, with cravings for both sweets and salt.

Caladium

This remedy may be helpful to a man whose genitals are completely limp, despite having sexual interest. Nocturnal emissions can occur without an erection, even if dreams are not sex-related. A person who needs this remedy often craves tobacco.

Causticum

This remedy may be indicated if physical pleasure during sex has diminished and sexual urges are reduced. The person feels tired and weak, and may experience memory loss, with a compulsive need to check things (to see that doors are locked, for example). Prostate problems may be associated with impotence, and urine may be lost when the person coughs or sneezes.

Lycopodium

People who need this remedy may have problems with erections because of worry, and can also be troubled by memory loss. They often lack self-confidence (though some may overcompensate by acting egotistically). People who need this remedy often have digestive problems with gas and bloating, and an energy slump in the late afternoon and evening.

Selenium metallicum

This remedy is often helpful to men who have diminished sexual ability, especially if the problem starts after a fever or exhausting illness. The person feels weak and exhausted, but interest is usually still present. Unusual hair loss (body hair or eyebrows) can also suggest a need for *Selenium*.

Staphysagria

Gentle-natured, quiet men with deep emotions may respond to this remedy. Problems with impotence often occur from embarrassment or shyness. People who need this remedy often have a history of emotional suppression and very sensitive feelings.

See p. 509 for Homeopathy: Dosage Directions.

Remedies for Indigestion and Gas

Indigestion and gas (p. 99) can be caused by poor eating habits, emotional tension, food allergies, imbalances in stomach acid or digestive enzymes, and many other factors. For moderate problems, homeopathy can offer a number of safe and gentle remedies. If discomfort is chronic and persistent or if symptoms are extreme, a doctor should be consulted.

Arsenicum album

This remedy may be indicated if a person feels anxious, restless yet exhausted, and is worse from the smell and sight of food. Burning pain in the stomach and esophagus may be experienced with relief from warmth and sitting up. Vomiting and diarrhea are possible. Upsets from spoiled food or from eating too much fruit will often respond to this remedy.

Bryonia

When this remedy is indicated, the stomach feels heavy, with rising acid and a bitter or sour taste. Pain and nausea are worse from motion of any kind. The person may have a dry mouth and be thirsty for long drinks, which may increase discomfort. *Bryonia* is strongly suggested if a person is grumpy and wants to stay completely still and not be touched or talked to.

Carbo vegetabilis

Sour belching bringing only small relief, burning pain in the stomach and abdomen, and flatulence after eating may be experienced when this remedy is needed. The person feels cold and faint, with a strong desire for fresh or moving air. Digestion may be slow and incomplete, with nausea or cramping.

Colocynthis

Cutting, cramping pain in the stomach and abdomen, with relief from hard pressure or from doubling over, indicates a need for this remedy. A bitter taste in the mouth, a feeling that the intestines are about to burst, or a sensation that stones are grinding together in the abdomen may be present. Indigestion may be worse when the person feels upset, especially after suppressing anger.

Lycopodium

This remedy is indicated for many digestive troubles. The person's appetite may be ravenous, but eating even a small amount can cause a feeling of fullness and bloating. Rumbling gas may form in the abdomen, pressing upward and making breathing difficult. The person often has a strong desire for sweets, is sleepy after meals, and feels worse in the late afternoon and evening.

Natrum carbonicum

This remedy can be helpful to mild people who have trouble digesting and assimilating many foods and have to stay on restricted diets. Indigestion, heartburn, and ulcers can occur if offending foods are eaten. Milk or dairy products can lead to flatulence or sputtery diarrhea that leaves an empty feeling in the stomach. Cravings for potatoes and sweets are common; also milk, but it makes these people sick, so they have usually learned to avoid it.

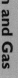

Natrum phosphoricum

A sour taste in the mouth, an acid or burning sensation in the stomach, sour vomiting, regurgitated bits of food, and a yellow coating on the tongue are all indications for this remedy. The person may have problems after consuming dairy products or too much sugar. Another indication for *Natrum phos* is a craving for fried eggs.

Nux vomica

This remedy is often useful for indigestion, and is especially suited to those who overindulge in stimulants, food, and alcohol. Chilliness, irritability, and sensitivity to odors, sound, and light are often seen. Pain and weight can be felt in the stomach, with cramps or constricting pains. The person often feels an urge to vomit or move the bowels and may strain to do so, feeling better if their efforts are successful.

Phosphorus

Burning pain in the stomach that feels better from eating ice cream or other cold, refreshing foods suggests a need for this remedy. The person is usually thirsty for cold drinks, but often feels nauseous or vomits once liquids warm up in the stomach. People needing *Phosphorus* may have a tendency toward easy bleeding and sometimes develop stomach ulcers.

Pulsatilla

Indigestion that is worse from eating rich and fatty foods, with a feeling of a lump or pulsation in the stomach, suggests a need for this remedy. Discomfort often is worse from warmth, especially in a stuffy room, and the person may feel better from gentle walking in open air. A bitter taste in the mouth can take the pleasure out of eating. A person who needs *Pulsatilla* usually does not feel thirsty and may be tearful and emotional.

See p. 509 for Homeopathy: Dosage Directions.

Remedies for Infection

Infection (p. 101) occurs when bacteria or viruses take hold in body tissues, and inflammation, swelling, fever, and other symptoms appear as the person's immune system works to overcome them. Homeopathic remedies can help the body work efficiently to fight acute infections, and also help improve immune response if a person's resistance is low. Other remedy descriptions can be found in sections discussing **common cold** (p. 41), **influenza** (p. 104), **ear infections** (p. 63), **bronchi-**tis, **urinary tract infections** (p. 160), **herpes** (p. 155), **boils**, and **yeast infections** (p. 169).

Aconitum napellus

This remedy is often indicated when fever and inflammation come on suddenly, sometimes after exposure to wind and cold, or after a traumatic experience. The person may be very thirsty and often feels fearful or anxious.

Belladonna

Intense heat, redness, swelling, throbbing, and pulsation indicate a need for this remedy. The person's face may be flushed and hot (though hands and feet may be cold) and the eyes are often sensitive to light. Thirst may be lower than expected during fever. Discomfort is worse from motion or jarring, and relieved by cold applications.

Bryonia

Feeling worse from even the slightest motion is a strong indication for this remedy. When ill, the person wants to stay completely still—to be left alone and not interfered with in any way. Fever with chills, a very dry mouth, and thirst are also likely. Local infections may be accompanied by tearing pains that feel worse from any motion, but improve from pressure if it adds stability.

Calcarea carbonica

People who need this remedy tire easily and have low stamina. They tend to feel chilly and sluggish, with clammy hands and feet (though their feet may heat up in bed at night, and their heads may perspire during sleep). Swollen lymph nodes, frequent colds, sore throats, ear infections, and skin eruptions are common. Children who need this remedy are often slow to walk and may have teething problems, frequent colds, and ear infections.

Calendula

This remedy is useful as a topical application for cuts, scrapes, and skin eruptions, to prevent and combat infection. It is usually used in unpotentized herbal form, as an ointment or tincture. *Calendula* can also be helpful potentized, when taken internally for boils or infections.

Ferrum phosphoricum

This remedy is indicated in the early stages of many inflammations. Taken at the very first sign of a cold or sore throat, it often helps a person throw the infection off and not get ill. Fever, pink-flushed cheeks, a general weariness, thirst, and moderate pain and swelling

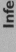

Infection

are typical symptoms suggesting *Ferrum phos* in illness or infection.

Graphites

This remedy may be useful when a person has unhealthy skin that tends toward cracking, oozing honey-colored discharge and crusts. Impetigo, herpes simplex, or infections involving the skin around the ears, the eyelids, nose, and sinuses are common—as are tendencies toward recurring colds and earaches. A feeling of sluggishness, slow waking, and difficulty concentrating are other indications for *Graphites*.

Hepar sulphuris calcareum

A person who needs this remedy may feel extremely sensitive and vulnerable when ill, especially if exposed to cold or drafts. Ear infections, sore throats, sinusitis, bronchitis, and skin eruptions are often seen, and cheesy-smelling discharge or offensive pus may be produced. Areas of inflammation can be very sore and sensitive, and splinter-like pains are often felt (in the tonsils when swallowing, in a boil when the skin is touched, etc.).

Mercurius solubilis

This remedy is needed when a person has swollen lymph nodes, offensive breath, and is extremely sensitive to any change in temperature. A tendency toward night sweats and profuse salivation during sleep are other indications. Infections of the gums, ears, sinuses, throat, and skin often respond to this remedy when the other symptoms fit.

Silicea (*also called* Silica)

A person who needs this remedy can be sensitive and nervous, with low stamina and poor resistance to infection—leading to swollen lymph nodes, frequent colds, sore throats, tonsillitis, sinusitis, bronchitis, and other illnesses. Boils, easy infection of wounds, and abscessed teeth are often seen. Although very chilly in general, the person may often perspire during sleep. Offensive foot sweat with an inclination toward fungal infections is also common.

Sulphur

This remedy is useful in many kinds of infection characterized by irritation, burning pain, redness of mucous membranes, and offensive odors and discharges. Skin problems are very common—eczema, acne, boils, lymphangitis, and inflammations on or around the genitals. Symptoms are often worse from warmth and worse after bathing. Colds, bronchitis, and other illnesses that have been neglected, or infec-

tions that drag on for a very long time, may be helped with this remedy

---

See p. 509 for Homeopathy: Dosage Directions.

Remedies for Influenza

Influenza (p. 104) refers to many strains of viral illness that are more intense than a common cold, and typically include fever, muscle aching, headache, and fatigue. Some kinds of flu have cold-like symptoms with sore throat or respiratory involvement; others focus on the digestive tract, with diarrhea, nausea, or vomiting. If a strain of flu with a characteristic set of symptoms is "going around," a remedy that matches them can often be used preventively. When a person is ill, a remedy should be chosen to match the specific symptoms.

Aconitum napellus

A flu that comes on suddenly and intensely—with fever, anxiety, constricted pupils, and strong thirst—is likely to respond to this remedy. The person may feel fearful or agitated, and the fever can alternate with chills. Symptoms are often worst around midnight. Exposure to cold wind or a shock of some kind often precedes the illness.

Apis mellifica

This remedy may be helpful if a person has facial flushing, dry fever that alternates with sweating, and a very sore throat with swollen tonsils. Pain may extend to the ears, and the eyelids may be swollen. Exposure to cool air and cold applications may bring relief. Despite the fever, thirst usually is low. The person can be very irritable, disliking interference.

Arsenicum album

A person who needs this remedy during flu feels chilly and exhausted, along with an anxious restlessness. The person may be thirsty, but often only takes small sips. Nausea with burning pain or vomiting and acrid diarrhea may occur, if the digestive system is involved. If the flu is respiratory, a watery, runny nose with sneezing paroxysms and a dry or wheezing cough are often seen. The person's head will often feel hot, while the rest of the body is chilly.

Belladonna

Sudden, intense symptoms—including fever, red face, hot skin, and extreme sensitivity to light and jarring—

Influenza

suggest a need for this remedy. The person may have a very red sore throat, a pounding headache, a nagging cough, or other throbbing and inflammatory symptoms. Despite high fever, the person's hands and feet may feel cold, or chills and heat may alternate.

Bryonia

When a person is very grumpy and feels miserable with the flu, wanting only to lie still and be left alone, this remedy is likely to be useful. Headache, muscle aches, and cough or stomach pain may be the major symptoms. Everything feels worse from even the slightest motion. The person's mouth may be dry, with a thirst for long cold drinks.

Eupatorium perfoliatum

Flu with deep pain occurring in the legs or back ("as if the bones would break") often responds to this remedy. Pain may be felt in the eyeballs, with a heavy sensation in the head. Illness often begins with chills and thirst, followed by high fever. Chills may be felt in the back and legs, and the aching in the bones is worse from motion. The person feels "wiped out" and miserable.

Ferrum phosphoricum

This remedy may be helpful during flu with fever, headache, rosy cheeks, and a feeling of weariness. Sensitive eyes, a short hard cough, strong thirst, and vomiting after eating are other indications. This remedy is often helpful in early stages of flu or fever, even if symptoms are not especially clear.

Gelsemium

Symptoms of fatigue and achiness that come on gradually, increasing over several days, may indicate a need for this remedy. The face feels heavy, with droopy eyes and aching. A headache may begin at the back of the neck and skull, and the person may feel chills and heat running up and down the spine. Anxiety, trembling, dizziness, perspiration, and moderate fever are other indications for *Gelsemium*.

Nux vomica

When this remedy is indicated in influenza, the person may have high fever, violent chills, strong nausea, and cramping in the digestive tract (or a painful cough and constricted breathing if the flu is respiratory). Headache usually occurs, along with oversensitivity to sound, bright light, and odors. A person who needs *Nux vomica* is often very irritable, feeling worse from exertion and worse from being cold in any way.

Oscillococcinum (*also called* Anas barbariae)

Oscillococcinum is one of the common names used for a remedy that is widely used for prevention and treatment of flu in the United States and Europe. Research suggests that it has strong antiviral effects.

Phosphorus

When this remedy is needed during flu, the person has a fever with an easily flushing face, and feels very weak and dizzy. Headache, hoarseness, sore throat, and cough are likely. If the focus is digestive, stomach pain and nausea or vomiting usually occur. A person who needs this remedy often has a strong anxiety, wanting others to be around to offer company and reassurance. Strong thirst, with a tendency to vomit when liquids warm up in the stomach, is a strong indication for *Phosphorus*.

Rhus toxicodendron

A person who needs this remedy during flu feels extremely restless. Fever is accompanied by bone and muscle aches. Sore throat, red tongue, a teasing cough, and nausea and bloating are other likely symptoms. Soreness and stiffness may be felt all over, with improvement from hot showers or from getting up and pacing. A person who needs *Rhus tox* will usually feel worse when waking up, after lying in bed, or from keeping still too long. Symptoms are relieved by rubbing and stretching, but warmth and movement are especially useful.

Sulphur

This remedy may be useful if a flu is very long-lasting or has some lingering symptoms—often after people have neglected to take good care of themselves. Symptoms, either digestive or respiratory, will often have a hot or burning quality. The person may feel hot and sweaty, with low fever and reddish mucous membranes. Heat aggravates the symptoms, and the person often feels worse after bathing.

See also Remedies for **Infection** (p. 548), **Common Cold** (p. 527), and **Cough** (p. 530).

See p. 509 for Homeopathy: Dosage Directions.

Remedies for Injuries

Homeopathic remedies are often very useful for soothing pain and promoting healing. A homeopathic first-aid kit is welcome when accidental falls or head bumps, fingertips shut in doors, scraped knees, a burn on the stove, a twisted ankle, or any number of minor mishaps occur. Remedies may also be used preventively for "expected" injuries that come from dental work or surgery, as well as sports-related bruising, or occupational injuries from strenuous or repetitive tasks. Homeopathy can also be used (along with medical care) for more serious or extensive injuries, to help control bleeding and tissue damage, relieve discomfort, and encourage healing. Any serious injury should have the care of a physician.

Aconitum napellus

This remedy can be helpful when a person feels extremely fearful or agitated after being injured. It may help to soothe anxiety and panic and reduce the chance of shock.

Arnica montana

This is the major remedy for new traumatic injuries—especially bruises, sprains, and concussions. Symptoms are worse from touch and motion. *Arnica* can be helpful for painful bruising and tissue damage caused by surgery and dental work—given preventively before an anticipated injury, and used to treat the soreness afterward. It is also helpful in preventing shock.

Bellis perennis

This remedy is useful for injuries to the trunk and deeper tissues, as from falls, car accidents, or surgery, especially if a feeling of stiffness or coldness develops in the injured area. If *Arnica* has been given for an injury—especially a strain or bruise—but has not had much effect, *Bellis perennis* may be helpful.

Calcarea phosphorica

This remedy is useful for bone bruises, old or slow-healing fractures, or any injury that leads to soreness in the bones, especially if the area feels cold or numb and improves with warmth. The muscles near the injury may ache or stiffen.

Calendula

This is a very helpful remedy for cuts and scrapes or other injuries involving broken skin. Potentized *Calendula* can be taken internally to prevent or combat infection if a cut or scrape becomes inflamed. Herbal calendula can be applied directly to wounds as an ointment, lotion, or diluted tincture.

Hypericum perforatum

This remedy is indicated for injuries to body areas with many nerves, such as fingertips and toes, the genitals, the spine and tailbone, and the eyeballs. Shooting pains, a feeling of "jangled nerves," and pains mixed with tingling and numbness are strong indications. People with concussions, nerve pain after surgeries and root canals, or bites and puncture wounds may benefit from *Hypericum*.

Ipecacuanha

This remedy can be helpful as first aid if heavy bleeding occurs after an injury, with a feeling of nausea and weakness. (Emergency care is crucial when serious bleeding occurs; pressure should be applied to a severely bleeding wound, and medical help should be found immediately.)

Ledum palustre

This remedy is indicated for injuries that lead to puffy swelling, especially when ice packs or cold applications bring relief. Sprained ankles or knees, bashed noses, black eyes, or any kind of bruising injury that is painful and very swollen may respond to *Ledum*.

Millefolium

Contusions or sprains that involve small broken blood vessels and lead to bruise-like bleeding beneath the skin suggest the use of this remedy. It is often also useful for nosebleeds after injury, and for bleeding in other parts of the body (for instance, after childbirth or surgery).

Phosphorus

When small wounds bleed easily, or a person has a tendency to bruise from minor injuries, this remedy can be helpful. It is also useful for nosebleeds.

Ruta graveolens

This remedy is helpful for injuries to tendons, joints, muscles, and to the coverings of the bones (the periosteum). Bone bruises, barked shins, or any injury that leads to stiffness and aching may respond. *Ruta* is often useful after *Arnica* for sprains, pulled muscles, and connective tissue injuries.

Symphytum officinale

This remedy is best known for its healing effect on broken bones, and is also good for bone bruises. It is valuable if blunt injury occurs to the eyeball (as from a rock, a stick, or a flying object). Any injury to the eye or eyeball should be examined by a doctor.

See also Remedies for **Bruising** (p. 520), **Broken Bones** (p. 518), and **Burns** (p. 521).

See p. 509 for Homeopathy: Dosage Directions.

Remedies for Insect Bites and Stings

Homeopathic remedies can be useful for relieving the pain and swelling of insect bites and stings. If a person

Insect Bites and Stings

is allergic to the venom of a stinging insect, or if a bite is from a poisonous spider, emergency medical attention is needed right away. (Remedies can still be used to reduce the early trauma and to help recovery.)

Aconitum napellus

This remedy can be helpful if a person feels fearful or panicked after being stung. Cutting, stabbing, or burning pain may be felt, along with swelling, tingling, or numbness. *Aconitum* should be used immediately, while symptoms are intense, and can be followed by another remedy, as indicated.

Apis mellifica

If a bite or bee sting causes puffy, tender swelling that is pink or red and hot to the touch, this remedy may be helpful. The area stings and burns, and cold applications bring relief. (If a person is allergic to insect venom, especially bee stings, *Apis* may help to reduce the swelling of the passages, given as first aid while on the way to emergency medical care.)

Cantharis

This remedy may be indicated if a bite or sting results in intensely burning, scalding pain. The area of inflammation is red, and blisters may develop.

Carbolicum acidum

This remedy is usually indicated in first-aid situations while medical help is being sought. The person feels sick and weak, and may have trouble breathing, with a dark or reddish face that looks pale around the mouth.

Hypericum perforatum

This remedy is known for its soothing effect on injuries to nerve-rich body areas. It is also useful after puncture wounds, including bites and stings. Shooting pains or pains with numbness and tingling often are experienced when *Hypericum* is needed.

Ledum palustre

Swelling that extends some distance from the bite—often with a bluish tinge, a feeling of cold and numbness, and aching pain—suggests the use of this remedy. If the swollen part seems cold, but the application of ice or cold water brings relief, *Ledum* is strongly indicated.

Urtica urens

Reddish blotches that burn and itch intensely (like a nettle sting) after insect bites may be relieved with this remedy. It is also a useful remedy for hives that sting and itch.

See p. 509 for Homeopathy: Dosage Directions.

Remedies for Measles

Measles is a contagious viral illness most often affecting children. Early measles symptoms resemble a common cold, with weakness, mild fever, watery eyes, a dry or hacking cough, and eyes that are very sensitive to light. Over the next few days, the fever rises and little white spots like grains of salt show up on the inner surface of the cheeks. On the fourth or fifth day, a blotchy pink rash breaks out—first on the face and neck, and later spreading to the chest and abdomen. Homeopathic remedies can be useful to soothe the fever and discomfort and to help recovery. Rarely, serious complications develop from a case of measles. If fever is very high or a painful pounding headache appears, if the cough is very painful with breathing problems, or if the person seems extremely ill in any other way, consult a doctor immediately.

Aconitum napellus

Sudden high fever with hot dry skin, pain in the eyes, strong thirst, and a fearful or panicky feeling are indications for this remedy. Symptoms often start near midnight, and may wake the person up.

Belladonna

Fever that comes on rapidly, with a red flushed face, hot skin, dilated eyes that are sensitive to light, and a throbbing headache that is worse from jarring are all indications for this remedy. The rash is red and may be hot to touch. Many children needing *Belladonna* have nightmares during fever and talk or cry out when apparently asleep.

Bryonia

This remedy can be indicated when the rash is slow to appear, and the chest is congested with a painful cough. The head hurts from coughing, and everything feels worse from motion, making the person want to stay completely still. Chills and shivering often come with fever, but warmth can make things worse. The mouth may be very dry, and a thirst for long, cold drinks is typical.

Euphrasia officinalis

When this remedy is indicated during measles, the eyes may be swollen, streaming, and very sensitive to light. The tears can irritate the face, and the person's nose may run with a bland and watery discharge. Headache may intensify with fever. The person has chills, feels worse from warmth, and prefers to stay in a darkened room.

Gelsemium

Fever with a drowsy, lethargic feeling, droopy eyes, and shaking chills running up and down the spine are strong indications for this remedy. The rash is itchy, hot, and dry. A headache that begins in the back of the head and neck is often seen when *Gelsemium* is needed.

Kali bichromicum

When this remedy is indicated in measles, cold symptoms worsen over time. Hoarseness, coughing up of stringy yellow mucus, earache, and sticky eyes may be experienced. Symptoms can be worse in the morning, and the person feels best from staying in bed and keeping warm.

Pulsatilla

This remedy is often indicated when the rash is slow to develop and the symptoms of a cold are prominent. A stuffy nose producing yellowish mucus, a gagging cough (most often dry at night and loose in the morning), and plugging or inflammation in the ears are common. The person does not feel thirsty, is worse from warmth and stuffy rooms, and improves in open air. People who need this remedy often want a lot of comforting and attention. (*Pulsatilla* is a very useful children's remedy.)

Rhus toxicodendron

An extremely itchy rash that feels better from applying heat may indicate a need for this remedy. The person is very restless, and may feel driven to get up and pace. Stiffness may be felt in all the muscles of the body—worse at night, from lying still in bed, and on waking in the morning. The person may have chills along with fever, and all symptoms are improved by warmth and motion.

See p. 509 for Homeopathy: Dosage Directions.

Remedies for Menopause Symptoms

When women reach the age of **menopause** (p. 118), hormonal shifts can cause both physical and emotional stress. Because of the inevitable but sometimes disconcerting signs of aging, as well as transitions involved with children growing up, a woman's life may be undergoing major changes at this time. Mood swings, depression, hot flashes, cold sweats, and irregular menstrual cycles—including missed periods and flooding—may all occur (over months to years) as the woman's body gradually adapts. Although these symptoms go away on their own in time, a correctly chosen homeopathic remedy will often help to ease them. A constitutional remedy, and the guidance of an experienced homeopath, can be reassuring and helpful for both physical and emotional aspects of menopause.

Belladonna

This remedy can be useful if flushes of heat during menopause are very sudden and intense. Pulsation or throbbing may be felt in the head, or any part of the body. A heavy flow of blood that feels very hot may appear with some periods. Although the woman may be fairly stable emotionally, short bursts of anger can occur during headaches or in stressful situations. Migraines, blood pressure fluctuations, and a craving for lemons or lemonade are often seen when this remedy is needed.

Calcarea carbonica

This remedy may be helpful to a woman with heavy flooding, night sweats and flushing (despite a general chilliness), as well as weight gain during menopause. People who need this remedy are usually responsible and hard-working, yet somewhat slow or plodding and can be easily fatigued. Anxiety may be strong, and overwork or stress may lead to temporary breakdown. Stiff joints or cramps in the legs and feet, and cravings for eggs and sweets are other indications for *Calcarea*.

Glonoinum

Women with intense hot flashes and flushing during menopause, along with feelings of pulsation or pounding in the head, may find relief with this remedy. Menstrual flow may start then stop too early—and be followed by palpitations, surging sensations, or headaches, accompanied by irritability and muddled thinking. Problems can be aggravated if the woman gets too warm or stays in the sun too long, and are often worse from lying down.

Graphites

A woman who is chilly, pale, and sluggish—with trouble concentrating, and a tendency toward weight gain during or after menopause—is likely to respond to this remedy. Hot flushing and sweats at night are often seen. A person who needs this remedy may also have a tendency toward skin problems with oozing cracked eruptions, and be very slow to become alert when waking in the morning.

Ignatia amara

Ignatia is often helpful for emotional ups and downs occurring during menopause. The woman will be very sensitive, but may try to hide her feelings—seeming guarded and defensive, moody, or hysterical. Headaches, muscle spasms, and menstrual cramps can occur, along with irregular periods. A heavy feeling in the chest, a tendency to sigh and yawn, and sudden outbursts of tears or laughter are strong indications for *Ignatia*.

Lachesis

Intense hot flashes with red or purplish flushing, palpitations, and feelings of pressure, congestion, and constriction may indicate a need for this remedy. Tight clothing around the neck and waist may be impossible to tolerate. A woman needing *Lachesis* is often very talkative, with strong emotions (often including jealousy and suspicion)—a "pressure cooker" needing an outlet both physically and emotionally.

Lilium tigrinum

A woman likely to respond to this remedy feels hurried, anxious, and very emotional—with a tendency to fly into rages and make other people "walk on eggs." She often has a sensation of tightness in her chest, and a feeling as if her pelvic organs are pressing out, which can make her feel a need to sit a lot or cross her legs.

Natrum muriaticum

A woman who needs this remedy may seem reserved, but has strong emotions that she keeps inside. She often feels deep grief and may dwell on the loss of happy times from the past or brood about hurts and disappointments. During menopause, she can have irregular periods accompanied by backaches or migraines. A person who needs this remedy often craves salt, and feels worse from being in the sun.

Pulsatilla

A person who needs this remedy is usually soft and emotional, with changeable moods and a tendency toward tears. Women are very attached to their families and find it hard to bear the thought of the children growing up and leaving home. They usually feel deeply insecure about getting older. A fondness for desserts and butter can often lead to weight problems. Changeable moods, irregular periods, queasy feelings, alternating heat and chills, and lack of thirst are com-

mon. Aggravation from stuffy rooms and improvement in open air may confirm the choice of *Pulsatilla*.

Sepia

This remedy can be helpful if a woman's periods are sometimes late and scanty, but heavy and flooding at other times. Her pelvic organs can feel weak and sagging, and she may have a craving for vinegar or sour foods. Women who need this remedy usually feel dragged-out and weary, with an irritable detachment regarding family members, and a loss of interest in daily tasks. Exercise, especially dancing, may brighten up the woman's mood and improve her energy.

Staphysagria

A person who needs this remedy usually seems mild-mannered, shy, and accommodating, but has many suppressed emotions. Women around the time of menopause may become depressed, or have outbursts of unaccustomed rage (even throwing or breaking things). Many people needing *Staphysagria* have deferred to a spouse for many years, or have experienced abuse in childhood.

Sulphur

This remedy is often helpful for hot flashes and flushing during menopause, when the woman wakes in the early morning hours and throws the covers off. She may be very anxious, weep a lot, and worry excessively about her health. A person needing *Sulphur* will often be mentally active (or even eccentric), inclined toward messy habits, and usually feels worse from warmth.

See p. 509 for Homeopathy: Dosage Directions.

Remedies for Menstrual Problems

Some women have very little trouble with their menstrual cycles, but others face a monthly ordeal with **PMS** (p. 141) or **Menorrhagia** (p. 120). An array of stressful symptoms—irritability, mood swings, headaches, bloating, water retention, soreness of the breasts—may occur with premenstrual syndrome. Periods can be irregular and troubled, with cramping, menorrhagia (abnormally heavy flow), and various discomforts. Homeopathic remedies will often bring relief in moderate situations. Menstrual problems that are chronic or severe are best addressed with the guidance of an experienced practitioner: a constitutional remedy can help to bring balance to a person's system on many levels. A woman with serious symptoms or extremely heavy bleeding should have an experienced physician's care.

See also Remedies for **Menstruation, Painful (Dysmenorrhea)** (p. 556).

Bovista

Premenstrual problems with puffiness in the extremities, fluid retention, and a bloated feeling often indicate a need for this remedy. The woman may feel very awkward and clumsy, and may constantly be dropping things because of swollen-feeling hands. Diarrhea occurring around the time of the menstrual period is a strong confirmation of this remedy choice.

Calcarea carbonica

PMS with fatigue, anxiety, and a feeling of being overwhelmed suggest a need for this remedy. The woman may have problems with water-retention and weight gain, tender breasts, digestive upsets, and headaches. Periods often come too early and last too long, sometimes with a flow of bright red blood. A general feeling of chilliness, with clammy hands and feet, and cravings for sweets and eggs are other indications for *Calcarea.*

Caulophyllum thalictroides

This remedy is often helpful to women with a history of irregular periods, difficulty becoming pregnant, or slow childbirth due to weak muscle tone of the uterus. Symptoms include discomfort during periods and a heavy flow of blood or other discharge. Drawing pains may be felt in the pelvic region, thighs, and legs. Stiffness or arthritis, especially in the finger joints, may also be seen when this remedy is needed.

Chamomilla

A woman likely to respond to this remedy can be very angry, irritable, and hypersensitive to pain. Cramping may come on, or be intensified, because of emotional upset. Flow can be very heavy, and the blood may look dark or clotted. Problems are often worse at night. Heating pads or exposure to wind may aggravate the symptoms, and motion (such as rocking or brisk walking) may help to reduce the tension and discomfort.

Cimicifuga (*also called* Actaea racemosa)

This remedy can be helpful for irregular and painful periods, with shooting pains that go down the hips and thighs, or cramps that feel like labor pains that are felt in the pelvic area. Headache with pain and stiffness in the neck and back will often occur with PMS. The woman is likely to be intense and talkative, becoming agitated, fearful, and depressed before a menstrual period.

Kreosotum

Headache, nausea, and a heavy flow that makes the genitals and surrounding skin feel irritated and swollen are indications for this remedy. *Kreosotum* is often indicated for women with PMS who feel irritable and uncomfortable, and have a strong dislike of sexual activity.

Lachesis

Women who need this remedy are usually intense, with a tremendous need for an outlet, both physically and mentally. Symptoms of PMS include congestion, headaches, flushing, surges of heat, and an intense outspoken irritability—often with strong feelings of suspicion or jealousy. When the flow arrives, it may be heavy, but brings relief of tension. Intolerance of restrictive clothing around the waist or neck is another indication for *Lachesis.*

Lilium tigrinum

This remedy may be helpful if a woman is inclined toward rage during PMS, makes other people "walk on eggs," and is extremely sensitive and irritable. Pressure in the rectum and in the pelvic region, with a sensation that the uterus is pushing out, may make her feel a frequent need to sit or cross her legs. Emotions and excitement aggravate the symptoms, and fresh air will often bring relief.

Lycopodium

PMS with a craving for sweets and a ravenous appetite (sometimes a bulimic tendency) suggests a need for this remedy. Digestive upsets with abdominal bloating and flatulence are often seen, with the person feeling worst in the late afternoon and evening. Menstrual periods may be delayed, followed by a heavy flow that goes on for extra days. A woman who needs this remedy will often wear a worried look and lacks self-confidence—although she may be irritable and bossy to pets and family members. A desire to be alone, but with someone in the other room, is another indication for *Lycopodium.*

Natrum muriaticum

A person who needs this remedy will usually seem reserved to others, but be deeply emotional inside. She may feel extremely sad and lonely, but gets affronted or angry if others try to console her or sympathize. Depression, anger over minor things, and a need to be

Menstrual Problems

alone to cry are often seen when *Natrum mur* is needed. Menstrual problems can be accompanied by migraines, or a backache that feels better from lying on something hard or pushing a solid object against the painful place. A craving for salt, strong thirst, and a tendency to feel worse from being in the sun are other indications for this remedy.

Nux vomica

When a woman with PMS is extremely impatient, pushy, and intolerant, this remedy may be of use. Uncomfortable, irregular menstrual periods can be experienced, often with a nagging urge to move the bowels before the flow begins. Constipation is common, and constricting pains may extend to the rectum or tailbone region. Anger, mental strain, physical exertion, and overindulgence in coffee, alcohol, or food can aggravate the problems. The woman often feels chilly and improves from warmth and rest.

Pulsatilla

This remedy can be helpful during many conditions involving hormonal changes and is often helpful to girls who have recently started having periods. PMS with irritability, moodiness, and weepiness is typical. Delay or suppression of the menstrual flow can be accompanied by queasy feelings, nausea, and faintness. Being too warm or in a stuffy room makes things worse, and fresh air can bring relief. The timing, amount, and nature of the menstrual flow are changeable—as are the woman's moods—when *Pulsatilla* is the remedy. The woman will often be emotional and needy, wanting a lot of attention and comforting.

Sepia

A woman who needs this remedy with PMS feels weary and dragged-out, wanting others (especially family members) to keep their distance. She may often feel taken for granted and overworked, becoming irritable or sarcastic if demands are made. Late periods or scanty flow with a feeling that the pelvic floor is weak, or as if the uterus is sagging, can indicate a need for *Sepia*. Dampness and perspiring may aggravate the symptoms. Warmth and exercise, especially dancing, often restore some energy and brighten up her mood.

Veratrum album

Menstrual periods with very heavy flow and cramping, with a feeling of exhaustion and icy coldness suggest a need for this remedy. Vomiting and diarrhea are often seen. Periods may start too early and go on too long. The woman typically feels worse at night, from exercise, and from drinking things that are warm. Cold drinks, small meals, and wrapping up in warm clothes or covers may help to bring improvement.

See p. 509 for Homeopathy: Dosage Directions.

Remedies for Menstruation, Painful (Dysmenorrhea)

Discomfort during menstrual periods can range from slightly annoying to agonizing. For many women, cramps, low back pain, aching legs, a heavy feeling in the abdomen and pelvis, digestive upsets, diarrhea, headaches, weakness, depression, and emotional stress can ruin several days each month. Homeopathic remedies can help to soothe these miseries, and may reduce a woman's tendency toward menstrual problems. If discomfort is not easily relieved, seek the guidance of an experienced homeopath. If pain or other symptoms seem to be serious, a physician's assessment is important.

Belladonna

Symptoms that are very intense and come and go suddenly, accompanied by a feeling of heat, will often indicate a need for this remedy. The menstrual flow is typically bright red, profuse, and may have begun too early. Pain and cramping are worse from jarring and from touch, yet applying steady pressure often brings relief. Walking or bending over can make things worse, and sitting may be the most tolerable position. A woman who needs this remedy may feel restless and flushed, with pulsing or pounding sensations, and eyes that are sensitive to light.

Bovista

Women needing this remedy tend to have problems with puffiness and edema during times of menstrual stress, and can feel very awkward and clumsy. Pain may be felt in the pelvic region, often with soreness near the pubic bone. Menstrual flow can increase at night (and may even be absent during the day). Diarrhea occurring at the time of the menstrual period is a strong indication for this remedy.

Caulophyllum thalictroides

Women with a history of weak uterine tone and irregular periods may find some relief in this remedy. Intense discomfort during periods, with drawing pains in the thighs and legs as well as the pelvic area, are strong indications. The woman may experience a heavy flow of blood or other discharge. Stiffness or arthritis, especially in the finger joints, may also be seen in a person who needs this remedy.

Chamomilla

This remedy is indicated when the person's mood and nerves are so sensitive that pains seem almost unbearable. Anger and irritability may be extreme (or pain and cramping may come on after the woman has been angry). The menstrual flow can be heavy, and the blood may look dark or clotted. Pain often extends from the pelvic area into the thighs, and may be worse at night. Heating pads or exposure to wind can aggravate the symptoms. Vigorous walking or moving around in other ways may help relieve the pain.

Cimicifuga (*also called* Actaea racemosa)

Cramping and pain that get worse as the flow increases, back and neck pain with muscle tension, and sharp pains like shocks that shoot upward, down the thighs, or across the pelvis, are all indications for this remedy. The woman is likely to be nervous, enthusiastic, and talkative by nature, yet feel pessimistic and fearful when unwell.

Cocculus

This remedy is indicated when a woman has cramping or pressing pain in the pelvic or abdominal region, along with weakness or dizziness. She may be inclined toward headaches or nausea, and parts of her body can feel numb or hollow. Feeling worse from standing up or from any kind of exertion and feeling better from lying down and sleeping are typical. *Cocculus* is often indicated when a person has not been sleeping well and then feels weak or ill.

Colocynthis

Sharp, cutting, tearing pains (that can make the person double over) bring this remedy to mind. Cramping may be felt throughout the pelvic area or be focused near the ovaries. The woman feels restless from the pain, but lying down and keeping hard pressure and warmth on the area may improve things. This remedy is often indicated if problems are worsened by emotional upsets, especially after feeling anger or suppressing it.

Lachesis

Women who have intense discomfort and tension before the menstrual period begins and feel much better when the flow is established may benefit from this remedy. Symptoms include a bearing-down sensation in the pelvis, flushes of heat, headache, and an inability to tolerate the touch of clothing around the waist or neck. A person who needs this remedy may feel "like a pressure cooker": intense and passionate, needing an outlet both physically and emotionally.

Lilium tigrinum

Indications for this remedy include great premenstrual irritability (making other people "walk on eggs") and cramping pain with a bearing-down feeling during periods. The woman may feel as if her uterus is pushing out, and may need to sit a lot or cross her legs. She is likely to feel worse from strong emotions or excitement and be better from fresh air.

Magnesia phosphorica

Painful cramps and pain in the pelvic region that are relieved by pressure and warmth are strong indications for this remedy. Periods may start too early, often with a dark or stringy discharge, and pain is usually worse on the right side of the body. The woman is sensitive and inclined toward "nerve pain"—feeling worse from being cold and also worse at night.

Nux vomica

This remedy may be indicated when a woman has irregular menstrual periods with constricting pains that can extend to the rectum or the area above the tailbone. The woman tends to be impatient, irritable, and easily offended. Chilliness and constipation are also common. Mental strain, anger, physical exertion, stimulants, strong foods, and alcohol are likely to make things worse. Warmth and rest will often help.

Pulsatilla

Delayed or suppressed menstrual flow, accompanied by nausea or faintness, suggests the use of this remedy. Getting too warm or being in a stuffy room may make things worse. Cramping pain with a bearing-down feeling, either with scanty flow or thick, dark, clotted discharge, can also occur. (Symptoms that are changeable often point to *Pulsatilla*.) The woman's moods are changeable as well, and a desire for attention and sympathy, along with a sensitive (even tearful) emotional state are typical. This remedy can be indicated during many conditions involving hormonal changes and is often helpful to girls who have recently started having periods.

Sepia

Indications for this remedy include painful, late, or suppressed menstruation, sometimes with a feeling that the pelvic floor is weak or as if the uterus is sagging. The woman may feel irritable, dragged out, and sad—losing interest temporarily in marital and family interactions, and wanting to be left alone. Dampness, perspiring, and doing housework may aggravate the symptoms. Warmth and exercise, especially dancing, often brighten the woman's outlook and restore some energy.

Veratrum album

Menstrual periods with a very heavy flow and cramping, along with feeling of exhaustion, chilliness, and even vomiting and diarrhea, are indications for this remedy. The periods may start too early and go on too long. Discomfort is often worse at night and also in wet, cold weather. Warm drinks, exercise, or moving the bowels may make things worse. Small meals, cold drinks, and wrapping up in warm clothes or covers will tend to bring relief.

See p. 509 for Homeopathy: Dosage Directions.

Remedies for Migraine Headaches

Migraines (p. 121) are extremely painful headaches that can be debilitating. Only one side of the head is involved in many cases. Circulation to the scalp and brain can be altered, which affects the person's perception, muscle tone, and mental function—causing weakness, nausea, vomiting, sweating, chills, and visual disturbances. A tendency toward migraines often runs in families, and allergic factors seem to be involved. Attacks can be triggered by hormonal shifts, emotional stress, and exposure to offending foods and additives (such as nitrates, nitrites, sulfites, MSG, and artificial sweeteners), or chemicals (such as air pollutants, chlorine, pesticides, colognes, and ingredients in cleaning products). Homeopathic remedies can help to soothe the pain and sickness, especially if taken in early stages. Long-term constitutional care, with the guidance of an experienced practitioner, often helps to reduce the frequency and severity of migraines.

Belladonna

Migraines that start in the back of the skull or upper neck and spread to the forehead and temple (especially on the right) may indicate a need for this remedy. Pain is throbbing or pounding, and worse from jarring, light, and noise. Headaches often begin in late morning or afternoon, and may be worst around 3:00 P.M. The face may be flushed and red, and the skin feels hot, although the feet and hands are often cold. The pupils may be dilated, with sensitivity to light, and the person may either feel delirious or drowsy.

Bryonia

This remedy can be helpful if a person has a heavy or "splitting" headache, with steady pain that settles over one eye (especially the left) or spreads to the entire head. Pain is worse from any motion, even from moving the eyes, and the person wants to lie completely still and not be talked to or disturbed. Nausea with a heavy feeling in the stomach and vomiting may occur. The person can have a very dry mouth and usually is thirsty.

Cimicifuga (*also called* Actaea racemosa)

This remedy is often indicated for migraines with throbbing pains ("as if the top of the head would fly open") or shooting pains in the eyes. Headaches are often associated with the menstrual period or come on after long-term study or worrying. The muscles of the neck are usually involved in the headache, feeling very stiff and painful. The person (normally talkative and energetic) feels mentally dull and gloomy, or even fearful, during a migraine. Pain is worse from motion and sometimes improved by eating.

Cyclamen

Migraines that start with flickering in the eyes, dim vision, or dizziness suggest a need for this remedy. Pain is often right-sided and may involve the ear—which can also ache or itch. The person feels very weak and sick (the nausea is often worse from fatty food) and is thirsty, very sensitive to cold, and worse from open air. People who need this remedy are sympathetic and emotional; they often have an anxious or remorseful feeling that they may have neglected some responsibility.

Gelsemium

When this remedy is indicated, the person feels weak and lethargic, with a heavy feeling in the face and eyes, and droopy eyes with diminished vision. Pain may be focused in the back of the head and muscles of the neck. The person may tremble, and heat or chills may run up and down the spine. Head pain may be relieved by urinating. Worry, fear, or dread of a stressful event may precipitate a headache.

Ignatia amara

This remedy is helpful for migraines in sensitive people, especially headaches after emotional upsets or caused by grief. The headache is often focused on one side of the head, and may feel as if a nail is driven in.

Twitching in the face or spasms in the muscles of the neck and back are likely to occur. The person often sighs or yawns and may sometimes weep or seem "hysterical."

Iris versicolor

Intense migraines with blurry vision and pain that extends to the face and teeth, along with vomiting and a burning feeling in the throat and stomach, can often be relieved with this remedy. The person tends to feel worse from resting and better from motion.

Kali bichromicum

Migraines with excruciating pain that is felt in little spots—or pain that settles over the eyebrows (or one eye)—suggest a need for this remedy. When the headache begins, the person is very sensitive to light, and vision gradually diminishes. Nausea and dizziness can be intense, but vomiting does not relieve the headache. The person may feel better from lying in bed and keeping warm.

Lachesis

Left-sided migraines with congested, pulsing pain that is worse from pressure or tight clothing may respond to this remedy. The person's face looks deeply flushed or blotchy. Headaches are often worse before the menstrual period and better once the flow begins. The person feels worse from sleeping (either in the daytime or at night) and is usually worse from heat.

Natrum muriaticum

Migraines (often on the right) that are worse from grief or emotional upsets, worse from too much sun, or occur just before or after the menstrual period, are likely to respond to this remedy. The headache can feel like "a thousand little hammers were knocking on the brain" and is often worse from eyestrain. The person may have numb or tingling feelings in the lips or face before the headache starts, and the eyes are very sensitive to light. The person often feels better lying in the dark and after sleeping.

Sanguinaria canadensis

Right-sided migraines with tension in the neck and shoulder, extending to the forehead with a bursting feeling in the eye, are often relieved with this remedy. Jarring, light, and noise can aggravate discomfort. The headaches improve after vomiting, as well as from burping or passing gas, and are often better after sleep. A person who needs this remedy often may come down with migraines after missing meals, and is likely to have digestive problems and allergies.

Sepia

Left-sided migraines with dizziness and nausea—worse from missing meals, and worse near menstrual periods or during menopause—often respond to this remedy. Pain may come in shocks or jerks, and the person may feel worse indoors and from lying on the painful side. People needing *Sepia* often feel weary, cold, and irritable, wanting no one to make demands on them.

Silicea (*also called* Silica)

Migraines that come on after mental exertion or near the menstrual period may indicate a need for this remedy—especially in a nervous person who is very chilly. Headaches are usually right-sided, starting in the back of the head and extending to the forehead, and can be worse from drafts or from going out in the cold without a hat. The person may feel better from lying down in a dark, warm room and also from covering the head.

Spigelia

Excruciating headaches on the left side of the head, with violent throbbing, or stitching pains above or through the eyeball, may respond to this remedy. Pain may extend through the face and can be worse from motion, touch, position changes, and jarring. The person may feel better from lying on the right side with the head supported, and keeping still.

See p. 509 for Homeopathy: Dosage Directions.

Remedies for Morning Sickness

Nausea during pregnancy, often called **morning sickness** (p. 126), can be miserable. At a time when many changes are occurring (enough to adapt to already), it is often very discouraging. Some women feel ill or queasy only in the morning, but for some it lasts all day and is even troublesome at night. Discomfort usually eases off by the third or fourth month, but not always. Homeopathic remedies can be very helpful to a woman with morning sickness and are safe to take, as indicated, during pregnancy. If discomfort is extreme, or the woman is unable to keep food and liquids down for an extended period of time, a physician should be consulted.

Asarum

This remedy is indicated when a woman feels very ill, with constant nausea and retching. She may be extremely sensitive to everything—especially noise, which can aggravate the nauseous feelings. She feels best when lying down and resting. Cool drinks or food may help, but it is usually hard for her to even think of eating.

Colchicum autumnale

Horrible nausea that is worse from the sight and smell of food (especially eggs or fish) often indicates this remedy. The woman may retch and vomit, and have a sore and bloated feeling in the abdomen. She has trouble eating anything—although she often craves things, when she tries to eat them they make her sick. She is likely to feel ill from many smells that others don't even notice.

Ipecacuanha

This remedy is indicated for intense and constant nausea that is felt all day (not only in the morning) with retching, belching, and excessive salivation. The woman may feel worse from lying down, but also worse from motion. Even after the woman vomits, nausea remains.

Kreosotum

When this remedy is indicated, the woman may salivate excessively and swallows so much that it makes her feel nauseous. She may also vomit up food that looks undigested, several hours after eating.

Lacticum acidum

This remedy is indicated for "classic morning sickness"—nausea worse immediately on waking in the morning and on opening the eyes. The woman may salivate a lot and have burning stomach pain. She will usually have a decent appetite and feels better after eating.

Nux vomica

Nausea, especially in the morning and after eating, may be relieved with this remedy—especially if the woman is irritable, impatient, and chilly. She may retch a lot and have the urge to vomit, often without success. Her stomach feels sensitive and crampy, and she may be constipated.

Pulsatilla

This remedy can be helpful if nausea is worse in the afternoon and evening (often in the morning, as well). The woman is not very thirsty, although she may feel better from drinking something cool. She can crave many different foods, but feels sick from many things (including foods she craves). Creamy foods or desserts may be appealing, but can cause discomfort and burp-

ing or bring on vomiting. A woman who needs this remedy will often be affectionate, insecure, and weepy—wanting a lot of attention and comforting.

Sepia

Gnawing, intermittent nausea with an empty feeling in the stomach suggests a need for this remedy. It is especially indicated for a woman who is feeling irritable, sad, worn out, and indifferent to her family. She tends to feel worst in the morning before she eats, but is not improved by eating and may vomit afterward. Nausea can be worse when she is lying on her side. Odors of any kind may aggravate the symptoms. Food often tastes too salty. She may lose her taste for many foods, but may still crave vinegar and sour things.

Tabacum

This remedy can be helpful to a woman who feels a ghastly nausea with a sinking feeling in the pit of her stomach. She may look extremely pale, feel very cold and faint, and need to lie very still keeping her eyes closed. If she moves even slightly, she may vomit violently—or break out in a cold sweat and feel "deathly ill".

See p. 509 for Homeopathy: Dosage Directions.

Remedies for Motion Sickness

Motion sickness (p. 126) often needs immediate attention, both to relieve the person's misery and to prevent disruption of a trip. Sometimes, as in the case of sea or air sickness, it is impossible to leave the vehicle—so bringing along a kit of remedies can be a good idea. (If vomiting is extreme or a person shows signs of dehydration, a physician should be consulted.)

Argentum nitricum

Indications for this remedy include dizziness, faintness, nausea, retching, and possibly balance or perception problems. The person may feel claustrophobic or be extremely anxious and excitable. Eating too much sweet or salty food may have contributed to the problem.

Arsenicum album

A person who needs this remedy is likely to be very anxious and feel both restless and exhausted. Nausea and vomiting can be accompanied by burning pain. The sight and smell of food, or odors of any kind, may make the nausea unbearable. The person may feel a burning sensation in the throat or stomach and want frequent sips of water.

Borax

Indications for this remedy include nausea, gas, and possibly diarrhea. The person has a fear of any downward motion (as is felt on a plane or roller coaster) and can be made sick by it. The person may also be very sensitive to noise, warm temperatures, and cigarette smoke.

Bryonia

A person needing this remedy usually wants to stay completely still and not be talked to or touched. Nausea and vomiting, with pain and pressure in the stomach, can be worse from even minor movements. The person may have a dry mouth and want cold drinks.

Cocculus

Indications for this remedy include dizziness, palpitations, headache, numbness, and an empty or hollow feeling in various parts of the body. The person may talk nervously, yawn, or tremble, and is likely to feel extremely weak. Problems are often worse after getting cold, and from not getting enough sleep.

Kali bichromicum

This remedy is indicated when vertigo and nausea are intense, and bright yellow fluid is vomited. The person feels worse from standing up, and can be very weak. Aching may be felt in facial bones or in small spots on the head. This remedy is often helpful during seasickness.

Petroleum

A feeling of empty nausea in the stomach, accompanied by cold sweat and excessive salivation can indicate this remedy. An ache in the back of the head and neck may be present. Food and warmth may bring some mild relief.

Sepia

This remedy is indicated when the person (often a woman or child) feels dizzy and irritable, and the nausea is made worse by lying on one side. A headache will often accompany these problems. The sight of food can intensify the nausea, although the person may still want sour things.

Tabacum

Indications for this remedy include violent nausea and vomiting with a terrible sinking feeling in the pit of the stomach, pale face, cold sweat, and icy feet and hands. Some relief may come from breathing cold, fresh air.

See p. 509 for Homeopathy: Dosage Directions.

Remedies for Mumps

Mumps is a viral infection in which the salivary glands, especially the large parotid gland in the cheek, become inflamed and swollen. Fever, headache, pain in front of and below the ears, and dry mouth (or sometimes excessive salivation) are common symptoms. The following homeopathic remedies can be helpful in many cases. Mumps in older children and adults can be serious, since ovaries and testicles can become inflamed or damaged. If areas other than the salivary glands are involved, if fever and headache are extreme, or if the person has abdominal pain and vomiting, consult a doctor right away.

Aconitum napellus

This remedy may be indicated in mumps if the fever comes on suddenly and the person is very agitated. Stabbing or tingling pain can be felt in the jaw or face. The person feels worse from warmth and better from fresh air, and is often very thirsty.

Apis mellifica

When this remedy is indicated, the face looks puffy, pink, and tender, and cool compresses are soothing. Even with fever, thirst is usually low. The person may be irritable, disliking interference.

Arsenicum album

Strong anxiety and restlessness, despite a feeling of exhaustion, suggest a need for this remedy. The head may feel hot and the rest of the body chilly. This remedy is sometimes helpful in preventing complications involving the ovaries or testicles.

Belladonna

When the illness comes on quickly with high fever, a hot flushed face, and eyes that are sensitive to light, this remedy may be indicated. Shooting pains can be felt in the swollen cheek (most often the right). The person may also have a throbbing headache.

Bryonia

This remedy is indicated when the person feels worse from any motion. Hard, tender swelling is felt in the cheek, and fever may be accompanied by headache. The person's mouth feels dry, with thirst for long cold

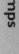

drinks. *Bryonia* may be helpful if the swelling abruptly disappears, but the person feels worse in general.

Calcarea carbonica

This remedy often helps during the mumps if the person's head perspires during sleep, the hands and feet feel cold and damp, and lymph nodes are also swollen. A person who needs this remedy often feels anxious and is easily fatigued. Children may feel hot, but adults often tend to be chilly.

Carbo vegetabilis

When this remedy is indicated, fever can develop slowly, and the person may feel chilled and faint. The stomach may also be upset, with gas and belching. The person may crave fresh air and often wants to be near a fan or open window. This remedy may help if testicles, ovaries, or breasts become involved in mumps, when the other symptoms fit.

Mercurius solubilis

This remedy can be helpful if hard, painful swelling of the salivary glands occurs below the chin, as well as in the cheeks, along with a large amount of salivation. The person may be very sensitive to temperature changes. Offensive breath, swollen lymph nodes, and perspiration during sleep are also seen.

Phytolacca

This remedy may be useful if swelling of the parotid gland is sore and tight, or if the breasts or other glands are becoming painful and swollen. The person may feel tired, dizzy, and sore all over. Relief may come from drinking something cold, but the person is often better from warmth in general.

Pulsatilla

Although this remedy is known for many kinds of children's illnesses, it can also be very helpful when adults come down with the mumps. Discomfort and swelling may be felt in the ovaries, breasts, or testicles. The person feels worse from warmth and in the evening and better from open air. Despite a fever, thirst is often low. A person who needs this remedy will tend to be emotional, wanting lots of sympathy and comforting.

Rhus toxicodendron

When swelling of the cheek looks reddish and the person feels achy, restless, and driven to get up and move around, this remedy may be helpful. Stiffness and aching are relieved by warmth and motion. This remedy may also help to prevent infection with the

mumps, and should be considered if older children or adults have been exposed.

See p. 509 for Homeopathy: Dosage Directions.

Remedies for Osteoarthritis

Osteoarthritis (p. 130) is an inflammation of the joints, involving breakdown of the cartilage at the ends of bones. Pain and inflammation, often from misalignment or overuse, can lead to thickening or bony deposits in these areas. Homeopathic remedies can be helpful during painful flare-ups. A constitutional remedy, chosen by an experienced practitioner to closely fit the individual, may help on deeper levels.

Aconitum napellus

This remedy may be helpful for pain and inflammation that comes on suddenly after exposure to cold wind and weather. The person is likely to feel fearful, panicked, or agitated.

Apis mellifica

This remedy can be helpful in acute conditions with redness, tenderness, and swelling. Joints feel hot and have stinging pain. The hands and knees are often affected. Warmth can aggravate the symptoms and cool applications bring relief.

Arnica montana

Chronic arthritis with a feeling of bruised soreness can indicate a need for this remedy. Pain is worse from touch, and may occur in joints that were injured in the past.

Belladonna

Sudden flare-ups of arthritis with a sensation of heat and throbbing pain may indicate a need for this remedy. The joints look red and inflamed, and the surface may feel hot to the touch.

Bryonia

This remedy can be useful for tearing or throbbing pain that is worse from any motion. Rest and pressure may bring relief (if the pressure adds stability), but movement is intolerable. Cold applications often reduce discomfort.

Calcarea carbonica

This remedy is often useful for arthritis in a person who is chilly, flabby or overweight, and easily tired by

Osteoarthritis *(vertical side tab)*

exertion. Inflammation and soreness are worse from cold and dampness, and weakness or cramping in the extremities are often experienced. Problems often focus on the knees when *Calcarea* is needed.

Calcarea fluorica

This remedy is often indicated for arthritic pains that are improved by heat and motion. Joints become enlarged and hard, and nodosities or bone spurs may develop. Arthritis after chronic injury to joints will often respond to *Calcarea fluorica*.

Calcarea phosphorica

Stiffness and soreness of the joints, worse from drafts and cold, may be relieved by this remedy. Aching in the bones and tiredness are common, and the person feels worse from exertion. Calcium deposits or bone spurs may develop, especially in the neck. A feeling of dissatisfaction and a strong desire for travel or a change of circumstances are often seen in individuals who need this remedy.

Cimicifuga (*also called* Actaea racemosa)

Severe aching and stiffness that is worse from cold may respond to this remedy, especially if the neck or larger joints are affected. Shooting pains or twitching can be felt in the area, and inflammation may be worse around the menstrual period.

Dulcamara

If a person has a flare-up of arthritis during cold damp weather, after getting wet and chilled, or when coming down with a cold, this remedy may be helpful. People who need this remedy are often stout, with a tendency toward allergies and back pain.

Kali carbonicum

If the joints have begun to get thickened or deformed, and discomfort is worse from cold and dampness, this remedy may help to bring relief. People who need this remedy are often dutiful and conservative, and tend to feel anxiety in the stomach.

Kalmia latifolia

Intense arthritic pain that appears quite suddenly may indicate this remedy—especially when the problems start in higher joints and extend to lower ones. Pain and inflammation often start in the shoulder, moving to the elbow, wrist, and hand. The knees are also frequently affected. Discomfort is worse from motion and often worse at night.

Ledum palustre

Arthritis that starts in lower joints and extends to higher ones suggests a need for this remedy. Pain and inflammation often begin in the toes and spread up through the ankles and knees. The joints may make cracking sounds and may be very swollen. Cold applications bring relief to both the pain and swelling.

Pulsatilla

Pain that moves unpredictably from one joint to another suggests a need for this remedy. The hips and knees are often affected, and pain may be felt in the heels. Symptoms tend to be worse from warmth, and better from cold applications and open air. A person who needs this remedy will often be moody and changeable, and usually wants a lot of attention and comforting.

Rhus toxicodendron

Arthritis with pain and stiffness that is worse in the morning and worse in cold, wet weather suggests a need for this remedy. The person may feel extremely restless. Both warmth and motion improve the symptoms in the joints, as well as the person's general state.

Ruta graveolens

Arthritis with a feeling of great stiffness and lameness—worse from cold and damp, and worse from exertion—may often be relieved by this remedy. Tendons and the capsules of the joints may be affected. Arthritis may have developed after overuse, from repeated wear and tear.

See also Remedies for **Bursitis** (p. 522), **Gout** (p. 540), **Fibromyalgia** (p. 538), and **Rheumatoid Arthritis** (p. 571).

See p. 509 for Homeopathy: Dosage Directions.

Remedies for Osteoporosis

Many factors can contribute to **osteoporosis** (p. 133), including the aging process (especially in women after menopause), inadequate exercise, dietary errors or deficiencies, and effects of certain drugs. Homeopathic remedies will not reverse existing bone loss, but can bring the body into better balance and help its minerals and nutrients be used efficiently. Remedies are also helpful for aching bones and prevention or healing of fractures.

Calcarea carbonica

This remedy is often helpful to individuals who are easily tired by exertion and tend to feel anxious and overwhelmed from work or stress. The person may be chilly, flabby or overweight, and feel worse from cold and dampness. Back pain, swollen joints, and a sweaty head at night are often seen. People who need this remedy often have strong cravings for both eggs and sweets.

Calcarea phosphorica

Stiffness, soreness, and weakness of the bones and joints often are experienced by those who need this remedy. Aching in the bones of the neck, upper back, and hips can be distressing. Deep tiredness frequently is felt, especially after exercise. Calcium deposits and bone spurs may develop, even while general bone loss is taking place, and fractures may be slow to heal. A feeling of dissatisfaction and a strong desire for travel or a change of circumstances are often seen in people who need *Calcarea phosphorica*.

Phosphorus

This remedy is often helpful to people who are sensitive, suggestible, imaginative, but easily tired or weakened physically. Bones may be less strong than normal, or be slow to heal after fractures. Weakness is often felt in the spine, with burning pain between the shoulder blades. People who need this remedy are often tall and thin with an easily flushing face. A desire for refreshing foods (especially ice cream) and strong thirst for cold or carbonated drinks are other indications for *Phosphorus*.

Silicea (*also called* Silica)

People who need this remedy are often nervous, easily tired, very chilly, and tend to sweat at night. They have a refined or delicate appearance, and often have weakness in the spine. Their injuries are slow to heal, and they tend to have a low resistance to infection. Moderate exercise often warms these people up and makes them feel more energetic.

Symphytum officinale

When osteoporosis is a problem, fractures often occur from mild trauma. This remedy can be useful for strengthening and healing bones when new fractures occur, and also helpful when pain persists in old, healed fractures.

See also Remedies for **Broken Bones** (p. 518).

See p. 509 for Homeopathy: Dosage Directions.

Remedies for Photosensitivity

Rashes that come on from exposure to sunlight are seen in the symptom pictures of several remedies.

Other remedies are suited to individuals who feel worse from the sun in general, having rashes, headaches, dizziness, tiredness, and other symptoms. If **photosensitivity** (p. 140) seems to be hereditary, a side effect of medication, or associated with an autoimmune condition such as lupus, the cause should be taken into account, and a doctor's care should be sought. Remedies listed here are sometimes helpful as first aid in moderate situations. Deep-seated or chronic problems are best approached through constitutional care, with the help of an experienced practitioner.

Aconitum napellus

If a rash breaks out suddenly and the person feels extremely anxious and apprehensive, this remedy may be indicated. Exposure to sunlight, or being out on a cold dry windy day, will often precipitate symptoms. The rash may feel numb or itch, and stimulants may reduce the itching.

Belladonna

This remedy may be indicated when a feeling of heat accompanies a bright red rash that comes on intensely and suddenly. The person's face is flushed, and pulsations may be felt in the head or other parts of the body.

Camphora

This remedy can be helpful for a rash that comes from sun exposure (and is sometimes also used in sunstroke). A guiding indication for this remedy is a feeling of general coldness and sensitivity, despite which the person does not want to be covered.

Natrum carbonicum

When this remedy is indicated, a blistery rash can come up in patches, and the person feels tired or ill from being in the sun. A person who needs this remedy also tends to be sensitive to weather changes and allergic to many foods, especially milk.

Natrum muriaticum

A person who needs this remedy may feel tired and weak after being in the sun, developing headaches and a blotchy or hive-like rash that itches and burns. Strong thirst, a craving for salt, and a private or reserved personality are other confirmations for this remedy choice.

Staphysagria

A blistery rash, with itching that changes locations from scratching, suggests the use of this remedy. *Staphysagria* is often suited to individuals who are

Photosensitivity

very sensitive emotionally and strongly affected by insults or embarrassment.

See p. 509 for Homeopathy: Dosage Directions.

Remedies for Postpartum Depression

Depression after childbirth, often called **postpartum depression**, is common, and usually lasts for several days. Many of the reasons for postpartum "blues" are physical—with many changes taking place in the mother's body during pregnancy, from the stress of labor and delivery, and due to hormonal shifts that occur once the baby is born. Emotional stress is also understandable: anxiety, insecurity, lack of confidence, and ambivalence about the sudden responsibility of motherhood can be completely normal. Some women have more serious problems at this time, including despair, delusions, hallucinations, or even destructive impulses toward their babies or themselves. If a woman's depression is deep, or her problems seem to be serious, it is very important that she have the help of a mental health professional, as well as loving care from family and friends. Homeopathic practitioners who specialize in pregnancy and childbirth may be able to choose a deeply acting remedy that closely fits the individual.

Arsenicum album

A woman who needs this remedy may feel extremely insecure about her situation, wanting constant help and support. She can be extremely picky and controlling toward others—or seem very restless, yet exhausted and incapable. Women who need *Arsenicum* sometimes feel despair from insecurity, with thoughts that deeply frighten them.

Aurum metallicum

When this remedy is indicated, depression can be dark and despairing. The woman may feel worthless and see little point in life. Problems may be worse at night, or when weather is dark and days are short. Women troubled by depression in the past (not necessarily related to pregnancy) are often likely to respond to *Aurum*. Professional help is needed if depression is severe.

Calcarea carbonica

This remedy can be helpful to a woman who is overwhelmed by working too hard and taking on too much responsibility. Weakness and fatigue may make her feel depressed. Anxiety, insomnia, and nightmares may develop. A person who needs this remedy often feels sluggish, cold, and easily tired by exercise.

Cimicifuga (*also called* Actaea racemosa)

This remedy is often useful when a woman is depressed for both emotional and hormonal reasons. She may feel "a dark cloud" has crept over her life and that everything is wrong. Extremely anxious and gloomy, she may start to think herself incapable of caring for the baby—or she may become excitable and talkative, saying and doing irrational things.

Ignatia amara

This remedy often is helpful if a mother feels tense, upset, or grief-stricken after childbirth. The grief may be based on an actual loss (for instance, the baby may have health problems)—but often occurs if the birth was difficult, and not as beautiful as she imagined. Defensiveness, hysterical behavior, sighing, sudden outbursts of tears or laughter, and insomnia are often seen when this remedy is needed.

Natrum muriaticum

This remedy can be helpful to a woman who feels sad and sensitive, and wants to be alone to cry. She may be brooding and withdrawn, anxious about her mothering abilities, or doubtful and discouraged about her relationship with the baby's father or other family members. Despite her sadness, she may seem angry or offended if anyone tries to console her. Women who need this remedy may also have headaches or palpitations when depressed.

Phosphorus

A woman who needs this remedy can have an active imagination with tremendous fear—thinking of every possible danger or misfortune that might occur. She may be very worried that she won't be able to cope if something happens, and terrified that harm might come to the baby, wanting constant company and feeling afraid to be alone. A woman who needs this remedy may also have a tendency toward easy bleeding and exhaustion, which may have added to her fear and nervousness.

Pulsatilla

This remedy is often indicated for women who are emotional, tearful, and sensitive in situations involving hormonal changes. The woman may feel extremely insecure and needy—wanting constant affection, reassurance, and nurturing. She is likely to feel worse when warm and in a stuffy room, improving after crying or from being out in open air.

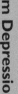

Postpartum Depression

Sepia

This remedy may be helpful to a mother who feels worn out and indifferent after childbirth, and does not want other people making demands or expecting anything of her. She may have trouble bonding with the baby, and may not even want to have it close to her. Most women who need this remedy feel resentful and overburdened (though some only feel exhausted, irritable, and sad). A feeling that the pelvic floor is weak or that the uterus is sagging are other indications for *Sepia*.

See also Remedies for **Depression** (p. 532) and **Anxiety** (p. 512).

See p. 509 for Homeopathy: Dosage Directions.

Remedies for Pregnancy and Delivery Support

Pregnancy (p. 143) is an absorbing and interesting time for most women, and also involves a lot of stress. Many emotional, hormonal, and physical changes take place as the baby grows and the woman prepares for motherhood. Homeopathic remedies can help a woman's body deal with various stresses, and help to maintain its balance as the pregnancy proceeds. Care and guidance from a competent, sympathetic physician or midwife are important during pregnancy—both for general support and to watch for complications.

Arnica montana

This remedy is often indicated for relief of soreness that comes from physical exertion and muscle strain. It is also useful for soreness after labor and delivery, and for hemorrhoids that follow childbirth.

Calcarea phosphorica

This remedy can help to strengthen a woman who tends toward easy tiredness, poor digestion, cold hands and feet, and poor absorption of nutrients. Some women who need this remedy find only "junk food" appealing during pregnancy, or have cravings for smoked and salty food. A history of easy tooth decay and aching bones and joints can also suggest a need for this remedy. A person who needs *Calc phos* is often irritable because of tiredness, and may long for travel or a change of circumstances.

Carbo vegetabilis

This remedy can be helpful to a woman who feels weak and faint during pregnancy, with poor circulation, a general feeling of coldness, and a craving for fresh or moving air. She may also have frequent digestive upsets with burning pain and a tendency to belch. A woman who is deeply tired from overwork, many pregnancies close together, or a previous illness may regain some strength with *Carbo vegetabilis*.

Caulophyllum thalictroides

This remedy may be helpful to women with weak muscle tone in the uterus. A history of irregular periods, slow and difficult labor with previous deliveries, or weakness of the cervix may bring this remedy to mind. The woman may feel erratic pains like sticking needles, or episodes of contracting pain. She typically feels nervous, shaky, and trembling (sometimes irritable as well).

Cimicifuga
(*also called* Actaea racemosa)

This remedy can be helpful to women who are nervous and talkative, with a tendency to feel fearful and gloomy during pregnancy. They may become over-agitated and fear a miscarriage—sometimes having pains that feel like labor pains too early, or pains that shoot from hip to hip and down the thighs.

Ferrum metallicum

A woman who has a sturdy build, but looks very pale and weary—flushing red from any exertion or emotion—may respond to this remedy. *Ferrum* is often helpful in correcting anemic tendencies.

Ferrum phosphoricum

This remedy can be helpful for nervous, sensitive women who often feel weak or tired, with easy flushing of the face and a tendency toward anemia. A woman who needs this remedy is likely to have a slender build and may develop frequent neck and shoulder stiffness.

Nux vomica

This remedy may be useful for indigestion, heartburn, stomach pain, and constipation during pregnancy. A woman who needs this remedy usually is impatient, irritable, and chilly.

Pulsatilla

This remedy is often helpful at times of strong hormonal changes, especially to women who are moody and emotional, and want a lot of affection and attention. They often crave desserts or butter and may overeat, which can lead to indigestion and nausea, or excessive weight gain. Pregnant women who need this remedy tend to feel uncomfortable in hot weather and in stuffy rooms, improving from gentle exercise in open air.

Sepia

Women who are tired, dragged-out, and irritable during pregnancy (feeling overburdened by demands of family members, or with little enthusiasm for the pregnancy) may benefit from this remedy. Poor circulation, nausea, constipation, a tendency toward accidental urine loss, and a feeling of sagging or weakness in the pelvic floor, and an energy boost from exercise are other indications for *Sepia*.

See also Remedies for **Morning Sickness** (p. 559).

See p. 509 for Homeopathy: Dosage Directions.

Remedies for Prostatic Hyperplasia, Benign

Men over fifty often experience swelling in the area of the prostate gland and a frequent need to urinate. These usually minor but annoying problems can be symptoms of **benign prostatic hyperplasia** (p. 145). Men with prostate conditions should have regular medical examinations, to make sure that deeper problems, such as serious infection or prostate cancer, are not involved.

Apis mellifica

Stinging pain during urination that is worse when the final drops are passing is a strong indication for this remedy. Discomfort may also involve the bladder. The prostate area is swollen and very sensitive to touch. The person may feel worse from heat and from being in warm rooms, with improvement from being out in open air or from cool bathing.

Causticum

Urine loss when the person coughs or sneezes often indicates a need for this remedy. Once urine has started passing, the person may feel pressure or pulsation extending from the prostate to the bladder. *Causticum* is also indicated when sexual pleasure during orgasm is absent or diminished.

Chimaphila umbellata

This remedy is often helpful when the prostate is enlarged, with urine retention and frequent urging. The person may have the feeling that a ball is lodged in the pelvic floor, or experience pressure, swelling, and soreness that are worse when sitting down.

Clematis

This remedy is often indicated when swelling of the prostate seems to have narrowed or tightened the urinary passage. Urine usually emerges slowly, in drops instead of a stream, with dribbling afterward.

Lycopodium

This remedy may be helpful if urine is slow to emerge, with pressure felt in the prostate both during and after urination. The prostate is enlarged, and impotence may also be a problem. People who need this remedy often suffer from digestive problems with gas and bloating, and have an energy slump in the late afternoon.

Pulsatilla

Prostate problems with discomfort after urination and pains that extend to the pelvis or into the bladder (often worse when the man is lying on his back) suggest a need for this remedy. There may also be a bland, thick, yellow discharge from the penis. *Pulsatilla* is usually suited to emotional individuals who want a lot of affection and feel best in open air.

Sabal serrulata

A man who has a frequent urge to urinate at night, with difficulty passing urine, and a feeling of coldness in the sexual organs, may respond to this remedy. It is sometimes also used in lower potencies for urinary incontinence in older men. This remedy is made from **saw palmetto** (p. 457) which is also used as an herbal extract for similar prostate problems.

Staphysagria

This remedy may be indicated if a man feels burning pain in his urinary passage even when urine is not flowing, and urine retention is troublesome. Men who are likely to respond to *Staphysagria* are often sentimental and romantic, and may also have problems with impotence (most often caused by shyness).

Thuja

When the prostate is enlarged, and the person has a frequent urge to urinate, with cutting or burning pain felt near the bladder neck, this remedy may bring relief. After urine passes, a dribbling sensation may be felt. A forked or divided urine stream is sometimes seen when this remedy is needed.

See p. 509 for Homeopathy: Dosage Directions.

Remedies for Psoriasis

Psoriasis (p. 147) is a chronic skin condition producing patches of silvery scales that cover areas of reddish skin. These often appear on the scalp, knees, elbows, buttocks, and back; sometimes the armpits, genitals, eyebrows, navel, nails, or other regions are involved. Psoriasis is a deep condition, and eruptions should not be suppressed with medications; they are best treated by restoring balance to the system. Descriptions below give brief information on some of the remedies that may help a person with psoriasis, when the remedy fits the individual on many levels. Like other chronic skin disorders, the treatment of psoriasis takes times and patience, and is best addressed with the guidance of an experienced practitioner.

Arsenicum album

People likely to respond to this remedy can be anxious, restless, and compulsively neat and orderly. They are often deeply chilly, experience burning pains with many physical complaints, and become exhausted easily. The skin is dry and scaly and may tend to get infected. Scratching can make the itching worse, and applying heat may bring relief.

Calcarea carbonica

This remedy is suited to people who are easily fatigued by exertion, sluggish physically, chilly with clammy hands and feet, and often overweight. Skin problems tend to be worse in winter. Typically solid and responsible, these people can be overwhelmed by too much work and stress. Anxiety, claustrophobia, and fear of heights are common. Cravings for sweets and eggs are often also seen when *Calcarea* is needed.

Graphites

People needing this remedy often have a long-term history of skin disorders. The skin looks tough or leathery, with cracks and soreness. Itching is often worse from getting warm, and the person may scratch the irritated places till they bleed. Trouble concentrating, especially in the morning, is also often seen when this remedy is needed.

Mercurius solubilis

People who seem introverted and formal—but are very intense internally, with strong emotions and impulses—may benefit from this remedy. They tend to have swollen lymph nodes and moist or greasy-looking skin, and are very sensitive to changes in temperature. The areas affected by psoriasis may become infected easily.

Mezereum

A person who needs this remedy tends to be serious, and often feels strong anxiety in the region of the stomach. Scaly plaques may itch intensely, thickening or crusting over if the person scratches them too much. Cold applications can relieve the itching (although the person feels generally chilly and improves with warmth). People who need this remedy often have a craving for fat, and feel best in open air.

Petroleum

This remedy is often indicated for people whose physical problems are aggravated by stressful emotional experiences. It is especially suited to individuals with extremely dry skin, and problems that involve the palms and fingertips. The person may feel a cold sensation after scratching, and the skin is easily infected and may look tough and leathery. Itching will be worse at night, and from getting warm in bed. People who need this remedy may also have a tendency toward motion sickness.

Rhus toxicodendron

When this remedy is indicated for a person with psoriasis, the skin eruptions are red and swollen, and often itch intensely. Hot applications or baths will soothe the itching—and also muscle stiffness, toward which these people often have a tendency. The person is restless, and may pace or constantly move around. A person who needs this remedy will often crave cold milk.

Sepia

This remedy may be helpful to a person who feels dragged out and irritable, often with little enthusiasm for work or family life. The person's skin may look dry and stiff. Psoriasis may appear in many places on the body, including the nails and genitals. Signs of hormonal imbalance are often seen (in either sex), and problems with circulation are common. Exercise often helps this person's energy and mood.

Staphysagria

This remedy may be helpful to individuals whose psoriasis has developed after grief or suppressed emotions. Any part of the body can be involved, but the scalp is often affected. People who need this remedy often seem sentimental, meek and quiet, and easily embarrassed—but often have a strong internal anger or deeply buried hurt.

Sulphur

Intensely burning, itching, inflamed eruptions that are worse from warmth and bathing suggest a need for this remedy. Affected areas often look bright red and irritated, with scaling skin that gets inflamed from scratching. This remedy is sometimes helpful to people who have repeatedly used medications to suppress psoriasis (without success).

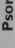

Psoriasis

See p. 509 for Homeopathy: Dosage Directions.

Remedies for Rashes

Rashes are often caused by contact with an irritating substance (such as oil from poison oak or ivy plants, ingredients in cleaning products and cosmetics, chemicals in swimming pools or hot tubs, or pollutants in the air and water). Some have viral causes (such as roseola, rubella, measles), and others appear for no apparent reason. If possible, the cause of a rash should be determined and removed. Homeopathic remedies can be useful in many cases, to soothe the itching, inflammation, and discomfort.

Anacardium orientale

This remedy is often helpful for rashes that come from poison oak, or other kinds of contact dermatitis. An intensely itching rash with swelling and fluid-filled blisters may appear. Itching is worse from applying heat or contact with hot water.

Apis mellifica

When a rash is the result of an allergic reaction and takes the form of hives, or if a rash is very pink and swollen with burning or stinging pain, this remedy may be useful. Discomfort and swelling are relieved by cold applications.

Belladonna

This remedy is useful for conditions with sudden onset that are hot, bright red, and throbbing. Rash may be accompanied by fever.

Bryonia

A bumpy, hot, dry rash may respond to this remedy. Discomfort may be worse from heat and touch, although applying pressure or lying on the affected side may soothe the itching. If illness accompanies the rash, the person often wants to lie completely still and be left alone.

Graphites

Rashes with eruptions that ooze a sticky golden fluid, then crust over, may be relieved with this remedy. Itching is often worse from warmth and worse at night.

Ledum palustre

This remedy is indicated for a puffy and swollen rash. Both the swelling and the itching tend to be relieved by cold applications.

Natrum muriaticum

This remedy is often helpful to people with chronic rashes at the margin of the scalp or in the bends of the knees and elbows. The skin is oily in most areas, but the rash looks dry and scaly. Itching is often worse from physical exertion and the person may feel worse from being in the sun. *Natrum muriaticum* can also help if hives break out during emotional stress, especially grief or romantic disappointment. A person who needs this remedy may have a tendency toward herpes.

Rhus toxicodendron

A blistery rash that burns and itches intensely, and is much improved by applying heat or bathing in hot water, may be relieved by this remedy. The person tends to be very restless, wanting to pace or constantly move around.

Sepia

Dry skin with a scaly reddish or brownish rash suggests a need for this remedy. The person may be chilly and better from keeping warm—but getting too warm under covers or clothing, and especially sweating, can make the itching worse.

Sulphur

Red, irritated, itchy, burning rashes that are aggravated by heat and washing may respond to this remedy. The touch of clothing, especially wool, can cause a rash or make it worse. Scratching seems irresistible, but disrupts and irritates the skin. Eruptions may be dry and scaly, or moist and infection-prone.

Urtica urens

Eruptions that resemble nettle rash, with blotches that sting and burn intensely, may be soothed by this remedy. Scratching can make the symptoms worse. Applying cold or water may aggravate the condition. Rashes that come out from eating shellfish, from being overheated, or along with rheumatism often bring this remedy to mind.

See also Remedies for **Eczema** (p. 535), **Shingles** (p. 572), and specific viral illnesses.

See p. 509 for Homeopathy: Dosage Directions.

Remedies for Raynaud's Disease

Raynaud's disease (p. 148) is a circulatory disorder involving spasms in small blood vessels in the

Raynaud's Disease

extremities. The tips of the fingers and toes turn pale or bluish, and tightness, numbness, and tingling are often felt. Warming up the affected area eventually restores the circulation and color. Raynaud's is usually brought on by exposure to cold, or by emotional stress, but is sometimes related to autoimmune disorders. Homeopathic remedies can help to relieve discomfort. The tendency toward episodes may be reduced with the help of a constitutional remedy and the guidance of an experienced practitioner.

Arsenicum album

This remedy can be useful when the tips of the extremities are icy cold, with a burning sensation that is much relieved by heat. The fingers or other affected areas may also look swollen and feel itchy. People who need *Arsenicum* are often perfectionistic, restless, anxious, and feel chilly generally.

Carbo vegetabilis

People who need this remedy have very cold extremities and often look pale and feel weak or faint, with a strong desire for moving air, and a tendency toward indigestion. Toes and fingertips may have a cramping sensation and sometimes overreact to circulation problems by turning red.

Chelidonium

This remedy may be helpful with Raynaud's disease if the person also has a tendency toward pain and tightness in the region of the shoulder blades and neck (especially on the right). A tendency toward right-sided headaches, indigestion, and liver problems also suggest the use of *Chelidonium*.

Hepar sulphuris calcareum

Individuals who need this remedy are extremely sensitive to drafts and cold, and often need to wear gloves and be warmly dressed, or even to stay indoors, to prevent unpleasant symptoms. People who need this remedy are often vulnerable in many ways, and can be very irritable and touchy.

Sepia

If a person with Raynaud's disease has cold extremities most of the time, and feels chronically worn out and irritable, this remedy may help. Circulation may be poor because the person's internal muscle tone is lax (including the tone of the blood vessels). The person may also experience chronic constipation or a weak or sagging feeling in the pelvic organs. Exercise often improves the symptoms, as well as the person's mood and energy.

Veratrum album

This remedy may be indicated for icy coldness and paleness—even blueness—with a sensation of cramping in the tips of the extremities. People who need this remedy often feel extremely cold and weak with other physical disorders, such as diarrhea and vomiting, or difficult menstrual periods.

See p. 509 for Homeopathy: Dosage Directions.

Remedies for Restless Legs Syndrome

People suffering from **restless legs syndrome** (p. 149) have a very unpleasant creeping sensation in the legs, with a nagging urge to move and stretch. Problems are often present in the day, but are usually worse at night—beginning shortly after the person goes to bed. Distress often interferes with sleep, putting further stress on the person's nervous system. Homeopathic remedies often help to relieve this disconcerting problem. If symptoms persist, a constitutional remedy and the guidance of an experienced homeopath may be valuable, to bring the system into better balance.

Aconitum napellus

If a person with restless legs syndrome is very anxious and tends to panic, this remedy may be soothing. Tingling or shooting pains are felt in the legs, and the nervous system is very agitated. The person may be unable to relax and fall asleep—or the sleep can be distressing and full of fearful dreams.

Arsenicum album

A person who needs this remedy feels simultaneously restless and exhausted, with feelings of weakness, heaviness, and trembling in the legs. Cramping and burning sensations may also be experienced. Anxiety and a feeling of insecurity may be pronounced. People who need this remedy are often deeply chilly and improved by warmth.

Causticum

This remedy can be helpful if a person has restless legs with sensations of burning and aching, and cramps in the calves and feet. Symptoms are worse in bed at night and often improve with warmth. People needing *Causticum* often have a tendency toward chronic problems with muscles and tendons, contractures, and muscle weakness. They are often very sensitive to other people's feelings, and are prone to nervous stress.

Ignatia amara

This remedy is indicated for sensitive, nervous individuals with a tendency toward twitching and spasms in the muscles. The legs and arms often jerk as the person falls asleep, and sleep may be extremely light. The person may frequently sigh and yawn, or burst into tears or laughter unexpectedly. Problems brought on by grief or emotional stress will often respond to this remedy.

Rhus toxicodendron

Overwhelming restlessness that makes a person want to constantly change position, or get up and pace the room at night, suggests a need for this remedy. The person may feel extremely apprehensive when trying to fall asleep and be unable to stay in bed. A tendency toward stiffness and soreness in many joints and muscles—feeling better from both warmth and motion—is a strong indication for *Rhus tox.*

Sulphur

A person who needs this remedy may experience a drawing feeling in the legs, with burning sensations and restlessness. The legs and feet may heat up during sleep, and the person may throw the covers off, or constantly move the legs to find a cooler spot. Jerking, twitching, and talking during sleep with frequent waking, are other indications for *Sulphur.*

Zincum metallicum

When restlessness in the legs is distressing and extreme, this remedy may be indicated. The person feels a constant need to move the legs, both at night and in the daytime (although night is usually worse), and the arms may be involved. Sleep is very agitated, with frequent starts and jerking. People who need this remedy are usually excitable and talkative, with active thoughts—although nervous overstimulation and loss of sleep can eventually lead to exhaustion or depression. Alcohol, especially wine, can aggravate the symptoms.

See p. 509 for Homeopathy: Dosage Directions.

Remedies for Rheumatoid Arthritis

Rheumatoid arthritis (p. 151) can come on gradually or suddenly, and usually develops simultaneously on both sides of the body—with painful inflammation, tender swelling, stiffness, contractures, and thickening or nodules around the joints. Homeopathy is often helpful for relieving pain and stiffness. A constitutional remedy, with the guidance of an experienced homeopath, is often the best approach for dealing with chronic conditions.

Arnica montana

Chronic arthritis with a feeling of bruising and soreness may be helped with this remedy. The painful parts feel worse from being moved or touched. (Herbal Arnica gels and ointments may also help to soothe arthritic pain when applied externally to areas of inflammation and soreness.)

Aurum metallicum

Wandering pains in the muscles and joints that are better from motion and warmth, and worse at night, suggest a need for this remedy. Deep pain may be felt in the limbs when the person tries to sleep, or discomfort may wake the person up. People who need this remedy are often serious and focused on work or career, with a tendency to feel depressed.

Bryonia

This remedy can be helpful for stiffness and inflammation with tearing or throbbing pain, made worse by even the smallest motion. The condition may have developed gradually, and is worse in cold dry weather. Discomfort is aggravated by being touched or bumped, or from any movement. Pressure brings relief (if it stabilizes the area) and improvement also comes from rest. The person may want to stay completely still and not be interfered with.

Calcarea carbonica

This remedy may be useful for deeply aching arthritis involving node formation around the joints. Inflammation and soreness are worse from cold and dampness, and problems may be focused on the knees and hands. Weakness in the muscles, easy fatigue from exertion, and a feeling of chilliness or sluggishness are common. A person who needs *Calcarea* is often solid and responsible, but tends to become extremely anxious and overwhelmed when ill or overworked.

Calcarea fluorica

This remedy is often indicated when arthritic pains improve with heat and motion. Joints become enlarged and hard, and nodes or deformities develop. Arthritis after chronic injury to joints may also respond to *Calcarea fluorica.*

Causticum

This remedy may be indicated when deformities develop in the joints, in a person with a tendency toward tendon problems, muscle weakness, and contractures. The hands and fingers may be most affected, although other joints can also be involved. Stiffness and pain are worse from being cold, and relief may come with warmth. A person who needs this remedy often feels best in rainy weather and worse when the days are clear and dry.

Dulcamara

If arthritis flares up during cold damp weather, or after the person gets chilled and wet, this remedy may be indicated. People needing *Dulcamara* are often stout, with a tendency toward back pain, chronic stiffness in the muscles, and allergies.

Kali bichromicum

When this remedy is indicated, arthritic pains may alternate with asthma or stomach symptoms. Pains may suddenly come and go, or shift around. Discomfort and inflammation are usually aggravated by heat, and worse when the weather is warm.

Kali carbonicum

Arthritis with great stiffness and stitching pains, worse in the early morning hours and worse from cold and dampness, may respond to this remedy—especially if joints are becoming thickened or deformed. People who need this remedy often have a rigid moral code, and tend to feel anxiety in the stomach.

Kalmia latifolia

Intense arthritic pain that flares up suddenly may respond to this remedy—especially when problems start in higher joints and extend to lower ones. Pain and inflammation may begin in the elbows, spreading downward to the wrists and hands. Discomfort is worse from motion and often worse at night.

Ledum palustre

Arthritis that starts in lower joints and extends to higher ones may respond to this remedy. Pain and inflammation often begin in the toes and spread upward to the ankles and knees. The joints may also make cracking sounds. *Ledum* is strongly indicated when swelling is significant and relieved by cold applications.

Pulsatilla

If rheumatoid arthritis pain is changeable in quality, or the flare-ups move from place to place, this remedy may be useful. The symptoms (and the person) feel worse from warmth, and better from fresh air and cold applications. People who need this remedy are

often emotional and affectionate, sometimes having teary moods.

Rhododendron

This remedy is strongly indicated if swelling and soreness flare up before a storm, continuing until the weather clears. Cold and dampness aggravate the symptoms. Discomfort is often worse toward early morning, or after staying still too long. The person feels better from warmth and gentle motion, and also after eating.

Rhus toxicodendron

Rheumatoid arthritis, with pain and stiffness that is worse in the morning and worse on first motion, but better from continued movement, may be helped with this remedy. Hot baths or showers, and warm applications improve the stiffness and relieve the pain. The condition is worse in cold, wet weather. The person may feel extremely restless, unable to find a comfortable position, and need to keep moving constantly. Continued motion also helps to relieve anxiety.

Ruta graveolens

Arthritis with a feeling of great stiffness and lameness, worse from cold and damp and worse from exertion, may be helped with this remedy. Tendons and capsules of the joints can be deeply affected or damaged. The arthritis may have developed after overuse, from repeated wear and tear.

See also Remedies for **Bursitis** (p. 522), **Gout** (p. 540), **Fibromyalgia** (p. 538), and **Osteoarthritis** (p. 562).

See p. 509 for Homeopathy: Dosage Directions.

Remedies for Shingles (Herpes Zoster)

Herpes zoster (p. 155), commonly known as shingles, is a viral infection that causes extremely painful blister-like eruptions to break out along the course of nerves. After a period of fever and malaise, the eruptions appear on parts of the rib-cage area (back, sides, or abdomen) or sometimes on the face. Homeopathic remedies are often very helpful for pain relief and recovery. Outbreaks near the eyes require medical attention.

Arsenicum album

If a person feels chilly, anxious, restless, and exhausted during fever—and the burning pain of the eruptions is relieved by heat—this remedy may be indicated. Discomfort is often worse around midnight.

Apis mellifica

Swollen, tender eruptions with burning, stinging pain and itching suggest a need for this remedy. Symptoms are aggravated by warmth, and relieved by cold applications or exposure to cool air. The person may be irritable and very sensitive to touch.

Clematis

Red, burning, blister-like eruptions with terrible itching, worse from washing or contact with cold water, may indicate a need for this remedy. The person feels worse at night and from the warmth of being in bed and feels better in open air. People who need this remedy may also have a tendency toward genito-urinary conditions.

Iris versicolor

This remedy is often helpful for herpes zoster infection that is accompanied by stomach problems with burning sensations and nausea. Eruptions may appear especially on the right side of the abdomen.

Mezereum

When this remedy is indicated, intense burning is followed by bright red eruptions that itch intolerably. The local pain of the eruptions is worse from heat and relieved by cold applications, and cool fresh air is soothing—although the person is often chilly in general and worse from getting cold.

Ranunculus bulbosus

This remedy is indicated for intensely itching shingles on the rib cage (either on the back or chest), which are also very sore, and worse from contact with clothing or any kind of touch. The blisters may look bluish. The person may feel worse from alcoholic beverages, and from exposure to cold air.

Rhus toxicodendron

This remedy may be indicated for a rash that begins with many small blisters, is red and intensely itchy, and is relieved by hot baths or hot wet compresses. Restlessness makes the person want to pace the room or constantly move around.

See p. 509 for Homeopathy: Dosage Directions.

Remedies for Sleeplessness

Sleep is an opportunity for the brain and body to rest and be restored. In addition, many functions important to good health take place during sleep at night. The amount of sleep that people need can vary widely. Infants may need up to 20 hours; many children need from 10 to 14 per night. The average requirement for adults is estimated at 6 to 8 hours, but many people need much more than that—and feel chronically stressed and compromised, both physically and mentally, because of insufficient sleep. Homeopathic remedies are useful during episodes of insomnia, and may also help individuals with long-standing sleep disorders. If problems are serious or very distressing, consult a professional homeopath.

Aconitum napellus

This remedy can be helpful if a person panics with insomnia. Fear and agitation come on suddenly when the person is drifting off to sleep, or may even wake a sleeping person up.

Arsenicum album

People who need this remedy are often anxious and compulsive about small details, and have trouble sleeping if they feel that everything is not in place. They are often deeply weary and exhausted, yet feel restless physically and mentally. Sleep, when it arrives, can be anxious and disturbed, with dreams full of fear and insecurity.

Calcarea phosphorica

This remedy is often helpful to children with growing pains, and also to adults who have aching in the joints and bones, or neck and shoulder tension that make it hard to fall asleep. The person lies awake for many hours, feeling upset and irritable—then has trouble waking in the morning, feeling deeply tired and weak.

Cocculus

This remedy is often helpful to those who feel "too tired to sleep" after long-term sleep loss—from getting up with an infant, taking care of someone who is ill, a disruptive work schedule, travel and jet lag, or chronic worry and insomnia. The person may feel weak and dizzy, have trouble thinking, and may be sleepy, irritable, or tearful.

Coffea cruda

Mental excitement and nervous stimulation that keep a person from sleeping suggest a need for this remedy.

Sleeplessness

Thoughts preventing sleep can be happy or distressing. The person may be looking forward to something that will happen in the morning, but feels stressed and exhausted as the night wears on. If the person falls asleep, it is usually very light with vivid dreams, and disturbed by any little noise or motion. (This remedy can also help if overuse of caffeine is the cause of sleeplessness.)

Ignatia amara

If insomnia is caused by emotional upset (grief or loss, a disappointment in love, a shock, or even an argument), this remedy may be helpful. The person is sensitive and nervous, and may often sigh and yawn in the daytime, yet find it hard to relax at night. As the person tries to fall asleep, the arms and legs may twitch or itch. If sleep arrives, it is usually light, with jerking of the legs and arms, or long and troubling nightmares.

Kali phosphoricum

A person with insomnia from nervous exhaustion caused by overwork or mental strain, or following a taxing illness, may respond to this remedy. The person is very weak and sensitive to everything (noise, lights, touch, and pain). Irritability, depression, and anxiety with an empty feeling in the stomach are often experienced.

Lycopodium

People who need this remedy often have no memory of dreams and may doubt that they have slept at all. Insomnia may set in primarily because of worry: lack of confidence can make them doubt their own abilities, although they are usually very capable. Insomnia caused by digestive trouble, especially gas, can also indicate a need for this remedy. The person feels drowsy after meals, but has trouble sleeping at bedtime. Ravenous night-time hunger that wakes the person up is another indication for *Lycopodium*.

Nux vomica

People who have insomnia after overindulgence in stimulants, food, and drink—or after overexertion, either physically or mentally—may benefit from this remedy. They may be able to drift off, but sleep is light, and they often awaken in the early morning (typically 3:00 A.M.) and lie awake for hours. On getting up, they are tense, impatient, and irritable, with a feeling that they sorely need more sleep.

Silicea (*also called* Silica)

This is a useful remedy for nervous people with low stamina who get too tired, then have insomnia. The person often goes to sleep at first, but awakens sud-

denly with a hot or surging feeling in the head—and finds it hard to fall asleep again. People who need this remedy usually have anxious dreams, and some (especially children) sleepwalk frequently.

Sulphur

This remedy may be helpful if insomnia comes from itching—or an increasing feeling of heat in bed, especially in the feet. The person is irritable and anxious, and often feels a need to throw the covers off. Lying awake between 2:00 and 5:00 A.M. is typical. Insomnia that develops because of a lack of exercise may also be helped with *Sulphur*.

Zincum metallicum

People who need this remedy often have insomnia from mental activity. They can get wound up from overwork—or be naturally inclined toward nervousness and just have trouble relaxing. Their legs and arms often feel extremely restless, and lying still in bed may be impossible. Even during the daytime, a person who needs this remedy may feel a constant need to move the muscles.

See also Remedies for **Restless Legs Syndrome** (p. 570).

See p. 509 for Homeopathy: Dosage Directions.

Remedies for Surgery and Recovery Support

Homeopathic physicians often suggest that a remedy for prevention of **bruising** (p. 28) and bleeding be taken the night before an operation, and that specific remedies (indicated by the person's symptoms and the type of surgery) be taken afterward. Homeopathic remedies are safe to use and do not interfere with surgical procedures or other medications. Their use should be discussed with the physician in charge. Remedies for emotional states such as **Anxiety** (p. 14) may also be helpful, taken days or weeks before the surgery.

Aconitum napellus

This remedy is indicated when people anticipating surgery are extremely agitated or panicked, especially if they fear that they will die. Easy startling, a sensitivity to light and noise, dry mouth, and thirst are other indications for *Aconitum*.

Arnica montana

This remedy is useful for all new injuries, and can help reduce soreness, bruising, tissue damage, and bleeding related to surgical procedures. *Arnica* can be taken the night before an operation, and is also helpful for bruising, swelling, and soreness during recovery.

Bellis perennis

This remedy is useful when bruising and trauma occur to deep internal tissues after surgery involving the abdomen, breasts, or trunk—especially if a feeling of stiffness or coldness has developed in the area.

China
(*also called* Cinchona officinalis)

If a person feels faint after loss of blood and fluids due to surgery, this remedy may be helpful. Ringing in the ears may also be experienced. *China* is also indicated for gas pains after an operation.

Ferrum phosphoricum

This remedy is helpful for early stages of any inflammation and may reduce the chance of soreness and infection after surgery.

Gelsemium

This remedy can be helpful to a person who feels nervous fear before an operation, with trembling, lethargy, and often diarrhea or headache.

Hamamelis virginiana

This remedy can help with passive bleeding if a person's veins are weak, and may also relieve discomfort after surgery on varicose veins and hemorrhoids.

Hypericum perforatum

This remedy is useful for injuries involving body parts that are rich with nerves. It can help reduce discomfort after surgeries that involve the spine, after dental surgery, and after amputation.

Ledum palustre

This remedy may help to relieve bruising and swelling around the eye after surgery. It is also useful for pain and swelling after surgery on varicose veins.

Phosphorus

This remedy may be helpful if a person has trouble recovering from the effects of anesthesia. Symptoms can include disorientation, stupor, weakness, nausea, and vomiting. The person may be thirsty but often vomits after drinking.

Rhus toxicodendron

This remedy is helpful for relief of stiffness, soreness, and restlessness after any surgery. It is often recommended after operations on tonsils and adenoids, appendectomy, and dental surgery.

Ruta graveolens

This remedy is often useful after surgeries involving tendons, connective tissue, cartilage, joints, and coverings of the bones. It can ease discomfort and promote recovery after surgery on knees, wrists, shoulders, elbows, ankles, hips, etc. It may also be soothing if deep stiffness is felt in joints and muscles after surgery.

Staphysagria

This remedy is useful when pain persists at the site of a surgical incision, or after procedures that involve the stretching of a sphincter muscle. It is also indicated after surgeries involving reproductive organs (such as prostate surgery, hysterectomy, C-section, episiotomy) or the abdomen, stomach, and rectum (including hemorrhoids). *Staphysagria* may also help after operations on traumatic injuries, such as stab or bullet wounds.

See p. 509 for Homeopathy: Dosage Directions.

Remedies for Teething

Teething is always uncomfortable, but some babies and toddlers feel more miserable than others. Episodes begin around 4 months of age and occur at intervals until age 2 or later. Babies are usually cranky or tearful, drool profusely, and feel a need to press their gums or bite down hard on toys. Sometimes a teething baby refuses to eat or nurse. The stress and discomfort of teething can lower a child's resistance to infection. Runny noses, rashes on the chin, spitting up of swallowed saliva, or mild diarrhea can occur without infection—but fever and symptoms of actual illness are not "just teething." Any illness needs attention of its own. Homeopathic remedies are a safe, nontoxic way to help relieve the pain and make the baby happier.

Aconitum napellus

If teething is very painful, and the baby seems agitated or fearful, this remedy can often bring relief. The baby's face may be flushed, the gums may look inflamed, and sleep can be very restless.

Belladonna

Intense inflammation and gum pain, with flushing of the face and a feeling of heat, often indicate a need for this remedy. The baby is restless, easily startled, and may tend to cry out during sleep.

Calcarea carbonica

If teething is late to begin, then slow and difficult, this remedy can be helpful. The baby may seem sad or

Teething

anxious with the pain, making chewing motions and pressing his gums together, often even while sleeping. Babies who need this remedy are usually chubby, slow to learn to crawl or walk, and their heads often sweat during naps or sleep at night.

Calcarea phosphorica

This remedy may be helpful to a child whose teeth are late to come in, with aching in the gums and trouble sleeping. Irritability, picky eating habits, and stomachaches are other indications. A child who needs this remedy may be allergic to many foods and may tend toward early tooth decay.

Chamomilla

This remedy is often indicated when a child seems extremely irritable or angry and the pain appears to be unbearable. Babies may feel agitated, scream and hit, and want to be rocked or carried constantly to distract them from the pain. The gums may be so tender that touching them is intolerable—or they may feel better from hard pressure and biting down on something cold. Greenish diarrhea that occurs because of teething stress is another indication for *Chamomilla*.

Coffea cruda

This remedy can be helpful when a child seems excitable and has trouble sleeping because of teething pain. Distressing pain in the gums may often be relieved by holding something cold on them.

Ignatia amara

If a child seems very emotional, upset, or sad because of teething, this remedy may bring relief. The baby's sleep may be light and restless, with jerking or twitching in the arms and legs.

Kreosotum

This remedy may be helpful if the child has irritating saliva and severe discomfort during teething. Teeth that decay soon after coming in will often indicate a need for *Kreosotum*.

Magnesia phosphorica

This remedy is often helpful for painful teething, relieved by pressing on the painful area and by heat. The baby may seem happier when drinking something warm from a cup or bottle, or when biting down on an object. A warm washcloth or hot water bottle held against the cheek may also help relieve the pain.

Phytolacca

This remedy may be indicated if a baby with teething pain constantly presses his or her gums together very hard, or tries to bite down on anything in reach.

Pulsatilla

A baby who is very tearful during teething, and wants to be constantly held and comforted, may respond to this remedy. Biting on something cold may help, and warmth increases discomfort. Cool food and drinks or being out in open air can also bring improvement.

Silicea (*also called* Silica)

Slow, difficult teething that makes the baby tired and nervous may be helped with this remedy. Children who need *Silica* often have fine hair and seem a little delicate, with low resistance to colds or other illnesses.

Sulphur

This remedy may be indicated if a reddish irritation or rash develops on the baby's chin or diaper area during teething episodes. Diarrhea (often whitish) may occur because of stress. The baby is often irritable and anxious, feeling worse from being warm.

See p. 509 for Homeopathy: Dosage Directions.

Remedies for Tinnitus (Ringing in the Ears)

Ringing, roaring, buzzing, and other noises in the ears (unrelated to external sounds) can be intermittent or continuous. **Tinnitus** (p. 158) can be very distracting and irritating, and is sometimes associated with partial hearing loss. Tinnitus can accompany other conditions related to the ears and nervous system, some of which need a physician's assessment and treatment. Homeopathic remedies often reduce the discomfort and frustration that come with tinnitus.

Calcarea carbonica

When this remedy is indicated, tinnitus may be experienced alone or with vertigo. The person may have hearing problems, or cracking and pulsing sensations in the ears. People who need this remedy are usually chilly, easily fatigued, crave sweets, and may feel overwhelmed and anxious when unwell.

Carbo vegetabilis

This remedy may be useful if ringing in the ears occurs during flu or other conditions involving vertigo and nausea. The symptoms may be worse in the evening and at night. The person may feel cold and faint, but usually has a craving for fresh and moving air. *Carbo vegetabilis* is also helpful when an illness has been prolonged or recovery is slow.

China (*also called* Cinchona officinalis)

This remedy is often helpful to people who feel touchy, weak, and nervous with sensitivity to noise and tinnitus. It is often indicated after fluids have been lost through vomiting, diarrhea, heavy sweating, and surgery or other conditions involving blood loss.

Chininum sulphuricum

Buzzing, ringing, and roaring sounds that are loud enough to impair the person's hearing suggest a need for this remedy. The person may also have a tendency toward chills and vertigo, during which the tinnitus is often worse.

Cimicifuga

People likely to respond to this remedy are very sensitive to noise, along with tinnitus, and often have pain and muscle tension in the neck and back. They are usually energetic, nervous, and talkative, but become depressed or fearful when not feeling well. Headaches and problems during menstrual periods are often seen in people who need this remedy.

Coffea cruda

This remedy may be helpful to an excitable, nervous person with tinnitus accompanied by extremely sensitive hearing and a buzzing feeling in the back of the head. People who need this remedy often have insomnia from mental overstimulation.

Graphites

This remedy may be beneficial to a person who has tinnitus with associated deafness. Hissing and clicking sounds are often heard in the ears (or even louder sounds like gunshots). People who need this remedy may also have a tendency toward constipation, poor concentration, and cracking skin eruptions.

Kali carbonicum

Tinnitus with ringing or roaring, accompanied by cracking noises and itching in the ears, may be relieved with this remedy. Vertigo experienced on turning is another indication. People who need this remedy are often quite conservative, with a rigid code of ethics. They tend to feel anxiety in the region of the stomach.

Lycopodium

A humming and roaring in the ears, along with impairment of hearing, suggest the use of this remedy. Sounds may also seem to echo in the ears. People needing *Lycopodium* often have a tendency toward ear infections with discharge, as well as chronic digestive problems or urinary tract complaints.

Natrum salicylicum

This remedy may be beneficial if ringing in the ears is like a low, dull hum. Loss of hearing related to bone conduction, as well as nerve interference and vertigo, may be involved. *Natrum salicylicum* is a useful remedy when tinnitus and tiredness occur after influenza or along with Ménière's disease.

Salicylicum acidum

This remedy is indicated for tinnitus with very loud roaring or ringing sounds, which may be accompanied by deafness or vertigo. The problem may have begun with flu, or occur in a person with Ménière's disease. *Salicylicum acidum* may also be helpful if tinnitus has been caused by too much aspirin.

See p. 509 for Homeopathy: Dosage Directions.

Remedies for Urinary Tract Infection

Homeopathic remedies are often helpful during **urinary tract infection** (p. 160), such as bladder infection (cystitis)—relieving discomfort and encouraging quick recovery. Symptoms include a frequent urge to urinate, with burning or stinging sensations, and sometimes aching in the bladder area. Offensive-smelling, cloudy, or discolored urine may be passed. Very uncomfortable or long-lasting urinary tract infections—especially those accompanied by fever, pain in the kidney region, or other serious symptoms—should be treated by a doctor.

Aconitum napellus

This remedy is often useful when a person feels anxious both before and during urination, with hot, scanty urine, and a burning or spasmodic feeling in the outlet of the bladder. It can also be helpful if retention of urine occurs after a person has been very cold and chilled, or after a shaking experience.

Apis mellifica

This remedy is indicated when the person frequently needs to urinate, but only small quantities are passed. Stinging and burning sensations are felt (especially with the last few drops) and the person may also experience soreness in the abdomen. Heat and touch make the symptoms worse, and cold applications, cool bathing, and open air may bring relief. A lack of thirst is another indication that *Apis* may be needed.

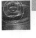

Belladonna

This remedy may be beneficial if urging to urinate is frequent and intense, and the bladder feels very sensitive. A cramping or writhing sensation may be felt in the bladder area. Small amounts of highly colored urine pass. (This remedy is sometimes helpful if a person passes small amounts of blood and no serious cause can be found on medical examination.)

Berberis vulgaris

Cystitis with twinges of cutting pain, or a burning feeling that extends to the urethra and its opening, may indicate a need for this remedy. The passage may also burn at times when no attempt at urination is being made. After emptying the bladder, the person may feel as if some urine still remains inside. Urging and discomfort are often worse from walking.

Borax

This remedy can be helpful for cystitis with smarting pain in the urinary opening and aching in the bladder, with a feeling that the urine is retained. Children may cry or shriek, afraid to urinate because they know the pain is coming. *Borax* is often indicated for people who are sensitive to noise and inclined toward motion sickness.

Cantharis

Strong urging to urinate—with cutting pains that are felt before the urine passes, as well as during and after—may indicate a need for this remedy. Only several drops pass at a time, with a scalding sensation. The person may feel as if the bladder has not been emptied, still feeling a constant urge to urinate.

Chimaphila umbellata

If a person has a troublesome urge to urinate, but has to strain (or even stand up and lean forward) to make it pass, this remedy may be useful. A scalding sensation may be felt while the urine flows, with a feeling of straining afterward.

Clematis

This remedy may be indicated if a person has to urinate frequently with only a small amount being passed. A feeling of constriction is felt in the urinary passage, and the flow may be interrupted, or there may be dribbling afterward. A tingling sensation may occur, lasting long after urination is finished.

Equisetum

If cystitis is accompanied by dull but distressing pain and a feeling of fullness in the bladder, even after urinating, this remedy may be helpful. Urging and discomfort are more intense when the bladder has recently been emptied, improving over time as the bladder becomes more full.

Lycopodium

This remedy may be helpful if a person has to urinate frequently during the night and passes large amounts of urine. Or the person may feel a painful urge, but has to strain to make the urine flow. Pain may be felt in the back before the urine passes. (If fever is present, the urine has a reddish color, or discomfort is felt in the kidney region, the person should see a doctor.)

Nux vomica

Irritable bladder with a constant need to urinate, passing only small amounts, suggests a need for this remedy. Burning or cramping pain may be felt in the bladder area, with an itching sensation in the urethra while the urine passes. The person may feel very irritable, impatient, and chilly. Symptoms may be relieved by hot baths or other forms of warmth.

Sarsaparilla

This remedy is often useful in cystitis and often helps when symptoms are unclear, or if other remedies have not been effective. Frequent urging is felt, with burning pain at the end of urination. Urine will pass when the person is standing up, but only dribbling occurs while sitting. Flakes or sediment are sometimes seen in the urine. (*Sarsaparilla* is sometimes helpful when stones are forming or the kidneys are involved; however, these conditions need a doctor's care.)

Sepia

This remedy may be helpful if a person has to urinate frequently, with sudden urging, a sense that urine will leak if urination is delayed, and small amounts of involuntary urine loss. The person may experience a bearing-down feeling in the bladder region, or pressure above the pubic bone. A person who needs this remedy often feels worn-out and irritable, with cold extremities, and a lax or sagging feeling in the pelvic area.

Staphysagria

This remedy is often indicated for cystitis that develops in a woman after sexual intercourse, especially if sexual activity is new to her, or if cystitis occurs after every occasion of having sex. Pressure may be felt in the bladder after urinating, as if it is still not empty. A sensation that a drop of urine is rolling through the urethra, or a constant burning feeling, are other indications. *Staphysagria* is also useful for cystitis that develops after illnesses with extended bed rest, or after the use of catheters.

See p. 509 for Homeopathy: Dosage Directions.

Remedies for Varicose Veins

When valves inside the veins are weak or absent, or return of blood from congested areas is inefficient, veins may become enlarged and swollen—and aching, itching, tenderness, and muscle cramping may occur. Varicose veins (p. 163) are most often seen in the legs, although they also occur in other areas. Hemorrhoids are varicose veins in the rectum; varicose veins in the legs and vulva often develop during pregnancy. Homeopathic remedies often help to relieve discomfort that comes with varicose veins, and may help to prevent their worsening. Individuals with serious cases may benefit from a constitutional remedy, prescribed by an experienced homeopath.

Arnica montana

When this remedy is indicated, the legs look bruised, or black and blue, and the swollen veins are very sore to touch. The legs feel deeply sore all over and are also worse from motion. Lying down may bring relief.

Calcarea carbonica

Varicose veins that hurt while the person is standing or walking may respond to this remedy. People who need this remedy often have poor circulation, with clammy hands and feet, and a general feeling of chilliness. They may have weak or flabby muscles, and be easily tired by exertion. Weight problems, cravings for sweets and eggs, and a tendency to feel anxious or overwhelmed when overworked are other indications for this remedy.

Carbo vegetabilis

Poor circulation with icy coldness of the extremities, and mottled skin with distended veins and a bruised or "marbled" look, may indicate a need for this remedy. The person's legs feel weak and heavy, and often itch and burn. Poor digestion, a feeling of faintness, and a craving for fresh or moving air are strong indications for *Carbo vegetabilis*. This remedy is often indicated for older people, or those who are slow to recover from an illness.

Hamamelis virginiana

This remedy can help when varicose veins are large and sore, and very weak and easily damaged, with a tendency to bleed. Pain is sore and bruise-like, and the legs look bruised and purple. A stinging feeling may be felt in the irritated veins. The muscles of the legs feel tired and are often cold. People who need this remedy may also develop varicose veins in the genital area or have a tendency toward bleeding hemorrhoids.

Lycopodium

When this remedy is indicated, drawing or tearing pains are felt in the legs, sometimes with a numb sensation. Symptoms are worse when the person is keeping still, and the legs may cramp at night in bed. People who need this remedy may have a worried facial expression along with digestive problems, sluggish liver function, and poor circulation.

Pulsatilla

Swollen veins in the legs, and sometimes even in the arms and hands, suggest a need for this remedy. Varicose veins in the legs feel hot and painful at night, with heaviness and weariness. Symptoms are worse when the legs are hanging down without support, and worse from warmth. Cold applications, motion, and cool fresh air may help. *Pulsatilla* is often helpful for varicose veins that develop during pregnancy.

Zincum metallicum

When this remedy is needed, the legs are fidgety and restless, with weakness in the muscles, crawling sensations, and a tendency to twitch. Large varicose veins may develop, with pain and soreness that are worse from touch. The person may feel worse from alcohol, especially wine.

See p. 509 for Homeopathy: Dosage Directions.

Remedies for Yeast Infection

Yeast infections (p. 169) are caused by the microorganism Candida albicans. This form of yeast is always present, but changes in the body's environment (acid/alkaline imbalance, antibiotics, poor nutrition, overconsumption of sugar, birth control pills, hormonal shifts, or compromised immune function) often provide a chance for yeast to proliferate. Vaginal yeast

Yeast Infection

infections are a common problem for women—with itching, burning, redness and irritation, and a discharge that is usually white or yellowish. Homeopathic remedies can soothe discomfort and help the body overcome infection without the use of toxic medicines. If a vaginal infection lasts longer than a week, has offensive-smelling discharge, or is accompanied by fever and a deeper feeling of illness, it is best to see a physician (in case the infection involves some organism other than simple yeast).

Borax

Yeast infections of the vagina with discharge resembling egg white, and a feeling that warm water is flowing out, suggest the use of this remedy. Vaginitis that responds to *Borax* usually appears midway between the menstrual periods. A person who needs this remedy is often nervous and very sensitive to noise.

Calcarea carbonica

When this remedy is indicated, burning and itching feelings may occur both before and after the menstrual period. Discharge from vaginitis is milky and acrid or thick and yellow. A person who needs this remedy is often chilly and stout, has a craving for sweets, and is easily tired by exertion.

Kali bichromicum

This remedy may be indicated in cases of vaginitis when discharge is yellow, tough, and sticky, and makes the vulva itch and burn. Symptoms may be worse in the morning. The person may feel better from resting and keeping warm.

Kreosotum

This remedy is strongly indicated for vaginitis with watery, thin, unpleasant-smelling, very irritating discharge that makes the vulva swell and itch. Symptoms

may be worse in the morning and worse when standing up. Infections are more likely to appear before the menstrual period or during pregnancy.

Natrum muriaticum

Vaginitis with discharge resembling egg-white, which itches and makes the vagina feel dry and irritated, is likely to respond to this remedy. A woman who needs this remedy will often seem reserved, yet is very emotional inside. A craving for salt and a tendency to feel worse from being in the sun are other indications for *Natrum muriaticum.*

Pulsatilla

When this remedy is indicated for yeast infections, symptoms may be changeable. A creamy white or yellowish discharge can appear, which can be either bland or irritating. The vagina may feel sore, and the labia may itch or burn. The woman will be moody, possibly tearful, wanting a lot of attention and affection. This remedy is often helpful for vaginitis during pregnancy.

Sepia

If yeast infections cause vaginal discharge that is yellow and itchy, or white and curd-like, this remedy may be indicated. A woman needing *Sepia* often feels worn down and irritable, with cold extremities and a weak or sagging feeling in the pelvic region. Discharge may be more profuse in the morning and increased by walking.

Sulphur

Discharge that looks yellowish, is offensive-smelling, and causes great burning and itching will bring this remedy to mind. Symptoms may be aggravated by warmth and bathing.

See p. 509 for Homeopathy: Dosage Directions.

Yeast Infection

Homeopathic Remedy Cross-Reference

Aconitum napellus

Alcohol withdrawal support (p. 510), Anxiety (p. 512), Bell's palsy (p. 517), Common cold (p. 527), Cough (p. 530), Ear infections (p. 534), Eye strain/eye injuries (p. 537), Infection (p. 548), Influenza (p. 549), Injuries (p. 550), Insect bites and stings (p. 551), Measles (p. 552), Mumps (p. 561), Osteoarthritis (p. 562), Photosensitivity (p. 564), Restless leg syndrome (p. 570), Sleeplessness (p. 573), Surgery and recovery support (p. 574), Teething (p. 575), Urinary Tract Infection (p. 577)

Actaea racemosa

See Cimicifuga (p. 516)

Aesculus hippocastanum

Backache (p. 516), Hemorrhoids (p. 542)

Agaricus

Bell's palsy (p. 517)

Agnus castus

Impotence (p. 546)

Allium cepa

Common cold (p. 527), Hay fever (p. 541)

Aloe

Hemorrhoids (p. 542)

Anacardium orientale

Rash (p. 569)

Antimonium crudum

Chicken pox (p. 525), Eczema (p. 535)

Antimonium tartaricum

Acne (p. 509), Bronchitis (p. 519), Chicken pox (p. 525)

Apis mellifica

Benign prostatic hyperplasia (p. 567), Chicken pox (p. 525), Conjunctivitis (p. 529), Edema (p. 536), Eye strain/eye injury (p. 537), Herpes simplex (p. 543), Herpes zoster (Shingles) (p. 572), Influenza (p. 549), Insect bites and stings (p. 551), Mumps (p. 561), Osteoarthritis (p. 562), Rashes (p. 569), Urinary tract infection (p. 577)

Argentum nitricum

Anxiety (p. 512), Conjunctivitis (p. 529), Diarrhea (p. 533), Eye strain/eye injuries (p. 537), High blood pressure (p. 544), Impotence (p. 546), Irritable bowel syndrome (p. 545), Motion sickness (p. 560)

Arnica

Athletic performance (p. 515), Backache (p. 516), Broken bone support (p. 518), Bruising (p. 520), Burns (p. 521), Bursitis (p. 522), Carpal tunnel syndrome (p. 524), Dental support (p. 532), Eye strain/eye injuries (p. 537), Fibromyalgia (p. 538), Gout (p. 540), Hemorrhoids (p. 542), Injuries (p. 550), Osteoarthritis (p. 562), Pregnancy and delivery support (p. 566), Rheumatoid arthritis (p. 571), Surgery and recovery support (p. 574), Varicose veins (p. 579)

Arsenicum album

Alcohol withdrawal support (p. 510), Allergies and Sensitivities (p. 510), Anxiety (p. 512), Asthma (p. 514), Boils (p. 518), Common cold (p. 527), Depression (p. 532), Diarrhea (p. 533), Eczema (p. 535), Hay fever (p. 541), Herpes simplex (p. 543), Herpes zoster (Shingles) (p. 572), Indigestion and gas (p. 547), Influenza (p. 549), Mumps (p. 561), Motion sickness (p. 560), Mouth ulcers (p. 523), Postpartum depression (p. 565), Psoriasis (p. 567), Raynaud's disease (p. 569), Restless leg syndrome (p. 570), Sleeplessness (p. 573)

Arum triphyllum

Eczema (p. 535)

Asafoetida

Irritable bowel syndrome (p. 545)

Asarum

Morning sickness (p. 559)

Aurum metallicum

Alcohol withdrawal support (p. 510), Depression (p. 532), High blood pressure (p. 544), Postpartum depression (p. 565), Rheumatoid arthritis (p. 571)

Baryta carbonica

Common cold (p. 527)

Belladonna

Boils (p. 518), Bursitis (p. 522), Chicken pox (p. 525), Colic (p. 526), Common cold (p. 527), Cough (p. 530), Dysmenorrhea (p. 556), Ear infections (p. 534), Gout (p. 540), High blood pressure (p. 544), Infection (p. 548), Influenza (p. 549), Measles (p. 552), Migraines (p. 558), Mumps (p. 561), Osteoarthritis (p. 562), Photosensitivity (p. 564), Rashes (p. 569), Teething (p. 575), Urinary tract infection (p. 577)

Bellis perennis

Athletic performance (p. 515), Broken bone support (p. 518), Bruising (p. 520), Injury (p. 550), Surgery and recovery support (p. 574)

Berberis vulgaris

Gallstones (p. 539), Gout (p. 540), Urinary Tract Infection (p. 577)

Borax

Herpes simplex (p. 543), Motion sickness (p. 560), Mouth ulcers (p. 523), Urinary tract infection (p. 577), Yeast infection (p. 579)

Bovista

Edema (p. 536), Menstrual problems and PMS (p. 554)

Bryonia

Backache (p. 516), Broken bone support (p. 518), Bronchitis (p. 519), Bursitis (p. 522), Chicken pox (p. 525), Colic (p. 526), Cough (p. 530), Constipation (p. 529), Diarrhea (p. 533), Measles (p. 552), Fibromyalgia (p. 538), Indigestion and gas (p. 547), Infection (p. 548), Influenza (p. 549), Measles

(p. 552), Migraines (p. 558), Motion sickness (p. 560), Mumps (p. 561), Osteoarthritis (p. 562), Rashes (p. 569), Rheumatoid arthritis (p. 571)

Cadmium iodatum

Chemotherapy support (radiation) (p. 525)

Cadmium sulphuratum

Bell's palsy (p. 517), Chemotherapy support (p. 525)

Caladium

Impotence (p. 546)

Calcarea carbonica

Acne (p. 509), Allergies and sensitivities (p. 510), Anxiety (p. 512), Backache (p. 516), Bronchitis (p. 519), Cataracts (p. 524), Constipation (p. 529), Depression (p. 532), Eczema (p. 535), Edema (p. 536), Fibromyalgia (p. 538), Gallstones (p. 539), High blood pressure (p. 544), Infection (p. 548), Menopause symptoms (p. 553), Mouth ulcers (p. 523), Mumps (p. 561), Osteoarthritis (p. 562), Osteoporosis (p. 563), Postpartum depression (p. 565), Psoriasis (p. 567), Rheumatoid arthritis (p. 571), Teething (p. 575), Tinnitus (p. 576), Varicose veins (p. 549), Yeast infection (p. 579)

Calcarea fluorica

Cataracts (p. 524), Gout (p. 540), Hemorrhoids (p. 542), Osteoarthritis (p. 562), Rheumatoid arthritis (p. 571)

Calcarea phosphorica

Allergies and Sensitivities (p. 510), Backache (p. 516), Broken bone support (p. 518), Bruising (p. 520), Carpal tunnel syndrome (p. 524), Injuries (p. 550), Osteoarthritis (p. 562), Osteoporosis (p. 563), Pregnancy and Delivery Support (p. 566), Sleeplessness (p. 573), Teething (p. 575)

Calendula

Boils (p. 518), Dental support (p. 532), Eczema (p. 535), Infection (p. 548), Injury (p. 550)

Calendula (topical)

Burns (p. 521), Dental support (p. 532)

Camphora

Photosensitivity (p. 564)

Candida albicans

Yeast infections (p. 579)

Cantharis

Burns (p. 521), Insect bites and stings (p. 551), Urinary tract infection (p. 577)

Carbo vegetabilis

Alcohol withdrawal support (p. 510), Allergies and sensitivities (p. 510), Asthma (p. 514), Colic (p. 526), Indigestion and gas (p. 547), Mumps (p. 561), Pregnancy and Delivery support (p. 566), Raynaud's disease (p. 569), Tinnitus (p. 576), Varicose veins (p. 579)

Carbolicum acidum

Insect bites and stings (p. 551)

Caulophyllum

Dysmenorrhea (p. 556), Menstrual problems and PMS (p. 554), Pregnancy and Delivery Support (p. 566)

Causticum

Bell's palsy (p. 517), Benign prostatic hyperplasia (p. 567), Bronchitis (p. 519), Burns (p. 521), Carpal tunnel syndrome (p. 524), Cataracts (p. 524), Constipation (p. 529), Depression (p. 532), Fibromyalgia (p. 538), Impotence (p. 546), Restless leg syndrome (p. 570), Rheumatoid arthritis (p. 571)

Chamomilla

Alcohol withdrawal support (p. 510), Asthma (p. 514), Bronchitis (p. 519), Colic (p. 526), Cough (p. 530), Dental support (p. 532), Diarrhea (p. 533), Dysmenorrhea (p. 556), Ear infections (p. 534), Menstrual problems and PMS (p. 554), Teething (p. 575)

Chelidonium majus

Gallstones (p. 539), Raynaud's disease (p. 569)

Chimaphila umbellata

Benign prostatic hyperplasia (p. 567), Urinary tract infection (p. 577)

China (Cinchona)

Surgery and recovery support (p. 574), Tinnitus (p. 576)

Chininum sulphuricum

Tinnitus (p. 576)

Cimicifuga

Backache (p. 516), Depression (p. 532), Dysmenorrhea (p. 556), Fibromyalgia (p. 538),

Menstrual problems and PMS (p. 554), Migraine (p. 558), Osteoarthritis (p. 562), Postpartum depression (p. 565), Tinnitus (p. 576)

Clematis

Benign prostatic hyperplasia (p. 567), Herpes zoster (Shingles) (p. 572), Urinary tract infection (p. 577)

Cocculus

Dysmenorrhea (p. 556), Motion sickness (p. 560), Sleeplessness (p. 573)

Coffea cruda

Alcohol withdrawal support (p. 510), Sleeplessness (p. 573), Teething (p. 575)

Colchicum

Gout (p. 540), Morning sickness (p. 559)

Colocynthis

Colic (p. 526), Diarrhea (p. 533), Dysmenorrhea (p. 556), Gallstones (p. 539), Indigestion and gas (p. 547)

Cuprum

Colic (p. 526)

Cyclamen

Migraine (p. 558)

Dioscorea

Colic (p. 526), Gallstones (p. 539)

Dulcamara

Backache (p. 516), Bell's palsy (p. 517), Bronchitis (p. 519), Common cold (p. 527), Herpes simplex (p. 543), Osteoarthritis (p. 562), Rheumatoid arthritis (p. 571)

Echinacea angustifolia

Boils (p. 518)

Eupatorium perfoliatum

Broken bone support (p. 518), Influenza (p. 549)

Euphrasia

Common cold (p. 527), Conjunctivitis (p. 529), Hay fever (p. 541), Measles (p. 552)

Ferrum metallicum

Edema (p. 536), Pregnancy and Delivery support (p. 566)

Ferrum phosphoricum

Bursitis (p. 522), Common cold (p. 527), Cough (p. 530), Ear infection (p. 534), Hay fever (p. 541), Influenza (p. 549), Pregnancy and Delivery support (p. 566), Surgery and recovery support (p. 574)

Gelsemium

Allergies and sensitivities (p. 510), Anxiety (p. 512), Chemotherapy support (p. 525), Dental support (p. 532), Diarrhea (p. 533), Hay fever (p. 541), Influenza (p. 549), Measles (p. 552), Migraines (p. 558), Surgery and recovery support (p. 574)

Glonoinum

High blood pressure (p. 544), Menopause symptoms (p. 553)

Graphites

Constipation (p. 529), Eczema (p. 535), Edema (p. 536), Hemorrhoids (p. 542), Herpes simplex (p. 543), Infection (p. 548), Menopause symptoms (p. 553), Psoriasis (p. 567), Rashes (p. 569), Tinnitus (p. 576)

Hamamelis

Hemorrhoids (p. 542), Surgery and recovery support (p. 574), Varicose veins (p. 579)

Hepar sulphuris calcareum

Acne (p. 509), Allergies and sensitivities (p. 510), Boils (p. 518), Bronchitis (p. 519), Burns (p. 521), Conjunctivitis (p. 529), Ear infections (p. 534), Eczema (p. 535), Herpes simplex (p. 543), Infection (p. 548), Mouth ulcers (p. 523), Raynaud's disease (p. 569)

Hypericum

Athletic performance (p. 515), Broken bone support (p. 518), Bruising (p. 520), Burns (p. 521), Carpal tunnel syndrome (p. 524), Dental support (p. 532), Injury (p. 550), Insect bites and stings (p. 551), Surgery and recovery support (p. 574)

Ignatia

Allergies and sensitivities (p. 510), Anxiety (p. 512), Backache (p. 516), Depression (p. 532), Hemorrhoids (p. 542), Menopause symptoms (p. 553), Postpartum depression (p. 565), Restless leg syndrome (p. 570), Sleeplessness (p. 573)

Ipecac

Asthma (p. 514), Chemotherapy support (p. 525), Cough (p. 530), Diarrhea (p. 533), Injuries (p. 550), Morning sickness (p. 559)

Iris versicolor

Herpes zoster (Shingles) (p. 572), Migraine (p. 558)

Kali bichromicum

Bronchitis (p. 519), Common cold (p. 527), Measles (p. 552), Migraines (p. 558), Motion sickness (p. 560), Rheumatoid arthritis (p. 571), Yeast infections (p. 579)

Kali carbonicum

Backache (p. 516), Edema (p. 536), Osteoarthritis (p. 562), Rheumatoid arthritis (p. 571), Tinnitus (p. 576)

Kali phosphoricum

Anxiety (p. 512), Chemotherapy support (p. 525), Depression (p. 532), Eye strain (p. 537), Sleeplessness (p. 573)

Kalmia latifolia

Bursitis (p. 522), Eye strain (p. 537), Fibromyalgia (p. 538), Herpes zoster (p. 572), Osteoarthritis (p. 562), Rheumatoid arthritis (p. 571)

Kreosotum

Menstrual problems and PMS (p. 554), Morning sickness (p. 559), Teething (p. 575), Yeast infection (p. 579)

Lachesis

Dysmenorrhea (p. 556), High blood pressure (p. 544), Menopause symptoms (p. 553), Menstrual problems and PMS (p. 554), Migraine (p. 558)

Lacticum acidum

Morning sickness (p. 559)

Ledum palustre

Athletic performance (p. 515), Bruising (p. 520), Edema (p. 536), Gout (p. 540), Injuries (p. 550), Insect bites and stings (p. 551), Osteoarthritis (p. 562), Rash (p. 569), Rheumatoid arthritis (p. 571)

Lilium tigrinum

Dysmenorrhea (p. 556), Irritable bowel syndrome (p. 545), Menopause symptoms (p. 553), Menstrual problems and PMS (p. 554)

Lycopodium

Allergies and sensitivities (p. 510), Anxiety (p. 512), Benign prostatic hyperplasia (p. 567), Constipation (p. 529), Edema (p. 536), Gallstones (p. 539), Impotence (p. 546), Indigestion and gas (p. 547), Irritable bowel syndrome (p. 545), Menstrual problems and PMS (p. 554), Sleeplessness (p. 573), Tinnitus (p. 576), Urinary tract infection (p. 577), Varicose veins (p. 579)

Magnesia phosphorica

Colic (p. 526), Dysmenorrhea (p. 556), Ear infection (p. 534), Teething (p. 575)

Mercurius solubilis

Boils (p. 518), Chicken pox (p. 525), Common cold (p. 527), Conjunctivitis (p. 529), Dental support (p. 532), Ear infection (p. 534), Herpes simplex (p. 543), Infection (p. 548), Mouth ulcers (p. 523), Mumps (p. 561), Psoriasis (p. 567)

Mezereum

Eczema (p. 535), Herpes zoster (Shingles) (p. 572), Psoriasis (p. 567)

Millefolium

Bruising (p. 520), Injuries (p. 550)

Natrum carbonicum

Allergies and sensitivities (p. 510), Depression (p. 532), Indigestion and gas (p. 547), Photosensitivity (p. 564)

Natrum muriaticum

Alcohol withdrawal support (p. 510), Backache (p. 516), Cataracts (p. 524), Common cold (p. 527), Conjunctivitis (p. 529), Edema (p. 536), Eyestrain (p. 537), Hay fever (p. 541), Herpes simplex (p. 543), High blood pressure (p. 544), Menopause symptoms (p. 553), Menstrual problems and PMS (p. 554), Migraine (p. 558), Mouth ulcers (p. 523), Photosensitivity (p. 564), Postpartum depression (p. 565), Rashes (p. 569), Yeast infection (p. 579)

Natrum phosphoricum

Indigestion and gas (p. 547)

Natrum salicylicum

Tinnitus (p. 576)

Natrum sulphuricum

Asthma (p. 514)

Nux moschata

Allergies and sensitivities (p. 510)

Nux vomica

Alcohol withdrawal support (p. 510), Allergies and sensitivities (p. 510), Asthma (p. 514), Backache (p. 516), Chemotherapy support (p. 525), Colic (p. 526), Common cold (p. 527), Constipation (p. 529), Dysmenorrhea (p. 556), Hay fever (p. 541), High blood pressure (p. 544), Indigestion and gas (p. 547), Influenza (p. 549), Irritable bowel syndrome (p. 545), Menstrual problems (p. 554), Mouth ulcers (p. 523), Pregnancy and delivery support (p. 566), Sleeplessness (p. 573), Urinary tract infection (p. 577)

Oscillococcinum

Influenza (p. 549)

Petroleum

Allergies and sensitivities (p. 510), Eczema (p. 535), Motion sickness (p. 560), Psoriasis (p. 567)

Phosphorus

Allergies and sensitivities (p. 510), Anxiety (p. 512), Bruising (p. 520), Burns (p. 521), Cataracts (p. 524), Common cold (p. 527), Cough (p. 530), Diarrhea (p. 533), High blood pressure (p. 544), Influenza (p. 549), Injuries (p. 550), Postpartum depression (p. 565), Surgery and recovery support (p. 574)

Phytolacca

Mumps (p. 561), Teething (p. 575)

Platinum metallicum

Bell's palsy (p. 517)

Plumbum

High blood pressure (p. 544)

Podophyllum

Diarrhea (p. 533), Gallstones (p. 539), Irritable Bowel Syndrome (p. 545)

Pulsatilla

Acne (p. 509), Anxiety (p. 512), Asthma (p. 514), Benign Prostatic hyperplasia (p. 567), Bronchitis (p. 519), Chicken pox (p. 525), Common cold (p. 527), Conjunctivitis (p. 529), Cough (p. 530), Diarrhea (p. 533), Dysmenorrhea (p. 556), Ear infection (p. 534), Edema (p. 536), Hemorrhoids (p. 542), Indigestion and gas (p. 547), Measles (p. 552), Menopause symptoms (p. 553), Menstrual problems and PMS (p. 554), Morning sickness (p. 559), Mumps (p. 561), Osteoarthritis (p. 562), Postpartum depression (p. 565), Pregnancy and delivery support (p. 566), Rheumatoid arthritis (p. 571), Teething (p. 575), Varicose veins (p. 579), Yeast infection (p. 579)

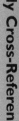

Homeopathic Remedy Cross-Reference

Ranunculus bulbosus

Fibromyalgia (p. 538), Herpes zoster (Shingles) (p. 572)

Rhododendron

Gout (p. 540), Rheumatoid arthritis (p. 571)

Rhus toxicodendron

Backache (p. 516), Bursitis (p. 522), Carpal tunnel (p. 524), Chicken pox (p. 525), Common cold (p. 527), Eczema (p. 535), Fibromyalgia (p. 538), Gout (p. 540), Herpes simplex (p. 543), Herpes zoster (Shingles) (p. 572), Influenza (p. 549), Measles (p. 552), Mumps (p. 561), Osteoarthritis (p. 562), Psoriasis (p. 567), Rashes (p. 569), Restless leg syndrome (p. 570)

Rumex crispus

Cough (p. 530)

Ruta graveolens

Athletic performance (p. 515), Backache (p. 516), Broken bone support (p. 518), Bruising (p. 520), Bursitis (p. 522), Carpal tunnel syndrome (p. 524), Eye strain (p. 537), Fibromyalgia (p. 538), Injuries (p. 550), Osteoarthritis (p. 562), Rheumatoid arthritis (p. 571), Surgery and recovery support (p. 574)

Sabadilla

Hay fever (p. 541)

Sabal serrulata

Benign prostatic hyperplasia (p. 567)

Salicylic acid

Tinnitus (p. 576)

Sanguinaria

Bursitis (p. 522), High blood pressure (p. 544), Migraine (p. 558)

Sarcolactic acid

Athletic performance (p. 515)

Sarsaparilla

Urinary tract infection (p. 577)

Selenium metallicum

Impotence (p. 546)

Sepia

Chemotherapy support (p. 525), Constipation (p. 529), Depression (p. 532), Dysmenorrhea (p. 556), Menopause symptoms (p. 553), Menstrual problems

and PMS (p. 554), Migraine (p. 558), Morning sickness (p. 559), Postpartum depression (p. 565), Pregnancy and delivery support (p. 566), Psoriasis (p. 567), Rashes (p. 569), Raynaud's disease (p. 569), Urinary tract infection (p. 577), Yeast infection (p. 579)

Silicea (Silica)

Acne (p. 509), Allergies and Sensitivities (p. 510), Anxiety (p. 512), Boils (p. 518), Bronchitis (p. 519), Cataracts (p. 524), Constipation (p. 529), Infection (p. 548), Migraine (p. 558), Osteoporosis (p. 563), Sleeplessness (p. 573), Teething (p. 575)

Spigelia

Migraine (p. 558)

Spongia tosta

Asthma (p. 514), Cough (p. 530)

Staphysagria

Alcohol withdrawal support (p. 510), Benign prostatic hyperplasia (p. 567), Depression (p. 532), Impotence (p. 546), Menopause symptoms (p. 553), Photosensitivity (p. 564), Psoriasis (p. 567), Surgery and recovery support (p. 574), Urinary tract infection (p. 577)

Sulphur

Acne (p. 509), Backache (p. 516), Bronchitis (p. 519), Burns (p. 521), Bursitis (p. 522), Chicken pox (p. 525), Conjunctivitis (p. 529), Constipation (p. 529), Cough (p. 530), Diarrhea (p. 533), Eczema (p. 535), Gout (p. 540), Hemorrhoids (p. 542), Influenza (p. 549), Irritable bowel syndrome (p. 545), Menopause symptoms (p. 553), Mouth ulcers (p. 523), Psoriasis (p. 567), Rashes (p. 569), Restless leg syndrome (p. 570), Sleeplessness (p. 573), Teething (p. 575), Yeast infections (p. 579)

Sulphuricum acidum

Allergies and sensitivities (p. 510), Bruising (p. 520)

Symphytum

Broken bone support (p. 518), Bruising (p. 520), Eye injury (p. 537), Injuries (p. 550), Osteoporosis (p. 563)

Tabacum

Morning sickness (p. 559), Motion sickness (p. 560)

Tarentula cubensis

Boils (p. 518)

Homeopathic Remedy Cross-Reference

Thuja occidentalis

Benign prostatic hyperplasia (p. 567)

Urtica urens

Burns (p. 521), Chicken pox (p. 525), Insect bites and stings (p. 551), Rashes (p. 569)

Veratrum album

Dysmenorrhea (p. 556), Menstrual problems and PMS (p. 554), Raynaud's disease (p. 569)

Viola odorata

Carpal tunnel syndrome (p. 524)

Wyethia

Hay fever (p. 541)

Zincum metallicum

Restless leg syndrome (p. 570), Sleeplessness (p. 573), Varicose veins (p. 579

Homeopathic Remedy Cross-Reference

Part Four: References

1. Linde K, Clausius N, Ramirez G, et al. Are the clinical effects of homeopathy placebo effects? A meta-analysis of placebo-controlled trials. Lancet 1997; 250: 834–43.

Analysis of 186 studies; concludes that positive results in subjects taking homeopathic medicines are 2.4 times more likely than with placebo.

2. Kleijnen J, Knipschild P, ter Riet G. Clinical trials of homeopathy. *Br Med J* 1991; 302: 316–23.

Review of 107 studies, 81 of which (77%) showed positive effects from homeopathic medicines; researchers concluded: "The evidence presented in this review would probably be sufficient for establishing homeopathy as a regular treatment for certain indications."

3. Summary and review of other recent homeopathic research studies, and other references, may be found in the following books:
- Jonas WB, Jacobs J. *Healing with Homeopathy*. New York: Warner Books, 1996.
- Ullman D. *The Consumer's Guide to Homeopathy*. New York: Tarcher/Putnam, 1995.

References and Resources: Professional

Allen HC. *Keynotes and Characteristics of the Materia Medica*. New Delhi: B. Jain (reprint), 1988.

Boericke W. *Materia Medica with Repertory*. Santa Rosa: Boericke and Tafel (reprint) 1988.

Borland D. *Homeopathy for Mother and Infant*. New Delhi: World Homeopathic Links (reprint).

Boyd H. *Introduction to Homeopathic Medicine*. Beaconsfield, England: Beaconsfield, 1981.

Hering C. *Guiding Symptoms of Our Materia Medica*. New Delhi: B. Jain (reprint), 1988, (Vol 1–10).

Herscu P. *The Homeopathic Treatment of Children*. Berkeley: North Atlantic, 1991.

Kent JT. *Lectures on Homeopathic Materia Medica*. New Delhi: B. Jain (reprint), 1980.

Kent JT. *Repertory of Homeopathic Materia Medica*. New Delhi: B. Jain (reprint), 1988.

Morrison R. *Desktop Guide to Keynotes & Confirmatory Symptoms*. Albany, CA: Hahnemann, 1993.

Nash EB. *Leaders in Homeopathic Therapeutics*. New Delhi: B. Jain (reprint), 1988.

Perko S. *Homeopathy for the Modern Pregnant Woman and Her Infant*. San Antonio: Benchmark Homeopathic Publications, 1997.

Schroyens F. *Synthesis Repertorium Homeopathicum Syntheticum*. London: Homeopathic Book Publishers, 1993.

Tyler M. *Drug Pictures*. Saffron Walden, Essex: CW Daniel, 1982.

Vithoulkas G. *Materia Medica Viva*. London: Homeopathic Book Publishers, 1992, 1995.

References and Resources: General

Castro M. *Complete Homeopathy Handbook*. New York: St. Martin's, 1991.

Castro M. *Homeopathy for Pregnancy, Birth, and Your Child's First Year*. New York: St. Martin's, 1993.

Cummings S, Ullman D. *Everybody's Guide to Homeopathic Medicines*. Los Angeles: Tarcher, 1991.

Lockie A. *Family Guide to Homeopathy*. New York: Fireside, 1993.

Panos M, Heimlich J. *Homeopathic Medicine at Home*. Los Angeles: Tarcher, 1980.

Ullman D. *Consumer's Guide to Homeopathy*. New York: Tarcher/Putnam, 1995.

Vithoulkas G. *Homeopathy: Medicine of the New Man*. New York: Avon, 1971.

Homeopathic History and Theory

Coulter HL. *Homeopathic Science and Modern Medicine: The Physics of Healing with Microdoses*. Berkeley: North Atlantic, 1987.

Coulter HL. *Divided Legacy: A History of the Schism in Medical Thought*. Berkeley: North Atlantic, 1975; 1977; 1981; 1994.

Hahnemann S., O'Reilly WB (ed.), Decker S. (translator). *The Organon of the Medical Art*, 6th Edition. Edmonds, WA: Birdcage Books, 1996.

Kent JT. *Lectures on Homeopathic Philosophy*. Berkeley: North Atlantic, 1979 (reprint).

Vithoulkas G. *The Science of Homeopathy*. New York: Grove, 1980.

Index

About the Authors

**Schuyler W. "Skye" Lininger, Jr., DC,
Contributor and Editor-in-Chief**

Dr. Skye Lininger is an acknowledged expert and popular speaker on nutritional therapeutics, computer technology, and the Internet. He has authored or coauthored a dozen computer books and written numerous technology-related and health-related articles. Healthnotes, Inc., which he founded in 1986, is the publisher of *Healthnotes Newsletter*, *Healthnotes Review of Complementary and Integrative Medicine*, and Healthnotes Online, and is the leading provider of high-quality, scientifically based information on natural medicine. A former instructor in nutrition, he gives regular seminars in both the United States and England and serves on the boards of several natural medicine colleges. He is also the editor-in-chief of *A–Z Guide to Drug-Herb-Vitamin Interactions* (Prima and Healthnotes, Inc., 1999).

**Alan R. Gaby, MD, Contributor
and Editorial Reviewer**

Dr. Alan Gaby, an expert in nutritional therapies, is the Contributing Medical Editor of the *Townsend Letter for Doctors*. He served as a member of the Ad-Hoc Advisory Panel of the National Institutes of Health Office of Alternative Medicine. He is the author of *B6: The Natural Healer* (Keats, 1987), *Preventing and Reversing Osteoporosis* (Prima, 1994), and *The Patient's Book of Natural Healing* (Prima, 1999). He is also a coauthor of *A–Z Guide to Drug-Herb-Vitamin Interactions* (Prima and Healthnotes, Inc., 1999). He is past-president of the American Holistic Medical Association. He has, along with Dr. Jonathan Wright, conducted nutritional seminars for physicians and has collected over 30,000 scientific papers related to the field of nutritional and natural medicine. He is currently the Endowed Professor of Nutrition at Bastyr University, Bothell, Washington, and is a frequent contributor to Healthnotes.

**Steve Austin, ND, Contributor and
Section Editor of Health Concerns
and Nutritional Supplements**

Dr. Steve Austin is a licensed naturopathic physician in Portland, Oregon. He is former Professor of Nutrition at the National College of Naturopathic Medicine. Dr. Austin has also headed the nutrition departments at Bastyr University and Western States Chiropractic College. He is the coauthor of *Breast Cancer: What You Should Know (But May Not Be Told) About Prevention, Diagnosis, and Treatment* (Prima, 1994) and *A–Z Guide to Drug-Herb-Vitamin Interactions* (Prima and Healthnotes, Inc., 1999), and a contributor to the *Textbook of Natural Medicine*, and nutrition editor for the *Healthnotes Review of Complementary and Integrative Medicine*.

**Donald J. Brown, ND, Contributor and
Section Editor of Herbal Remedies**

Dr. Donald Brown is a naturopathic physician and one of the leading authorities in the United States on evidence-based herbal medicine. A graduate and former associate professor of the Bastyr University of Natural Health Sciences in Seattle, he is the founder and director of Natural Product Research Consultants, Inc. and serves on the Advisory Board of the American Botanical Council and the President's Advisory Board of Bastyr University. Dr. Brown has served as an adviser to the Office of Dietary Supplements at the National Institutes of Health. He is the editor-in-chief of the *Healthnotes Review of Complementary and Integrative Medicine* (formerly the *Quarterly Review of Natural Medicine*), author of *Herbal Prescriptions for Better Health* (Prima, 1996), and coauthor of *A–Z Guide to Drug-Herb-Vitamin Interactions* (Prima and Healthnotes, Inc., 1999).

Jonathan V. Wright, MD, Contributor

Dr. Jonathan Wright practices nutritional medicine at the Tahoma Clinic in Kent, Washington. He is regarded as one of the world's finest preventive medical doctors. He is the author of *Dr. Wright's Book of Nutritional Therapy* (Rodale, 1979), *Dr. Wright's Guide to Healing with Nutrition* (Keats, 1990), and *Natural Hormone Replacement: for Women Over 45* (Smart, 1997). He contributes regularly to *Healthnotes* and authors the newsletter *Nutrition and Healing*.

Alice Duncan, DC, CCH, Contributor and Section Editor of Homeopathic Remedies

Dr. Alice Duncan is a certified classical homeopath and chiropractic physician, practicing in Oregon. She is the author of *Your Healthy Child: A Guide to Natural Healthcare* (JP Tarcher, 1990; Sanicula, 1995), former editor of the professional homeopathic journal, *Simillimum*, and a frequent contributor to *Healthnotes*.

Eric Yarnell, ND, Contributor

Dr. Eric Yarnell works as a naturopathic physician and is chair of the department of botanical medicine at the Southwest College of Naturopathic Medicine. He is treasurer of the board of the Botanical Medicine Academy and research editor for the *Journal of Naturopathic Medicine*. He is a contributor to the *Healthnotes Review of Complementary and Integrative Medicine* and coauthor of *A–Z Guide to Drug-Herb-Vitamin Interactions* (Prima and Healthnotes, Inc., 1999).

James Gerber, DC, Contributor

Dr. James Gerber is Associate Professor of Clinical Sciences at Western States Chiropractic College (WSCC) in Portland, Oregon, and also teaches postgraduate courses for several other colleges. He graduated from WSCC in 1981, received his Master's degree in Nutrition from the University of Bridgeport in 1986, and is board-certified in Nutrition and Orthopedics. Dr. Gerber is the author of *Handbook of Preventive and Therapeutic Nutrition* (Aspen, 1993) and a contributor to *Conservative Management of Sports Injuries* (Williams & Wilkins, 1997). In addition to contributing to Healthnotes Online, he is the scientific editor for the *Healthnotes Newsletter*.

Ronald G. Reichert, ND, Contributor

An expert in European phytotherapy, Dr. Ronald Reichert resides in Vancouver, BC, where he has an active medical practice. He regularly contributes articles to lay and professional publications in Canada. In addition to his regular herbal research columns, he provides professional review of German translations for the *Healthnotes Review of Complementary and Integrative Medicine*.

Trina Seligman, ND, Contributor

Dr. Trina Seligman is a graduate of Bastyr University and has completed a one-year residency with Jonathan Wright, MD. She currently practices at Moss Bay Center for Integrative Medicine in Bellevue, Washington. Dr. Seligman also works for the research department of Bastyr University assisting in both the design of research protocols and the administration of clinical trials.

Tori Hudson, ND, Contributor

Dr. Tori Hudson is a nationally known expert on women's health. Her column appears in the *Townsend Letter for Doctors*. A popular speaker, she is the author of *Women's Encyclopedia of Natural Medicine* (Keats, 1999) and a regular contributor to *Healthnotes*.

Lauri M. Aesoph, l.c., ND, Contributor

Dr. Lauri Aesoph, cofounder of the Aesoph Group in Sioux Falls, South Dakota, specializes in healthcare education through writing, training, and consulting. Dr. Aesoph is the author of *Your Natural Health Makeover* (Prentice Hall, 1998) and *How to Eat Away Arthritis* (Prentice Hall, 1996); she has also contributed to *Alternative Medicine* and *A Textbook of Natural Medicine*. She is a former editor for the *Journal of Naturopathic Medicine* and is founding president of the South Dakota Association of Naturopathic Physicians. Dr. Aesoph is a regular contributor to Healthnotes Online and over the past twelve years has published hundreds of articles in publications such as *Woman's World*, *Nutrition Science News*, and *Let's Live*.

Chris Meletis, ND, Contributor

Dr. Chris Meletis is a licensed naturopathic physician and a graduate of the National College of Naturopathic Medicine, Portland, Oregon. He is in private practice at the Natural Health Center in Portland and serves as the Dean of Clinical Education, Chief Medical Officer, and Medicinary Director at his alma mater. Dr. Meletis has authored several books, including *Better Sex Naturally* (HarperCollins, February 2000), and coauthored *Comprehensive Guide to Drug-Nutrient and Nutrient-Nutrient Interactions* (Eclectic Publishing, 1999). He is a regular columnist and contributor to numerous magazines and books.

Editorial Staff

Victoria Dolby Toews, MPH, Managing Editor

Mrs. Victoria Dolby Toews writes about health issues, with a special focus on nutritional supplements. Her articles appear regularly in several magazines. She is the coauthor of *The Common Cold Cure* (Avery, 1999) and *The Green Tea Book* (Avery, 1998). She is the managing editor for Healthnotes Online and *A–Z Guide to Drug-Herb-Vitamin Interactions* (Prima and Healthnotes, Inc., 1999) and the editor-in-chief of the *Healthnotes Newsletter*.

Rick Wilkes, Chief Technology Officer

Mr. Rick Wilkes is an Internet and electronic publishing specialist from Deep Creek Lake, Maryland. For over 20 years he has focused on building supportive, interactive online communities; and publishing enabling software and newsletters to help clients apply complex computer technology more effectively. He graduated from Johns Hopkins University, Baltimore, Maryland, where he now serves on the Computer Science Advisory Board.

Healthnotes, Inc., Team

Skye Lininger (President/CEO), Tim O'Connor (General Manager), Cheryl Bottger (Director of Marketing and Product Development), Mike Shriner (Director of Business Development), Rick Wilkes (Chief Technology Officer), Rachel Gaffney (Accounting Manager), Geoff Lay (Internet Product Manager), Tara Schweig (National Retail Sales Manager), Cindy Hambly (National Accounts Manager), Brent Blomgren (National Accounts Manager), Karen Considine (Inside Sales Representative), Caroline Petrich (Marketing Manager), Janet Jaffee (Marketing Assistant), Autumn Moore (Customer Care Manager), Jim Garner (Customer Care Specialist), Dan Widger (Technical Support Specialist), JoAnn DeVischer (Office Manager), Debbie Cheney (Fulfillment Specialist), Annette LaBarge (Accounts Receivable Specialist), Sally S. K. Lee (Bookkeeper) Judy Robinson (Executive Assistant), Marcia Barrentine (Creative Services Manager), Nichole Klaes (Graphic Designer); Loren Jenkins (Programmer), Marianne Bhonslay (Editorial Manager), Victoria Dolby Toews, MPH (Managing Editor), Jenny Morrison and Richard Walsh (Copy Editors); Legal and Accounting: Curt Gleaves and Jim Baker; U.K. Team: Michael Peet, Taylor, Gareth Zeal, and Nigel Perkins.

Also Available from Healthnotes

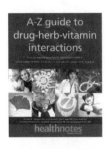

The *A–Z Guide to Drug-Herb-Vitamin Interactions* (Prima Health and Healthnotes, Inc., 1999), by Schuyler Lininger, Jr, DC, (editor-in-chief), Alan R. Gaby, MD, Steve Austin, ND, Forrest Batz, PharmD, Eric Yarnell, ND, Donald J. Brown, ND, and George Constantine, RPh, PhD.

Finally, a book that details the interactions—both positive and negative—between prescription and nonprescription drugs and vitamins and herbs. The other companion volume to Healthnotes Online, *A–Z Guide to Drug-Herb-Vitamin Interactions* catalogs more than 4,500 interactions. Learn how some herbs help drugs work better; learn which drugs deplete your body of crucial nutrients; learn which drugs and supplements should never be taken together; and learn which drug side effects can be reduced by taking the right vitamin or herb. (*$19.95*)

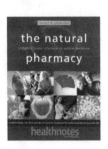

The Natural Pharmacy: Complete Home Reference to Natural Medicine CD-ROM (Healthnotes, Inc., 1999). With this companion to *The Natural Pharmacy*, you'll have a wealth of information literally at your fingertips. This Macintosh or Windows compatible CD-ROM has fully referenced information on Health Concerns, Nutritional Supplements, Herbal Remedies, Homeopathic Remedies, and Diets and Therapies.

Take home—for personal or family use—this fascinating and comprehensive database, and increase your understanding of herbs and vitamin supplements. Requires an Internet browser (such as Microsoft Internet Explorer version 3.x or later, or Netscape 3.x or later) and a CD-ROM drive. Does not require Internet access. (*$24.95*)

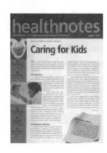

Healthnotes Newsletter (Healthnotes, Inc., 1999) This four-page, monthly newsletter focuses on specific health concerns and related natural remedies. Fully referenced articles are easy to understand and informative. Topics for 2000 include: Managing Medications for Seniors; Sports Nutrition; Women and Hormones (PMS and Menopause); Digestive Health; Antibiotic Overuse; Cold and Flu Prevention; and Thyroid Health. To register online to receive the newsletter via e-mail every month go to http://www.healthnotes.com, and click on "*Healthnotes Newsletter.*"